Clinical
Veterinary
Toxicology

Clinical Veterinary Toxicology

Konnie H. Plumlee, DVM, MS, Dipl ABVT, ACVIM

Arkansas Diagnostic Laboratory
Livestock and Poultry Commission
Little Rock, Arkansas

Illustrated, including 58 color plates

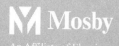 Mosby

An Affiliate of Elsevier

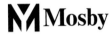

An Affiliate of Elsevier

11830 Westline Industrial Drive
St. Louis, Missouri 63146

CLINICAL VETERINARY TOXICOLOGY   0-323-01125-X
Copyright © 2004, Mosby, Inc. All rights reserved.

NOTICE

Veterinary medicine is an ever-changing field. Standard safety precautions must be followed, but as new research and clinical experience broaden our knowledge, changes in treatment and drug therapy may become necessary or appropriate. Readers are advised to check the most current product information provided by the manufacturer of each drug to be administered to verify the recommended dose, the method and duration of administration, and contraindications. It is the responsibility of the licensed prescriber, relying on experience and knowledge of the patient, to determine dosages and the best treatment for each individual patient. Neither the publisher nor the author assumes any liability for any injury and/or damage to persons or property arising from this publication.

Library of Congress Cataloging-in-Publication Data

Clinical veterinary toxicology/[edited by] Konnie H. Plumlee.
    p. cm.
    Includes bibliographical references.
    ISBN 0-323-01125-X
    1. Veterinary toxicology. I. Plumlee, Konnie.

SF757.5.C65 2003
636.089'59—dc22
                                    2003061495

Publishing Director: Linda L. Duncan
Senior Editor: Liz Fathman
Managing Editor: Teri Merchant
Publishing Services Manager: Patricia Tannian
Project Manager: Sarah Wunderly
Designer: Julia Dummitt

Printed in United States

Last digit is the print number: 9 8 7 6 5 4 3 2 1

Contributors

Jay C. Albretsen, DVM, PhD, Dipl ABT, ABVT
Study Director, Toxicology
Covance Laboratories Inc.
Madison, Wisconsin

Jeremy Allen, BVSc, BSc, PhD
Principal Veterinary Toxicologist
Animal Health Laboratories
Western Australian Department of Agriculture
South Perth, Australia

Neal Bataller, ME, DVM
Regulatory Policy Analyst
Division of Compliance
Center for Veterinary Medicine
Food and Drug Administration
Rockville, Maryland

Karyn Bischoff, DVM, MS, Dipl ABVT
Resident, Anatomic Pathology
Veterinary Toxicologist
Department of Pathobiology
University of Florida
College of Veterinary Medicine
Gainesville, Florida

Dennis J. Blodgett, DVM, PhD, Dipl ABVT
Associate Professor
Biomedical Sciences and Pathobiology
Virginia-Maryland Regional College of Veterinary Medicine
Virginia Tech
Blacksburg, Virginia

Gary O. Bordson, BS, MS
Senior Organic Analytical Chemist
Illinois Waste Management and Research Center
Illinois State Department of Natural Resources
Champaign, Illinois

George Burrows, BS, DVM, PhD, Dipl ABVT
Professor of Toxicology, Emeritus
Oklahoma State University
Stillwater, Oklahoma

Thomas L. Carson, DVM, PhD, Dipl ABVT
Veterinary Toxicologist
Department of Veterinary Diagnostic and Production Animal Medicine
College of Veterinary Medicine
Iowa State University
Ames, Iowa

Stan W. Casteel, DVM, PhD, Dipl ABT
Professor of Toxicology
Veterinary Medical Diagnostic Laboratory
University of Missouri
Columbia, Missouri

Peter D. Constable, BVSc, MS, PhD, Dipl ACVIM
Associate Professor
Veterinary Clinical Medicine
University of Illinois
Urbana, Illinois

Robert Coppock, DVM, MS, PhD, Dipl ABVT, ABT
Adjunct Professor
Agriculture, Food and Nutritional Science
Faculty of Agriculture, Forestry and Home Economics and Public Health Sciences
Faculty of Medicine
University of Alberta
Edmonton, Alberta, Canada

Rosalind Dalefield, BVSc, PhD, Dipl ABVT, ABT
Principal Scientist, Study Direction
Mammalian Toxicology
Covance Laboratories Inc.
Vienna, Virginia

David Dorman, DVM, PhD, Dipl ABVT
Adjunct Professor, Toxicology
Department of Molecular Biomedical Sciences
College of Veterinary Medicine
North Carolina State University
Raleigh, North Carolina

Margita M. Dziwenka, DVM
Research Veterinarian
Department of Toxicology and Environmental Health
Alberta Research Council
Vegreville, Alberta, Canada

Steve Ensley, DVM, PhD, Dipl ABVT
Canine Study Director
Department of Toxicology
Bayer CropScience LP
Kansas City, Kansas

TIM J. EVANS, DVM, MS, PHD, DIPL ACT, ABVT
Assistant Professor, Toxicology
Department of Veterinary Pathobiology
Veterinary Toxicologist
Veterinary Medical Diagnostic Laboratory
College of Veterinary Medicine
University of Missouri
Columbia, Missouri

SCOTT D. FITZGERALD, DVM, PHD, DIPL ACVP, ACPV
Professor
Department of Pathobiology and Diagnostic Investigation
Diagnostic Center for Population and Animal Health
College of Veterinary Medicine
Michigan State University
East Lansing, Michigan

RICHARD L. FREDRICKSON, JR., DVM, MS
Assistant Professor
Veterinary Diagnostic Laboratory
University of Illinois
Urbana, Illinois

FRANCIS D. GALEY, DVM, PHD, DIPL ABVT
Dean
College of Agriculture
University of Wyoming
Laramie, Wyoming

SHARON GWALTNEY-BRANT, DVM, PHD, DIPL ABVT, ABT
Adjunct Instructor
Department of Veterinary Biosciences
College of Veterinary Medicine
University of Illinois
Manager, Veterinary Toxicology Training
ASPCA Animal Poison Control Center
Urbana, Illinois

JEFFREY O. HALL, DVM, PHD, DIPL ABVT
Associate Professor and Diagnostic Toxicologist
Department of Animal, Dairy, and Veterinary Sciences
Utah State University
Logan, Utah

WILLIAM R. HARE, DVM, MS, PHD, DIPL ABVT, ABT
Veterinary Medical Officer
USDA—ARS-ANRI
Beltsville Agricultural Research Center
Beltsville, Maryland

WILLIAM C. KELLER, DVM, MS, DIPL ABVT, ABT
Retired Director
Division of Surveillance
Center for Veterinary Medicine
Food and Drug Administration
Rockville, Maryland

ANTHONY P. KNIGHT, BVSc, MS, MRCVS, DIPL ACVIM
Professor
Clinical Sciences
Colorado State University
Fort Collins, Colorado

CAMILLA LIESKE, DVM, MPVM
Toxicology Resident
College of Veterinary Medicine
University of Illinois
Urbana, Illinois

SHAJAN A. MANNALA, BSc, BVSc, MS, PGD
Toxicologist
Human Safety Division
Veterinary Drug Directorate
Health Canada
Ottawa, Ontario, Canada

MILTON M. McALLISTER, DVM, PHD, DIPL ACVP
Associate Professor
Department of Veterinary Pathobiology
University of Illinois
Urbana, Illinois

CHARLOTTE MEANS, DVM, MLIS
Consulting Veterinarian in Clinical Toxicology
ASPCA Animal Poison Control Center
Urbana, Illinois

GAVIN L. MEERDINK, DVM, DIPL ABVT
Clinical Professor and Head, Diagnostic Toxicology
Veterinary Diagnostic Laboratory
University of Illinois
Urbana, Illinois

VALENTINA MEROLA, DVM
Resident in Veterinary Toxicology
Department of Veterinary Biosciences
College of Veterinary Medicine
University of Illinois
Urbana, Illinois

ROBERT B. MOELLER, JR., DVM
Associate Professor, Clinical Veterinary Pathology
California Animal Health and Food Safety Laboratory
System
University of California—Davis
Tulare, California

SANDRA E. MORGAN, DVM, MS, DIPL ABVT
Associate Professor and Veterinary Toxicologist
Department of Physiological Sciences
Oklahoma Animal Disease Diagnostic Laboratory
College of Veterinary Medicine
Oklahoma State University
Stillwater, Oklahoma

SHERRY J. MORGAN, DVM, PhD, DIPL ACVP,
ABT, ABVT
Scientific Director
Preclinical Safety
Abbott Laboratories
Abbott Park, Illinois

CARLA K. MORROW, DVM, MS, DIPL ABVT
Veterinary Toxicology Resident
Veterinary Biosciences
University of Illinois
Urbana, Illinois

STEVEN S. NICHOLSON, DVM, DIPL ABVT
Extension Specialist and Associate Professor
of Veterinary Toxicology
Veterinary Science Department
Louisiana State University AgCenter
School of Veterinary Medicine
Louisiana State University
Baton Rouge, Louisiana

GENE NILES, DVM, MS, DIPL ABVT
Illinois Department of Agriculture
Animal Disease Laboratory
Centralia, Illinois

FRED OEHME, DVM, PhD, DIPL ABVT
Professor, Toxicology, Pathobiology, Medicine and
Physiology
Director, Comparative Toxicology Laboratories
College of Veterinary Medicine
Kansas State University
Manhattan, Kansas

GARY OSWEILER, DVM, MS, PhD, DIPL ABVT
Professor
Department of Veterinary Diagnostic and
Production Animal Medicine
Iowa State University
Ames, Iowa

KIP E. PANTER, PhD
Adjunct Professor
Animal, Dairy and Veterinary Science Department
Utah State University
Logan, Utah

MUKUND PARKHIE, DVM, PhD
Consultant, Drug Regulatory Affairs
Germantown, Maryland

KATHLEEN HENRY PARTON, BS, DVM, MS
Senior Lecturer
Institute of Veterinary, Animal and Biomedical Sciences
Massey University
Palmerston North, New Zealand

MICHAEL E. PETERSON, DVM, MS
Section Head, Toxicology
Reid Veterinary Hospital
Albany, Oregon

JOHN A. PICKRELL, DVM, PhD, DIPL ABT
Associate Professor and Environmental Toxicologist
Diagnostic Medicine/Pathobiology
College of Veterinary Medicine
Kansas State University
Manhattan, Kansas

KONNIE H. PLUMLEE, DVM, MS, DIPL ABVT,
ACVIM
Director
Veterinary Diagnostic Laboratory
Arkansas Livestock and Poultry Commission
Little Rock, Arkansas

ROBERT POPPENGA, DVM, PhD, DIPL ABVT
Associate Professor of Veterinary Toxicology
Chief, Toxicology Laboratory
New Bolton Center
Department of Pathobiology
School of Veterinary Medicine
University of Pennsylvania
Kennett Square, Pennsylvania

LYNN POST, MS, DVM, PhD, DIPL ABVT
Director, Division of Surveillance
Center for Veterinary Medicine
Food and Drug Administration
Rockville, Maryland

BIRGIT PUSCHNER, DVM, PhD, DIPL ABVT
Assistant Professor, Veterinary Toxicology
California Animal Health and Food Safety Laboratory
System
School of Veterinary Medicine
University of California—Davis
Davis, California

JILL RICHARDSON, DVM
Associate Director
Consumer Relations and Technical Services
The Hartz Mountain Corporation
Secaucus, New Jersey

JOSEPH D. RODER, DVM, PhD, DIPL ABVT
Manager, Livestock Technical Services
Schering-Plough Animal Health Corporation
Canyon, Texas

MARCY ROSENDALE, DVM
Veterinary Medical Officer
USDA-APHIS
Fresno, California

GEORGE E. ROTTINGHAUS, PhD
Associate Professor
Veterinary Medical Diagnostic Laboratory
University of Missouri
Columbia, Missouri

WILSON K. RUMBEIHA, DVM, PhD, DIPL ABT, ABVT
Veterinary Clinical Toxicologist
Pathobiology and Diagnostic Investigation
College of Veterinary Medicine
Michigan State University
East Lansing, Michigan

MARY MICHAEL SCHELL, DVM
Consulting Veterinarian in Clinical Toxicology
ASPCA Animal Poison Control Center
Urbana, Illinois

GEOFFREY W. SMITH, DVM, MS, PhD
Assistant Professor, Ruminant Medicine
Department of Population Health and Pathobiology
North Carolina State University
Raleigh, North Carolina

WAYNE SPOO, DVM, DIPL ABT, ABVT
Assistant Research Director
Center for Life Sciences and Toxicology
RTI International
Research Triangle Park, North Carolina

ERIC L. STAIR, DVM, PhD, DIPL ABVT, ABT
Veterinary Pathologist/Toxicologist
Veterinary Diagnostic Laboratory
Arkansas Livestock and Poultry Commission
Little Rock, Arkansas

BRYAN STEGELMEIER, DVM, PhD, DIPL ACVP
Veterinary Pathologist
USDA/ARS Poisonous Plant Research Laboratory
Logan, Utah

PATRICIA A. TALCOTT, MS, DVM, PhD, DIPL ABVT
Associate Professor
Department of Food Science and Toxicology
University of Idaho
Moscow, Idaho

RONALD J. TYRL, PhD
Professor, Botany
Curator of Herbarium
Department of Botany
Oklahoma State University
Stillwater, Oklahoma

DAVID VILLAR, DVM, MS, PhD, DIPL ABVT
Adjunct Instructor, Toxicology
Veterinary Diagnostic Laboratory
Iowa State University
Ames, Iowa

PETRA A. VOLMER, DVM, MS, DIPL ABVT, ABT
Assistant Professor, Toxicology
Department of Veterinary Biosciences
Veterinary Diagnostic Laboratory
University of Illinois
Urbana, Illinois

DIANN L. WEDDLE, DVM, PhD
Pathologist
Department of Pathology, Preclinical Safety
Abbott Laboratories
Abbott Park, Illinois

SHERRY WELCH, DVM
ASPCA Animal Poison Control Center
Urbana, Illinois

DENNIS W. WILSON, DVM, PhD, DIPL ACVP
Professor
Department of Pathology, Microbiology, and Immunology
School of Veterinary Medicine
University of California—Davis
Davis, California

Tina Wismer, DVM, Dipl ABVT
Veterinary Toxicologist
ASPCA Animal Poison Control Center
Urbana, Illinois

Leslie W. Woods, DVM, PhD, Dipl ACVP
Associate Professor
California Animal Health and Food Safety Laboratory
School of Veterinary Medicine
University of California—Davis
Davis, California

In memory of my grandmother
Edith Plumlee
who always told me,
"You can do anything you set your mind to."

Veterinary toxicology is a difficult subject because poisons can affect animals differently depending on species, breed, age, gender, health status, or reproductive status. This book is a comprehensive text to be used as a teaching tool for veterinary students and as a reference for clinical practitioners treating pets, livestock, or birds.

ORGANIZATION

The book is divided into three parts.
- PART ONE: PRINCIPLES OF TOXICOLOGY. This part provides the basic information needed to understand how poisons affect the body, how the body responds to a foreign substance, how poisonings are diagnosed, and how poisonings are treated.
- PART TWO: MANIFESTATIONS OF TOXICOSES. This part provides differential diagnoses and pathologic findings associated with toxic effects on each body system. The pages in this section are edged in gray to make the section easy to find.
- PART THREE: CLASSES OF TOXICANTS. This part classifies poisons by type or source and provides detailed information regarding synonyms, sources, toxicokinetics, mechanism of action, toxicity, risk factors, clinical signs, clinical pathology, lesions, diagnostic testing, treatment, prognosis, and prevention and control. Several toxicants fall into more than one category; to prevent redundancy, each toxicant was placed in the most logical category.

The plant chapter was the most difficult to organize, with options including plant family, genus name, or common name. The decision was made to classify the plants by toxin so there would be a unified discussion of all plants that cause the same disease. Plants with undescribed toxins are categorized under "Unknown Toxins." Of course, some plants cause more than one toxic problem, and the reader is referred to the index to locate all page references for any given plant.

FUNCTION

This book is designed to be a comprehensive and unique text that meets the needs of the veterinary student as well as the clinician. It can be used either to study groups of poisons or as a resource for developing a differential diagnosis for poisoned animals.

PART THREE categorizes the poisons by type (metals, mycotoxins, etc.) or source (feed-associated, household, etc.) to assist the reader in grouping the poisons in a logical manner. This allows the veterinarian, when confronted with a known poison, to determine the class of toxicant, its mechanism of action, and the proper course of treatment. However, the veterinarian is often confronted with a patient that is intoxicated with an unknown poison. The reader can refer to PART TWO to find a list of potential toxicants based on the clinical signs or lesions that the patient is exhibiting. From there, the reader can refer to PART THREE to read about the specific poisons so that the list of possible etiologies can be narrowed further.

Konnie H. Plumlee

Acknowledgments

Throughout my years as a veterinary student, a clinician, and finally a toxicologist, I wondered why a comprehensive textbook devoted to veterinary toxicology was not available. About a year into the writing of this book, I understood why! Organizing the contents of the book and the multitude of authors was a daunting task. I owe a great deal of gratitude to the contributing authors, who graciously share their knowledge and expertise on the pages of this book. Special thanks to everyone at Elsevier who worked on this project, especially Linda Duncan for understanding my vision for the book, and Teri Merchant for her infinite patience and words of encouragement.

Konnie H. Plumlee
Little Rock, Arkansas

Contents

Detailed Contents

PART ONE

PRINCIPLES OF TOXICOLOGY

1

Concepts and Terminology

Wayne Spoo

Toxicology is the study of poisons, including their chemical properties and biological effects. Diagnosis and treatment of organisms that are affected by poisons are included in this study. A poison is any solid, liquid, or gas that interferes with life processes, ranging from the molecular level, to the organism level, to the population level. The study of toxicology has rapidly evolved during the twentieth century into a specialty area of scientific research. Its early beginnings primarily focused on describing the appearance of a toxic effect and perhaps how to treat it, with not much emphasis on why the toxic effect occurred in the first place. Currently, veterinary toxicologists not only provide valuable descriptive toxicology on a wide range of metals (cadmium, mercury, lead), organics (2,3,7,8-tetrachlorodibenzo-dioxin, polychlorinated biphenyls, and water disinfection by-products, such as chloroform), drugs (sulfonamides, aminoglycosides), and man-made products (asbestos), but they also provide much needed mechanistic information down to the molecular and genetic level. These veterinary toxicologists are valuable contributors in veterinary preventive health issues and in new research areas such as genomics and proteomics.

DEFINITIONS

The following are basic concepts and definitions related to toxicology:

- *Toxicant.* An alternative term for poison.
- *Toxin.* A poison that originates from biological processes; also called a *biotoxin*. Mycotoxins (fungal toxins) and zootoxins (animal toxins) are common examples of biotoxins. Many plants are also known to be toxic when consumed by specific types of animals.
- *Toxicity.* The quantity or amount of a poison that causes a toxic effect. "Toxicity" and "toxicosis" are often mistakenly used interchangeably.
- *Toxicosis.* A disease state that results from exposure to a poison.
- *Dose.* The amount of toxicant that is received per animal.

- *Dosage.* The amount of toxicant per unit of animal mass or weight. It can also be expressed as the amount of toxicant per unit of mass or weight per unit of time. For instance, a dog could receive a dosage of chemical at the rate of 2 mg/kg/day. When conducting traditional acute, subacute, subchronic, or chronic studies (defined later in this section), the length and frequency of exposure are also noted. For instance, rats may receive a chemical dosage of 2.5 mg/kg/day for 2 years.
- *Route of exposure.* The route of exposure is an important component of assessing the toxicity of a chemical or drug. The most common routes of exposure are inhalation, oral, and dermal, with some variations for each. In oral exposure, for example, a known amount of the chemical may be offered in drinking water, via gavage, or by introducing it into the stomach via gastrostomy, depending on what the investigator needs to learn about the specific toxicant. Dermal exposure may involve putting a known amount of chemical onto a patch of skin and leaving it occluded (covered) or unoccluded (uncovered and open to the air). Intravenous studies are more commonly used during toxicokinetic studies. Less frequently used routes of exposure include rectal, sublingual, subcutaneous, and intramuscular.
- *Threshold dose.* The highest dose of a toxicant at which toxic effects are not observed.
- *Lethal dose (LD).* When a new drug or chemical is first being examined for possible use, investigators often know little about how this entity behaves in a mammalian system. Acute toxicity studies determine the effects of the drug or chemical observed over a wide range of doses. One such effect is the potential of the drug or chemical to cause death. The dose at which 50% of the animals die during some period of observation is termed the *lethal dose 50%,* or LD_{50}. LD can also be expressed as other percentages such as LD_{10} (dose at which 10% lethality occurs in test animals) or LD_{90} (dose at which 90% lethality occurs in test animals).

- *Lethal concentration (LC).* Similar to an LD, an LC is the lowest concentration of a chemical or drug in a matrix (usually feed or water) that causes death. If the chemical was present in water, the dose that killed half of the animals may be expressed as unit of chemical per unit of water (e.g., 50 mg chemical/100 ml water) and would be expressed as the LC_{50}. LCs are most commonly used when expressing lethality for fish or wildlife species.
- *Median lethal dose (MLD).* A term used interchangeably with the LD_{50}.
- *NOEL* and *NOAEL.* Acronyms for *no observed effect level* and *no observed adverse effect level.* An NOEL is defined as the highest dose at which a significant effect could not be found. Similarly, an NOAEL is the highest dose at which a significant *adverse* effect could not be found. The difference between an NOEL and an NOAEL is significant when performing risk assessment estimates. Suppose a study tested a chemical at dosages of 1, 5, 10, 50, and 100 mg/kg/day for 30 days via the drinking water. After the data were analyzed and the dose per animal was corrected for water intake, no effects were found at the 1 and 5 mg/kg/day dosages. However, a 2% increase in body weight (BW) occurred at 10 mg/kg/day, a 7.5% increase occurred at 50 mg/kg/day, and an 11% increase in BW occurred at 100 mg/kg/day. Two questions arise: (1) Is an increase in BW an adverse effect? (2) If so, at what level is it considered an adverse effect? If this particular study defined BW as not a significant effect, then the NOEL is 100 mg/kg/day. However, if BW gain can be considered an adverse effect, but a 2% gain is not adverse whereas a 7.5% gain is considered adverse, then the NOEL is 5 mg/kg/day and the NOAEL is 10 mg/kg/day.
- *LOEL* and *LOAEL.* Acronyms for *lowest observed effect level* and *lowest observed adverse effect level.* An LOEL is defined as the lowest dose at which a significant effect could be found. Similarly, an LOAEL is the lowest dose at which a significant *adverse* effect could be found. As with NOELs and NOAELs, the difference between a LOEL and LOAEL can be significant. Suppose again that a study tested a chemical at dosages of 1, 5, 10, 50, and 100 mg/kg/day for 30 days via the drinking water. After the data were analyzed and the dose per animal was again corrected for water intake, no toxicologic effects were found at the 1 and 5 mg/kg/day dosages. A 2% increase in BW was noted at the 10 mg/kg/day dosage, an increase of 7.5% was noted at 50 mg/kg/day, and an increase of 11% in BW was noted at 100 mg/kg/day. If BW gain was considered a significant adverse effect, then by definition the LOAEL is 10 mg/kg/day. If BW gain was classified as just an effect (but not considered adverse), the LOEL is 10 mg/kg/day. This example also illustrates that there can be overlap in doses between NOELs, NOAELs, and LOELs, depending on the data being examined.

- *Effective dose (ED).* The dose of drug or toxicant that produces some desired effect in 50% of a population.
- *Therapeutic index (TI).* Defined by the equation $TI = LD_{50}/ED_{50}$, the TI is a unitless estimate that characterizes the relative safety of a drug or chemical. The larger the TI, the more "safe" a chemical is relative to another with a smaller TI. For example, if chemical X has an LD_{50} of 1000 mg/kg and an ED_{50} of 10 mg/kg, the TI would be 100 (the mg/kg units cancel). Compare this to chemical Y, which has an LD_{50} of 50 mg/kg and an ED_{50} of 40 mg/kg. The TI of chemical Y is 1.25, a much less safe chemical when compared with chemical X.
- *Standard safety margin (SSM)* or *margin of safety (MoS).* Defined by the equation $SSM = LD_1/ED_{99}$, the SSM, like the TI, is a unitless estimate that characterizes the relative safety of a drug or chemical, but much more conservative data are used. The larger the SSM, the more safe the chemical tends to be relative to other chemicals with smaller SSMs.
- *Exposure duration.* The length of time an animal is exposed to a drug or chemical. In general, there are four subgroups:
  - Acute. Exposure to a single or multiple doses during a 24-hour period. The LD_{50} is often determined during acute exposure studies.
  - Subacute. Exposure to multiple doses of a toxicant for greater than 24 hours but for as long as 30 days.
  - Subchronic. Exposure lasting from 1 to 3 months.
  - Chronic. Exposure for 3 months or longer. Chronic duration carcinogenicity studies in rats can last up to 2 years (104 weeks), whereas chronic duration (life-span) studies in dogs can last several years.
- *Hazard (risk).* Hazard, or risk, is the likelihood that a chemical or drug will cause harm under certain conditions. Risk assessment is a specialized area of toxicology that is of great importance to health assessors and government regulators.

TOXICOLOGY VERSUS PHARMACOLOGY

Toxicology and pharmacology can be thought of as the same discipline on two different ends of the spectrum (Fig. 1-1).

Pharmacology is the study of chemicals (drugs) used at doses to achieve therapeutic (beneficial) effects on an organism. Toxicology is the study of chemicals (toxicants) that produce a harmful (detrimental) effect on an organism. Using a hypothetical chemical such as shown in Fig. 1-1, the effect is largely determined by how much of a chemical the organism receives. In this illustration, little effect is noted until a dosage of 125 mg/kg/day is reached. As the dosage increases through 250 mg/kg/day, more effect is produced. In this example, the beneficial effects of decreasing the heart rate by 5% (125 mg/kg/day) and by 10% (200 mg/kg/day) was followed by decreasing serum cholesterol by 20% (250 mg/kg/day). If all of these effects are considered to

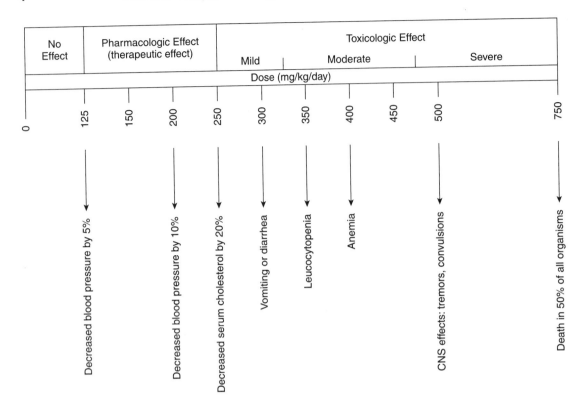

Fig. 1-1 Linearized plot of the dose-response to a chemical.

be desirable, then they are considered therapeutic effects. However, as the dosage increases to more than 250 mg/kg/day, the therapeutic effects are thwarted by a series of toxic effects, such as vomiting and bloody diarrhea (300 mg/kg/day), leukocytopenia (350 mg/kg/day), anemia (400 mg/kg/day), and central nervous system effects, including tremors and convulsions (500 mg/kg/day). As the dosage climbs higher, exposure to this chemical ultimately results in death of 50% of the organisms when the dosage reaches 750 mg/kg/day. Fig. 1-1 portrays the basic concept of the dose-response relationship.

THE DOSE-RESPONSE RELATIONSHIP

The dose-response relationship is the most basic and most important fundamental concept in the field of toxicology because so many health and economic assessments, as well as regulatory decisions, often depend on the integrity of this relationship. In a true dose-response relationship, there is some measurable effect that is proportional to the amount of the chemical received. Three general assumptions must be considered when evaluating the dose-response relationship:

1. The chemical interacts with a molecular or receptor site to produce a response.
2. The production of the response, or the degree of response, is correlated to the concentration of the chemical at that receptor site.
3. The concentration of the chemical at the receptor site is related to the dose of chemical received.[1]

There is a varied response as to which or to how many receptor sites a given chemical will affect. Much of this response depends on the toxicokinetic properties of the chemical (see Chapter 2). Some chemicals may be absorbed quickly and distributed to a large number of tissues, but they may only affect one or a few specific tissues, whereas other chemicals may have similar or identical properties but affect many cells and tissues throughout the body. Conversely, other chemicals may be poorly absorbed and distributed within the body, and may affect just one, a few, or many tissues. Others may be absorbed with little or no immediate effect, but may increase the risk of cancer in some tissues many years later.

Exposure to a toxicant assumes that one or more cells, tissues, or organs are susceptible to being disrupted by this chemical. The area of the body that is most often affected by this chemical is usually referred to as the *target organ* and may or may not cause pathognomonic lesions that indicate its presence. The route of exposure also plays a role in determining the target organ. For example, oral exposure to cadmium results in renal lesions with little effect on the lungs, whereas inhalation exposure affects the lungs first, with possible involvement of the kidneys. Dermal exposure produces little if any toxicity, even after prolonged exposure. Again, toxicokinetics plays a role. More chemical is needed to produce more effect. One route of exposure may provide a larger amount of chemical over the same exposure period than another route of exposure, providing more chemical and hence more effect and more toxicity. Species differences in

TABLE 1-1   Model Mortality Data for Two Chemicals Administered to a Group of Animals.

Dosage (mg/kg/day)	Number of Animals Exposed (per Chemical)	Chemical A		Chemical B	
		Number of Animals that Died	(% Mortality)	Number of Animals that Died	(% Mortality)
500	10	0	0	0	0
600	10	1	10	3	30
700	10	3	33	1	10
800	10	7	70	4	40
900	10	9	90	1	10
1000	10	10	100	0	0

absorption, distribution, metabolism, and excretion, as well as interspecies susceptibility may play integral roles in determining the toxicity of a specific chemical.

For example, consider the dose-response to "chemical A" and "chemical B" shown in Table 1-1 and graphically represented in Fig. 1-2.

The key question that must be answered is this: Does increasing the exposure dosages of these chemicals result in a corresponding increase in mortality? Dose-response curve A shows increasing amount of mortality as the dose of the chemical increases. Therefore, if the assumptions stated earlier in this section are true, then the logical conclusion is that this chemical causes increasing mortality as the dose increases. Dose-response curve B, however, suggests this is not the case. Mortality is not correlated to either increased or decreased amounts of this chemical, suggesting that mortality is not definitively linked to exposure to this chemical.

The dose-response curve for any number of chemicals can be altered by a number of factors: selective toxicity, interspecies differences, and individual (intraspecies) differences.

- **Selective Toxicity.** This type of toxicity produces injury to one kind of organism (or part of an organism) and not to another. Selective toxicity may be due to a number of

reasons, including the presence or absence of the target receptor in one species and not another. Selective toxicity can be used to a toxicologist's advantage when designing drugs and chemicals with specific species use in mind. For example, toxicologists in the agrochemical industry may take advantage of selective toxicity and manipulate test chemicals so as to enhance the selective toxicity of their pesticides toward a specific pest while minimizing (to the greatest extent possible) the toxic effects in nontarget species, such as pets, food animals, wildlife, and humans. Many of the very early forms of the organophosphate pesticides had powerful insecticidal effects but also produced toxicosis in animals that were not the intended target species, including humans. Today, chemical manipulations of the basic organophosphate molecules have resulted in higher affinity toward the target species and less toxic effects in workers exposed to these pesticides.

Another classic example of selective toxicity is the sulfonamide class of antimicrobials. Bacteria cannot absorb folic acid, so they must manufacture folic acid. Mammals, on the other hand, cannot synthesize folic acid, so they must absorb the needed folic acid from the diet. Veterinarians routinely take advantage of this information when administering sulfonamides for susceptible bacterial infections. Sulfonamides act as competitive antagonists with *para*-aminobenzoic acid, a critical intermediate in the formation of folic acid in the bacterial cell. Hence, sulfonamides block the production of folic acid in the bacterial cell, but because mammals derive their source of folic acid from the diet and not through intracellular manufacturing, normal cell processes can continue in the mammalian cell.

- **Interspecies Differences.** Both quantitative and qualitative differences occur between species as to the toxicity of a particular chemical or drug, both in the intensity of the toxic response and perhaps even the target organ affected. A good example of species differences in toxicity is acetaminophen use in canines versus felines. The toxic dose of acetaminophen in felines is 50 to 100 mg/kg, whereas the toxic dose for the canine is 600 mg/kg.[2] Canines can tolerate 6 to 12 times the dose on a

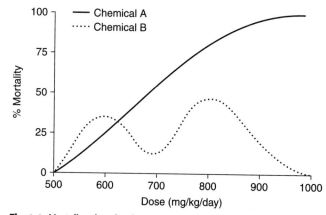

Fig. 1-2 Mortality plot of a chemical used to calculate the LD_{50}.

milligram per kilogram basis than can felines. Why such a dramatic difference between species? The increased sensitivity to acetaminophen in felines is related to how the drug is metabolized. In dogs (and humans), acetaminophen is metabolized via phase II metabolism by hepatic glucuronide, sulfate, or cysteine conjugation, with glucuronidation being the primary form of conjugation. This conjugate is then excreted and toxicosis is averted. Felines, however, possess limited glucuronidation metabolic capabilities, hence they must rely on the two other, less-efficient pathways. As more acetaminophen is absorbed and taken to the liver for metabolism, hepatic necrosis ultimately occurs. Methemoglobinemia, Heinz body formation, cyanosis, anorexia, hemolysis, and icterus are all consequences of the feline's inability to glucuronidate acetaminophen to any appreciable extent. Conversely, dogs have a more developed glucuronidation capability and can, therefore, withstand much higher doses of acetaminophen on a milligram per kilogram basis than felines.

- **Individual (Intraspecies) Differences.** Whereas toxicity differences between species can be profound, differences between individuals within a species can also be significant.

Few good examples of intraspecies variations in toxicity can be found in the veterinary literature. Intraspecies differences in toxicity to a chemical or drug have drawn the most attention in human toxicology and pharmacology. Hereditary polymorphism, or hereditary differences in a single gene, has been the subject of research in recent years. For example, transgenic mice that possess a copy of the mutated p53 gene (i.e., the "tumor suppressor gene") are at increased risk of developing some types of cancer when compared with those mice with two normal copies of the same gene. As research expands in this area, intraspecies differences of veterinary importance will no doubt surface.

USEFUL VALUES AND CALCULATIONS

Veterinary toxicologists often have to calculate the amount of toxicant that an animal is or was exposed to in order to construct dose-response curves or to estimate exposure. Table 1-2 lists common conversion factors and units used in day-to-day toxicologic calculations.[2]

Toxicologists routinely have to answer two questions: How much did the animal receive of the toxicant (or potential toxicant)? Will the animal suffer ill effects from the dose of the toxicant received? Sample calculations are demonstrated below:

SAMPLE CALCULATION 1

Chemical X is present in horse feed at 50 parts per million (ppm). What is the concentration of Chemical X expressed in mg/kg and g/ton?

TABLE 1-2 Conversion Factors Used in Veterinary Toxicology

Unit	Symbol	Equivalent
Parts per million	ppm	mg/kg
		0.91 g/ton
		0.0001%
		µg/ml
Weight Measurements		
1 ounce	oz	28.35 g
1 gram	g	15.43 grains
1 pound	lb	453.6 g
1 milligram	mg	0.001 g
		1/1,000,000 kg
1 kilogram	kg	2.205 lb
1 ton		907.2 kg
	ton	2000 lb
1 metric ton	ton	1000 kg
Liquid Measurements		
1 ounce	oz	29.6 ml
1 quart	qt	0.946 L
		57.75 cubic inches
1 gallon	gal	3.785 L
1 gallon (pure water)	gal	8.35 lb
1 cubic foot	cu ft	7.48 gal
		28.32 L
1 bushel	bu	9.31 gal
1 liter	L	1.057 qt
		0.264 gal
1 teaspoon	tsp	5 ml
1 tablespoon	T	15 ml
1 acre-foot		3.259×10^5 gal
Dry Measurements		
1 bushel	bu	8 gal
		35.24 L
		1.24 cu ft
1 cubic meter	m³	35.3 cu ft
Length		
1 inch	in	2.54 cm
1 yard	yd	91.44 cm
1 meter	m	39.37 in
1 centimeter	cm	0.3937 in
1 millimeter	mm	1×10^{-3} m
1 micron	µm	1×10^{-6} m
		1×10^{-3} mm
Area		
1 acre	acre	43,560 sq ft
1 hectare	hectare	2.471 acres
		10,000 m²

Modified from Osweiler GD: *Toxicology*, Philadelphia, 1996, Williams & Wilkins.

SOLUTION:

Table 1-2 states that 1 ppm is equivalent to 1 mg/kg, hence 50 ppm = 50 mg/kg, which completes the first requirement for expression of exposure in mg/kg.

Table 1-2 also states that 1 ppm is equivalent to 0.91 g/ton (or 1 g/ton = 1.1 ppm). Therefore, 50 ppm = 45.5 g/ton.

SAMPLE CALCULATION 2

Chemical X is known to induce hepatic necrosis at 100 mg/day in feed and causes central nervous system (CNS) depression at 700 mg/day. If an animal consumes 12 lb of feed that contains 25 mg/kg of the toxicant, what toxic effects can be expected to occur?

SOLUTION:

First convert pounds to kilograms:

12 lb × 0.45 kg/lb = 5.4 kg of feed consumed per day

Next, calculate the amount of toxin consumed per day:

5.4 kg feed × 25 mg/kg toxin = 135 mg total toxin consumed per day

Because 100 mg < 135 mg < 700 mg, then hepatic necrosis can be expected, but not CNS depression.

SAMPLE CALCULATION 3

A 350-g female rat on a routine toxicology screening study is to receive a dose of 50 mg/kg twice a day of a chemical suspected of disrupting estrogen production. The rat will receive the chemical via gavage using corn oil as the vehicle. If the corn oil solution contains 45 mg/ml of chemical, how much of the solution should the animal receive per day?

SOLUTION:

First, determine how much total chemical the rat should receive:

350 g × 1 kg/1000 g = 0.35 kg rat

0.35 kg × 50 mg/kg/dose period = 17.5 mg of chemical per dosing period

Next, determine the dose volume per dose period:

45 mg/1 ml = 17.5 mg/x

x = 0.39 ml

So, this rat will receive 0.39 ml of the solution per dose period. Because there are two dose periods, then 0.39 × 2 = 0.78 ml per day.

SUMMARY

Toxicology has evolved into an exciting and specialized field of study. The veterinary toxicologist must have a complete understanding of the basic concepts of toxicology and how these concepts are applied in real-world situations for both humans and animals. Interpretation of dose-response curves is a critical task that must be performed in order to determine NOEL, NOAEL, LOEL, LOAEL, target organ toxicity, and LD_{50}, which in turn provide valuable information about the toxicity of the chemical or drug. All of this information is compiled to provide the best information possible to determine the risk of drugs and chemicals to both animals and humans.

REFERENCES

1. Eaton DL, Klaassen CD: Principles of toxicology. In Klaassen CD, editor: *Casarett and Doull's toxicology: the basic science of poisons*, ed 5, New York, 1996, McGraw-Hill.
2. Osweiler GD: *Toxicology*, Philadelphia, 1996, Williams & Wilkins.

2

Toxicokinetics

Wayne Spoo

Xenobiotic metabolism and kinetics involve the understanding of how a xenobiotic (or chemical) is absorbed, distributed, metabolized, and excreted within the framework of a biological system. If the xenobiotic is used for a pharmacologic purpose, then the *pharmacokinetics* must be studied and clearly defined before it can be used in humans or animals. However, if a xenobiotic is introduced into the body in a quantity that could produce toxicosis, then the *toxicokinetics* of this xenobiotic is important information that is needed both to determine the risk to the animal and to devise treatment protocols.

Pharmacokinetics and toxicokinetics are also important concepts regarding food residue and safety issues as well as drug withdrawal times in food-producing animals. In 1982, the U.S. Department of Agriculture (USDA) Extension Service began involvement in an educational/service project to further enhance the safety of animal-derived foods. The Residue Avoidance Program, which was initially founded by the USDA Food Safety and Inspection Service (FSIS), targeted the area of xenobiotic residues. The aim of the Residue Avoidance Program was to reduce the rate of animal residue violations through education rather than enforcement. As part of this program, the Food Animal Residue Avoidance Databank (FARAD) program was developed by pharmacologists and toxicologists at the University of California (Davis), University of Florida, North Carolina State University, and the University of Illinois. FARAD is a computer-based decision support system designed to provide livestock producers, extension specialists, and veterinarians with practical information on how to avoid drug, pesticide, and environmental contaminant residue problems. More information on FARAD is available at *http://www.farad.org/index.html.*

DEFINITIONS

A chemical must gain access to the systemic processes of the body before it can exert a toxic effect. The amount of the chemical that enters the animal determines the type of effect (if any) that occurs and how intense that effect will be; this is the dose-response (see Chapter 1).

Once the animal has been exposed to a chemical, four events take place: absorption, distribution, metabolism, and excretion (commonly known as ADME). *Absorption* defines how much of a chemical passes into the body over a period of time. Different routes of exposure produce different absorption patterns, which can vary both within a species (intraspecies variation) and between different species (interspecies variation). Once absorbed, the chemical is then distributed to different organs within the body, based again on a number of variables. *Distribution* varies widely from chemical to chemical, but it is sometimes possible to predict the distribution of a chemical based on its physiochemical properties or based on its structural similarities to related chemicals for which the ADME has been characterized. Some chemicals remain in the body water, whereas others are distributed within adipose tissue. Once distributed, the chemical can then be metabolized. *Metabolism* of chemicals varies, ranging from simple hydrolysis, to glutathione conjugation, to no metabolism at all. The liver is usually thought of as the major metabolic organ of the body. Other organs, however, such as skin, kidney, and gastrointestinal tract, also possess significant metabolic powers. Once metabolism (or lack of metabolism) takes place, the chemical is then eliminated from the body. *Elimination* usually occurs via the kidney (urine), gastrointestinal tract (feces), or lungs (exhalation of volatile chemicals); however, other excretory mechanisms do exist (e.g., tears, sweat, skin exfoliation).

Specific terms are required to provide an accurate description of the ADME characteristics of a chemical. Table 2-1 lists terms and definitions used in this process. Some of these terms are used herein; other terms are commonly used in scientific literature that describes ADME characteristics for many chemicals.

ABSORPTION

For a xenobiotic to exert a toxic effect, it must reach its site of actions. In doing so, it must gain access to the body by crossing any number of body membranes (e.g., skin, lung, gastrointestinal tract, and red blood cell membranes). Cell

TABLE 2-1 **Common Terms Used to Describe the ADME Characteristics of Chemicals**

Term	Abbreviation	Definition
Concentration	C_p	Concentration of a chemical in plasma (p) at a specific time (t).
Time	t	Chronologic measurement of a biological function.
Half-life	$t_{1/2}$	Time required for exactly 50% of a drug to undergo some defined function (i.e., absorbed, distributed, metabolized, or excreted).
Volume of distribution	V_d	Unitless proportionality constant that relates plasma concentration of a chemical to the total amount of that chemical in the body at any time after some pseudoequilibrium has been attained.
Volume of distribution (steady-state)	$V_{d(ss)}$	Same as V_d, except measured when the chemical has reached a steady-state in the body.
Area under the curve	AUC	Total area under the plasma chemical concentration curve from t = 0 to t = ∞ after the animal receives one dose of the chemical.
Body clearance of a chemical	Cl_B	The sum of all types of clearance from the body.
Renal clearance of a chemical	Cl_R	Volume of chemical that is completely cleared by the kidneys per unit of time (ml/min/kg).
Nonrenal clearance of a chemical	Cl_{NR}	Volume of chemical that is completely cleared by organs other than the kidneys per unit of time (ml/min/kg).
Dose	D	The amount of chemical that is administered to an animal. Can be further defined as the total dose, that total dose the animal was exposed to, or the absorbed (effective) dose, that being the fraction of the total dose that was actually absorbed by the animal.
Bioavailability	F	Also known as *systemic availability of a chemical*. The quantity or percentage portion of the total chemical that was absorbed and available to be processed (DME) by the animal. In the case of intravenous administration, F = 100%.

membranes are typically composed of phospholipid bilayers with embedded proteins and pores of various sizes, all potential routes of entry into a cell. Composition of these membranes varies, resulting in various levels of resistance to penetration. For example, the skin barrier generally offers more resistance to penetration because of the thick layers of stratum corneum than does the thin membrane of the lung alveolar surface.

Absorption can be described in terms of bioavailability (F), which is the quantity or percentage portion of the total chemical that is absorbed and available to be processed (DME) by the animal. In the case of intravenous administration, F = 100% because all of the xenobiotic enters the animal. For other routes of entry, the amount of xenobiotic that enters the animal can be measured (or at least estimated using mathematical expressions), and the F can be determined.

Inhalation, oral, and dermal are the three usual routes of exposure to xenobiotics. Each route has specific characteristics that allow a xenobiotic to gain access to the rest of the body.

INHALATION (PULMONARY)

Inhalation exposure to chemicals occurs when the chemical is dissolved in the ambient air inhaled by the animal. The chemical first reaches the nasal passages, when some absorption (and perhaps some metabolism) can take place before it enters the trachea, bronchi, and finally the alveoli. Once in the alveolus, the chemical can cross the very thin alveolar wall and enter the blood where it can then be distributed. Solubility of the chemical in the blood depends largely on the physiochemical properties, specifically the blood/gas partition coefficient. In most cases, not all of the chemical partitions into the blood and is exhaled.

ORAL (GASTROINTESTINAL)

Chemicals can enter the gastrointestinal tract in either contaminated food or water sources. Some inhaled substances can also enter the gastrointestinal tract via the mucociliary escalator and be swallowed; however, this is normally a minor route of exposure. Again, depending on the physicochemical properties of the chemical, several events can occur. For example, some chemicals are unstable in the stomach's acidic environment and can be destroyed to varying degrees, resulting in decreased absorption. On the other hand, some chemicals are readily absorbed from the stomach. Other chemicals enter the small intestine, where they may undergo enzymatic degradation or absorption through the intestinal mucosa and then into the blood. Portal circulation delivers them to the liver, a major metabolic organ of the body. Larger molecules that do not undergo degradation may not be absorbed and continue into the lower small intestine and into the large bowel, where they can be degraded by large intestine bacteria or be eliminated in feces.

DERMAL (PERCUTANEOUS)

Dermal absorption of chemicals has been largely ignored or considered to be insignificant in the past; however, the role of percutaneous absorption has been recognized as a significant route of exposure in many scenarios. Three key events must occur for percutaneous absorption to take place. First, the chemical must be soluble in the vehicle (solvent) that is applied to the skin. Second, it must be able to penetrate the thick keratin layer of the epidermis. Finally, it must make its way through the lower cells of the epidermis and into a blood vessel.

Percutaneous absorption is an important risk factor when applying certain pesticides on hot summer days. If workers in the hot sun enter a field whose foliage is still wet with pesticide and if that pesticide is water soluble, then the pesticide may be transferred from the water vehicle of the application solvent into the sweat on the skin of the worker. Absorption across the keratin and remaining epidermis is largely by passive transport, governed by the physiochemical properties of the chemical. The greater the ability of the chemical to cross a lipid membrane, the greater its likelihood of being absorbed. Percutaneous absorption can be modulated in a number of ways; more comprehensive information can be found elsewhere.[1]

Xenobiotics can pass through body membranes by either passive transport or active transport.

1. **Passive transport.** Passive transport requires no energy expenditure on the body's part to transport the xenobiotic across a cell membrane. According to Fick's law, the diffusion rate is directly proportional to the concentration gradient across a membrane. Passive transport is a nonsaturable process and is driven by concentration gradients across membranes. Passive transport occurs via two distinct mechanisms: simple diffusion and filtration.
   a. *Simple diffusion.* Most chemicals pass through biological membranes via this mechanism. Simple diffusion depends on both the lipid solubility and the size of the molecule. In general, lipid-soluble molecules and lipid-insoluble molecules of small size can pass through a membrane via simple diffusion. In biological matrices, most xenobiotics exist in a solution as either an ionized or un-ionized form. Un-ionized (uncharged) molecules have greater lipid solubility than the ionized forms and can thus traverse the phospholipid bilayers with much greater ease than charged (ionized) molecules.

      To predict whether a xenobiotic will penetrate a body membrane, three facts must be known: (1) whether the xenobiotic is a weak acid or a weak base, (2) the pH of the biological matrix that the xenobiotic will exist in, and (3) the association constant of the xenobiotic (or pK_a, the pH at which 50% of the xenobiotic is ionized and 50% is un-ionized). Once this information is known, the Henderson-Hasselbalch equation for either a weak acid or a weak base can be applied. For a weak acid:

      $$pK_a - pH = \log \frac{[\text{un-ionized}]}{[\text{ionized}]}$$

      For a weak base:

      $$pK_a - pH = \log \frac{[\text{ionized}]}{[\text{un-ionized}]}$$

      The higher the ratio of un-ionized:ionized, the greater the potential for absorption across a lipid membrane.

   b. *Filtration.* Filtration relies on the patency of a membrane. When water flows in bulk across a porous membrane, any solute that is small enough to pass through the pores flows with it. Xenobiotics that are small enough cross the cellular membrane and gain access to the biological matrix on the other side of the membrane.

2. **Active transport.** Active transport mechanisms usually require an energy expenditure on the body's part to transport the xenobiotic across a cell membrane.
   a. *Active transport* is a saturable process and is not driven by concentration gradients across membranes; rather, active transport moves xenobiotics against concentration gradients.
   b. *Facilitated transport* expends energy on xenobiotic transport, but it does not occur against a concentration gradient.
   c. *Pinocytosis* is another type of active transport mechanism that involves the ability of cells to engulf small masses of xenobiotic and carry it through the cell membrane.

DISTRIBUTION

Once absorbed across one of the body's barriers, the chemical enters the blood so that it can be distributed to the body's organs and tissues. The chemical leaves the blood and enters the tissues at varying rates, depending on a number of factors: (1) rate of blood flow (generally, the higher the blood flow, the more potential distribution to the organ), (2) the ability of the chemical to traverse the capillary endothelial wall, and (3) the physiochemical properties of the chemical, such as lipid solubility. For example, lindane is a lipid-soluble chemical that easily enters adipose tissue and remains sequestered there for an extended length of time. Conversely, ethanol is water soluble and remains in tissues that have significant amounts of water rather than distributing into the fat.

The extent of distribution within an animal can be described by the volume of distribution (V_d), which is a proportion between the amount of a chemical found in the blood to the total amount of drug in the body at any given time.[2] The equation is

$$V_d = A_{C(t)}/C_B$$

where $A_{C(t)}$ is the total amount of the chemical in the body at time t and C_B is the concentration of the chemical in the blood (B). The V_d does not specify a concentration of a chemical in a specific organ or describe which organ would accumulate the chemical; rather, it defines the volume of fluid that would be required to contain the amount of a chemical in the body if that concentration were to be equal to that found in the blood.

Knowing the V_d is clinically useful because it can give relative information about the potential of a chemical to distribute throughout the body. Examining the V_d equation, the higher the numerator or the lower the denominator, the higher the V_d. Restated, the higher the total chemical in the body or the lower the concentration in the blood, the higher

<table>
<tr><td colspan="2">

BOX 2-1 V_Ds OF THREE CHEMICALS
</td></tr>
</table>

CHEMICAL	V_D
Pentobarbital	1.8
Propranolol	3
Chlorpromazine	20

the V_d. Therefore, the higher the V_d, the higher the distribution from the blood to the tissues. Any number of factors may prevent a chemical of low V_d from distributing out of the blood compartment, including a high amount of binding to plasma proteins, being unable to cross the capillary endothelial cell layer into tissues, and animal to animal variation.

Box 2-1 shows that pentobarbital has a lower V_d than either propranolol or chlorpromazine, indicating that less pentobarbital would be expected to distribute into tissues than either propranolol or chlorpromazine. Chlorpromazine has the greatest potential to distribute out of the blood and into tissues, but the number does not give any indication about which tissues it would distribute to or in what quantity.

METABOLISM (BIOTRANSFORMATION)

Almost all organs have some ability to metabolize at least one xenobiotic, but the liver possesses the most metabolism capacity, regardless of species. However, other organs such as the kidneys, gastrointestinal tract, skin, heart, and brain also have considerable metabolic capabilities.

Numerous potential metabolic pathways exist for xenobiotics.[3,4] The ideal metabolic system should produce metabolites that are water soluble to allow for efficient excretion in the urine or bile. In addition, the metabolites should themselves be nontoxic. The enzymes used to produce the metabolites should have a broad enough substrate specificity to properly handle any newly encountered xenobiotic.

The metabolism of a xenobiotic usually occurs in several steps. As stated earlier, a key component of metabolism is to convert the xenobiotic into a water-soluble form (if it is not already) so it can be excreted from the body. To accomplish this, metabolic conversion can be categorized into two steps or phases, classically known as phase I and phase II. Phase I metabolism converts apolar, lipophilic xenobiotics into more polar and more hydrophilic metabolites via introduction or liberation of functional groups that can be used during phase II. Phase I metabolism uses a wide assortment of reactions that processes the xenobiotic via hydrolysis, oxidation, or reduction pathways. Phase II conjugates either the xenobiotic itself or its metabolite formed during phase I metabolism with a functional group that results in a multifold increase in water solubility. A xenobiotic may undergo phase I only,

<table>
<tr><td colspan="2">

BOX 2-2 COMMON BIOTRANSFORMATION PATHWAYS IN MAMMALIAN SYSTEMS
</td></tr>
</table>

PHASE 1

Reaction	Enzyme
Hydrolysis	Carboxylesterase
	Peptidase
	Epoxide hydrolase
Oxidation	Alcohol dehydrogenase
	Aldehyde dehydrogenase
	Aldehyde oxidase
	Xanthine oxidase
	Monoamine oxidase
	Diamine oxidase
	Prostaglandin H synthase
	Flavin-monooxygenases
	Cytochrome P-450
Reduction	Azo-reduction/nitro-reduction
	Carbonyl reduction
	Disulfide reduction
	Sulfoxide reduction
	Quinone reduction
	Reductive dehalogenation

Phase 2
Glucuronidation
Sulfation
Amino acid conjugation
Acylation
Methylation

phase II only, or both phase I and II, depending on the xenobiotic. Box 2-2 lists the most common metabolic reactions and the enzymes involved for each phase of metabolism.

Mammalian systems have a number of potential pathways for metabolizing xenobiotics; however, not all species have equal capabilities to do so. For example, most species of animals have the ability to glucuronidate xenobiotics during phase II metabolism, except for felines (e.g., domestic cats, lynxes, and lions). The major pathway for metabolism of acetaminophen is via glucuronidation. Unless acetaminophen is glucuronidated, the cytochrome P-450 system metabolizes this compound into *N*-acetybenzoquinoneimine, which binds to hepatic proteins and leads to centrilobular necrosis. Therefore, cats that receive a dose of acetaminophen can die of widespread hepatic failure within a few days.

Even when the correct metabolic enzyme is present, the presence of other xenobiotics can inhibit its function. An example of this is the cytochrome P-450 system of phase I metabolism, which metabolizes a number of therapeutic drugs, including phenytoin, piroxicam, and warfarin. Xenobiotics such as sulfaphenazole and sulfinpyrazone can inhibit CYP2C9 function, resulting in slower metabolism of the drugs and potential toxic side effects if inhibition continues for an extended period of time. Conversely, rifampin is a known CYP2C9 inducer, which can accelerate the metabolism of these drugs and decrease their clinical efficacy.

EXCRETION

Excretion is the last toxicokinetic step for a xenobiotic and involves removing the xenobiotic out of the body by a number of passages. Removing the xenobiotic via the urine is the most common route of excretion; however, other pathways do exist and are important alternates for some chemicals.

One of the alternate pathways is fecal excretion. Not all xenobiotics are completely absorbed, particularly via oral exposure. If absorption is less than 100%, the xenobiotic can continue down the gastrointestinal tract and either be metabolized by gut microbes or be passed unmetabolized out of the body via feces. Even if absorbed, some xenobiotics may be metabolized, excreted via the bile, and removed from the body in the feces. Enterohepatic circulation, which occurs when a xenobiotic is excreted in the bile and then reabsorbed later in a more distal part of the gastrointestinal tract, can occur with some chemicals and can lead to a prolonged half-life and potential toxicity. The intestinal tract itself can also push xenobiotics into the lumen of the tract and allow them to pass out of the body.

Other nonrenal routes of excretion include milk (particularly important because of the potential for residues in milk), cerebrospinal fluid, sweat, and saliva. Toxicants that are distributed to the skin can be detected in the keratin layer several days after exposure, followed by normal sloughing of the skin, which can rid the body of the xenobiotic. Exhalation is an important route of elimination, particularly when xenobiotics are inhaled or are volatile. For example, dogs administered small amounts of ethanol intravenously have detectable amounts of ethanol exhaled.

Excretion of a xenobiotic is generally broken down into two broad categories: renal and nonrenal. Determining the sum of clearance pathways can be defined by the following equation:

$$CL_B = CL_R + CL_{NR}$$

where CL_B is the total amount of xenobiotic and its metabolites, CL_R is the amount cleared via the urine, and CL_{NR} is the sum of all nonrenal pathways.

First order and *zero order kinetics* are terms used to describe how the body eliminates xenobiotics. Assuming a one-compartment model (i.e., the xenobiotic change in concentration in the plasma accurately reflects changes in tissue concentration), most xenobiotics are eliminated via first order kinetics. First order kinetic processes state that the rate of

TABLE 2-2   First Order Kinetics for Chemical X, 4 Hours after an Intravenous Dose

Dose (mg)	Amount Remaining (mg)	Amount Eliminated (mg)	Amount Eliminated (as % of Dose)
1	0.36	0.64	64
10	3.6	6.4	64
20	7.2	12.8	64
40	14.4	25.6	64
80	28.8	51.2	64
160	57.6	102.4	64

TABLE 2-3   Zero Order Kinetics for Chemical Y, after One 100-mg Intravenous Dose

Time (Hour after Administration)	Chemical Y Remaining (mg)	Chemical Y Eliminated (mg)	Chemical Y Eliminated (as % Remaining)
0	100	0	0
1	80	20	20
2	60	20	25
3	40	20	33
4	20	20	50
5	0	20	100

elimination (meaning both biotransformation and excretion) at any time point is proportional to the amount of the chemical in the body at that time. First order kinetics generally consist of nonsaturable pathways. Table 2-2 illustrates a data set that reflects first order kinetics.

Zero order kinetics are used to describe the elimination of xenobiotics through pathways that are saturable, meaning that the metabolic pathway can only eliminate a finite amount of chemical per unit of time. Table 2-3 demonstrates a data set that reflects zero order kinetics.

REFERENCES

1. Riviere JE, Spoo JW: Dermatopharmacology: drugs acting locally on the skin. In Adams HR, editor: *Veterinary pharmacology and therapeutics*, ed 8, Ames, Iowa, 2001, Iowa State University Press.
2. Brown SA: Pharmacokinetics: disposition and fate of drugs in the body. In Adams HR, editor: *Veterinary pharmacology and therapeutics*, ed 8, Ames, Iowa, 2001, Iowa State University Press.
3. Medinsky MA, Klaassen CD: Toxicokinetics. In Klaassen CD, editor: *Casarett and Doull's toxicology: the basic science of poisons*, ed 5, New York, 1996, McGraw-Hill.
4. Oesch F, Arand M: Xenobiotic metabolism. In Marquardt H, Schafer S, McClellan R, Welsch F, editors: *Toxicology*, San Diego, 1999, Academic Press.

3

Treatment

Robert Poppenga

In many situations, even when there is a strong suspicion of intoxication, no specific toxicant can be identified and no exposure determined. Ultimately, the advice to "treat the patient and not the toxicant" is sound. Most intoxicated patients recover with close monitoring, appropriate symptomatic intervention, and good nursing care.

Once a determination is made that an animal has been exposed to a potentially toxic amount of a substance or is intoxicated, a general approach to case management should adhere to the following principles:

Stabilize vital signs

Obtain a history and clinically evaluate the patient

Decontaminate to prevent continued systemic absorption of the toxicant

Administer an antidote if indicated and available

Enhance elimination of absorbed toxicant

Provide symptomatic and supportive care

Closely monitor the patient[1,2]

Each situation is unique and one or more of the steps may be eliminated. For example, there may not be an antidote for a given toxicant or a way to significantly enhance its elimination once systemically absorbed.

STABILIZATION OF VITAL SIGNS

Specific approaches to stabilization of vital signs are discussed more thoroughly elsewhere.[3,4] Briefly, attention should be paid to maintaining a patent airway and providing adequate ventilation, maintaining cardiovascular function with attention to appropriate fluid and electrolyte administration, maintaining acid-base balance, controlling central nervous system signs such as seizures, and maintaining body temperature. In some situations, it may be critical to administer an antidote quickly. For example, in suspected cholinesterase-inhibiting insecticide intoxication (organophosphates or carbamates), administration of atropine may be critical to control life-threatening muscarinic signs such as bronchospasm and bronchorrhea before proceeding with subsequent management steps.

EVALUATION OF THE PATIENT

Once vital signs are stable, a thorough history should be obtained while the animal is being further evaluated. If blood or urine samples are obtained for clinical evaluation, appropriate portions should be set aside for possible toxicologic testing. A minimum database in suspected toxicologic cases includes complete blood count, blood urea nitrogen, creatinine, serum electrolytes, glucose, liver enzymes, electrocardiogram, blood gases, pulse oximetry, urinalysis, and body temperature. Abdominal radiographs should be considered to detect ingested metal objects.

DECONTAMINATION

The goal of decontamination is to prevent continued absorption of the toxicant. A number of factors should be considered in deciding the best approach to decontaminating a toxicant-exposed patient. These factors include consideration of the substance and amount of exposure, whether multiple agents are involved, the time since exposure, whether attempts at decontamination have been undertaken before presentation, the species of animal involved, number of individuals exposed, and whether there is any known underlying organ dysfunction, especially affecting the liver or kidneys.

TOXICITY

If a substance is nontoxic or has relatively low toxicity, then extensive decontamination procedures are generally not necessary. An exposure assessment should always be attempted to estimate the dose; this estimate should be compared with known toxicity information when possible. If the dose approaches a toxic dose, then more vigorous decontamination procedures are warranted. For example, if a dog has recently ingested an amount of an anticoagulant rodenticide that is well below reported toxic doses (less than or equal to one tenth of an LD_{50}, as a general rule), then close monitoring at home for several days may be sufficient. Ingestion of higher doses may warrant administration of an adsorbent such as activated charcoal (AC), with or without a cathartic, followed by close monitoring in the hospital. In many situations, toxicity information is not available for the specific toxicant ingested, or, if such information is available, it may have been determined only in a laboratory species such as a rat or mouse. In the latter case, extrapolation of toxicity data to the affected species can be problematic. It is probably better to be conservative and institute decontamination procedures as soon as possible.

TYPE OF SUBSTANCE

The nature of the substance should be considered. For example, if a volatile organic hydrocarbon has been ingested, the high risk of aspiration of material into the lungs following emesis precludes the routine administration of an emetic. If a product containing several potentially toxic substances was ingested, all ingredients in the formulation need to be considered when selecting an appropriate decontamination plan. Volatile petroleum hydrocarbons can be vehicles for a variety of pesticides. Therefore, the risks associated with aspiration of the hydrocarbons should be considered when assessing the toxicity and amount of active ingredient ingested.

TIME SINCE EXPOSURE

The time since exposure is critical. Numerous studies have shown that the amount of material retrieved from the stomach following induction of emesis or performance of gastric lavage (GL) declines dramatically with time.[5,6] In most situations, induction of emesis or performance of GL more than 1 hour after ingestion may not retrieve a clinically significant amount of material and may delay the administration of an adsorbent such as AC. If toxicant-induced emesis has occurred or if emesis was successfully induced at home before presentation, there is little to be gained from further attempts to remove material from the stomach.

SPECIES AFFECTED

The species of animal is an important consideration, both physiologically and logistically. Some species do not readily vomit, and if such animals are exposed to toxicants, the administration of emetics is contraindicated. The performance of GL is less likely to be worth the time and effort in a ruminant because of the large volume of contents in the rumen.

UNDERLYING DISEASE

A history of cardiac disease or epilepsy may prohibit the use of gastric evacuation in dogs and cats. Underlying organ dysfunction may preclude use of such techniques as forced diuresis or urinary pH manipulations.

TOPICAL DECONTAMINATION

Exposure to potential toxicants other than via the oral route may necessitate specific decontamination procedures such as ocular irrigation or bathing. Large volumes of warm water and a mild detergent should be used to thoroughly wash hair and skin; multiple cycles of washing and rinsing may be necessary. Severely depressed or comatose patients require close monitoring to avoid hypothermia or aspiration of water and detergent. Whatever decontamination procedure is undertaken, it is important to protect oneself and others from toxicant exposure.

GASTROINTESTINAL DECONTAMINATION

Gastrointestinal decontamination (GID) is a critical component of case management. Appropriate and timely decontamination may prevent the onset of clinical signs or significantly decrease the severity or shorten the course of intoxication.

In recent years, a critical reappraisal of GID approaches in human intoxications has occurred that is relevant for the management of intoxicated animals.[7] A movement away from gastric evacuation (induction of emesis or GL) followed by the administration of an adsorbent toward the administration of only the adsorbent has been recommended, especially in mild to moderate intoxications. Early administration of AC alone has been shown to be as efficacious as the combination of gastric evacuation followed by AC. The advantages to the administration of AC alone compared to gastric evacuation procedures followed by AC administration include the more rapid administration of AC and subsequent adsorption of toxicant, the rapid movement of an AC slurry through the pylorus to the small intestine where systemic absorption of the majority of toxicants occurs, and the effectiveness of AC to adsorb most commonly ingested toxicants.[8]

The case for or against the inclusion of a cathartic with AC is less clear-cut but the administration of a single dose of a cathartic along with the initial dose of AC is currently recommended.[9] Those AC formulations that include a cathartic such as sorbitol should be administered only once, followed by AC alone if repeated doses of AC are indicated.

Gastric evacuation

Emesis. Approaches to gastric evacuation include induction of emesis with emetics such as syrup of ipecac, 3% hydrogen peroxide, apomorphine, or xylazine. Syrup of ipecac and 3% hydrogen peroxide are often available in the home and should be considered for inducing emesis if there is a delay in bringing an animal to the hospital (see Table 3-1 for recommended dosages). Three percent hydrogen peroxide can be administered relatively easily; if emesis does not occur within 10 minutes, the dose can be repeated once. Emesis is often more effectively induced when the stomach is full; therefore, instructing the owner to feed a small amount of food before induction can improve efficacy. The primary disadvantage of 3% hydrogen peroxide is its inconsistent efficacy. Owners may have difficulty administering syrup of ipecac to cats because of its objectionable taste. Disadvantages of syrup of ipecac include prolonged emesis and adsorption by AC. The latter is undesirable because the

TABLE 3-1 **Common Decontamination Agents**

Agent	Indication	Dosage
Syrup of ipecac	Emesis	Dogs: 1 to 2 ml/kg PO Cats: 3.3 ml/kg PO diluted 50:50 with water
3% hydrogen peroxide	Emesis	1 to 2 ml/kg PO; if no emesis, repeat once
Apomorphine	Emesis	Dogs: 0.03 mg/kg IV or 0.04 mg/kg IM. If conjunctival route is used, place $\frac{1}{4}$ to one 6- mg tablet in the conjunctival sac and dissolve using an ophthalmic irrigating solution. Thoroughly flush any remaining tablet from the sac when emesis begins. Do not use in cats.
Activated charcoal	Adsorption	All animals: 1 to 4 g/kg PO as an aqueous slurry (~1 g per 5 ml water); may be repeated at 4- to 6-hr intervals
Sodium or magnesium sulfate	Catharsis	Dogs: 5 to 25 g mixed in AC slurry Cats: 2 to 5 g mixed in AC slurry; give only once
Sorbitol	Catharsis	Often included in AC formulations; if not, give 3 ml/kg PO of 70% sorbitol
Polyethylene glycol	Whole bowel irrigation	Not established for animals; however, young children are given 20 to 40 ml/kg/hr until clear rectal effluent is noted
Sodium bicarbonate	Urine alkalinization	Generally, 1 to 2 mEq/kg administered every 3 to 4 hr; goal is to achieve urine pH of 7 or greater
Ammonium chloride	Urine acidification	Dog: 100 mg/kg PO bid Cat: 20 mg/kg PO bid

AC, Activated charcoal.

administration of AC may have to be delayed to allow the emetic action of syrup of ipecac to occur.

In a clinical setting, apomorphine is the emetic of choice for dogs.[1,3] Apomorphine stimulates dopaminergic receptors in the chemoreceptor trigger zone (CRTZ) and the emetic center. Stimulation of the CRTZ induces emesis, whereas stimulation of the emetic center suppresses emesis. Therefore, it is important that apomorphine reaches the CRTZ before the emetic center. This is accomplished by rapidly administering apomorphine intravenously (IV), intramuscularly (IM), or via instillation in the conjunctival sac. Oral administration is less efficacious. Apomorphine is not recommended for use in cats. As an alternative, xylazine can be used. Although apomorphine and xylazine induce emesis quickly, they also cause central nervous system (CNS) depression and bradycardia, which are unwanted side effects. Naloxone can reverse the CNS and respiratory effects of apomorphine, whereas yohimbine can be used to reverse the respiratory depression and bradycardia associated with xylazine use.[3,10]

Table salt, liquid dish detergent, and dry mustard should not be used as emetics because of their questionable efficacy and potential for side effects. In the case of repeated administration of table salt, iatrogenic hypernatremia can be a serious sequela.

Gastric lavage. GL can be used when gastric evacuation is indicated but administration of an emetic is contraindicated (presence of seizures, severe depression or coma, loss of normal gag reflex, hypoxia, species unable to vomit, and known prior ingestion of corrosives or volatile petroleum products). In a conscious animal, GL requires anesthesia. Airway protection is necessary whenever GL is performed. As large a gastric tube as possible with terminal fenestrations is introduced into the stomach. Tube placement is confirmed by aspiration of gastric contents or air insufflation with a stethoscope placed over the stomach. After the tube is placed, the mouth should be kept lower than the chest. Tepid tap water or normal saline (5 to 10 ml/kg) is introduced into the stomach with minimal pressure application and is withdrawn by aspiration or allowed to return via gravity flow. The procedure is repeated until the last several washings are clear; numerous cycles may be required. AC (with or without cathartic) can be administered via the tube just before its removal. The initial lavage sample should be retained for toxicologic analysis.

Adsorbents

The only adsorbent routinely used in veterinary medicine is AC, which is available as a powder, an aqueous slurry, or combined with cathartics such as sorbitol. It is formed from the pyrolysis of various carbonaceous materials such as wood, coconut, or peat. The material is treated with high temperatures and oxidizing agents to form a maze of pores to increase its surface area.[11] Adsorption of chemicals occurs as a result of noncovalent binding (ion-ion, dipole, and van der Waal's forces). Rate of adsorption is dependent on external surface area, whereas the adsorptive capacity is dependent on internal surface area.[12] In rare instances, other adsorbents such as Fuller's earth or bentonite may be suggested for specific toxicants such as paraquat.[8] AC is an effective adsorbent for a number of toxicants with several notable exceptions. Substances not well adsorbed to AC include strongly ionized and dissociated salts such as sodium chloride and small, highly polar, hydrophilic compounds such as alcohols, strong acids, alkalis, and bromide, and metals such as lead, iron, and lithium.[11,13] In situations in which there is a high suspicion of significant toxicant ingestion but a specific toxicant cannot be identified, AC should be administered.

AC given repeatedly (multiple dose AC, or MDAC) is effective in interrupting enterohepatic recycling of a number of toxicants, and the continued presence of AC in the gastrointestinal tract may allow the tract to serve as a sink for trapping toxicant passing from the circulation into the intestines.[14,15] MDAC has reportedly increased the elimination of digitoxin, phenobarbital, carbamazepine, phenylbutazone, dapsone, methotrexate, nadolol, theophylline, salicylate, cyclosporine, propoxyphene, nortriptyline, and amitriptyline.[11] MDAC is beneficial when large amounts of toxicant are ingested, when dissolution of toxicant is delayed (masses of capsules), when the toxicant has a delayed or prolonged release phase, and when the toxicant undergoes extensive enterohepatic recirculation. Empirically, a loading dose of 1 to 2 g/kg of AC is administered, followed by 0.25 to 0.50 g/kg every 1 to 6 hours. The total dose administered may be more important than the actual dosage protocol. There is little hazard to repeated administration of AC, although cathartics should be given only once. On rare occasions, constipation or intestinal obstruction can occur with MDAC, particularly in a dehydrated patient.[11]

AC should be administered as soon as possible after toxicant ingestion. In a recent summary of 115 human volunteer studies in which reduction in drug absorption by a single dose of AC given at various times after drug administration was assessed, the mean reduction when AC was given within 60 minutes of drug ingestion was approximately 64% compared with only approximately 33% when AC was given more than 60 minutes after drug administration.[12]

Cathartics

Both saline (sodium sulfate or magnesium sulfate or citrate) and saccharide (sorbitol) cathartics are available. Cathartics hasten the elimination of unabsorbed toxicant via the stools. In general, cathartics are safe, particularly if used only once. However, repeated administration of magnesium-containing cathartics can lead to hypermagnesemia manifested as hypotonia, altered mental status, and respiratory failure.[9] Also, repeated administration of sorbitol can cause fluid pooling in the gastrointestinal tract, excessive fluid losses via the stool, and severe dehydration. Table 3-1 lists the most commonly used cathartics and appropriate doses. Contraindications to the use of cathartics include absence of bowel sounds, intestinal obstruction or perforation, recent bowel surgery, volume depletion, significant electrolyte imbalance, and ingestion of a corrosive substance.[9] The use of a cathartic

is questionable in a patient that presents with toxicant-induced diarrhea. Additionally, cathartics should be used cautiously in very young or old animals. Bulk and lubricant laxatives such as methylcellulose and mineral oil, respectively, are not recommended because of their relatively slow onset of action. Irritant or stimulant laxatives such as castor oil and phenolphthalein are also not recommended. The efficacy of administering mineral oil to horses exposed to toxicants has not been demonstrated and its use in lieu of more accepted methods of gastrointestinal decontamination (AC plus osmotic cathartic) is difficult to justify.

Whole bowel irrigation

One newer approach to human GID is whole bowel irrigation (WBI), which involves the oral administration of large volumes of an electrolyte-balanced solution until a clear rectal effluent is produced.[16] A polyethylene glycol solution is routinely used to cleanse the gastrointestinal tract for surgical or radiographic procedures in humans. WBI is efficacious when an ingested toxicant is poorly adsorbed to AC or when sustained-release medications have been ingested. Another potential use for WBI is in those instances after small metal objects or lead-based paint has been ingested. WBI has been well tolerated in human pediatric patients. The utility of WBI in veterinary medicine has not been determined, but the need to administer large volumes of liquid may limit its use.

Endoscopy

Endoscopic removal of foreign objects is a viable decontamination procedure. Removal of potentially toxic metallic objects such as zinc-containing pennies, galvanized metal or lead objects, or button batteries from the stomach may prevent or minimize morbidity or mortality.

ANTIDOTES

Antidotes are therapeutic agents that have a specific action against the activity or effect of a toxicant. Although no classification scheme is ideal, antidotes can be broadly classified as chemical or pharmacologic antidotes. Chemical antidotes specifically interact with or neutralize toxicants. For example, metal chelators such as calcium disodium edetate ($CaNa_2EDTA$) or succimer combine with metals to form soluble metal-chelator complexes that are subsequently eliminated via the kidneys. Pharmacologic antidotes neutralize or antagonize toxicant effects. Such antidotes can prevent formation of toxic metabolites (fomepizole), compete with or block the action of a toxicant at a receptor site (naloxone), or help restore normal function (N-acetylcysteine).

Antidotes should be administered if indicated and available. Because of the costs associated with keeping a full range of antidotes on hand, many veterinarians may not have ready access to all of those that are clinically useful. Table 3-2 lists antidotes that should be immediately available for case management; this list is based on the frequency with which intoxications occur (as reported by animal poison control statistics). Table 3-3 lists antidotes that may be needed less frequently. It is recommended that a source such as a human hospital or pharmacy be identified for obtaining the latter antidotes before they are needed.

TABLE 3-2 **Antidotes for Common Intoxications**

Antidote	Indication	Dosage	Comments
N-Acetylcysteine (NAC)	Acetaminophen	Loading dose of 140 to 280 mg/kg PO or 140 mg in 5% dextrose/water followed by maintenance dose of 70 mg/kg PO qid for 2 to 3 days.	A suggested alternative is sodium sulfate at 50 mg/kg of a 1.6% solution IV every 4 hr for 6 treatments.[26] Clinical efficacy not proven. Use of ascorbic acid or methylene blue not shown to be better than use of NAC alone.
Atropine sulfate	OP/carbamate insecticides	0.1 to 0.5 mg/kg (given until muscarinic signs controlled), ¼ initial dose given IV with the remainder given IM or SQ. Administered as needed.	Glycopyrrolate can be used in lieu of atropine. Onset of action is slower than that of atropine but duration of action is longer. Drug of choice for use in horses.
CaNa$_2$EDTA	Lead, zinc	25 mg/kg SC qid as a 1% solution (in 5% dextrose/water) for 5 days. Provide 5- to 7-day rest period between courses of treatment to minimize potential for nephrotoxicity.	No veterinary formulation; human formulation can be used in small animals, but use in large animals requires compounding. Succimer is the chelator of choice for treating small animals. Doses for exotic species are empirical.
Calcitonin	Cholecalciferol	4 to 6 IU SC bid to qid	Pamidronate may be more efficacious and convenient, and is associated with fewer side effects.
Ethanol (20%)	Ethylene glycol—cat, dog	Dog: 5.5 ml/kg IV every 4 hr for five treatments then every 6 hr for four treatments. Cat: 5 ml/kg IV qid for five treatments then tid for four treatments. Effective oral dose is estimated to be 2 to 3 ml of 80 proof (40% ethanol) product.	Many disadvantages to use of ethanol: CNS and respiratory depression, metabolic acidosis, hypocalcemia, hyperosmolality, and osmotic diuresis. In dogs, fomepizole is the antidote of choice.
4-methylpyrazole (fomepizole)	Ethylene glycol—dog, possibly cat	Initial dose: 20 mg/kg slow IV in a 5% solution followed by 15 mg/kg at 12 and 24 hr and then 5 mg/kg at 36 hr. In a limited study in cats, 125 mg/kg IV at 1, 2, and 3 hr following ethylene glycol ingestion and 31.25 mg/kg at 12, 24, and 36 hr in conjunction with continuous IV fluid therapy prevented renal failure after administration of ethylene glycol at 1.7 g/kg PO.[27]	Direct inhibitor of alcohol dehydrogenase. Feline alcohol dehydrogenase may not be as effectively inhibited by fomepizole, thus requiring higher doses in cats than in dogs. Mild (CNS) depression was noted in cats given high doses of fomepizole.
Pralidoxime chloride (2-PAM)	OP insecticides	20 mg/kg IM, SC, or slow IV bid	Not necessary in carbamate intoxications. If in doubt as to whether exposure is to OP or carbamate, administer 2-PAM (except carbaryl). Probably not cost effective for use in livestock.
Succimer	Lead, arsenic	10 mg/kg PO tid for 5 days followed by 10 mg/kg PO bid for 2 wk	Orally effective, which makes its use on an outpatient basis possible.
Vitamin K$_1$	Anticoagulant rodenticides	First generation anticoagulants: 1 mg/kg PO for 4 to 6 days. Second generation anticoagulants: 2.5 to 5 mg/kg PO for 2 to 4 wk	Close monitoring for recurrence of coagulopathy is critical following cessation of vitamin K$_1$. Vitamin K$_3$ is not effective.

CNS, Central nervous system; OP, organophosphate.

TABLE 3-3 **Less Commonly Used Antidotes**

Antidote	Indication	Dosage	Comments
Ammonium tetra-thiomolybdate	Copper intoxication of sheep	1.7 to 3.4 mg/day given IV or SC every other day for three treatments.	Used for treating acutely symptomatic animals. Ammonium molybdate can be administered at 200 mg/day PO for 3 wk to treat nonacutely symptomatic animals. Not approved for use in food animals. Withdrawal period of 30 days if used in food animals.
Sodium thiosulfate	Arsenic, cyanide	30 to 40 mg/kg of a 20% solution IV, may be repeated.	No withdrawal time in food animals.
D-penicillamine	Copper, lead	Copper: 10 to 15 mg/kg/day PO (for treatment of chronic copper storage disease in dogs). Lead: 110 mg/kg/day PO for 1 to 2 wk, reevaluate animal 1 wk after initial course, additional treatment may be necessary.	Not approved for use in food animals.
Sodium nitrite	Cyanide	16 mg/kg of a 1% solution IV, given only once.	No withdrawal time in food animals.
Deferoxamine mesylate	Iron	Not determined. For humans, suggested dose is 5 g of a 5% solution given orally, then 20 mg/kg IM every 4 to 6 hr. If shock is present, dose is 40 mg/kg by IV drip over 4 hr, which is repeated 6 hr later and then 15 mg/kg by IV drip every 8 hr.	Little clinical benefit if treatment is begun more than 12 hr after iron ingestion. Chelation therapy should continue until serum iron concentration is less than 300 mg/dl or is less than serum iron binding capacity. Urine turns reddish-brown.
Digoxin Fab fragments	Cardiac glycosides (i.e., digoxin; plants such as *Digitalis, Nerium* spp., and *Bufo* spp)	Dosing in animals is empirical. In humans it is suggested that 1.7 ml (of Digibind) be administered IV per 1 mg of digoxin ingested. If ingested dose is unknown, then 400 mg Digibind is given IV.	Administered over 30 minutes unless cardiac arrest is imminent, in which case a bolus is given. Monitor for anaphylaxis and hypokalemia. Based on human use, patient should improve quickly.
Pamidronate	Cholecalciferol	Not determined, although in dogs, 1.3 mg/kg IV in 150 ml normal saline 1 and 8 days after ingestion of a toxic dose of cholecalciferol was effective in decreasing hypercalcemia.	Theoretical advantages over calcitonin include more convenient dosage, fewer side effects, and better efficacy.
Methylene blue	Nitrites, chlorates	Dogs: 8.8 mg/kg of a 1% solution given by slow IV drip. Cats: not recommended Ruminants: 4 to 15 mg/kg IV; may be repeated in 6 to 8 hr.	Possible carcinogen; therefore, withdrawal time is extended if used in food animal (180 days).
Naloxone	Opioids	Not determined. In children, a dose of 2 mg is given IV. If there is no response, a second dose of 2 mg is given. This dose is repeated every 2 min until there is a clinical response or 10 to 20 mg has been given (if no response to this dose, opioid overdose has been ruled out).	Patients should be monitored for relapse because duration of effect for naloxone may be less than that of the ingested opioid. Very safe.

Continued

TABLE 3-3 **Less Commonly Used Antidotes**—cont'd

Antidote	Indication	Dosage	Comments
Antivenins (coral snake antivenom, *Latrodectus* spp. antivenom, polyvalent Crotalidae antivenom, and scorpion antivenom)	Venomous spiders, snakes, fish, and marine invertebrates	Follow specific antivenin recommendations.	Dose is based on estimated amount of venom injected and not on body weight of the individual. Expensive. Anaphylactic reactions can occur, so close monitoring of patient after administration is critical.
Dimercaprol (BAL)	Arsenic, mercury	2.5 to 5 mg/kg of a 10% solution in oil IM every 4 hr for 2 days then bid for the next 10 days or until recovery.	Injection can be painful because of peanut oil formulation. Should not be given IV or SC.
Tolazoline	Xylazine, amitraz	Dogs: 4 mg/kg IV. Cats: not determined.	Tachycardia and arrhythmias are most common side effects.
Yohimbine	Xylazine, amitraz	Dogs: 0.1 to 0.125 mg/kg IV. Cats: not determined.	Tachycardia, agitation, and tremors are most common side effects.

In some cases, antidotes need to be compounded by the veterinarian or a compounding pharmacy. This is particularly true for large animal antidotes such as $CaNa_2EDTA$. See reference 17 for an excellent review of the current status of antidotes for food animal use.

The use of some antidotes in food animals can result in food safety concerns.[17] Because of these concerns, extended withdrawal times have been established for ammonium salts for treatment of copper intoxicated sheep (30 days) and for methylene blue for treatment of nitrate/nitrite intoxication in ruminants (180 days).

In many cases, appropriate dosages of antidotes for various species have not been determined with precision and recommended protocols may vary depending on the source consulted.

CALCITONIN

Calcitonin is widely recommended for the treatment of cholecalciferol (vitamin D)-induced hypercalcemia, although controlled studies of its efficacy are lacking. Regardless of its efficacy, the use of calcitonin has two major disadvantages. The recommended protocol is to administer 4 to 6 IU every 6 hours for up to 3 weeks; this requires considerable nursing care.[18] In addition, administration of calcitonin can be associated with side effects such as anorexia, anaphylaxis, and emesis. Recently, a specific inhibitor of bone resorption called pamidronate disodium has been investigated for its efficacy in correcting cholecalciferol-induced hypercalcemia in dogs.[18,19]

PAMIDRONATE

Pamidronate is a diphosphonate analogue of pyrophosphate that is efficacious for the treatment of hypercalcemia associated with several human diseases including hypercalcemia of malignancy and Paget's disease of bone. Experimentally, it appears to be efficacious in dogs, needs to be administered less frequently than calcitonin (although as a slow IV infusion), and is associated with few side effects. Thus, pamidronate or other diphosphonate drugs may become the antidotes of choice to treat cholecalciferol or vitamin-D analogue (calcipotriol) intoxication.

FOMEPIZOLE

Fomepizole has replaced ethanol as the antidote of choice for treating ethylene glycol–intoxicated dogs. It is a better inhibitor of alcohol dehydrogenase than ethanol, and its administration is not associated with significant side effects. However, fomepizole has not been shown to be efficacious for treating ethylene glycol–intoxicated cats using similar dosages as those used in dogs, possibly because of the less effective inhibition of alcohol dehydrogenase in cats.[20] Higher doses of fomepizole may be effective in cats, but this has not yet been demonstrated.

SUCCIMER

Succimer is the chelator of choice for the treatment of lead-intoxicated small companion animals. Advantages of using succimer over $CaNa_2EDTA$ include oral effectiveness, allowing treatment of animals on an outpatient basis, more specific chelation of lead, and fewer potential side effects. However, a recently published study in cockatiels raised some concerns regarding the therapeutic index of succimer in that bird species.[21] Succimer is probably not economically justifiable for use in food animals such as cattle. In livestock, $CaNa_2EDTA$ is still the chelator of choice, although currently no available veterinary formulation exists. Recipes have been published for making solutions of $CaNa_2$ EDTA or compounding pharmacies can be used to make formulations.[22]

N-ACETYLCYSTEINE

N-Acetylcysteine (NAC) is antidotal for acetaminophen intoxication. In humans, NAC treatment is based on serum/plasma acetaminophen concentrations, which are not readily available for guiding veterinary therapy. Ideally, the first dose of NAC should be administered within 8 hours of exposure.[23] It can be administered either orally or intravenously. Oral administration has not been associated with adverse effects in humans, whereas intravenous administration has resulted in urticaria, anaphylactoid reactions, and, rarely, death. Any orally administered dose vomited within 1 hour should be repeated. Although NAC is adsorbed to AC, evidence suggests that such adsorption is not clinically significant.

ENHANCED ELIMINATION

Various methods of increasing the elimination of absorbed toxicants have been advocated. The advantages and disadvantages of these methods are discussed in this section.

ACTIVATED CHARCOAL

AC, especially MDAC, may provide a gastrointestinal "dialysis" effect. Evidence for such a dialysis effect is derived from dog and human studies in which the clearance of marker drugs given intravenously is increased after oral administration of AC.[14,15] In studies using dogs, multiple doses of AC given orally enhanced the elimination of IV-administered theophylline.[15] It was hypothesized that theophylline, passing from the circulation into the lumen of the gastrointestinal tract, was adsorbed, thus preventing its reabsorption. MDAC was also shown to dramatically decrease the serum half-life of IV-administered phenobarbital in healthy human volunteers.[14]

FORCED DIURESIS

Forced diuresis via the IV administration of sodium-containing solutions is often recommended to hasten the elimination of many toxicants via the kidneys.[3,24] However, administration of high volumes of fluid runs the risk of volume overload with resultant pulmonary and cerebral edema. The potential for volume overload and the unproven efficacy of forced diuresis in the management of the intoxicated patient has led most human medical centers to abandon its use.[25]

ION-TRAPPING

Facilitating the removal of absorbed toxicants via the urine by ion-trapping may be indicated in several specific situations. For example, alkalinization of the urine to a pH of 7 or greater with sodium bicarbonate has been shown to enhance the urinary elimination of weak acids such as ethylene glycol, salicylates, phenobarbital, and the herbicide 2,4-D.[25] This degree of alkalinization may be difficult to achieve in the presence of a metabolic acidosis and acidemia, which can occur in salicylate intoxication.

The administration of ammonium chloride to acidify the urine (pH of 5.5 to 6.5) may enhance the elimination of weak bases such as amphetamine and strychnine. However, urinary acidification as a means to eliminate such toxicants should be abandoned because it does not enhance their elimination to a degree that alters clinical outcome and there is a substantial risk of causing or exacerbating an existing metabolic acidosis.[25]

PERITONEAL DIALYSIS

Peritoneal dialysis has also been advocated to enhance the elimination of water-soluble, low-molecular-weight, poorly protein-bound compounds with a small volume of distribution such as alcohols, lithium, salicylate, and theophylline.[3] Although peritoneal dialysis is relatively simple to perform, it is considered to be too slow to be clinically useful.[25] Other methods for hastening elimination of an absorbed toxicant, such as charcoal hemoperfusion and hemodialysis, are less practical and less available in veterinary medicine.

SYMPTOMATIC AND SUPPORTIVE CARE

As mentioned earlier, many intoxicated patients recover if attention is paid to appropriate symptomatic and supportive care. For example, even if GID is not possible after ingestion of strychnine, effective control of muscle rigidity with pentobarbital often results in complete recovery from intoxication. Attention to patient monitoring to institute appropriate symptomatic treatment in a timely manner cannot be overemphasized.

REFERENCES

1. Beasley VR, Dorman DC: Management of toxicoses. In Beasley VR, editor: *The Veterinary Clinics of North America: toxicology of selected pesticides, drugs, and chemicals,* Philadelphia, 1990, WB Saunders.
2. Shannon MW, Haddad LM: The emergency management of poisoning. In Haddad LM, editor: *Clinical management of poisoning and drug overdose,* ed 3, Philadelphia, 1998, WB Saunders.
3. Hackett T: Emergency approach to intoxications, *Clin Tech Sm Anim Prac* 15:82, 2000.
4. Drellich S, Aldrich J: Initial mmanagement of the aacutely poisoned patient. In Peterson ME, Talcott PA, editors: *Small animal toxicology,* Philadelphia, 2001, WB Saunders.
5. American Academy of Clinical Toxicology and the European Association of Poison Centres and Clinical Toxicologists: Position statement: ipecac syrup, *J Toxicol Clin Toxicol* 35:699, 1997.
6. American Academy of Clinical Toxicology and the European Association of Poison Centres and Clinical Toxicologists: Position statement: gastric lavage, *J Toxicol Clin Toxicol* 35:711, 1997.
7. Perry H, Shannon M: Emergency department gastrointestinal decontamination, *Pediatr Ann* 25:19, 1996.
8. Oehme FW, Mannala S: Paraquat. In Peterson ME, Talcott PA, editors: *Small animal toxicology,* Philadelphia, 2001, WB Saunders.

9. American Academy of Clinical Toxicology and the European Association of Poison Centres and Clinical Toxicologists: Position statement: cathartics, *J Toxicol Clin Toxicol* 35:743, 1997.

10. Plumb DC: *Veterinary drug handbook*, ed 2, Ames, Iowa 1995, Iowa State University Press.

11. Howland MA: Antidotes in depth: activated charcoal. In Goldfrank LR, et al, editors: *Toxicologic emergencies*, ed 6, Norwalk, Conn, 1994, Appleton & Lange.

12. American Academy of Clinical Toxicology and the European Association of Poison Centres and Clinical Toxicologists: Position statement: single dose activated charcoal, *J Toxicol Clin Toxicol* 35:721, 1997.

13. Kulig K: Gastrointestinal decontamination. In Ford MD, et al, editors: *Clinical toxicology*, Philadelphia, 2001, WB Saunders.

14. Berg M et al: Acceleration of the body clearance of phenobarbital by oral activated charcoal, *N Engl J Med* 307:642, 1982.

15. Kulig KW et al: Intravenous theophylline poisoning and multiple-dose charcoal in an animal model, *Ann Emerg Med* 16:842, 1987.

16. American Academy of Clinical Toxicology and the European Association of Poison Centres and Clinical Toxicologists: Position statement: whole bowel irrigation. *J Toxicol Clin Toxicol* 35:753, 1997.

17. Post LO, Keller WC: Current status of food animal antidotes. In Osweiler GD, Galey FD, editors: *The Veterinary Clinics of North America, food animal practice*, Philadelphia, 2000, WB Saunders.

18. Rumbeiha WK et al: Use of pamidronate disodium to reduce cholecalciferol-induced toxicosis in dogs, *Am J Vet Res* 61:9, 2000.

19. Rumbeiha WK: Cholecalciferol. In Peterson ME, Talcott PA, editors: *Small animal toxicology*, Philadelphia, 2001, WB Saunders.

20. Connally HE et al: Inhibition of canine and feline alcohol dehydrogenase activity by fomepizole, *AJVR* 61:450, 2000.

21. Denver MC et al: Comparison of two heavy metal chelators for treatment of lead toxicosis in cockatiels, *AJVR* 61:935, 2000.

22. Baker JC, Poppenga RH: Lead poisoning in cattle, *AHDL Veterinary Diagnostic Newsletter* 6:1, 1989.

23. Anker A: Acetaminophen. In Ford MD et al, editors: *Clinical toxicology*, Philadelphia, 2000, WB Saunders.

24. Peterson M: Toxicologic decontamination. In Peterson ME, Talcott PA, editors: *Small animal toxicology*, Philadelphia, 2001, WB Saunders.

25. Goldfarb DS, Pond SM: Principles and techniques applied to enhance elimination of toxins. In Goldfrank LR et al, editors: *Toxicologic emergencies*, ed 6, Norwalk, Conn, 1998, Appleton & Lange.

26. Savides MC et al: Effects of various antidotal treatments on acetaminophen toxicosis and biotransformation in cats, *Am J Vet Res* 46:1485, 1985.

27. Thrall MA et al: Ethylene glycol. In Peterson ME, Talcott PA, editors: *Small animal toxicology*, Philadelphia, 2001, WB Saunders.

4

Diagnostic Toxicology

Francis D. Galey

oisoning cases make up a small fraction of the cases presented to veterinarians. As with other types of diseases, an accurate and speedy diagnosis is necessary to provide adequate treatment for affected animals and prevent new cases from developing. However, poisoning cases require special effort because, in addition to diagnosis and treatment, clinicians are often confronted with owner emotion, publicity, and medicolegal issues. Diagnosis depends heavily on a systematic approach that includes proper sample collection and handling. Such cases require piecing together a "diagnostic puzzle" that includes a complete case history, clinical signs, clinicopathologic findings, postmortem findings, results from chemical analyses, and occasionally bioassay findings.

In addition to the need to obtain the best diagnostic result, the potential litigious nature of many toxicology-related cases necessitates careful sampling and sample handling. The initial investigation should identify the animal, the owner, and the environment around the affected animal. Careful records should be kept. If a case has medicolegal implications, the chain of custody (written documentation of custody) of all samples must be recorded.

HISTORY

In a possible poisoning case, the environmental and time-related conditions surrounding an event must be carefully studied. The primary goal of the history is to identify possible sources of a toxicant. Sources are found by examining the environment, reviewing management practices, and recording the movement and fate of animals, feed, water, and bedding. Even if a specific toxicant is not immediately isolated, early identification of a possible toxic source allows the veterinarian to terminate exposure and prevent additional cases. Clients should be told not to discard, disrupt, or give away samples (e.g., back to feed companies or other agencies) until the investigation is done.

Anyone with information pertinent to the case should be interviewed. Animals, feeds, water, and bedding should be located and traced. Both the local (feed, available plants, water sources, management practices) and regional (nearby industry, other farms) environments can be investigated. Management practices should be reviewed with all involved (e.g., owners, ranch hands). For feeds other than pasture, the lots, time of acquisition, visible condition, any changes, composition, and time and amount of feeding should be recorded.

The type of case that is presented depends in part on the type of animal involved. The small animal toxicology case centers on individual animals. However, in the case of the roaming pet, its recent whereabouts may not be known and are thus difficult to document. Conversely, equine and food animal toxicology cases usually involve animals from a known environment (e.g., pasture) and roaming is less of a concern. For the food animal case, however, the concern is often for the herd and economics as much as it is for treatment of the individual animal. The wildlife toxicology case is characterized by concerns for both the individual and the population (like food animals). The immediate past environmental history of the wildlife patient may also not be known to the clinician.

The chronologic outline of events will help match the onset of signs with other environmental factors. Useful epidemiologic information includes the case information (incidence rates, geographic location, and movement of affected and nonaffected animals), management (employee actions, neighbors), signalment (species, age, gender, breeds), and past and present history. The investigation of the individual animals should review the history of vaccinations, feeding, onset of signs, specificity of signs, severity and progression of signs, and response to treatment. Recent medication history should be recorded, including information about the substances given, time of administration, amount used, reason for use, and individuals treating the animal.

SAMPLE COLLECTION AND STORAGE

Samples for toxicology testing fall into three general categories: environmental, antemortem, and postmortem. Toxicology testing is often time consuming, expensive, and sensitive to sampling and storage conditions. Thus, a proper strategy for collecting samples is critical to obtain the best results from a diagnostic laboratory (Table 4-1). Toxicology specimens are often best collected and held until other testing can be completed because results from other tests (e.g., histology, bacteriology) can give information about the organ that is affected and perhaps the poison itself. Once lesions or alterations are identified, appropriate toxicology testing can be assigned.

All samples should be labeled regarding the date, case, source, description, and the clinician taking the sample. As long as size and volume allow, critical samples should be split before storage or at least before shipment to a laboratory so that additional samples are available in case initial samples are lost in the mail or further testing is necessary. Samples should not be pooled unless they are from the same lot or bunk of feed. Otherwise, dilution from pooling can decrease the amount of toxicant found or even make finding the toxicant impossible.

Many poisons are fragile, necessitating proper sample care to obtain the most reliable results. If in doubt, fresh samples should be frozen for toxicology as soon as possible after they are obtained. Exceptions to the freezing requirement include very dry samples such as hay or grain, which should be kept cool and dry, and whole blood samples, which may be refrigerated for most tests. All serum and plasma samples should be spun and removed from the clot as soon as possible. The serum or plasma should be labeled and frozen. Blood samples should be kept out of sunlight and the heat. Environmental and tissue samples are frozen in separate cups, jars, or bags. Samples should not be stored or shipped in rectal examination sleeves or gloves, which can leak and result in contamination of the sample with other substances or samples.

ENVIRONMENTAL SAMPLES

Many toxicants are not detectable in tissues. Thus, environmental samples (e.g., source materials, feeds) are critical to diagnosis in a poisoning case as well as being important for identifying and removing the source of a poison.

FEED SAMPLES

To avoid dilution, samples should not be pooled between lots, shipments, feed bunks, or animal pens. Pooling is desirable, however, if done *within* the same lot of feed or stack of hay from one field to ensure that the sample is representative of the lot. For example, mold toxins (e.g., aflatoxin in grain or nitrate from weeds) in a lot of hay occur in "hot spots," or isolated portions of a lot or bag. Thus, one grab sample from one part of a bin may miss the toxin, but multiple samples from different parts of the bin have a greater chance of locating the toxin. Samples are individually labeled. Sample sizes vary, but the optimal size in most

instances is about 500 g of material (about 1 lb). Some samples may be considerably larger to ensure adequate representation of the lot in question. Moist samples should be frozen. Feeds to be kept dry should be stored in a cool, dry environment in containers that discourage condensation and mold growth (plastic bags promote decay).

WATER SAMPLES

Water samples are obtained at the source (well, canal, pond), in transit (piping, tankers), in storage tanks, and at the site of exposure. Spills are sampled if animals are exposed to the materials. The history should include recent occurrences regarding the water (tides, storage). Some chemicals are toxic in water even when present in very low concentrations. Thus, two 1-L samples should be obtained from each site. Glass preserving jars (1 L) are useful for water samples. Plastic and metal containers should be avoided. Metal and salt samples can be covered with plastic wrap and then the lid; organic chemical samples should be covered with foil and then the lid. For extremely sensitive tests, the jars can be rinsed with acetone (nail polish remover) and then the source water itself before filling with the sample. Small samples of blue-green algae can be mixed half and half with 10% neutral buffered formalin for identification, with larger samples (up to 5 gallons) being saved in plastic buckets for possible toxin identification using bioassay or instrumental techniques.

PLANT SAMPLES

Many plant poisonings still rely on plant identification for diagnosis. Pastures should be examined, with plants being identified as the investigation proceeds. Grabbing a single flake of hay at random and sending for plant identification is usually unrewarding. Several bales should be opened until suspicious weeds are found (if present). The amount of the weeds in the bale, stack, or lot should be estimated, and then the weeds can be sent to a laboratory for identification if needed. Assistance with identification of plants can be found from a number of sources. Occasionally, a specialist from a herbarium or agricultural extension can be found to walk a field. If local experts are available, representative specimens of fresh plants (including flower, greenery, and roots) are obtained, wrapped with wet newspaper, and taken for identification. If local help is unavailable, samples can be catalogued, pressed in folds of newspaper under heavy books, and then shipped to a diagnostic service for identification. Rapid plant identifications can be attempted by pressing a plant on a high-quality office copier and transmitting the copy by FAX for identification.

Identification of a potentially toxic plant is not usually definitive; it only suggests an opportunity for exposure. Diagnosis of plant poisoning also requires evidence of consumption of a plant by the animal. That evidence may include an abundance of the plant in the field, indications of grazing (stripped stalks or topped plants), or the finding of

TABLE 4-1   **Samples for Analytical Toxicology Testing**

Sample Type	Amount	Description	Examples
Environmental			
Concentrate feeds or baits	500 g plus composites	In paper or plastic bags, glass jars	Pesticides, heavy metals, salts, additives, antibiotics, ionophores, mycotoxins, hormones, nitrates, sulfate chlorate, cyanide, plant toxins, plants, botulinum, vitamins A, D, or E
Plants	Entire plant	Press and dry or freeze	Identification; alkaloids, tannins, cardenolides, cardiac glycosides (oleander)
Mushroom	Whole	Keep cool and dry in paper bag	Identification; identification of cyclic peptide hepatotoxin
Water	1 L	Preserving jar	Pesticides, salts, heavy metals, blue-green algae identification, sulfate, nitrate
Environment	Source/bait	Freeze in bag	Try to obtain label and send also, variety of toxicants
Live Animal			
Whole blood	5-10 ml	EDTA Anticoagulant	Lead, arsenic, mercury, molybdenum, manganese, selenium, cholinesterase, anticoagulants, cyanide, some organic chemicals
Serum	5-10 ml	Spin and remove clot; special tube for zinc	Copper, zinc, iron, magnesium, calcium, sodium, potassium, drugs, nitrates, ammonia, alkaloids, tannins, vitamins A and E, antifreeze
Urine	50-100 ml	Send in plastic, screw-cap vial	Drugs, heavy metals, alkaloids, tannins, cantharidin, fluoride, paraquat
Milk	30 ml	Do not freeze	Antibiotics, organochlorines, polychlorinated biphenyls (PCBs)
Ingesta/feces	100 g plus	Freeze	Heavy metals, organic compounds, some plant toxicants, oleander
Biopsy specimens	e.g., Liver	Freeze, package to allow retrieval	Metals
Hair	10 g	Tie mane or tail hair so origin is noted	Selenium toxicosis
Postmortem			
Ingesta	1 kg	Frozen	Heavy metals, plants, oleander, cardenolides, alkaloids, tannins, insecticides, drugs, nitrates, cyanide, ammonia, pesticides, cantharidin, avitrol, petroleum hydrocarbons, antifreeze
Liver	200 g	Smaller samples for small patients OK; freeze	Heavy metals, insecticides, anticoagulant rodenticides, some plant toxins, some drugs, vitamins A and E
Kidney	200 g	Smaller samples for small animals OK; freeze	Heavy metals, calcium, some plant toxins, antifreeze
Brain	½ of brain	Sagittal section; leave midline in formalin for pathologist	Sodium, cholinesterase, organochlorine insecticides
Fat	100 g	Smaller sample OK for biopsy samples	Organochlorine insecticides, PCBs
Ocular fluid	1 eye		Nitrate, potassium, ammonia, magnesium
Injection site	100 g		Some drugs, other injectables
Miscellaneous	100 g	Special tests	Special tests, e.g., spleen (barbiturates), lung (paraquat)

plant material in the gut contents of the victim. Some tests identify plant exposure chemically for some plant toxins such as alkaloids, oleander toxin, cardenolides (e.g., azaleas), and oak tannins in ingesta or body fluids.

After the environmental history and samples are recorded, the clinician can concentrate on affected animals. Before doing complete examinations and initiating therapy (other than that needed to preserve life), an attempt should be made to deduce likely sources of the poisoning and remove those sources from animals.

ANTEMORTEM SAMPLES

The obvious toxicology case involves sudden onset of disease or death in a number of animals. Other cases may involve a more insidious onset of signs, or perhaps merely a decrease in production. Finding of common feed or environmental conditions helps support a suspicion of poisoning. Clinical signs may be absent altogether, such as for residues, testing for nutritional adequacy, or drug testing for forensic or regulatory purposes (e.g., horse racing or livestock shows).

The next step in investigating a toxicology case is to examine the affected animals. Clinical effects of toxicants vary, depending on the organs involved, route of exposure, species and host characteristics (e.g., age, past history, environment, use), and dose. The incidence rate, the nature and speed of onset, and the progression of clinical signs can be examined.

Numbers of affected animals can be compared with time of clinical onset. A pattern may indicate a possible poisoning. For example, some poisons may lead to acute signs in multiple animals in a short time after a single exposure. For example, ingestion of oleander plants may lead to collapse within hours. Conversely, toxicants that have a longer period from exposure to onset of signs have incidence rates spread over longer periods of time. For example, clinical pyrrolizidine alkaloid poisoning may not appear until after weeks of exposure, or even after exposure has ended. The incidence rates end abruptly for acute toxicants as the source of poisoning is recognized and removed, yet those with a longer latent period may continue to appear for days to months.

Clinical signs range from specific to nondescript. Specific clinical entities can include paralysis from botulism or staggering and knuckling from "cracker heels" caused by ingestion of some vetches. Conversely, pyrrolizidine alkaloids from a variety of plants such as the *Senecio* sp. may cause presentation for nonspecific wasting and illthrift. Many toxicants (e.g., ionophore antibiotics) may cause sudden death with little clinical evidence. The primary goal for the clinician in these instances is to avoid focusing too intensely on toxicology and to rule out all possible causes of the illness. Unwary owners may miss a high incidence of a virulent infectious pneumonia that may appear to have caused "sudden death."

In the food animal, veterinarians and producers must also be concerned about the potential for residues. Any exposure to a poison should be reviewed to determine whether a residue hazard exists. Items to consider include withdrawal times for drugs, elimination times for chemicals, time when milk or meat can be marketed, and fate of carcasses when animals have died. Residue hazards may exist in exposed animals regardless of whether clinical signs were present.

Clinical testing that can be performed includes serum biochemistry, complete blood count (CBC), and chemistry analysis. Serum biochemistry and CBC data are critical to help identify affected organ systems. Special testing of some biochemical parameters, such as clotting factors (e.g., prothrombin time is prolonged by anticoagulant rodenticides) or cholinesterase (inhibited by pesticides), is useful as indicators of exposure to poisons. Some chemistry analyses are possible for samples from live animals and can be useful in diagnosing a poisoning. Samples that may be of use include blood, serum, urine, hair, ingesta, and biopsies (see Table 4-1).

Whole blood and serum samples are used for a variety of tests (see Table 4-1). Whole blood is preferred using EDTA (ethylenediaminetetraacetic acid) as an anticoagulant if possible. Heparinized blood is acceptable, but heparin tends to break down under the rigors of storage and transport. If samples clot in the tubes, tests are ruined. Whole blood samples should be refrigerated until analysis can be done. Serum is required for other tests because some analytes are destroyed on contact with red cells. Others, such as phosphorus and potassium, increase in concentration on contact with decaying erythrocytes. Therefore, for analytical toxicology it is critical that the serum and plasma be rapidly removed from the clot. Separated serum is frozen until analyzed. Some analyses need special attention to obtain valid results. Rubber contains zinc, which can contaminate the sample. Therefore, nutritional analyses that include zinc should be drawn, spun, and stored in a manner that avoids contact with rubber. (Syringe plungers and tops of red-topped clot tubes are made with rubber.) Sera for trace elements such as zinc can be drawn in royal blue–topped clot tubes using a vacuum system, spun, and decanted into plastic vials before freezing and shipment. Vitamins and some other organic compounds are sensitive to both heat and light. Therefore, blood tubes can be wrapped in foil when filled. After the samples have clotted, they are decanted with serum tubes and then wrapped in foil and frozen until testing.

Urine is tested for drugs and some plant toxins. Like water, however, urine often has physiologically active chemicals in extremely low concentrations. So, large sample sizes (100 ml or more) provide optimal results. No sample (urine, serum, or otherwise) should be supplied in a syringe. Syringes leak, are dangerous to receiving personnel, and are not secure. It is difficult to analyze packing material for drugs after a syringe leaks in the pack. In addition, many shipping companies, including the U.S. Postal Service, take a dim view of leaky containers and may refuse to accept further materials from repeat offenders for shipment to laboratories.

Hair is generally an unreliable sample for toxicology testing with a few exceptions, such as testing for chronic selenium poisoning. In such cases, whole blood may have high but not excessive levels of selenium. Ambient dust may have metals such as arsenic or selenium in near physiologic-appearing concentrations. Therefore, the sample must be carefully obtained. One technique is to wash and rinse (using de-ionized water, *not* selenium shampoos) a section of hair. Then the hair in that region can be shaved (1 to 2 g) with a clean razor into a collection vial, sealed, and tested. Longer hairs can be sampled in such a manner as to retain orientation of growth, allowing estimation of time and duration of exposure to selenium.

Testing of ingesta and feces is valuable to determine exposure to a variety of toxicants. The value of these matrices lies in the likelihood that toxicants may be present in high enough levels to be detected when compared with other body fluids and substances. For example, many compounds are diluted and metabolized after absorption. Thus, a compound is at its highest concentration in the rumen or stomach content.

Biopsies are invasive and are done only when other diagnostic options are limited. Liver is the most common tissue that is biopsied for toxicology analysis. Fat is also biopsied when a lipophilic food residue must be assessed. Liver tissue can be split, with a portion placed in formalin for histology and another bit frozen in an accessible vial for chemistry analysis. Histology may help identify organ specificity of disease. Histologic examination can be diagnostic for pyrrolizidine alkaloid poisoning (megalocytosis, biliary hyperplasia, and periportal fibrosis) or aflatoxicosis. Fresh biopsy specimens, if properly obtained and frozen, can be used for heavy metal analysis (e.g., copper, lead, zinc). Fat biopsy specimens should be placed in acetone-rinsed foil and sealed frozen for organic chemical analyses.

POSTMORTEM SAMPLES

A toxicology case frequently depends on the postmortem examination for a diagnosis. Although practitioners are trained to perform a necropsy to identify disease and traumatic conditions, it may be advisable to refer extensive cases to a veterinary diagnostic laboratory if possible. The diagnostic laboratories usually have board certified pathologists with specialized training in accepted procedures for investigating this type of case.

If the case is accepted, a complete necropsy should be done, not a partial, "keyhole" necropsy. Such an incomplete job may cause a practitioner to miss an essential sample or observation, perhaps leading to professional and legal embarrassment. If an animal is insured, the insurance company should be contacted before the examination to find out what samples, testing, observations, or procedures must

be conducted. Photographs of the animal and findings may be helpful in assessing the case. Animals submitted for necropsy should be positively identified (record or save ear tags, identify brands and other markings) to help track results.

The necropsy itself is conducted systematically. These cases may involve a great deal of emotion and money. Thus, it is imperative for the clinician to keep an open mind and not to focus on only one diagnosis or on poisoning possibilities alone. Each system should be examined thoroughly. The clinician should look for evidence of struggle (e.g., head injuries, damage to corrals), and search the subcutis and muscles for bruising and trauma.

Once the body cavity is opened, samples that might be contaminated (e.g., microbiology) should be obtained before the full examination begins. Next, the urine should be sampled using a syringe. The urine is put into a plastic or glass container; it is not left in the syringe. Even in dead animals, the urine is still the best sample possible to test for drugs. All major organ systems, including the central nervous system, are critically evaluated. The clinician attempts to determine whether lesions occurred antemortem or from postmortem changes. One of the most sensitive and accurate analytical instruments is the clinician's eye. The clinician carefully visualizes all of the organs and the ingesta, noting the character, volume, and consistency of gut content and body fluids. All of the ingesta is closely examined. Leaves, insects (e.g., blister beetles), chunks of metal, and other items from those gut contents are collected.

Samples of tissue should be fixed in formalin for histology testing, appropriately preserved for microbiological testing, and frozen fresh in separate containers for toxicology testing. Formalin-fixed tissue is usually useless for toxicology testing. However, fixed tissue should be collected for histology examination, which is also critical to a toxicology diagnosis. Because toxicology laboratories differ in some tests and test methods, a veterinary toxicologist and the state or regional laboratory should be consulted about proper sampling before an investigation is initiated.

All samples should be saved despite any initial findings. It is much easier to clean out a freezer later than it is to produce a new sample after the carcass has been disposed of. For the legal case, duplicate samples should be frozen to compensate for shipping losses and such. Each sample is labeled as to origin, tissue type, date, animal, and clinician.

Toxicants cause a variety of lesions ranging from no lesions to specific changes in tissue structure. No lesions at all may be present for some poisoning (e.g., some neurotoxins) or residue cases. Lesions may be lacking also in animals that die peracutely, before visible morphologic changes occur. Some toxicants cause nonspecific lesions. For example, hemorrhagic gastroenteritis may result from a variety of toxicants such as arsenic or even salt poisoning. However, the large intestine may look just the same in a case of severe septicemic shock. More specific lesions may result from other toxicants. A pale, streaked heart may result from a few, more defined etiologies such as selenium deficiency, monensin toxicosis, or exposure to a plant such as white snakeroot (*Eupatorium rugosum*). At the other end of the spectrum, some lesions are specific for a given toxicant. For example, megalocytosis, periportal fibrosis, and biliary hyperplasia in combination are suggestive of pyrrolizidine alkaloid poisoning. In addition to the pattern and type of lesions, the chronicity of those lesions can also yield clues about the nature of the toxin and exposure pattern.

Once the examination is complete, it may help to refer to a checklist prepared before the examination to be sure all organ systems were properly examined and sampled. A preliminary diagnosis may be given after all laboratory testing is complete. For example, gross findings and an initial check on the history may be misleading and could be embarrassing later if a diagnosis is made too soon. A written history and description of signs and lesions should be included with the samples to help the laboratory diagnostician provide the best advice regarding selection of tests and interpretation of findings.

ANALYTICAL TOXICOLOGY

Many poisons can be identified in environmental samples or tissues. As mentioned, no single analysis can identify one of the thousands of diverse chemicals that may be toxic. Toxicology test methods range from simple visualization (e.g., identification of plant parts) to modern analytical chemistry methods.

Analyses for metals are done using spectroscopy. Spectroscopy is rapid and accurate, allowing for analysis of lead in liquids (e.g., blood) within a few hours. Tissue analysis requires additional time for digestion of the sample to free the metals before analysis.

Analyses for organic compounds such as some plant poisons, drugs, or pesticides are done using chromatography. Chromatography is separation of compounds based on characteristic chemical properties in liquid (high performance liquid chromatography), solid (thin layer chromatography), or gas (gas chromatography). After separation, chemicals are detected by analyzing for chemical properties, including absorption of ultraviolet light, fluorescence, oxidation and reduction, electron transfer, and mass weight. In general, chromatography is more time consuming than spectroscopy because extraction of the sample with solvent and purification are needed before testing is done. Some methods (e.g., for cyanide) rely on use of chemical reaction charac-

teristics for analysis. Assay for cholinesterase can be done in hours to assess significant exposure to a cholinesterase inhibitor such as an organophosphorous or carbamate insecticide. Sometimes multiple tests must be done to confirm the presence of a poison in a sample. Thus, testing of tissues and environmental samples may take from a few hours to weeks depending on the method and sample type to be tested.

Diagnosis in some instances may rely on bioassay. Two types of bioassay are used in veterinary diagnostics. The most common bioassay is to monitor patients for response to a treatment or known antidote. The other type of bioassay is to feed a suspected toxic feed in a controlled setting to laboratory animals or livestock to demonstrate its toxicity. The latter type of bioassay is not conducted unless all other avenues for diagnosis have been exhausted. In that instance a suspected toxic source may be fed to prove toxicity and, therefore, help prevent additional cases of poisoning. That is also the first step for further investigations about the causative agent, its effects, and, ultimately, techniques for diagnosis and treatment.

In most competent diagnostic laboratories analytical findings are interpreted by a veterinary toxicologist to determine significance in light of historical, clinical, and pathologic findings. A veterinary toxicologist also provides consultation about possible toxic rule-outs for a case, treatment of affected animals, and prevention of additional cases.

Once all the information is available, a complete summary of the findings can be provided to the client. When the procedures outlined herein are followed, including a systematic approach to collecting all the evidence (historical, clinical, pathologic, and analytical), proper sampling techniques, and good communication between the clinician and the client and laboratory, the usefulness of the toxicology investigation is most fruitful.

RECOMMENDED READING

Blodgett D: The investigation of outbreaks of toxicologic disease, *Vet Clin North Am* 4:145, 1988.

Galey FD: Diagnostic toxicology. In Robinson NE, editor: *Current therapy in equine medicine*, ed 3, Philadelphia, 1992, WB Saunders.

Galey FD: Diagnostic toxicology for the small animal veterinarian, *California Vet* Sept-Oct:7, 1994.

Galey FD: Diagnostic and forensic toxicology, *Vet Clin North Am: Equine Pract* 11:443, 1995.

Hancock DD et al: The collection and submission of samples for laboratory testing, *Vet Clin North Am: Food Anim Pract* 4:33, 1988.

Johnson BJ:, Forensic necropsy. In Robinson NE: *Current therapy in equine medicine*, ed 3, Philadelphia, 1992, WB Saunders.

5

Regulatory Toxicology

Lynn O. Post, Neal Bataller, Mukund Parkhie, and William C. Keller

This chapter is organized into three sections. "Regulatory Agencies" describes the pertinent federal agencies, including processes, organizational structure and mission, and selected programs. "Testing Methods" describes the toxicology studies required by regulatory agencies and, to a limited extent, food safety regulatory programs. "Pharmacovigilance" describes the emerging area of monitoring for unintended harmful effects of marketed animal health products.

This chapter is an introduction to a complex, dynamic area that is continually changing as a result of competing interests that result in new legislation, legal precedents, animal health products, and issues. More detailed and recently updated information can be found on Internet home pages of federal agencies and other reliable organizations, which are cited in the text.

REGULATORY AGENCIES

STATUTES, REGULATIONS, AND GUIDELINES

Federal statutes are the laws that provide the authority for regulatory agencies to operate; these laws are passed by Congress and signed by the President.

Regulations are basic tools for achieving a regulatory agency's goals, such as consumer or environmental protection. Regulations inform the affected industries and the public of statutory requirements and the agency's procedures. Regulations interpret the law and spell out the details needed to implement the general provisions in the statutes. For instance, regulations describe the product-approval process for many individual products or set forth required standards of product composition or performance.

Change is constant and agencies must issue new regulations and amend or revoke old ones. All regulations must be authorized by statute, and the rulemaking procedures must conform to requirements of the Administrative Procedures Act, which applies to all executive branch departments and agencies of the federal government. The administrative process for establishing regulations is referred to as *notice and comment rulemaking.*

New and amended regulations and other notices are disseminated by publication in the *Federal Register* (*http://www.access.gpo.gov/su.doc/aces/aces140.html*), issued daily by the federal government. Regulations are codified in the Code of Federal Regulations (CFR), which is updated annually. Preparing and issuing a regulation is a complex and lengthy process because agencies must be sure any new rule is needed and well conceived. Stake holders, such as affected industry, and consumers generally must be given an opportunity to participate through the notice and comment rulemaking process. Ordinarily, this is done by publishing in the *Federal Register* a notice of proposed rulemaking and inviting comments within a specified timeframe, typically 60 or 90 days. In appropriate cases public hearings are also held. The written and public hearing comments must then be reasonably responded to before issuing a final regulation. After reviewing all comments, an agency publishes the final rule in the *Federal Register* and announces the effective date of the regulation. The regulation then becomes part of the CFR (*http://www.access.gpo.gov/nara/cfr/index.html*). A regulation in this context is considered to be a part of and to carry the legal weight of the law.

Guidelines establish practices of general applicability and do not include decisions or advice on specific product situations. Guidelines are not legal requirements, but they may be relied on with the assurance that they are acceptable procedures or standards. A guideline represents the formal position of the agency on a matter and obligates the agency to follow it until it is amended or revoked. The guideline development process is similar to the regulation publication process. Draft guideline availability and request for comments are typically announced in the *Federal Register* and comments are considered when developing final guidelines.

FREEDOM OF INFORMATION

The Freedom of Information Act (FOIA) became effective in 1967. It provides access to information in government files and requires that each government agency publish descriptions of its operations and procedures. Each agency must also make available opinions, orders, and statements of public policy that affect the public.

Any person can obtain information through an FOIA request. Certain types of information are not available under FOIA. For example, national security information, trade secrets and commercial information, and personnel and medical files are exempt. Agencies are given a certain period of time to process requests, typically within 20 days of receipt. A fee may be charged. The key to obtaining the desired information is to make the request sufficiently detailed and specific to allow identification of the records.

Information important to veterinarians include adverse reaction information for animal drugs, regulatory letters written by the agency, Compliance Policy Guidelines (to direct Food and Drug Administration (FDA) field staff in enforcement activities), and guidelines implementing regulations. Most of this information is available on federal agency Internet home pages. For instance, warning letters to manufacturers for violations of Good Manufacturing Practices and livestock producers or veterinarians involved in causing violative drug residues may be viewed on FOIA Internet site. Summary information on reports of adverse drug reactions is available on the FDA Center for Veterinary Medicine (CVM) home page.

FDA AND ANIMAL DRUGS

Creation and organization of the FDA CVM

Animal drugs and medical devices are regulated by the FDA CVM under the Federal Food, Drug and Cosmetic Act (FFDCA). FDA is an agency within the Department of Health and Human Services. The senior official within FDA is the FDA Commissioner. The agency is organized by product responsibility into centers such as CVM and the Center for Food Safety and Nutrition (CFSAN), and geographically into regional offices and component districts where FDA field staff are assigned.

The first federal FDA act was passed in 1906. It prohibited interstate shipment of adulterated or misbranded food, drink, and drugs and was administered by the U.S. Department of Agriculture (USDA) Bureau of Chemistry. In 1938, landmark broader legislation was passed requiring manufacturers to provide evidence of product safety before distributing new drugs. This legislation also provided authority to conduct manufacturing site inspections, establish tolerances for unavoidable contaminants, and use court injunctions as enforcement tools. In 1940, the FDA was transferred from USDA, ultimately becoming part of the Department of Health, Education, and Welfare (DHEW), which subsequently became the Department of Health and Human Services (DHHS). During the early 1950s, a veterinary branch, which subsequently developed into a division, was established within the FDA Bureau of Drugs.

Subsequently, two major amendments to the FFDCA were passed. The Food Additive Amendments of 1958 expanded the FDA's authority over animal food additives and drug residues in animal-derived foods. The Kefauver-Harris Drug Amendments of 1962 brought major changes to the FFDCA, requiring manufacturers to test new drugs for effectiveness before marketing them and to report adverse events promptly to the FDA. These requirements were also applied through a modified process to products already on the market. Recognizing the importance of animal health products, the FDA established the Bureau of Veterinary Medicine (all bureaus became centers in 1984) in 1965. However, animal drugs were still regulated under three different sections of the FFDCA, either as new drugs, antibiotics, or, if labeled for food animals, as food additives. Because this situation produced a regulatory scheme for

BOX 5-1	**RECENT MAJOR ANIMAL HEALTH PRODUCT–RELATED AMENDMENTS TO THE FFDCA**
Amendment	**Summary of Changes**
Generic Animal Drug and Patent Term Restoration Act (GADPTRA)	Enacted 1988. Provides for approval of generic copies of animal drug products that have been previously approved and shown to be safe and effective. Provides for prescription status for animal drugs.
Animal Drug Use Clarification Act of 1994 (AMDUCA)	Allows veterinarians to prescribe extralabel uses of approved animal drugs and approved human drugs for animals under certain conditions. Allows FDA to restrict extralabel use in certain circumstances. Allows FDA to establish a safe level for a residue for such extralabel use by regulation or order and require the development of analytical methods for residue detection.
Animal Drug Availability Act of 1996 (ADAA).	Amends the definition of substantial evidence of effectiveness. Creates a new category of drugs: "veterinary feed directive drugs." Permits a range of doses to appear on animal drug product labeling, rather than one optimum dose. Provides for licensing of feed mills and eliminates the requirement for medicated feed applications.

FDA, Food and Drug Administration.
From FDA Center for Veterinary Medicine, Rockville, Md: Specific subject index, 2000. http://www.fda.gov/cvm/fda/mappgs/specificsubj.html.

animal drugs that was confusing and more complex than for human drugs, the Animal Drugs Amendments of 1968 were passed, consolidating the various sections of the FFDCA that applied to animal drugs in one section (512) of the FFDCA. More complete discussions of the history of the FFDCA and CVM are available.[1,2] More recent animal health product–related amendments to the FFDCA are listed in Box 5-1.[3]

Approving and monitoring animal drugs

Under the FFDCA, the CVM is responsible for ensuring that animal drugs and medicated feeds are safe and effective for their intended uses and that food from treated animals is safe for human consumption. To accomplish this, the CVM is organized into premarket review, postmarket monitoring, and research components. In addition, FDA field staff conducts inspections of FDA-regulated animal health industries and products. Before a product is marketed, it must have an approved New Animal Drug Application (NADA). In order for an NADA to be approved there must be substantial evidence that the new animal drug is effective as well as safe for its intended uses under the conditions of use prescribed, recommended, or suggested in the proposed labeling. In addition, methods, facilities, and controls used for the manufacturing, processing, and packaging the drug must be shown to be adequate to preserve its identity, strength, quality, and purity.

For food animal products, safety includes safety of drug residues in animal-derived food. This is achieved by establishing tolerances for drug residues (see discussion of tolerances under "Pesticide Residues in Food" in this section and under "Testing Methods: FDA-Required Toxicologic Testing in Food-Producing Animals"). FDA animal drug tolerances may be found in 21 CFR 556, *Tolerances for Residues of New Animal Drugs in Food*. The USDA Food Safety Inspection Service monitors animal-derived food for overtolerance residues and notifies the FDA for enforcement action when violations occur. Safety also includes an assessment of the effects of the proposed animal drug on the environment and on human health. After approval, products are monitored to ensure that safety and effectiveness are maintained under actual conditions of use.

ENVIRONMENTAL PROTECTION AGENCY

Creation of the EPA

The Environmental Protection Agency (EPA) is the newest of the federal agencies that regulate animal health products. During the 1960s, activists became increasingly effective in focusing attention on environmental and public health issues. Rachael Carson's book, *Silent Spring* (1962), provided a worldwide view of the effects of indiscriminate use of pesticides. By 1969, the word *ecology* had become part of American culture. Under criticism that his environmental committees were largely ceremonial bodies, President Nixon

appointed a White House committee in December 1969 to consider whether there should be a separate environmental agency. About the same time, Congress sent the National Environmental Policy Act (NEPA) to the president, which he signed on January 1, 1970. It was against the background of environmental activism that Reorganization Plan No. 3 was sent to Congress by the Nixon administration. Under Reorganization Plan No. 3, the EPA was formed in 1970 to establish and enforce environmental protection standards, to conduct environmental research, to provide assistance to other agencies in combating environmental pollution, and to assist in developing and recommending new policies for environmental protection. The regulatory activities for environmental protection were consolidated from 15 components of five executive departments and independent agencies into a single agency—the EPA. Certain pesticide regulatory functions were transferred from the FDA and USDA to the EPA. The enactment of major new environmental laws and important amendments since 1970 have expanded and refined the role of the EPA (Box 5-2).

The EPA is organized into major offices headed by assistant EPA administrators who develop and implement policies and programs. For instance, the Office of Prevention, Pesticides and Toxic Substances (OPPTS) develops national strategies for toxic substance control and promotes pollution prevention and the public's right to know about chemical risks. A component office, the Office of Pesticide Programs (OPP), regulates the use of all pesticides in the United States and establishes maximum levels for pesticide residues in food. The EPA also has geographically organized regions. Each EPA regional office is responsible within selected states for the execution of the agency's programs, considering regional needs, and implementing federal environmental laws.[4]

Federal Insecticide, Fungicide and Rodenticide Act

The Federal Insecticide, Fungicide and Rodenticide Act (FIFRA) has a major impact on the practice of veterinary medicine because it provides the EPA with the authority to regulate pesticide use in animals. Under FIFRA, the term *pesticide* includes products such as insecticides, fungicides, rodenticides, insect repellants, weed killers, antimicrobials, and swimming pool chemicals. Pesticides are intended to prevent, destroy, repel, or reduce pests of any sort. If a pesticide can be used with "reasonable certainty of no harm," it is granted a "registration" that permits its sale and use according to requirements set by the EPA to protect human health and the environment. During its evaluation of a proposed pesticide, the EPA considers the toxicity of the pesticide, the quantity and frequency of pesticide application, and the amount of pesticide that remains on food by the time it is marketed.

The FIFRA was enacted in 1947 as a consumer protection statute to regulate the manufacture, sale, distribution, and use of pesticides. The USDA administered FIFRA. Pesticide registration was required before marketing in

BOX 5-2	MAJOR STATUTES THAT FORM THE BASIS FOR THE PROGRAMS OF THE EPA

STATUTE OR LAW	DESCRIPTION
Federal Food, Drug, and Cosmetic Act, Delaney Clause (1958)	FFDCA prohibits any manmade chemical in food that caused cancer in any animal, including humans.
National Environmental Policy Act (1969)	NEPA is the basic national charter for protection of the environment.
Clean Air Act (1970)	CAA is the comprehensive federal law that sets standards and regulates air emissions from area, stationary, and mobile sources.
Occupational Safety and Health Act (1970)	OSHA ensures worker and workplace safety from hazards, such as exposure to toxic chemicals, excessive noise levels, mechanical dangers, heat or cold stress, or unsanitary conditions.
Federal Insecticide, Fungicide and Rodenticide Act (1972)	FIFRA provides federal control of pesticide distribution, sale, and use and requires users (farmers, utility companies, and others) to register when purchasing pesticides.
Endangered Species Act (1973)	ESA provides a program for the conservation of threatened and endangered plants and animals and the habitats in which they are found.
Safe Drinking Water Act (1974)	SDWA was established to protect the quality of drinking water in the United States.
Resource Conservation and Recovery Act (1976)	RCRA gives the EPA the authority to control hazardous waste during the generation, transportation, treatment, storage, and disposal of hazardous waste.
Toxic Substances Control Act (1976)	TSCA gives the EPA the ability to track approximately 75,000 industrial chemicals produced or imported into the United States.
Clean Water Act (1977)	CWA gives the EPA the authority to set effluent standards on an industry basis (technology based) and continues the requirements to set water quality standards for all contaminants in surface waters.
Comprehensive Environmental Response Compensation and Liability Act (1980)	CERCLA creates a tax on the chemical and petroleum industries and provides broad federal authority to clean up abandoned hazardous waste sites (Superfund).
Emergency Planning and Community Right-to-Know Act (1986)	EPCRA was enacted by Congress as the national legislation on community safety.
Superfund Amendments and Reauthorization Act (1986)	SARA amended CERCLA and reflects EPA's experience in administering the complex Superfund program.
Pollution Prevention Act (1990)	PPA encourages industry to control toxic emissions by using cost-effective changes in production.
Oil Pollution Act (1990)	OPA streamlines and strengthens the EPA's ability to prevent and respond to catastrophic oil spills through a tax on oil.
Food Quality Protection Act (1996)	FQPA amended FIFRA and FFDCA.

From FDA Center for Veterinary Medicine. Rockville Md. A historical perspective of CVM, 1999. http://www.fda.gov/cvm/fda/mappgs/aboutcvm.html

interstate commerce, and the pesticide product had to bear a label with the manufacturer's name and address, name brand and trademark of the product, net contents, ingredient list, warning statements to prevent injury, and directions for use. Subsequent amendments added more product classes, including nematicides, plant regulators, defoliants, and desiccants (1959), and a requirement that all pesticide labels contain a federal registration number and safety information words, such as "warning," "danger," "caution," and "keep out of reach of children" (1964).

In 1970, authority for FIFRA was transferred from the USDA to the newly created EPA. Another amendment in 1972 provided the EPA with authority to regulate pesticides to prevent unreasonable adverse effects on the environment. The 1972 amendment changes included the following.

- Requirements to follow the label
- Requirements for heavy fines for violations
- Classification of pesticides as "restricted use" or "general use"
- Requirements for state certification, manufacturer registration, and inspection by the EPA
- Requirements for scientific evidence that the product is effective and safe for humans, crops, and animals

Subsequent clarifying amendments provided for significant changes to improve the registration process, including establishing generic standards for the active ingredient rather than for each formulated product, re-registration of all products registered before 1975, conditional registration in which efficacy data may be waived, state enforcement authority, and definition of the phrase "to use any registered pesticide in a manner inconsistent with its labeling." In 1988, the EPA was required to re-register existing pesticides that were originally registered before current scientific and regulatory standards were formally established. The Food Quality Protection Act (FQPA) of 1996 is the most recent significant amendment to FIFRA.

Pesticide residues in foods

When pesticides are used in producing food, they may remain in small amounts called *residues*. To protect the public from potentially harmful effects caused by pesticide residues on food, the EPA regulates the amount of each pesticide that may remain on or in each food. The EPA regulates pesticides under two major federal statutes. Under FIFRA, the EPA registers pesticides for use in the United States and prescribes labeling and other regulatory requirements to prevent unreasonable adverse effects on health or the environment. Under FFDCA, the EPA establishes tolerances (maximum legally permissible levels) for pesticide residues in food. Tolerances are established as part of the premarket registration process. Exceeding the tolerance initiates enforcement actions wherein the commodity may be subject to seizure. Tolerance limits apply to both domestic and imported food. Some foods do not require tolerances because the exposure and toxicity data show that the food is safe when the pesticide is used according to the directions on the label.

Several other government agencies enforce the EPA's pesticide tolerances in food. The FDA tests food produced in the United States and imported food. State agencies also test food produced in the United States. The USDA tests milk, meat, and eggs. The USDA and FDA have programs designed to develop statistically valid information on pesticide residues in foods (see "USDA Food Safety Inspection Service"). This information is provided to the EPA for use in

risk assessments for pesticides. When the USDA detects violations of tolerances in their data collection program, it notifies the FDA for possible enforcement action.

The EPA has responded to both large and small environmental disasters during the past 30 years. Less visible but just as important is the EPA's present effort to reassess all the pesticide and other ingredient tolerances and exemptions that were in effect as of 1996 when the FQPA of 1996 was passed. It amended both the FIFRA and the FFDCA. These amendments changed the way the EPA regulates pesticide residues. Examples of FQPA changes include the following:

- Setting a single residue safety standard of "a reasonable certainty of no harm"
- Requiring an explicit determination that pesticide tolerances are safe for children (an additional safety factor)
- Limiting consideration of benefits when setting tolerances to nonthreshold (e.g., carcinogenic) effects
- Requiring review of existing pesticide tolerances within 10 years
- Requiring new data, including potential endocrine effects
- Imposing of civil penalties
- Expediting review of safer pesticides

USDA AND VETERINARY BIOLOGICS

Regulatory authority and mission

The authority for regulating veterinary biologics in the United States is provided in the Virus-Serum-Toxin Act (VSTA), enacted in 1913 and amended in 1985. It requires (with some exceptions) that all veterinary biologics be licensed. The Licensing and Policy Development (LPD) unit in the Center for Veterinary Biologics (CVB), Veterinary Services, Animal and Plant Health Inspection Service (APHIS), United States Department of Agriculture (USDA) enforces the VSTA. The act authorizes the Secretary of the USDA to prescribe regulations governing the preparation and marketing of veterinary biologics shipped into, within, or from the United States. The VSTA makes it unlawful to sell worthless, contaminated, dangerous, or harmful veterinary biologics or to ship veterinary biologics in or from the United States unless they are prepared in a licensed establishment in compliance with USDA regulations. It requires the issuance of a permit by the USDA before the importation of a veterinary biologic product and gives the department the authority to test veterinary biologic products before importation, if desired. In case of violation, the act permits the USDA to remove or suspend establishment or product licenses and permits. It also gives authority for detention, seizure, and condemnation of products and injunctions against products or establishments.

Definition and functions

The regulations in 9 CFR 101.2 (w) define veterinary biologic products to be "All viruses, serums, toxins, and analogous products of natural or synthetic origin that are intended for use in the diagnosis, treatment, or prevention of diseases of animals." The products include diagnostics, antitoxins, vaccines, live or killed microorganisms, and their antigenic or immunizing components. The LPD reviews license applications for production facilities, biologic products, and importation. It reviews production methods, labels, and supporting data involved in the licensing and permit process and issues licenses and permits. An exemption from this licensing provision is given for products prepared by (1) a person solely for administration to that person's own animals, (2) a veterinarian for use in his or her own licensed practice under a veterinarian-client-patient relationship, and (3) a person operating a state-licensed facility solely for distribution of product within the state of production in a state that has a USDA-approved state regulatory control program for veterinary biologics. The VSTA provides for the issuance of conditional or special licenses for products to meet emergency conditions (*www.aphis.usda.gov/vs/cvb/lpd/index.html*).

USDA FOOD SAFETY INSPECTION SERVICE

The USDA Food Safety Inspection Service (FSIS) is the federal agency responsible for ensuring the safety and wholesomeness of poultry, processed eggs, and meat. The FSIS is organized into a number of subordinate offices including Field Operations, which is divided into geographic districts for managing and coordinating meat and poultry inspection staff activities. The original basis for FSIS inspection activities was the Meat Inspection Act of 1906. This act provided for comprehensive inspection including antemortem and postmortem inspection of individual animals, continuous inspection during processing, and control of meat entering food channels. The Poultry Products Inspection Act, passed in 1957, and the Wholesome Meat Act of 1967 further expanded and strengthened FSIS meat and poultry inspection authority. FSIS also maintains extensive agreements with states for performing inspections.

FSIS staff inspect animals delivered to slaughter facilities and processing establishments through visual examination and sampling of edible tissues collected from livestock, poultry, and processed eggs to ensure that these edible products do not contain illegal levels of drugs, pesticides, or environmental contaminants. Inspectors check animals before and after slaughter, examining carcasses for visible defects including evidence of recent medication that may affect food safety and quality. FSIS laboratories test samples submitted by inspection operations staff, who carry out these responsibilities in more than 6000 privately owned U.S. commercial facilities.

The FSIS National Residue Program includes a comprehensive program to monitor meat and poultry for residues that exceed legal limits (tolerances) to ensure that the nation's animal-derived food is free of potentially harmful chemical residues. The program includes monitoring and surveillance activities designed to develop profile information on various residues and livestock classes for the purpose of designing detection and mitigation strategies. It also includes individual enforcement testing designed to identify and remove individual animals with violative residues from food channels (see "Testing Methods: Tolerances").[5,6]

DRUG ENFORCEMENT ADMINISTRATION

Mission and public health impact

Illegal drug use is a widespread problem in the United States. In 1998, an estimated 13.6 million Americans used an illicit drug at least once during the 30 days before being interviewed. During the same period, nearly 1 in 10 youths aged 12 to 17 years was an illicit drug user, and 130,000 were current users of heroin. The Drug Enforcement Administration (DEA) was established on July 1, 1973. Its mission is to enforce the controlled substances laws and regulations of the United States and to bring to the criminal justice system, or any other competent jurisdiction, those organizations and principal members of organizations who are involved in the growing, manufacture, or distribution of controlled substances in the United States.

Illicit veterinary drugs of public health concern

Approved veterinary scheduled drugs that are illicitly used in humans include boldenone (Equipoise), ketamine, stanozolol (Winstrol), and trenbolone (Finajet). Veterinary products containing anabolic steroids that are exclusively intended for administration through implants to cattle or other non-human species and that have been approved by the FDA CVM are excluded from all schedules.[7,8]

Ketamine hydrochloride, known as "special k" and "k," is a general anesthetic for human and veterinary use. Ketamine produces effects similar to those of phencyclidine (PCP or "angel dust"). Ketamine sold on the streets comes from diverted legitimate supplies, primarily veterinary clinics. Its appearance is similar to that of pharmaceutical grade cocaine, and it is snorted, placed in alcoholic beverages, or smoked in combination with marijuana. The incidence of ketamine abuse is increasing. Ketamine was placed in Schedule III of the Controlled Substances Act (CSA) in August 1999.[9,10]

Concerns over a growing illicit market and prevalence of abuse combined with the possibility of harmful long-term effects of steroid use led Congress in 1991 to place anabolic steroids into Schedule III of the CSA. The CSA defines anabolic steroids as any drug or hormonal substance chemically and pharmacologically related to testosterone (other than estrogens, progestins, and corticosteroids) that promotes muscle growth. Most illicit anabolic steroids are sold at gyms, competitions, and through mail operations. For the most part these substances are smuggled into the United States. Those commonly encountered on the illicit market include boldenone (Equipoise), fluoxymesterone (Halotestin), methandriol, methandrostenolone (Dianabol), methyltestosterone, nandrolone (Durabolin, Deca-Durabolin), oxandrolone (Anavar), oxymetholone (Anadrol), stanozolol (Winstrol), testosterone, and trenbolone (Finajet). Physical side effects include elevated blood pressure and cholesterol levels, severe acne, premature balding, reduced sexual function, and testicular atrophy. In males, abnormal breast development (gynecomastia) can occur. In females, anabolic steroids have a masculinizing effect, resulting in more body hair, a deeper voice, smaller breasts, and fewer menstrual cycles. Several of these effects are irreversible. In adolescents, abuse of these agents may prematurely stop the lengthening of bones, resulting in stunted growth.[7,8]

DEA regulatory requirements for veterinarians

Federal DEA regulations are contained in 21 CFR 1300-1316. Clinicians who are authorized to prescribe controlled substances may do so for legitimate medical purposes in the context of a valid veterinary-client–patient relationship. Under these regulations, the prescribing practitioner is held responsible in case the prescription does not conform to the regulations for records and reports (21 CFR 1304), submitting proper ordering forms (21 CFR 1305), and for meeting the requirements for prescriptions [21 CFR 1306 (1)]. Requirements for prescribing Schedule II drugs are more stringent than for Schedules III, IV, and V. For example, an oral order or refilling of the prescription for Schedule II drugs is prohibited under the CSA. DEA has divisional offices in various regions, including Atlanta, Boston, Chicago, Dallas, Denver, Detroit, El Paso, Houston, and Los Angeles. In addition, each division has several district offices.

Veterinarians should write to the DEA Office of Diversion Control, 600 Army Navy Drive, Arlington, VA 22202, for additional information regarding registration and drug schedules. The web address of the DEA is *www.usdoj.gov/dea/*. It is advisable to contact the divisional office for a prompt response. A written request can be made to the Information Services Section, DEA, 700 Army Navy Drive, Arlington, VA 22202.

OCCUPATIONAL SAFETY AND HEALTH ADMINISTRATION

Organization and mission

Harmful chemical compounds in the form of vapors, fumes, mists, gases, liquids, and solids are encountered in the workplace by inhalation, absorption (through direct skin contact), or, to a lesser extent, ingestion. Airborne chemical hazards have great occupational health significance. The degree of worker risk from exposure to any given substance depends on the nature and potency of the chemical's toxic effects and on the duration and intensity of exposure.[11]

In 1970, Congress passed the Occupational Safety and Health Act.[12] The act requires employers to maintain a safe workplace and created the Occupational Safety and Health Administration (OSHA). This agency's mandate includes regulatory responsibility for establishing mandatory occupational exposure standards, as well as related research, training, education, and enforcement. OSHA is part of the Department of Labor and is headed by the Assistant Secretary of Labor for Occupational Safety and Health. Major OSHA programs are administered through directorates such as the Directorate for Safety Standards Programs, which provides workplace standards and regulations to ensure safe working conditions. Programs are carried out by regional offices and district offices. Under the act, many states have OSHA-approved occupational safety and health programs that function in lieu of OSHA programs or standards. OSHA has broad workplace safety responsibilities that pertain to physical hazards such as electromagnetic radiation, temperature, noise and vibration, ergonomic hazards such as repeated motions or heavy lifting, and biological hazards including bacterial and viral pathogens, in addition to the chemical hazards that are the primary subject of this section. The act also established the National Institute for Occupational Safety and Health (NIOSH) within the Department of Health and Human Services (HHS). NIOSH is authorized to develop and establish recommended occupational safety and health standards by conducting research and experimental programs for the development of new and improved occupational safety and health standards.

Exposure limits

OSHA limits occupational exposure to hazardous chemicals by establishing exposure limits and directing changes in employer work processes or equipment; when that is not feasible, OSHA requires personal protective equipment. Unlike for drugs, biologics, pesticides, and food additives, evidence of safety does not have to be provided by industry, nor does approval need to be obtained before manufacturing and marketing new products that may entail occupational exposure to hazardous chemicals. Thus, exposure limits may be adopted after the chemical has entered the occupational environment. The act specifies that, for regulating toxic chemicals, OSHA must adopt standards that most adequately assure, to the extent feasible, on the basis of the best available evidence, that no employee will suffer material impairment of health or physical capability. Thus, some consideration must be given to the issue of technologic achieveability for industry in promulgating standards.

OSHA standards are called *permissible exposure limits* (PELs). They are legal standards that may not be exceeded. PELs have been controversial and susceptible to successful legal challenges. Thus, many chemicals do not have PELs. In the absence of OSHA PELs, employers use recommended occupational exposure limits established by acknowledged sources to meet OSHA's requirements for worker safety. NIOSH has *recommended exposure limits* (RELs). The American Conference of Governmental Industrial Hygienists Threshold Limit Values (TLVs) for Chemical Substances and Physical Agents in the Work Environment are widely used.[13] TLVs refer to airborne concentrations of substances and represent conditions under which it is believed that nearly all workers may be repeatedly exposed day after day without adverse health effects. There are three categories of occupational exposure limits:

1. Time-weighted average (TWA)—the time-weighted average concentration for a conventional 8-hour workday and 40-hour workweek, to which it is believed that nearly all workers may be repeatedly exposed, day after day, without adverse effect.
2. Short-term exposure limit (STEL)—the concentration to which it is believed that workers can be exposed for a short period of time without suffering from irritation, tissue damage, or narcosis. It is not a separate exposure limit but supplemental to the TWA and limited to a 15-minute TWA.
3. Ceiling—the concentration that should not be exceeded during any part of the working exposure.[14]

The OSHA Hazard Communication Standard (29 CFR 1910.1200), also called the Right to Know Law, ensures that the hazards of all chemicals are evaluated and the information concerning their hazards is transmitted to employers and employees. It requires chemical manufacturers and importers to obtain or develop a material safety data sheet (MSDS) for each hazardous chemical they produce or import. Distributors are responsible to ensure that their customers are provided a copy of these MSDS forms. An MSDS must contain information describing the physical and chemical properties, health hazards, routes of exposure, precautions for safe handling and use, emergency procedures, and control measures. The MSDS has become a well-established document for disseminating health and safety information about chemical products.[15] The *NIOSH Pocket Guide to Chemical Hazards* is another useful document for health and safety information about hazardous chemicals.[16]

TESTING METHODS

The FDA and EPA have developed extensive, detailed guidelines for conducting studies required to obtain approval to market products. This section provides a brief description of the animal safety and efficacy studies and human safety studies that may be performed. They are provided to familiarize the reader with the general scope of information required for product approval, not to provide guidance in designing studies for product approval. The specific pertinent agency guideline should be consulted before designing a study protocol. This section also contains an overview of the regulatory process for monitoring and limiting violative residues.

TARGET ANIMAL SAFETY TESTING

FDA animal safety and product efficacy

A veterinary drug sponsor must show that a drug is safe to use as described in the proposed labeling [21 CFR 514.1 (b)(1) and 512 (d) of the FFDCA].[17] The information

needed to determine product safety in the target species depends on many factors: proposed use, type of product, chemistry, intended species, breed, class of animal (calves versus mature ruminants), claims, and previous use history. Existing data collected from previous studies are used to develop and refine protocols for toxicity studies. A CVM target animal safety guideline provides general guidance for acquiring essential information. However, all the data requirements for a standard target animal safety study are not required for every product, and special circumstances may require the collection of additional data that are not specified for the standard study.

Good laboratory practices and general study requirements. Laboratory studies in animals, including target animals, are conducted according to Good Laboratory Practice (GLP) regulations (21 CFR Section 58). Target animal safety studies are also subject to GLP regulations. The GLP regulations ensure that study methods and procedures for collecting, processing, and reporting data are standardized and verified. GLPs ensure an adequate level of accuracy and quality control. Many GLP requirements are inherent in any well-designed scientific study.

Because animal husbandry requirements often differ for laboratory animals and domestic animals, clinical studies for domestic animals are not conducted under GLP conditions. In conducting these studies, appropriate diagnostic tests, vaccinations, prophylactic, and therapeutic treatments are completed before the treatment phase of the study. During this initial phase, a complete physical examination is also performed and a qualified person collects baseline data. The test product formulation must be identical to the proposed marketed product. The route of administration should be the same as the proposed labeling; however, the toxicity or nature of the product may require a different type of administration than that of the final product. For example, in the case of feed refusal, a drench of a product may be required instead of delivery of the drug through a medicated feed.

Data are collected at predetermined intervals during the study. Clinical observations are recorded at specified intervals, usually twice a day, 7 days a week during the entire study or modified according to the study protocol. During the study, appropriate clinical pathology procedures are conducted in all test groups, usually involving half of the animals selected at random from each group at predetermined intervals.

Histopathologic examinations may be required from all or a portion of the animals. Tissues from the highest treatment and control groups must be examined. If microscopic lesions are observed, corresponding tissues from the next lower treatment group are examined until a no observed effect level (NOEL) is established.

Drug tolerance test. The drug tolerance test is often done as a preliminary study using a multiple of the proposed label dose. Usually, up to 10 times (10×) the maximum proposed clinical dose is administered. The toxic dose (10×)

may be reduced or increased in order to manifest toxic signs without causing death. The main purpose of the tolerance test is to characterize toxic signs, which can be used to develop toxicity study protocols at lower doses (1×, 3×, and 5×). The toxicity studies are used to design the clinical efficacy study protocol. Under controlled conditions, the target animal response to a toxic dose is characterized by clinical signs. Clinical signs include changes in behavior and appearance and gross lesions in animals that die during the study. Clinical pathology and histology data reveal physiologic functions that are most readily affected by the drug. The duration of the toxicity studies may range from acute to chronic.

Although systemic toxicity testing is required for new products or new chemical entities and additional animal species, it is not required for drugs administered locally, such as otic, ophthalmic, intramammary, or intraarticular preparations. This exception does not apply to generalized dermal or topical drugs that may act systemically. The market formulation of a drug must be administered according to the proposed conditions of use. If volume or palatability becomes a limiting factor for administration, gavage, intravenous, multiple sites, or incremental doses may be used. A vehicle control group must be included in the experimental design.

Toxicity study. The objectives of toxicity studies in target animal species are (1) to demonstrate safety of the drug product under conditions of use, (2) to demonstrate signs and effects associated with toxicity, and (3) to demonstrate a margin of safety at 5× or below. If the drug has a narrow margin of safety with an intended use in debilitated animals, safety studies in diseased animals may be necessary. This may require more animals per treatment group because of greater variability. Special studies may be requested by the FDA, involving, for example, lameness, reproduction, dermal irritation, specific routes of administration, tissue disposition, and combination drugs. The CVM *Guideline for Target Animal Safety Studies* may be found on the CVM Internet home page at *http://www.fda.gov/cvm/fda/TOCs/guideline33.html.*

FDA efficacy studies. Efficacy trials or studies are clinical studies. The purpose of an efficacy study is to evaluate the response of the test article under actual conditions of use. Clinical studies to establish efficacy are also important to the overall safety assessment of the product. GLP regulations do not apply because clinical studies are conducted in a clinical environment under actual conditions of use rather than in a rigorously controlled laboratory setting. For example, veterinary practitioners may enroll their client's dogs in a nonsteroidal antiinflammatory study, and food animal producers may participate in a production drug study. In efficacy studies, special care must be exercised in handling animals to avoid undue stress, which may alter the response to the drug, affecting the study results. Laboratory samples should be collected from all animals at specified times in order to minimize bias.

The design of the efficacy trial is flexible and depends on the species, breed, drug, class of production animal, and data endpoints. In some instances, such as for production drugs, many animals are required per treatment group for the efficacy trial because of variability from environmental conditions and in the test animals. For typical therapeutic products, the number of subjects used for an animal drug clinical trial is about one tenth to one twentieth of the number required for an equivalent human drug clinical trial. Additionally, although toxicity is not the objective of these studies, animals are observed periodically (usually daily) for clinical signs and abnormalities. These observations give valuable information for designing additional safety study protocols or reveal information that should appear in the safety information on the product label. Some animals may be necropsied at the end of the study if animals exhibit signs of toxicity. On the other hand, the drug may also be discontinued in an animal exhibiting toxic signs.

Even though the efficacy studies are non-GLP, the test methods and procedures for administering the test article are verified and monitored throughout the study. This ensures that the drug is being delivered to the animals according to the protocol. For example, an oral drug may be administered with or without food, or the mixing procedure for dispersing a production drug in feed must be periodically validated.

After all requirements have been met, FDA approval of the product allows it to be legally marketed and promoted as a new animal drug. The label must contain the product claims, pharmacology, side effects, precautions, and warnings. After approval, the drug is monitored through periodic and special industry drug experience reports (DERs) to the CVM. These reports include adverse experiences and may result in label changes related to product safety (see "Pharmacovigilance").

EPA companion animal safety testing

Companion animal safety studies for EPA-registered pesticides apply only to dogs and cats because of widespread use of these external products for pests.[18] The companion animal safety study is not a study that is required for pesticide registration. Companion animal safety studies for pesticide formulations for the treatment of external pests are intended to demonstrate that an adequate margin of safety exists with overuse or misuse (40 CFR Section 792 and 40 CFR 160, Good Laboratory Practice Standards). Data from companion animal safety studies for pesticides serve as a basis for product labeling. The study can be compared to an acute dermal toxicity study and is limited in scope because an NOEL is not required. External pesticide products include collars, sprays, dips, shampoos, and spot treatments.

The design of a companion animal safety study should reflect the product label (method of administration, species and age group, and frequency of application). The criteria for use of the product should be used in the study. A control group should receive a concurrent vehicle at the 5× level. The vehicle should contain the inert ingredients at the maximum levels that would appear in the 5× formulation. Negative (untreated) control subjects may occasionally be used to determine whether adverse effects are due to the inert ingredients in a formulation. The test formulation is applied to several groups of (sex) experimental animals at the label dose and multiples of this dose (3× and 5×). For exaggerated doses (3× and 5×), products specifically prepared for this type of study that contain higher concentrations of the active ingredient are preferred. If the drug cannot be formulated at the 3× or 5× concentration because of volume constraints, multiple treatments at frequent intervals may be necessary. If the high-dose level (at least 5×) produces no evidence of drug-related toxicity, a full study (three dose levels) may not be necessary. Multiple pesticides formulated into a single product may also be evaluated. Depending on the severity of signs of toxicity, products with less than 5× margin of safety may be considered for registration. The route of administration of these product studies should be topical. The skin or hair should not be prepared in any manner unless such directions appear on the label. If the product label recommends several treatments, multiple treatments at frequent intervals are included in the study design based on label claims and instructions for use.

The species recommended for treatment on the product label is included in the study. Studies are performed on representative classes of healthy dogs and cats by size, weight, sex, and age based on label claims. For instance, if only adults older than 6 months of age are the label population of animals to receive treatment, only adults are enrolled in the study. If the product is registered for puppies and kittens, the label should state a minimum age for this group and this class should be included in the study. An equal number of animals per sex are used at each dosage level. Animals are appropriately examined and prepared during the acclimation period.

Clinical observations are conducted at hourly intervals for at least 4 hours after the last treatment and twice daily for the duration of the study. If adverse reactions are observed, the observation period on the day of treatment is extended to a time at which no toxic signs are observed. Observations should include all systems. Special attention is directed to observations of central nervous system signs of seizures, tremors, and salivation and of gastrointestinal signs of vomiting and diarrhea. Observations and measurements are reported for a minimum of 14 days after treatment and longer if appropriate. Various samples and measurements are collected throughout the study. Individual body weights and food consumption are measured during acclimation and periodically during the study. Animals that die or are euthanized in a moribund state are subjected to a gross necropsy, and abnormal tissues are examined histopathologically to determine the cause of death. Routine poststudy necropsy is not required. Clinical pathology samples, including red cell cholinesterases when appropriate, are

assessed before treatment, 24 hours posttreatment, and on day 7 of treatment.

FOOD SAFETY TESTING

FDA-required toxicologic testing in food-producing animals

FDA general requirements and specific study protocol recommendations are described in the guidance documents contained in the *Redbook 2000*, formally titled *Toxicologic Principles for the Safety of Food Ingredients (www.cfsan.gov/redbook/red-toct.html)*. These studies must be conducted according to GLPs. For compounds used in food-producing animals, CVM is concerned with intermittent and chronic exposure of humans to relatively low concentrations of residues. CVM tailors the type of toxicologic testing needed to show safety for a specific compound. Factors that are considered include the proposed use and the potential human exposure of the parent compound, its residues, or both, as deduced by structure-activity relationships. Some compounds need only a minimum of testing; others may need extensive studies in a number of diverse biologic systems.

The purpose of the toxicology studies is to define the biologic effects of the sponsored compound and its quantitative limits. The CVM generally asks that the sponsor, at a minimum, determine a dose of the compound that produces an adverse biologic effect in test animals and a dose that does not produce any significant toxicologic or pharmacologic effect (the NOEL). The spacing of the doses should provide an assessment of the dose-response relationship.[19]

Testing requirements. The CVM generally believes that the following studies are the minimum necessary for each sponsored compound:

- A battery of genetic toxicity tests. Positive results indicate the drug may be a carcinogen.
- A 90-day feeding study in both a rodent species (usually the rat) and a nonrodent mammalian species (usually the dog).
- A two-generation reproduction study with a teratology component in rats. Two litters should be produced in each generation. If toxicity occurs at a lower dose, with a higher incidence, or with greater intensity in the second generation as compared to the first, then the study should include a third generation. Additional information is given under EPA Chronic Toxicity Testing of Pesticides.

The FDA may require the following additional studies, which should be conducted using an approved protocol:

- Chronic bioassays for oncogenicity in each of two rodent species when indicated by positive results in genetic toxicity tests. Additional information is given under EPA Chronic Toxicity Testing of Pesticides.
- One-year feeding studies in a rodent species (usually the rat) and in a nonrodent species (usually the dog) are needed when human residue exposure exceeds 25 μg/kg body weight/day. This daily intake is equivalent to 1 ppm

in a total solid diet of 1500 g, normally consumed by a 60-kg human subject. The CVM calculates permissible exposure when evidence indicates that the residue bioaccumulates in the tissues of target animals.

- A teratology study in a second species when the compound is structurally related to a known teratogen, when the compound has hormonal activity that may affect the fetus, or when the compound shows adverse effects in the reproduction or teratology study indicating that the compound may be a teratogen.
- Other specialized testing as necessary to define the biological effect of the compound. Examples of specialized studies include testing for neurotoxicity, immunotoxicity, hormonal activity, toxicity after in utero exposure, or for toxicity from a "biomass" product.

If the testing shows that the sponsored compound is a carcinogen, the CVM applies the "no-residue" requirement of section 409(c)(3)(A), 512(d)(1)(H), or 706(b)(5)(B) of the FFDCA as operationally defined in 21 CFR subpart E of Part 500. The FDA calculates the concentration of residue, giving no significant risk of cancer from the tumor data using a statistical extrapolation procedure. In the absence of information establishing the mechanism of carcinogenesis for a particular chemical, the CVM uses a nonthreshold, linear-at-low dose extrapolation procedure that determines the upper limit of the risk.[20,21] In the extrapolation, the CVM uses the upper 95% confidence limit on the tumor data and a permitted maximum lifetime risk to the test animal of 1 in 1 million.

Acceptable daily intake and safety factors.   For other toxicologic endpoints, the CVM calculates the acceptable daily intake (ADI) from the results of the most sensitive study in the most sensitive species. From that study, the ADI is the highest dose showing no observed effect divided by the appropriate safety factor (Box 5-3).

Sex steroids.   Although not all sex steroids are demonstrated carcinogens, the evidence supports the CVM's conclusion that all endogenous sex steroids and synthetic compounds with similar biological activity should be regarded as suspect carcinogens and that the endogenous sex steroids are not genotoxic agents. If these compounds produce an oncogenic response in experimental animals, the mechanism of action is not related to a direct chemical interaction with

DNA, but tumor development is a consequence of hyperproliferation of endocrine-sensitive tissue resulting from persistent overstimulation of the hormonal system.

Based on this mechanism of action, the safety of endogenous sex steroids and their simple ester derivatives can be assured without additional animal study data. Large quantities of these compounds are produced by de novo synthesis in humans and in food-producing animals. The CVM has concluded that no physiologic effect occurs in individuals ingesting animal tissues that contain endogenous steroids equal to 1% or less of that produced daily in the population with the lowest production. In the case of estradiol and progesterone, prepubertal boys synthesize the least; in the case of testosterone, prepubertal girls synthesize the least. The product is considered safe within the meaning of the act, if data acceptable to the CVM demonstrate that under the proposed conditions of use the residue concentration of the endogenous sex steroid in treated food-producing animals does not exceed the permitted increase at the time of slaughter.

Synthetic sex steroids.   In addition to the standard requirements, CVM recommends the following additional test: a 180-day study in rhesus monkeys or another suitable subhuman primate to assess the effect of the sponsored compound on various parameters including ovulation, menstrual cycle, circulating levels of gonadotropins, and sex steroids. The study should establish a dose that gives a no observed hormonal response.

The CVM also normally uses a safety factor of 100 for the study in subhuman primates. If a carcinogenic response is observed in a nonendocrine-sensitive tissue, the CVM determines the dose that will satisfy the "no residue" requirement of the act using the tumor data from that tissue and a statistical extrapolation procedure.

EPA chronic toxicity testing of pesticides

The EPA requires a variety of toxicity testing before registration of pesticides. The 870 Series Final Guidelines describe study protocols that meet testing requirements of the FIFRA and the Toxic Substances Control Acts (TSCA). Reproduction and fertility (870.3800) and Combined Chronic Toxicity/Carcinogenicity (870.4300) studies are described.

Reproduction toxicity testing.   The two-generation reproduction study provides information on the effects of a test substance on the male and female reproductive systems. EPA and FDA *(Redbook)* recommendations for this study are similar. The study should be conducted in accordance with the Good Laboratory Practice Standards stipulated in 40 CFR Part 160 (FIFRA) and 40 CFR Part 792 (TSCA). The test substance is administered to parental (P) animals before and during their mating, during the resultant pregnancies, and through the weaning of their F1 offspring. The substance is then administered to selected offspring during their growth into adulthood, mating, and production and

BOX 5-3	HUMAN FOOD SAFETY STUDIES AND SAFETY FACTORS	
TYPE OF STUDY		**SAFETY FACTOR**
Chronic		100
Reproduction/teratology (100 for a clear indication of maternal toxicity; 1000 for other effects)		100 or 1000
90-day		1000

weaning of a subsequent generation. The rat is the most commonly used species for testing. Each control group should contain a sufficient number of mating pairs to yield approximately 20 pregnant females. Each test group should contain a similar number of mating pairs. At least three dose levels and a concurrent control should be used. The dose levels should be spaced to produce a gradation of toxic effects. The highest dose should be chosen to induce some reproductive or systemic toxicity but not death or severe suffering. The intermediate dose levels should produce minimal observable toxic effects. The lowest dose level should not produce any evidence of either systemic or reproductive toxicity. The highest dose tested should not exceed 1000 mg/kg/day (or 20,000 ppm in the diet), unless potential human exposure data indicate the need for higher doses. A concurrent control group should be used. The test substance is usually administered by the oral route (diet, drinking water, or gavage). The animals should be given the test substance on a daily basis. Daily administration of the test substance to the parental males and females should begin when they are 5 to 9 weeks old, and that administration to the offspring should begin at weaning. Daily doses should begin at least 10 weeks before the mating period and continue until termination of the study.

The endpoints measured should provide data regarding the performance of the male and female reproductive systems including gonadal function, the estrous cycle, mating behavior, conception, gestation, parturition, lactation and weaning, and growth and development of the offspring. The study may also provide information about the effects of the test substance on neonatal morbidity, mortality, target organs in the offspring, and preliminary data on prenatal and postnatal developmental toxicity, as well as serve as a guide for subsequent tests. Additionally, because the study design includes in utero as well as postnatal exposure, it provides the opportunity to examine the susceptibility of the immature or neonatal animal. For further information on functional deficiencies and developmental effects, additional study segments can be incorporated into the protocol using the guidelines for developmental toxicity or developmental neurotoxicity.[22,23]

Combined chronic toxicity and carcinogenicity testing. The objective of the combined chronic toxicity and carcinogenicity study is to determine the effects of a substance in a mammalian species after prolonged and repeated exposure. The design and conduct should allow for the detection of neoplastic effects and a determination of the carcinogenic potential as well as general toxicity, including neurologic, physiologic, biochemical, and hematologic effects and exposure-related morphologic (pathology) effects.[24]

Preliminary studies providing data on acute, subchronic, and metabolic responses should be conducted. The route of exposure is generally oral, dermal, or inhalation. For the combined chronic toxicity and carcinogenicity study, the rat is the species of choice for oral and inhalation studies, whereas the mouse is the species of choice for the dermal route. The choice of the route of administration depends on the physical and chemical characteristics of the test substance and the product exposure in humans. The duration of studies should be at least 18 months for mice and hamsters and 24 months for rats. The following general requirements apply to all combined chronic toxicity and carcinogenicity studies regardless of the route of administration. Testing should be started with young healthy animals as soon as possible after weaning and acclimatization, but no later than 8 weeks of age. At commencement of the study, the weight variation of animals used should be within 20% of the mean weight for each sex. At least 100 rodents (50 males and 50 females) should be allotted randomly to each dose level and concurrent control group. At least 20 additional rodents (10 males and 10 females) should be used for satellite dose groups and the satellite control group. The purpose of the satellite group is to allow for the evaluation of chronic toxicity after 12 months of exposure to the test substance. The number of animals in any group should not go below 50% during the course of the study at 15 months in mice and 18 months in rats, so that a meaningful and valid interpretation of negative results can be achieved. Survival in any group should not go below 25% at 18 months in mice and 24 months in rats.

Tolerances

Increased consumer and federal agency interest in eliminating potentially unsafe residues from food has resulted in animal producers and food animal practice veterinarians receiving increased regulatory scrutiny and in some cases being subjected to FDA regulatory action. The basis of regulatory action is generally a pattern of violative tissue residues. Violative tissue residues are those residues that exceed the tolerance.

The tolerance is the legal enforcement level for a residue. It is generally identified as the parent drug or a specific metabolite occurring in a specific tissue of a specific species. For example, for florfenicol in cattle, a tolerance of 3.7 ppm of florfenicol amine in liver has been established. Tolerances and safe levels of residues are codified in 21 CFR 556. Meat with residues greater than the tolerance (illegal residues) that result from misuse of a drug is considered adulterated under the FFDCA, section 402(a)(2)(C).

The USDA FSIS routinely monitors residues in tissue samples. Violations are traced back to the animal origination. The FSIS notifies the owner of the violation and recommends measures to prevent future violations. The information is reported to the FDA for possible regulatory action.

After completion of toxicity studies to establish an ADI, residue chemistry studies are conducted to establish a tolerance and withdrawal time. These studies generally include total residue and metabolism studies, comparative metabolism studies, and residue depletion studies. The total residue and metabolism study is conducted in the target species and is intended to show drug deposition, metabolism, and elimination. It is conducted using radiolabeled drug and monitors all drug-derived residues. Analytical technology is used to separate the total residue into its components and to identify and quantify individual drug-derived compounds. Total residues after administration are compared with the safe concentration established in the toxicity studies to determine whether a withdrawal time is needed. If total residues exceed the respective safe concentration, then a preslaughter drug withdrawal time is required and a tolerance must be established. The target tissue is the edible tissue selected to monitor for total residue and is usually the last tissue with total residue to deplete to the safe concentration. The marker residue is a residue whose concentration is in a known relationship to the concentration of total residue in the last tissue to deplete to the safe concentration. The target tissue and marker residue are selected so that when the depletion of the marker residue in the target tissue is less than a designated concentration (tolerance), no other tissues will contain unsafe residues. Comparative metabolism studies are conducted in the toxicologic species to confirm that the animals used for toxicity testing were exposed to the same metabolites that occur in the target (food animal) species. If a withdrawal time is required, a residue depletion study is conducted using the commercial product under field conditions. The study monitors the marker residue in the target tissue as it depletes to the tolerance level using a method developed by the sponsor and accepted by the FDA. A statistical method that provides a wide margin of safety is used to establish the withdrawal time to ensure that even those animals that fall outside the predictive model do not contain residues that exceed the tolerance.[19,25]

ANIMAL CARE AND WELFARE REQUIREMENTS

Researchers who conduct studies funded by the federal government are subject to a number of animal care requirements imposed by various federal agencies. The Animal Welfare Act (AWA) is administered by the USDA APHIS Animal Care Program.[26] It applies specifically to dogs, cats, and a number of other listed species as well as to any other warm-blooded animals designated by the Secretary. It requires covered facilities to register and comply with AWA regulations. Examples of types of requirements established to implement the AWA include living space, lighting, heating, ventilation, drainage, transportation, feeding and watering, and veterinary care. The AWA establishes the requirement for an Institutional Animal Care and Use Committee, which must include a veterinarian and an external member. This committee reviews the program and inspects the facility periodically and reviews protocols for research conducted within the facility. It does not apply to animal agriculture or nonresearch horses. It does apply to dealers and exhibitors. Federal agencies such as the

National Institutes of Health may impose additional requirements.

As a practical approach to ensuring that their programs and facilities meet these requirements, many organizations participate in the Association for Assessment and Accreditation of Laboratory Animal Care (AAALAC) International's accreditation process. The AAALAC was founded in 1965 to address laboratory animal welfare issues. AAALAC International is a nonregulatory, nonprofit corporation.[27] Its mission is to promote high standards for animal care, use, and welfare and to enhance life sciences research and education through its accreditation process. For updated or additional information, contact the AAALAC at *www.aaalac.org.*

PHARMACOVIGILANCE

Pharmacovigilance consists of the means and methods for monitoring and ensuring the safety and efficacy of marketed medicinal products. (Note: In this section, the term *pharmaco* is used to encompass not only drugs but also all types of medicinal products.) Pharmacovigilance is made necessary by the limitations of preapproval or preregistration studies for animal medicinal products. Economic and practical considerations limit the number of animals included in safety and efficacy studies. Furthermore, many of the animals used during the testing phase consist of experimental animals that are homogenous in age, breed, and genetics. More variation is obtained when the drug is tested in clinical studies, but these types of studies generally have few animals. Thus, even though premarketing studies may be adequate in demonstrating efficacy and common adverse drug reactions, they generally have limited power to detect less frequently occurring adverse events that may occur when the product is finally used under actual conditions of use in the general veterinary community.

Veterinary pharmacovigilance within the federal government is typically based on the receipt of spontaneous reports involving complaints of product performance. *Spontaneous* refers to reports that are voluntarily submitted by veterinarians, animal producers, and animal owners. The reports may be submitted by mail, phone, fax, or e-mail. The reports may be originally submitted to the drug company, a federal agency, or even a third-party reporting organization, such as to the U.S. Pharmacopeia (USP) or to the American Society for the Prevention of Cruelty to Animals (ASPCA) Animal Poison Control Center (APCC). Product complaints might involve a suspected animal injury, failure of the product to perform (or ineffectiveness), or a product defect. A complaint of this nature associated with the use of an animal medicinal product is referred to as an adverse event (AE), which is synonymous with a suspected adverse reaction.

The key to understanding the spontaneous AE reporting process is in recognizing and appreciating the word *suspected.*

Any complaint evaluation must start with the establishment of an actual AE because any one spontaneously reported AE might be misrepresented, or perhaps not exist at all. A certain level of bias is automatically introduced when the reporter associates the AE with the administration of a specific drug. Because evidence that unquestionably documents and supports the AE occurrence is nearly always lacking, information criteria must be established for accepting an AE into a pharmacovigilance system. This information should include an identifiable reporter, an identifiable animal, an identifiable product, and an adequately described adverse event.

In the case of the existence of an actual AE, a reporter lodges a complaint in the form of an adverse event report (AER). The AER is the mechanism through which all relevant aspects of the AE are described. The main goal of the pharmacovigilance program receiving an AER should be to ensure that all needed data elements are accurately and fully described. In many cases, follow-up information may be needed to augment the original AER. Even if the most accurate information is obtained for an AE, the possibility of one or more alternative non–drug-related explanations for the AE occurrence cannot be discounted.

This approach establishes some level of assurance that the drug under question was "associated" with the reported AE. Strength of association is often determined by using objective-based guidelines. The main strength of the spontaneous reporting system is in detecting the occurrence of drug-related adverse effects that are uncommon and cannot be detected by premarketing studies, which generally have low statistical power. Once a trend or suspected adverse reaction is detected, other methods may be used to investigate the suspected AE and determine the most appropriate course of action. For instance, the drug company may be requested to provide more information or to conduct studies investigating the specific issue, or expert opinions may be sought from relevant veterinary specialists. Recommended actions might include labeling changes, recall of specific batches of product, or even removal of the product from the market.

The three federal agencies responsible for regulating animal health products (FDA, EPA, USDA) all maintain surveillance programs for monitoring products after they are marketed. Because the laws that provide regulatory authority (and thus the regulatory goals, regulations, and approach by these three agencies) are different, the pharmacovigilance programs used for monitoring the safety and efficacy of marketed animal medicinal products are different. The spontaneous reporting system for each of the agencies are discussed, as is the role of the USP and ASPCA APCC in contributing to pharmacovigilance efforts.

FDA/CVM ADVERSE DRUG EVENT REPORTING SYSTEM

The regulations that specifically address the spontaneous reporting obligations of the drug sponsors of FDA-approved animal drugs are contained in 21 CFR §510.300 ("Records and reports concerning experience with new animal drugs for which an approved application is in effect"). Reporting of AEs is mandatory for the pharmaceutical industry. It is voluntary for veterinarians.

For industry reporting, the regulations categorize AERs into three categories: significant product defect reports that should be submitted to CVM immediately [21 CFR §510.300(b)(1)]; AERs involving unexpected animal injury and unexpected product ineffectiveness that should be submitted within 15 working days [21 CFR §510.300(b)(2)]; and the remaining types of AERs and product defects, which should be submitted at periodic intervals [21 CFR §510.300(a)]. All categories of complaints are required to be submitted by the drug sponsor on Form FDA 1932 ("Veterinary Adverse Drug Reaction, Lack of Effectiveness, Product Defect Report").

Significant product defects are those involving either label mixups or a significant departure of the product from approved specifications, wherein the product defect may result in immediate harm to animals. Corrective action is accomplished through the FDA field office responsible for the manufacturing site.

The types of AERs requiring 15-day submissions include
- Any unexpected side effects, injury, toxicity
- Any unexpected sensitivity reaction
- Any unexpected incidence or severity
- Any unusual failure to exhibit expected pharmacologic activities (ineffectiveness)

Unexpected refers to either information that is not contained either on product labeling or as part of the approved FDA application. Regulations further require reporting of unexpected adverse events that are associated with clinical use, studies, investigations, or tests, whether or not determined to be attributable to the suspected drug. CVM expects the drug sponsor to submit all AERs rather than only those reports the firm believes are associated with the AE. CVM considers selective report submission (filtering) to introduce a bias that confounds the evaluation of submitted AERs.

All AERS submitted to CVM are evaluated by a staff of veterinarians assigned to this task. All relevant information is extracted from the AERs and entered into the appropriate fields of a relational database using standard terminology. A six-step algorithm evaluation process is used to assign a score that represents the strength of the veterinarian's opinion that the use of the drug was associated with the adverse clinical sign.

The database is used by product managers, who are veterinarians assigned to monitor the safety and efficacy of specific products. When a potential problem is identified, the Monitored Adverse Reaction Committee (MARC) is convened to assist in evaluating information related to the potential problem. The MARC also recommends appropriate regulatory action if the problem is considered significant. AER information is released to the public by means of summary report publication on the CVM website. Additional requests for AER information can be made through the freedom-of-information officer.

AER submission is required only from companies marketing FDA-approved animal drugs. There are no requirements for submitting AERs for human drugs used in animals or unapproved products labeled for animals. The CVM has limited ability to monitor the performance of these drugs in animals.

Veterinarians are encouraged to report AEs directly to the manufacturer or sponsor. The manufacturer should record the information and send a report of their investigation to the CVM. Another reporting option is to call the CVM AE

hotline (1-888-FDA-VETS) to report AEs. An FDA veterinarian will return the telephone call. The reporter can also either call or write the CVM to obtain a postage-paid reporting form.

AE reporting to CVM has significantly increased over the last decade. Examples of recent AERs and FDA actions are listed in Box 5-4. During the early 1990s, the CVM received approximately 1000 AERs each year. The CVM received about 20,000 AE reports for the year 2000. Reasons for the increase are numerous and include the new types of drugs approved for use in companion animals, label information provided for contacting drug companies, and the interest of the public in reporting perceived product problems.

EPA ADVERSE EFFECTS INFORMATION REPORTING

The EPA OPP has regulatory responsibility for pesticides. Regulatory authority is derived from section 6(a)(2) of FIFRA. The regulations that specifically address reporting of adverse effects of pesticides are contained in 40 CFR §159 ("Reporting Requirements for Risk/Benefit Information"). Reporting of AEs is mandatory for industry.

The EPA collects information on pesticide use, whether exposure was intended or unintended. Adverse effects information may include information on human or animal injury, plant injury, or environmental contamination. All adverse effects information is accepted regardless of the registered label use of the product.

Specific industry reporting requirements for adverse effects information depend on the category of the information. Reports of human death should be submitted within 15 calendar days as an individual report. A variety of other information, including suspected product defects, human epidemiology and exposure studies, and pest resistance reports should be submitted within 30 calendar days as individual reports. Reports involving major and moderate human injury, major injury to plants and wildlife, water contamination, and public health product ineffectiveness should be submitted after a 1-month accumulation as individual reports.

Animal reports receive lower priority. Reports involving any type of domestic animal injury and some minor types of human, plant, and wildlife injury should be reported within 2 months, after a 3-month accumulation of reports. The information may be submitted in an aggregate format. An aggregate report for a specific time period includes a count of domestic injuries within categories of assessed seriousness. Information concerning the specific details of each individual AER is not included in an aggregate report. The EPA, however, may request additional information for any AERs that involved the death of an animal.

The OPP gathers AE information from other sources. Information and complaints may be submitted directly to the EPA. Information may also be obtained through the National Pesticide Communications Network based at

BOX 5-4	**REPORTED ADVERSE REACTIONS AND AGENCY/SPONSOR ACTION**
DRUG/SPECIES	**REGULATORY ACTION**
Quest/horse	Various label sections revised, drug delivery system redesigned
Acepromazine/dog	Adverse reaction revised to include aggression
Dichlorophene/toluene/dog	Serious adverse reactions added to label
Otomax/dog	Adverse reactions section revised to include possible deafness
Program/dog	Adverse reactions section revised
Vitamin E/selenium/cattle	Adverse reactions section revised to include cardiovascular collapse
Rimadyl and Etogesic/dog	Adverse reactions extensively revised, Dear Doctor Letter, Client Information Sheet
Baytril/cat	Dear Doctor Letter, dosage change, adverse reactions section revised to include blindness
Posilac/cattle	Adverse reactions section revised
Heartgard and Interceptor/dog	Adverse reactions section revised
Bovi-Cu/cattle	Product recall, approval withdrawn
Warbex/cattle	Contaminated lots recalled, United States Department of Agriculture coordinated program to withhold animals from slaughter for extended time

Oregon State University, the USP Practitioner's Reporting Network, the National APCC, and other sources. Much of this information may be entered into the EPA Incident Data System. Some aggregate reports may also be entered into the system.

Various product divisions within OPP review the AE information. A complete review of product-related information is performed for re-registration. A special review may be set in motion when the EPA has reason to believe that the use of a pesticide may result in unreasonable adverse effects, including acute toxicity to domestic animals. Subsequent regulatory actions may range from removal of the product from the market to changes in permitted uses.

Because the OPP regulates all pesticides, jurisdictional AE issues resulting from extralabel use are not a consideration. Furthermore, the mission of the OPP is to monitor the safety of pesticides in humans and animals regardless of the intended use. Evaluation of domestic animal AERs involving pesticides labeled for therapeutic use on animals is given the same attention as a pesticide labeled for use on plants. Intended use is more likely to affect what regulatory actions may be subsequently taken to improve the overall safety of product use.

USDA ANIMAL IMMUNOBIOLOGIC VIGILANCE PROGRAM

Regulation of animal immunobiologics is centralized within the APHIS CVB. Adverse events associated with vaccines may be particularly difficult to verify. Vaccines are generally used for the prevention of disease. The real or perceived failure of a vaccine to perform may be dependent on a number of factors and difficult to assess. Suspected vaccine failure in individuals is particularly difficult to assess. Furthermore, assessing AERs involving adverse events that are manifested some time after vaccine administration can be complicated. In addition to the "active ingredient," vaccines can include other ingredients, such as preservatives, stabilizers, and adjuvants that can affect product performance. Vaccinovigilance may require additional information from formal studies to verify suspected problems.

The USDA currently has no regulations that require the immunobiologic industry to routinely submit AERs to the CVB. Because the immunobiologic industry is not required to submit AERs, the CVB has limited ability to monitor AERs involving animal safety. The USDA may at times request companies to voluntarily submit AERs that are related to a particular safety issue. Although the USDA does not presently mandate specific AER record-keeping practices, the USDA does have the ability to conduct investigations at the immunobiologic manufacturing site.

The CVB may receive AERs from a variety of sources other than industry. The USDA publishes a toll-free number for reporting AEs directly to the CVB. The USDA received approximately 100 direct reports in 1999. The majority of

AERs come through the USP Practitioner's Reporting Network (PRN). In 1999, approximately 1000 AERs were submitted to the CVB by the USP.

Regulatory actions may result in the removal of the licensed product from the market. Other actions may include manufacturing changes or label revisions.

USP VETERINARY PRACTITIONER'S REPORTING PROGRAM

The USP is primarily involved with setting product standards for use by the drug industry. Other USP endeavors include developing authoritative drug information monographs using an evidence-based expert committee process and receiving reports of suspected adverse drug experiences in the clinical setting. In 1994, this latter program was expanded to specifically include AERs involving animal medicinals, the USP Veterinary Practitioner's Reporting Program (VPRN). USP VPRN provides a third-party reporting option for veterinarians and animal owners who do not wish to report AEs directly to either industry or the regulatory agency.

The primary goal of the USP VPRN is to facilitate reporting of AERs to the appropriate regulatory authority. It has provided valuable information to each of the federal regulatory agencies of animal medicinal products. For animal immunobiologics, the USP VPRN is the primary means by which the CVB is made aware of AEs. The USP VPRN is an important source of AERs to the FDA CVM for adverse effects in animals involving human drugs and unapproved animal drugs. For the EPA, the USP VPRN is an additional source of information.

ASPCA ANIMAL POISON CONTROL CENTER

The APCC is an operating division of the ASPCA. The APCC provides for-fee, 24-hour-a-day, 7-day-a-week telephone assistance in cases of animal poisoning. The goal of the APCC is to aid animals exposed to potentially hazardous substances by providing 24-hour veterinary diagnostic and treatment recommendations. The APCC also promotes animal health through toxicology educational programs and nontraditional research.

The APCC is not required to submit AERs to either the industry or to federal regulators. However, the APCC may enter into financial agreements to act as a company's agent in receiving reports of AEs and provides these AERs to the product manufacturer. In some circumstances, the APCC acts as an official part of the company's pharmacovigilance program, collecting and submitting AERs on behalf of the company to appropriate regulatory agencies. The APCC does not submit AERs directly to regulatory agencies outside of these contracts.

FUTURE DIRECTIONS OF ADVERSE EVENT REPORTING

Adverse event reporting requirements differ substantially from country to country. Missions, goals, resources, admin-

---

BOX 5-5	PHARMACOVIGILANCE AGENCY/ORGANIZATION CONTACT INFORMATION

AGENCY/ORGANIZATION (PHONE)	INTERNET ADDRESS
FDA/CVM (1-888-FDA-VETS	http://www.fda.gov/cvm/fda/TOCs/adetoc.html
USDA (1-800-752-6255)	http://www.aphis.usda.gov/vs/cvb/ic/aiv.htm
EPA (1-800-858-7378)	http://www.epa.gov/pesticides/fifra6a2.htm
USP (1-800-4-USPPRN)	http://www.usp.org/reporting/vprp.htm
ASPCA APCC (1-888-4ANI-HELP)	http://www.napcc.aspca.org/
VICH	http://vich.eudra.org/

istrative procedures, and AER sources vary considerably. The variations reflect the fundamental differences in the agencies and the laws they administer. The International Cooperation on Harmonization of Technical Requirements for Registration of Veterinary Medicinal Products (VICH) is a trilateral (Europe-Japan-United States) program aimed at harmonizing technical requirements for animal medicinal product registration. The VICH was officially launched in 1996. One of the goals of the VICH is the harmonization of pharmacovigilance reporting requirements, including standardized pharmacovigilance definitions, reporting time periods, data fields, reporting forms, electronic submission protocols, and medical nomenclature.

Successful efforts of VICH will lead to the timely transmission of AER information among all parties and organizations involved in animal pharmacovigilance. Electronic reporting standards would also be established to allow for reporters to submit their complaints electronically, directly to the appropriate reporting system. Worldwide AER information would also be readily available for examination and analysis by all interested parties.

Pharmacovigilance agency contact information is provided in Box 5-5.

REFERENCES

1. Food and Drug Administration Center for Veterinary Medicine, Rockville, Md: A historical perspective of CVM, 1999. *http://www.fda.gov/cvm/fda/mappgs/aboutcvm.html.*
2. Teske RH: In Adams RH, editor: *Veterinary pharmacology and therapeutics*, ed 7, Ames, Iowa, 1995, Iowa State University Press.
3. Food and Drug Administration Center for Veterinary Medicine, Rockville, Md: Specific subject index, 2000. *http://www.fda.gov/cvm/fda/mappgs/specificsubj.html.*
4. U.S. Environmental Protection Agency, Washington, DC: Programs, June 20, 2000. *http://www.epa.gov/epahome/programs.htm.*
5. U.S. Department of Agriculture: *Agricultural Fact Book 98,* Chapter 9, *http://www.usda.gov/news/pubs/fbook98/chart9.htm.*
6. Paige JC et al: In Tollefson L, editor: *Veterinary clinics of North America food animal practice,* Philadelphia, 1999, WB Saunders.
7. Code of Federal Regulations 21: Drug Enforcement Agency, Department. of Justice, Chapter II, parts1300-1316, April 1, 2000, Superintendent of Documents, Mail Stop SSOP, Washington, DC 20402-9328.
8. U.S. Drug Enforcement Agency: *List of scheduling actions and controlled substances,* July 1999, Office of Diversion Control, Drug and Chemical Evaluation Section, Washington, DC 20537.
9. U.S. Drug Enforcement Agency: *Drugs of abuse,* 1997, Superintendent of Documents, Mail Stop SSOP, Washington, DC 20402-9328.
10. U.S. Drug Enforcement Agency, Washington, DC: Schedules of controlled substances: placement of ketamine into Schedule III, 64FR(133): 37673-37675, July 13, 1999.
11. Occupational Safety and Health Administration, Washington, DC: OSHA 3143 *Informational booklet on industrial hygiene,* 1998. *http://www.osha-slc.gov/Publications/OSHA3143/OSHA3143.html.*
12. Occupational Safety and Health Administration, Washington, DC: *The Occupational Safety and Health Act of 1970 and amendments, http://www.oshaslc.gov/OshAct_toc/OshAct_toc_by_sect.html.*
13. National Oceanographic and Atmospheric Administration, Washington, DC: *Occupational exposure limits,* 1998. *http://www.noaa.gov.*
14. The American Conference of Governmental Industrial Hygienists, 2000 Threshold Limit Values (TLVs) for Chemical Substances and Physical Agents and Biological Exposure Indices. Cincinnati, Ohio. *http://www.acgih.org.*
15. Occupational Safety and Health Administration, Washington, DC: *Salt Lake Technical Center brochure, technical assistance,* 2000. *http://www.osha-slc.gov/dts/sltc/brochure/hyperlinks/technical assistance.html.*
16. National Institute for Occupational Safety and Health, Cincinnati, Ohio: *1997 NIOSH pocket guide to chemical hazards. http://www.cdc.gov/niosh/npg/npg.html.*
17. Food and Drug Administration Center for Veterinary Medicine, Rockville, Md: *Target animal safety guidelines for new animal drugs,* 1989. *http://www.fda.gov/cvm/fda/TOCs/guideline33.html.*
18. U.S. Environmental Protection Agency, Washington, DC: *Health effects test guidelines, OPPTS 870.7200, companion animal safety, prevention, pesticides and toxic substances,* August 5, 1998. *http://www.epa.gov/OPPTS Harmonized/870 Health Effects Test Guidelines.*
19. Food and Drug Administration Center for Veterinary Medicine, Rockville, Md: *General principles for evaluating the safety of compounds used in food-producing animals guidelines,* 1994. *http://www.fda.gov/cvm/fda/TOCs/guideline3toc.html.*
20. Gaylor DW, Kodell RL: Linear interpolation algorithm for low dose risk assessment of toxic substances, *J Environ Pathol Toxicol* 4:305, 1980.
21. Farmer JH et al: Estimation and extrapolation of tumor probabilities from a mouse bioassay with survival/sacrifice components, *Risk Analysis* 2:27, 1982.
22. U.S. Environmental Protection Agency: *Subpart E-Specific organ/tissue toxicity: reproduction and fertility effects, 40CFR 798.4700,* Washington, DC, 2000, U.S. Government Printing Office.

23. U.S. Environmental Protection Agency, Washington, DC: Reproductive toxicity risk assessment guidelines, *Fed Reg* 61 FR 56274, 1996.

24. Weingand K et al: Harmonization of animal clinical pathology testing in toxicity and safety studies. *Fund Appl Toxicol* 29:198, 1996.

25. Friedlander LG et al: In Tollefson L, editor: *Veterinary clinics of North America food animal practice*, Philadelphia, March 1999, WB Saunders.

26. U.S. Department of Agriculture, Washington, DC: *APHIS animal care program publications*, June 2000. *http://www.aphis.usda.gov/ac/publications.html.*

27. AAALAC International, Rockville, Md: *About AAALAC. http://www.aaalac.org.*

PART TWO

MANIFESTATIONS OF TOXICOSES

Cardiovascular System

6

DIFFERENTIAL DIAGNOSIS

Konnie H. Plumlee

Most cardiovascular toxicoses are caused by accidental ingestion of pharmaceutical agents; however, several plants also can cause cardiovascular disease as well. Most plant toxicoses occur in herbivores that inadvertently ingest toxic plants.

Regardless of the etiology, most patients with cardiovascular disease have similar clinical signs; therefore, determining the etiology often depends on finding the source of the poison. Postmortem lesions can assist in narrowing the list of possible poisons. Animals that die acutely after plant ingestion may have identifiable pieces of plant material in the stomach or rumen.

Table 6-1 lists poisons that have direct effects on the cardiovascular system.

TOXIC RESPONSE OF THE CARDIOVASCULAR SYSTEM

Diann L. Weddle and Sherry J. Morgan

SUSCEPTIBILITY

Structure and function, and their relationship to each other, play a vital role in determining the susceptibility of an organ to toxicants and its response to tissue damage. These factors, in turn, influence the findings that the clinician or pathologist observes.

The cardiovascular system is composed of the heart and the vascular network. The heart is a four-chambered pump, whose chambers are composed of a dense array of muscle fibers separated by valves and activity governed by appropriate innervation and an elaborate conduction system. The combined, organized efforts of these features drive the circulatory system in the distribution of life-giving nutrients and oxygen. The right side of the heart receives blood that is spent of its oxygen and some nutrients. This blood also carries potential waste products and metabolites such as carbon dioxide. The blood continues on to the pulmonary system where exchange of the carbon dioxide and oxygen occurs. This reoxygenated blood enters the left side, which then supplies the systemic circulation and the cardiovascular system itself.

Heart

Anatomic considerations. The heart is composed of the epicardium, myocardium, and endocardium. The epicardium is the visceral layer of the serous pericardial sac, whereas the subpericardial region is composed of connective tissue, adipose, vessels, lymphatics, and nerves. The endocardium is the inner lining layer with the subendothelial region also composed of connective tissue, vessels, nerves, and Purkinje fibers. The muscular wall or myocardium is the workhorse of the heart. It is the region composed of elongated myocytes joined together by intercellular junctions and embedded in a connective tissue matrix along with a network of blood vessels and capillaries. Ultrastructurally, myocytes have a limiting membrane known as the *sarcolemma*, which is composed of the plasma membrane and the external lamina. These muscle cells have one to two oblong, centrally located nuclei. Highly ordered arrays of contractile elements known as *myofibrils* surround the nuclei. These contractile elements occupy 50% of the cytoplasm. The remaining cytoplasm is filled by mitochondria, sarcoplasmic reticulum, T-tubules, rough endoplasmic reticulum, moderate amounts of glycogen, lysosomes, and phagosomes. As evidence of the heart's need for large amounts of energy, mitochondria constitute 35% of the cell volume.[1]

Myocytes communicate with the environment via a network of tubular invaginations of the sarcolemma known as the *T-system*. The T-system serves in the exchanging of ions with the interstitium, the coupling of excitation-contraction in the ventricles, and the facilitating of the spread of electrical events. Intercellular junctions that connect neighboring myocytes end to end (intercalated discs) and side to side (lateral junctions) mediate intercellular adhesions and transmission of electrical impulse. In general, atrial and ventricular myocytes are very similar. However,

TABLE 6-1   **Toxicants that Cause Cardiovascular Disease**

Plants	Species	Mechanism
Avocado	Rabbits, goats, caged birds, ostriches, horses	Cardiomyopathy with edema of the head, neck, brisket; acute pulmonary edema
Calcinogenic glycosides	Livestock	Soft tissue mineralization
Cardiac glycosides	All	Inhibit Na^+/K^+ ATPase
Gossypol	Swine, preruminal ruminants	Myocardial necrosis; conduction abnormalities
Grayanotoxins	All	Stabilize sodium channels
Taxine alkaloids	All	Inhibit ion channels
Tremetone	Cardiovascular signs most common in horses	Cardiomyopathy
Tropane alkaloids	All	Parasympathetic effects on heart
Pharmaceuticals	**Species**	**Mechanism**
Antibiotic antineoplastics	Pets most commonly exposed	Cardiomyopathy
Bronchodilators	Pets most commonly exposed	Beta receptor agonist
Calcium channel blocking agents	Pets most commonly exposed	Conduction blockade
Cardiac glycosides	Pets most commonly exposed	Inhibit Na^+/K^+ ATPase
Ionophores	Any species; horses most susceptible	Increase ion transport across membranes
Methylxanthines	Pets most commonly exposed	Antagonism of adenosine receptors
Tilmicosin	Livestock most commonly exposed	Negative inotropic actions
Tricyclic antidepressants	Pets most commonly exposed	Inhibition of myocardial sodium channels
Miscellaneous	**Species**	**Mechanism**
Bufo toads	Dogs most commonly exposed	Inhibit Na^+/K^+ ATPase
Fireflies	Frogs and lizards	Inhibit Na^+/K^+ ATPase
Sodium fluoroacetate	All	Myocardial necrosis; interferes with tricarboxylic acid cycle
Cholecalciferol rodenticide	All	Soft tissue mineralization

atrial myocytes are arranged in a less regular pattern than myocytes of the ventricles. In addition, atrial myocytes contain cytoplasmic granules composed of regulatory hormones (atrial natriuretic peptides) that promote natriuresis and diuresis in response to elevated vascular volume.

Myocardial contraction is controlled by the conduction system, which is composed of the sinoatrial node, internodal pathways, atrioventricular node, bundle of His, left and right bundle branches, and the Purkinje fibers (cardiac conducting fibers). These components of the conduction system represent modified cardiac myocytes with the inherent property of automaticity.

Susceptibility of the heart. With respect to the heart, several features must be kept in mind: (1) its level of energy and nutrients needed, (2) its level of exposure to toxicants, (3) its relatively limited protective metabolic systems, and (4) its limited ability to handle structural loss.

First, in order for the heart to adequately perform, the myocardium is dependent on a steady supply of nutrients (oxygen, energy substrates, adenosine triphosphate [ATP], calcium, and other electrolytes), properly functioning organelles (mitochondria), contractile elements, and conduction system. Energy is generated almost exclusively via the oxidation of substrates, necessitating adequate blood flow for the delivery of oxygen and substrates and a large number of mitochondria within individual myocytes. To provide for this energy need, the heart esentially feeds itself first via coronary arteries that exit the aorta just distal to the aortic valve and then branch into small vessels and an extensive microcirculatory network. Although myocytes compose approximately 90% of the volume of the myocardium, they are only responsible for 25% of the total number of cells. The remaining 75% are the endothelial cells, predominantly those of the aforementioned capillary network, and connective tissue cells.[2] Oxygen and energy substrates (e.g., glucose, lactate, fatty acids) allow mitochondria to produce ATP via the tricarboxylic acid cycle and oxidative phosphorylation. Appropriate electrolyte levels, including calcium, must be present to maintain resting potential and allow depolarization and repolarization for action potentials to occur. This influx of sodium and calcium also results in the depolarization of the sarcoplasmic reticulum and release of intracellular stores of calcium. ATP and calcium allow proper interaction of myosin and actin filaments for contraction. Cytosolic calcium binds regulatory proteins, tropomyosin, and troponin in the thin actin filament. Myosin ATPase is activated and hydrolyzes ATP for energy to form the cross-bridges between actin and myosin, resulting in contraction.

Second, for practical purposes, the heart receives all of the systemic circulation. This results in the heart being exposed to a toxicant and its metabolites at potentially high concentrations for a potentially protracted period of time. In addition, unlike some organ systems, the exposure potential of the heart is far less likely to be influenced by route of administration.

Third, oxygen radical species are produced in cells as a consequence of general metabolism and can also be formed in the metabolism of a toxicant or via the agent's toxic mechanism. In fact, oxygen radical species play an important role in the mechanism of many toxic agents. Oxygen radicals, via a process termed *oxidative stress*, can damage cellular and organellar membranes and lead to lipid peroxidation with resultant impaired membrane integrity, dysfunction of mitochondria and sarcoplasmic reticulum, and then altered calcium homeostasis. Cells have protective mechanisms for the removal of these radical species including catalases and glutathione peroxidases. However, these systems are limited in the myocardium, making the myocardium potentially vulnerable to oxidative stress.[3]

Fourth, cardiac muscle, except in neonates, does not have the ability to regenerate as does skeletal muscle. Lost myocytes are replaced by fibrosis, and remaining myocytes enlarge to compensate for this loss.

Vascular system

Anatomic considerations. The heart's ventures are accomplished in concert with the vascular system, a network of arteries, veins, capillaries, and lymphatics. These structures are essentially tubes lined by endothelium with various mural patterns that accommodate potentially changing volume and pressure relationships. The vascular wall is organized into the tunica intima, tunica media, and tunica adventitia. The tunica intima is subdivided into the endothelium and a subendothelial region composed of connective tissue, fibroblasts, and the internal elastic membrane, which separates the intima from the media. The tunica adventitia is the outer region and is composed of the external elastic membrane and fibroelastic connective tissue. The innermost region of the wall is the media and is the most variable region of vascular anatomy. This region is minimal to nonexistent in veins and lymphatics. The region varies in thickness and composition in the arterial branch of the vascular system, depending on size. In large arteries (aorta, common carotid), the region is dense and is composed of smooth muscle and elastic fibers. There is a decrease in the amount of elastic fibers, with smooth muscle taking more prominence as the arteries become smaller and terminate toward the capillary beds. The capillaries of the microcirculation are tiny tubes in which the endothelium may be arranged in a continuous, discontinuous, or fenestrated pattern. These patterns are designed to facilitate the exchange of gases, ions, fluids, and metabolic products at the cellular level.

For the cardiovascular system to perform properly, the heart must continually pump in a regular, organized manner while the vascular system remains patent and adjusts to changing pressures.

Susceptibility of the vascular system. Key features influence the susceptibility of the vascular system: (1) its level of distribution and heterogeneity within an organism, (2) its level of exposure to toxicants, (3) its level of metabolism of toxicants.

First, the vascular system extends throughout an organism and intimately associates with all other organ systems. Toxicants that affect the vascular system can potentially have widespread effects.

Second, like the heart, the vasculature is exposed to most toxicants that gain access to the systemic circulation. It must be a dynamic system and able to react, potentially acutely, to changing needs. The vascular system is heterogeneous with respect to anatomy and function. Susceptibility to a toxicant can be influenced by whether the location is a vein, an artery, or the capillaries. In addition, increasing evidence shows that vessels vary in pharmacologic and toxicologic responses.[1] This variation is not only present between veins and arteries but also between different circulatory regions. Toxicants may preferentially affect vessels of a given organ or tissue and be classified and discussed with respect to that organ or tissue. Another important factor with respect to the level of exposure of a vascular system to a given toxicant is understanding the influence of blood composition on this relationship. Binding of poisons by plasma proteins may limit exposure.[3] Alternatively, changes in plasma protein concentrations can increase exposure to a poison.

Third, the influence of metabolism on the level of exposure is an important feature of vascular system susceptibility. Metabolic inactivation of toxins is one common process for the vascular system to limit its exposure; however, alterations in this capacity can render the system susceptible.

MECHANISMS OF ACTION

Mechanisms of toxicosis may be described as direct or indirect. Direct-acting mechanisms are those that have a primary effect on the physiologic and functional or biochemical properties of the vascular system. Indirect mechanisms are those that arise from an exaggerated pharmacologic effect of an agent on the vascular system or to the vascular system being secondarily affected as a result of toxicosis to another system.

Mechanisms in the heart

With respect to the heart, direct mechanisms can be loosely divided into those that relate to alterations in the physiologic aspects of cardiac function, biochemical properties, or cell structure; however, many of the specific pathologic processes overlap among these general categories. Generally, no one single physiologic or biochemical process can account for the mechanism by which an agent is toxic toward a given system.

Alteration of conduction. Coordinated and sustained action of the heart is initiated and controlled by specialized cells of the sinoatrial node and the conducting tissue. Slow response fibers are located in the sinoatrial and atrioventricular nodes. Fast response fibers are present in the remaining portions of the conduction system and in the atria and ventricles. Toxicants that alter sensitive ion gradients and fluxes involved in the initiation or propagation of cardiac impulse can produce arrhythmias. Alterations of these gradients and fluxes can occur by a number of mechanisms, often in concert together: inhibition of the function of sodium or calcium channels, alteration in the level of ions available, and perturbation of cell and organellar membranes by oxidative stress. Erythromycin can cause cardiac dysrhythmias by blockade of fast sodium channels. Amphotericin B has been proposed to cause cardiodepression by decreasing activation of slow calcium channels and inhibition of sodium influx.[4]

The presence of reactive oxygen species can result in lipid peroxidation in the sarcolemma and organellar membranes. This oxidative stress can lead to increased membrane permeability, fluidity, and loss of membrane integrity. Oxygen radicals can result in disrupted ion gradients by altering Na^+/K^+ ATPase or calcium homeostasis or by modifying Na^+/Ca^{++} exchange and Ca^{++} transport of the sarcoplasmic reticulum. The antineoplastic anthracycline drug doxorubicin has been associated with electrocardiographic abnormalities and cardiomyopathy.[4] Among the many proposed mechanisms of its toxicity is the generation of oxygen radicals resulting from its quinone-like structure and subsequent redox cycling.[5] Superoxide generation has been proposed to occur between complexes I and III of the respiratory chain in the inner mitochondrial membrane.

Alteration of contractile ability. Alterations in contractile elements (myofibrils), disruption in the inactivation of myosin and actin, inhibition of myosin ATPase, or disturbances in calcium levels can result in limited or increased contractility. In addition to producing other effects, cobra venom is proposed to disrupt myofibrils via alteration of calcium homeostasis.[1] Endotoxin can depress contractility through altered calcium homeostasis, and halothane has been suggested to modify responsiveness of contractile regulatory proteins by calcium.[4,6] Disturbances in ATP synthesis via inhibition of oxidative phosphorylation can result in alteration of contractile ability. Hydrolysis of ATP is needed for cross-bridge formation between actin and myosin for contraction.

Alteration of metabolism. The heart is dependent on chemical energy, stored in the form of ATP, for continual contraction. Energy sources (glucose, lactate, triglycerides, fatty acids) are converted to substrates that enter the tricarboxylic acid cycle. Electron sources generated via this cycle are then used in oxidative phosphorylation to generate ATP. In this process, electrons are transferred within the respiratory assembly to molecular oxygen. This process generates energy, which is then used to make ATP. Toxicants can either influence formation or use of ATP. Toxicants that disturb ATP formation may do so via inhibition of a given step of the respiratory assembly or disruption of mitochondrial ultrastructure. As examples, antimycin A inhibits electron transport between coenzyme Q and cytochrome c, whereas cyanide inhibits electron transfer from cytochrome oxidase to oxygen.[4] Oxidative stress can influence either formation of ATP via disruption of mitochondria or utilization by disruption of important ATPases such as Na^+/K^+ ATPase or Ca^{++} ATPase. Disturbances of the Ca^+ ATPase, which is responsible for transport of Ca^{++} by the sarcoplasmic reticulum, can alter Ca^{++} homeostasis. Calcium overload can impair mitochondrial energy production and activate phospholipases and neutral proteases whose degradative properties can inhibit membrane-bound Na^+/K^+ ATPase. Proposed mechanisms of the toxic effects of catecholamines have included both oxidative stress and calcium overload.[4]

Alteration in ultrastructure. The ultrastructure of a cell can be defined as the sublight microscopic anatomy. These structures include, among others, the membranes, the various organelles, and the nucleus. With regard to cardiotoxicity, several organelles should be kept in mind: myofibrils, sarcoplasmic reticulum, and mitochondria. Myofibrils contract the heart. Sarcoplasmic reticulum releases and stores calcium and is important in calcium homeostasis. Mitochondria take substrates and generate ATP, in addition to acting as a long-term calcium buffer against potential calcium overload.[7]

Indirect mechanisms. Drug-induced toxicity associated with exaggerated pharmacologic effects has been well documented, especially that of catecholamines. In addition, toxicants that produce effects in other organ systems or concurrent disease in other systems can induce negative outcomes in the heart. Hemodynamic alterations associated with hypovolemia secondary to systemic vasodilation can induce reflex tachycardia and myocardial damage. Acid-base disturbances associated with renal disease can impair conduction and contractility of the heart.

Mechanisms in the vascular system

Three general categories are discussed: alterations in metabolism, alterations in structure, and immunologic mechanisms.

Alteration in metabolism. Two of the most important cell types to consider in vascular toxicosis are the endothelium and smooth muscle cells. Both are metabolically active. These cells can metabolically inactivate poisons. However, the opposite is also true. Several systems present in these cells can be responsible for the bioactivation of poisons: amine oxidases, cytochrome P-450 monoamine oxidases, and prostaglandin synthetase. In addition, deficiencies can be present in the capacity of a target cell to detoxify an agent or manage oxidative stress. Oxygen radicals can arise during the metabolism of an agent and be generated secondary to reperfusion injury and inflammatory mediators. These oxygen radicals can injure endothelial cells, alter permeability, and alter responsiveness of vasoactive substances.

Alteration in structure and function. Toxicants can cause structural alterations in components of vessels. Hypertonic solutions such as those containing sodium chloride, urea, or mannitol can alter normal metabolism and cause shrinkage of endothelial cells and an increase in permeability of the endothelium. Agents such as endotoxin that damage or injure endothelial cells can result in thrombosis via activation of the thrombolytic pathway. Alteration in vascular tone is an important mechanism of some toxicants. These substances can produce systemic or local vasodilation or vasoconstriction, which can then lead to profound hemodynamic changes and indirect effects in other organ systems. For an example, ergotamine results in prolonged vasoconstriction in peripheral arteries and ischemic necrosis of tissue serviced by those arteries.

Immunologic mechanisms. Biosynthetic peptides and proteins will become increasingly important as therapeutic agents. Sensitization to proteins or haptens can induce a type III hypersensitivity vasculitis secondary to deposition of soluble immune complexes within the vessel wall and the activation of the complement cascade. This mechanism has been proposed for treatment complications with penicillin and sulphonamides in humans.[1,3]

Indirect mechanisms. Endothelial permeability can be influenced by hydrostatic and oncotic pressures and by molecular concentration gradients. Alterations in plasma protein levels can influence not only the oncotic pressure but also the exposure level of the vascular system to toxicants via decreased binding. Agents that result in alterations in the number of platelets or homeostasis of clotting factors can influence hemodynamics.

RESPONSE TO TOXIC INJURY

Responses in the heart

Conduction disturbances. Disturbances of impulse initiation and conduction or excitation and contraction can result in arrhythmias and heart block. Arrhythmias are among the most serious and life-threatening complications of cardiac toxicosis. Alterations in ionic events, signaling through adrenergic receptors, and decreases in energy supply or utilization can result in changes in contractility. Numerous plant species contain cardiac glycosides that can increase force of contraction by inhibiting Na^+/K^+ ATPase, which is responsible for maintaining transmembrane ion concentration and membrane potential of myofibers.[8] Monensin in horses and pigs (simple-stomached animals) increases force of contraction by increasing Na^+ influx by creating artificial sodium channels in the sarcolemma.[1]

Degenerative changes. Given the continual activity of the heart, there is a great liability for the myocardium to undergo degenerative changes. Several forms of degenerative changes are recognized: myocytolysis, hydropic degeneration, fatty change, and lipofuscinosis. Myocytolysis is associated with sublethal injury of myocytes. Affected cells, histologically, have loss of striations, with hyalinized cytoplasm. An example of this lesion is seen in furazolidone toxicosis in birds. Hydropic degeneration has indistinct vacuolization associated with initial distention of elements of the sarcoplasmic reticulum and can lead to eventual lysis of contractile material. Grossly, these lesions can appear dull gray. A more serious change than hydropic degeneration is that of fatty change. Histologically, myocytes have accumulation of lipid vacuoles within the sarcoplasm, and patchy, pale yellow foci within the myocardium may be present. Atrophy is another form of degeneration that may be present in aged or cachectic animals. In some cases, it may be accompanied by a brown pigment termed *lipofuscinosis*. Histologically, this pigment is represented by granules that are intralysosomal accumulations of membranous and amorphous debris. This pigment has been reported in Ayrshire cattle as a hereditary condition.[1]

Necrosis. Degenerative changes can lead to necrosis, or cell death. Necrosis can be caused by direct injury of a cell or by ischemia. Although agents that cause arrhythmias and altered contractile ability may not produce a gross or histologic lesion, cellular damage associated with depleted energy reserves and altered ionic states can result and produce necrosis if the animal survives long enough. Toxicants known to produce myocardial necrosis in animals include gossypol in pigs and young ruminants, thallium in dogs, saccharated iron in pigs, and fluoroacetate in dogs and ruminants.[8] Grossly, necrosis appears as multifocal or patchy, pale tan foci.

Two types of necrosis are recognized in myocardium: coagulation and contraction band necrosis. Ischemia greater than 20 minutes in duration can lead to irreversible damage and necrosis. The more central regions of the focus exhibit coagulation necrosis, whereas the periphery exhibits contraction band necrosis. Contraction band necrosis is characterized by hypercontraction of myofibrils and is generally associated with the entry of large amounts of calcium ions secondary to partial reperfusion of peripheral zones. Contraction band necrosis can be a common result of toxicosis secondary to catecholamines and vasodilatory antihypertensive therapeutic agents.

Consequences of necrosis can include interstitial edema, inflammation, and dystrophic mineralization. An example of dystrophic mineralization is organomercurial poisoning in cattle resulting in necrosis of Purkinje fibers with deposition of calcium salts. Myocardial cells do not regenerate; therefore, resolving necrotic foci are replaced by fibroblasts and may be grossly evident as a white band or scar. In addition, remaining myocytes may enlarge (hypertrophy) to compensate for the loss of neighbors.

Cardiomyopathies. Two forms of cardiomyopathy are recognized: hypertrophic and dilatory. With respect to toxicants in animals, the hypertrophic form of cardiomyopathy has more relevance for discussion. Agents that alter hemodynamics, inducing hypertension and increased workload, can lead to an enlargement of the heart over time. Grossly, these hearts have an increase in weight and a thickness of the muscular wall.

Neoplastic changes. Tumors of endocardial origin are described infrequently in laboratory rodent species that have been experimentally exposed to chemicals such as carbamates and nitrosamines. Two forms of tumors have been described: schwannomas arising from endocardial mesenchymal cells and hemangiosarcomas in the microvasculature of the pericardium or myocardium.[1] We are not aware of toxin-induced tumors arising in animals under nonexperimental situations.

Responses in the vascular system

As in the heart, some of the more important outcomes of toxic exposure can result in no apparent lesion within the vascular system. Examples of such conditions include altered hemodynamics (systemic vasodilation or constriction) or increased permeability (interstitial edema). Responses of the vascular system may be acute (necrosis) or chronic (medial proliferation). In addition, a response may be more common in a given type of vessel or within a given tissue organ or region of the circulatory system.

Necrosis. Necrosis and hemorrhage of the medial smooth muscle in arteries has been associated with the administration of vasodilatory agents. Another potential response in arteries or veins is necrosis of the wall with accumulation of serum proteins and fibrin termed *fibrinoid necrosis*. Histologically, the walls of these vessels have complete loss of architecture and the individual vessel in cross section appears as an amorphous, eosinophilic focus.

Intimal and medial proliferation. Vascular responses can be chronic in nature, such as with intimal or medial proliferation. Both of these changes occur in arteries. Intimal proliferation is associated with the induced proliferation of fibroblasts and smooth muscle cells within the subendothelial region. Medial proliferation occurs in arteries and arterioles and is characterized by proliferation of smooth muscle cells within the tunica media. This change is associated with sustained hypertension. Pyrrolizidine alkaloids and ergot alkaloids are toxins that can produce this response.[1,8]

Capillary injury. Ergot alkaloids can also cause peripheral vasoconstriction, leading to capillary endothelial damage with thrombosis and subsequent ischemic necrosis of extremities, particularly the hind limbs of grazing cattle.

Mineralization. In vessels, dystrophic mineralization can occur within arteries with hemorrhage, degeneration, or necrosis. Metastatic mineralization is a well-known sequela to toxins that produce hypercalcemia or hyperphosphatemia. This condition results in calcium and phosphorus deposition adjacent to elastic fibers within the vascular wall. In smaller vessels, a concentric ring of mineralization may be produced. Examples of toxicants that result in hypercalcemia are agents containing 1,25-dihydroxycholecalciferol (vitamin D): plants, including *Cestrum diurnum* and *Solanum malacoxylon;* excess supplementation in rations; and cholecalciferol rodenticides. Whether the condition is dystrophic or metastatic, affected vessels may be rigid and hard grossly. This is particularly true for metastatic mineralization. Histologically, with dystrophic mineralization, the mineral is deposited in the wall in association with necrosis and hemorrhage. If metastatic in origin, the mineral is deposited in the wall among the elastic fibers, and osseous metaplasia is possible in large arteries.

Neoplastic. Hemangiosarcomas have been reported to occur as a consequence of toxicants. As in the heart, these are primarily in experimental situations.

GROSS LESIONS

Gross lesions in the heart, as in other tissues, are characterized by alterations in consistency, size, shape, or color. Alterations in consistency may be the result of fatty infiltration, edema, excessive flaccidity, or firmness. The latter two characteristics may indicate a change in size and shape. Ventricular wall widths can be measured; the heart itself can be weighed. These measurements vary by species and can be compared with normal reference ranges. Reference values for heart weights and ventricular ratios for various species have been determined.[8] With respect to color, hemorrhage appears red to brown depending on chronicity; necrosis appears pale tan; fibrous tissue appears white; mineralization appears white and chalky. In the vascular system, this is also true; however, because of the relative size of the tissue, some gross lesions may be difficult to discern. In the vascular system, it may be more important to be aware of the potentially larger, more readily discernible secondary lesions associated with vascular insult (e.g., gangrenous necrosis with ergot alkaloids). The absence of gross lesions can be important for the diagnosis.

Few if any poisons exhibit gross lesions that would be considered pathognomonic. For example, metastatic mineralization is characteristic for vitamin D poisoning; however, renal disease can produce a similar lesion. Some lesions such as neoplasms rarely occur in association with toxicants under natural conditions.

HISTOPATHOLOGY

As with gross lesions, few if any toxicants exhibit histologic lesions that are considered pathognomonic. The heart and vascular systems have only a limited number of morphologic responses to any form of insult. The absence of histologic lesions can be important. Knowledge of the site or sites of predilection of a given poison is invaluable in interpreting histologic findings. An accurate history including signalment, clinical signs, and treatment are imperative.

REFERENCES

1. Haschek WM, Rousseaux CG: *Fundamentals of toxicologic pathology*, San Diego, 1998, Academic Press.
2. Schoen FJ: In Cotran RS et al: *Robbins pathologic basis of disease*, ed 6, Philadelphia, 1999, WB Saunders.
3. Isaacs KR: In Turton J, Hooson J, editors: *Toxic organ pathology: a basic text*, Bristol, Pa, 1998, Taylor & Francis.
4. Ramos KS et al: In Klaassen CD, editor: *Casarett and Doull's toxicology: the basic science of poisons*, ed 5, New York, 1996, McGraw-Hill.
5. Powis G: Free radical formation by antitumor quinines. *Free Radic Biol Med* 6:63, 1989.
6. Bosnjak ZJ: In Blanck TJ, Wheeler DM, editors: *Mechanisms of anesthetic action in skeletal, cardiac, and smooth muscle*, New York, 1991, Plenum Press.
7. Baskin SI, Behonick GS: In Ballantyne B, Marrs TC, Syversen T, editors: *General and applied toxicology*, vol 2, ed 2, New York, 1999, Grove's Dictionaries.
8. Robinson WF, Maxie MG: In Jubb KVF, Kennedy PC, Palmer N, editors: *Pathology of domestic animals*, vol 3, ed 4, San Diego, 1993, Academic Press.

7

Dermal System

DIFFERENTIAL DIAGNOSIS

Konnie H. Plumlee

The extent of effects on the dermal system by poisons ranges from hair discoloration to sloughing of skin. Most of the toxic effects are a result of either primary or secondary photosensitization.

Photosensitizing agents enable long-wave ultraviolet and visible radiation to interact with biological molecules in the skin. Primary photosensitization occurs when a photosensitizing agent enters the body by an oral, topical, or parenteral route and directly causes the skin to become more sensitive to light. Secondary, or hepatogenous, photosensitization is more common. It occurs when hepatobiliary damage prevents the body from removing phylloerythrin, a metabolite of dietary chlorophyll. Normally phylloerythrin is cleared by the liver and excreted in the bile so that it does not accumulate in the systemic circulation. Phylloerythrin acts as the photosensitizing agent in all cases of secondary photosensitization.

Regardless of the type of photosensitizing agent, clinical signs are basically the same. Pigmented skin is typically unaffected, whereas areas of light-colored skin and hairless skin (e.g., the nose, udder, tongue, eyelids, and vulva) become damaged. Affected skin initially is red and edematous and then follows a progression of exudation, crust formation, hardening, cracking, and sloughing. Animals are photophobic and seek shade. Pruritus can become severe and induce self-inflicted trauma. Lacrimation, conjunctivitis, and keratitis can occur, possibly followed by scar formation of the cornea. Tongue lesions in cattle are typically confined to the tip of the tongue and the underside of the tongue, which become exposed to sunlight during prehension of food.

Table 7-1 lists the poisons that have direct effects on the dermal system.

TABLE 7-1 Toxicants that Affect the Dermal System

Effect	Species	Toxicant	Comment
Dry gangrene	Livestock, especially cattle	Ergot Fescue	Sloughing of skin, tail, ears, and hooves caused by vasoconstriction
Hyperkeratosis	Cattle	Chlorinated naphthalene	Decreased serum vitamin A precedes onset of lacrimation, salivation, and weight loss
		Iodine (EDDI)	Chronic exposure also causes exfoliative dermatosis and alopecia
Granulomatous dermatopathy	Cattle, horses	Vicia villosa	Accompanied by systemic granulomatous lesions
Epithelial necrosis	Any	Trichothecenes Stachybotrys	Radiomimetic lesions, especially around the mouth
Contact dermatitis	Any	Turpentine Mineral spirits Essential oils Phenols Pine oils Acids Alkalies	Severity ranges from mild dermatitis to skin sloughing, depending on the volume and concentration of the agent

Continued

TABLE 7-1 **Toxicants that Affect the Dermal System—cont'd**

Effect	Species	Toxicant	Comment
Hair changes	Cattle primarily	Molybdenum	Lightening of hair from copper deficiency
	Cattle, swine, horses	Selenium	Lightening of hair color; alopecia, especially of the mane and tail
Hoof deformities	Cattle, horses, swine	Selenium	Separation of hoof at coronary band; horizontal hoof cracks
Primary photosensitization	Livestock	Furanocoumarins Phenothiazine Sulfonamide antibiotics Tetracycline antibiotics	
Secondary photosensitization	Livestock	Red clover, alsike clover Quinones Steroidal saponins Tetradymia, *Artemisia* sp. Sporidesmin Forage-induced photosensitization *Microcystis* spp. Phomopsins	Concurrent hepatobiliary disease

8

Endocrine System

DIFFERENTIAL DIAGNOSIS

Konnie H. Plumlee

Very few poisons have direct effects on hormones. Table 8-1 lists the poisons and the hormones that they affect.

TABLE 8-1 **Toxicants that Affect the Endocrine System**

Hormone	Toxicant	Species	Clinical Findings
Thyroid hormones (decreased)	Iodine Glucosinolates	Livestock	Goiter
Prolactin (decreased)	Ergot Fescue	Livestock	Agalactia
Estrogen (increased)	Phytoestrogens	Ruminants	Infertility, irregular estrus, follicular cysts, dystocia
	Zearalenone	Prepubertal gilts	Hyperestrogenism
		Nonpregnant sows	Anestrus, pseudopregnancy
		Pregnant sows	Embryonic death
		Cows	Infertility

Gastrointestinal System

9

DIFFERENTIAL DIAGNOSIS

Konnie H. Plumlee

Determining the etiology of gastrointestinal (GI) disease can be difficult. Several factors can contribute to the challenge of making a diagnosis.

A wide array of poisons, bacteria, viruses, and parasites affect the GI tract. Even nutritional deficiencies and stress can result in GI signs.

Animals can exhibit GI signs secondary to other diseases. Liver disease, kidney disease, and neurologic disease can result in nonspecific signs such as vomiting and diarrhea.

Clinical signs of the gastrointestinal tract are limited. Anorexia and diarrhea are common signs in all species. Vomiting frequently develops in dogs and cats. Ruminants and birds can regurgitate their ingesta. Colic is a frequent manifestation of GI disease in horses. Toxicants that irritate the upper alimentary tract can cause excess salivation, gagging, and coughing.

Box 9-1 lists the poisons that directly affect the GI system. The plants, except for the insoluble calcium oxalates, cause varying degrees of gastroenteritis. The pharmaceutical agents, mycotoxins, and metals also cause gastroenteritis. The insoluble calcium oxalates and many of the household agents affect the upper alimentary tract, resulting in lesions that vary from mild mouth irritation to esophageal perforation, depending on the type of agent and its concentration.

BOX 9-1	TOXICANTS THAT HAVE PRIMARY EFFECTS ON THE GASTROINTESTINAL SYSTEM

PLANTS	HOUSEHOLD AND INDUSTRIAL
Chinaberry	Acids and alkalies
Colchicine	Batteries
Cycad (sago) palms	Bleaches
Diterpene esters	Boric acid
Escin saponins	Detergents
Glucosinolates	Dipyridyl herbicides
Grayanotoxins	Essential oils
Insoluble calcium oxalates	Fertilizers
Lectins	Naphthalene
Ligustrum spp.	Petroleum products
Lycorine	Phenols
Mayapple	Pine oil
Oak	Turpentine
Phoradendron	
Protoanemonin	
Sesquiterpene lactones	
Titerpenoid saponins	

PHARMACEUTICALS	METALS
5-fluorouracil	Arsenic
Lincomycin	Iron
Methotrexate	Lead
Methylxanthines	Mercurial salts
Nonsteroidal antiinflammatory drugs	Molybdenum
	Zinc

MYCOTOXINS	MISCELLANEOUS
Patulin	Blister beetles
Stachybotrys	Variety of mushrooms
Trichothecenes	

10

Hematic System

DIFFERENTIAL DIAGNOSIS

Konnie H. Plumlee

A variety of toxicants affect the formation or function of blood (Table 10-1). Some suppress the bone marrow and inhibit its ability to form normal blood components. Other poisons cause destruction of red blood cells. Some poisons prevent the blood from performing its normal clotting functions. Asphyxiants inhibit ability of the blood to carry oxygen to the tissues.

TABLE 10-1 **Poisons that Affect the Hematic System**

Clinical Effect	Toxicant	Species
Hemolytic anemia	*Allium* spp.	All
	Brown recluse spider	All
	Copper	Sheep most susceptible; other ruminants and some breeds of dogs
	Dimethyl disulfide	Ruminants
	Methylene blue	Cats most susceptible
	Naphthalene	All
	Phenols	Cats most susceptible
	Propylene glycol	Dogs and cats
	Red maple	Horses
	Vitamin K_3	Horses
	Phenothiazine	Horses
	Zinc	All
Methemoglobinemia	3-chloro-p-toluidine hydrochloride	All
	Acetaminophen	Primarily cats; dogs at high doses
	Chlorate	All
	Nitrate	Ruminants
	Phenols	Cats most susceptible
Suppression of bone marrow or red blood cell formation	5-fluorouracil	Dogs most commonly exposed
	Chloramphenicol	Cats and humans most susceptible
	Methotrexate	Dogs most commonly exposed
	Ptaquiloside	Ruminants
	Sulfonamides	All
	Vincristine	Dogs most commonly exposed
	Lead	All, especially waterfowl; in dogs, basophilic stippling and nucleated red blood cells are common

Continued

TABLE 10-1 **Poisons that Affect the Hematic System—cont'd**

Clinical Effect	Toxicant	Species
Coagulopathy	Anticoagulant rodenticides	All
	Brown recluse spider	All
	Coumarin glycosides	All
	Pit vipers	All
	Sulfonamides	All
	Aspirin	All
Asphyxiation	Hydrogen sulfide	All
	Nitrogen dioxide	All
	Carbon dioxide	All
	Carbon monoxide	All
	Methane	All
	Cyanide	All
	Cyanogenic glycosides	All

Hepatobiliary System

11

DIFFERENTIAL DIAGNOSIS

Konnie H. Plumlee

Liver disease often causes clinical signs that are nonspecific and similar to signs related to other organ systems. Depression, anorexia, and vomiting are commonly observed. In animals, icterus and weight loss may develop, depending on the chronicity of the disease.

As the function of the liver decreases, several secondary problems can develop. Coagulopathy may develop because the liver synthesizes many coagulation factors. As the liver loses the ability to metabolize the end products of nitrogen, hyperammonemia can develop and result in hepatic encephalopathy. The liver can lose the ability to metabolize phylloerythrin, a metabolite of chlorophyll, resulting in secondary photosensitization in herbivores. Hepatic damage also makes the animal more susceptible to drugs and poisons that are ordinarily metabolized by the liver (Table 11-1).

TOXIC RESPONSE OF THE HEPATOBILIARY SYSTEM

Robert B. Moeller, Jr.

The liver is essential for life and has a vast reserve, which assists in maintaining homeostasis in an animal. Damage to the liver can result in profound physiologic and metabolic disturbances, which can affect both the liver and other organ systems in the body. Consequently, mild to moderate liver damage may occur with the animal demonstrating little or no response to the injury. However, once extensive damage has occurred, serious life-threatening problems usually develop.

Many therapeutic and industrial compounds, toxins, and heavy metals alter hepatocellular and biliary function. These agents can lead to severe hepatocellular dysfunction or necrosis, resulting in catastrophic consequences to the animal. To understand hepatocellular toxic injury, one must first understand the structure of the liver, the major functions of the liver, and the process of bile formation and excretion. All of these aspects of hepatocellular dynamics contribute to the vulnerability of the liver to a toxic insult.

STRUCTURE

Models

The structure of the liver is based on two fundamental models: the hepatic lobule or the hepatic acinus.[1,2]

Lobular model. The lobular unit model is based on a hexagonal lobule with a portal venule, hepatic artery, and bile duct (forming the portal triad) at the edge of the lobule. The portal triads ring the lobule that is composed of chords of hepatocytes lined by endothelial-lined sinusoids. The sinusoids carry the blood, nutrients, and toxins to the hepatocytes, and drain toward a central terminal hepatic vein (central vein). The lobules are divided into three different regions. The periportal region involves hepatocytes adjacent to the portal triad. The midzonal region involves hepatocytes in the area midway between the portal triad and the central vein. The centrilobular region consists of hepatocytes adjacent to the central vein.

Acinar model. The hepatic acinar unit model is based on an individual portal triad with the acinar unit formed by the portal venule and hepatic artery bridging to the next portal triad by the penetrating venules.[2] The acinar unit is composed of three zones. Zone 1 region consists of hepatocytes that are closest to the penetrating venule near the portal triads. Zone 2 region is midway between the penetrating venules and the terminal hepatic vein. Zone 3 region is the area adjacent to the terminal hepatic vein. These zones of the acinar model are very similar anatomically to the regions of the lobular unit model.

Blood supply

The liver has two blood supplies: the hepatic artery and the portal vein. The hepatic artery provides oxygen and nutrients to the liver. The portal vein provides food-laden material and other substances (vitamins, metals, xenobiotics, endotoxins, and bacteria) from the gastrointestinal tract for hepatocellular metabolic conversion or removal.[2,3]

In all mammalian species, the lobular architecture of the liver allows the blood flowing from the portal vein and

TABLE 11-1　**Poisons that Affect the Hepatobiliary System**

Source	Toxicant	Species
Plants	Alsike clover	Horse
	Cycad (sago) palms	Dogs most commonly exposed
	Forages that induce photosensitization	Livestock
	Pyrrolizidine alkaloids	Livestock
	Quinones	Livestock
	Red clover	Horse
	Steroidal saponins	Primarily ruminants
	Tetradymia spp. and *Artemisia* spp.	Primarily sheep
	Xanthium	Primarily swine; also ruminants and horses
Mycotoxins	Aflatoxins	All
	Fumonisin	All
	Phomopsins	Sheep and cattle
	Sporidesmin	Sheep
Pharmaceuticals	Acetaminophen	Dogs primarily; cats at high doses
	Arsenical antihelminthics	Dogs
	Ketoconazole	Primarily cats
	Nonsteroidal antiinflammatory drugs	All
Toxins	Amatoxins (mushrooms)	All
	Microcystin (blue-green algae)	All
	Nodularin (blue-green algae)	All
Metal	Copper	Primarily in sheep and susceptible breeds of dogs
	Iron	All

hepatic artery to mix in the penetrating venules at the periphery of the lobule. The blood then enters the fenestrated, endothelial-lined hepatic sinusoids and moves along the hepatic cords to the terminal hepatic venule (central vein). Blood flowing from the terminal hepatic venule connects with sublobular hepatic veins that eventually connect to the posterior vena cava and drain into the heart.

Hepatocytes

The hepatic cords are composed of rows and columns of hepatocytes, which have a variety of functions. Normally, hepatocytes undergo cell division to replace lost cells. Hepatic stem cell production appears to be located in the area of the canals of Hering where the bile canaliculi and the bile ducts meet. These stem cells, called *oval cells,* can differentiate toward either hepatocytes or bile ductal epithelium. As hepatocytes mature, the cells move along the cords to the centrilobular region where they remain until they are displaced, because of either natural cell death or a toxic event.[4]

The metabolic actions and functions of hepatocytes vary depending on their location within the lobule. Different hepatic enzymes and hepatic functions are observed in different regions of the hepatic lobule, allowing hepatic injury from a toxic event to be exhibited in a zonal pattern in different regions of the lobule. Hepatocytes closest to the portal region are rich in mitochondria. These cells have major functions in gluconeogenesis, fatty acid oxidation, and ammonia detoxification. Hepatocytes near the terminal hepatic venule are important in detoxification and transformation of various xenobiotics and other toxic substances into less toxic metabolites for clearance in the bile or urine. Cells in this region have abundant phase 1 and phase 2 enzymes, which are important in the biotransformation of many xenobiotics. Of particular importance are the cytochrome P-450–related enzymes and numerous oxidative and reductive enzymes (reductases and dehydrogenases).[5,6]

Sinusoids

Blood, nutrients, and various hepatotoxic substances flow through hepatic sinusoids that are lined by endothelial cells lacking a basement membrane. The endothelial-lined sinusoids are fenestrated with numerous pores that allow an exchange of fluids and various molecules between the sinusoids and the perisinusoidal space of Disse.[6,7]

Residential macrophages (Kupffer cells) reside in the sinusoidal spaces that closely adhere to the endothelial cells.

These cells function in the ingestion and degradation of particulate matter, endotoxins, and bacteria in the circulatory system. These cells are also responsible for the production of major inflammatory mediators (interleukin [IL]-1, IL-6, and tumor necrosis factor-α). Macrophages in the periportal region tend to be more active in phagocytosis of foreign material and bacteria. Kupffer cells also have the capacity to assist in the destruction of some metastatic tumors.[6]

Ito cells (satellite cells or fat storage cells) are located in the perisinusoidal space of Disse. These cells contain lipid droplets, store vitamin A, and synthesize collagen. During injury and inflammation in the liver, these cells become myofibroblast-like cells and are important in laying down collagen for repair of hepatocellular injury.[6,7]

Pit cells are large granular lymphocytes that are attached by pseudopodia to the sinusoidal endothelium. These cells are believed to function as natural killer cells and play a significant roll in tumor cell destruction. They are also believed to be important in granuloma formation in the liver.[7]

Biliary system

The biliary system begins in the bile canaliculi, which are formed by specialized regions in the plasma membrane between hepatocytes in the hepatic cords. These canaliculi have tight junctions, which prevent leakage of bile into the perisinusoidal space of Disse and sinusoids. Bile is transported in the bile canaliculi through the canal of Hering to the bile ducts by contraction of the pericanalicular cytoskeleton. Bile ducts join the larger intrahepatic bile ducts and finally leave the liver through the hepatic duct. The gall bladder (not present in all animals) is located adjacent to the hepatic duct. This structure is important in the storage of bile, which is excreted during digestion.

Toxicants that damage hepatocytes may cause damage to the tight junctions between the hepatocytes resulting in separation and damage to the bile canaliculi. This results in leakage of bile salts into the circulatory system. Damage to the pericanalicular cytoskeleton adjacent to the bile canaliculi can lead to bile stasis and plugging.[8,9]

FUNCTION

The complex nature of the liver allows it to have multiple functions, which, if altered, can have serious adverse effects on other organ systems. The major functions of the liver are excretion of waste products (ammonia and hemoglobin); bile formation and secretion; storage of glycogen, lipids, heavy metals, and vitamins; synthesis of clotting factors; and phagocytosis of foreign material and bacteria. The liver is also essential in detoxification of various substances through conjugation, esterification, and other biotransforming enzymes that prepare metabolites of poisons for excretion by the biliary system or the kidneys.[7,10,12] These various functions appear to be regionalized to different areas of the hepatic lobule. In the periportal region, hepatocytes appear to be involved in gluconeogenesis, bile salt formation and

excretion, oxidative energy metabolism, amino acid catabolism, and ureagenesis from amino acid catabolism.[10] In the centrilobular region of the hepatic lobule, hepatocytes are primarily involved in biotransformation of xenobiotics, ureagenesis of ammonia, glycolysis, and liponeogenesis.[10]

One major function of the liver, seen primarily in the fetus (occasionally in adults) is hematopoiesis. The fetal liver is the major organ in which hematopoietic stem cells develop prior to seeding the bone marrow. Injury to hematopoietic stem cells located in the hepatic sinusoids of the fetal liver can have serious effects in fetal and neonatal development. In adults, damage to the hematopoietic elements in the bone marrow may lead to hematopoiesis in the liver with the expansion or development of hematopoietic stem cells in the sinusoids of the hepatic lobules.

RESPONSE TO INJURY

Each cell type in the liver may respond to a toxic insult. The cell response may vary from minor cytoplasmic variations to cell death. In many cases, the liver may not undergo an identifiable response to xenobiotics. However, when the hepatocytes and other cells in the liver (Kupffer cells and Ito cells) are overwhelmed by a particular poison or metabolite of that poison, alterations in various hepatic functions may take place.

Gross or microscopic hepatic changes resulting from hepatic damage from various poisons may occur as hepatic lipidosis, necrosis, nodular regeneration, fibrosis, atrophy, or changes in pigmentation.

Hepatic lipidosis

Hepatic lipidosis or fatty liver is a common change found in some domestic animals (Fig. 11-1). The cause of this lesion is the accumulation in the hepatic cytoplasm of membrane-bound vacuoles containing triglycerides. The cause of hepatic lipidosis is primarily due to an imbalance in the uptake of fatty acids by the hepatocytes and their secretion of very low-

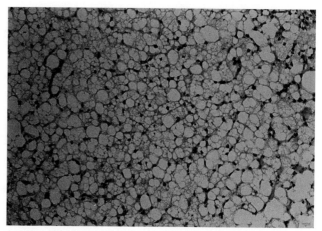

Fig. 11-1 Fatty liver in a cow with ketosis. Hepatocytes are filled with variably sized vacuoles.

density lipoproteins. The reasons for this imbalance are excessive intake or oversupply of triglycerides to hepatocytes; interference with the triglyceride formation cycle; increased synthesis of fatty acids or the decrease in fatty acid oxidation; and the decreased synthesis or secretion of low-density lipoproteins.[13-17]

On gross examination, hepatic lipidosis is characterized by an enlarged swollen liver with prominent rounded edges. The liver may be light brown to yellow. The hepatic parenchyma may be friable and easily ruptured when pinching the tissue. In some cases the hepatocytes may be so heavily laden with lipid that the tissue floats in formalin.

Microscopically, hepatic lipidosis is characterized by variably sized vacuoles in the cytoplasm of hepatocytes that may displace the nucleus to the periphery of the cell. The affected hepatocytes are most commonly observed in the centrilobular region of the hepatic lobule or diffusely scattered throughout the hepatic lobule. In severe cases these vacuoles become large, filling the cytoplasm of hepatocytes. The hepatocytes may rupture if they rapidly accumulate these lipids. If lipid accumulation is slower, the vacuoles are multiple and small, filling the hepatic cytoplasm without hepatocellular rupture. In these cases the nucleus is usually not displaced to the periphery of the cell.

In poison-induced hepatic lipidosis, hepatocellular death does not necessarily result. However, because of the disturbances in triglyceride metabolism, the affected liver is more susceptible to additional toxic insults. However, a fatty liver does not necessarily indicate toxic insult to the liver. Other causes involving other organ systems need to be evaluated when attempting to determine whether the causative agent is caused by a hepatocellular poison or to other metabolic disturbances (e.g., diabetes mellitus, ketosis, and hypoxia caused by anemia).[18-22]

Hepatocellular necrosis

Hepatocellular necrosis may take the form of centrilobular necrosis, midzonal necrosis, periportal necrosis, or massive necrosis.

Centrilobular necrosis. Centrilobular necrosis is the most common hepatotoxic injury observed. Hepatocytes in this region have a high concentration of mixed function oxidases (cytochrome P-450) and other associated enzymes. Consequently, these cells are the most active in the biotransformation of toxic substances and xenobiotics into less toxic intermediates or metabolites that can be excreted in either the bile or urine.[5,10,11] Because of the high enzymatic activity of hepatocytes, it is easy for these cells to become overwhelmed and damaged by metabolites or toxic products resulting from biotransformation of the intermediate products.

Grossly, centrilobular necrosis may be variable in appearance and is often dependent on whether hemorrhage is present. The affected tissues may have a mottled appearance varying from pale brown to yellow areas surrounded by normal dark brown parenchyma. If hemorrhage has occurred in the areas of centrilobular necrosis, the liver has dark red areas surrounded by normal dark brown parenchyma or light brown to yellow parenchyma. These areas of damage are small, usually 1 mm or less in diameter (easier to observe with a magnifying lens).

Histologically, centrilobular necrosis is characterized by necrotic hepatocytes surrounding the central vein (Fig. 11-2). In this type of necrosis, the majority of centrilobular regions are usually affected throughout the hepatic parenchyma. The areas of necrosis are usually well demarcated and associated with coagulative necrosis of the hepatocytes. In cases of coagulative necrosis, the hepatocytes maintain their normal architecture and become hypereosinophilic with pale and distinct nuclei. Occasionally, severe damage to the hepatic parenchyma is characterized by disassociation of hepatocytes from the hepatic chords with loss of hepatocytes. The effects of the necrosis on sinusoidal endothelium are variable. When the sinusoidal epithelium remains intact, it rarely hemorrhages into the centrilobular region. However, if the endothelium is damaged, then pooling of blood into the empty spaces caused by the hepatocellular loss is possible.

Centrilobular necrosis is usually repaired rapidly with the damaged liver parenchyma being replaced with viable hepatocytes. Consequently the damaged area can be repaired within several days, resulting in the damaged region showing little or no evidence of a previous insult. However, if the sinusoidal endothelium is damaged, some fibrosis occurs, particularly in the area adjacent to the central vein region.

Hepatotoxic agents are not the only cause of centrilobular necrosis. Centrilobular necrosis is a common finding with hypoxia resulting from circulatory collapse, acute anemia, and blood loss. Thus, when evaluating centrilobular necrosis of the liver, one must be sure to evaluate the animal for cardiac lesions or possibly acute blood loss. Cardiotoxic agents or toxicants that damage erythroid elements also have the potential for developing centrilobular hepatic necrosis that

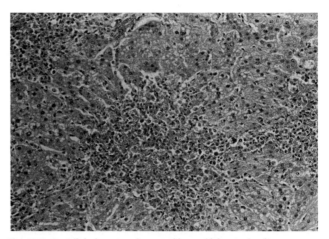

Fig. 11-2 Centrilobular necrosis caused by cocklebur toxicosis.

would be difficult to differentiate histologically from hepatotoxic agents.

Midzonal necrosis. Midzonal necrosis is the least common form of hepatocellular necrosis. Histologically, the necrosis is usually coagulative and equidistant between portal triads and the central vein. This type of lesion is difficult to observe grossly.

Periportal necrosis. Necrosis of periportal hepatocytes is also rarely observed. This pattern of necrosis is characterized by necrosis of hepatocytes surrounding the portal triads. Affected hepatocytes usually undergo coagulative necrosis with the hepatic architecture remaining intact. Rarely is hemorrhage observed. Because this region is usually associated with young hepatocytes, necrosis of these young cells often results in an increase in portal fibrosis, which is noted during the reparative process. Bile duct proliferation (from the canal of Hering) near the limiting plate and portal regions is a common finding early in repair of the damaged region. However, the bile duct proliferation eventually resolves.

Grossly, periportal necrosis looks very similar to centrilobular necrosis. Usually this lesion is presented as a mottled parenchyma consisting of light brown to yellow regions surrounded by normal, darker brown parenchyma. This pattern is easier to see with the help of a magnifying lens. This lesion has no discerning features that would make it easy to separate from centrilobular necrosis.

Massive necrosis. Massive necrosis is a term used to describe necrosis of the entire hepatic lobule. This type of lesion is usually extensive and affects the entire lobular architecture. Grossly, a large, pale, swollen liver characterizes massive necrosis. Usually, the parenchyma has scattered brown or yellow areas of viable tissue surrounded by red collapsed areas of necrosis. The dark red areas of necrosis may be extensive or regional depending on the severity of the hepatotoxin present. The hepatic parenchyma is friable and easily ruptured when pinched. If the hepatocellular insult does not kill the animal, the liver attempts to repair itself. In these cases the liver becomes irregularly depressed and firm as a result of collapse and fibrosis of the hepatic parenchyma.

Histologically, massive necrosis is characterized by necrosis of the entire hepatic lobule including the limiting plate. Massive necrosis may be coagulative, but often it is lytic, with the loss of hepatocytes, collapse of lobular architecture, and hemorrhage into the parenchymal spaces. Usually not all of the lobule is affected. In most cases consistent bridging necrosis is characterized by coagulative or lytic necrosis from the central vein to the portal triad or limiting plate. If the lobule is completely lost, no regeneration of the hepatic lobule occurs and the tissue collapses upon itself with abundant hemorrhage. If portions of the lobule remain, attempts to repair the damage occur. Because sinusoidal endothelial cells have also been damaged, regenerative attempts cannot mimic the normal hepato-

cellular architecture, resulting in nodular regeneration and fibrosis.

When studying necrosis, one must also be aware of *apoptosis,* or programmed cell death. Apoptosis is distinguished from necrosis in that necrosis of cells is not a natural event in the life cycle of the cell. Occasionally, apoptotic bodies are present histologically in the centrilobular region of the liver. These cells are individual hepatocytes that are condensed and deeply eosinophilic with either dense or fragmented nuclei. These are always found adjacent to normal cells and are not associated with inflammation. These apoptotic bodies occasionally are phagocytized by adjacent macrophages or hepatocytes and are seen in the cytoplasm of these cells as acidophilic bodies.[23,24]

Nodular regeneration

Nodular regeneration is a reparative process seen after severe hepatotoxic insults. It usually is noted after a toxic insult has caused massive necrosis of the hepatic lobules, with viable portions of the hepatic lobule remaining. Because most of the endothelial-lined sinusoids have been damaged, a normal lobular architectural pattern cannot be completed. Consequently, the hepatocytes proliferate in a random fashion, forming variably sized nodules in the parenchyma.

Grossly, these lesions appear as micronodular or macronodular raised areas over the capsular of the liver. On cut surfaces, scattered rounded nodules can also be observed in the parenchyma. Because the areas of regeneration have undergone some fibrosis, the hepatic tissue is usually firmer than normal.

Histologically, nodular areas of hepatocytes, which fail to form organized cords and have no sinusoidal architecture leading to a central vein, characterize nodular regeneration. These nodular areas may vary in size. Portions of the lobule that maintained normal architecture may remain adjacent to these areas of regeneration. Fibrosis is variable, but is usually associated with the areas of nodular regeneration. The adjacent portal triads also have some increase in fibrous connective tissue.

Liver atrophy

Hepatocellular atrophy is a rare finding and is usually not associated with hepatotoxic injuries. The most common cause of hepatic atrophy is starvation; however, prolonged cachexia caused by a toxic compound could have similar results. Because liver size is reduced from shrinkage of hepatocytes and not from toxic injury, these cells will remain biologically active with normal liver functions. Hepatic atrophy can also occur as a result of reduced blood flow from damage to the circulatory system. Circulatory damage to a lobe of the liver may result in atrophy of that portion of the lobe while the remaining liver may be normal. Biliary obstruction can also lead to damage to the hepatic circulation by causing additional fibrosis of portal areas. This type of damage may be regionalized to a lobe or generalized depending on where the biliary obstruction takes place. Previous insults caused by circulatory toxins that affect the biliary system need to be considered when looking at hepatic atrophy.

Macroscopically, the entire liver or a lobe of the liver may be smaller than normal with the hepatic parenchyma a dark brown. The parenchyma is usually firmer than normal and may be difficult to rupture when pinching the tissue. Because of shrinkage of the liver parenchyma, the capsular surface may be easily wrinkled when handled.

Histologically, the normal architectural pattern of the hepatic lobule is still present. The lobules appear smaller than normal with the portal areas and the terminal hepatic veins appearing closer. Hepatocytes in the lobules are usually reduced in size and contain scant cytoplasm.

Pigmentation

Pigmentation of the liver can be an important indicator of liver injury. Knowledge of these changes to hepatocytes both grossly and histologically may assist in identifying a toxic event. When there is damage to the biliary tract, either from cholestasis or biliary obstruction, accumulation of bile pigment often produces a light olive green to yellow-green liver. Histologically, a yellow pigment fills and distends canaliculi between hepatocytes as well as bile ducts (Fig. 11-3). If the bile canaliculi rupture, the yellow bile pigment can be observed in hepatocytes and Kupffer cells. Special stains for bile pigments are commonly used in histological examination of these tissues to differentiate the bile pigments from other pigments.

Iron and copper pigmentation can often be seen histologically in hepatocytes. These pigments accumulate in hepatocytes and Kupffer cells as yellow to yellow-brown material in the cytoplasm. Special stains such as Pearls iron stain and Rhodanine method for copper help in differentiating these pigments.[25] If iron and copper are responsible for toxic insult, these elements may be released by the hepatocytes through necrosis, with the newly regenerated

hepatocytes lacking excessive levels of these elements, and little pigment accumulation is noted. In these cases the liver may demonstrate elevated but nontoxic levels of these elements (particularly copper). If copper toxicosis is suspected, kidney copper levels as well as liver copper levels should be evaluated to determine whether a toxic event has occurred because copper, once released by the liver, is excreted by the kidney.

Lipofuscin is another common yellow-brown pigment found in hepatocytes. This pigment is associated with cells that are undergoing senile changes and that are unable to completely break down old, damaged organelles in the cytosol (lysosomal accumulation of poorly digested lipids). This pigment may be difficult to distinguish histologically from iron pigment; however, with special stains for iron, the lipofuscin pigments can be easily differentiated from iron pigments.

Melanin pigment can occasionally be observed in livers and is not associated with disease or toxic insults. Affected liver is usually mottled with black pigment seen on the capsular surface or in the parenchyma. Histologically, the melanin pigment is observed in hepatocytes, Kupffer cells, and the portal connective tissue.

Megalocytosis

Hepatic megalocytosis is observed with certain toxic insults, particularly pyrrolizidine alkaloid toxicosis and aflatoxin toxicosis. This lesion is not observed grossly and must be reviewed histologically. In these cases, enlarged hepatocytes with markedly enlarged nuclei (Fig. 11-4) are observed. This lesion is caused by an impaired ability of the cell to divide; consequently, the nucleus and cytoplasm enlarge.

In some aged animals (particularly aged mice), random megalocytosis of hepatocytes is a common finding. These enlarged hepatocytes are randomly scattered throughout the hepatic parenchyma and usually contain either single enlarged nuclei or double nuclei. This change is considered age related and is not due to exposure to a toxic insult.

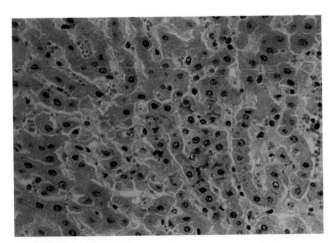

Fig. 11-3 Bile canalicular stasis caused by sporidesmin toxicosis.

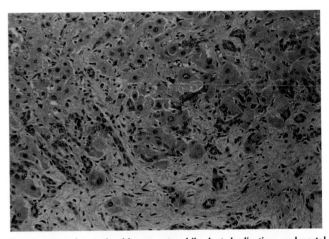

Fig. 11-4 Megalocytosis of hepatocytes, bile duct duplication, and portal fibrosis resulting from pyrrolizidine alkaloid toxicosis.

Biliary system damage

Toxic injury to the biliary duct system usually results in cholestasis involving the bile canaliculi or bile ducts. With cholestasis, the liver has a yellow to yellow-green color because of the bile. The yellow or yellow-green liver may remain normal in size or may become enlarged and swollen. Cholestasis may occur as a result of extrahepatic obstruction of the bile duct (i.e., neoplasia or cholelithiasis) or intrahepatic alterations that affect the bile canaliculi or intrahepatic bile ducts. Causes of canalicular bile stasis include damage to the hepatocellular cytoskeleton responsible for the transport of bile in the canaliculi or membrane damage in hepatocytes resulting in abnormal bile acid accumulation and bile salt transport.[8,9,26]

Toxic injury to the bile duct epithelium may result in necrosis of the biliary epithelium and plugging of the bile duct with cellular debris and bile. Histologically, dilatation of bile ducts with necrosis and sloughing of biliary epithelium into the lumen of the ducts characterize bile duct necrosis. Edema and inflammatory cells are variable in the affected portal triads depending on the extent of damage to the bile ducts. Bile may be present in the bile ducts of the portal triads; however, bile canaliculi in the periportal regions are often distended with bile (see Fig. 11-3).

Regeneration of the bile duct is usually rapid because surviving epithelium proliferates in the affected ducts. The amount of bile duct hyperplasia depends on the severity and duration of injury. The proliferation of the epithelium in the canal of Hering causes multiple ducts to appear near the limiting plate and adjacent portal triad. As the damage heals, the proliferating bile ducts regress and a normal portal system reappears.

Hepatic neoplasia

Neoplasms occasionally arise after exposure to certain hepatotoxins. These neoplasms often occur months or years after exposure to a particular hepatotoxin. Tumors that arise in the liver are hepatomas and hepatocellular carcinomas, bile duct adenomas and adenocarcinomas, and vascular endothelial-derived neoplasms (hemangiosarcomas).

Hepatocellular neoplasms are occasionally observed in animals. It is often difficult to distinguish hepatocellular adenomas from hepatocellular carcinomas by gross examination; however, most hepatocellular adenomas are usually single, firm, nodular masses that are dark red. Hepatocellular carcinomas can appear as single nodular masses or metastatic tumors. Many hepatocellular carcinomas have areas of necrosis and hemorrhage in the parenchyma. Occasionally, these neoplasms can be a grayish white from fibrosis. Prolonged exposure to aflatoxins causes hepatomas and hepatocellular carcinomas. These tumors occur long after exposure to the toxin. Androgenic substances that are commonly used in bodybuilding also cause hepatocellular tumors.[27,28]

Bile duct adenomas and adenocarcinomas are also noted in the liver. Grossly, adenomas are nodular, firm, white masses that may contain multiple fluid-filled cysts. Biliary adenocarcinomas are often firm nodular masses with variable amounts of hemorrhage and necrosis present. Occasionally, some of these masses are umbilicated. Biliary carcinomas can metastasize to other regions of the liver as well as to other organs. These carcinomas are often difficult to distinguish from other metastatic carcinomas grossly. The causes of biliary carcinoma are not known; however, repeated irritation of the bile duct from biliary flukes has been associated with this neoplasm. Consequently, continued bile duct irritation and necrosis from poisons may lead to neoplasia.

Primary hepatic endothelial neoplasms (hemangiomas and hemangiosarcomas) are uncommon in animals. Most hemangiosarcomas seen in the liver are metastatic masses from other organs (e.g., spleen, skin, right ventricle of the heart). Grossly, these masses can be variably sized nodular masses with a dark red to a mottled red and white appearance. Hemorrhage from the mass is common, with the animal dying of acute blood loss into the peritoneal cavity. Substances known to cause vascular neoplasms are vinyl chloride and arsenic.[28]

REFERENCES

1. Rappaport AM: The microcirculatory hepatic unit, *Microvasc Res* 6:212, 1973.
2. Rappaport AM: Hepatic blood flow: morphologic aspects and physiologic regulations; liver and biliary tract physiology 1, *Int Rev Physiol* 21:1, 1980.
3. Lautt WW, Macedo MP: Hepatic circulation and toxicology, *Drug Metab Rev* 29:369, 1997.
4. Sigal SH et al: The liver as a stem cell and lineage system, *Am J Physiol* 263:G139, 1992.
5. Lee WM: Review article: drug induced hepatotoxicity, *Aliment Pharmacol Ther* 7:477, 1993.
6. Jungermann K, Kietzmann T: Zonation of parenchymal and nonparenchymal metabolism in liver, *Annu Rev Nutr* 16:179, 1996.
7. Laskin DL: Nonparenchymal cells and hepatotoxicity, *Semin Liver Dis* 10:293, 1990.
8. Erlinger S: Review article: new insights into the mechanism of hepatic transport and bile secretion, *J Gastroenterol Hepatol* 11:573, 1996.
9. Phillips MJ et al: Biology of disease: mechanism of cholestasis, *Lab Invest* 6:593, 1986.
10. Jungermann K, Katz N: Functional hepatocellular heterogeneity, *Hepatology* 2:385, 1982.
11. Caldwell J: Biological implications of xenobiotic metabolism. In *The liver: biology and pathobiology*, ed 2, New York, 1988, Raven Press.
12. Bell DR: An overview of the symposium on "Peroxisomes: Biology and Role in Toxicology and Diseases," Aspen, Colorado, USA, June 28-July 2, 1995, *Hum Exp Toxicol* 14:846, 1995.
13. Hansen RJ, Walzem RL: Avian fatty liver hemorrhagic syndrome: a comparative review, *Adv Vet Sci Comp Med* 3:451, 1993.
14. Lombardi B: Fatty liver, considerations on the pathogenesis of fatty liver, *Lab Invest* 15:1, 1966.
15. Neuschwander-Tetri BA, Bacon BR: Nonalcoholic steatohepatitis, *Med Clin North Am* 80:1147, 1996.

16. Alpers DH, Sabesin SM: In *Disease of the Liver,* ed 1, Philadelphia, 1982, JB Lippincott.
17. Lundquist G et al: A case control study of fatty liver disease and organic solvent exposure, *Am J Indust Med* 35:132, 1999.
18. Reid IM, Collins RA: The pathology of post-parturient fatty liver in high yielding dairy cows, *Invest Cell Pathol* 3:237, 1980.
19. Bogin E et al: Biochemical changes associated with the fatty liver syndrome in cows, *J Comp Pathol* 98:337, 1988.
20. Thornburg LP et al: Fatty liver syndrome in cats, *J Am Anim Hospt Ass* 18:397, 1982.
21. Ludwig J et al: Metabolic liver diseases. Review: nonalcoholic steatohepatitis, *J Gastroenterol Hepatol* 12:398, 1997.
22. Jeffcott LB, Field JR: Current concepts of hyperlipaemia in horses and ponies, *Vet Rec* 116:461, 1985.
23. Schulte-Hermann R et al: Active cell death (apoptosis) in liver biology and disease, *Progr Liver Diseases* 13:1, 1995.
24. Searle J et al: The significance of cell death by apoptosis in hepatobiliary disease, *J Gastroenterol Hepatol* 2:77, 1987.
25. Prophet EB: In *Laboratory method in histotechnology,* Washington, DC, 1992, Armed Forces Institute of Pathology.
26. Tsukada N et al: The structure and organization of the bile canalicular cytoskeleton with special reference to actin and actin-binding proteins. *Hepatology* 21:1106, 1995.
27. Piolot HC, Dragon YP: In *Cassarett and Doull's toxicology: the basic science of poisons,* New York, 1996, McGraw-Hill.
28. Farrell GC: In *Drug induced liver disease,* New York, 1994, Churchill Livingstone.

Musculoskeletal System

DIFFERENTIAL DIAGNOSIS

Konnie H. Plumlee

Most of the poisons that affect the musculoskeletal system are toxic to the muscles themselves rather than to the bone or cartilage (Table 12-1). Some of the poisons that affect the skeletal muscles also affect cardiac muscle. Those poisons are also listed in Chapter 6, Cardiovascular System. Toxicants that cause fetal musculoskeletal damage are discussed in Chapter 14, Reproductive System.

TABLE 12-1 Poisons that Affect the Musculoskeletal System

Area Affected	Toxicant	Species	Comments
Bone or teeth	Fluoride	All	Bone lesions; teeth mottling
	Vitamin A	All	Fusion of physeal region of long bones, vertebrae, and sternum
Hoof	Black walnut	Horses	Laminitis
	Ergot	Livestock	Dry gangrene
	Fescue		
	Hoary alyssum	Horses	Laminitis and limb edema
	Selenium	Livestock	Abnormal hoof growth; separation of coronary band
Joints	Fluoroquinolones	Young animals	Arthropathy
	Zinc	Foals	Epiphyseal swelling; lameness
Muscle	Brown recluse spider	All	Muscle necrosis
	Hops	Dogs	Malignant hyperthermia-like syndrome
	Tremetone	Ruminants, horses	Muscle tremors
	Thermopsis montana	Ruminants	Myopathy
	Senna	Ruminants, horses	Myopathy
	Macadamia nuts	Dogs	Transient muscle weakness
	Ionophores	Ruminants, swine, horses, dogs, birds	Muscle necrosis
	Vitamin D	All	Soft tissue mineralization
	Calcinogenic glycosides	Livestock	Soft tissue mineralization
	Cholecalciferol	Pets most commonly exposed	Soft tissue mineralization

Nervous System

DIFFERENTIAL DIAGNOSIS

Konnie H. Plumlee

Disease of the nervous system produces the largest variety of clinical signs as compared to the other organ systems. Tables (Tables 13-1 through 13-5) list toxicants in general categories. Even though the tables are intended to assist the veterinarian in forming a differential diagnosis based on clinical signs, several other factors must be considered:

1. Some poisons affect multiple areas of the nervous system.
2. The clinical signs can vary with dose, route of exposure, and toxicity of compound.
3. The clinical signs can vary depending on the species of animal.
4. The poison can cause a progression of clinical signs that begin in one category and end in another. For example, a given poisoning may begin with signs of a depressed central nervous system, but progress to seizures.

Therefore, the information in the tables should be used as a general guideline.

TOXIC RESPONSE OF THE NERVOUS SYSTEM

Sherry J. Morgan and Diann L. Weddle

SUSCEPTIBILITY

The nervous system has unique qualities that influence its susceptibility to damage and potential repair. To familiarize the reader with the basic cell types of the central and peripheral nervous system, the following discussion describes functions and structures of the major cellular components.

Cell types

Neurons are the primary cell type in the nervous system, being responsible for the propagation of impulses. The portions of the neuron include the cell body and processes, axons, and dendrites. The cell body contains the nucleus and multiple subcellular organelles, including rough endoplasmic reticulum, free ribosomes, Golgi, lysosomes, smooth endo-

plasmic reticulum, neurofilaments, and microtubules. Axons, which are frequently myelinated, consist of a single process that extends a variable length from the cell body before branching. In contrast, dendrites are not myelinated, are typically multiple, and extend only a short distance from the cell body before branching. The flow of nerve impulses extends from the axon, to the cell body, to the dendrites, then to the axon of a different neuron. Cell-to-cell networks are intricate, and a deleterious effect on one neuron may result in a secondary effect on anatomically diverse neurons.

Neurons may undergo some degree of differentiation and migration in the postnatal period (particularly in animals that are born with incomplete development of motor skills, for example, puppies and kittens), and repair or regeneration of some neuronal processes (axons, dendrites) is possible. However, the adult neuron does not divide, making the nervous system particularly vulnerable.

In the central nervous system, the axonal myelin is provided by an oligodendroglia, whereas the Schwann cell provides myelin in the peripheral nervous system. The peripheral nervous system is more likely to undergo regeneration than is the central nervous system. At least a portion of this difference in potential for repair lies in the relationship of the myelin-providing cell to the axon. In the central nervous system, the oligodendroglia tends to supply myelin for several axons; thus, a variable but relatively high number of the axons are located a considerable distance from the myelin-providing cell. In contrast, in the peripheral nervous system, the Schwann cell tends to provide myelin for only a single axon and is located adjacent to the axon for which it provides myelin. Thus, if there is damage with subsequent loss of myelin, it is logistically simpler for remyelination to occur in the peripheral nervous system than in the central nervous system. If the myelin cannot be regenerated to serve as a coating over the axon, degeneration of the axon itself occurs.

Blood supply

Approximately 20% to 25% of cardiac output goes directly to the brain. This high percentage of blood flow to a tissue that

TABLE 13-1 Poisons that Stimulate the Central Nervous System

Source	Toxicant	Comments
Pesticides	4-Aminopyridine	
	Anticholinesterase insecticides	Seizures occur with highly toxic compounds
	Bromethalin	Stimulant at high doses; depressant at low doses
	DEET	
	Metaldehyde	
	Organochlorine insecticides	
	Pyrethrins	
	Sodium fluoroacetate	
	Zinc phosphide	
Feed-related	Ammoniated feed	
	Non-protein nitrogen	
Drugs	5-Fluorouracil	
	Amphetamines	
	Antihistamines	Stimulant at high doses; depressant at low doses
	Cocaine	
	Decongestants	
	Methylxanthines	Stimulant at high doses; gastrointestinal signs at low doses
	Nitrofurazone	
	Serotonergic drugs	
	Tricyclic antidepressants	
Metals	Lead	Signs of excitation may be intermittent with depression
	Sodium	
Plants	*Asclepias* spp.	
	Water hemlock	
Tremorgens	Tremorgenic forages	
	Penitrem A and Roquefortine	
	Annuals	

makes up a relatively small percentage of the total mass of an animal has several implications that are directly associated with susceptibility to injury. The high blood flow indicates that the tissue requires a continual high level of oxygen and nutrient supply to maintain function. This unique need is thought to be related to the necessity for maintaining ionic gradients across membranes.[1] If this high blood flow is interrupted, even briefly, significant damage may result. The areas of damage depend on the distribution and extent of the blood flow disturbance. Even if the disruption in blood flow affects the entire body, there are still differential effects because of the varying requirements for oxygen and energy supply between cell types, and even between neurons themselves.

Within the variety of cell types, it is generally accepted that the neuron is the most sensitive to hypoxic and anoxic injury, followed by astrocytes, oligodendroglia, microglia, and blood vessels. The reason for the relative resistance of the glial cells as opposed to neurons is likely multifactorial, both

related to the significant energy demand of the neuron and the presence of high levels of pentose shunt enzymes in the glia.

Barriers

The brain is extremely susceptible to fluctuations in its local environment; without a mechanism for minimizing these fluctuations, the brain would not function properly. Specialized barriers exist within the brain: the blood-brain barrier and the blood–cerebrospinal fluid barrier. These barriers are relatively effective for many compounds, except those that are nonpolar or actively transported.

The blood-brain barrier is dependent on a specialized feature of the central nervous system capillaries. The endothelial cells form tight junctions in contrast to the capillary structure in other tissues, which have fenestrations or other forms of transmembrane channels. Other unique features of the endothelial cells of the central nervous system include the presence of a high number of mitochondria, which may be

TABLE 13-2 **Poisons that Depress the Central Nervous System**

Source	Toxicant	Comments
Household-industrial	Alcohol	
	Essential oils	Cats are most susceptible; ataxia, tremors, salivation, hypothermia
	Turpentine	
Drugs	Antihistamines	Depressant at low doses; stimulant at high doses
	Barbiturates	
	Bromide	
	Macrolide endectocides	
	Marijuana	
	Opiates	
	Piperazine	
	Propylene glycol	
Pesticides	Amitraz	
	Bromethalin	Depressant at low doses; stimulant at high doses
	Starlicide	
Mycotoxin	Fumonisin	Leukoencephalomalacia in horses
Metals	Lead	Depression may be intermittent with excitation
	Organic alkyl mercury	Blindness, ataxia, paralysis, coma
Snake toxins	Coral snake	Ataxia, tremors, paresis
Plants	*Centaurea* spp.	Nigropallidal encephalomalacia in horses
	Stipa robusta	Primarily affects horse, but also ruminants
	Thiaminase	Depression, ataxia, paralysis
Liver toxicants		Hepatic encephalopathy secondary to liver disease

TABLE 13-3 **Poisons that Affect the Spinal Cord or Peripheral Nerves**

Source	Toxicant	Comments
Plants	Cycad palm	Demyelination of the spinal cord white matter
	Hypochaeris radicata	Hyperflexion of hindlimbs in horses; left laryngeal hemiplegia reported in Australia
	Karwinskia spp.	Progressive ascending polyneuropathy
	Lathyrus	Neurolathyrism of peripheral nerves in ruminants, horses, and chickens; horses also have degeneration of vagus and recurrent laryngeal nerves
	Nitropropanol glycosides	Spinal lesions in cattle, sheep, and horses; also brain lesions
	Sorghum spp.	Flaccid posterior paralysis and cystitis in horses
	Tryptamine alkaloids	Spinal lesions in sheep and cattle; also brain lesions
Metals	Lead	Paralysis of the recurrent laryngeal nerves in horses
	Pentavalent organic arsenicals	Demyelination of peripheral nerves, especially in swine
	Selenium	Focal, symmetrical poliomyelomalacia in swine
Chemicals	Triaryl phosphates	Axonopathy
Bacteria	Botulinum	Blocks release of acetylcholine at neuromuscular junctions
	Tetanus	Inhibition of release of glycine and GABA from Renshaw cells in spinal cord

TABLE 13-4 **Poisons that Affect the Autonomic Nervous System**

Mechanism of Action	Toxicant	Comments
Cholinesterase inhibitors	Anatoxin-a(s) Carbamate insecticides Organophosphate insecticides Solanum-type steroidal alkaloids	
Parasympathomimetic	Anatoxin-a Meliatoxins Muscarinic mushrooms Nicotine Piperidine alkaloids Pyridine alkaloids Slaframine	Nicotinic agonist Exact mechanism is unknown, but appears to be similar to nicotine Muscarinic agonist Stimulates nicotinic receptors at low doses, but blocks them at high doses Stimulate nicotinic receptors at low doses, but blocks them at high doses Stimulate nicotinic receptors at low doses, but blocks them at high doses Muscarinic agonist
Parasympatholytic	Diterpene alkaloids Quinolizidine alkaloids Tropane alkaloids	Block nicotinic acetylcholine receptors Primarily block nicotinic acetylcholine receptors, but can also block muscarinic receptors Inhibit acetylcholine at postganglionic neuroeffector sites

TABLE 13-5 **Poisons that Affect Behavior**

Source	Toxicant	Comments
Metals	Lead Sulfur	Hysteria, aggression, or dementia are possible Polioencephalomalacia in ruminants
Plants	Indolizidine alkaloids	Locoism in horses
Mushrooms	Ibotenic acid Muscimol Psilocybin	Delirium and hallucinations in humans; spasms, head pressing, and incoordination in dogs Hallucinations in humans

both a "blessing and a curse," because the high number of mictochondria may help to maintain the integrity of the blood-brain barrier while at the same time leaving brain capillaries uniquely susceptible to hypoxia. Some areas of the central nervous system, such as the pituitary gland, portions of the hypothalamus, and the pineal gland, do not have these specialized types of endothelial cells and so are not protected by the "blood-brain barrier."[2]

The blood–cerebrospinal fluid barrier is dependent on tight junctions formed by choroid plexus epithelial cells, somewhat like those formed by the endothelial cells that make up the blood-brain barrier.[3] No effective brain–cerebrospinal fluid barrier exists. Once a substrate gains access to the cerebrospinal fluid, no significant restriction prevents the free exchange of constituents with the extracellular fluid.[4]

Although the anatomic structures noted earlier play integral roles in the maintenance of the barriers, characteristics of the solute and carrier-mediated transport systems also play roles in the existence or disruption of complete barrier function. Molecule size is of utmost importance, with small molecules entering the brain more rapidly than large molecules. With an intact blood-brain barrier, large proteins and substances bound to albumin do not enter the cerebrospinal fluid. Lipid solubility is also of importance, with CO_2, O_2, volatile anesthetics, and other highly lipid-soluble compounds easily traversing the blood-brain barrier.[2] Many substances that are not lipid soluble but are necessary components for normal brain function (glu-cose, amino acids, ions) can make use of carrier-mediated transport systems to gain access to the central nervous system.

MECHANISMS OF ACTION

The mechanism of action of a toxicant may be direct or indirect. Direct actions result in direct neuronal toxicosis, whereas indirect actions include those that result in a change in metabolism or blood supply, with a secondary neuronal toxicosis.

Various factors may result in damage to the nervous system via inhibition of neuronal oxidative metabolism. These factors include interference with blood supply (hypoxia and ischemia), hypoglycemia, and damage to cell ion homeostasis.

Hypoxia

Hypoxia- and ischemia-induced neuronal injury is one of the major mechanisms by which damage may occur. The susceptibility of neurons varies considerably between different anatomic locations, with certain neuronal groups of the hippocampus and granule cells, for example, being particularly susceptible to hypoxic-ischemic injury. Toxicants could result in hypoxic-ischemic damage by several mechanisms: reaction to systemic hypotension, cerebral infarction, or reaction to vascular injury.

Hypoglycemia

Hypoglycemia may also result in neuronal damage. As is the case with hypoxia- and ischemia-induced neuronal injury, hypoglycemia typically results in damage to certain subsets of cells, including dentate and granule cells as well as large neurons. Although the reasons for the different susceptibility of various neurons is not completely understood, it may lie in part with local differences in energy demands and the variability in sensitivity to excitatory neurotransmitters.

Ion balance disruption

The brain, neurons in particular, is extremely sensitive to fluctuations in ion balance. Thus, agents that result in disruption or damage of ion homeostasis are frequent nervous system toxicants. The excessive intracellular accumulation of calcium is of most concern. Although the cell does have some mechanisms for sequestering excessive calcium (in the plasma membrane, mitochondria, and endoplasmic reticulum), these storage facilities are easily overwhelmed. Once there is excessive free cytosolic calcium, a cascade of deleterious effects occurs as a result of the activation of phospholipases and proteases. The damage may be sublethal, or it may result in extensive mitochondrial damage, endoplasmic reticulum swelling, and cell death.

Cytoskeleton damage

Changes in the integrity of the cytotoskeleton may also result in neural toxicosis because the cytoskeleton is an all-important component of the transmission of impulses from one neuron to another. The primary site of injury is in the axon or peripheral nerve because this is where these cytoskeleton components function. Damage occurs within the distal aspects of the axon or peripheral nerve first because these portions are most subject to alterations in membrane permeability. Their distance from the cell body and the energy source of the cell makes them more vulnerable. The damage then progresses toward the cell body, being termed a "dying-back" degeneration. The myelin sheath remains intact until the axon itself retracts; once the axon retracts, the myelin degenerates (known as secondary demyelination in which the loss of myelin is secondary to axon loss).

If within the peripheral nervous system the axon does not regenerate, the Schwann cells eventually degenerate as well. Schwann cells of the peripheral nervous system tend to reside relatively close to the axons they support and only support one or a few axons; if their axon is lost, they readily degenerate. In contrast, oligodendroglia of the central nervous system reside a considerable distance from the multitude of axons they support; thus, it takes loss of a greater number of widely distributed axons in the central nervous system to create a significant loss of oligodendroglia. However, the myelin sheath is readily lost once the axon retracts, just as is the case in the peripheral nervous system.

Decreased protein synthesis

Other mechanisms that may result in damage to the nervous system include interference with protein synthesis. Without the constant production of the multitude of proteins that are integral to normal function, the integrity of neuronal transmission and other important functions are impaired. Cell changes include a loss of rough endoplasmic reticulum. In neurons, this is characterized by a loss of Nissl substance, which is represented by a clearing of the cytoplasm with peripheral displacement of the nucleus. Central chromatolysis may be reversible, depending on the duration and extent of the injury, or it may be irreversible with eventual cell death. Another typical change includes the presence of an increased number of neurofilaments in the cytoplasm caused by failure of normal axonal transport because transport is dependent on production of several cytosolic proteins. Examples of compounds that may result in damage via this pathway include ricin and some antineoplastic drugs (doxorubicin and cisplatin).

Glial cell damage

Glial cells may react in unique ways to particular toxicants. For example, some forms of hepatic toxicosis result in excessive accumulation of ammonia within the blood and the animal may exhibit "hepatic encephalopathy," an abnormal condition of the brain caused by hepatic change. The clinical signs vary but generally include depression, head pressing, and the possibility of progression to coma and death. The changes center around the astrocyte because the astrocyte contains abundant glutamine synthetase, which converts glutamate to glutamine by using ammonia as a substrate. A unique morphologic change ensues, with the astrocytic nuclei becoming enlarged, vesicular, and lobulated. These cells are termed *Alzheimer type II astrocytes*.

Other changes to glial cells may include damage to the oligodendroglia, the myelin-providing cell of the central nervous system. Triethyltin is one poison that can cause such damage.

RESPONSE TO INJURY

In general, damage to the nervous system more frequently results in irreversible morphologic and functional changes than occur in most other organ systems. As is the case in other tissues, damage to individual cellular components can be reversible or irreversible. Chromatolysis (or loss of Nissl substance) is a potentially reversible change. Also, axons and dendrites can regenerate as long as the neuronal cell body is intact. However, once a neuron is severely damaged, there may be significant functional deficits as a result of the inability of the adult neuron to divide. If neuronal loss is not extensive, proliferation of neuronal processes with reorganization of pathways may occur. Also, regeneration and proliferation of supporting structures including capillaries and glial cells is a possibility, depending on the extent of the injury. However, if a significant number of neurons are lost, persistent neurological deficits may result.

The following classification of responses to injury is based on cellular target sites, as described by Spencer and Schaumburg.[5] This classification separates the responses into those that affect the neuron, axon, myelin, neuromuscular endplate and synaptic transmission, and blood vessels.

Neuron

With those responses that affect the neuron, the target site is the neuronal cell body. These neuronopathies are subdivided into selective and diffuse neuropathies.

Selective neuropathies. These have a wide variation. For example, the toxicosis caused by yellow star thistle *(Centaurea solstitialis)* is highly selective because there is necrosis only of the substantial nigra and globus pallidus (hence, the condition is termed *nigropallidal encephalomalacia).* Other selective neuronopathies are not as selective as those noted with yellow star thistle. For example, carbon monoxide and cyanide result in damage to particular portions of the brain, but the damage is more widespread. Carbon monoxide, which has greater affinity for hemoglobin than does oxygen, results in hypoxic damage with resultant edema and laminar necrosis of the cerebral cortex, hippocampus, globus pallidus, and, less frequently, other sites within the brain. With cyanide toxicosis, the injury is considered to be secondary to inhibition of cytochrome oxidase (the terminal enzyme in the electron transport chain that uses oxygen derived from oxyhemoglobin). Here, the injury consists of a demyelination involving the cerebrum, corpus callosum, basal ganglia, and optic tracts.[6] Therefore, despite relatively similar end results (deficient oxygen supply), considerable variation exists between the morphologic changes noted in carbon monoxide and cyanide toxicosis.

Diffuse neuronopathies. These tend to affect a wide variety of types and locations of neurons. However, considerable variation exists within this classification. For example, methylmercury, although classified as causing a diffuse neuropathy, exerts its primary effect on granule cells of the visual cortex and cerebellum as well as sensory neurons of the dorsal root ganglion. It is thought that the sensitivity of these small neurons to methylmercury is largely related to the extensive binding of the compound to cytoplasmic components, particularly ribosomes and rough endoplasmic reticulum, with a resultant inhibition of protein synthesis.

This toxicant can also have an indirect effect on neurons, because it may cause damage to the endothelium with resultant damage to the blood-brain barrier.

With some toxicants, the damage is diffuse. For example, in the neuronopathy noted with locoweed toxicosis, there is widespread vacuolation of cells within the central and peripheral nervous system. The pathogenesis is related to inhibition of lysosomal alpha-mannosidase. With prolonged or excessive ingestion of the toxic plant *(Astragalus, Oxytropis,* or *Swainsona* spp.), neuronal necrosis and axonal degeneration may occur.

Axon

The site of axonal damage varies with the particular toxicant involved and is subdivided into proximal and distal axonopathies, depending on the targeted site of injury. Distal axonopathies are more frequently encountered.

Proximal axonopathy. One example of a proximal axonopathy includes the toxicosis noted with 3,3'-iminodiproprionitrile, which results in axonal swelling secondary to a defect in slow axonal transport with resultant excessive accumulation of neurofilaments. Secondary changes occur in both the neuronal cell body and the distal axon, with degeneration and necrosis in the former and atrophy in the latter.

Distal axonopathy. Toxicants that may cause a distal axonopathy include hexacarbons (n-hexane, 2,5-hexanedione, and methyl n-butyl ketone) and organophosphates. The axonopathy induced by hexacarbons is a sensory motor axonopathy characterized by the presence of giant axonal swellings caused by aggregations of neurofilaments. Organophosphate axonopathy is associated with a delayed form of toxicosis secondary to inhibition of neurotoxic esterase. This toxicosis primarily affects long or large-diameter myelinated fibers of the spinal cord and peripheral nerves. A dying-back degeneration of the axon occurs, with the proximal portion of the axon undergoing degeneration after damage and degeneration to the proximal axon.

Endplate and synaptic transmission

Other toxicants may cause neuromuscular endplate and synaptic transmission deficits. Such toxicants include those that are produced by *Clostridium botulinum* (botulism) and *Clostridium tetani* (tetanus).

With botulism, the toxicant binds to presynapatic axon terminals, with resultant interference of the supply or action of calcium and secondary impairment of release of acetylcholine. Because the molecule does not cross the blood-brain barrier, the primary effect is at the level of the skeletal muscle itself, with resultant flaccid paralysis. The initial site of involvement generally varies with the type of botulism toxicosis and the species affected. For example, in horses with type B and, less frequently, type C botulism, one of the first detectable signs is dysphagia. Death generally results from respiratory paralysis.[7]

In contrast to botulism in which the primary effect is at the level of the skeletal muscle, tetanus affects the central nervous system. The toxin reaches the central nervous system by means of retrograde transport along spinal nerves. Within the spinal cord and brain stem, the toxin binds to presynaptic terminals with the predominant effect on inhibitory synapses. The result is excessive stimulation with ensuing tonic spasms, opisthotonus, and seizures. Death is caused by respiratory failure.

Myelin

Toxicants may also exert their effect on myelin, with secondary deficits in neural transmission. The loss of myelin may be considered primary or secondary, with the initial effect being on the cells that provide or support myelin (oligodendroglia or Schwann cells in the central or peripheral nervous system, respectively). Examples of primary myelinopathies include those caused by triethyltin and hexachlorophene. The resultant lesions consist of edema and status spongiosus of the white matter.

Secondary myelinopathies include swayback of lambs and carbon monoxide toxicosis. In swayback, lesions including demyelination of the brain and spinal cord are predominant and considered secondary to the loss of oligodendroglia. The pathogenesis of carbon monoxide toxicosis is less clear, but it is hypothesized that prolonged low levels of oxygen to the brain may have an adverse effect on oligodendroglia.

Vasculature

Many toxicants may induce their deleterious effects on the central or peripheral nervous system through their effects on the vasculature. With lead toxicosis, the neuron is considered to be both directly[8] and indirectly (via its effect on the vasculature) affected. The pathogenesis of lead toxicosis is thought to be related to the effect of lead on the endothelial cell, with resultant endothelial swelling, proliferation, and necrosis with secondary vascular thrombosis and hyalinization. As a result of the vascular damage, there is extensive neuronal degeneration with reactive gliosis and astrocytic proliferation. Studies indicate that the initial effect on the endothelial cell is at least in part related to the inhibition of endothelial cell glucose metabolism.[9]

GROSS LESIONS

Gross lesions in the central nervous system are characterized by changes in color, contour, or consistency of the tissue. Even though hemorrhage presents as a shade of red or brown, depending on the chronicity of the change, necrosis that is devoid of significant hemorrhage likely appears somewhat yellow to tan. Changes in contour are generally associated with swelling of the tissue, which by nature of the location (within the confines of the cranium or spinal canal), is somewhat limited. Lesions with significant necrosis or hemorrhage may also be softer than the normal neural tissue.

Unfortunately, gross changes associated with damage by a toxicant can only infrequently be distinguished from those associated with a traumatic or infectious etiology. However, in most cases, metabolic or toxic neurologic diseases have at least some degree of bilateral symmetry.

A limited number of toxins exhibit gross changes that are considered pathognomonic. For example, *Phalaris* sp. intoxication results in bilaterally symmetrical, greenish pigmented areas in the gray matter of brain stem and diencephalon along with a greenish tinge between the cortex and medulla of the kidney.[10] The gross appearance of a horse brain that is affected with yellow star thistle (*C. solstitialis*) toxicosis is characterized by the presence of changes in color and consistency of the substantia nigra and globus pallidus (nigropallidal encephalomalacia). In carnivores the presence of bilaterally symmetrical regions of discoloration (frequently red) in the brain stem nuclei is suggestive of thiamine deficiency.

Although the presence of laminar softening and discoloration of the gray matter in a ruminant is consistent with polioencephalomalacia (gray matter necrosis), polioencephalomalacia is a general term and such a change can be seen with other diseases such as lead toxicosis, hypoxia, or other conditions.[10]

HISTOPATHOLOGY

As is the case with gross changes, histologic changes associated with a toxic condition affecting the central nervous system are only rarely specific for poisons. Phalaris toxicosis is one of the few conditions that is associated with a highly specific histologic change (greenish pigment in the cytoplasm of neurons). The central nervous system has only a limited number of ways that it can respond to an injury, whether that injury is from an infectious agent, a traumatic incident, or a poison. Knowledge of the site of predilection for a specific toxic entity as well as the information that is provided by the practitioner are essential. Thus, it is imperative that a complete history including clinical signs, treatment, and previous health status be provided.

REFERENCES

1. Iversen LL: The chemistry of the brain, *Sci Am*, Sept 1979.
2. Betz et al: In Siegel GJ, editors: *Basic neurochemistry: molecular, cellular, and medical aspects*, ed 4, New York, 1989, Raven Press.
3. Nag S: In Davis RL, Robertson DM, editors: *Textbook of neuropathology*, ed 2, Baltimore, 1991, Williams & Wilkins.
4. Ramsay DA, Robertson DM: In Davis RL, Robertson DM: *Textbook of neuropathology*, ed 2, Baltimore, 1991, Williams & Wilkins.
5. Schaumburg HH, Spencer PS: Classification of neurotoxic responses based on vulnerability of cellular sites, *Neurol Clin* 18(3):517, 2000.
6. Salkowski AA, Penney DG: Cyanide poisoning in animals and humans: a review, *Vet Hum Toxicol* 36(5):455, 1994.

7. Kinde H et al: *Clostridium botulinum* type-C intoxication associated with consumption of processed alfalfa hay cubes in horses, *Am J Vet Res* 199(6):742, 1991.

8. Kim JS et al: The effects of thiamine on the neurophysiological alterations induced by lead, *Vet Hum Toxicol* 32(2):101, 1990.

9. Ahrens FA: Effects of lead on glucose metabolism, ion flux, and collagen synthesis in cerebral capillaries of calves, *Am J Vet Res* 54(5):808, 1993.

10. Odriozola E et al: Neuropathological effects and deaths of cattle and sheep in Argentina from *Phalaris angusta, Vet Hum Toxicol* 33(5):465, 1991.

14

Reproductive System

DIFFERENTIAL DIAGNOSIS

Konnie H. Plumlee

Disease of the reproductive system can affect the male reproductive system, the female reproductive system, the embryo or fetus, or a combination of these. Many functions of the reproductive system are vulnerable: hormone production, spermatogenesis, follicular development, implantation, and placentation, among others. Determination of the steps of the reproductive process that have been affected assists the clinician in narrowing down the list of potential toxicants.

Many diseases can cause reproductive losses as a result of stress, decreased food intake, or hypoxia. However, a limited number of toxicants directly affect the reproductive system. The clinician is often faced with a diagnostic challenge when trying to determine whether reproductive losses are primary or secondary. Therefore, it can be difficult to determine whether a toxicosis is directly responsible for reproductive disease, especially abortions, or whether reproductive losses are secondary to a toxicosis or other disease. Tables 14-1 through 14-4 are limited to those poisons that directly affect the reproductive system.

TABLE 14-1 Toxicants that Affect the Male Reproductive System

Effect	Species	Toxicant	Comments
Loss of libido	Swine	Zearalenone	Caused by estrogenism
Decreased spermatogenesis	Cattle	Gossypol	Detrimental effects on the seminiferous tubules

TABLE 14-2 Toxicants that Affect the Female Reproductive System

Effect	Toxicant	Species	Comments
Estrogenism	Phytoestrogens Zearalenone	Ruminants Prepubertal gilts Nonpregnant sows Pregnant sows Cows	Infertility, irregular estrus, follicular cysts, dystocia Hyperestrogenism Anestrus, pseudopregnancy Embryonic death Infertility
Lactation	Avocado Ergot Fescue	Horse, cow, goat, rabbit Horse Cow, swine	Noninfectious mastitis, agalactia Agalactia Decreased milk production, infertility
Prolonged gestation	Ergot Fescue	Horse	Large foal, dystocia, retained placenta

TABLE 14-3 **Toxicants that Cause Teratogenic Effects**

Toxicant	Species	Abnormality
Piperidine alkaloids Pyridine alkaloids	Cattle, goats, sheep, pigs	Cleft palate, arthrogryposis, scoliosis, kyphosis, torticollis, limb contracture
Quinolizidine alkaloids	Cattle	Cleft palate, arthrogryposis, scoliosis, kyphosis, torticollis, limb contracture
Jervanine alkaloids	Sheep primarily; cattle	Cyclops, craniofacial malformations
Selenium	Waterfowl	Underdeveloped feet and legs, malformed eyes and beak

TABLE 14-4 **Toxicants that Cause Abortions**

Toxicant	Species	Gestation Period	Comments
Isocupressic acid	Cattle primarily; also sheep, goats, llamas, buffalo	Last trimester	May also include premature udder development and milk production, vulvar swelling, vaginal discharge, retained fetal membranes
Gutierrizia spp.	Cattle; sheep	Any	Vulvar swelling and udder development occur several days before abortion
Phomopsins	Sheep; cattle	Late pregnancy	Embryonic loss and decreased lambing rates also reported in sheep

15

Respiratory System

DIFFERENTIAL DIAGNOSIS

Konnie H. Plumlee

Direct toxic effects on the respiratory system include irritation, edema, emphysema, and fibrosis. Table 15-1 also lists poisons that cause asphyxiation and aspiration pneumonia, both of which prevent oxygen from being delivered to the tissues.

TOXIC RESPONSE OF THE RESPIRATORY SYSTEM

Leslie W. Woods and Dennis W. Wilson

The respiratory tract is the primary site of entry for, the first barrier of defense from, and the primary target organ for pneumotoxic agents, which can exert their harmful effects through several mechanisms including displacement asphyxia, oxygen transport asphyxia, toxin absorption, and local irritation.[1] Displacement asphyxia occurs with gases such as carbon dioxide, nitrogen, and methane, which cause hypoxia through displacement of oxygen in inspired air. On the other hand, carbon monoxide and cyanide are gases that cause hypoxia by interfering with oxygen transport. However, some toxicants, such as mercury, are absorbed through the lungs but cause damage to other organs. This section on respiratory toxicologic pathology concentrates primarily on toxicants that exert local effects on the respiratory tract and on the reaction of the respiratory tract to toxic injury.

In addition to having respiration capabilities, the lungs have extensive metabolic capabilities. Total cardiac output passes through the lungs, with a large volume of blood present in the lungs at any given moment.[2] The lung is ideal, then, not only for exchange of gases but also for rapid and efficient metabolic activity, making the lungs highly vulnerable to blood-borne toxicants. Therefore, exposure of the respiratory tract to poisons may occur via inhalation or systemically via the pulmonary circulation.

Pulmonary defenses that protect the lungs against toxic and microbial insults include a mucous barrier, filtration and

TABLE 15-1 Poisons that Affect the Respiratory System

Toxic Effect	Toxicant	Species
Asphyxiation	Carbon dioxide	All
	Carbon monoxide	
	Cyanide	
	Cyanogenic glycosides	
	Hydrogen sulfide	
	Methane	
Irritation of the upper tract	Ammonia	All
	Nitrogen dioxide	
Pulmonary edema	Fumonisins	Swine
	Paraquat	All
	Nitropropanol glycosides	Ruminants
	Furans	Cattle
	Tryptophan	Cattle
	Hydrogen sulfide	All
	Nitrogen dioxide	All
	Pine oil	Cats most susceptible
	Patulin	All
Pulmonary emphysema	Nitropropanol glycosides	Ruminants
	Furans	Cattle
	Tryptophan	Cattle
	Hydrogen sulfide	All
	Nitrogen dioxide	All
Fibrosis	Paraquat	All
Aspiration pneumonia	Petroleum hydrocarbons	All
	Turpentine	All
Increased secretions	Iodine (EDDI)	Cattle
	Anticholinesterase insecticides	All

clearance of foreign particles, an active mucosal immune system, and neutralization and metabolism of potentially pathogenic substances.[3] These defense mechanisms are partly responsible for the variation in susceptibility to toxic injury among specific regions or cell populations of the respiratory tract.

Toxicants may selectively induce damage to specific tissues or cell populations. Tissue or cellular tropism may be related to the physicochemical nature of the poison and its anatomic location as well as the physical and metabolic features of the susceptible tissues or cells. For example, water-soluble gases such as formaldehyde and sulfur dioxide are mostly trapped in the upper respiratory tract where air approaches 100% humidity.[1] Ciliated cells are targeted in this region because their excessive membranous surface area makes them highly susceptible to oxidant injury.[4]

Some pneumotoxins have direct toxic effects as parent compounds, whereas others require bioactivation to toxic metabolites. Cells that have metabolizing enzymes may be injured when nontoxic parent compounds are metabolized to toxic metabolites. Cytochrome P-450–dependent monooxygenases have been demonstrated in nonciliated bronchiolar epithelial cells (Clara cells) and in alveolar endothelium in some species.[3] Therefore, these cells are preferentially injured when 3-methylindole, which is produced in the bovine rumen after ingestion of forage high in tryptophan, is converted to 3-methoxindole by local mixed function oxidases.[5]

Species variability exists with regard to susceptibility to toxins, target organs, or cellular tropism.[3] Species differences can sometimes be attributed to the variable distribution of cells with xenobiotic metabolizing enzymes. Differences in species susceptibility to poisons may also be associated with anatomic configuration and regional variation in cell populations. For example, the simple anatomic configuration of the human nasopharynx can make humans far more susceptible to the deep lung effects of a toxic gas than animals with more complicated nasal cavities.[6]

The unique anatomic configuration and cell populations of the nasopharynx, trachea, and lungs contribute to the variation in susceptibility to toxicants and in the different patterns of cellular injury. Additionally, repair mechanisms and cell renewal in each of these regions are different and account for the variable histopathology findings in injured tissue. Therefore, the regions of the upper and lower respiratory tract are discussed separately.

NASOPHARYNX

Turbulent air flow in the nasal turbinates in conjunction with mucus production traps particles larger than 10 μm as well as highly soluble gases.[1,3] Hygroscopic gas droplets enlarge as they progress through the 100% humidity of the nasal region and become entrapped. For example, formaldehyde and sulfur dioxide are absorbed in the nasopharynx during nasal breathing in some species.[4] Species differences in the degree of anatomic complexity and the extent of nasal breathing alter regional effects of these toxins. Additionally, the extensive vascular network in the region affects airway caliber and therefore resistance and turbulence of air flow. Mucus

physically traps and chemically inactivates foreign substances. Mucociliary clearance in the nasal cavity moves entrapped particles retrograde toward the pharynx.

Four types of epithelium are present in the nasal cavity. They are distributed rostrocaudally as stratified squamous, transitional, ciliated respiratory, and olfactory epithelium.[3]

Ciliated respiratory epithelium

Ciliated respiratory epithelium is a stable population of cells composed of pseudostratified ciliated, mucous, nonciliated, and basal cells. This population of cells has a continual low turnover rate. Ciliated cells are highly susceptible to injury because of their excessive membranous surface area and because they slough early in injury. These cells have no regenerative capacity. However, mucous cells, nonciliated cells, and sometimes basal cells are progenitor cells that assist epithelial repair by regeneration and differentiation into ciliated cells.

Initial changes that occur with acute injury are subtle and can be seen by transmission electron microscopy. Ultrastructural changes are likely to occur initially in the ciliated cell and include blebbing and eventual loss of cilia.[4] Extensive deciliation can be seen by light microscopy. As injury progresses, degeneration and sloughing of ciliated cells occur, followed by mucous cell proliferation. Early termination of the insult with rapid repair results in a return of normal structure and function. However, continued injury triggers inflammation that may be grossly visible as mucosal hyperemia and a granular appearance with adherent exudate. Chronic exposure to poisons may lead to mucous cell hyperplasia with excessive mucus production that may be apparent as excessive mucus on the mucosal surface. Squamous metaplasia and, ultimately, fibrosis may be the end result.

Olfactory epithelium

Olfactory epithelium includes olfactory sensory cells that are rich in cytochrome P-450 monooxygenases, which catabolize toxic drugs, pesticides, and carcinogens. This characteristic feature also makes this cell population more susceptible to poisons that require bioactivation to reactive intermediates.[3] Responses of the olfactory mucosa to toxic injury include degeneration, regeneration, postdegenerative atrophy, inflammation, respiratory metaplasia, and basal cell hyperplasia.[7]

Degeneration is the earliest morphologic change and is characterized by single cell necrosis and loss of sensory and sustentacular cells, giving the mucosa a vacuolated appearance. Regeneration is characterized by basal cell hyperplasia and usually occurs concurrent with degeneration. Depending on the duration of exposure, dose, and physical and chemical nature of the toxicant, full recovery to original function and structure may occur, or metaplasia and fibrosis may result. When extensive injury occurs, postdegenerative atrophy results in the olfactory mucosa being replaced by a thin pseudostratified layer of nonciliated, flattened to cuboidal cells with little evidence of regeneration. [7] Inflammation is seldom seen with toxic injury to the olfactory mucosa, but when it does occur, it typically accompanies extensive erosion and ulceration of the mucosa. Replacement by respiratory epithelium or basal cells may also be seen.

AIRWAYS

Dichotomous branching is the primary difference between the intrapulmonary airways and the trachea. Sharper angles accommodate easy impact of particles. Laminar flow in the trachea changes to turbulent flow in smaller branching airways and almost ceases at the bronchiolar-alveolar junction as the airways open up, resulting in a sudden increase in cross-sectional area. [3] Larger particles of 10 micrometers or greater impact in more proximal airways of the respiratory tract, whereas smaller particles penetrate deeper into the respiratory tract. At the bronchiolar-alveolar junction, particles less than 2 micrometers settle out by gravity as the linear velocity of air decreases. [3]

A gradation of injury is apparent in the response to respired gaseous irritants. The upper airways (trachea and mainstem bronchi), by virtue of being exposed to the highest concentrations, are most injured. [4] The more distal airways are protected until the last generations. These terminal airway regions are a second site of injury as a result of slower airflow, a thinner surface layer of mucus, and the transition to alveolarized airways at the beginning of the parenchymal region of the lung.

Mucociliary escalator

The trachea and mainstem bronchi share similarities in structure and response to injury with the nasal respiratory ciliated epithelium. [3] Mucus traps foreign substances in the trachea as it does in the nasal cavity, but is also a part of a unique defense mechanism, the mucociliary escalator. Mucus derived from the surface mucous cells and submucosal gland cells overlies a nonviscous solution that bathes cilia. The cilia move in unidirectional waves, forcing mucus, which contains entrapped foreign substances and macrophages that have phagocytized debris in the deep lung, up to the pharynx to be swallowed.

The distribution of secretory cells in the bronchi and bronchioles varies between species and airway generation. Mucus-secreting cells are most prominent in the upper airways, whereas the secretory cell of the lower airways, the nonciliated bronchiolar epithelial cell (NCBE or Clara cell) secretes a less viscous product (Fig. 15-1, *A*). [3]

Response to injury

The ciliated cell population is most sensitive to injury as a result of the large surface area of membrane available for oxidative interaction. [4] In the early stages of injury, ciliated cell degeneration may be reflected morphologically as swollen, fractured, or lost cilia and may result in individual ciliated cell necrosis. Excess mucus overlying the airway mucosa may be visible on gross examination.

The response to oxidant injury includes ciliogenesis, sometimes inflammatory cell transmigration, and proliferative repair. Ciliogenesis occurs by synthesis of new basal bodies from aggregates of deuterosome precursors. With more severe, sustained injury, cilia cell necrosis occurs, followed by proliferative repair. Repair is accomplished by proliferation of secretory and basal cells (Fig. 15-1, *B*). [3,4] Secretory cells dedifferentiate and migrate to cover any denuded epithelial spaces. Secretory cells then undergo ciliogenesis and transdifferentiate to ciliated cells in the

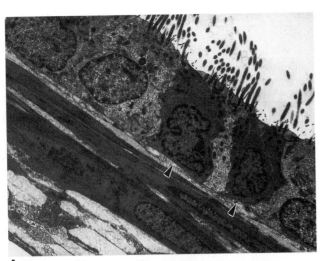

A

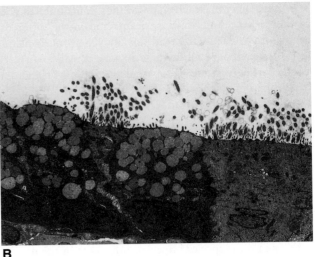

B

Fig. 15-1 A, Transmission electron photomicrograph of normal small airway epithelium in the rat. Ciliated and nonciliated *(arrows)* bronchiolar epithelial cells form a simple low columnar epithelium overlying a basal lamina and bronchiolar smooth muscle. **B,** Transmission electron photomicrograph demonstrating mucous cell hyperplasia in small airway epithelium of a rat after injury with 3-methylindole. (From Woods LW et al: Structural and biochemical changes in lungs of 3-methylindole-treated rats, *Am J Pathol* 142:129, 1993.)

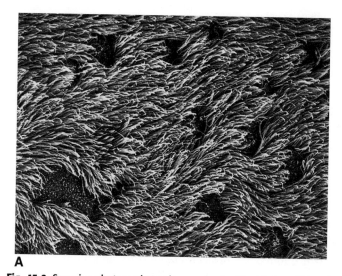

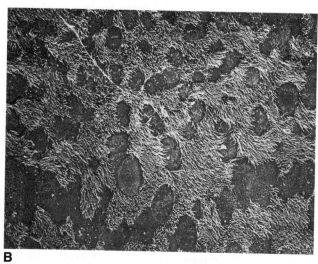

A

B

Fig. 15-2 Scanning electron photomicrograph of oxidant-induced loss of respiratory cilia in the trachea of a monkey exposed to ozone for 7 days. **A,** Normal respiratory surface has regular long cilia arranged in parallel arrays. Secretory cells with surface microvilli are interspersed in large regions of cilia. **B,** Airways exposed to ozone have irregularly shortened and randomly oriented cilia. (From Woods LW et al: Structural and biochemical changes in lungs of 3-methylindole-treated rats, *Am J Pathol* 142:129, 1993.)

process of reforming a pseudostratified respiratory epithelium. In chronic exposures, adaptational responses include markedly shortened cilia with a consequently smaller membrane surface area (Fig. 15-2) and squamous metaplasia. Mucus hypersecretion, mucous cell metaplasia, and mucous gland hypertrophy may also be seen. The process appears to be similar in both large and small airways except that small airways tend not to have basal cells and the repair process is dependent only on secretory cells. The secretory product of small airway cells may also alter from the normal serous, protein-rich product to the more viscous glycoproteins of mucous cells. This mucous cell metaplasia is a hallmark of chronic bronchitis and occurs in response to any number of inflammatory stimuli.[4]

Disruption of the mucociliary apparatus either by ciliastasis, deciliation, or cilia cell necrosis ultimately leads to bacterial bronchopneumonia. For example, ammonia intoxication is one of the most common irritant gas intoxications seen in veterinary medicine. High ammonia levels are commonly encountered in poorly maintained, poorly ventilated poultry facilities, and bronchopneumonia is the most common sequela. Lungs may be red, wet, and consolidated with exudates visible in the major airways. Exposure to ammonia also induces keratitis. Therefore, when concurrent keratitis and bronchopneumonia are apparent on necropsy of multiple animals housed in an enclosed facility, then high environmental ammonia should be suspected. Exposure to extremely high ammonia concentrations occurs as a result of industrial accidents and can result in desquamation of airway epithelium, laryngeal edema, and pulmonary edema and hemorrhage. Bronchitis and bronchiectasis may be long-term effects of ammonia intoxication in survivors.[1] Other gases such as SO_2, NO_2, O_3, and NH_4 cause paralysis of cilia at low doses and deciliation at higher doses.[8]

Bioactivation

Nonciliated bronchiolar epithelial cells (NCBEs, or Clara cells) in some species have high cytochrome P-450 monooxygenase activity and can activate many xenobiotic compounds to toxins that cause injury. NCBE cells can be found from the trachea to the distal bronchioles; the distribution varies according to species. Acute changes of discrete NCBE cell necrosis may be too subtle for examination by light microscopy and may require transmission electron microscopy. NCBE cells are expelled outward by bronchoconstriction and are replaced by progenitor cells. Chronic changes are more visible by light microscopy and can include mucous cell metaplasia or squamous metaplasia.

Extensive research into the relationship between metabolism and the NCBE cell cytotoxic responses to chemicals demonstrates a strong association between the presence of specific P-450 isozymes and the susceptibility to chemically induced NCBE cell necrosis. These differences in metabolic capabilities appear to account for much of the species and location differences in cytotoxic responses. Experimentally, clear selective necrosis of NCBE cells is evident. Despite considerable understanding of these mechanisms, the clinical implications of NCBE cell necrosis seem relatively insignificant. Speculation exists that NCBE cell necrosis could contribute to bronchitis in horses (Fig. 15-3), but other animal disease syndromes consequent to NCBE cell toxicosis have not been described. The more likely concern for metabolic activity in NCBE cells is the potential for bioactivation of carcinogens, causing neoplasia.

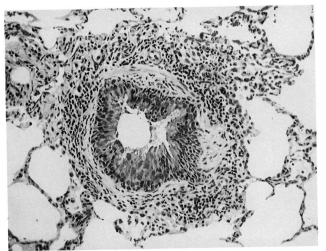

Fig. 15-3 Light photomicrograph of chronic bronchitis in a horse with clinical signs of chronic obstructive pulmonary disease. The small airways are surrounded by lymphocytic inflammation, the smooth muscle is prominent, and the lumen contains mucus admixed with neutrophils. The airway epithelium is hyperplastic.

ALVEOLI

With few exceptions, toxic injury to the deep lung typically manifests as a diffuse interstitial pneumonia. Interstitial pneumonia is easily distinguished from a bacterial bronchopneumonia on gross examination. Interstitial pneumonias typically involve the entire lung, whereas bronchopneumonias affect primarily the cranial-ventral portions of the lungs with lesions clearly centered around airways. Interstitial pneumonias may be multinodular and random or have a diffuse pattern of injury.

Diffuse alveolar damage

Lungs of animals that die with acute diffuse alveolar damage are uniformly affected, red-purple, meaty, and wet. In cows the interlobular septa and pleura may be emphysematous as a result of poor collateral ventilation (Fig. 15-4). It is not possible to grossly distinguish toxin-induced interstitial pneumonias from diffuse interstitial pneumonias caused by other etiologies. Chronically affected lungs that have progressed to diffuse interstitial fibrosis are contracted, pale, and firm.

Pneumotoxins are a few of several known causes of diffuse alveolar damage that result in adult respiratory distress syndrome (ARDS). In addition to pneumotoxins (3-methylindole, 4-ipomeanol, oxygen, nitrogen dioxide, paraquat, and other irritants), septic shock, shock associated with trauma, hemorrhagic pancreatitis, and burns are just a few events associated with ARDS.[9] Distinguishing between ARDS induced by pneumotoxins and damage associated with other events by gross or microscopic pathology is therefore not possible.

Three principle target cell populations are present in the alveolar parenchyma: the capillary endothelial cell, the type I or squamous alveolar epithelial cell, and the type II or cuboidal epithelial cell. Type I alveolar epithelial cells are most susceptible to injury because of their large membrane surface area in relation to a limited cytoplasmic volume and lack of organelles for antioxidant defenses.[3] Injury of type I epithelium is repaired by proliferation and migration of type II cells (Fig. 15-5, *A* and *B*), which then transdifferentiate into type I cells.[1]

The sequence of diffuse alveolar damage can vary with the poison. Type I cell necrosis is the initial response to metabolically activated respiratory toxins such as 3-methylindole and

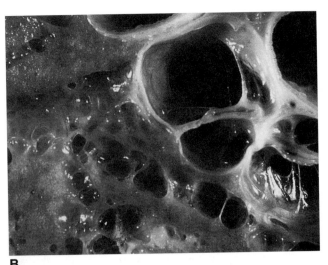

Fig. 15-4 A, Gross photograph of interstitial emphysema in a cow. Although potentially present in any cow with respiratory difficulty, the trapping of air in interstitial connective tissue is especially prominent in cows with diffuse alveolar damage induced by toxins such as 3-methylindole or 4-ipomeanol. **B,** Higher magnification demonstrating multiple gas pockets that dilate the interlobular septa, leaving strands of connective tissue traversing gas-filled spaces.

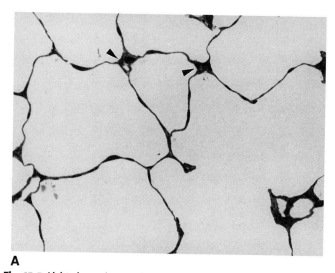

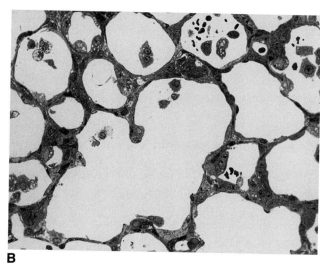

A

B

Fig. 15-5 Light photomicrograph of normal **(A)** and regenerating lung **(B)** in experimental diffuse alveolar damage induced by 3-methylindole in the rat. **A,** Alveolar type II cells are evident in the branching corners of alveoli of control lungs *(arrows)*. **B,** Three days after administration of 3-methylindole, the alveolar walls are markedly thickened by type II cells, which have proliferated to replace type I cells that have been lost by necrosis. There is an increase in alveolar macrophages and interstitial cells in the alveolar walls.

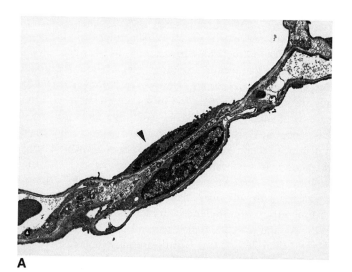

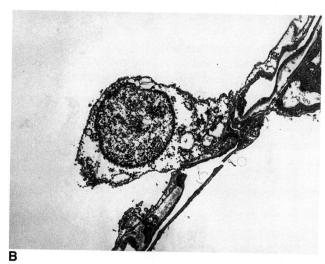

A

B

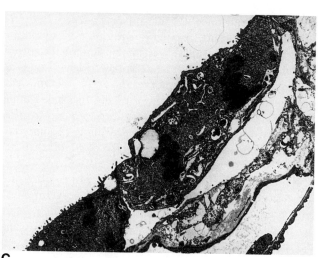

C

Fig. 15-6 A, Transmission electron photomicrograph of normal alveolar wall. Note how the (partially collapsed) alveolar capillaries overlie a thin connective tissue stroma to protrude slightly into the alveolar lumen. The squamous or type I pneumocyte *(arrow)* extends across the alveolar surface with cell membranes only slightly separated by scant amounts of cytoplasm. **B,** Transmission electron photomicrograph of type I pneumocyte necrosis in a rat with experimental 3-methylindole. The epithelial cell cytoplasm is dilated with electron-lucent spaces and the cell membrane is discontinuous. The nucleus is also swollen with dispersed chromatin. **C,** Transmission electron photomicrograph of type II cell undergoing mitosis in postinjury regeneration in a rat with 3-methylindole toxicosis. Note the characteristic surface microvilli and occasional lamellar granules.

4-ipomeanol (Fig. 15-6, *A* and *B).*[10-13] However, endothelial cells appear to be the first target with oxygen toxicosis, in diffuse alveolar damage associated with systemic inflammatory disease, and from toxicosis resulting from the antineoplastic agent bleomycin.[13] Type I cell injury quickly follows the endothelial injury.[9] Therefore, the progression of events then becomes identical despite the different primary target cells.

In the acute stage, endothelial cell and type I cell injury leads to vascular leakage, interstitial and intraalveolar edema, fibrin exudation, and formation of hyaline membranes (Fig. 15-7). Loss and dilution of surfactant leads to atelectasis. Type I alveolar epithelial cell necrosis also stimulates vascular and interstitial leukocytosis. Type I pneumocyte necrosis and sloughing exposes the basement membrane and leads to the next phase of proliferation, which is type II alveolar epithelial cell hyperplasia and interstitial inflammation. In this proliferative phase, type II pneumocytes undergo division and migration to cover the exposed basement membrane (see Fig. 15-6, *C*). Type II pneumocytes eventually differentiate into squamous Type type I cells.

Natural toxins that cause diffuse pulmonary parenchymal damage in animals include 3-methylindole (associated with ingestion of forage high in tryptophan), perilla mint ketone, toxin from moldy sweet potato (4-ipomeanol) (Fig. 15-8), stinkwood poisoning, and toxin from moldy garden beans.[3] Crofton weed has been associated with proliferative interstitial pneumonia in horses.

Nitrogen dioxide generated in corn silos has caused numerous deaths in humans and has been suspected but never proven in animals.[1] Animals trapped in burning buildings that survive asphyxiation may die days after exposure with widespread epithelial parenchymal necrosis and exudation from the combined chemical and heat effects of smoke.

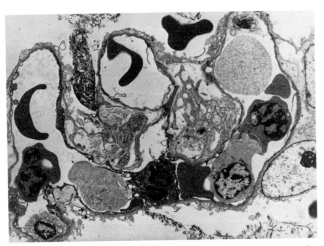

Fig. 15-7 Adult respiratory distress syndrome in a cynomolgus monkey that died of sepsis. Fibrin is forming both intracapillary thrombi and fibrillar lamellae along the epithelial surface of the alveolus. Intracapillary accumulation of degranulated neutrophils and densely staining degenerate endothelial cells are prominent.

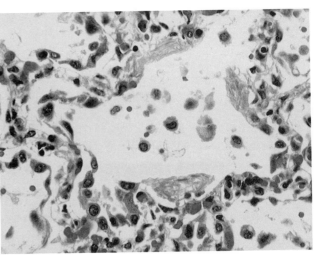

Fig. 15-8 Alveolar inflammation and early repair in a cow with moldy sweet potato (4-ipomeanol) poisoning. Accumulations of fibrin in the alveoli form thick inspissated layers consistent with hyaline membranes. Migrating immature type II pneumocytes cover much of the alveolar surface. (From Woods LW et al: Structural and biochemical changes in lungs of 3-methylindole-treated rats, *Am J Pathol* 142:129, 1993.)

Birds are exquisitely sensitive to pneumotoxic gases and were used as sentinels for early detection of gas leaks in coal mines. Aerosol sprays, cooking gas, carbon monoxide, tobacco smoke, and fumes from burning foods and cooking oils are known to be toxic to birds. Oxygen causes a diffuse pattern of injury to the alveolar wall, but there are species differences in susceptibility to oxygen toxicosis. Chickens do not appear to be susceptible to hyperoxia. In one study, chickens that were exposed to 100% oxygen at 1 atm for a prolonged period did not develop clinical signs or lesions associated with pulmonary damage.

Polytetrafluoroethylene-coated (Teflon) pans undergo pyrolysis, and toxic particulates are released when overheated (greater than 260° C).[14, 15] Birds are most sensitive to these toxic degradation products, but a flulike syndrome called *polymer-fume fever* has been reported in humans as well.[1] Guinea pigs and mice did not appear to be affected after experimental exposure. A rapid progression from dyspnea to death is the typical clinical presentation in birds exposed to degradation products of polytetrafluoroethylene. Lungs are severely congested and hemorrhagic, and sometimes sink when placed in formalin. Microscopically, major and minor airways, including air capillaries, are filled with and are often obliterated by hemorrhage. Epithelial lining is sometimes sloughed from the basement membrane of parabronchi and air capillaries.

Repair after diffuse alveolar damage can result in full recovery of structure and function, or an aberrant repair process can lead to metaplasia and fibrosis ultimately resulting in death. A few factors that may affect the outcome include expediency of repair, inflammatory mediators, and whether or not damage includes progenitor stem cells. It is generally thought that if injury is quickly followed by repair, there is little to no residual tissue damage and normal function is restored.[16,17] If injury to cells is extensive and repair is delayed, or if stem cell populations are destroyed, then tissue damage is more extensive and may progress to chronic irreparable damage and loss of function. Epithelial repair is a late event with cytostatic drugs. Diffuse pulmonary fibrosis sometimes follows use of the chemotherapeutic agents cyclophosphamide and 1,3-bis(2 chloroethyl)-1-nitrosourea (BCNU) (cCarmustine).[17] Paraquat injures both type I epithelial cells and the progenitor type II pneumocytes and commonly results in diffuse pulmonary fibrosis and death.[13]

Pneumoconiosis

This defense mechanism of the lungs is the key to toxicity resulting from cytotoxic particulate pneumotoxins such as silicates.[1,9] Macrophages remove particles that have deposited in the lung and are carried out via the mucociliary escalator or through lymphatic clearance. This clearance system fails when inhaled cytotoxic particles induce macrophage death and trigger subsequent granulomatous inflammation. Crystalline silicates are highly toxic to macrophages, forming crystalline arrays at the cellular membrane.

Human patients with silicosis exhibit many immunologic abnormalities. Rheumatoid factor and antinuclear antibodies are often present in the serum.[9] It is unknown whether animals exhibit these same characteristics, but experimental studies in animals have demonstrated that silica acts as an immunosuppressive agent for B- and T-cell functions.[3]

Silicosis is most important in horses.[3,18] Lesions are characterized by multiple foci of granulomatous inflammation with interstitial fibrosis (Figs. 15-9 and 15-10, *A)*. Necrosis and mineralization are sometimes seen in the granulomatous centers and refractile crystals can be seen

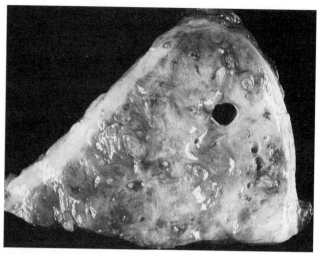

Fig. 15-9 Granulomatous pneumonia caused by silicosis in a horse. Section of lung has thickened pleura overlying parenchyma consolidated by coalescing granulomas. The remaining parenchyma is firm, pale, and disrupted by bands of fibrosis.

within the granulomas (Fig. 15-10, *B)*. The variable crystalline structures of the silicates affect the pathogenicity and the ultimate distribution in the lungs. Variable structures, in turn, are highly determined by geographic location, which is why silicosis is more commonly seen in animals in some regions as opposed to others.[18]

Asbestos, a specialized crystalline silicate, causes similar granulomatous and fibrotic changes, but has also been associated with mesotheliomas, tumors of the pleura in humans.[1,9] Mesotheliomas associated with asbestos exposure and demonstration of asbestos bodies in the lungs have also been reported in dogs.[19]

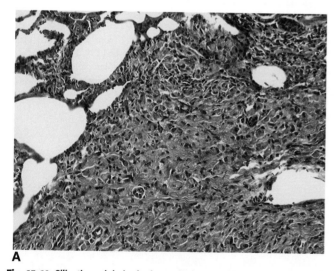

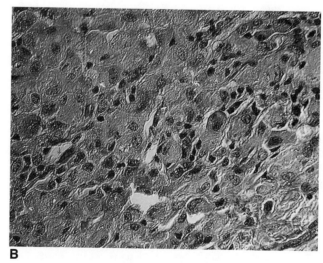

Fig. 15-10 Silicotic nodule in the lung of a horse. At low magnification **(A)**, coalescing granulomatous inflammation with extensive fibrosis obliterates much of the alveolar parenchyma. At higher magnification **(B)**, the extensive, largely mononuclear population of activated macrophages has fine intracellular crystals evident by interference contrast microscopy.

Hypersensitivity pneumonitis

A wide variety of substances generally associated with occupational exposures cause immune-mediated interstitial inflammation in the lungs of people. Hypersensitivity pneumonitis can develop after exposure to inhaled antigens, which can include some metals, inert substances, and organic products of some organisms.

A syndrome occurs in cattle and horses similar to "farmer's lung" of humans, in which inhalation of exogenous organic dusts and spores of fungi from various foods and bedding triggers allergic pneumonitis, which may progress to granulomatous inflammation and fibrosis.[20] The syndrome is commonly associated with *Micropolyspora faeni* in humans but has also been associated with exposure to *Aspergillus* sp. During the early phase of the syndrome, cut surfaces of the lungs of horses and cattle have miliary, yellow-grey nodules distributed irregularly in the ventral portion of the cranial lobes in cattle and in the diaphragmatic lobes in the horse. Microscopically, alveolar spaces are flooded with protein-rich exudation admixed with desquamated alveolar epithelial cells followed by bronchiolar and epithelial hyperplasia. Changes are lobular in the apical and cardiac lobes and the subpleural region of the diaphragmatic lobes. Nodular or diffuse lymphocytic and eosinophilic inflammatory cell infiltrates progress to multifocal granulomatous inflammation with epithelioid macrophages and multinucleated giant cells

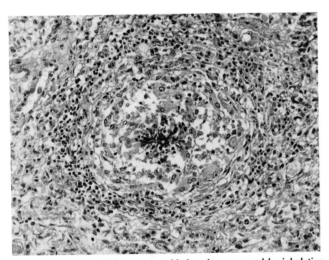

Fig. 15-11 Hypersensitivity pneumonitis in a horse caused by inhalation of mold. Granulomatous inflammation includes a significant component of lymphocytes suggestive of activation of cell-mediated immunity. In this instance, a unitized granuloma surrounds a fragment of inhaled mycelium.

(Fig. 15-11). Fibrosis and smooth muscle hyperplasia develop in chronic stages of the disease. Nodules are typically associated with disease bronchioles placed centrally in the mass of inflammatory cells. Dust particles or fungi can sometimes be seen within epithelioid cells or multinucleated giant cells.

REFERENCES

1. Graham DR: In Gaum GL, Wolinsky E, editors: *Textbook of pulmonary diseases,* ed 5, Boston, 1994, Little, Brown.
2. Berne RM, Levy MN: *Cardiovascular physiology,* ed 2, St Louis, 1972, CV Mosby.
3. Dungworth DL: In Jubb KVF et al, editors: *Pathology of domestic animals,* San Diego, 1993, Academic Press.
4. Dungworth DL: In McClellan RO, Henderson RF, editors: *Concepts in inhalation toxicology,* New York, 1988, Hemisphere Publishing.
5. Smith L, Benoit N: In Cohen GM, editors: *Target organ toxicology,* Boca Raton, 1986, CRC Press.
6. Plopper CG, Pinkerton KE: In Parent RA, editor: *Comparative biology of the normal lung,* Boca Raton, 1992, CRC Press.
7. Hardisty JR et al: Histopathology of nasal olfactory mucosa from selected inhalation toxicity studies conducted with volatile chemicals. *Toxicol Pathol* 27:618, 1999.
8. Last JA: In Witschi H, Nettesheim P, editors: *Mechanisms in respiratory toxicology,* Boca Raton, 1982, CRC Press.
9. Cotran RS et al: *Robbins pathologic basis of disease,* ed 4, Philadelphia, 1989, WB Saunders.
10. Woods LW et al: Structural and biochemical changes in lungs of 3-methylindole-treated rats, *Am J Pathol* 142:129, 1993.
11. Bray RM, Carlson JR: Role of mixed function oxidase in 3-methylindole-induced acute pulmonary edema in goats, *Am J Vet Res* 40:1268, 1979.
12. Yost GS: Mechanisms of 3-methylindole pneumotoxicity, *Chem Res Toxicol* 2:273, 1976.
13. Gram RE: Chemically reactive intermediates and pulmonary xenobiotic toxicity. *Pharmacol Rev* 49:297, 1997.
14. Wells RE: Fatal toxicosis in pet birds caused by an overheated cooking pan lined with polytetrafluoroethylene, *J Am Vet Med Assoc* 182:1248, 1983.
15. Wells RE et al: Acute toxicosis of budgerigars (*Melopsittacus undulatus*) caused by pyrolysis products from heated polytetrafluoroethylene: clinical study, *Am J Vet Res* 43:1238, 1982.
16. Witschi H: Proliferation of type II alveolar cells: a review of common responses in toxic lung injury, *Toxicology* 5:267, 1976.
17. Witschi H et al: Pulmonary toxicity of cytostatic drugs: cell kinetics, *Fund Appl Toxicol* 8:253, 1987.
18. Schwartz LW et al: Silicate pneumoconiosis and pulmonary fibrosis in horses from the Monterey-Carmel Peninsula, *Chest* 80:82S, 1981.
19. Harbison ML, Godleski JJ: Malignant mesothelioma in urban dogs, *Vet Pathol* 20:531, 1983.
20. Pauli B et al: In de Haller R, Suter F, editors: *Aspergillosis and farmer's lung in man and animal,* Bern, 1974, Hans Huber Publishers.

16

Sudden Death

DIFFERENTIAL DIAGNOSIS

Konnie H. Plumlee

Establishing a death as "sudden" can be challenging. To veterinarians sudden death typically means that the animal died acutely with few or no previous clinical signs. Animal owners are usually emotional in these situations, especially if more than one animal has died. Therefore, obtaining an accurate history can be difficult and the veterinarian must ask pointed questions to avoid any misconceptions:

1. The animal may have been ill for one or more days before death, but the illness was not observed, so the owner makes the assumption that the death was sudden. Establishing a timeline is important in these cases. The owner may state that the animal was perfectly healthy the last time he or she saw the animal; however, it may have been 2 or more days since the owner saw the animal closely.

2. The owner may not have recognized the prior clinical signs. The ability of animal owners to determine that an animal is ill early in the course of a disease varies widely. Some clinical signs can be subtle and easily missed.

3. The owner may have recognized the presence of clinical signs, but dismissed them as minor. Clinical signs such as a depressed appetite or mild gastrointestinal signs are not unusual from time to time, and the owner may not have taken them seriously. Feelings of regret are natural after the animal's death and may make an owner reluctant to admit that the animal had been sick before death.

Most poisons that cause sudden death prevent the heart from distributing blood, produce seizures, or prevent oxygen from being released to tissues. Therefore, most poisons that cause sudden death affect the cardiovascular system, the nervous system, the respiratory system, or the hematic system (Table 16-1).

TABLE 16-1 **Poisons that Can Cause Sudden Death**

Source	Toxicant	Species
Plants	Diterpene alkaloids	Cattle primarily; also sheep and horses
	Cardiac glycosides	All
	Taxine alkaloids	All
	Nitropropanol glycosides	Cattle and sheep
	Cevanine alkaloids	Sheep primarily; also cattle and horses
	Quinolizidine alkaloids	Sheep
	Pyridine alkaloids	Livestock
	Carboxyatractyloside	Swine primarily; also cattle and sheep
	Avocado	Goats, caged birds, rabbits
	Tropane alkaloids	Swine primarily, but any species
	Chinaberry	All
	Hops	Dogs
	Cicutoxin	All
	Tryptamine alkaloids	Sheep
	Cyanogenic glycosides	All
	Gossypol	Swine

Continued

TABLE 16-1 **Poisons that Can Cause Sudden Death—cont'd**

Source	Toxicant	Species
Feed-related toxicants	Ionophores	Horses most susceptible
	Nitrate	Ruminants
	Nonprotein nitrogen	Ruminants
	Sodium	All
Toxins	Bufo toads	Dogs most often exposed
	Fireflies	Lizards and frogs
	Blue-green algae	All
	Blister beetles	Horses
Asphyxiant gases	Hydrogen sulfide	All
	Nitrogen dioxide	
	Carbon dioxide	
	Carbon monoxide	
	Cyanide	
	Methane	
Insecticides	Anticholinesterase	All
	Metaldehyde	
	Organochlorines	
Rodenticides	Strychnine	All
	Zinc phosphide	
	Sodium fluoroacetate	
Pharmaceuticals	Tricyclic antidepressants	All
	Tilmicosin	
	Serotonergic drugs	
	Amphetamines	
	Ephedrine	
	Heart medications	

17

Urinary System

DIFFERENTIAL DIAGNOSIS

Konnie H. Plumlee

Most toxic effects in the urinary system involve the kidney. Very few poisons affect the lower urinary tract. Clinical signs are similar regardless of the type of poison (Table 17-1).

TOXIC RESPONSE OF THE URINARY TRACT

Scott D. Fitzgerald and Wilson K. Rumbeiha

KIDNEY

Susceptibility

The kidney is susceptible to toxicants because of its high relative blood flow—approximately 25% of total cardiac output—compared with its low percentage of total body weight (approximately 0.5% in mammals, approaching 1% in some birds).[1,2] The renal cortex receives nearly 90% of the total renal blood flow, whereas the medulla receives 6% to 10% of the blood flow, and the papilla receives approximately 2%.[3] Therefore, blood-borne toxicants tend to be delivered at highest rates to cortical tissues, whereas the medullary and papillary regions are exposed to the highest luminal concentrations of toxicants and for longer periods of time.

The kidney also has high metabolic demands, accounting for approximately 10% of the body's total oxygen consumption.[1] The kidney serves vital roles, including excretion of metabolic wastes, metabolism and excretion of xenobiotics, regulation of extracellular fluid volume, maintenance of electrolyte composition, and regulation of acid-base balance. Many of these functions rely on active transport mechanisms, which can be inhibited by toxicants. Given the diversity of kidney functions, toxicant damage to renal tissues results in a variety of systemic abnormalities.

Different portions of the kidney vary in their susceptibility to toxicant damage. The functional unit of the kidney is the nephron, which is composed of the glomerulus, proximal tubule, loop of Henle, distal tubule, and collecting duct. The proximal tubule is highly involved in active transport of substances and is the most sensitive portion of the nephron to both hypoxia and toxicosis. The principal function of the proximal tubule includes resorption of water, electrolytes, glucose, amino acids, and small peptides. Active resorption of solutes such as glucose, amino acids, and organic acids is dependent on Na/K-adenosine triphosphatase within tubular epithelial cells.[3] Enzymes important in the metabolism of xenobiotics, including mixed function oxidases, are present in high concentrations in the proximal tubule epithelium. Prostaglandins are produced in highest concentrations in medullary collecting ducts, predisposing the inner medullary and papillary regions to nonsteroidal antiinflammatory drug damage as a result of their inhibitory effect on prostaglandins.[3]

The glomerulus contains a tuft of specialized capillaries. The fenestrated endothelium, the glomerular basement membrane, and the visceral epithelial cell foot processes are the three components constituting the glomerular filtration membrane (GFM). Twenty percent to 40% of the blood volume flowing to the glomeruli is filtered through the GFM, which forms the ultrafiltrate.[3]

Despite the kidney's susceptibility to numerous toxicants, it also possesses enzymes for detoxification, some ability to regenerate, and considerable reserve capacity before developing clinical renal failure. Cytochrome P-450s and other enzymes that metabolize xenobiotics are found in highest concentrations in the proximal convoluted tubular epithelium. Even though glomeruli are not capable of regeneration, renal tubules may regenerate if their basement membranes remain intact following injury. In regard to reserve capacity, between 50% and 70% of nephrons must be damaged before elevations in serum renal markers (blood urea nitrogen [BUN], creatinine) occur.[3]

Mechanisms of action

Even though the list of nephrotoxicants is long, the response of the kidney is limited to only five categories (four in the

TABLE 17-1   Poisons that Affect the Urinary System

Source	Toxicant	Species
Plants	Calcinogenic glycosides	Livestock
	Lily	Cats
	Oak	Cattle, sheep
	Oxalates	Livestock
	Pigweed	Swine, cattle
	Ptaquiloside	Primarily cattle, but also other ruminants
Mycotoxins	Citrinin	All
	Ochratoxin	All
	Oosporein	Chicks, turkeys
Other toxins	Blister beetles	Primarily horses, but also cattle
	Cortinarius spp. (mushrooms)	All
	Pit vipers	All
Metals	Arsenic	All
	Mercurial salts	All
Pesticides	3-chloro-p-toluidine hydrochloride	Birds
	Cholecalciferol rodenticide	All
	Diquat	All
	Paraquat	All
Household and industrial	Ethylene glycol	All
	Phenols	Cats most susceptible
	Pine oil	Cats most susceptible
	Toluene	All
Pharmaceuticals	Alkylating antineoplastics	All
	Aminoglycosides	All
	Amphotericin B	All
	Cisplatin	All
	NSAIDs	All
	Sulfonamides	All
	Tetracyclines	All
	Vitamin D	All
	Vitamin K$_3$	Horses

kidney, the fifth affecting predominantly the lower urinary tract) based on anatomic site and reaction (Box 17-1).

Glomerular lesions. Glomerular lesions are among the most common renal lesions reported in animals. These lesions are primarily associated with immune complex deposition in glomerular basement membranes and are caused by a variety of infectious and immune-mediated diseases. However, toxic injury of the glomeruli is infrequently recognized in veterinary medicine. The single, well-recognized, toxicant-induced syndrome with direct glomerular effects is caused by snake venom. Envenomation by poisonous snakes results in a variety of toxic effects, including local reactions at the site of the wound, systemic effects such as shock, disseminated intravascular coagulopathy (DIC), and specific organ effects.[4] Venom from viperid snakes, such as Russell's vipers, and crotalid snakes,

such as rattlesnakes, may cause renal lesions. Both glomeruli and the renal tubules are affected by snake envenomation. Renal tubular necrosis is thought to be caused by a combination of factors, including myoglobinuria from muscle breakdown, ischemia caused by shock, and DIC, and only partly caused by direct toxic effects of venom components. The glomerular lesions result from toxin damage directed toward the glomerular capillary endothelium and the supporting mesangial structures.[5,6] The specific venom components involved and their specific mode of action on glomerular tissues remain an active area of research.

Nephrosis. Acute tubular necrosis, also called tubular nephrosis, is by far the most commonly recognized form of toxicant-induced renal damage.[3] Toxicosis produced by a wide range of xenobiotics manifests itself by this lesion, including antimicrobial drugs, antineoplastic drugs, herbi-

---

| BOX 17-1 | PRINCIPAL ANATOMIC SITES AFFECTED BY AND REACTIONS TO NEPHROTOXINS |

I. KIDNEY

Glomerulus (mesangiolysis)
Snake venoms

Renal tubules (acute tubular necrosis)
Antimicrobials
Antineoplastic drugs
Anesthetics
Chlorinated hydrocarbons
Herbicides
Immunosuppressants
Solvents
Metals
Mycotoxins
Plants: Oxalate-containing and other toxins
Endogenous nephrotoxins

Renal mineralization
Vitamin D
Cholecalciferol-type rodenticides
Plants with vitamin D–like activity

Renal papilla and crest necrosis
Antiinflammatory drugs

II. RENAL PELVIS AND LOWER URINARY TRACT

Contact irritant
Cantharidin

Hemorrhage and neoplasia
Bracken fern (Pteridium aquilinum)

Hemorrhage secondary to other causes
Vitamin D
Anticoagulant rodenticides

---

obstruction of the tubules as well as tubular epithelial necrosis.[1]

Inorganic mercury is a heavy metal that produces tubular necrosis. Mercury binds to various enzyme systems, partly because of its affinity for protein sulfhydryl groups, subsequently resulting in mitochondrial dysfunction.[3] Mercury also produces oxidative stress through lipid peroxidation.

Mineralization. A third type of nephrotoxic response is renal mineralization or nephrocalcinosis. Sources for this type of toxicant include excessive supplementation of vitamin D_3, ingestion of plants containing vitamin D_2, or exposure to the recently developed cholecalciferol-type of rodenticides. Cholecalciferol is metabolized in the liver to a monohydroxy metabolite that is subsequently metabolized by the renal tubular epithelial cells to the dihydroxy metabolites including calcitriol, which is the most active metabolite.[7] Calcitriol then results in increased blood calcium by stimulating calcium absorption in the gut and resorption of calcium from bones, resulting in dystrophic mineralization and damage to renal tubules, glomeruli, and blood vessels.

Papillary necrosis. The fourth type of nephrotoxic response is ischemic necrosis of the inner portion of the renal medulla, the renal papilla, or the renal crest, depending on the host species. Drugs such as acetaminophen and nonsteroidal antiinflammatories (aspirin, ibuprofen, indomethacin, phenylbutazone) produce their therapeutic effects through inhibition of prostaglandin synthesis.[3] The renal papilla receives relatively small amounts of the total renal blood flow, and so when locally produced prostaglandins, which act as vasodilators, in the papillary region are suppressed, the result is even lower local blood flow and ischemia. Although single exposure frequently produces a reversible lesion, repeated exposures result in irreversible necrosis of the medullary loops of Henle and the capillaries, with subsequent papillary fibrosis.

Organ response to injury

The three basic clinicopathologic manifestations of renal injury caused by toxicant damage are discussed in the following paragraphs.

Minimal alterations. The kidney may continue to function using its reserve capacity with only minimal alterations being found on urinalysis, such as inability to concentrate urine (isosthenuria) and increased protein leakage (proteinuria). These abnormalities are indications of mild damage and may be completely reversible.

Acute renal failure. Acute renal failure is a more severe consequence of nephrotoxicity, and is characterized by significant decrease in glomerular filtration rate and elevations in BUN and creatinine (azotemia). Acute renal failure results in marked decrease in urine production (oliguria) or anuria, proteinuria, aminoaciduria, and glucosuria. Common systemic sequelae include dehydration, metabolic acidosis, and hyperphosphatemia.[1] With proper therapy, acute renal failure can be reversed in many cases.

cides, heavy metals, and several classes of plant-related toxins (see Box 17-1). As previously mentioned, the proximal tubule is the portion of the nephron most severely affected by tubular necrosis for most compounds; however, the exact mechanism varies with the xenobiotic. Individual mechanisms for the various compounds are described in greater detail elsewhere in this book; only examples are cited here.

Aminoglycoside antibacterials are water-soluble, low-molecular-weight compounds and are eliminated unmetabolized, primarily by glomerular filtration. They are present in high concentrations in the renal tubules and are reabsorbed by proximal tubule epithelium cells. Aminoglycosides produce renal nephrosis by inhibiting phospholipases, leading to lysosomal dysfunction and eventually lysis.[1,3]

Oxalate toxicants, originating as metabolites from ingested ethylene glycol or directly from ingestion of oxalate-containing plants, produce tubular necrosis by chelating calcium and forming calcium oxalate crystals within renal tubules. The calcium oxalate crystals cause mechanical

Chronic renal failure. Chronic renal failure is a result of prolonged renal damage and is manifested after the reserve capacity is exhausted. It represents a progression of renal damage toward end-stage kidneys and is frequently irreversible. Chronic renal failure is characterized by polyuria, isosthenuria, and elevations in BUN and creatinine. Progressive renal failure is not dependent on continued or repeated toxicant exposure. The kidneys react with compensatory mechanisms, following even a single toxicant exposure, and these compensatory mechanisms themselves may lead to continued and progressive renal damage.

Gross lesions

Mild cases of nephrotoxicosis are generally not associated with gross lesions. Kidneys suffering from more severe acute toxicoses, resulting in acute renal failure, are swollen and excessively moist on cut section. The renal parenchyma may be paler than normal and striations normally visible in the renal tissue become less clearly defined. Cases associated with diffuse vascular congestion or with pigments such as hemoglobin may present with a diffusely dark or reddened kidney. Linear pale streaks in the cortex or medulla are often grossly visible in cases associated with tubule crystal deposition or parenchymal mineralization. Papillary necrosis may present grossly as a zone of pale ischemic tissue within the inner papilla and crest; however, in chronic cases the entire papilla and crest may appear as a sharply delineated mass of dry, dark necrotic tissue.

Chronic renal failure generally results in more obvious gross lesions. End-stage kidneys are often smaller than normal, exhibiting asymmetry of size and shape between the two kidneys. The subcapsular surface tends to be pitted and irregular, and it is difficult to peel off the renal capsule as a result of multifocal fibrous adhesions. The kidney may be difficult to section because of increased interstitial fibrosis, and it may be gritty because of partial mineralization of

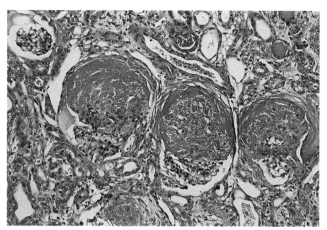

Fig. 17-2 Photomicrograph of canine renal tissue after exposure to snake venom. Three glomeruli have varying degrees of hemorrhage and necrosis (mesangiolysis). (10×)

tissues. On cut section, the end-stage kidney may have marked variation in cortical and medullary tissue thickness, single or multiple renal cysts, and radiating pale streaks within the cortex representing interstitial fibrosis (Fig. 17-1).

Histopathology

As previously stated, despite the long list of toxicants that have primary renal effects, nephrotoxicants can be divided into five basic categories based on anatomic site and reaction (see Box 17-1).

Mesangiolysis. One of the least frequently reported forms of nephrotoxicosis in veterinary species is mesangiolysis, which involves necrosis and destruction of the glomerulus. Envenomation by poisonous snakes, including viperidae and crotalidae, results in a variety of toxic renal effects. In the kidney, glomerular alterations include damage to the endothelium, formation of hemorrhagic cysts, and destruction of the mesangial matrix, hence the term *mesangiolysis* (Fig. 17-2).[5,6] These changes vary from mild to severe, and the more mildly affected individuals that survive may develop mesangial proliferative glomerulonephritis. In addition, tubular necrosis in snake envenomation cases is frequent, which is believed to be caused by a combination of direct toxic tubular effects of venom fractions, as well as myoglobinuria and ischemia caused by systemic effects of the toxins.

Nephrosis. By far the most common form of toxic nephropathy is acute tubular necrosis, also referred to as nephrosis. Microscopically, this tends to affect the proximal tubules most severely, and is characterized by degeneration and necrosis of the proximal convoluted tubular epithelium (Fig. 17-3). Epithelial cells swell, developing intracytoplasmic vacuolation or hypereosinophilia. The nuclei become pyknotic and then lyse (karyolysis). Eventually, entire cells slough and undergo lysis, and the cytoplasmic remnants accumulate within the dilated tubular lumens forming granular or cellular casts.

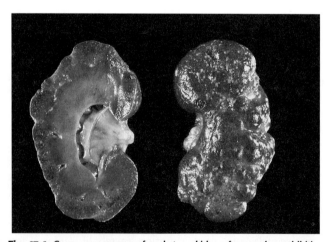

Fig. 17-1 Gross appearance of end-stage kidney from a dog exhibiting chronic renal failure. The capsular surface is pitted and irregular *(right)*. The cut section shows the uneven thickness of the cortical tissue *(left)*.

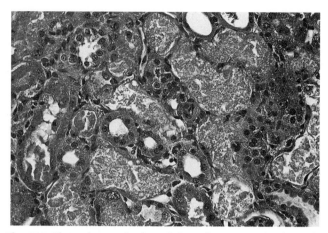

Fig. 17-3 Photomicrograph of renal tissue from a rat experimentally dosed with mercuric chloride. Multiple proximal tubules exhibit acute tubular necrosis characterized by loss of nuclei, and lumens filled with hypereosinophilic cellular debris. Admixed are relatively normal appearing distal tubules and collecting ducts. (40×)

Differentiation between acute tubular necrosis as a result of poisons or ischemia is sometimes possible, particularly in acutely affected individuals. Ischemia tends to cause a patchy epithelial necrosis as compared with the more extensive necrosis associated with toxicants.[1] Ischemia also produces a more severe necrosis that disrupts the tubular basement membrane, whereas poisons usually leave the basement membrane intact (at least until tubular swelling results in secondary localized ischemia). Through the use of either periodic acid-Schiff reaction or one of the many silver stains available, basement membranes can be evaluated microscopically to attempt differentiation between toxic and ischemic-induced tubular necrosis.

Mineralization. Renal mineralization or nephrocalcinosis may occur as a result of a variety of toxicants or as a secondary feature of renal failure. Deposits of calcium salts in the kidney tend to occur along basement membranes first, such as those lining the renal tubules, blood vessels, and glomerular tuft and capsule (Fig. 17-4). Histologically, mineral appears as thin basophilic, slightly refractile material with routine hematoxylin and eosin staining. Special stains for calcium, such as Von Kossa's stain, can be used to confirm the microscopic diagnosis. As mineralization progresses, the tubular epithelial lining becomes mineralized and degenerates, until cells exfoliate and result in tubular obstruction. Because mineral is harder than the surrounding soft tissues, the microtome blade tends to cause a shattering effect, resulting in sharp and angular bits of basophilic material, lending a distinctive microscopic appearance to mineral.

Papillary necrosis. The final category for toxicant-induced change in the kidney is necrosis of the renal papilla or crest. This portion of the kidney receives the least blood flow, and agents that tend to further restrict blood flow locally result in this type of damage. The entire inner portion of the renal medulla becomes ischemic, resulting in poorly stained necrotic tubules, whereas the surrounding area maintains normal staining affinity and may show varying degrees of vascular congestion (Fig. 17-5). Subsequently, the ischemic tissue may undergo complete coagulative necrosis and may become partially mineralized as well.

LOWER URINARY TRACT

Susceptibility

The lower urinary tract, consisting of the ureters, urinary bladder, and urethra, is more resistant to toxic-induced injury than the kidney. Perhaps this reduced susceptibility is because urinary wastes travel through this portion of the tract relatively rapidly, and the transitional epithelium lining these regions is less metabolically active than renal tissues. For this discussion, the renal pelvis is also considered part of

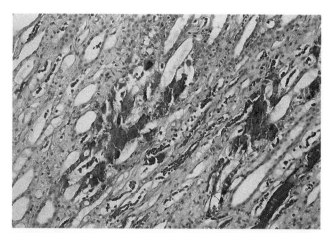

Fig. 17-4 Photomicrograph of renal tissue from a dog experimentally dosed with cholecalciferol. Multiple renal tubules contain partially mineralized epithelium which appears dark and angular (nephrocalcinosis). (20×)

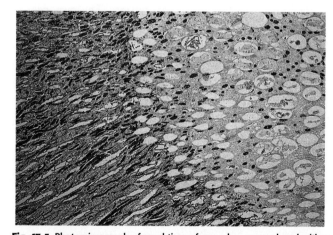

Fig. 17-5 Photomicrograph of renal tissue from a horse overdosed with a nonsteroidal antiinflammatory agent. Note the clear line of demarcation between the normal congested portion of the proximal papilla (*left*), and the pale-stained necrotic tubules in the distal papilla (*right*). (4×)

the lower urinary tract. It is anatomically part of the kidney, but its transitional lining and toxic responses are similar to those of the lower urinary tract. The portion of the lower urinary tract that is most commonly affected by toxicants is the urinary bladder because it acts as the holding chamber for urinary wastes between voidings. If toxicants are present in the urine, they have more prolonged exposure to the bladder lining.

Mechanisms of action

Hemorrhage of the lower tract is the most frequently seen response to toxic injury. Several poisons act systemically and damage blood vessels or interfere with blood clotting, so the resulting hemorrhages found in the urinary bladder are nonspecific, as with vitamin D toxicosis and anticoagulant rodenticides. On the other hand, the mechanism of action of cantharidin from ingestion of hay contaminated with blister beetles *(Epicauta* sp.) is that of a contact irritant. Even though all levels of the urinary tract, from the renal pelvis down through the urethra, can hemorrhage, the risk of hemorrhage is generally most severe in the urinary bladder.[1]

The mechanisms involved in enzootic hematuria, caused by ingestion of bracken ferns *(Pteridium aquilinum)* by ruminants, are more complicated. Toxins present in bracken ferns include a thiaminase, an unidentified bleeding factor, and multiple carcinogens (quercetin, shikimic acid, prunasin, ptaquiloside, aquilide A).[1] Although hemorrhages may be present throughout the lower urinary tract, they are most easily seen in the bladder mucosa. These hemorrhages are caused by the acute effect of the toxin on bone marrow, causing a pancytopenia and thrombocytopenia. With more prolonged ingestion, the chronic activity of the carcinogens results in multiple epithelial or mesenchymal neoplasms in the bladder, which frequently ulcerate and bleed into the bladder lumen.

Organ response to injury

Toxicants within the urine cause damage to the transitional epithelium lining the lower urinary tract. The responses of the transitional epithelium are limited, and include multifocal hemorrhage, ulceration, inflammation (ureteritis, cystitis, urethritis), squamous metaplasia, and neoplastic transformation into a variety of epithelial tumors.

Gross lesions

The most common gross lesions in urinary bladders in response to toxicants are multifocal petechial, ecchymotic, or suffusive hemorrhages. Large patches of the urinary bladder lining may become diffusely reddened and roughened in response to contact irritants. In response to chronic bracken fern ingestion, single or multiple polypoid tumors arise from the bladder wall and protrude into the lumen. These bladder tumors resulting from exposure to carcinogens within the urine most frequently develop in the trigone area, or along the ventral and lateral fundic bladder walls, because these sites have the most prolonged contact with urine.[8]

Histopathology

Microscopic alterations in the urinary bladder are consistent with the organ responses previously described. Hemorrhages within the mucosa are commonly seen. Cystitis varies from acute with associated ulcerations of the epithelium and variable leukocyte infiltrates, to chronic with subepithelial fibrosis. Transitional epithelium, when chronically irritated, tends to become initially hyperplastic and then undergoes metaplasia to squamous epithelium. Following neoplastic transformation, the epithelium may give rise to papillomas, transitional cell carcinomas, or squamous cell carcinomas, The underlying mesenchymal tissues may give rise to fibromas, fibrosarcomas, hemangiomas, hemangiosarcomas, leiomyomas, or leiomyosarcomas.[1,8]

REFERENCES

1. Maxie GM: The urinary system. In Jubb KVF et al, editors: *Pathology of domestic animals*, ed 4, San Diego, 1993, Academic Press.
2. King AS, McLelland J: Urinary system. In *Birds, their structure and function*, ed 2, London, 1984, Bailliere Tindall.
3. Goldstein RS, Schnellmann RG: Toxic responses of the kidney. In Klaassen CD, editor: *Casarett & Doull's toxicology: the basic science of poisons*, ed 5, New York, 1996, McGraw-Hill.
4. Sitprija V, Chaiyabutr N: Nephrotoxicity in snake envenomation. *J Nat Toxins* 8:271, 1999.
5. Swe TN et al: Russell's viper venom fractions and nephrotoxicity. *Southeast Asian J Trop Med Public Health* 28:657, 1997.
6. Morita T et al: Mesangiolysis: an update. *Am J Kid Dis* 31:559, 1998.
7. Tepperman J, Tepperman HM: Hormonal regulation of calcium homeostasis. In *Metabolic and endocrine physiology*, ed 5, Chicago, 1987, Year Book Medical Publishers.
8. Nielsen SW, Moulton JE: Tumors of the urinary system. In Moulton JE, editor: *Tumors in domestic animals*, ed 3, Berkeley, 1990, University of California Press.

PART THREE

CLASSES OF TOXICANTS

18

Biotoxins

BACTERIA

Joseph D. Roder

BOTULISM

Synonyms. Botulism, limber neck (avian), and shaker foal syndrome (horses) are names used for the disease caused by toxins produced by *Clostridium botulinum*.

Sources. *C. botulinum* is an anaerobic, gram-positive, spore-forming rod that is commonly found in soil. Seven distinct antigenic botulinum toxins include A, B, C, D, E, F, and G.[1] In the United States, type A toxin is found mostly in the west and type B toxin is typically found in the mid-Atlantic states and Kentucky. The toxin is heat labile; however, the spores of the bacteria are resistant to drying and normal environmental temperatures.

Mechanism of Action. The toxin is comprised of a heavy chain (100-kD) and a light chain (50-kD) that are linked together by disulfide bonds and noncovalent forces.[1] Following ingestion of the toxin, the heavy chain binds a specific presynaptic vesicle protein, synaptotagmin. The botulinum toxin is then internalized via endocytosis and the disulfide bond linking the heavy and light chains is cleaved. The light chain of the botulinum toxin cleaves neuronal proteins associated with docking and release of the acetylcholine vesicles. There are differences in specific protein binding of the light chain depending on the toxin. The light chains of botulinum toxins A and E cleave a synaptosome-associated protein of 25 kD (SNAP-25).[2] The light chains of botulinum toxin B, D, F, and G cleave a specific substrate vesicle-associated membrane protein (VAMP or synaptobrevin), whereas the light chain of botulinum toxin C cleaves both SNAP-25 and syntaxin (a synaptic membrane-associated protein).[3]

The cumulative result of the proteolytic actions of the botulinum toxins is a disruption of the protein scaffolding within the presynaptic terminus that is responsible for the docking, fusion, and release of the acetylcholine vesicles. The botulinum toxins block the release of acetylcholine from the presynaptic neuron of the neuromuscular junction, resulting in flaccid paralysis.

Toxicity and Risk Factors. Botulism occurs from one of three mechanisms: ingestion of preformed toxin, ingestion of spores, or contamination of wounds with spores. Toxico-infectious botulism (shaker foal syndrome) occurs in foals that ingest spores, which result in an overgrowth of the organism in the gastrointestinal system. Wound botulism occurs in deep puncture sites or surgical sites such as castration or hernia repair.

Ingestion of preformed toxin is most common in cattle, adult horses, and birds. Outbreaks of botulism caused by ingestion of preformed toxin can occur in livestock after consumption of improperly ensiled poultry litter, small grain haylage, alfalfa silage, or alfalfa hay cubes. Other sources of preformed toxin are poultry litter or hay contaminated with decaying carcasses of chickens, rodents, or cats.[4] Waterfowl are at increased risk of intoxication when eating rotten vegetation in shallow waters.

Cattle are most commonly affected by toxins B, C, and D in North America. Horses are most commonly affected by type B, but can also be affected by types A and C. Both domestic and wild avian species are most commonly affected by type C. Swine, dogs, and cats are reported to be less sensitive to botulism.

Clinical Signs. The classic clinical syndrome attributable to botulism is a progressive flaccid paralysis. Animals suffering from clinical botulism commonly exhibit weakness and ataxia. These signs may be more pronounced when the animal is excited or forced to move. Acute death may be the first clinical sign noted and large numbers of animals may die in a short period, especially waterfowl. Weakness of the muscles of the tail are often noted and may be used to identify an affected animal. Exercise intolerance and ataxia are common findings in horses.[5] Affected animals may also exhibit difficulties with prehension and swallowing. Other gastrointestinal signs may include ileus, constipation, or ruminal atony. Death is generally thought to be due to respiratory paralysis.

Unique symptoms occur in foals, which develop tremors (shaker foal syndrome), and in waterfowl, which develop a profound weakness in the neck (limber neck).

Diagnostic Testing. Analysis of serum, gastrointestinal contents, and feedstuffs for the preformed toxin may support a clinical diagnosis of botulism. Ruminal fluids may be obtained from animals exhibiting acute death and analyzed for botulism toxins.[6] A mouse bioassay is available in most diagnostic laboratories. An enzyme-linked immunosorbent assay technique is available at some laboratories, but it is currently specific for only one toxin type, which limits its usefulness as a screening method.

Treatment. The initial step in treatment is to remove any feedstuffs that may be causing the disease. Individual treatment of affected animals may include antitoxin therapy if a correct clinical diagnosis can be made early in the course of disease. Antitoxin, antibiotics (penicillin), and debridement of wounds may be beneficial for animals suffering from wound botulism.[7] Animals should also receive symptomatic and supportive care; small animals may require artificial respiration.

Prognosis. The prognosis in animals exhibiting clinical signs is guarded to poor. If a contaminated feedstuff is the source of intoxication, many animals may die. Botulism-related mortality has been reported to continue for 17 days after a single-day exposure to contaminated feedstuffs.[8]

Prevention and Control. Vaccination against the *C. botulinum* toxins with toxoid can prevent clinical disease. Evaluation and management of feedstuffs is essential. Proper ensiling of poultry litter with mixing to allow the surface material to be exposed to elevated temperatures is required. All feeds should be examined for evidence of decaying carcasses.[4,5] A rodent control program reduces the number of mice or rats in stored feeds. Proper disposal of any dead animals (deep burial) reduces exposure to botulism toxin.

TETANUS

Synonyms. Tetanus is also known as "lockjaw."

Sources. A neurotoxin, tetanospamin, is produced by *C. tetani*.[1,2] The clostridial organism is a gram-positive, strictly anaerobic bacteria. The bacteria are shed in the feces and sporulates, and remain in the environment for long periods. The organism also produces a cytolysin, called tetanolysin, which induces pore formation in a variety of cells to aid in the replication of the tetanus organism locally at the wound site.[3]

Mechanism of Action. Tetanus toxin prevents the release of inhibitory neurotransmitters, particularly glycine, from neurons in the central nervous system, which results in uncontrolled muscular contractions. Tetanus toxin is generated from the clostridial organisms in the anaerobic wound environment. To gain entry into neurons, the tetanus toxin interacts with gangliosides (GT1b, GD1b) on the surface of neurons. It is thought that these gangliosides are associated with a tetanus toxin receptor.[1] The tetanus toxin is then internalized into the neuronal cell and the disulfide bonds that hold the heavy and light chains of the toxin are cleaved. The toxin enters into the cytoplasm of peripheral neurons, is incorporated into endocytic vesicles, and travels retroaxonally to the central nervous system.[2] The light chain of the tetanus toxin is a zinc endopeptidase that cleaves VAMP.[1,2] This results in an interruption of translocation and exocytosis of neurotransmitters from inhibitory neurons at the spinal cord.

Toxicity and Risk Factors. The persistent spores are ubiquitous in the feces and soil in areas where animals are raised. Spores of the organism are introduced into a wound. Animals at greater risk include those that have had recent field surgeries, castrations, shearing, or retained placentas. Horses and ruminants are more susceptible to tetanus than are cats and dogs.[4] It has been suggested that species sensitivity to tetanus may be due to differences in the gangliosides on the neurons.[2]

Clinical Signs. Affected animals exhibit generalized musculoskeletal stiffness. The nictitating membrane ("third eyelid") is often elevated and fine motor muscles of the eyelids may be affected, resulting in abnormal blinking response. In carnivores, contraction of the muscles of the lips produces a "sardonic grin." These clinical signs may progress to more severe muscular rigidity, leading to the classic "sawhorse stance," a fixed stare, erect ears, a reluctance to eat or drink because of a "locked jaw," an elevated tail, and flared nostrils. As the disease progresses, an increase in muscular rigidity may cause the animal to become recumbent and unable to rise. In all species, convulsions may occur; death is caused by marked contraction of the muscles of respiration. These episodes of muscular contraction can be induced by external stimuli such as a sudden loud noise or a flashing light.

Lesions. No lesions are characteristic of tetanus intoxication in animals.

Diagnostic Testing. A diagnosis can be made by finding the organism *C. tetani* in a culture of the wound. Attempts to identify the toxins from affected animals is generally unrewarding.

Treatment. The treatment should include antibiotic therapy (penicillin) to eliminate the bacterial replication at the wound site, antitoxin therapy, and cleaning of the wound. Individual animals may be managed by placing them in dark, quiet areas to minimize convulsions from external stimuli.[4] Additionally, the use of tranquilizers to control convulsions may need to be considered.

The antitoxin is an equine-derived product from healthy horses that have been hyperimmunized with repeated doses of *C. tetani* toxin. Treatment is 10,000 to 50,000 units of antitoxin subcutaneously or intramuscularly to horses and cattle; 3,000 to 15,000 units to sheep and swine. Repeated doses of antitoxin may be required 7 to 10 days later as clinical judgment warrants. Serum hepatitis (Theiler's disease) is possible following antitoxin administration. Animals suffering from this adverse reaction may exhibit subcutaneous edema, icterus, elevation of hepatic-specific enzymes, and possibly death.[5,6]

Prognosis.   The prognosis for animals showing clinical signs is guarded to poor.

Prevention and Control.   All attempts should be made to prevent the introduction of the organism into any wounds or surgical sites. Good husbandry practices include using clean needles and clean blades for vaccination, tagging, and castration.

Optimal tetanus protection includes a vaccination program, especially for farms or operations with a history of tetanus. In general, the manufacturers' recommendation for bacterin or toxoid for an unvaccinated animal is two injections separated by 2 to 4 weeks. Furthermore, a preventive, presurgical dose of 1500 units of antitoxin administered subcutaneously or intramuscularly should be considered on farms where there is a history of tetanus or if the animal's tetanus vaccination status is unknown. The tetanus antitoxin may be used concurrently with toxoid vaccination. However, these products should be given in different injection sites to prevent any possible interaction.

BLUE-GREEN ALGAE

Joseph D. Roder

Synonyms.   Cyanobacteria is another name for blue-green algae.

Sources.   Not all algae produce toxins. Cyanobacteria intoxication is most commonly associated with ingestion of water with excessive growth of *Anabaena* sp., *Aphanizomenon* sp., *Oscillatoria* sp., which produce the neurotoxins anatoxin-a and anatoxin-a(s); *Microcystis* sp., which produces the hepatotoxin microcystin; or *Nodularia* sp., which produces the hepatotoxin nodularin.[1-3]

Toxicokinetics.   The cyanobacteria ingested with water can be rapidly broken down in the gastrointestinal tract. In the acidic environment of the stomach, the bacteria are lysed with the resulting release of toxins.[2] Free toxins can be rapidly absorbed from the small intestine. The microcystins are transported to the liver and enter this organ using a bile acid transporter.[3]

Mechanism of Action.   The hepatotoxic microcystins and nodularin alter the cytoskeleton of liver cells. Microcystin action relates to its ability to inhibit serine/threonine phosphatases type 1 and type 2A (PP1 and PP2A).[3,4] The microcystins bind covalently to and inhibit the function of the protein phosphatases, which regulate the phosphorylation and dephosphorylation of regulatory intracellular proteins. In vitro, microcystins act on intermediate filaments (vimentin or cytokeratin), microtubules, and microfilaments causing

altered structural integrity of these cytoskeletal elements.[5] Microcystins have also induced apoptosis in a variety of mammalian cells in vitro.[4] Microcystin causes immediate blebbing of the cell membranes, shrinkage of cells, organelle redistribution, chromatin condensation, DNA fragmentation, and DNA ladder formation.[4]

The neurotoxin anatoxin-a, most commonly produced by *Anabaena flos-aquae*, is a bicyclic secondary amine that causes depolarization of nicotinic membranes.[1,6] The depolarization of neuronal nicotinic membranes is rapid and persistent and can lead to respiratory paralysis.

The neurotoxin anatoxin-a(s) inhibits acetylcholinesterase in the peripheral nervous system. This toxin does not appear to cross the blood-brain barrier.

Toxicity and Risk Factors.   The environmental risk factors most commonly associated with intoxication include warm weather, increased nutrients in the body of water, and wind. A rapid increase in the growth of the algae, or a "bloom," is more commonly noted in warm weather during the late summer and early fall. This rapid growth is enhanced by increased nitrogen and phosphorus in the water, which may be more prevalent in ponds that receive runoff from fertilized fields. Increased wind activity concentrates the cyanobacteria along the shoreline of the pond or lake, thereby increasing the risk of intoxication.

Clinical Signs.   Ingestion of water that contains cyanobacteria or their associated toxins may result in acute death with few clinical signs.[7]

Within 1 to 4 hours, animals that ingest microcystin or nodularin can present with a myriad of clinical signs that generally relate to damage of the liver: lethargy, vomiting, diarrhea, gastrointestinal atony, weakness, and pale mucous membranes.[2,3,8] Death often occurs within 24 hours, but may be delayed several days. In animals that survive the initial toxicosis, secondary photosensitization may develop.[2]

Animals that ingest anatoxin-a may present acutely with muscle tremors, rigidity, lethargy, respiratory distress, and convulsions.[1] Death from respiratory paralysis can occur within 30 minutes from the onset of clinical signs.

Following ingestion of anatoxin-a(s) animals may present with signs consistent with inhibition of cholinesterase: increased salivation, urination, lacrimation, and defecation as well as tremors, dyspnea, and convulsions.[1] Death from respiratory arrest can occur within 1 hour.

Clinical Pathology.   Animals intoxicated with microcystin-producing cyanobacteria have elevated serum concentrations of hepatic enzymes.[3,8] Anatoxin-a(s) depresses the blood cholinesterase activity, but not the brain cholinesterase activity because it does not cross the blood-brain barrier.

Lesions.   Microcystin results in an enlarged liver that is congested and dark in color (hemorrhagic).[1,2,8] Hepatic enlargement is thought to be a result of intrahepatic hemorrhage. Histologic examination of the liver reveals a centrilobular to midzonal necrosis and hemorrhage.[2,7,8]

Gross and microscopic lesions are typically not noted following intoxication with the anatoxins or saxitoxin.

Diagnostic Testing. A water sample should be carefully taken from the area of greatest concentration of algae. Examination of fresh or formalin-preserved samples using light microscopy identifies the toxin-producing cyanobacteria. A sample of the water might be used in a mouse bioassay; however, this bioassay is not universally available in diagnostic laboratories. Water samples may also be examined by a few laboratories using high-performance liquid chromatography (HPLC)/thin-layer chromatography (TLC) or gas chromatography-mass spectrometry (GC-MS) to identify the causative toxin.

Recently a colorimetric assay has been developed to identify the presence of microcystin-LR in water.[9] This method can detect microcystin-LR at concentrations of 1 μg/L and may be used as a screening tool to identify potentially positive samples with additional confirmation by HPLC or MS methods.

Treatment. None of the cyanobacteria have antidotes; therefore, therapy is directed toward symptomatic and supportive therapy. Decontamination of dogs includes emesis, activated charcoal, and a cathartic as well as bathing if algae remains on the haircoat. Decontamination in large animals is limited to activated charcoal, a cathartic, and possibly bathing.

Animals that present with signs associated with the hepatotoxic algae should be aggressively treated with fluids, corticosteroids, and other elements of shock therapy. Animals that present with signs associated with the neurotoxic algae require aggressive respiratory support and seizure control as needed. Additionally, animals with anatoxin-a(s) toxicosis may be treated with atropine to reverse muscarinic signs.

Prognosis. Animals that exhibit clinical signs of intoxication have a poor to grave prognosis, depending on the amount of toxin consumed.

Prevention and Control. The key control measure is to limit or eliminate animal exposure to water containing the algae. If possible, the animals should be moved to a different pasture or the water source fenced off and an alternate water supply provided. The use of copper sulfate as an algaecide in ponds with a cyanobacterial bloom may be beneficial. After treatment with copper sulfate, animals must be removed from the water source for a period of 3 to 7 days to allow for the degradation of the cyanobacterial toxins.[3]

INSECTS

BLISTER BEETLES

Eric L. Stair and Konnie H. Plumlee

Synonyms. The disease caused by blister beetles is referred to as cantharidin toxicosis or cantharidiasis. Cantharidin has been used for centuries as a treatment for a variety of illnesses and as a supposed aphrodisiac known as Spanish fly.[1-3]

Sources. Cantharidin is a bicyclic terpenoid (sesquiterpene) vesicant found in the hemolymph and genitalia of blister beetles.[1,4,5] Production of cantharidin is believed to act as a chemical defense against predation.[1,3] Hundreds of beetle species exist; however, those that produce cantharidin are in the Meloidae family, especially in the *Epicauta* genus.[5] Only males synthesize the vesicant, which they transfer to females during copulation.[1-3,5]

Adult beetles feed primarily on plant floral parts; some beetles, particularly the *Epicauta* spp., eat leaves as well. Most cases of blister beetle toxicosis occur when livestock eat alfalfa hay produced in the semiarid regions of the United States, especially Texas and Oklahoma, where the three-striped blister beetles *(Epicauta temexa* and *Epicauta occidentalis)* are the most common species associated with toxicosis.[1,3,6]

Mechanism of Action. Cantharidin is rapidly absorbed from the gastrointestinal tract and excreted in the urine.[5] Because of the vesicant properties of cantharidin, irritation characterized by acantholysis and vesicle formation leading to ulcers or erosions occurs where the compound contacts a mucosal surface. The exact mechanism for this action is unclear; however, cantharidin results in an increased mitotic rate in epithelial cell tissue cultures.[5] It is thought to interfere with the oxidative enzyme systems that are involved with active transport across the mitochondrial membrane, resulting in permeability changes.[5] Disruption of the membrane results in acantholysis and vesicle formation.[5] In mouse studies, cantharidin inhibits protein phosphatase 2A, which controls cell proliferation, modulates phosphatases and protein kinases involved in cell function, and plays a role in the activity of cellular membrane channels and receptors.[1]

Toxicity and Risk Factors. Adult blister beetles feed principally on lush alfalfa fields as the alfalfa plants mature and bloom. Some blister beetle species are gregarious, congregating in large numbers, especially near field margins. Livestock poisoning usually is a result of ingestion of alfalfa hay that has had beetle swarms baled into the hay. Therefore, blister beetles that exhibit this swarming behavior are of greatest concern because of the greater risk of a large number of beetles becoming trapped in a small amount of hay.[1] The species most commonly recognized for its swarming characteristic is the three-striped blister beetle, *Epicauta lemniscata.* However, many other species (*E. occidentalis, E. temexa, E. pennsylvanica, E. maculata, E. vittata*) are commonly associated with cantharidin toxicosis of livestock.

Modern hay harvesting practices (e.g., hay crimping) increase the likelihood that blister beetles are incorporated into hay.[1,5] Cantharidin is released when adults are crushed and can contaminate hay even if the beetles are not found in the hay. Cantharidin is a colorless, odorless, and stable chemical. Chemically killing the beetles does not diminish the toxin's activity. Even the remains or dried juices from crushed beetles in the hay may cause severe digestive and urinary tract disease in livestock. Toxicity is not affected by storage time of the hay.[5]

Even though cantharidin toxicosis is usually localized in the southern United States where alfalfa is grown, toxicosis has been reported from Florida to Arizona and as far north as Illinois.[5,6] However, poisoning can occur anywhere because of the transport of alfalfa hay contaminated with cantharidin.[3] Processed alfalfa products, such as alfalfa pellets, green chop, cubes, or silage, may also contain cantharidin because the compound is heat stable; however, toxicosis from these sources is unlikely presumably because of dilution during processing.

Cantharidin toxicosis is most commonly reported in horses, which may be more susceptible to the toxic effects than other livestock.[1,6] However, cases have also been reported in sheep and cattle.[1,6] Toxicosis occurred in emu chicks that ingested *Pyrota insulata*, which is a species of blister beetles found in Texas and Oklahoma and whose main food source is blooms of mesquite trees.[2]

Studies on common blister beetle species indicate widely varying amounts of cantharidin, from less than 1% to more than 5% of dry weight.[3,6] Such variation in cantharidin content of beetles within the same species makes it difficult to determine the number of beetles necessary to result in toxicosis.

The toxicity of blister beetles to horses is estimated at a minimum lethal dose of 1 mg or less of cantharidin/kg of body weight.[1,5,6] The number of beetles necessary to provide a lethal dose of cantharidin depends on the amount of cantharidin present in the beetles and the weight of the horse (Table 18-1).

Clinical Signs.   The severity of clinical signs varies according to the dose of cantharidin consumed. Signs can range from depression and discomfort to severe colic.[5] Animals ingesting high doses may experience severe shock and death within several hours.[7] An apparently healthy animal may be found dead with little or no signs of struggle after being fed contaminated hay the night before.[7]

In horses, the most frequent signs are related to colic: restlessness, depression, sweating, congested mucous membranes, increased heart rate, and increased respiratory rate. Horses with gastric lesions may submerge their muzzles or play in water. Other common signs include fever, pollakiuria, and diarrhea. Blood is usually not seen in the feces; however, feces are frequently positive for occult blood.[5] Less common signs include oral lesions, salivation, stiff gait, and blood-tinged urine. Synchronous diaphragmatic flutter and muscle fasciculations are believed to be caused by hypocalcemia.

Clinical Pathology.   The packed cell volume is typically elevated. The serum protein concentration may be normal or elevated early in the disease, but frequently goes below normal in horses that survive longer than 24 hours.[5] Increased creatine kinase occurs in some horses; persistently increasing levels indicates a poor prognosis.[5] The urine specific gravity is often low even in dehydrated horses.[5]

Decreased serum total calcium occurs in many horses; however, a normal or slightly reduced serum ionized calcium has been reported.[5] Serum magnesium is significantly decreased in many horses. In experimental toxicosis, hypocalcemia and hypomagnesemia were the most persistent findings even after all other values had returned to baseline levels.[4] Potassium is usually within a normal range, but mild or transient hypokalemia has been reported.[5]

Lesions.   Large doses of cantharidin may result in sudden death without gross lesions.[4,7] However, because of the irritant nature of cantharidin, some animals display gross lesions throughout the urinary tract and gastrointestinal tract, possibly including the lips and oral cavity. Lesions are most common in the terminal portion of the esophagus, stomach, and intestines.[5,7] Classic lesions consist of areas of ulceration or erosion. However, lesions may be limited to reddening of the mucosal lining of the gastrointestinal tract and urinary bladder.[7] Streaks of ventricular myocardial necrosis occur occasionally.[1,5]

Diagnostic Testing.   Samples of urine or intestinal contents (500 ml each) are the preferred diagnostic specimens and may be submitted for analysis by HPLC or GC-MS.[1,5,6] Detection of cantharidin at any level is considered clinically significant.[1] Urine samples should be collected for analysis as early as possible because renal clearance of cantharidin is rapid (3 to 4 days).[1,5] Liver, kidney, and serum samples have also been used for chromatographic analysis, but they are not the specimens of choice.

Treatment.   Treatment of cantharidin toxicosis should focus on enhancing fecal and urinary elimination of cantharidin, correcting dehydration, managing serum calcium and magnesium abnormalities, and controlling pain.[7] Intensive supportive treatment may be required for 3 to 10 days depending on the severity of illness.[7]

Mineral oil should be administered to provide a lipid-soluble substrate to possibly bind cantharidin and to hasten movement of poison through the intestinal tract. Repeated doses of mineral oil may be beneficial. Activated charcoal may also bind cantharidin.

Commonly prescribed analgesics may not provide adequate pain relief. Therefore, α_2-adrenergic agonists may need to be administered in horses. Acepromazine maleate is contraindicated because it may potentiate shock.[5]

Fluid therapy should be established to adequately rehydrate the horse, decrease serum cantharidin levels, and increase toxin excretion via the kidneys.[5] Serum calcium and magnesium levels should be monitored frequently during treatment and fluids supplemented with these electrolytes if indicated. Calcium preparations should be diluted in isotonic fluids that do not contain sodium bicarbonate and administered slowly.[5]

TABLE 18-1 **Estimated Number of Beetles Necessary to Provide a Lethal Dose of Cantharidin (Assuming the Lethal Dose Is 1 mg/kg)**

Cantharidin Content (mg/beetle)	Horse Weight (lbs)	
	550	1100
1	250	500
2	125	250
3	83	166
4	63	126
5	50	100

Prognosis. A prognosis of poor to guarded is warranted in most cases, depending on the amount of cantharidin ingested. A more favorable prognosis may be given if the animal is diagnosed early and responds to aggressive treatment. Experimental cantharidiasis resulted in a higher incidence of nonsurvival when a persistent increase in pulse and respiratory rate or an increasing creatine kinase level was observed.[4]

Prevention and Control. Prevention centers on feeding alfalfa hay that is free of beetles. Contaminated hay is usually the result of beetles being crushed before baling. Beetles disperse in the field as the cut hay dries. However, beetles are often crushed during harvesting especially if the swather is equipped with a crimper to speed drying of the hay. Beetle body parts may be concentrated in small portions of bales and consumed by livestock. Suggested means of combating blister beetle problems in alfalfa include the following:

1. Feed small rectangular bales instead of large round bales so that individual flakes make be hand inspected before feeding.
2. Cut hay early before the bloom stage so that plants do not attract adult blister beetles. First-cutting hay and late cuttings of hay (especially after the first frost) often escape contamination because they are produced before and after peak periods of beetle activity.
3. Cut hay without using crimpers. This suggestion does not usually interest producers, because drying time of hay is increased when crimping is not used.
4. Use a sickle bar mower without conditioner, which is generally slower and does not crimp.
5. Avoid wheel traffic on standing or cut hay. This can be difficult because mowers often require driving the tractor over previously cut hay. However, some mowers or conditioners allow the swath to be straddled by subsequent wheel traffic.

6. Scout fields before and during harvest. Beetles disperse when encountered, so swarms can be detected just in front of the harvester. Drivers spotting swarms can stop and allow swarms to disperse before proceeding with the harvesting.

FIREFLIES

Konnie H. Plumlee

Sources. Fireflies of the genus *Photinus* contain steroidal pyrones called lucibufagins, which are structurally related to the cardiotoxic bufodienolides of toads and cardenolides of plants. Lucibufagins protect fireflies against predators such as spiders and birds.[1]

Mechanism of Action. The mechanism of action is unknown. However, because of their structural similarity to bufodienolides and cardenolides, it is likely that lucibufagins are also cardiotoxic.

Toxicity and Risk Factors. Toxicosis has been reported in two bearded dragons, an African chameleon, two White's tree frogs, and a *Lacerta derjugini* lizard that were kept as pets and fed fireflies by their owners.[1]

Clinical Signs. Signs that have been reported by owners are summarized in Table 18-2.

Lesions. Postmortem examination of two bearded dragons revealed no gross internal lesions.[1]

Treatment. Because of the acute onset of signs, veterinary care could not be instituted before death in any animals so far.[1]

TABLE 18-2 **Course of Disease in Animals That Have Ingested Fireflies**

Animal	Number of Fireflies Ingested	Onset of Signs after Ingestion	Clinical Signs
Bearded dragon	About 9	30 minutes	Head-shaking, oral gaping, dyspnea; color change to black on dorsal trunk and nape; died about 60 minutes after ingestion
Bearded dragon	1	60-90 minutes	Oral gaping; color change to black on ventral neck, abdomen, tail; died at unknown time
African chameleon	5-6	Unknown	Clinical signs not described; died at unknown time
White's tree frog	About 3	Unknown	Found dead next morning
Lacerta derjugini (lizard)	1	5 minutes	Oral gaping, regurgitation; died 15 minutes following ingestion

Data from reference 1.

REPTILES

Michael E. Peterson

CORAL SNAKES

Sources. Coral snakes belong to the reptilian family Elapidae. Two genera of coral snakes are indigenous to the United States. The Sonoran coral snake *(Micururoides euryxanthus)* inhabits central and southeastern Arizona and southwest New Mexico. The other genus is composed of several subspecies of *Micrurus fluvius*, including the Texas coral snake *(M. f. tenere)*, the Eastern coral snake *(M. f. fulvius)*, and the South Florida coral snake *(M. f. barbouri)*. The Eastern coral snake inhabits eastern North Carolina south to central Florida, west to Alabama and Mississippi, and throughout eastern Louisiana to the Mississippi River. The South Florida coral snake is found in southern Florida. The Texas coral snake inhabits eastern and south central Texas north into southern Arkansas and Louisiana.

Coral snakes are relatively uncommon, generally shy, and often nocturnal. The Sonoran coral snake is rarely significant medically. This snake is small, nocturnal, burrowing, nonaggressive, and shy, which limits exposure to dogs and cats. Bites to livestock are unlikely. Their venom potency is relatively low.[1]

Coral snakes belonging to the genera *Micrurus* are generally small mouthed, diurnal, and reclusive. In North America they can be identified by their bright coloration of fully encircling bands beginning with a black head then alternating yellow, red, and black color pattern. The yellow bands may be a bright primary yellow to an almost white or cream color. Several species of tricolored kingsnakes mimic the coral snake color pattern; however, they have yellow and black bands touching. The identifying key for North American coral snakes is the yellow (caution) and red (danger) colored bands touching.

These snakes have small heads, round pupils, and a relatively primitive and inefficient venom delivery apparatus with fixed front fangs.[2] They are known to bite pugnaciously, employing a vigorous chewing action to facilitate venom delivery; human victims often have to manually remove the biting snake (often describing a separating Velcro sound).[2]

Toxicokinetics. Coral snake venom is composed of many small polypeptides and possibly cholinesterase. Acetylcholine and some poorly defined enzymatic fractions to the venom may be involved.

The toxicokinetics are poorly understood. Onset of neurologic signs is often delayed up to 12 or more hours and binding at the site of action seems irreversible. Unlike curare, the onset of action is slow and the duration of the syndrome is prolonged. The venom can take up to 14 days to totally clear the body.[3] In envenomated cats, clinical improvement began at 36 hours and the cats were able to move their limbs after 48 hours.[4]

Mechanism of Action. Neurotoxins affect the postsynaptic motor nerve membranes with a curare-like action. The multiple neurotoxic fractions combine to induce a nondepolarizing postsynaptic neuromuscular blockade. This activity is clinically manifested as vasomotor instability, muscle paralysis, and central nervous system depression.

The enzymatic fraction can cause local tissue damage, and in dogs can cause hemolytic anemia with a resultant hemoglobinuria.[5,6] Phospholipase A may trigger damage to red blood cell membranes. In cats, myoglobin release can be induced as a result of enzymatic effects.

Intravenous (IV) injection of venom can cause a dramatic decrease in blood pressure as cardiac output declines as a result of vasodilatation in the primary shock organs of the victim species.[7]

Toxicity and Risk Factors. The severity of the envenomation is directly related to the size of the victim and amount of venom injected. The amount of venom available to be injected is directly related to the size of the snake.[8] The volume of venom injected is proportional to the motivation of the snake (defensive vs. offensive bite) along with the duration of the bite and intensity of the chewing action.

Clinical Signs. Clinical signs vary depending on the victim species. In cats, the primary clinical issues are neurologic with ascending flaccid quadriplegia, reduced nociperception, and central nervous system depression. Decreased blood pressure, respiratory depression, loss of spinal reflexes in all limbs, anisocoria, and hypothermia can also manifest. There is no evidence of intravascular hemolysis in envenomated cats, but significant release of myoglobin does occur.[4]

Canine patients also exhibit central nervous system depression, decreases in spinal reflexes in all limbs, and respiratory depression. Additionally, they may vomit and salivate excessively, and hypotension and ventricular tachycardia may develop. Hemolysis can occur within the first 72 hours with hemoglobinuria, anemia, and alterations of red cell morphology.[5]

The usual cause of death is respiratory collapse. Additionally, dysfunctional swallowing facilitates the primary complication of aspiration and subsequent pneumonia.[9]

Clinical Pathology. Early elevations of fibrinogen or creatine kinase can be indicators that envenomation has occurred.[4] In canines, intravascular hemolysis, anemia, and hematuria can occur. Dogs can exhibit burring and sphereocytosis of red blood cells.[5] Feline patients can exhibit increased myoglobin and alkaline phosphatase as a result of rhabdomyolysis.

Lesions. Local lesions are primarily small (often bleeding) puncture wounds with minimal tissue swelling.

Diagnostic Testing. No specific diagnostic test is available to identify envenomation by coral snakes. Diagnosis relies on witnessing the bite (snake attached to victim), onset of clinical signs, or educated supposition based on circumstances (e.g., location, probability of snake interaction).

Treatment. Recommended field management is primarily rapid transport to veterinary care. The use of a compression bandage around and over the bite site is advocated in Elapid bites in other countries. This method of first aid is often precluded in veterinary patients with their proclivity for receiving bites to the head. The key to medical management of coral snake envenomations is to be aware that onset of clinical signs may be delayed 12 hours. The primary medical goal with a coral snakebite victim is to institute therapy before the onset of clinical signs if possible.

On arrival at the veterinary facility, the patient should have pretreatment blood samples collected and evaluated including a complete blood count and serum chemistries to establish a baseline and identify underlying disease processes. Red blood cells should be examined for alterations in morphology that might be indicative of envenomation. The patient should be hospitalized for observation for a minimum of 24 hours. In anticipation of progression of the envenomation syndrome, the clinician should be prepared to respond to possible respiratory collapse, dysphagia, and aspiration pneumonia. Often this requires transporting the victim to a 24-hour intensive care facility with the capacity for vigilant observation and ability to supply ventilatory support.

The only definitive treatment for coral snake envenomation is the use of specific antivenin. Antivenin (*M. fulvius*, equine origin) is manufactured by Wyeth Laboratories of Marietta, PA, and is effective against the venom of all coral snakes in North America except the Sonoran coral snake (*Micruroides euryxanthus*).[10] Antivenin can block further action of venom but is less effective against venom components already attached to receptor sites. Early administration of the antivenin is important for maximum effectiveness; clinical signs can progress rapidly and are difficult to reverse after they manifest.

Antivenin is reconstituted with the provided sterile diluent; it can be swirled but should not be shaken. Warming the diluent to body temperature facilitates the reconstituting process, which usually takes 10 to 15 minutes. The antivenin should only be administered intravenously; this can be facilitated by mixing the reconstituted antivenin in crystalloid fluids at a rate of one vial to 100 to 250 ml of fluid (depending on patient size). Administration should be slow initially, and the patient should be monitored for allergic reactions such as nausea, hyperemia of the pinna, fluffing of the tail hair, and pruritus. If no reaction occurs within the first 5 minutes then the infusion rate can be increased to allow the entire dose to be given over a 30-minute period. Multiple vials may be necessary; smaller patients often require higher dosages and progression of the envenomation syndrome is the indicator for additional administration.[5] A single vial binds 2 mg of coral snake venom; a large coral snake could deliver a venom load of 20 mg.

Antivenin contains equine antiglobin IgG (T) and a significant amount of other proteins; approximately 50% of the final product is equine albumin. The veterinarian should be prepared to respond to an allergic reaction caused by the extraneous protein content of this product. Allergic reactions to the antivenin can be exhibited in one of three forms: true anaphylaxis (which is rare), complement-mediated anaphylactoid (more common secondary to rapid administration of foreign protein), and delayed serum sickness (rare). Anaphylactoid reactions should be treated by stopping the infusion of antivenin, administering diphenhydramine, waiting 5 minutes, and then restarting the antivenin infusion at a slower rate. If delayed serum sickness occurs 1 to 2 weeks after infusion, it can be treated with corticosteroids and antihistamines. Anaphylaxis should be treated with intravenous fluids for volume support and epinephrine.

If antivenin is not available or its administration is delayed for a significant time period, respiratory support may be needed. Patients can be placed on a ventilator until the respiratory effect of the venom is cleared, but this may require 48 to 72 hours or longer.[11]

Broad-spectrum antibiotics are generally recommended in veterinary patients.[12,13] Corticosteroid use is unjustified in the treatment of coral snake envenomations.

Treatment of Sonoran coral snake envenomations is limited to providing adequate supportive care and responding to clinical signs as they appear.[14,15]

Prognosis. The prognosis is fairly good with early medical intervention. Patients sometimes need prolonged supportive care, and complete resolution of neurologic signs can take months. The major complication is aspiration pneumonia, which worsens the prognosis.

LIZARDS

Source. Two thousand species of lizards exist, but only two are venomous. The North American continent is home to the only poisonous lizards in the world. Both are members of the genus *Heloderma*, which comprises two species and five subspecies. The Gila monsters (*Heloderma suspectum*) are found in Arizona, parts of New Mexico, southern Utah, parts of Nevada, and portions of southern California. In Mexico, they are found in the state of Sonora west to the Gulf of Mexico. The other, larger lizard is the Mexican beaded lizard (*Heloderma horridum*), which inhabits parts of Mexico and Guatemala.[1]

These lizards are large (maximum size Gila monster is 55 cm; Mexican beaded lizard is larger) and stout bodied. The snout is rounded, the muzzle is flat and large, and the mandibles are heavily muscled. They generally are slow moving and lethargic but can strike rapidly and aggressively when disturbed. They have thick, beadlike scales over their bodies. Gila monsters are colorful with an orange-yellow to pink background, a black banded tail, and a dark, reticular body pattern. Mexican beaded lizards are dark brown or black and are less regularly banded.

The lizards generally inhabit desertlike environments, living around small shrubs, cacti, and rocks. In the cooler times of the year, the lizards are diurnal, but they are nocturnal during the hotter summer months. They hunt in burrows or protected shady areas looking for their primary food sources including bird eggs, young birds, and mammals.

Unlike other venomous reptiles, these lizards use their venom for defensive purposes only. They do not have the ability to inject their venom, but rather infuse the venom as they bite, holding on tenaciously and chewing to allow the venom to mix with the saliva into the wound. The venom is released from two venom glands on the lower jaw, onto the gums, and then flows up the grooved teeth by capillary action.[2] The teeth are extremely sharp, arch backward, and are fragile, often breaking off in the bite wound. Because of the method of venom delivery, the severity of the envenomation is directly related to the duration of the bite. The lizards are so pugnacious that often the victim is presented for veterinary care with the lizard still attached.

Mechanism of Action. The venom is a mixture of biologically active proteins. *Heloderma* venoms do not have neurotoxins and generally do not affect coagulation. The venom contains multiple proteins, including an extremely active kallikrein, arginine ester hydrolase, phospholipase A_2, very active hyaluronidase, gilatoxin, helothermine, and helospectin.[3,4]

Kallikrein releases bradykinins, inducing pain and hypotension. Gilatoxin is a glycoprotein with a lethal dose 50 (LD_{50}) similar to the crude venom itself. Another venom component is arginine ester hydrolase, which hydrolyzes amino acid esters. One of these esters can cause massive hemorrhage experimentally in several organs of laboratory animals, but this hemorrhage has not been seen in clinical cases. Phospholipase A_2 is present and has more than 50% homology with bee venom phospholipase. Helodermin and helospectin are peptides similar to mammalian vasoactive intestinal peptides. Helothermine is found in the Mexican beaded lizard, causing hypothermia, lethargy, and rear limb weakness in mice.[3,4]

Hyaluronidase is prominent in this venom and very active. Hyaluronidase is called the spreading factor because of its ability to break down connective tissue attachments by cleaving hyaluronic acid, thus allowing the penetration of the venom components deeper into the victim's tissues.[5]

Toxicity and Risk Factors. The LD_{50} in mice ranges from 0.4 to 1.4 mg/kg injected subcuticularly and 0.4 to 2.7 mg/kg injected intravenously. The minimal toxic dose calculated for humans has been estimated at 8 mg of venom (dry weight).[6] The venom yield of a Gila monster is 15 to 20 mg dry weight; however, the venom delivery system of the lizard is poor. The toxic dose for dogs and cats is unknown. I am aware of fatalities in two dogs.

Clinical Signs. The bite site is extremely painful. Intense pain usually reaches its peak by one hour after the bite and often persists 24 hours. There can be significant bleeding from the bite wound secondary to multiple lacerations from the sharp teeth, which often break off in the wound. The area around the bite site can become edematous. Regional tenderness and lymphadenitis may occur. Hypotension and tachycardia can occur with resultant weakness. Feline victims can exhibit tachypnea, tachycardia, and vomiting, most likely the result of pain. Muscle fasciculations can occur regionally. Tissue necrosis is rare, but secondary infection can be a sequela, particularly if broken teeth are embedded in the wound.

Clinical Pathology. Clinical laboratory values are generally within normal limits. Occasionally a stress leukocytosis develops.

Lesions. The bite wound is the only apparent lesion.

Treatment. It is not uncommon for the patient to be presented for veterinary care with the lizard still attached. There are several methods for extracting the lizard, but prying the mouth open with some instrument is recommended. Victims should be hospitalized for a few hours to monitor for progression of the envenomation syndrome. No specific antivenin is available.

Treatment is largely supportive. Intravenous fluid administration for volume support may be necessary to treat systemic hypotension. Pain control may be achieved with narcotics or fentanyl drip. Nonsteroidal antiinflammatory drugs may not be aggressive enough to control pain and might affect coagulation. The wound should be irrigated with lidocaine and, using a 25-gauge needle, probed for broken lizard teeth. Broad-spectrum antibiotics are indicated to combat secondary infection.

Prognosis. As a general rule, the prognosis is good; however, fatalities do occur in smaller animals such as dogs and cats. The single largest predictor of the prognosis is the duration of the bite. The longer the bite, the more venom delivered, thereby worsening the prognosis. Patients with underlying cardiac or pulmonary conditions are at higher risk of negative outcomes from venomous lizard bites.

Prevention and Control. These lizards are federally protected; therefore, controlling domestic animals is the best prevention.

PIT VIPERS

Synonyms. The pit vipers belong to one of three genera: *Crotalus* with at least 26 subspecies of rattlesnakes; *Sistrurus* with three subspecies of pygmy rattlesnakes *(S. miliaris)* and three subspecies of massassauga *(S. catenatus)*; and *Agkistrodon* with three subspecies of water moccasins or cottonmouths *(A. piscivorus)* and five subspecies of copperheads *(A. contortrix)*.

Source. Identification of pit vipers can be made by their characteristic morphologic traits. These snakes have elliptical pupils, bilateral heat sensing "pits" between the eye and nostril, a single row of subcaudal scales distal to the anal plate, triangular shaped heads, and retractable front fangs. The rattlesnakes have keratin rattles on the caudal end of their tails; however, they do not always rattle before striking. The pit viper's heat-sensing pit can sense a temperature change of 0.003° Celsius at a distance of more than 12 inches.

The majority of snakebites are inflicted by snakes less than 20 inches in length. The snakes are heavy bodied and muscular, which allows them to strike up to one half the length of their body at a speed of 8 feet per second. The pit vipers deliver their venom by rotating the retractable front fangs downward and stabbing forward. Muscular contractions of the venom glands then force the venom through the hollow fangs and into the victim. The snake, through this muscular activity, can control the amount of venom it injects. A "dry" bite in which no venom is injected occurs in approximately 25% of strikes.[1,2]

Every state in the United States, except Hawaii, Maine, and Alaska, is home to at least one species of pit viper. Approximately 8000 pit viper bites occur annually in people in the United States. Most of the bites (5000) are inflicted by copperheads, which live in close association to human habitation throughout the southeastern United States. The venom potency of copperheads is less than that of the rattlesnakes.[1] The water moccasins (cottonmouths), also southeastern inhabitants, are pugnacious and have a reputation for being somewhat territorial and aggressive.

Pit viper bites account for 99% of all the snakebites to animals in North America. The true incidence of venomous snakebites is unknown, but I estimate that approximately 150,000 cats and dogs are bitten annually in the United States. The incidence in livestock has not been estimated. Bites are more common in hotter summer months when the snakes are more active and venom yields are increased.

Toxicokinetics. The venom contains multiple toxins that act on the victim's various tissues and are metabolized with their metabolites interacting with each other. The net effect is a complex toxic stew, varying with each envenomation. Toxicokinetics of individual venom fractions have not been fully elucidated. More than 50 venom components have been identified and any single venom contains a minimum of 10 (Table 18-3). The venoms contain several nonenzymatic polypeptides, the "killing fractions," which are up to 50 times more toxic than the crude venom. These fractions are some of the first regenerated after envenomation.

Rattlesnake venom fractions have been identified in the victim's circulation for weeks after envenomation. The nadir of venom-induced thrombocytopenia in humans not receiving antivenin is approximately 80 hours.

Mechanism of Action. The primary purpose of pit viper venom is to immobilize prey and predigest victim's tissues. The enzymatic fraction of the venom breaks down connective tissue.[2-4] Hyaluronidase is called the *spreading factor* because it cleaves hyaluronic acid in collagen, allowing rapid penetration of the other venom components into the victim's tissues.[3] Myotoxins destroy muscle tissue, sometimes incurring permanent damage.[6] The lower weight myotoxins act by opening sodium channels through the muscle cellular membrane with the resultant destruction of the muscle cell.[5] Phospholipase A can cause the rupture of myofibrils by inducing hypercontraction of the plasma membrane.[5]

The venoms often contain multiple hemorrhagic toxins that affect the coagulation ability of the victim in many ways. Both hypercoagulation and hypocoagulation are possible, depending on the venom involved.[8] Additionally, some venoms do not specifically affect clotting but induce hyperfibrinolysis and dissolve clots as they form. True disseminated intravascular coagulation is possible but rare.[20] Some venoms, such as those of the western diamondback rattlesnake younger than the age of 30 days, usually completely defibrinate their human victims.

Cardiotoxic components have been identified as myocardial depressor factors in the venom of western and eastern diamondback venom.[12] Hypotension nonresponsive to intravenous fluid therapy is manifest in only the most severe envenomations.

Venom kallikrein-like activity and metalloproteinase (with zinc cofactor) induce marked local pain, tissue necrosis, and significant systemic hypotension.[13-15] A combination of the aforementioned venom factors and cardiovascular active

TABLE 18-3 **Partial List of North American Pit Viper Venom Fractions**

Classification	Venom Fractions
Enzymes	Proteinases, collagenase, proteolytic trypsinlike enzyme, arginine ester hydrolase, and hyaluronadases.[2-4]
Myotoxins	Phospholipase A2, phospholipase B, phosphodiesterase, and L-amino acid oxidase. Also the low-molecular-weight proteins crotamine and myotoxin a.[5-7]
Hemorrhagic/coagulation	Fibrinogenases, plasminogen activators, platelet aggregators/inhibitors, thrombinlike venom enzymes, and protein C activator.[5,8]
Neurotoxins	Generally presynaptic: phospholipase A2, and Mojave toxin.[9-11]
Cardiotoxins	Myocardial depressant factor.[12]
Cardiovascular	Kallikrein-like activity and metalloproteinase with zinc cofactor.[13-15]
Lipids	Caprylic, capric, lauric, linoleic, myristic, oleic, palmitic, palmitoleic, stearic, and arachidonic acids.[16]
Nucleosides/nucleotides	NAD nucleotidase[17]
Organic acids	Citrate[18]
Cations	Zinc[17,19]

components, including those that markedly affect clotting, are responsible for the primary systemic pathophysiologic clinical manifestation of hypotension. All these components can combine to produce a profound hypotension. For example, a 2-cm increase in the circumferential measurement of the swelling in an envenomated human thigh can remove up to one third of the body's circulating fluid volume and thereby compound the hypotensive event. Differing amounts of metalloproteinase inhibitors are the primary reason for varying mammalian resistance to pit viper venoms.[21]

The nonenzymatic polypeptides in the venom include the "killing fraction," which is more than 50 times more toxic than the crude venom. The lipid fraction in cobra venoms potentiates the toxicity by a factor of 50%; however, their impact in pit viper venoms has not been totally elucidated.[16]

Some pit viper venoms include potent presynaptic neurotoxins, whereas other pit vipers only have neurotoxic venoms (Table 18-4).[9-11] These toxins act triphasically by binding to the presynaptic nerve membrane, inhibiting neurotransmitter release. Then phospholipase increases the release of neurotransmitter and a final block occurs when the transmitter is depleted.[5]

In general, three venom types in North American rattlesnakes have been defined. The classic diamondback rattlesnake venom causes marked tissue destruction, coagulopathy, and hypotension. Mojave A rattlesnake venom causes virtually no tissue destruction or coagulation defects, but it induces a severe neurotoxicosis. The third venom class is an intergrade found in multiple species of rattlesnakes that have interbred, resulting in venoms that contain both the neurotoxins and the classic venom components (e.g., Mojave A/B and tiger rattlesnakes).

TABLE 18-4 Rattlesnake Species with Neurotoxic Venom

Latin Name	Common Name
Crotalus horridius atricaudatus	Canebreak rattlesnake
Crotalus lepidus klauberi	Banded rock rattlesnake
Crotalus mitchellii mitchellii	San Lucan speckled rattlesnake
Crotalus tigris	Tiger rattlesnake
Crotalus vegrandis	Uracoan rattlesnake
Crotalus durissus durissus	Central American rattlesnake
Crotalus durissus terrificus	South American rattlesnake
Crotalus viridis abyssus	Grand Canyon rattlesnake
Crotalus viridis concolor	Midget faded rattlesnake
Crotalus scutulatus scutulatus (A)	Mojave A rattlesnake
Crotalus scutulatus salvini	Huamantlan rattlesnake
Sistrurus catenatus catenatus	Eastern massasauga

Data from reference 22.

Toxicity and Risk Factors. The toxicity and risk factors depend on the snake and the victim. The snake factors include species of snake, size of the snake, time of year, attitude of snake (affecting volume of venom injected, e.g., defensive vs. offensive strike), age of the snake, and time since last bite (quantity of venom fractions reconstituted). Victim-related factors are species (natural immunity), size, bite site, time elapsed from bite to medical care, amount of physical activity after the bite, preexisting medical conditions, and medications.

Studies over the years have given a wide range of LD_{50}s and venom yields that highlight the individual variations in these levels regardless of snake species. Therefore, Table 18-5 is primarily useful for comparisons of toxicity between species. How dangerous a particular species is relates not only to the toxicity of the venom but also the total venom yield available. The analysis is additionally affected by both the circumstances of the bite situation (offensive vs. defensive) and the proclivity of that particular snake species to bite and inject venom. Some snake species (e.g., eastern and western diamondback rattlesnakes) are aggressive and strike readily, whereas other species (e.g., speckled rattlesnake) are docile and need a higher level of stimulation to be induced to bite and envenomate.

Clinical Signs. The initial clinical sign is usually marked regional swelling resulting from increased vascular permeability. Ecchymosis and petechiation may become evident, and discoloration of the skin often occurs within hours of the bite if coagulation factors are affected. The intensity of pain at the bite site is significant and the onset of pain is almost immediate.

Venomous snakebite is not always easy to diagnose, particularly when swelling and a heavy haircoat obscure puncture wounds. Clipping the hair in the region of an unknown swelling often helps in locating the bite site. Usually, painful, bleeding puncture wounds can be found consistent with a pit viper bite. Single or multiple punctures may be present from an individual bite or the victim may have received multiple bites.

The severity of the envenomation cannot be judged solely by assessing the local tissue response. Life-threatening envenomations with severe systemic manifestations can occur with little to no local tissue pathology. As a general rule, the severity of systemic clinical signs is most severe with the rattlesnakes, followed by water moccasins and copperheads. In species with only neurotoxic venom, the signs may be limited to puncture wounds and neurologic deficits.

TABLE 18-5 Approximate LD_{50} and Venom Yields of Selected North American Pit Vipers

Snake	LD_{50}	Venom Yield (mg)
Eastern diamondback (C. adamanteus)	1.68	590
Western diamondback (C. atrox)	2.18	500
Timber rattlesnake (C. horridus)	2.69	140
Copperhead (A. contortrix)	10.92	60
Cottonmouth (A. piscivorus)	4.17	130
Mojave A rattlesnake (C. scutulatus)	0.23	113

Bite site has a significant part to play in the severity of a given bite, primarily because of regional differences in systemic venom uptake. Most bites in dogs are to the head or front legs. As local swelling increases, alterations in regional vascular supply begin to slow venom uptake. Swelling from bites to a horse's muzzle can occlude the nares and the victim can die of the subsequent anoxia. Envenomations to the body wall allow venom to be absorbed more rapidly. Bites to the tongue are equivalent to intravascular envenomations, usually resulting in rapid and devastating results.

Onset of significant clinical signs may be delayed for several hours. This phenomenon cannot be overemphasized. One report of a human victim describes resolution of mild swelling over 3 hours, at which time he was discharged. The patient returned to the emergency department 12 hours later with severe pain, swelling, and a marked coagulopathy.[23] Traditionally, 40% of severe human envenomations are graded as mild to nonenvenomating at some point in the envenomation syndrome.[24] Twenty-five percent of all rattlesnake bites are nonenvenomating, and another 20% are mild envenomations.[1,25]

Marked hypotension often develops early, but can be delayed. Swelling is progressive for up to 36 hours after envenomation. Additional clinical signs can include tachycardia, shallow respirations, lethargy, nausea, obtundation, muscle fasciculations, increased salivation, and enlarged, painful regional lymph nodes.

Clinical Pathology. Initial diagnostic testing should include a baseline complete blood count with serum chemistries to identify not only the possible effects of the venom but also highlight any underlying disease processes in the patient. Repeated laboratory testing at 6, 12, and 24 hours is recommended. Early high elevations of creatine phosphokinase (more than 1000 on entry) can be an indicator of severe envenomation.

Coagulation parameters including activated partial thromboplastin time, prothrombin time, fibrinogen, fibrin split products, and platelet counts should be monitored at baseline, 6, 12, and 24 hours or as indicated by the progression of the envenomation syndrome.

Urinalysis should be performed to examine for signs of hematuria or rhabdomyolysis. This should be repeated at 6 and 12 hours, or more often if the case dictates.

Lesions. The characteristics of the local lesions depend on several factors, such as the species of snake, amount of venom injected, bite site, and time to medical care. Water moccasin bites create significant tissue necrosis. On the other hand, multiple species of rattlesnakes have subpopulations that have a neurotoxin (Mojave A) in their venom, which results in only a local lesion from the puncture wounds.[26-28]

Tissue necrosis and sloughing in the region of the bite site can be severe, particularly in areas with minimal muscle mass such as over the carpus. Systemic lesions often revolve around the primary shock organ of the victim species. Feline patients can have severe pulmonary hemorrhage. In dogs, the hepatosplenic vascular bed is primarily affected.

In horses, the bites most frequently occur on the nose, and marked tissue necrosis is possible. Cattle are often bitten on the muzzle or tongue. Tissue necrosis and secondary infection is a major problem in large animals that have not had a bite identified until several days after envenomation. One study implies persistent cardiac damage in prairie rattlesnake (*C. viridis viridis*) envenomated horses.[29]

Diagnostic Testing. A non-EDTA blood smear or one drop of blood mixed with a drop of saline should be examined microscopically, looking for evidence of echinocytosis, which has been reported in many pit viper envenomations during the first 12 hours.[30] The presence of echinocytosis greatly increases the probability that the victim has been envenomated.[31] However, a negative test does not preclude envenomation.

Treatment. Many first aid measures have been advocated for early field treatment of pit viper bites, but none have proven to lessen mortality or morbidity.[32] In particular, cold packs, ice, tourniquets, incision and suction, electroshock, and alcohol are to be avoided. Additionally, a significant period of time can be consumed trying to use questionable first aid measures when time would be better spent transporting the victim to a veterinary facility where specific medical therapy can be instituted. The key principle in first aid is to do no additional harm. Therefore, the victim should be kept calm, the bitten extremity should be maintained below heart level if possible, and the victim should be rapidly transported to a veterinary facility.

Circumferential measurements above, below, and at the bite site should be measured hourly for the first 6 hours and then as indicated. This allows the clinician to objectively monitor regional swelling and the progression of the envenomation locally. Temperature, respiration rate, pulse, and blood pressure should be monitored hourly for the first few hours after admission and then as dictated by the progression or resolution of the envenomation.

The use of a severity score system is helpful in monitoring the severity of the snakebite, the progression of the envenomation, and the success of the treatment (Box 18-1). This system has been validated in the human model and has been used successfully in veterinary cases to allow an objective systemic evaluation of the patient.[33] I am aware of several fatal envenomations that had entry severity scores as low as 2. Therefore, it is important to view these envenomations as a progressive syndrome. In general, severity score sheets should be completed at baseline (entry) and at 6, 12, and 24 hours after hospital admission.

General medical management of pit viper envenomations should combat specific venom-induced pathophysiology. Therefore, intravenous crystalloid fluid therapy should be started to combat the third spacing of fluids and the resultant hypovolemic crisis.[34] The primary cause of death is cardiovascular collapse resulting from hypovolemic shock.

Broad-spectrum antibiotics are not routinely recommended in human snakebite victims. However, I recommend their use in veterinary patients, particularly in species highly susceptible to clostridial infections. One should avoid selecting antibiotics that may negatively affect renal function.

BOX 18-1	SNAKEBITE SEVERITY SCORE

Pulmonary System

0   Signs within normal limits
1   Minimal: slight dyspnea
2   Moderate: respiratory compromise, tachypnea, use of accessory muscles
3   Severe: cyanosis, air hunger, extreme tachypnea, respiratory insufficiency or respiratory arrest from any cause

Cardiovascular System

0   Signs within normal limits
1   Minimal: tachycardia, general weakness, benign dysrhythmia, hypertension
2   Moderate: tachycardia, hypotension (but tarsal pulse still palpable)
3   Severe: extreme tachycardia, hypotension (nonpalpable tarsal pulse or systolic blood pressure <80 mm Hg), malignant dysrhythmia or cardiac arrest

Local Wound

0   Signs within normal limits
1   Minimal: pain, swelling, ecchymosis, erythema limited to bite site
2   Moderate: pain, swelling, ecchymosis, erythema involves less than half of extremity and may be spreading slowly
3   Severe: pain, swelling, ecchymosis, erythema involves most or all of one extremity and is spreading rapidly
4   Very severe: pain, swelling, ecchymosis, erythema extends beyond affected extremity, or significant tissue slough

Gastrointestinal System

0   Signs within normal limits
1   Minimal: abdominal pain, tenesmus
2   Moderate: vomiting, diarrhea
3   Severe: repetitive vomiting, diarrhea, or hematemesis

Hematologic System

0   Signs within normal limits
1   Minimal: coagulation parameters slightly abnormal, PT <20 sec, PTT <50 sec, platelets 100,000-150,000/mm^3
2   Moderate: coagulation parameters abnormal, PT 20-50 sec, PTT 50-75 sec, platelets 50,000-100,000/mm^3
3   Severe: coagulation parameters abnormal, PT 50-100 sec, PTT 75-100 sec, platelets 20,000-50,000/mm^3
4   Very severe: coagulation parameters markedly abnormal with bleeding present or the threat of spontaneous bleeding, including PT unmeasurable, PTT unmeasurable, platelets < 20,000/mm^3.

Central Nervous System

0   Signs within normal limits
1   Minimal: apprehension
2   Moderate: chills, weakness, faintness, ataxia
3   Severe: lethargy, seizures, coma

Total Score Possible   0 to 20

Hypoalbuminemia can be treated with plasma infusion; however, coagulopathies are particularly difficult to treat with blood products that are rapidly consumed by the venom.

Coagulopathies generally respond well to intravenous antivenin administration. Resolution followed by recurrence of thrombocytopenia may occur in up to 30% of severely thrombocytopenic patients.[35] However, the recurrent thrombocytopenia is usually less severe than the baseline level and may not require additional antivenin administration.

Topical application of dimethyl sulfoxide (DMSO) to the bite site in envenomated horses increases the speed of venom uptake systemically and is not recommended.

Corticosteroids should not be used and have no place in the treatment of venomous snakebites (Glen J: Veterans Administration Medical Center Venom Research Laboratories, personal communication, 1990).[36-51] Some studies revealed increases in mortality with the use of corticosteroids.[52,53] They can be used in the treatment of allergic reactions to antivenin if it occurs.

Administration of diphenhydramine (10 to 25 mg SC or IV) aids in calming fractious or painful animals and may be used to pretreat the patient against possible allergic reactions to antivenin. However, antihistamines have no direct effect against the snake venom or its action.

The only proven treatment against pit viper envenomation is intravenous administration of antivenin, which stops progression of swelling, reverses coagulopathy, reverses thrombocytopenia, and improves muscle strength in patients with weakness and paralysis.[54-60] Thrombocytopenia induced by *Crotalus horridus horridus* venom may not reliably respond to antivenin because of the presence of a novel platelet-aggregating protein in the venom.

Two antivenins are available in North America for use against pit viper venoms. The only licensed veterinary antivenin product is produced and distributed by Fort Dodge Laboratories, Ames, Iowa (Antivenin [Crotalidae] Polyvalent—equine origin). Approximately 50% of the total protein in each vial is equine albumin and severe allergic reactions are possible; however, true anaphylaxis occurs in less than 1% of all patients receiving this product. The immunizing snake venoms present in this antivenin are eastern diamondback rattlesnake (*C. adamanteus*), western diamondback rattlesnake (*C. atrox*), fer-de-lance (*Bothrops atrox*), and the South American rattlesnake (*C. durissus teriffcus*). This antivenin is the least effective against Southern Pacific rattlesnake (*Crotalus viridis helleri*) venom.

The other antivenin available in the United States is manufactured by Protherics, Nashville, Tennessee (CroFab [Crotalidae polyvalent immune Fab] ovine origin). This product is currently approved by the Food and Drug Administration for human use and is in the final stage of U.S. Department of Agriculture approval for the veterinary market. The immunizing snakes are all indigenous to North America: eastern and western diamondback rattlesnakes (*C. adamanteus* and *C. atrox*, respectively), water moccasin (*A. piscivorus*), and Mojave A rattlesnake (*C. scutulatus scutulatus*). Because the purification process removes extraneous protein and the Fc antibody fragments, the risk of anaphylaxis or serious allergic reactions is minimized (although not completely removed). Large-scale clinical trials of CroFab have been completed in dogs with results comparable to those obtained in human snakebite victims. This antivenin has proven its effectiveness against a wide range of pit viper venoms and is capable of binding Southern Pacific rattlesnake (*C. viridis helleri*) venom.[60]

Regardless of which antivenin is used, the earlier it is administered, the more effective its action. Epinephrine should be available and the clinician should be prepared to respond to an anaphylactic event. More commonly, particularly with the Fort Dodge antivenin, anaphylactoid reactions occur. Discontinuing the infusion of antivenin, administering diphenhydramine, waiting 5 minutes, and then restarting the antivenin infusion at a slower rate usually solves this complication. Delayed serum sickness can occur in 7 to 10 days, but is rare in dogs and cats. The incidence of delayed serum sickness is more prevalent in the equine-origin, multiple-protein antivenin (Fort Dodge); it was not identified in a CroFab antivenin trial of 115 dogs.

Infusion of antivenin can be facilitated by mixing each vial of antivenin with approximately 200 ml of crystalloid fluid (limited by the victim's body weight). Infusion rates are much easier to control when mixed in this manner, and the patient can be monitored for any possible adverse reaction (e.g., redness of pinna, fluffing of the tail, nausea).

The typical dose of antivenin is a single vial. Critics of antivenin use have claimed that because the dosage required in a human averages 12 vials, that a single vial in a dog would be insignificant to the treatment. However, results from clinical trials with the CroFab antivenin revealed the same 6- and 12-hour severity scores with a single vial as their human counterparts averaging 13 vials.[61] The difference in the effective dosage is due to the natural immunity of various species, all having different levels of antimetalloproteinases. For example, wood rats (Neotoma micropus) are 120 times more refractory to the pit viper venoms than are Balb/C mice.[20] Occasionally multiple vials of antivenin are required, and repeat administration may be indicated depending on monitoring of deteriorating severity scores, clinical signs, or serial laboratory values.

Antivenin should only be administered intravenously because intramuscular or bite site injection delays uptake of the antivenin by several hours.[62] If coagulation parameters continue to deteriorate (even as long as 72 hours after envenomation), venom components are still active and antivenin should be administered. Antivenin cannot correct necrotic tissue damaged by venom; therefore, early administration is recommended.

Prognosis. With early medical intervention, most snake-bitten dogs and cats survive. Large animals often survive the initial venom effect; however, by the time they are recognized as having been envenomated they are at risk of death from secondary tissue damage and infection.

SPIDERS

Joseph D. Roder

BLACK WIDOW

Synonyms. The black widow spider (*Lactrodectus mactans*) is also known as the brown widow, the red-legged spider,

and the murderer. This spider earned its name as a result of the female behavior in which she consumes her mate.

Sources. The characteristic red hourglass-shaped marking is found on the ventral abdomen of these spiders. This is not to be confused with nonvenomous species that use mimicry with an orange or red hourglass on the dorsal aspect of their abdomen. The black widow spiders are generally shy and are found in garages or outside in brush or wood piles. The spiders generally envenomate if their web or egg sack is disturbed. The female of the species causes envenomation because the males have small jaws and are unable to penetrate the skin.

Toxicokinetics. The venom of the black widow is potent, much more so than the venomous snakes. It is thought that picomolar concentrations of the venom can result in clinical intoxication.[1]

Mechanism of Action. The toxin primarily responsible for clinical signs is generally thought to be α-latrotoxin, which is a labile, large (120 to 130 kD) protein neurotoxin.[2] The three-dimensional structure has recently been identified as a tetramer of molecules in the presence of cations (calcium and magnesium).[3] The toxin binds to at least two different neuronal receptors: neurexins and CIRL (Ca++-independent receptor for α-latrotoxin) also known as latrophilin.[4,5] Binding of α-latrotoxin to these receptors serves to recruit the toxin to the synapse, specifically the presynaptic neuronal membrane,[4] which leads to the release of neurotransmitters by calcium-dependent (catecholamines) and calcium-independent (acetylcholine, GABA, glutamate) mechanisms.[4]

In the presynaptic nerve terminals, the α-latrotoxin performs several functions. Dimers of the toxin form tetramers in the presence of divalent cations with the newly formed tetramers binding to the CIRL receptor, which is coupled to a G protein. The binding CIRL receptor protein is calcium independent and activates phospholipase C, leading to inositol triphosphate–induced calcium mobilization.[1] The α-latrotoxin also binds to neurexin receptor proteins when in the presence of calcium. The neurexin receptor proteins then bind to membrane-bound kinases that are involved in synaptic vesicle trafficking. Furthermore, the α-latrotoxin tetramer forms a stable transmembrane pore that allows calcium influx into the presynaptic nerve terminal.[1,2] These actions of α-latrotoxin are not exclusive; they all work in concert to increase the movement of neurotransmitter-laden synaptic vesicles to the membrane for exocytosis.

Toxicity and Risk Factors. All mammalian species are susceptible to α-latrotoxin; however, limited literature reports of clinical envenomation are found in species other than dogs, cats, and humans. Cats are more sensitive to envenomation.[6]

Clinical Signs. The clinical signs associated with black widow spider envenomation are generally related to the nervous or muscular systems. The signs include muscle fasciculation and rigidity, abdominal pain, ataxia, and flaccid paralysis. This may progress to an ascending paralysis that involves the muscles of respiration. If the respiratory muscles are involved, the animal exhibits dyspnea and altered breathing mechanics.

Clinical Pathology.   Elevation of enzymes indicating skeletal muscle damage (creatine kinase, aspartate transaminase) may be noted in envenomated animals.

Treatment.   Supportive and symptomatic therapy is essential initially to stabilize the patient. The therapeutic plan should include respiratory and cardiovascular monitoring as well as pain management. In humans, pain management is a key element in the management of *Latrodectus* envenomation. Opioids (fentanyl) or benzodiazepines (diazepam) have been recommended for the control of pain.

Specific therapy for black widow envenomation includes calcium gluconate to reverse the signs of muscle fasciculation and weakness. A 10% calcium gluconate solution is given at a dose of 5 to 15 ml for cats and 10 to 30 ml for dogs.

A specific antidote for black widow evenomation is available: Antivenin *(Latrodectus mactans),* Equine Origin, Merck & Co., Inc. This antivenin may be obtained from most hospital pharmacies or located through a regional poison control center. If the clinician believes the patient's condition warrants the use of antivenin, generally a single vial is required for a cat or dog. An intradermal injection of the antivenin is recommended before administration to determine whether the patient is hypersensitive to the product. The antivenin is diluted in normal saline (10 to 50 ml) and is given intravenously over 15 minutes.[6]

Prognosis.   Most animals respond to supportive and symptomatic therapy and return to normal within a few days. In severe clinical cases, complete recovery may take weeks.

BROWN RECLUSE

Limited information is available concerning brown recluse envenomation in veterinary patients. Most of the following information is derived from information and cases of human envenomation.

Synonyms.   The brown recluse spider *(Loxosceles* spp.) is also known as the brown spider, fiddleback spider, or violin spider.

Sources.   Thirteen different species of *Loxosceles* are found in the United States.[1] The most commonly reported species associated with toxicosis is *Loxosceles reclusa.*[1] The brown recluse spider is more commonly found in the southern half of the United States. These spiders have a characteristic dark marking of the dorsal aspect of the cephalothorax that resembles a violin or fiddle. They have long, thin legs compared to their body and are reclusive as their name suggests. They are commonly found in corners, closets, or attics, and envenomation generally occurs when the spider is disturbed or threatened.

Toxicokinetics.   The venom from a single bite is sufficient to cause intoxication. It has been estimated that during an envenomation, 40 µg of venom-proteins are introduced into the victim.[2]

Mechanism of Action.   The venom of the brown recluse spider is a complex mixture of enzymes. The component of the venom most commonly associated with dermal necrosis is a 32-kD protein, sphingomyelinase.[1,3] This component of the venom interacts with the plasma membrane of a variety of cells: endothelium, erythrocytes, and platelets. The protein causes a disruption of these membranes with resulting microvascular damage and platelet aggregation. Sphingomyelinase D may also act as a chemotactic factor for neutrophils, resulting in recruitment of inflammatory cells to the wound. The influx of neutrophils with accompanying platelet aggregation results in intravascular coagulation in the capillaries surrounding the wound and leads to dermal necrosis.

Additionally, recent in vitro and in vivo studies of the venom of *Loxosceles intermedia* have shown degradation of basement membrane components, specifically heparan sulfate proteoglycan and laminin-enactin, of endothelial cells.[2,4] This action of the venom was noted in the absence of neutrophils and may cause an altered organization and adhesion of endothelial cells.[2,4] Other components of venom include hyaluronidase for venom spreading, lipase, alkaline phosphatase, esterases, and proteases.[1] In addition to the components of the venom previously described, the fangs of the brown spider may introduce clostridial organisms into the wound.[5] There may be some synergistic effect of the venom with the toxins liberated by the growing clostridial organisms.[5]

Toxicity and Risk Factors.   All mammalian species are susceptible to the venom of brown recluse spiders. Dogs and cats are more likely to come into contact with these spiders and be presented for veterinary care.

Clinical Signs.   The clinical signs associated with brown recluse envenomation are grouped into local and systemic signs. The local signs relate to the ability of the venom to cause dermal necrosis. In humans, the dermal lesions develop within a few hours to several days after envenomation.[1] Rabbit models of envenomation and dermal necrosis are the most commonly referenced animal information in the literature.[5] No clinical reports of envenomation in veterinary patients are in the literature. In humans, the progression of the dermal lesion generally starts with a central blister at the wound site with surrounding edema and erythema. The lesion progresses to one with a darkened center and the development of a vesicle. The central area of the wound may become necrotic with the development of an eschar.[6] In humans, systemic signs of envenomation are uncommon: hemolysis, nausea, vomiting, fever, and generalized malaise.[6]

Clinical Pathology.   A complete blood count and serum chemistry evaluation may show evidence of a Coombs-negative hemolytic anemia.

Treatment.   Most human patients envenomated by the brown recluse spider do not require treatment.[1] Treatment of brown recluse envenomation is controversial in the human literature because there is a lack of well-controlled clinical studies of treatment efficacy. Animals with suspected brown recluse bites should be treated conservatively with general wound care and observed for any generalized symptoms. A broad-spectrum antibiotic may be indicated because bacteria may be introduced into the wound by the fangs of the spider.[5]

No specific antidote for brown recluse envenomation exists. Antivenin therapy is experimental and the antivenin is not commercially available.

Anecdotal treatment for human envenomation includes dapsone, wound excision, and hyperbaric oxygen therapy. The rationale for dapsone treatment is that it inhibits the influx of neutrophils to the site of envenomation. It is recommended that this drug be used within 36 hours of the envenomation. The probable delay in presentation of veterinary patients as well as the propensity of dapsone to induce methemoglobinemia would reduce the effectiveness of this possible therapy. Excision of the wound and hyperbaric oxygen therapy have not been shown to be reliably effective in controlled experimental settings. In addition to being unnecessary, aggressive wound excision may prolong the healing of the necrotic area.

Prognosis. In human cases of envenomation, uncomplicated dermal necrosis is associated with a good prognosis. The time for complete healing of the necrotic area of skin depends on the size of the lesion. In humans, the healing time ranges from 1 to 7 weeks. The prognosis becomes guarded if systemic signs occur.

TOADS

Joseph D. Roder

Synonyms. *Bufo marinus* (cane or marine toad) and *Bufo alvarius* (Colorado River toad) are the most toxic toads in North America.

Sources. These toads are primarily located in Florida, Texas, Colorado, Arizona, and Hawaii.

Toxicokinetics. When these toads are mouthed or bitten by a dog, the parotid glands located on the toad's dorsum release toxins that are absorbed via the buccal mucous membranes of the dog.[1] The secretions from these glands may contain a variety of substances including epinephrine, serotonin, ergosterol, and bufodienolides (bufogenins).

Mechanism of Action. The bufotoxins are cardiac glycosides. They bind to and inhibit sodium-potassium ATPase in a manner similar to other cardiac glycosides, such as digoxin and digitoxin. The inhibition of the sodium-potassium ATPase results in an increased extracellular concentration of potassium and an increased intracellular concentration of sodium. The increased sodium concentration is a powerful driving force to increase the influx of calcium into the cytosol.

These changes alter the resting membrane potential of excitable cells resulting in a depressed electrical conduction, which leads to an inhibition of myocardial conduction and function.

Toxicity and Risk Factors. The toxicity of bufotoxin has been reported to be 100 mg of crude toxin for a dog weighing 9 to 14 kg.[2] Dogs are the most commonly poisoned species.[1-3] The risk of intoxication is greater during the spring, summer, and fall at dusk or dawn or after a rainfall.

Clinical Signs. Hypersalivation, vomiting, and anxiety are common initial signs in dogs after biting a toad. The majority of animals in one study presented with neurologic abnormalities, including convulsions, ataxia, nystagmus, stupor, or coma.[3] The mucous membranes of the oral cavity may be hyperemic.[3] The onset of clinical signs is rapid and death may occur 15 minutes after the onset of clinical signs.[1]

Diagnostic Testing. The diagnosis of toad intoxication depends on clinical signs and a history of exposure to toads.

Treatment. Initial treatment of toad intoxication should focus on decontamination of the oral cavity. The dog's mouth should be immediately flushed with copious volumes of running water unless the animal is seizing or unconscious. If the animal presents with seizures, diazepam (0.5 mg/kg IV) may be administered as an anticonvulsant.[3] An initial cardiac examination should include auscultation, determination of heart rate, and evaluation of perfusion. If the animal has arrhythmias or signs of shock, it should be monitored by electrocardiogram. If bradycardia is noted, the animal may be treated with IV atropine at 0.02 mg/kg.[3] Sustained tachycardia can be treated with beta-antagonists. Atropinization should be reserved for animals with marked bradycardia and not used as a symptomatic treatment for hypersalivation. If hyperkalemia is present, treat with an infusion of insulin, glucose, and sodium bicarbonate to drive potassium back into cells. Administration of calcium is contraindicated in animals suffering from bufotoxicosis.

Digoxin-specific Fab-fragment (Digibind) has been successfully used experimentally in mice and clinically in humans.[4,5] Even though this antidote has been used for digoxin toxicosis in a dog, it has not been evaluated in clinical cases of toad intoxication.[6]

Prognosis. Most animals recover if treated with early decontamination and appropriate symptomatic therapy.

REFERENCES

Bacteria

BOTULISM
1. Huang W et al: Pharmacology of botulism toxin, *J Am Acad Dermatol* 43:249, 2000.
2. Washbourne P et al: Botulinum neurotoxin E-insensitive mutants of SNAP-25 fail to bind VAMP but support exocytosis, *J Neurochem* 73:2424, 1999.
3. Rossetto O et al: Bacterial toxins with intracellular protease activity, *Clin Chim Acta* 291:189, 2000.

4. Galey FD et al: Type C botulism in dairy cattle from feed contaminated with a dead cat, *J Vet Diagn Invest* 12:204, 2000.
5. Galey FD: Botulism in the horse, *Vet Clin North Am Equine Pract* 17(3):579, 2001.
6. Heider LC et al: Presumptive diagnosis of *Clostridium botulinum* type D intoxication in a herd of feedlot cattle, *Can Vet J* 42:210, 2001.
7. Bernard W et al: Botulism as a sequel to open castration in a horse, *J Am Vet Med Assoc* 191:73, 1987.
8. Ortolani EL et al: Botulism outbreak associated with poultry litter consumption in three Brazilian cattle herds, *Vet Human Toxicol* 39:89, 1997.

TETANUS
1. Williamson LC et al: Neuronal sensitivity to tetanus toxin requires gangliosides, *J Biol Chem* 274 (35):25173, 1999.
2. Pellizzari R et al: Tetanus and botulinum neurotoxins: mechanism of action and therapeutic uses, *Philos Trans R Soc Lond B Biol Sci* 354(1381):259, 1999.
3. Raya SA et al: Cytolysins increase intracellular calcium and induce eicosanoids release by pheochromocytoma PC12 cell cultures, *Nat Toxins* 1:263, 1993.
4. Baker JL et al: Tetanus in two cats. *J Am Anim Hosp Assoc* 24:159, 1988.
5. Messer NT, Johnson PJ: Serum hepatitis in two brood mares, *J Am Vet Med Assoc* 204:1790, 1994.
6. Guglick MA et al: Hepatic disease associated with administration of tetanus antitoxin in eight horses, *J Am Vet Med Assoc* 206:1737, 1995.

Blue-Green Algae

1. Beasley VR et al: Diagnostic and clinically important aspects of cyanobacterial (blue-green algae) toxicoses, *J Vet Diagn Invest* 1:359, 1989.
2. Puschner B et al: Blue-green algae toxicosis in cattle, *J Am Vet Med Assoc* 213:1605, 1998.
3. Bischoff K: The toxicology of microcystin-LR: occurrence, toxicokinetics, toxicodynamics, diagnosis and treatment, *Vet Hum Toxicol* 43:294, 2001.
4. McDermott CM et al: The cyanobacterial toxin, microcystin-LR, can induce apoptosis in a variety of cell types, *Toxicon* 36:1981, 1998.
5. Khan SA et al: Microcystin-LR and kinetics of cytoskeletal reorganization in hepatocytes, kidney cells, and fibroblasts, *Nat Toxins* 4:206, 1996.
6. Molloy L et al: Anatoxin: a is a potent agonist of the nicotinic acetylcholine receptor of bovine adrenal chromaffin cells, *Eur J Pharmacol* 289:447, 1995.
7. Frazier K et al: Microcystin toxicosis in cattle due to overgrowth of blue-green algae, *Human Toxicol* 40:23,1998.
8. DeVries SE et al: Clinical and pathologic findings of blue-green algae (*Microcystis aeruginosa*) intoxication in a dog, *J Vet Diagn Invest* 5:403, 1993.
9. Heresztyn T, Nicholson BC: A colorimetric protein phosphatase inhibition assay for the determination of cyanobacterial peptide hepatotoxins based on the dephosphorylation of phosvitin by recombinant protein phosphatase, *Environ Toxicol* 16:242, 2001.

Insects

BLISTER BEETLES
1. Guglick MA et al: Equine cantharidiasis, *Compend Contin Educ Pract Vet* 18:77, 1996.
2. Barr AC et al: Cantharidin poisoning of emu chicks by ingestion of *Pyrota insulata*, *J Vet Diagn Invest* 10:77, 1998.
3. Edwards WC et al: Cantharidin content of two species of Oklahoma blister beetles associated with toxicosis in horses, *Vet Hum Toxicol* 31:442, 1989.
4. Shawley RV, Rolf LL: Experimental cantharidiasis in the horse, *Am J Vet Res* 45: 2261, 1984.
5. Schmitz DG: Cantharidin toxicosis in horses, *J Vet Int Med* 3:208, 1989.
6. Ray AC et al: Etiologic agents, incidence, and improved diagnostic methods of cantharidin toxicosis in horses, *Am J Vet Res* 50:187, 1989.
7. Helman RG, Edwards WC: Clinical features of blister beetle poisoning in equids: 70 cases (1983-1996), *J Am Vet Med Assoc* 211: 1018, 1997.

FIREFLIES
1. Knight M et al: Firefly toxicosis in lizards, *J Chemical Ecology* 25:1981,1999.

Reptiles

CORAL SNAKES
1. Lowe C Jr, Limbacher H: *Micruroides euryxanthus*, the Sonoran coral snake, *A Z Med* 8:128, 1961.
2. Kitchens C, Van Mierop L: Envenomation by the eastern coral snake (*Micrurus fulvius fulvius*): a study of 39 victims, *JAMA* 258:1615, 1987.
3. Weis R, McIsaac R: Cardiovascular and muscular effects of venom from coral snake, *Micrurus fulvius*, *Toxicon* 9: 219, 1971.
4. Chrisman C et al: Acute, flaccid quadriplegia in three cats with suspected coral snake envenomation, *J Am Anim Hosp Assoc* 32:343, 1996.
5. Marks S et al: Coral snake envenomation in the dog: report of four cases and review of the literature, *J Am Anim Hosp Assoc* 26:629, 1990.
6. Ellis M: *Venomous and non-venomous snakes. Dangerous plants, snakes, arthropods and marine life: toxicity and treatment*, Hamilton, Ill, 1978, Drug Intelligence Publications.
7. Ramsey H et al: Mechanism of shock produced by an elapid snake (*Micrurus f. fulvius*) venom in dogs, *Am J Physiol* 222:782, 1972.
8. Fix J: Venom yield of the North American coral snake and its clinical significance, *South Med J* 73:737, 1980.
9. Parrish H, Klan M: Bites by coral snakes: report of 11 representative cases, *Am J Med Sci* 253:561, 1967.
10. *Antivenin* (Micrurus fulvius) (*equine origin*). Drug circular. Marietta, Pa, 1983, Wyeth Laboratories.
11. Moseley T: Coral snake bite: recovery following symptoms of respiratory paralysis, *Ann Surg* 163:943, 1966.
12. Kerrigan K et al: Antibiotic prophylaxis for pit viper envenomation: prospective, controlled trial, *World J Surgery* 21:369, 1997.
13. Clark R et al: The incidence of wound infection following crotalid envenomation, *J Emerg Med* 11:583, 1993.
14. Russell F: Bites by the Sonoran coral snake *Micruroides euryxanthus*, *Toxicon* 5:39, 1967.
15. Russell F, Lauritizen L: Antivenins, *Trans R Soc Troop Med Hyg* 60:797, 1966.

LIZARDS
1. Bogert C, del Carpo R: The gila monster and its allies. The relationships, habits, and behavior of the lizards of the family *Helodermatidae, Bull Am Mus Nat Hist* 1:109, 1956.
2. Fox H: In Leob L, editor: *The venom of heloderma*, Washington, DC, 1953, Carnegie Institution.
3. Mebs D, Raudonat H: Biochemical investigations of Heloderma venom, *Mem Inst Butantan Sao Paulo* 33:907, 1966.
4. Tu A, Murdock D: Protein nature and some enzymatic properties of the lizard *Heloderma suspectum suspectum* (Gila monster) venom, *Comp Biochem Physiol* 22:389, 1967.
5. Tu A, Hendon R: Characterization of lizard venom hyaluronidase and evidence for its action as a spreading factor, *Comp Biochem Physiol* 76B:377, 1983.
6. Phisalix M: Note sur les effects mortels reciproques des morsures de l'*Heloderma suspectum* cope et de la *Vipera aspis* laur et sur les caracte'res diffe'rentiels de leurs venins, *Bull Mus Hist Nat Paris* 17:485, 1911.

PIT VIPERS
1. Russell FE, Carlson RW, Wainschel J, Osborne AH: Snake venom poisoning in the United States, *JAMA* 233:341, 1975.
2. Barrett AJ: In Dalling MJ, editor: *Plant proteolytic enzymes,* Boca Raton, Fla, 1986, CRC Press.
3. Meyer K, Hoffman P, Linker A: In Boyer PD, Lardy H, Myrback K, editors: *The enzymes,* New York, 1960, Academic Press.
4. Iwanaga S, Suzuki T: In Lee CY, editor: *Snake venoms,* Berlin, 1979, Springer.
5. Ownby C: In Shier WT, Mebs D, editors: *Handbook of toxinology,* New York, 1990, Marcel Decker, p 601.
6. Tu A: *Handbook of natural toxins,* vol 5, New York, 1991, Marcel Decker.
7. Kitchens CS, Hunter S, Van Mierop LHS: Severe myonecrosis in a fatal case of envenomation by the cane break rattlesnake (*Crotalus horridus atricaudatus*), *Toxicon* 25:455, 1987.

8. Markland FS: Inventory of A– and B– fibrinogenases from snake venoms, *Thrombo Haemostas* 65:438, 1991.

9. Gopalakrishnakone P, Hawgood BJ, Holbrooke SE: Sites of action of Mojave toxin isolated from the venom of the Mojave rattlesnake, *Br J Pharmacol* 69:421, 1980.

10. Jansen PW, Perken RM, Van Stralen D: Mojave rattlesnake envenomation: prolonged neurotoxicity and rhabdomyolysis, *Ann Emerg Med* 21: 322, 1991.

11. Valdes JJ, Thompson RG, Wolff VL: Inhibition of calcium channel dihydropyridine receptor binding by purified Mojave toxin, *Neurotoxicol Teratol* 11:129, 1989.

12. Harris J: In Harvey AL: *Snake toxins,* Oxford, 1991, Pergamon Press.

13. Mebs D: A comparative study of enzyme activities in snake venoms, *Int J Biochem* 1: 335, 1970.

14. Tu AT: Local tissue damage (hemorrhage and myonecrosis) toxins from rattlesnake and other pit viper venoms, *J Toxicol Toxin Rev* 2:205, 1983.

15. Bjarnason JB, Fox JW: Hemorrhagic metalloproteinases from snake venoms, *Pharmacol Ther* 62:325, 1994.

16. Cooke ME, Odeh GV, Hudiburg SA et al: *Analysis of fatty acids in the lipid components of snake venoms,* Proceedings of the 2nd American Symposium on Animal, Plant, and Microbial Toxins, Tempe, Ariz, 1986.

17. Bieber L: In Lee CY, editor: *Snake venoms,* Berlin, 1979, Springer.

18. Freitas MA, Geno PW, Summer LW: Citrate is a major component of snake venoms, *Toxicon* 30:461, 1992.

19. Bjarnason J, Tu A: Hemorrhagic toxins from western diamondback rattlesnake *(Crotalus atrox)* venom: isolation and characterization of five toxins and the role of zinc in the hemorrhagic toxin E, *Biochemistry* 17:3395, 1978.

20. Hasiba U, Rosenbach L, Rockwell D, Lewis J: DIC-like syndrome after envenomation by the snake *Crotalus horridus horridus, N Engl J Med* 292:505, 1975.

21. Perez JC, Haws WD, Garcia VE, Jennings BM: Resistance of warm blooded animals to snake venoms, *Toxicon* 16,375, 1978.

22. Glen J, Straight R: Distribution of proteins immunologically similar to Mojave toxin among species of *Crotalus* and *Sistrurus, Toxicon* 23:28, 1985.

23. Guisto J: Severe toxicity from crotalid envenomation after early resolution of symptoms, *Ann Emerg Med* 26:387, 1995.

24. Swindel G, Seaman K, Arthur D: The six hour observation rule for grade I crotalid envenomation: is it sufficient? *J Wilderness Med* 3:168, 1992.

25. Curry SC, Horning D, Brady P: The legitimacy of rattlesnake bites in central Arizona, *Ann Emerg Med* 18:658, 1989.

26. Weinstein S, Smith L: Preliminary fractionation of tiger rattlesnake *(Crotalus tigris)* venom, *Toxicon* 28:1447, 1990.

27. Glen J, Straight R: Mojave rattlesnake *(Crotalus scutulatus scutulatus)* venom: variations in toxicity with geographical origin, *Toxicon* 16:81, 1978.

28. Glen J, Straight R, Wolff T: Regional variation in the presence of Canebrake toxin in *Crotalus horridus* venom, *Comp Biochem Physiol C Pharmacol Toxicol Endocrinol* 107:337, 1994.

29. Dickinson CE, Traub-Dargatz JL, Dargatz DA: Rattlesnake venom poisoning in horses: 32 cases, 1973-1993, *J Am Vet Med Assoc* 208:1866, 1996.

30. Walton RM, Brown DE, Hamar DW: Mechanisms of echinocytosis induced by *Crotalus atrox* venom, *Vet Pathol* 34:442, 1997.

31. Brown DE, Meyer DJ, Wingfield WE: Echinocytosis associated with rattlesnake envenomation in dogs, *Vet Pathol* 31:654, 1994.

32. Stewart M, Greenland S, Hoffman J: First-aid treatment of poisonous snakebite: are currently recommended procedures justified? *Ann Emerg Med* 10:331, 1981.

33. Dart RC, Hurlburt KM, Garcia R: Validation of a severity score for the assessment of crotalid snakebite, *Ann Emerg Med* 27:321, 1996.

34. Schaeffer RC Jr, Carlson R, Puri VR, Callahan B, Russell F, Weil MH: The effects of colloidal and crystalloidal fluids on rattlesnake venom shock in the rat, *J Pharmacol Exp Ther* 206:687, 1978.

35. Boyer L, Seifert S, Clark R, McNally J, Williams S, Nordt S, Walter F, Dart R: Recurrent and persistent coagulopathy following pit viper envenomation, *Arch Intern Med* 159(7):706, 1999.

36. Clark R: Cryotherapy and corticosteroids in the treatment of rattlesnake bite, *Mil Med* 136:42, 1971.

37. Grace T, Omer G: Management of upper extremity pit viper wounds, *J Hand Surg* 5:168, 1980.

38. Russell FE: Snake venom poisoning in the United States, experiences with 550 cases, *JAMA* 233:341, 1975.

39. Van Mierop L: Snake bite symposia, *J Florida Med Assoc* 63:101, 1976.

40. Arnold R: Treatment of snake bite, *JAMA* 236:1843, 1976.

41. Arnold R: Controversies and hazards in the treatment of pit viper bites, *South Med J* 72:902, 1979.

42. Gennaro JF Jr: In Keegan HL, MacFarlane WV, editors: *Venomous and poisonous animals and noxious plants of the Pacific region,* Oxford, 1963, Pergamon Press.

43. Schottler WHA: Antihistamine, ACTH, cortisone and anesthetics in snake bite, *Am J Trop Med* 3:1083, 1954.

44. Allam NW, Weiner D, Lukens FDW: In Buckley EE, Porges N: *Venoms.* Washington, DC, 1956, American Association for Advancement of Science.

45. Russell FE, Emery JA: Effects of corticosteroids on lethality of *Ancistrodon contortrix* venom, *Am J Med Sci* 241:135, 1961.

46. Russell FE: Effects of cortisone during immunization with *Crotalus* venom. A preliminary report, *Toxicon* 3:65, 1965.

47. Visser J, Chapman DS: *Snakes and snake bite,* Cape Town, South Africa 1978, Purnell & Sons.

48. Reid HA, Thean PC, Martin WJ: Specific antivenene and prednisone in viper bite poisoning, a controlled trial, *BMJ* 2:1378, 1963.

49. Reid HA: Snake bite. Part 2. Treatment, *Trop Doctor* 2:159, 1972.

50. Wood JT, Hoback W, Green TW: Treatment of snake venom poisoning with ATCH and cortisone, *Virg Med Month* 82:130, 1955.

51. Carlson R, Schaeffer R Jr, Russell FE, Weil M: A comparison of corticosteroid and fluid treatment after rattlesnake venom shock in rats, *Physiologist* 18:160, 1975.

52. Cunningham ER, Sabback MS, Smith RM, Fitts CT: Snake bite: role of corticosteroids as immediate therapy in an animal model, *Am Surg* 45(12):757, 1979.

53. Russell FE: Shock following snake bite, *JAMA* 198:171, 1966.

54. Gurierrez J, Rojas G, Lomonte B: Comparative study of edema forming activity of Costa Rican snake venoms and its neutralization by a polyvalent antivenom, *Comp Biochem Physiol* 85C:171, 1986.

55. Lomonte B: Short communication: Edema forming activity of Bushmaster *(Lachesis muta stenophyrys)* and Central American rattlesnake *(Crotalus durissus durissus)* venoms and neutralization by a polyvalent antivenom, *Toxicon* 23:173, 1985.

56. Minton S: Polyvalent antivenom in the treatment of experimental snake venom poisoning, *Am J Trop Med Hyg* 3:1077, 1954.

57. Riffer E, Curry SC, Gerlun R: Successful treatment with antivenin of marked thrombocytopenia without significant coagulopathy following rattlesnake bite, *Ann Emerg Med* 16:1297, 1987.

58. Garfin S, Castilonia R, Mubarak S: The effect of antivenin on intramuscular pressure elevations induced by rattlesnake venom, *Toxicon* 23:677, 1985.

59. Dart R, McNally J: Efficacy, safety, and use of snake antivenoms in the United States, *Ann Emerg Med* 37(2):181, 2001.

60. Russell F, Ruzic N, Gonzalez H: Effectiveness of antivenin (Crotalidae) polyvalent following injection of Crotalus venom, *Toxicon* 11:461, 1973.

61. USDA Study Report: Crofab antivenin in treatment of rattlesnake envenomations in dogs, Nashville, submitted December 2002, Protherics Inc.

62. Kocholaty W, Billings T, Ashley B, Ledford W, Goetz J: Effect of the route of administration on the neutralizing potency of antivenins, *Toxicon* 5:165, 1968.

Spiders

BLACK WIDOW

1. Saibil HR: The black widow's versatile venom, *Nat Struct Biol* 7:3-4, 2000.

2. Grishin E: Polypeptide neutrotoxins from spider venoms, *Eur J Biochem* 264:276, 1999.

3. Orlova EV et al: Structure of α-latrotoxin oligomers reveals that divalent cation-dependent tetramers form membrane pores, *Nat Struct Biol* 7:48, 2000.
4. Sudhof TC: Alpha-latrotoxin and its receptors: neurexins and CIRL/latrophilins, *Annu Rev Neurosci* 24:933, 2001.
5. Bittner MA et al: A Ca2+-independent receptor for alpha-latrotoxin, CIRL, mediates effects on secretion via multiple mechanisms, *J Neurosci* 18:2914, 1998.
6. Twedt DC et al: Black widow spider envenomation in a cat, *J Vet Intern Med* 13:613, 1999.

BROWN RECLUSE
1. Walter FG et al: Envenomations, *Crit Care Clin* 15:353, 1999.
2. Veiga SS et al: *In vivo* and *in vitro* cytotoxicity of brown spider venom for blood vessel endothelial cells, *Thromb Res* 102:229, 2001.
3. Tambourgi DV et al: Sphingomyelinases in the venom of the spider *Loxosceles intermedia* are responsible for both dermonecrosis and complement-dependent hemolysis, *Biochem Biophys Res Commun* 251:366, 1998.
4. Veiga SS et al: Effect of brown spider venom on basement membrane structures, *Histochem J* 32:397, 2000.

5. Monteiro CL et al: Isolation and identification of *Clostridium perfringens* in the venom and fangs of *Loxosceles intermedia* (brown spider): enhancement of the dermonecrotic lesion in loxoscelism, *Toxicon* 40:409, 2002.
6. Bond GR: Snake, spider, and scorpion envenomation in North America, *Pediatr Rev* 20:147, 1999.

Toads

1. Otani A et al: Pharmacodynamics and treatment of mammals poisoned by *Bufo marinus* toxin, *Am J Vet Res* 30:1865, 1969.
2. Palumbo NE et al: Experimental induction and treatment of toad poisoning in the dog, *J Am Vet Med Assoc* 167:1000, 1975.
3. Roberts BK et al: *Bufo marinus* intoxication in dogs: 94 cases (1997-1998), *J Am Vet Med Assoc* 216:1941, 2000.
4. Brubacher JR et al: Efficacy of digoxin specific Fab fragments (Digibind) in the treatment of toad venom poisoning, *Toxicon* 37:931, 1999.
5. Brubacher JR et al: Treatment of toad venom poisoning with digoxin-specific Fab fragments, *Chest* 110:1282, 1996.
6. Ward DM et al: Treatment of severe chronic digoxin toxicosis in a dog with cardiac disease, using ovine digoxin-specific immunoglobulin G Fab fragments, *J Am Vet Med Assoc* 215:1808, 1999.

19

Feed-Associated Toxicants

AMMONIATED FEED

Sandra E. Morgan

Synonyms. The terms *bovine bonkers, bovine hysteria,* and *ammoniated feed syndrome* have all been used to describe a hyperexcitability syndrome seen in cattle after ingestion of toxic ammoniated hay, ammoniated liquid molasses, and protein and molasses blocks. This syndrome has also been seen in nursing calves and lambs that have had no access to toxic feed.

Sources. Ammoniation is a process by which feed stuffs are treated with anhydrous or aqueous ammonia to increase the protein content. The ammonia can be injected directly into the bales, but uneven ammoniation may result. Anhydrous ammonia is more commonly used with the "stack method," in which round bales (or square bales) are stacked in rows two to three bales high. An empty barrel is placed in the middle of the stack with plastic tubing in it that is connected to the anhydrous ammonia tank. The stack is covered with black plastic and sealed around the edges with dirt. The anhydrous ammonia is then pumped into the barrel, which helps it disperse, filling the plastic like a balloon. The amount of time it takes to ammoniate the hay depends on the ambient temperature. If the ambient temperature is greater than 80° F (26.6° C), it can take less than 1 week, but if the temperature is less than 40° F (4.4° C), then it can take more than 8 weeks. A variety of feeds have been associated with bovine bonkers. The earliest reports were associated with ammoniated molasses. Experiments and feeding trials in the 1950s resulted in so many affected animals that further research was not attempted for more than 30 years. The same syndrome was seen again during the 1980s from ammoniated hay and protein blocks made with urea and molasses. It was suspected at that time that the calves were getting the poison through the milk.[1]

Ammoniated hay has been the source most often reported. During the 1980s, ammoniation of poor-quality roughage became popular as a means of increasing the nutritive value and reducing the spoilage of high-moisture hay. The ammoniation process increased palatability, digestibility of crude protein and crude fiber, and the rate of gain and efficiency of feed utilization. It could replace up to 40% of protein-derived nitrogen with nonprotein nitrogen. Spoilage was reduced because the ammonia prevented heating and the subsequent microbial proliferation, fermentation, and mold formation.[2]

Bovine bonkers was not reported until higher quality forages were ammoniated, such as wheat hay instead of wheat straw. Alfalfa, Bermuda grass, forage sorghums, orchard grass, brome, and fescue have all been associated with the disease. Rice straw and wheat straw have actually been reported to cause the disease, but the incidence is much lower. The amount of grain left in the straw is a factor, in that an ample amount of soluble reducing sugars are necessary for the toxicosis to occur. Corn silage, corn stalks, and small grains have not been implicated because of their low level of soluble sugars.

Toxicokinetics. The route of exposure in each instance has been oral. The cattle have either ingested the toxic feed or the nursing calves have received it via the milk. Because the exact toxin or combination of toxins has not been found, the dose of toxin has not been established. Nursing calves have often been reported as the only animals affected in a group. Also, because of the variability of the substance in the hay, a toxic dose is difficult to determine. One farm that had death loss in nursing calves fed 4 kg of ammoniated barley greenfeed to each animal (charolais-cross cows) per day.[2] Other affected farms have fed ammoniated hay free choice to their lactating cows. Cattle had access to the protein-molasses blocks at all times, although they were formulated for 2 lb per head per day.

Mechanism of Action. Pyrazines and imidazoles (2-methyl and 4-methylimidazole) were found in toxic hay by gas chromatography/mass spectrophotometry (GC/MS) in the 1980s. The imidazoles were found to be convulsing agents and were formed by a nonenzymatic browning reaction (Maillard reaction) caused by the condensation with an amino group with a reducing compound. The amino acids from ammonia or urea and reducing sugars from high-quality hay in ammoniated feeds go through a series of reactions that are dependent on temperature, pH, and water content. Because ammoniated molasses, ammoniated hay, and protein-molasses blocks all contain these essential ingredients, they can all potentially form the same toxins. Water is necessary for the initial reaction to take place; then only reducing sugars can provide the necessary carbonyl groups to take part in a Maillard reaction. The higher the temperature and pH, the more rapidly the reaction takes place.[1]

Initial research pointed toward 4-methylimidazole (4-MeI) as the most potent convulsant responsible for the clinical signs but low levels of this compound in milk and plasma from poisoned sheep suggested that other agents may be involved. Because of the toxicity of the milk to the nursing calves and lambs, it was believed that the toxic compounds were readily transported and possibly concentrated in the milk, even more so in the colostrum. This suggested a lipophilic character or a basic character because of the lower pH value of milk compared with that of plasma. With this in mind, an analytical approach was designed to include all compounds that might contribute to the toxicity of ammoniated forage, in contrast to previously published analysis, which was aimed at finding 4-MeI. Along with 4-MeI and 2-MeI previously identified, the following imidazoles have been isolated from forage and milk: 1,2-dimethyl-, 1,4-dimethyl-, 1,5-dimethyl-, 2,4-dimethyl-, and 2-ethyl-4-methylimidazole.[3] These new compounds have not been found to be more toxic than 4-MeI in mice, and their concentrations in milk and ammoniated forage are in lower concentrations than 4-MeI. The toxins or combinations that cause this syndrome may still be a mystery.[4]

Toxicity and Risk Factors.   The formation of toxins during the ammoniation process is temperature dependent. If temperatures remain less than 70° C during ammoniation, hyperexcitability does not occur. This is sometimes difficult because of the exothermic reactions involved. Square bales stacked under black plastic and ammoniated during excessive ambient temperatures caused hyperexcitability if they were on the outside of the stack nearest the black plastic, whereas bales on the inside of the stack were not toxic. Thermoammoniation ovens can ammoniate one round bale in 23 hours with controlled temperatures.

Excessive ammonia may be a contributing factor to the formation of toxins. The weight of ammonia applied should be equal to 3% to 4% of the dry weight of the straw. The underestimation of moisture content may have led to over-application of ammonia with subsequent toxin formation.[2]

Lactating cows or ewes fed high-quality forages, ammoniated during excessive ambient temperatures with excess ammonia, are at a high risk for passing a toxin through the milk to their calves.

Clinical Signs.   Ammoniated feed toxicosis was nicknamed bovine bonkers because normal cattle have been observed to start trembling, then stampede wildly into anything in their way regardless of the pain involved, and then moments later appear calm and begin eating again.

The syndrome of hyperexcitability has included the following symptoms: nervousness, rapid blinking, involuntary ear twitching, dilation of the pupils, trembling, ataxia, rapid respiration, salivation, apparent impairment of vision, frequent urination and defecation, frothing at the mouth, sweating, bellowing, convulsions, and stampeding, with normal behavior between episodes. Cattle have been found outside of their destroyed pens with broken bones. The onset of clinical signs is rapid. When the toxic feed is removed, the recovery is rapid, if the animal has not injured itself.

Clinical Pathology.   Clinical pathology tests are not helpful for confirming the diagnosis of ammoniated feed toxicity. Tests done on affected animals have ruled out viral or bacterial meningitis and calcium, magnesium, or glucose deficiency.

Lesions.   Lesions associated with this syndrome are those that occur as a result of the physical trauma following the hyperexcitability episodes.

Diagnostic Testing.   Whenever central nervous system (CNS) signs are observed, a differential list should be made that includes, for example, lead, herbicides, pesticides, urea, polio, hypocalcemia, hypomagnesemia, and other CNS toxins. Most of these toxins can be ruled out by diagnostic testing of appropriate samples. Diagnostic laboratories with GC/MS capabilities should be able to test milk, serum, and forage samples for the various imidazoles, but this may not be routinely done.[4]

At this time, history of access to ammoniated feed or protein-molasses blocks with appropriate clinical signs associated with bovine hysteria and the ability to rule out other CNS toxins is the best way to make a diagnosis.

Treatment.   Many animals exhibiting symptoms have not responded to any treatments. Calves treated with acepromazine (0.045 mg/kg and 0.045 mg/kg intramuscularly) and thiamine hydrochloride (1.14 mg/kg intravenously and 1.14 mg/kg intramuscularly) survived. The sedation may have prevented self-mutilation.[3] Removal of the suspect feed should be done as soon as possible. Milking out cows that have affected calves may prevent further exposure.

Prognosis.   The prognosis is good in adults if the feed is removed quickly and the animals do not injure themselves. The prognosis for nursing calves or lambs may be guarded. It is not known whether they are more sensitive to the toxin or they are receiving a higher dose based on body weight.

Prevention and Control.   The best prevention is education of clients about the ammoniation process. Clients should only ammoniate poor-quality roughage (straw verses hay), be as accurate as possible when calculating ammonia and estimating moisture content, and ammoniate during the cooler seasons.

The protein-molasses blocks associated with the death of 13 nursing calves occurred during an extremely wet, hot spring. The conditions may have been ideal for the formation of toxins, but in general, this is not a common occurrence.

Sandra E. Morgan

Source. Cotton is grown in warm climates around the world and is best known for its fiber and oil. When the cotton is harvested, the cottonseeds are removed. Whole cottonseed (WCS) is the seed with the hull still on it. WCS is commonly fed to livestock as a source of protein and fiber. When cottonseed oil is extracted from the seeds, one of the by-products is cottonseed hulls (CSHs), which are removed and used in livestock feed primarily as a source of fiber. The oil can be extracted from the seeds by various methods, which affect the use of the other by-product, cottonseed meal (CSM).

Like any feed ingredient, all factors must be considered when formulating a complete ration. The best qualities of cottonseed are that it is high in protein, high in fiber, very digestible, and economical, making it one of the most widely used protein sources in the livestock feed industry. A ration with cottonseed must be balanced because it is low in the essential amino acids lysine and tryptophan; deficient in calcium, vitamin A, and vitamin D; contains high levels of phosphorus; and contains varying levels of the toxin gossypol. Because WCS still has oil in it, rancidity can also be a factor.

Gossypol is a yellow polyphenolic pigment found in most parts of the cotton plant, but it is concentrated in glands in the seed. It makes the cotton plant more insect resistant. Glandless cottonseed has been developed but has never become popular because it lacks insect resistance. The amount of gossypol in a cotton plant depends on a variety of factors, including genetics, climate, growing season, fertilizer, and soil composition, among others.

Other pigments in cottonseed are considered to be more toxic than gossypol, but they are present in such small quantities that most of the focus is on gossypol.[1]

Gossypol is more readily available in CSM than WCS because the seed is broken open and the glands are ruptured.

Toxicokinetics. Gossypol is classified as a cardiotoxin and an antifertility agent. The two forms of gossypol are free and bound. The bound form is less toxic. The route of exposure is always oral. In ruminants gossypol is bound to proteins in the rumen, thus making them more resistant to gossypol toxicosis than monogastric animals. Gossypol has been found to accumulate in plasma, heart, liver, kidney, muscle, and testes, but not milk. More research is needed regarding metabolism and elimination.

Mechanism of Action. The mechanism of action is still not fully understood. In adult ruminants large amounts of free gossypol are detoxified in the rumen by binding to protein. Gossypol toxicosis can occur if there is not enough available protein or the cottonseed contains high levels of gossypol. Once free gossypol is absorbed, it gradually accumulates in the body and exerts cardiotoxic and repro-ductive effects. It has also been shown to cause lysis of erythrocytes.

The cardiotoxic effects are a gradual destruction of the cardiac musculature and interference with the conduction system by affecting the movement of potassium (K^+) across the cell membrane. In China, hypokalemia developed in men using gossypol as a sterility agent; supplemental potassium could not reverse the hypokalemia.[2] This interference with potassium could account for the sudden deaths without any ongoing symptoms or gross lesions seen at necropsy. The gradual heart failure accounts for the fluid buildup in the rest of the body.

More research is being done on the antifertility aspect of gossypol toxicosis. It has resulted in irregular estrous cycles and reduced pregnancy rates in laboratory rodents. Sows have had reduced conception rates, abortions, or reduced litter size. Gossypol is believed to suppress progesterone and estradiol during the implantation period in rats; it is also believed to affect the follicular development, embryo recovery and production, and corpus luteum function in superovulated heifers.[2]

In male ruminants gossypol inhibits sperm motility and adversely affects sperm production by damaging the spermatogenic epithelium and causing reduced germinal cell layers. Vitamin E supplementation improved libido in bulls fed CSM.[2]

Toxicity and Risk Factors. After so many poultry and swine died from gossypol toxicosis in the early 1900s, their feed was regulated and was not allowed to contain more than 100 ppm free gossypol. The amount of gossypol is not regulated in cattle rations because of the large number of factors that influence it. This is also why the toxic dose is difficult to determine. The age, diet, and amount of stress are important factors to consider. It is generally not used as the protein source in calf and lamb starter rations because they are not considered to have a fully functional rumen.

Except for monogastric animals, newborn dairy calves raised on a bottle and calf starter ration are probably at the highest risk. Thousands of animals died in the 1980s when the type of oil extraction changed from a heat-press to a solvent extraction. The heat increased the binding of free gossypol, making it less toxic. The solvent extraction did not use heat. The solvent extraction method is still used because it extracts the most oil, but an expander-extruder process is also used, which involves heat.

More research is needed regarding gossypol in horses. Even though they are monogastric, there is not much information concerning gossypol toxicosis.

Clinical Signs. Two syndromes affect the heart. One is sudden death in animals that were believed to be healthy. Lambs that died suddenly were often misdiagnosed as "overeating." The other syndrome is a chronic labored breathing syndrome that does not respond to antibiotics. This was called *thumping* in pigs and has been mistaken for pneumonia in lambs and calves. These animals gradually become anorexic, develop a rough hair coat, become chronic poor-doers, and die. Adult dairy cattle have been reported to have decreased heat tolerance, hemoglobinuria, abomasitis, and anorexia.

Clinical Pathology. The most significant clinical pathology findings are increased erythrocyte fragility resulting in decreased packed cell volume. Liver enzymes are elevated.

Lesions. The animals that die suddenly without any previous clinical signs may not have any lesions. Most gross lesions are a result of chronic heart failure with buildup of excessive fluid in the thoracic and peritoneal cavities and edema of the lymph nodes, mesentery, intestine, and other organs. The lungs are uniformly heavy and wet. The pericardial sac may have excessive clear to red-tinged fluid with fibrin clots. The heart may be enlarged and flabby with dilated ventricles and edematous valves. The cardiac musculature may be streaked, pale, or mottled. Pale, swollen, friable nutmeg livers have been observed and are often icteric along with the rest of the animal. Congestion of kidneys and spleen, pale muscles, abomasitis, and red urine have also been seen.

Primary histopathologic findings are myocardial degeneration, centrilobular liver necrosis and congestion, and pulmonary edema. Renal tubular necrosis, abomasitis, and enteritis have also been seen.

Diagnostic Testing. Cottonseed should be tested only at a laboratory that is certified by the American Oil Chemists Society or the Association of Official Analytical Chemists. Because it is a pigment, other pigments can interfere with analysis. Mixed rations like "baby beef" have other feed ingredients that interfere with the gossypol analysis. The most accurate analysis of the level of gossypol in feed must be from the WCS or CSM before it is mixed in a complete ration. The results are reported as free, bound, or total gossypol. Some researchers believe that bound gossypol becomes unbound in the intestine, so a total gossypol value is all that is needed and it is a less expensive test. Others believe that most of the gossypol in the kernel is in the free form so free and total values are similar. The results are in parts per million (ppm), which is mg of gossypol/kg of feed. The interpretation of the results also depends on whether the gossypol is from the kernel or whole seed and whether the level reported is on an "as received" or "dry matter" basis. The results can then be converted to milligrams of gossypol per kilogram body weight or grams per head per day that an animal would consume.[4]

Treatment. No antidote or treatment for gossypol toxicosis is available. The feed source that contains CSM or the WCS should be removed immediately along with any other stress factors. It may take several weeks to months for the animal to return to normal, but it is possible if animals are not severely affected.

Prognosis. The prognosis for gossypol toxicosis is guarded. It depends on the age of the animal, amount and duration of gossypol ingestion, and severity of lesions.

Prevention and Control. The following recommendations have been made concerning the use of cottonseed that has not been tested for gossypol levels. Preruminant calves and lambs (8 to 16 weeks) should not be fed cottonseed prod-

ucts until more research has been done. Young bulls and rams used for breeding should be limited to 10% or less WCS and 5% CSM in their total diet. Beef cows and range bulls can be fed cottonseed meal (2 lb/head/day of direct solvent extracted; 4 lb/head/day of expander or screw-press processed meal; or 4 to 6 lb/head/day of WCS) and not pose any practical problems for fertility. In embryo transfer programs, other protein sources could be used if a more conservative approach is desired.[5]

When the levels of gossypol are known, recommendations for feeding WCS and CSM are reported as the "Maximum Safe Level for Free Gossypol in the Total Diet" for the following: cattle (preruminants)—100 ppm CSM and WCS; growing steers and heifers—200 ppm CSM, 900 ppm WCS; young developing bulls—150 ppm CSM, 600 ppm WCS; mature bulls (during breeding season, about 120 days)—200 ppm CSM, 900 ppm WCS; mature cows—600 ppm CSM, 1200 ppm WCS.[6]

IONOPHORES

Jeffrey O. Hall

Synonyms. Ionophores, scientifically described as polyether acid ionophore antibiotics, are a large class of antibiotics that are produced by filamentous branching bacteria of the order Actinomycetales. This class of antibiotics originated with the discovery of three compounds in 1951.[1] Pressman established the common name of this antibiotic class as ionophores, by identifying that they could bind and transport ions down concentration gradients through biologic membranes.[2]

Sources. Three primary forces resulted in the rapid expansion of this antibiotic class: their extensive use in biologic research, their effective anticoccidial properties, and their enhancement of feed efficiency and rate of weight gain in ruminants. Several ionophores have been approved by the Food and Drug Administration for use in domestic animals as coccidiostats and growth promotants. Thus, the concentration of an ionophore to which an animal may be exposed can range from the amount in labeled-use products up to the percent concentrations found in premixes or concentrates.

Extensive use of ionophores has resulted in animal poisonings in both target species, ones for which ionophores are approved, and nontarget species, ones for which the ionophores are not approved. Although these antibiotics are safe when included at appropriate concentrations in diets of species for which they have been labeled, poisonings can occur with overdoses. Ionophore poisonings are most commonly associated with ingestion by nontarget species, but feeding excessive dietary concentrations has resulted in poisonings in species for which the feed was intended. For nontarget species the most common ionophore exposures are from ingestion of ionophore-medicated feeds resulting from feed mixing errors, ingredient contamination, or feeding of labeled feed to inappropriate species. For target species, poisonings occur with ingestion of excessive doses after feed mixing errors or overfeeding of medicated feeds. Field cases of ionophore toxicosis have been reported in horses, cattle, sheep, turkeys, pigs, dogs, cats, rabbits, white-tailed deer, guinea fowl, ostriches, and chickens.[3-38]

Common and trade names of ionophores approved for use as coccidiostats in broiler replacement layer chickens, turkeys, sheep, and bobwhite quail include narasin (Maxiban, Monteban), salinomycin (Coxistat, Biocox, Saccox), lasalocid (Avatec), monensin (Coban), semduramicin (Aviax), and maduramicin (Cygro).[39,40] The ionophores approved for use as growth promotants in cattle include monensin (Rumensin), lasalocid (Bovatec), and laidlomycin propionate (Cattlyst). Several of these ionophores have multiple approvals, including a variety of combinations with other drugs.

Toxicokinetics. Very little literature on the absorption kinetics of the ionophores is available. Monensin was found to have greater than 95% oral bioavailability in rats, with either lesser availability (50% to 60%) or a much lower systemic metabolism in steers.[41] In comparison, in chickens, salinomycin had a systemic oral bioavailability of 73.02% with an absorption half-life of 3.64 hours.[42] The onset of clinical effects from toxic doses of the various ionophores can be within a few hours, indicating that these drugs are bioavailable and have a moderate absorption rate.

Ionophores are widely distributed in the body once they are absorbed. The only true distribution parameters found were for salinomycin in chickens, in which it had a volume of distribution of 3.28 L/kg and serum protein binding of 19.78%.[42] In a variety of other reported studies, ionophores have been quantified in a variety of tissues in chickens and cattle, including serum, lung, liver, muscle, fat, kidney, skin, and heart.[41-45] Liver concentrations tend to be the greatest for each ionophore in the species tested. Overall, these studies tend to indicate that the ionophores, as a rule, have a large volume of distribution.

Extensive metabolism of ionophores occurs in species that have been tested.[41,43,46-49] Glutathione and P-450 metabolic pathways play a role in the metabolism of ionophore antibiotics. Numerous metabolites can be produced via these pathways, with monensin-dosed rats having greater than 50 metabolites. In addition, interaction of other drugs with these pathways caused enhancement of the ionophore toxicity via competitive or inhibitory enzyme kinetics.[47-49]

Ionophore elimination is via biliary elimination with no renal elimination having been demonstrated. The elimination of the ionophores has been shown to occur relatively quickly; thus, they have short slaughter withdrawal times. However, a slower terminal elimination that may be accounted for by accumulation of parent compound in adipose tissues has been observed.[41]

Mechanism of Action. The mechanisms by which ionophores induce toxicosis are primarily related to their ability to form lipid-soluble complexes with and transport ions across biologic membranes, but they can include the transport of catecholamines. This transport can be between the extracellular and intracellular spaces or between extraorganelle and intraorganelle spaces. Lasalocid was shown to have relative binding-transport rates of Ca^{++} and $Cs^+ > Ba^{++} >$ ethanolamine, Sr^{++}, Rb^+, and $Na^+ >$ norepinephrine > epinephrine and isoproterenol.[50] In comparison, salinomycin has been shown to bind ions preferentially as follows: $Rb^+ > Na^+ > K^+ >>> Cs^+$, Mg^{++}, Ca^{++}, and Sr^{++}.[51] Laidlomycin preferentially transported monovalent ions with a higher propensity for potassium than sodium, with a much lower affinity for divalent ions.[52] And, monensin transports $Na^+ >> K^+$, but did not transport Ca^{++} or Mg^{++}.[53] Narasin has been shown to preferentially bind and transport $Na^+ > K^+ = Rb^+ > Cs^+ > Li^+$, and was shown to transport NH_4^+.[54] By complexing with a cation, the weak organic acid ionophores can maintain a neutral charge and be lipid soluble. Although the ionophores have ion selectivity with preferential binding to specific ions, the ionophore-associated transport must proceed down concentration gradients. And the ionophore must bind another cation to recross the membrane. Thus, the movement of ions results in transfer of one ion into the cell or organelle and another one out.

The ion transport of ionophores results in a net cellular imbalance of sodium, potassium, calcium, and hydrogen. These effects are the direct result of the ionophore-associated transport and the cellular ionic movement that is attempting to regain normal ion balance. These same effects occur in organelles, resulting in functional damage caused by the ion imbalance. Of specific importance is the effect in the mitochondria, where the ionic imbalance results in the loss of adenosine triphosphate (ATP) production via the electron transport chain.

Experimentally, the ionophore-induced changes in metabolic activity can be monitored in intact mitochondria. Narasin and monensin decreased mitochondrial ATPase activity.[54] Salinomycin and lasalocid caused a pH-dependent inhibition of both coupled and uncoupled respiration as well as ATPase activity.[55,56] Also, lasalocid inhibited glutamate oxidation and induced changes in mitochondrial membrane potential of intact mitochondria.[56,57] These effects result in the net loss of mitochondrial function and loss of the ability of the cell to perform oxidative metabolism. Loss of mitochondrial integrity is key in the subsequent tissue damage associated with ionophore poisoning.

Toxicity and Risk Factors. The toxicity of ionophores varies greatly among the ionophores and among species for a single ionophore (Table 19-1). The general toxicity and toxic syndromes induced by ionophores, as well as those specifically of monensin and lasalocid, have been reviewed.[57,70,71] Reviews of laboratory animal toxicology studies have been published for narasin and monensin.[60,61] However, it must be noted that field cases of ionophore poisoning (Table 19-2) and dosage studies (see Table 19-1) indicate that lethality from multiple exposures is at lower exposures than those reported for acute lethality studies. This indicates a cumulative effect with multiple doses or daily exposure. Because of the nonuniformity that occurs in some feed, the concentrations identified in field cases may or may not represent the actual concentrations that the animals ate at the time of poisoning.

TABLE 19-1 **Reported LD$_{50}$s and Toxic Doses of Lasalocid, Monensin, Narasin, Salinomycin, Laidlomycin, and Maduramicin**

Ionophore	Animal	Route	Acute LD$_{50}$s (mg/kg)	Toxic Dose
Lasalocid	Chicken	Oral	71.5	
	Mouse	Oral	100 to 146	
	Mouse	IP	40	
	Rat	Oral	122 to >130	
	Rat	IP	8	
	Rabbit	Oral	40	
	Swine	Oral		Toxic at 35 mg/kg; lethal at 58 mg/kg
	Cattle	Oral		5 of 6 died at 50 mg/kg
	Horse	Oral	21.5	
Monensin	Chicken	Oral	200	
	Mouse	Oral IP	70 to 96	
	Mouse	Oral	10	
	Rat	IP	28.6 to 100	
	Rat	Oral	15	
	Rabbit	Oral	41.7	
	Dog	Oral	>10	5 mg/kg/day was toxic
	Pig	Oral	16.7 to 50	
	Sheep	Oral	11.9	
	Goat	Oral	26.4	
	Cattle	Oral	26.4	7.6 mg/kg/day was lethal
	Horse		2 to 3	
Narasin	Mouse	Oral	15.8 to 36.7	
	Mouse	IP	7	
	Rat	Oral	18.5 to 40.8	
	Rabbit	Oral	11.9 to 15.5	Toxic at 1.2 mg/kg/day
	Dog	Oral	>10	Toxic at 2 mg/kg/day 61
Salinomycin	Mouse	Oral	50	
	Mouse	IP	18	
	Turkey	Oral	0.6	22 mg/kg of feed in adults
	Horse	Oral		
Laidlomycin Propionate	Rat	Oral	63	Toxic at 8 mg/kg/day
	Dog	Oral		Toxic at 1.5 mg/kg/day
	Cattle	Oral `		Toxic at 5.5 mg/kg
Maduramicin	Chicken	Oral		Toxic at 9 mg/kg of feed
	Rat	Oral		Lethal at 3 mg/kg of feed
	Dog	Oral		Toxic at 12 mg/kg of feed
	Horse	Oral		Toxic at 55 mg/kg of feed

Data from references 1, 7, 29, 53, 57-63, 65-69.

Adult turkeys are sensitive to the toxic effects of some ionophores. But, age is an important risk factor in the sensitivity of turkeys.[23,75] Adult turkeys have a much greater sensitivity to the toxic effects of some ionophores than young birds, with lasalocid being an exception to this effect.[76]

Drug and compound interactions with ionophores pose an additional risk for ionophore poisoning. Most of the toxic interactions are due to competition for the enzymes of metabolism. Dihydroquinoline antioxidants were toxic in combination with salinomycin, narasin, monensin, and maduramycin at concentrations that independently were advantageous.[77,78] Similarly, monensin, maduramicin, and salinomycin have toxic interactions with tiamulin in poultry and pigs.[29,79-81] However, no interactive effects were observed between lasalocid and either tiamulin in turkeys or dihydroquinoline antioxidants.[73,78,82] The tiamulin effect could be explained by findings that it inhibits P-450 metabolism, which could result in decreased metabolism of the

TABLE 19-2 **Reported Lethal Doses from Field Cases of Ionophore Poisoning**

Ionophore	Animal	Route	Lethal Doses
Lasalocid	Chicken	Oral	Lost egg fertility and hatchability 105-150 mg/kg of food or 15-20 mg/kg/day
	Dog	Oral	166-210 mg/kg of food or 10-15 mg/kg/day
	Cattle	Oral	1010-1700 mg/kg of feed or 17-28 mg/kg/day
Monensin	Chicken	Oral	161-325 mg/kg of feed or 16-32 mg/kg/day
	Turkey	Oral	200 mg/kg of feed or 15-20 mg/kg/day
	Dog	Oral	165 mg/kg of feed or 6-7 mg/kg/day
	Pig	Oral	7 mg/kg/day
	Sheep	Oral	83-650 mg/kg of feed or 2.2-26 mg/kg/day
	Cattle	Oral	440 mg/kg of feed or 10 mg/kg/day
	Horse	Oral	235-300 mg/kg of feed
Narasin	Turkey	Oral	28-70 mg/kg of feed or 3-8 mg/kg/day
	Rabbit	Oral	30-35 mg/kg of feed or 3-5 mg/kg/day
	Pig	Oral	58-1057 mg/kg of feed
Salinomycin	Turkey	Oral	15-56 mg/kg of feed or 1-6 mg/kg/day
	Cat	Oral	13-21 mg/kg of feed
	Pig	Oral	166-720 mg/kg of feed
	Horse	Oral	190-500 mg/kg of feed
Maduramicin	Sheep	Oral	2.5-6.1 mg/kg of poultry litter feed
	Cattle	Oral	2.5-6.1 mg/kg of poultry litter feed

Data from references 4-7, 9, 10, 12, 16, 18-23, 25-27, 28-30, 34, 35, 37, 38, 72-74.

ionophores.[49] Thus, any drug that competes with or inhibits the metabolism of the ionophores could enhance their toxicity.

Clinical Signs. The clinical syndromes of ionophore toxicosis are somewhat consistent among ionophores, but have slight differences among species. Clinical signs are related to cellular and subcellular ion imbalances causing deficits in the function of excitable tissues: neurologic, musculoskeletal, cardiac, or smooth muscle. But, in all species, death can occur without observation of any other clinical signs.

The clinical syndrome of ionophore toxicosis in equids is similar for those that have been reported. The more common onset of clinical signs is less than 24 hours, but it can be as long as several days.* Feed refusal is frequently the first clinical sign noted, but often occurs after sufficient feed has been ingested to result in toxicosis.[4-7,69,83-86] However, horses that refuse to eat the concentrate portion of their diet continue to eat hay. The more common clinical signs that occur include some degree of weakness, ataxia and incoordination, tremors, stumbling, exaggerated stepping, hesitance to move or turn, tachycardia, congested mucous membranes, hypotension, dyspnea, hyperpnea, sweating, recumbency, and death.† Less frequently reported clinical signs or ones that occur just before death are prolonged capillary refill, jugular pulse, increased or

decreased borborygmus, audible arrhythmias, bladder distention, pitting edema, and electrocardiographic (ECG) changes. Death from ionophore poisoning can occur within the first 24 hours or can be delayed. Death can occur months after a poisoning incident as a result of residual tissue damage. The long-term clinical effects of ionophore poisoning are due to cardiovascular damage that occurs with the initial poisoning. Horses can present for unthriftiness, poor performance, poor exercise tolerance, arrhythmias, pitting edema, hyperpnea, or death.[3,4] Because horses can die suddenly as a result of the cardiac damage of ionophores, any horse that has had ionophore poisoning is a high-risk animal.

The clinical syndrome of ionophore toxicosis in cattle is dose dependent and can vary in severity from decreased feed intake to severe cardiac, skeletal muscle, and gastrointestinal effects. Lasalocid and monensin toxicoses in cattle cause varying degrees of anorexia, depression, muscle tremors, weakness, incoordination and ataxia, tachycardia, tachypnea, labored respiration, watery diarrhea, rumen atony, dehydration, and death.[9-15,58,63,87-90] Diarrhea and reluctance to eat the concentrate portion of the ration are the earliest clinical signs to develop. A dose-related severity and duration of signs are expected. Other signs that occur with less frequency include dragging of the rear legs, recumbency, jugular pulse, subcutaneous edema, ECG changes, and nasal discharge. Death generally occurs more than 2 days after exposure, but it can occur in some cases weeks after the ingestion. Development of congestive heart failure can occur as a sequela to an acute ionophore poisoning.

*References 5, 7, 8, 59, 69, 83, 84.
†References 4, 5, 7, 8, 59, 69, 84, 85.

Ionophore poisoning in sheep generally mimics the clinical signs observed in cattle. Administration studies and field cases of ionophore poisoning in sheep are limited to monensin. Initial clinical signs include anorexia and depression, which are followed by diarrhea, abdominal pain, weakness, a humped stance, incoordination, muscular stiffness, reluctance to move, knuckling, posterior paresis, muscle wasting, dyspnea, recumbency, and death.[16-18,91,92] In clinically affected sheep that do not die, poor weight gain, poor condition, and ataxia may last up to 3 months.[17]

Ionophore toxicosis in pigs generally is characterized by gastrointestinal and neuromuscular effects. Clinical signs of ionophore-poisoned pigs include stiffness, tremors, reluctance to move, knuckling, diarrhea, anorexia, lethargy, ataxia, dyspnea, recumbency, myoglobinurea, ECG changes, and death.* But there was no observed effects in piglets suckling sows fed narasin.[25] Clinical signs can begin within 24 hours and deaths can continue for weeks after a poisoning incident. Various studies suggest that the clinical syndrome does not vary among the ionophores in pigs.

The clinical syndrome induced by ionophores in dogs and cats seems to reflect primarily neurologic or muscular dysfunction. Field cases of ionophore poisoning in dogs presented with clinical signs that included depression, weakness, ataxia, paresis, myoglobinuria, recumbency, paraplegia, quadriplegia, dysuria, fecal and urinary incontinence, partial anorexia, constipation, weight loss, and dyspnea.[26,27] In comparison, cats in a field case of ionophore poisoning displayed weakness, paresis, paralysis, dysphonia, loss of spinal reflexes with intact conscious pain perception, dyspnea, and death.[28] Similar clinical syndromes have been produced in toxicity trials with narasin, monensin, laidlomycin propionate, and maduramicin.[60,61,66-68] Onset of clinical signs can be as early as 6 to 12 hours after ingestion, with the duration of effects lasting weeks to months.

The clinical signs of ionophore-poisoned rabbits are similar to those observed in other species. Clinical signs of ionophore toxicosis in research trials included weakness, ataxia, depression, anorexia, hypoactivity, and diarrhea.[61] The onset and duration of clinical signs were variable, with some rabbits succumbing within hours and others dying days to weeks later. Similar clinical signs were reported in field cases, with additional clinical signs of sialorrhea, opisthotonus, tonic-clonic muscle spasms, torticollis, paralysis (especially of the hind limbs), and recumbency.[29,30]

Clinical signs induced by various ionophore toxicoses tend to have a similar presentation in different birds. Ionophore toxicosis in chickens results in severe anorexia, diarrhea, depression, squatting, sternal recumbency, ataxia, drooped heads, drooped wings, weight loss, weakness, proprioceptive deficits, paralysis, and death.[34,35,95,96] The syndrome has an onset of less than 1 day to several days, and the birds that survived gradually improved over a period of several days to weeks. In comparison, monensin-poisoned mature ostriches became ataxic and recumbent before death.[33] The clinical signs of ionophore-poisoned turkeys can include decreased feed intake, diarrhea, drowsiness, polydipsia, tachypnea, dyspnea, incoordination, weakness, locomotor disorders, paraly-

sis, recumbency, weight loss, and death.[19-24,96-98] The clinical course in turkeys has an onset range of up to 3 days and deaths continued for several days after an ionophore-containing diet was removed. Attempts to reproduce ionophore toxicosis were initially unsuccessful when young turkeys were used, but the syndrome was reproduced using adult turkeys. Thus, the clinical syndrome of ionophore toxicosis in different avian species is almost identical.

Another significant clinical sign of ionophore poisoning in laying birds is the loss of egg production, fertility, or hatchability, without observation of other clinical signs of toxicosis in the layers.[23,35-38,99] Infertile eggs, early embryonic death, bacterial contamination, deformed embryo, leg weakness and ataxia in hatched chicks, and inability to break out of the shell by mature chicks also has been observed. In field cases, normal fertility has returned after the contaminated feed was discontinued for 2 to 3 weeks. Thus, an important component of ionophore toxicosis in birds is the effect on egg production and development.

Clinical Pathology.   Clinical pathologic alterations reported with ionophore poisoning must be applied to clinical cases cautiously. Although serum chemistry changes can occur, a lack of abnormal findings does not rule out ionophore poisoning. The changes discussed in this section frequently have sporadic occurrence or occur less than 24 hours before an animal dies. Thus, an animal may have normal serum biochemistry readings for a week or longer after an ionophore ingestion before clinical pathologic changes occur. Better application of clinical pathology can be made by testing groups of animals.

In horses, the clinicopathologic changes induced by ionophores are generally associated with muscle and liver damage, as well as electrolyte abnormalities. However, in field cases and research studies, serum electrolyte changes occurred late in the clinical syndrome, were variable in occurrence, or were not detected.[8,85,86] Clinicopathologic abnormalities that have been reported from field cases and administration studies include increased serum values for alkaline phosphatase, aspartate aminotransferase (AST), lactate dehydrogenase (LDH), creatine phosphokinase (CPK), creatinine, indirect bilirubin, BUN, glucose, hematocrit, serum osmolality, and phosphorus; decreased values for serum Ca^{++} and K^+; and decreased urine osmolality that was accompanied by increased urine volume.[3,7,8,59,85] Although abnormalities occur variably, increases in LDH, AST, CPK, and bilirubin were more consistently identified.

Clinicopathologic changes observed with lasalocid or monensin toxicosis are attributed to dehydration, electrolyte changes, and muscle damage. Changes identified in monensin administration studies were as follows: leukocytosis; increased serum AST, CPK, and protein; decreased serum K^+, Na^+, and Ca^{++}; and increased urine glucose, protein, myoglobin, and hemoglobin, as well as decreased specific gravity and pH.[88,90] The occurrence and degree of change were somewhat dose dependent, but more a function of the time of sample collection. For example, the greatest increases in AST and CPK occurred within 1 day of death, even when death occurred several days after ingestion. Lasalocid toxicosis induced the following abnormalities: increased red blood cell count, hemoglobin, hematocrit, and leukocyte count;

*References 25, 62, 72, 73, 93, 94.

increased serum CPK, LDH, sorbitol dehydrogenase (SDH), BUN, creatinine, total protein, albumin, and total bilirubin; and increased urine specific gravity and decreased urine pH.[58] Similar changes were observed in a monensin treatment group used as a positive control. A single affected animal in a case of monensin toxicosis had increased BUN, creatinine, K^+, AST, SDH, LDH, and CPK, whereas Ca^{++} and Na^+ were decreased.[12] In dosing studies, animals within treatment groups are not uniform in their clinicopathologic changes. Thus, clinicopathologic effects of the ionophores may be used for overall monitoring, but changes may not be observed in an individual animal because of a very high degree of animal-to-animal variability.

Clinicopathologic alterations in pigs are related to skeletal muscle damage. Massive increases in AST and CPK can occur by 1 day after ingestion and stay increased for several days.[62,93,94] The isoenzymes of CPK should indicate primarily the MM (skeletal muscle origin) isotype. In addition, pigs may have decreased serum vitamin A and E as a result of increased serum and tissue lipid peroxidation.[99]

Reported clinicopathologic parameter changes in sheep are limited. Changes that have been reported to occur include increased CPK, increased AST, increased SDH, decreased calcium, myoglobinuria, and a stress leukogram.[16,18,91,92] However, there can be a highly variable onset and increases are not necessarily dose dependent.

Milder clinicopathologic changes are more typical for ionophore toxicoses in dogs. Transient increases in AST, CPK, and ALT were observed in chronic and subchronic studies with monensin.[60] In comparison, dogs from field cases of monensin toxicosis had increased serum LDH, AST, urinary protein, and urinary white blood cell count, as well as myoglobinuria.[27] Lasalocid toxicosis resulted in polycythemia, mildly increased CPK, and mildly increased LDH.[26] In chronic and subchronic studies with narasin, transient increases in both AST and CPK were identified.[61] In a subchronic study with laidlomycin propionate, increased BUN, AST, ALT, LDH, and globulin were found.[67]

The only clinicopathologic aberrations of ionophore toxicosis that have been reported in birds are associated with muscle damage. Increases in CPK and AST occur before the detection of light microscopic lesions.[20] Chickens may have decreased serum vitamin A and E as a result of increased serum and tissue lipid peroxidation associated with muscle damage.[99]

Lesions. Both gross and histologic lesions associated with ionophore poisoning are somewhat dependent on the species involved. No matter what species is involved, it is not uncommon for lesions to be absent in animals that die quickly after the ingestion. Lesions are more likely to be identified in animals that survive for more than 24 hours. Therefore, in cases of ionophore toxicosis, it is important to evaluate tissues from more than one animal to maximize the likelihood for identification of tissue damage.

Gross pathology. In the horse, gross lesions caused by ionophores are generally associated with the heart and the secondary effects of heart failure. However, it is not uncommon for lesions to be absent.[6,69,83,86] A variety of gross lesions have been reported from ionophore-poisoned horses, including epicardial and endocardial hemorrhage,

paleness or pale streaking of the ventricular myocardium, increased myocardial friability, loss of heart tone, accentuated hepatic lobular pattern, hydropericardium, hydrothorax, ascites, pulmonary congestion and edema, systemic congestion, and subcutaneous fluid accumulation.* Less commonly identified lesions include a shrunken spleen, splenomegaly, hepatomegaly, distention of the bladder, hyperemic kidneys, and pale skeletal musculature.[3,7,59,83]

Ionophore-poisoned cattle and sheep typically have gross lesions associated with heart damage and skeletal muscle damage. But, an absence of gross lesions is not uncommon. Frequently identified lesions are paling of the myocardium, myocardial streaking, petechia and ecchymosis of the myocardium, enlarged hearts, pulmonary congestion, pulmonary edema, hepatic congestion and occasional hepatomegaly, hydropericardium, hydrothoracic, ascites, subcutaneous edema, streaking and hemorrhage of the skeletal muscles, and pale skeletal muscles.† In general, skeletal lesions are more commonly identified in sheep than in cattle, but both have more frequent skeletal lesions than do horses. Also, in sheep, gastrointestinal mucosal congestion or hemorrhage, muscle wasting, and renal congestion have been observed.[16-18] The severity of lesions is variable and some animals may have minimal to no gross lesions.

Gross lesions in pigs involve skeletal muscles and a systemic congestion. Common gross lesions include white areas within skeletal muscle groups, hydropericardium, pulmonary congestion and edema, skin congestion, generalized congestion, mottling of the epicardium and myocardium, and myoglobinuria; however, gross lesions are often absent.[25,62,72,73] The gross lesions of the heart are much less frequent and skeletal lesions are more common than in horses or ruminants.

Minimal gross lesions have been described in cats or rabbits and none have been described in dogs. Paling of the myocardium was the only gross lesion observed in salinomycin-poisoned cats.[28] In rabbits, narasin caused minimal gross lesions of altered muscle color, and this was difficult to see.[30]

Macroscopic lesions in poultry include gastrointestinal, skeletal muscle, cardiac, and liver damage, as well as systemic congestion. Gross lesions include emaciation, small pale spleens, pale kidneys, cardiac enlargement, loss of myocardial tone, pale myocardium, hydropericardium, ascites, pulmonary congestion, hepatic congestion, and enteritis.[21,23,34,35,101] An absence of gross lesions is common.

Histopathology. Histologic lesions in most species are most commonly found in the skeletal or cardiac muscles. However, lesions in neurologic, hepatic, and renal tissues also may be identified. The location of primary tissue damage is somewhat species dependent.

Microscopic tissue evaluation of ionophore-poisoned horses generally reveals some degree of myocardial damage, but can include hepatic and renal damage as well. However,

---

*References 3, 4, 7, 8, 59, 69, 83.
†References 9, 11-14, 16, 18, 88, 92, 100.

no lesions may be identified in animals that die quickly after a toxic ingestion. Lesions that may be identified include swollen myocardial fibers with loss of striations, foci of myocardial necrosis, myocardial intracytoplasmic vacuolization, myocardial hyaline degeneration, myocardial mineralization, congestion and edema in a variety of tissues, hepatocellular necrosis, hepatocyte vacuolization, and renal tubular necrosis.* Swelling and dissociation of Purkinje fibers also have been observed.[6,7] In animals that survive for an extended period after the poisoning incident, fibrous connective tissue replacement of lost myocardial cells can be seen.[3] In horses, the most prominent muscle necrosis observed is myocardial, with skeletal muscle lesions being much less common.

Cattle, sheep, and rabbits have histologic lesions that are similar to those described in horses. The similarities include the myocardial, skeletal muscle, hepatic, and Purkinje cell necrosis, as well as the congestion and edema of various tissues.† Additional findings include loss of pancreatic zymogen granules, rumenitis, cellular infiltrates in the areas of tissue necrosis, mineralization of necrotic foci, and fibrous connective tissue repair of muscle necrosis.[16,17,88,91,100] In comparison to the horse, cattle and sheep have a greater occurrence of skeletal muscle lesions.

Swine typically have a predominance of skeletal muscle necrosis, with some findings of myocardial necrosis.[25,62,72,94] With time, the skeletal muscle lesions progress from acute necrosis to myocellular regeneration. In addition, renal tubular nephrosis with casts occurs as a result of myoglobin release from the damaged musculature.

Histopathologic lesions in ionophore-poisoned dogs are both neurologic and muscular in nature. As in pigs, the predominant muscular necrosis is of skeletal muscles, but occasional myocardial lesions can be seen.[60,61] Focal degeneration of intramuscular nerves, retinal atrophy, or a significant peripheral neuropathy also can be observed.[61,66-68]

In the only reported observation of ionophore-poisoned cats, the primary lesion was of a distal polyneuropathy, but myocardial and skeletal muscle lesions also occurred.[28] The acute lesions were described as swelling, fragmentation, and loss of axons. This was followed by collapse and loss of the myelin sheaths. Changes occurred to both the sensory and motor nerves.

Avian species also have light microscopic myocyte, myocardial, hepatic, and renal tissue lesions, as well as tissue congestion and edema.[20-22,24,33-35,38,101] Mineralization of damaged muscle tissue, enteritis, and pancreatic necrosis are occasionally observed. In addition, neurologic lesions of axonal swelling with fragmentation in sciatic nerves, as well as degenerating axons and myelin sheaths in the spinal cord, have been described.[38,96]

Diagnostic Testing. Diagnosis of ionophore toxicosis is primarily based on clinical signs, clinical pathology, pathologic lesions, and identification of compatible ionophore concentrations in the diet. However, an absence of clinical pathology or lesions is not uncommon if animals die quickly

after the ingestion. Additionally, if there is nonuniformity of the feed, the analyzed concentration may not truly represent the concentration ingested.

Feed and tissue analyses for the ionophores are available from most diagnostic laboratories or may be provided by the manufacturer. But identification of an ionophore in tissues only provides evidence that an animal was exposed and does not necessarily indicate that such exposure was the cause of death. Feed being used at the time is the best analytic sample, but if many bags or containers of feed are available, then it is wise to test several. A variety of thin layer, liquid, and gas chromatographic methods have been developed for ionophore analysis.[102-108]

Other diagnostic testing that assists in cases of ionophore poisoning are ECG and echocardiography. A variety of ECG alterations have been described in horses, cattle, pigs, and dogs. Abnormalities identified in horses include prolongation of atrial and ventricular depolarization, prolonged repolarization, increased S wave amplitude, depression of the S-T segment, absence of P wave, increased T wave, intermittent premature ventricular contractions, ventricular tachycardia, transient arrhythmias, AV block, atrial fibrillation, and ventricular fibrillation.[3,5,7,8,83] In comparison, ionophore-poisoned cattle were found to have abnormal ST segments, Q-T interval prolongation, QRS interval prolongation, first degree heart block, infrequent premature atrial beats, and increased T-wave amplitude.[14,88] Pigs have widening of the P wave, notched P wave, long Q-T intervals, ventricular parasystole, nodal beats, and sinus arrest.[62,94] The only ECG changes noted in dogs were premature ventricular contractions and bradyarrhythmia or tachyarrhythmia.[109,110] However, caution must be maintained when using ECG evaluations, because abnormalities vary dramatically among animals or can be absent in some animals that have myocardial lesions. For example, an individual animal may have only one or no ECG changes that have been reported for that species. This is likely due to damage that is not interfering with the plane of electrical current being measured. Echocardiographic evaluation also may be used to identify abnormal ventricular function in ionophore-poisoned horses.[111] Changes in fractional shortening of the ventricular myocardium have been reported in ionophore-poisoned horses, but the ability of this method to rule out ionophore-associated damage has not been evaluated. Thus, the presence of ECG or echocardiographic abnormalities provides additional evidence that ionophore poisoning is possible, but their absence does not rule out myocardial damage or ionophore poisoning.

Treatment. Currently, there is no specific antidote for ionophore-poisoned animals, but some beneficial therapeutics may be used. The first course of treatment in animals that have recently ingested high doses of ionophores is gastric decontamination. Emesis can be induced in dogs or cats to empty the stomach. Activated charcoal with a cathartic to bind and enhance removal of the ionophore should be used in cases in which the ionophore ingestion was very recent. Treatment with vitamin E or selenium to help minimize the secondary oxidative tissue damage has shown some limited benefit in cattle and pigs, especially

---

*References 4, 6-8, 59, 69, 83, 96.
†References 9, 12-14, 16-18, 29, 30, 88, 90-92, 100.

when given before development of clinical signs.[62,92] Other than decontamination and antioxidants, the primary treatments are supportive. This includes fluids to maintain hydration and enhance elimination or prevent renal casting by myoglobin. Keeping animals quiet and minimizing stress may help limit the cardiac damage from the ionophores. Good nutritional and husbandry support also should be provided.

Prognosis. The prognosis is guarded to poor for any animal that has the potential for myocardial damage. Even if the animal survives the acute phase of a poisoning incident, a great potential exists for long-term cardiac problems. These effects may range from poor performance or exercise intolerance to congestive heart failure, shortened life expectancy, or death. Horses with breeding potential may be used, but if myocardial damage is present, the stresses of breeding or foaling may be life threatening. Food-producing animals that survive can often be maintained and salvaged for slaughter, but their performance (e.g., feed efficiency, weight gain) may be decreased. Ionophore-poisoned dogs recover over weeks to months, but heart damage should still be of concern even though myocardial effects are somewhat less in dogs.

Prevention and Control. Ionophore-containing feeds should be used only in species for which they were formulated to prevent nontarget species from being exposed. In addition, feed mills or individuals should carefully store ionophore premixes or concentrates and carefully calculate and mix feed formulations.

NITRATE

Stan W. Casteel and Tim J. Evans

Synonyms. Nitrate poisoning or intoxication also has been referred to as *nitrite* or *nitrate/nitrite* poisoning because it is generally the toxic effects of the nitrite anion, produced from ingested nitrate in the gastrointestinal tract, that is responsible for the clinical syndrome.

Sources. Nitrate or nitrite poisoning can occur in all animals. However, ruminants are most susceptible to nitrate toxicosis because of the nitrate-reducing ability of rumen microbes. Poisoning is most often a drought-associated problem in ruminants consuming plants with an accumulated excess of nitrate. Nitrate-based fertilizer is another source; animals consume the granular formulation after gaining access to storage areas or to piles accidentally deposited on the ground. Ingestion of nitrate-based fertilizers also may cause gastrointestinal irritation in most animals, and methemoglobin formation in ruminants and monogastrics. Water containing several hundred parts per million of nitrate is another possible source of toxic exposure. In an unusual case, three cats and two dogs suffered nitrite intoxication from excessive sodium nitrite used to preserve a commercial pet food.[1]

BOX 19-1	WEEDS AND CROPS WITH NITRATE-ACCUMULATING POTENTIAL

GENUS, SPECIES, AND COMMON NAMES OF WEEDS

Ambrosia spp.	Ragweed
Amaranthus spp.	Pigweed, Carelessweed
Carduus nutans	Musk thistle
Chenopodium spp.	Lambsquarters
Cirsium arvense	Canada thistle
Gnaphalium spp.	Cudweeds
Helianthus annuus	Annual sunflower
Kochia scoparia	Kochia, Fireweed
Lygodesmia spp.	Skeleton-plants
Malva parviflora	Cheeseweed
Melilotus officinalis	Sweetclover
Polygonum spp.	Smartweeds
Rumex spp.	Docks
Salsola pestifer	Russian thistle
Silybum marianum	Milk thistle
Solanum spp.	Nightshades
Sorghum halepense	Johnsongrass
Viguiera spp.	Golden-eyes

GENUS, SPECIES, AND COMMON NAMES OF CROPS

Avena sativa	Oat
Beta vulgaris	Beet
Brassica spp.	Rape, Turnip
Glycine max	Soybean
Hordeum spp.	Barley
Linum usitatissimum	Flax
Medicago sativa	Alfalfa
Pennisetum typhoides	Pearl millet
Secale cereale	Rye
Sorghum vulgare	Sorghum sudan grass
Triticum aestivum	Wheat
Zea mays	Corn

Box 19-1 lists nitrate-accumulating plants. The combination of plant stress and high levels of soil nitrate is conducive to nitrate accumulation in many other species of weeds and normally acceptable forages. Crops injured by stress, such as frost, drought, herbicides, or hail, have reduced capability for photosynthesis, a process primarily restricted to the leaves. Roots and stems generally are unaffected and continue to supply nitrate to the upper plant portions. Damage to the photosynthetic machinery reduces the efficiency of nitrate incorporation into other plant constituents, thereby leading to accumulation of toxic levels. Nitrate concentrations are likely to remain elevated until new leaf growth facilitates an increased level of photosynthesis to utilize the accumulated nitrate. If forage is harvested for hay, the accumulated nitrate concentration is retained, thereby remaining a toxic hazard. Cornstalks left in Nebraska fields had an average decrease of just 30% potassium nitrate approximately 90 days after harvest.[2]

Toxicokinetics. As a component of the nitrogen cycle, nitrates are present in all plants and represent a continuous source of exposure for herbivores. Rumen microorganisms reduce nitrate to nitrite, the proximate toxin responsible for induction of methemoglobinemia. The reduction of nitrate to nitrite occurs rapidly in the rumen, whereas the large bowel of horses provides an environment intermediate in nitrate-reducing activity between that of ruminants and other monogastric animals.[3] However, documented nitrate toxicosis in horses is rare.[4] Pregnant and open mares have ingested forage containing nitrate concentrations of 2.5% to 3.5% percent for several months and suffered no adverse effects. In other cases, both pregnant and open mares tolerated forage that was lethal to cattle.

Nitrate and nitrite anions are readily absorbed from the gastrointestinal tract into the bloodstream. Peak methemoglobin levels occur in cattle approximately 3 hours after intraruminal administration or drenching with nitrate. In dogs, most absorbed nitrate is eliminated in the urine, whereas ruminants eliminate a comparatively small portion. Like monogastric animals, preruminant calves also excrete large quantities of nitrate in urine. The elimination half-life for nitrate in dogs is 44.7 hours, in sheep 4.2 hours, and in ponies 4.8 hours. The nitrite elimination half-life in dogs is 0.5 hour, in sheep 0.475 hour, and in ponies 0.57 hour.[3] In adult cattle, the elimination half-life for nitrate is estimated to be 9 hours, whereas the half-life for nitrate is more than 24 hours in the bovine fetus.[2]

Experimental and anecdotal evidence supports the view that nitrate induces abortion as a sequela of nitrate toxicosis in the dam.[3] In general, this is consistent with sequelae to severe upsets in maternal homeostasis; however, nitrite also passes the placental barrier to act on fetal erythrocytes. Elevated ocular nitrate concentrations in aborted fetuses are often used to support the diagnosis of nitrate-induced abortion.[5] High levels of methemoglobinemia in stillborn calves from cows receiving a high-nitrate ration also have been reported. Experimentally, cows infused intravenously for 30 minutes with nitrite at doses up to 12 mg/kg body weight (BW) had a dose-related increase in methemoglobin concentration to a maximum of 35% about 1.5 hours after infusion commenced.[6] This effect was accompanied by an immediate onset of decreasing arterial blood pressure with a maximum decrease of up to 50% attained at the end of nitrite infusion. The combined adverse effects resulted in significant depression of fetal oxygenation (30% to 40%), but were of insufficient magnitude to kill the fetus. These results indicate that fetal lethality may require higher or more sustained exposures to nitrate or nitrite.

Mechanism of Action. Although poisoning from the various forms of nitrate is referred to as *nitrate poisoning,* the nitrate ion itself has a low order of toxicity compared with the nitrite anion. In the anaerobic environment of the rumen, ingested nitrate is reduced to the directly toxic nitrite anion, which then undergoes further reduction to ammonia for incorporation into microbial protein. The reduction of nitrate to nitrite occurs much more rapidly in the rumen than does the reduction of nitrite to ammonia. Consequently, when ruminants consume plants high in nitrate, some fraction of nitrite formed in the rumen enters the bloodstream where it oxidizes ferrous iron (Fe^{+2}) in blood

hemoglobin to ferric iron (Fe^{+3}), which by definition is methemoglobin. This destroys the oxygen-carrying capacity of affected hemoglobin, and the animal ultimately suffers from oxygen deprivation as methemoglobin levels increase. Mild clinical signs of intoxication, such as exercise intolerance, may begin to show when methemoglobin levels reach 30% to 40%, whereas methemoglobin concentrations exceeding 80% are lethal.[7] Both nitrate and nitrite are also vasoactive compounds capable of reducing vascular tone and further compromising delivery of oxygen to the tissues. Prussic acid (cyanide) produced in tandem in *Sorghum* species also causes death by tissue asphyxiation, but by a different process. In general, nitrate poisoning is a more common problem, because cyanide occurs in early plant growth and dissipates on curing of harvested forages.

Toxicity and Risk Factors. All plants contain some nitrate-nitrogen with potentially toxic levels accumulating in forage grown under stressful circumstances. Conditions associated with nitrate accumulation and retention by plants include adverse environmental influences during growth, large amounts of nitrate available for plant uptake, herbicide application, plant species, plant part, and post-harvesting storage methods.[8] Moisture stress, unusually high ambient temperatures, unusually cool, cloudy weather, leaf-damaging hail, frost, and herbicide application are all conditions hindering the photosynthetic activity required for appropriate nitrate use. Consumption of the stalk portion of *Sorghum* species (e.g., grain sorghum, sorghum sudan hybrids, Johnsongrass) and corn (*Zea mays*) deprived of water are classically responsible for nitrate intoxication in ruminants. Water deprivation of forage results in inhibition of enzyme-mediated nitrate reduction required for synthesis of plant proteins and other nitrogen-containing compounds. The primary site for the nitrate reduction reaction is the green leaf actively engaged in photosynthesis. Consequently, the highest concentration of nitrate is in the lower stalks and stems that transport nitrate absorbed by the roots. Because nitrate is translocated from the soil up the stalk and stems, leaf material and grain or seeds do not accumulate significant nitrate levels. Plants with a high stem-to-leaf ratio are most likely to be problematic.[8,9]

Nitrate poisoning occurs in animals throughout the world. Cattle are most susceptible to nitrate intoxication, especially when on a low-energy ration. Sheep are less sensitive than cattle to dietary nitrates because of their slower rate of intake and shorter nitrate elimination half-life.[9] Nitrate poisoning in horses induced by ingestion of high nitrate plants has not been reliably documented, and it is a common misconception that horses are as susceptible to nitrate poisoning as ruminants.[4] Monogastric animals such as horses, poultry, pigs, dogs, and cats require much higher levels of nitrates than ruminants to produce clinical signs of nitrate intoxication.

Acute nitrate poisoning most likely occurs in cattle when forage nitrate exceeds 10,000 ppm (1%) on a dry-weight basis. Forage containing less than 5000 ppm (0.5%) nitrate is generally considered safe for all classes of livestock, whereas concentrations in the 5000 to 10,000 ppm range should not be fed to pregnant cattle. Nitrates may accumulate to concentrations of several percent in plants, with the toxicity of high-nitrate forage unaltered by drying. Conversely, ensiling of forages results in a large reduction of nitrate concentration from the microbial activity during the following 30 to 60 days.

Susceptibility of cattle to nitrate toxicosis depends on several risk factors including amount and rate of intake, variations in gastrointestinal nitrate reduction capability (adaptation), low-carbohydrate diet, and metabolic state of the animal (age, pregnancy, disease).[10] Cattle that are hungry and cold may consume a great deal of high-nitrate hay in a short time. This is often the situation when cattle have been consuming high-nitrate forage for days to weeks with no apparent problem, and a sudden change in weather (usually a winter cold front) precedes clinical intoxication and sudden death. Aggressive eaters are often the first victims.

The estimated safe level for nitrate concentration in water for livestock ranges from a few hundred to more than 1000 ppm.[11] Acute nitrate intoxication has resulted from the additive sources of drinking water containing more than 500 ppm and feed containing 5000 ppm.[12]

Clinical Signs. Ruminants are commonly poisoned because of their nature as foraging herbivores and their high level of nitrate-reducing microbes in the rumen. Furthermore, having the predilection to lick, mouth, and chew on various objects often leads to ingestion of many unusual substances, including nitrate-based fertilizer. Rapid ingestion of high-nitrate material may induce onset of clinical intoxication in 1 to 4 hours. Clinical signs reflect tissue oxygen deprivation and include exercise intolerance, dyspnea, weakness, ataxia, tachycardia, depression, tremors, muddy or cyanotic mucous membranes, collapse, and terminal convulsions. Fertilizer ingestion also is likely to induce diarrhea as a result of gastrointestinal irritation. Clinical intoxication becomes apparent when methemoglobin levels reach between 30% and 40% in blood. Undisturbed animals do not always show oxygen deprivation but are exercise intolerant. The severity of signs worsens until the lethal level of about 80% methemoglobin is reached.[7] Forced movement or restraint of severely intoxicated animals may prove fatal because of increased oxygen demand. Death may occur 6 to 24 hours after the onset of signs, depending on the total dose and rate of consumption. Left untreated, many intoxicated animals recover because of the red blood cells' NADPH-dependent reduction of ferric iron in methemoglobin back to functional ferrous iron in hemoglobin.

Abortion in ruminants is a sequela of sublethal nitrate intoxication in the dam. Anecdotal and experimental evidence have shown that abortions usually occur 3 to 7 days after exposure of dams to toxic levels of nitrate.[3] High levels of methemoglobinemia have been measured in stillborn calves from cows fed a high-nitrate ration. Fetal death and abortion were induced in cattle given potassium nitrate.[13] Field cases of bovine abortion have been associated with forage containing as little as 0.52% nitrate and are usually reported to occur with feeds containing 0.61% to 1% nitrate.[6] A cow consuming 3% of her body weight in forage containing 0.5% nitrate would receive a dose of 150 mg nitrate/kg BW. Intravenous infusion of nitrite doses up to 12 mg/kg BW in cows in the last trimester did not

substantially increase the risk of premature delivery or abortion. However, because increases in methemoglobin and decreases in maternal blood pressure are dose-dependent, it is plausible that, with higher infusion rates of nitrite, the increased impairment in fetal oxygenation would result in intrauterine death.[6] Placental transfer of oxygen may be reduced severely with consequent hypoxia and intrauterine death of the fetus in nitrate-poisoned cows. Further adverse effects of nitrite include its vasodilatory action and the consequent reduction in mean arterial blood pressure and partial oxygen tension. Hypoxemia in late-gestation fetuses results in increased cortisol and adrenocorticotropic hormone concentrations in fetal plasma. Nitrite-induced fetal hypoxemia could result in abortion caused by anoxic death of the fetus as well as activation of the fetal hypothalamic-pituitary-adrenal axis. Sodium nitrite given intravenously to pregnant cows at a dosage of 20 mg/kg BW was fatal to two of eight fetuses within 24 hours. Nitrate concentration in postmortem fetal ocular fluid of cesarean-delivered fetuses equaled or exceeded the 20 µg NO_3^-/ml (20 ppm) perinatal concentrations found in specimens generally considered diagnostic for excessive nitrate exposure.[2]

Lesions. Chocolate-colored blood and the consequent brownish cast to all tissues is the hallmark of nitrate poisoning. Detection of methemoglobin in dead cattle is possible only when observations are made within a few hours of death. The postmortem instability of methemoglobin results from its spontaneous reduction back to hemoglobin, thereby precluding direct observation of chocolate-colored tissues.[3] Nonspecific findings include congestion of ruminal or abomasal mucosae. Signs of gastrointestinal irritation are especially consistent with ingestion of nitrate fertilizer.

Diagnosis. Clinical signs consistent with oxygen deprivation, muddy-colored tissues, chocolate-colored blood, lesions, history of exposure to high-nitrate source, and chemical analysis are required for diagnosis of nitrate poisoning. Definitive diagnosis requires finding excess nitrate in plasma, serum, blood, heart blood from fetus or dam, forages, urine, or aqueous humor. Because of its longer half-life, nitrate is usually easier to detect than nitrite in biological samples. Specimens should be collected and shipped refrigerated or frozen to a diagnostic laboratory. Plasma or serum is an acceptable antemortem sample; postmortem ocular fluid concentrations correlate well with serum values and clinical signs while remaining stable for at least 24 hours at room temperature and 1 week in a refrigerator.[14]

Although 35% lower than the concentration values in serum, ocular fluid nitrate concentration is a reliable indicator of poisoning. Some reports indicate that ocular fluid nitrate levels greater than 10 ppm from cattle suggest excessive nitrate exposure, whereas nitrate concentrations greater than 20 ppm in these animals are diagnostic for poisoning.[9] However, weak neonatal or stillborn calves born within 2 weeks of their expected calving date present a potential diagnostic dilemma. Normal ocular fluid nitrate levels in these calves may approach 20 ppm.[15] In light of this fact, ocular fluid nitrate concentrations slightly greater than

20 ppm in weak or stillborn calves are only suggestive of excessive maternal exposure to dietary nitrates. Higher ocular fluid nitrate concentrations, possibly greater than 30 ppm, or additional diagnostic information such as elevated forage nitrate levels, may be necessary to confirm nitrate poisoning as a cause of fetal death or neonatal intoxication in cattle.

Rumen contents are not diagnostically useful because of postmortem instability caused by microbial activity. Methemoglobin analysis is neither recommended nor practical because blood samples must be collected within 2 hours of death and immediately frozen or preserved with phosphate buffer. Neither is the presence of methemoglobin specific for nitrate intoxication a useful indicator because there are other chemicals capable of oxidizing hemoglobin, such as copper and chlorates. Furthermore, few diagnostic laboratories offer such an analysis because of the rapid postmortem regeneration of hemoglobin. The diphenylamine spot test for nitrate in forage is especially useful for rapid identification of potentially toxic plant material; this test also has been adapted for screening biological fluids for elevated nitrate levels.[9] Other causes of methemoglobinemia in livestock include copper and sodium chlorate herbicides. Ingestion of wilted red maple (Acer rubrum) leaves is a much more likely cause of methemoglobinemia in horses than nitrate intoxication.[4,16]

Treatment. Because severely hypoxic animals are subject to sudden death, stress associated with handling must be minimized. Methylene blue is the specific antidote to be delivered intravenously at 5 to 15 mg/kg BW as a 1% solution in physiologic saline. If improvement is not apparent, lower doses can be repeated.[7] The dose of methylene blue is dictated by the severity of clinical signs and the likelihood of further nitrite absorption. The safety margin for methylene blue in cattle is substantial so that the likelihood of overdosing with a 1% solution is minimal. Rumen lavage with cold water and oral penicillin may slow the continuous reduction of nitrate to nitrite in the rumen.

Prognosis. From a clinical standpoint, prognosis for intoxicated cattle is speculative. Without knowing the amount and rate of consumption of high-nitrate material or the observed phase of the intoxication syndrome, there is no reasonable degree of certainty in these situations. Undisturbed animals may not show any evidence of clinical intoxication. Cattle that live beyond 24 hours following intake are likely to survive. Most lethal intoxications occur within the first 6 to 8 hours after onset. However, the same cannot be assumed for the conceptus of exposed cows. Abortion may occur 3 to 7 days after sublethal intoxication in the dam.

Prevention and Control. Cattle that are not pregnant should not be permitted to subsist on forage containing greater than 1% nitrate. Pregnant cattle should not be fed forage containing greater than 0.5% nitrate. Several forage samples should be tested to establish a reliable index of nitrate concentration for the entire lot. Forage containing 1% nitrate or greater is potentially lethal to cattle and cannot be guaranteed safe under all conditions. Several management strategies are available to reduce the risk associated with

feeding high-nitrate forage. One should allow for a period of adaptation when bringing cattle onto a full ration over the course of at least a week. One should not allow extremely hungry cattle unlimited access to high-nitrate forage; this increases the rate of intake and amount ingested. The forage ration should be split, making half available in the morning and the other half in the afternoon to reduce the risk of intoxication, or supplement with low-nitrate forage or high-carbohydrate feed to enhance tolerance.

Cattle grazing high-nitrate forages should be fed low-nitrate hay or concentrates before release. When forage or a crop is grown under conditions conducive to nitrate accumulation, harvesting should be delayed until conditions improve to allow nitrate levels in stalks to decrease, or raise the harvesting cutter bar to 18 inches, leaving the lower portion with the highest nitrate in the field. Drought-stressed corn plants reduce normal growth after adequate rainfall allowing nitrate levels to return to normal in 3 to 4 days. Drought-damaged forage also may be ensiled to allow microbial degradation a chance to reduce nitrate to acceptable concentrations. This may require at least 30 days to reduce concentrations by one third; ensiled samples should be tested before feeding.

Some strains of propionibacteria can rapidly reduce nitrate to nontoxic nitrogen compounds. Rumen inoculation with nitrate-protective strains can reduce ruminal nitrite and blood methemoglobin concentrations by 40% or 50%.[17] This product is available as a feed additive or gel paste. The feed additive must be fed for a minimum of 8 days and livestock must not be allowed access to high-nitrate forage for at least 10 days from the time treatment ends to allow establishment of a sufficient population of propionibacteria in the rumen.

NONPROTEIN NITROGEN

Camilla Lieske and Petra A. Volmer

Synonyms. Ammonia toxicosis and urea poisoning are names used for the disease caused by overconsumption of nonprotein nitrogen.

Sources. Nonprotein nitrogen (NPN) includes all nitrogen sources that are not part of a polypeptide. Although NPN is a component of most grains and forages,[1] the ability of ruminants to use NPN as a substitute for natural proteins has resulted in other NPN sources to be commonly used in ruminant rations. Feed grade urea is the most common source, but other sources include urea phosphate, biuret, ammonium polyphosphate, and ammonium salts such as diammonium phosphate, monoammonium phosphate, and ammonium acetate (Table 19-3). Ammoniated forages (especially rice hulls, beet pulp, molasses, hay, or silage) are also often used.

Supplements are most often mixed into feed rations (especially into the concentrate portion). Liquid supplements mixed with molasses are popular, but access must be controlled (such as by using a "lick-tank" or adding phos-

TABLE 19-3 **Common Nonprotein Nitrogen Sources and Their Comparative Toxicity**

Compound	Formula	% Nitrogen Content	% Crude Protein*	Comparative Toxicity (g/kg body weight)†
Urea–feed grade	$CO(NH_2)_2$	42-46	262-287	1
Biuret–feed grade	NH_2-CO-NH-CO-NH_2	35-37	219-231	8
Diammonium phosphate	$(NH_4)_2HPO_4$	21	131	2
Ammonium sulfate	$(NH_4)_2SO_4$	21	131	3
Monoammonium phosphate	$NH_4H_2PO_4$	12	75	2

*% crude protein = 6.25 × % nitrogen content (assumes protein contains 16% N).
†Toxicity is based on an acclimated ruminant[4].

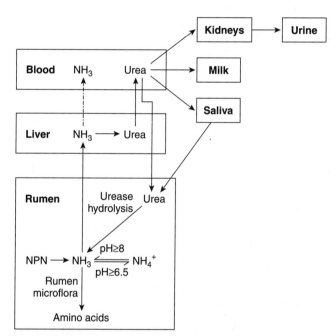

Fig. 19-1 General metabolic and distribution pathway for urea and nonprotein nitrogen. Ammonia (NH_3) increases in blood when the detoxification cycle in the liver is overwhelmed *(dotted line)*.

phoric acid) or else overconsumption may occur. Urea has been added to some mineral blocks, but this method is not recommended because it is difficult to ensure the daily intake. Livestock may also be exposed from consuming ammonium or urea-containing fertilizers.

Toxicokinetics. The toxicity of NPN is due to ammonia (NH_3) production following hydrolysis of the NPN source in the rumen (Fig. 19-1). Ammonia is used by rumen microflora to produce amino acids. At a rumen pH of less than 7, ammonia is predominantly converted to ammonium (NH_4^+) through the addition of a proton. This charged ammonium ion does not move readily across the rumen wall, and thus is not well absorbed. As NH_3 continues to be converted to NH_4^+, the rumen pH increases. As the rumen pH increases and fewer protons are available, the conversion to NH_4^+ slows down and the reaction shifts back toward producing NH_3. When the rumen pH is around 8, the ratio of NH_3 to

NH_4^+ favors NH_3. Rumen NH_3 is absorbed into the portal circulation and detoxified in the liver by conversion to urea, which is excreted in the urine or recycled to the rumen either directly via blood or in saliva. Recycled urea constitutes 11% to 70% of the protein intake[2] depending on the amount of NH_3 present in the rumen (urea does not pass back into the rumen from the blood if rumen NH_3 is high). If the ammonia detoxification pathway in the liver is overwhelmed and blood NH_3 levels increase, signs of a toxicosis may be seen. Urea itself is relatively nontoxic; animals with low or no urease activity in the gut show little effect. Ruminants do have ample urease activity in the rumen and thus are susceptible to a urea toxicosis. Urease activity in the cecum of horses is 25% of that in ruminants. The hydrolysis of urea to ammonia by urease is optimum under conditions in which pH is 7.7 to 8 and temperature is 49° C.[3] Changes in rumen pH are most commonly seen with urea exposure. Nonprotein nitrogen sources such as ammonium acetate act as a buffer in the rumen, decreasing the fluctuation of pH.[4]

Ammoniated forages are associated with a specific hyperexcitability syndrome (sometimes termed "bovine bonkers") not associated with free ammonia.[5,6] It is believed that this syndrome may be due to imidazoles that are formed as a byproduct of the ammoniation process. This toxicosis is described in a separate chapter.

Mechanism of Action. It is believed that ammonia depletes α-ketoglutarate needed to run the citric acid cycle resulting in the inhibition of the cycle, increased lactate (acidosis), and a decrease in ATP production. Neurotoxicity is frequently found with ammonia toxicosis.

Toxicity and Risk Factors. Relative toxicities of different NPN sources to ruminants are listed in Table 19-3. The solubility of the NPN is important in the comparative toxicity. Although biuret is a urea source, it is less soluble than feed-grade urea, is released slowly into the rumen, and thus is less toxic. Feed labels may list the percent NPN content; however, the percent from each NPN source may not be individually broken down. Thus to determine toxic exposure, the percent protein equivalent from all NPN sources can be combined and a "urea exposure" calculated. (Even if the percent urea is listed, using the total percent NPN for the calculation results in a more conservative estimate of exposure because toxicity is due to ammonia production and not just the amount of urea consumed.) This exposure calculation is based on the relationship that an average protein contains 0.36 parts urea. Box 19-2 shows how to calculate the urea exposure. In an unacclimated animal, toxicosis is seen at 0.2 to 0.5 g urea/kg BW, although the acclimated ruminant can tolerate up to 1 g urea/kg body weight.[5] Acclimation can be lost within 1 to 3 days of withholding urea. Because of lack of rumen flora, very young calves are less susceptible than adults to urea. However, after rumen development, young animals may be more susceptible to a urea toxicosis than older ones. In ponies, urea was lethal at 4 g/kg BW.[7] Ammonium salts at 1.5 g/kg BW may be lethal to pigs, horses, and young calves.[3]

Risk of NPN toxicosis in ruminants is increased by the following:

1. A lack of acclimation of an individual to urea
2. Anything that increases the alkalinity of the rumen
3. Rations that are high in roughage and low in carbohydrate (i.e., low-energy rations)
4. Animals that are in poor body condition
5. Poorly mixed rations
6. Unrestricted access to palatable supplements

Feeding unprocessed grain with urea has been shown to delay signs of toxicity compared to feeding grain processed by extrusion.[8] Adding molasses with NPN source may decrease rumen pH and increase nitrogen use by microflora, resulting in decreased rumen ammonia concentrations.[4] Negative reproduction effects (e.g., increased time to conception and decreased embryo viability) were seen in both cattle and sheep on high urea supplementation diets. This may be an effect of nitrogen surplus.[9,10]

Clinical Signs.   Clinical signs can be seen in ruminants anywhere between 20 minutes and 4 hours after ingestion (usually within 20 to 60 minutes in cattle or 30 to 90 minutes in sheep). After onset of signs, progression is often rapid. Terminal convulsions and death are often seen within 2 hours in cattle, 4 hours in sheep, and 3 to 12 hours in horses. Animals may simply be found dead. Clinical signs include uneasiness, muscle and skin tremors (face and ears),

dyspnea, tachypnea, frequent urination and defecation, stiffening of the front legs, and prostration when blood ammonia is greater than 0.7 to 0.8 mg/dl.[4] Both increased and decreased salivation have been reported.[4,11] Other signs include colic, rumen atony, bloat, regurgitation, cardiac arrhythmias, cyanosis, and a marked jugular pulse. In horses, head pressing has been seen.

Lesions.   No characteristic lesions are found with an ammonia toxicosis. Rumen pH greater than 8, bloat, and rapid decomposition are indicative of NPN toxicosis.

Diagnostic Testing.   Analysis for ammonia nitrogen (NH_3N) can be done on rumen fluid, CNS fluid, vitreous fluid, serum, or whole blood. Samples should be collected in suitable clean or sterile containers and frozen until analysis. In affected animals, rumen NH_3 content is greater than 80 mg/dl. Samples from the rumen should be taken from several different areas because the ammonia concentration may not be uniformly distributed. Normal CNS, vitreous, blood or serum NH_3N levels are less than 0.5 mg/dl. Clinical signs may be seen at levels around 1 mg/dl, and death may be seen at levels around 3 to 6 mg/dl.[3,5]

Elevations should be seen in all three areas (rumen, blood or serum, vitreous or CSF) for confirmation of postmortem diagnosis. Postmortem changes including acidification of the rumen and breakdown of natural proteins to ammonia may complicate diagnosis. Animals dead more than 12 hours in moderate climates have undergone too much autolysis for diagnostic value. Analysis of the feed for NPN content can also be performed.

Treatment.   Treatment of an ammonia toxicosis is often impossible because of the rapid progression of clinical signs. Infusing the rumen with 5% acetic acid (vinegar) to decrease the pH is effective. Two to 8 L should be given in cattle, and 0.5 to 2 L should be given to sheep or goats. Up to 40 L of cold (0° C to 4° C) water can be given to cattle (and a proportionate amount to smaller ruminants). This decreases the temperature of the rumen, thus decreasing the activity of urease as well as diluting the contents of the rumen. This treatment may need to be repeated if signs return. A rumenotomy to replace rumen contents with hay slurry may also be beneficial. Survivors generally recover in 12 to 24 hours with no sequelae.[3,5]

Prognosis.   Ammonia toxicosis is highly fatal. Animals recumbent or moribund generally have a poor prognosis.

Prevention and Control.   Toxicosis can be avoided with careful formulation and feeding. It is recommended that NPN constitute less than one third of the total nitrogen in the ration. NPN should also constitute less than 3% of the concentrate. It is important to slowly acclimate the animals to the increased NPN in the diet over many days to weeks. Acclimation is lost if an animal stops eating the NPN for 1 to 3 days.

SULFUR

Milton M. McAllister

Synonyms. Excessive sulfur intake can result in polio-encephalomalacia (PEM) in ruminants.

Sources. Sulfur is an essential nutrient that is generally consumed within organic complexes. Most sulfur in the body is in protein, so sulfur deficiency is nearly synonymous with protein deficiency. Monogastric animals must consume sulfur-containing amino acids (cystine, cysteine, and methionine) and vitamins (biotin and thiamine). In ruminants, microbial synthesis of protein and vitamins can reduce dietary requirements for these organic constituents, as long as the ration contains sufficient energy, inorganic nitrogen, and inorganic sulfur.

Forms of dietary sulfur may include protein or amino acid supplements such as methionine or inorganic forms such as elemental sulfur (flowers of sulfur), sodium sulfate (Glauber's salt), magnesium sulfate (Epsom salt), ammonium sulfate, calcium sulfate (gypsum), and sulfur dioxide. The various forms of inorganic sulfur may be used as folk remedies, fertilizer, laxatives, urinary acidifiers, as an amendment to restrict feed intake, or to balance the nitrogen-to-sulfur ratio in ruminant diets. One of the most common sources of excessive sulfur is high-sulfate water, particularly in the Great Plains of the United States and Canada.[1,2] Molasses-based diets for feedlot cattle, frequently used in countries that produce sugar cane, often have high levels of sulfates as a result of the manufacturing process. Such diets are associated with a high incidence of PEM, also called "molasses drunkenness."[3,4] Inhalation of hydrogen sulfide gas, released from a manure slurry, has caused PEM in cattle.[5]

Toxicokinetics. Most of the deleterious effects of sulfur toxicosis appear to result from excessive production of sulfide by the ruminal microflora. Organic and inorganic forms of sulfur are normally reduced to the sulfide anion (S^{-2}) by ruminal bacteria before incorporation or reincorporation in sulfur-containing amino acids and bacterial protein.[6] In experimentally induced PEM in cattle, the rate of sulfur reduction increased significantly 10 or 12 days after introduction to a high-sulfate diet, and ruminal sulfide concentrations were correspondingly elevated.[7] In cattle that do not develop PEM, ruminal sulfide concentrations later decrease as the microflora apparently adapt; in a feedlot with high-sulfate water, ruminal sulfide concentrations decreased sometime between 3 weeks and 2 months after cattle entered the feedlot.[1] This period of increased ruminal sulfide concentration, between approximately 10 and 30 days after introduction to a high-sulfur diet, coincides with the period of greatest risk of PEM in both experimental and natural circumstances.[1,7,8] However, in one catastrophic case, sheep became ill within 2 hours of being moved to a pasture that had been fertilized with elemental sulfur.[9] Experimental administration of sodium sulfide to sheep induces clinical signs consistent with PEM in as little as 20 minutes and causes typical gross and microscopic lesions.[10]

Mechanism of Action. The exact mechanisms by which sulfide induces PEM have not been proven. Sulfide inhibits cellular respiration, in a manner similar to cyanide, by blocking activity of cytochrome c oxidase in the electron transport chain.[11] It is speculated that sulfide, produced in the rumen and absorbed into the blood, can inhibit energy metabolism of neurons and that this either directly causes neuronal necrosis or leads to necrosis by interfering with local cerebral blood flow and creating regional ischemia.[12] The latter possibility correlates well with the typical pattern of necrosis and with causes of cerebral vasospasm.[13] Another possible pathogenic effect of sulfide includes the generation of free radicals. The most important route of sulfide absorption is not known; absorption across the gastrointestinal mucosa and pulmonary absorption after inhalation of eructated hydrogen sulfide gas are both possible. Most evidence indicates that sulfur-associated PEM does not involve reduced concentrations of thiamine in blood or tissues,[1,4,6,8,14] nor reduced activity of transketolase, a thiamine-dependent enzyme.[4,14]

Toxicity and Risk Factors. Induction of sulfur toxicosis in ruminants is a complex phenomenon that is difficult to predict and incompletely understood. The most frequently documented consequence of sulfur toxicosis is PEM. Toxicity appears to be dependent on the dose of sulfur, rate of dietary change, dietary form of sulfur, age of animals, dietary factors apart from sulfur, and even ambient temperature.

Although past teaching has emphasized the role of altered thiamine metabolism in the pathogenesis of PEM, in the last 2 decades most published reports have been associated with excessive dietary sulfur or occasionally with lead poisoning.[15] Feedlot cattle fed diets containing gypsum or other sulfate salts, which were added to restrict daily feed consumption when feed was provided ad libitum, had a fortyfold increased risk of PEM compared with cattle fed diets without added sulfate.[16] Outbreaks of PEM in cattle and sheep have been associated with high-sulfate water,[1,17-20] sulfur fertilization of pasture,[9] the feeding of ammonium sulfate to prevent urolithiasis,[21] or other types of high-sulfur diets.[22,23] In retrospect, it is apparent that molasses diets, associated with a 15% incidence of PEM,[3] have excessive sulfate.

The National Research Council (NRC) specifies that 0.40% dietary sulfur (dry matter) is the maximum tolerated amount for cattle. Although this is a useful rule-of-thumb, sulfur toxicosis can occur in cattle consuming less than 0.40% dietary sulfur.[8] Conversely, there are many instances in which cattle consume greater than this amount without ill effect.[24,25]

Clinical Signs. Clinical signs of sulfur-associated PEM include visual impairment, lethargy, ear twitching and drooping, anorexia, bruxism, head pressing, recumbency, convulsions, coma, and death. The breath, especially on eructation, may smell like hydrogen sulfide (like rotten eggs), or this odor may be detected in the rumen of a fresh carcass. However, the odor is transient and may be gone soon after the onset of clinical signs and anorexia, or by the time of death.

Excessive production of sulfide in the rumen may have deleterious consequences other than induction of PEM. In sheep administered high doses of sodium sulfide, hepatic necrosis developed in addition to PEM.[10] Hepatic necrosis was also observed in a lamb during an outbreak of sulfur-associated PEM.[22]

The effect of excessive dietary sulfur may be only subclinical, as manifested by reduced feed intake or rate of gain.[25,26] Excessive sulfur can also reduce the absorption of copper, thereby contributing to the occurrence of copper deficiency.[27] In pigs, high sulfate content of drinking water has a laxative effect, although it is not clear whether this decreases performance.[28,29]

There is at least one report of intoxication of horses following ingestion of as much as 400 g of elemental "flowers of sulfur" as a tonic.[30] Variable symptoms were observed in 12 of 14 horses, including lethargy, colic followed by diarrhea, jaundice, frothing from the nostrils, and abnormally deep breathing. Two horses died after 2 days. One horse had elevated AST and a prolonged bromsulfophthalein excretion test, which returned to normal over a 4-month period.[30]

Lesions.   In some cases, the ruminal ingesta or ruminal mucosa may be dark gray or black, as a result of the formation of black iron and copper sulfides. Cerebral lesions include swelling, flattening, and softening of cerebral gyri, multifocal pale-yellow discoloration of the ribbon of cortical gray matter, and occasional herniation of the cerebellum into the foramen magnum.[31] In most instances, necrotic areas exhibit autofluorescence when illuminated with ultraviolet light, which may also reveal necrotic foci in the thalamus or midbrain. Chronic cases may exhibit malacia or cavitation.

Diagnostic Testing.   Pathologic concentrations of sulfide are transient in ruminal fluid and ruminal gas and are usually depleted by the time clinical signs are noticed in naturally occurring cases, so diagnosis of sulfur toxicosis is often made by retrospective dietary analysis. However, measurement of sulfide concentrations in clinically normal herdmates during an outbreak of PEM may be helpful.[6] Although accurate measurement of sulfide in ruminal fluid is laborious, a commercially available system for the immediate estimation of H_2S concentrations in the ruminal gas cap has been adapted. Gas is collected through a needle inserted percutaneously into the rumen.[32] During an outbreak of PEM, H_2S concentrations in four of six clinically normal pen mates were above 2000 ppm, a concentration that can precede the development of PEM.[6]

Treatment.   Treatment of PEM is largely supportive. The reported mortality is highly variable. Many authors recommend thiamine injections; although the efficacy is not clear, no harm is done. Other treatments include removal of the source of sulfur intoxication, provision of roughage to animals on high-concentrate diets, the possible administration of corticosteroids or other treatments to reduce cerebral edema, and general supportive care such as administration of oral fluids and nutrients.

Prevention and Control.   Prevention of sulfur-associated PEM involves reducing dietary sulfur concentrations, if possible, to less than 0.40% and preferably less than 0.30%. When urinary acidification is desired, care should be taken to evaluate the total sulfur intake before adding ammonium sulfate to the diet. Ammonium chloride may be a safer alternative. Although unproven, it is likely that gradual adaptation to a high-sulfur diet, rather than sudden introduction, could reduce the incidence of PEM or prevent depression of weight gains. Addition of trace metals (iron, copper, and zinc) that form insoluble metal sulfides has been proposed to prevent PEM by reducing absorption of sulfide.[12] However, excessive dietary sulfur is present in molar concentrations that greatly exceed that which can be achieved by the addition of even maximum quantities of trace metals. In one study, PEM developed in two of three steers when fed a high sulfate diet, despite the addition of the NRC guidelines of maximum tolerable concentrations of copper, iron, and zinc.[12] The ruminal ingesta and ruminal mucosa turned black, indicative of the formation of iron and copper sulfides. However, the ingesta turned pale-yellow when it reached the abomasum, because the metal sulfides dissolved in gastric acid.

REFERENCES

Ammoniated Feed

1. Haliburton JC: In Burrows GE, ed: *Veterinary clinics of North America: food animal practice,* Philadelphia, 1989, Saunders.
2. Brazil TJ et al: Ammoniated forage toxicosis in nursing calves: a herd outbreak, *Can Vet J* 5:45, 1994.
3. Morgan SE: In Howard JL, Smith RA, eds: *Current veterinary therapy 3: food animal practice,* Philadelphia, 1993, Saunders.
4. Muller L et al: Ammoniated forage poisoning: isolation and characterization of alkyl-substituted imidazoles in ammoniated forage and in milk, *J Agric Food Chem* 46:3172, 1998.

Gossypol

1. Morgan SE: In *Veterinary clinics of North America: food animal practice,* Philadelphia, 1989, Saunders.
2. Randell RD et al: Effects of diets containing free gossypol o follicular development, embryo recovery and corpus luteum function in brangus heifers treated with bFSH, *Theriogenology* 45:911, 1996.
3. Velasquez-Pereira J et al: Reproductive effects of gossypol and vitamin E in young bulls, *J Anim Sci* 76:2894, 1998.
4. Morgan SE: In Howard JL, Smith RA, eds: *Current veterinary therapy 4: food animal practice,* Philadelphia, 1998, Saunders.
5. Lusby K et al: "Recommendation statement" on feeding cottonseed and cottonseed meal to beef cattle in Texas and Oklahoma, *Proc Natl Cottonseed Products Assoc* 1991, pp 93.
6. Rogers GM, Poore MH: Optimal feeding management of gossypol-containing diets for beef cattle, *Vet Med* 10:994, 1995.

Ionophores

1. Berger J et al. The isolation of three new crystalline antibiotics from *Streptomyces, J Am Chem Soc* 73:5295, 1951.
2. Pressman BC et al: Antibiotic-mediated transport of alkali ions across lipid barriers, *Proc Nat Acad Sci* 58:1949, 1967.
3. Muylle E et al: Delayed monensin sodium toxicity in horses, *Equine Vet J* 13:107, 1981.
4. Nava KM: Mysterious horse deaths at Bonita Valley Farms, *Calif Vet* 32:27, 1978.
5. Nel PW et al: Salinomycin poisoning in horses, *J S Afr Vet Assoc* 59:103, 1988.
6. Rollinson J et al: Salinomycin poisoning in horses, *Vet Rec* 121:126, 1987.
7. Van Amstel SR, Guthrie AJ: Salinomycin poisoning in horses: case report, *Proc Am Assoc Equine Pract* 31:373, 1985.
8. Whitlock RH et al: *Monensin toxicosis in horses: clinical manifestations,* Proceedings of the 24th Annual Convention AAEP 473, 1978.
9. Blanchard PC et al: Lasalocid toxicosis in dairy calves, *J Vet Diagn Invest* 5:300, 1993.
10. Buck WB: Rumensin can be toxic to swine and cattle, *Nebraska Extension Newsletter* 8:104, 1979.
11. Collins EA, McCrea CT: Monensin sodium toxicity in cattle, *Vet Rec* 103:386, 1978.
12. Geor RJ, Robinson WF: Suspected monensin toxicosis in feedlot cattle, *Aust Vet J* 62:130, 1985.
13. Janzen ED et al: Possible monensin poisoning in a group of bulls, *Can Vet J* 22:92, 1981.
14. Schweitzer D et al: Accidental monensin sodium intoxication of feedlot cattle, *J Am Vet Med Assoc* 184:1273, 1984.
15. Shlosberg A et al: The chronic course of a probable monensin toxicosis in cattle, *Vet Hum Toxicol* 28:230, 1986.
16. Bourque JG et al: Monensin toxicity in lambs, *Can Vet J* 27:397, 1986.
17. Nation PN et al: Clinical signs and pathology of accidental monensin poisoning in sheep, *Can Vet J* 23:323, 1982.
18. Newsholme SJ et al: Fatal cardiomyopathy in feedlot sheep attributed to monensin toxicosis, *J S Afr Vet Assoc* 54:29, 1983.
19. Davis C: Narasin toxicity in turkeys, *Vet Rec* 113:627, 1983.
20. Griffiths GL et al: Salinomycin poisoning in point-of-lay turkeys, *Aust Vet J* 66:326, 1989.
21. Halvorson DA et al: Ionophore toxicity in turkey breeders, *Avian Dis* 26:634, 1982.
22. Salyi G et al: Narasin poisoning in turkeys, *Acta Vet Hung* 36:107, 1988.
23. Stuart JC: An outbreak of monensin poisoning in adult turkeys, *Vet Rec* 102:303, 1978.
24. Stuart JC: Salinomycin poisoning in turkeys, *Vet Rec* 113:597, 1983.
25. Van Halderen A et al: An outbreak of narasin poisoning in swine, *J S Afr Vet Assoc* 64:43, 1993.
26. Safran N et al: Paralytic syndrome attributed to lasalocid residues in a commercial ration fed to dogs, *J Am Vet Med Assoc* 1993;202:1273.
27. Wilson JS: Toxic myopathy in a dog associated with the presence of monensin in dry food, *Can Vet J* 21:3, 1980.
28. Van Der Linde-Sipman JS et al: Salinomycin-induced polyneuropathy in cats: Morphologic and epidemiologic data, *Vet Pathol* 36:152, 1999.
29. Osz M et al: Narasin poisoning in rabbits, *Vet Bull* 59:416 (abstr 2985), 1989.
30. Salles MS et al: Ionophore antibiotic (narasin) poisoning in rabbits, *Vet Hum Toxicol* 36(5):437, 1994.
31. Glover GL, Wobeser G: Monensin toxicity in a captive white-tailed deer (*Odocoileus virginianus*), *J Zoo Anim Med* 14:13, 1983.
32. Reece RL et al: Investigations of toxicity episodes involving chemotherapeutic agents in Victorian poultry and pigeons, *Avian Dis* 29:1239, 1985.
33. Gregory DG et al: A case of monensin poisoning in ostriches, *Vet Hum Toxicol* 34:247, 1992.
34. Chalmers GA: Monensin toxicity in broiler chickens, *Can Vet J* 22:21, 1981.
35. Howell J et al: Monensin toxicity in chickens, *Avian Dis* 24:1050, 1980.
36. Jones JE et al: Reproduction responses of broiler-breeders to anticoccidial agents, *Poult Sci* 69:27, 1990.
37. Patten BE: The effect of the accidental feeding of lasalocid sodium to breeder birds, *Aust Vet J* 64:217, 1987.
38. Perelman B et al: Effects of the accidental feeding of lasalocid sodium to broiler breeder chickens, *Vet Rec* 132:271, 1993.
39. Bennett K: *Compendium of veterinary products,* 3rd ed, Port Huron, Mich, 1995, North American Compendiums.
40. McDougald LR, Roberson EL: Antiprotozoan drugs. In Booth NH, McDonald LE, eds: *Veterinary pharmacology and therapeutics,* 6th ed, Ames, Iowa, 1988, Iowa State University Press.
41. Donoho A et al: Metabolism of monensin in the steer and rat, *J Agric Food Chem* 26:1090, 1978.
42. Atef M et al: Kinetic disposition, systemic bioavailability and tissue distribution of salinomycin in chickens, *Res Vet Sci* 54:179, 1993.
43. Herberg R et al: Excretion and tissue distribution of [14C] monensin in cattle, *J Agric Food Chem* 26:1087, 1978.
44. Stipkovits L, Juhasz S: Assay of lasalocid and monensin residues in chicken lung and serum samples of small quantity, *Acta Vet Hung* 35:237-244, 1987.
45. Stipkovits L et al: *In vitro* testing of the anti-mycoplasma effect of some anti-coccidial drugs, *Vet Microbiol* 15:65, 1987.
46. Donoho AL: Biochemical studies on the fate of monensin in animals and in the environment, *J Anim Sci* 58:1528, 1984.
47. Mezes M et al: Effect of acute salinomycin-tiamulin toxicity on the lipid peroxide and antioxidant status of broiler chicken, *Acta Vet Hung* 40(4):251, 1992.

48. Horvath CJ et al: Effects of monensin on selenium status and related factors in genetically hypo- and hyperselenemic growing swine, *Am J Vet Res* 53:2109, 1992.

49. Witkamp RF et al: Tiamulin selectively inhibits oxidative hepatic steroid and drug metabolism *in vitro* in the pig, *J Vet Pharmacol Ther* 17:317, 1994.

50. Pressman BC, De Guzman NT: New ionophores for old organelles, *Ann N Y Acad Sci* 227:380, 1974.

51. Mitani M et al: Salinomycin: a new monovalent cation ionophore, *Biochem Biophys Res Commun* 66:1231, 1975.

52. Grafe U et al: Monovalent cation specificity of passive transport mediated by laidlomycin and 26-deoxylaidlomycin, *J Basic Microbiol* 29:391, 1989.

53. Gad SC et al: Thirteen cationic ionophores: Their acute toxicity, neurobehavioral, and membrane effects, *Drug Chem Toxicol* 8:451, 1985.

54. Wong DT et al: Ionophorous properties of narasin, a new polyether monocarboxylic acid antibiotic, in rat liver mitochondria, *Biochem Pharmacol* 26:1373, 1977.

55. Mitani M et al: Salinomycin effects on mitochondrial ion translocation and respiration, *Antimicrob Agents Chem* 9:655, 1976.

56. Estrada OS et al: Model translocators for divalent and monovalent ion transport in phospholipid membranes. II. The effects of ion translocator X-537A on the energy-conserving properties of mitochondrial membranes, *J Membr Biol* 18:201, 1974.

56. Pereira de Silva L et al: Inhibition of ruthenium red-induced Ca^{2+} efflux from liver mitochondria by the antibiotic X-537A, *Biochem Biophys Res Commun* 124:80, 1984.

57. Galitzer SJ, Oehme FW:. A literature review on the toxicity of lasalocid, a polyether antibiotic, *Vet Hum Toxicol* 26:322, 1984.

58. Galitzer SJ et al: Lasalocid toxicity in cattle: acute clinicopathological changes, *J Anim Sci* 62:1308, 1986.

59. Hanson LJ et al: Toxic effects of lasalocid in horses, *Am J Vet Res* 42:456, 1981.

60. Todd GC et al: Comparative toxicology of monensin sodium in laboratory animals, *J Anim Sci* 58:1512, 1984.

61. Novilla MN et al: The comparative toxicology of narasin in laboratory animals, *Vet Hum Toxicol* 36(4):318, 1994.

62. Van Vleet JF et al: Acute monensin toxicosis in swine: effect of graded doses of monensin and protection of swine by pretreatment with seleniun-vitamin E, *Am J Vet Res* 44:1460, 1983.

63. Potter EL et al: Monensin toxicity in cattle, *J Anim Sci* 58:1499, 1984.

64. Berg DH, Hamill RL: The isolation and characterization of narasin, a new polyether antibiotic, *J Antibiot* 31:1, 1978.

65. Miyazaki Y et al: Salinomycin, a new polyether antibiotic. *J Antibiot* 27:814, 1974.

66. Syntex, Inc., Palo Alto, CA: *Material safety data sheet*, July, 1991.

67. NADA Number 141-025. Laidlomycin propionate. Freedom of Information Office, Center for Veterinary Medicine, FDA, Rockville, Md, 1994.

68. NADA Number 139-075. Maduramicin ammonium. Freedom of Information Office, Center for Veterinary Medicine, FDA, Rockville, Md, 1994.

69. Hall JO: *Mechanisms of ionophore toxicoses: laidlomycin propionate toxicosis in the horse, laidlomycin propionate, laidlomycin, and monensin in muscle cell cultures,* Ph.D. Dissertation, University of Illinois, 1997.

70. Novilla MN: The veterinary importance of the toxic syndrome induced by ionophores, *Vet Hum Toxicol* 34:66, 1992.

71. Langston VC et al: Toxicity and therapeutics of monensin: a review, *Vet Med* 80:75, 1985.

72. Kavanagh NT, Sparrows DSH: Salinomycin toxicity in pigs, *Vet Rec* 118:73, 1990.

73. Plumlee KH et al: Acute salinomycin toxicosis in pigs, *J Vet Diagn Invest* 7:419, 1995.

74. Fourie N et al: Cardiomyopathy of ruminants induced by the litter of poultry fed rations containing the ionophore antibiotic, maduramicin. I. Epidemiology, clinical signs, and clinical pathology, *Onderst J Vet Res* 58:291, 1991.

75. Potter LM et al: Salinomycin toxicity in turkeys, *Poult Sci* 65:1955, 1986.

76. Lodge NJA et al: Safety of lasalocid in turkeys and its compatibility with tiamulin, *Vet Rec* 122:576, 1988.

77. Varga I et al: Potentiation on ionophorous anticoccidials with dihydroquinolones: battery trials against *Eimeria tenella* in chickens, *Int J Parasitol* 24:689, 1994.

78. Prohaszka L et al: Growth depression in broiler chicks caused by incompatibility of feed ingredients, *Acta Vet Hung* 35:349, 1987.

79. Laczay P et al: Potentiation of ionophorous anticoccidials with dihydroquinolones: reduction of adverse interactions with antimicrobials, *Int J Parasitol* 24:421, 1994.

80. Miller DJS et al: Tiamulin/salinomycin interactions in pigs, *Vet Rec* 118:73, 1986.

81. Weisman Y et al: Acute poisoning in turkeys caused by incompatibility of monensin and tiamulin, *Vet Res Commun* 4:231, 1980.

82. Comben N: Toxicity of the ionophores, *Vet Rec* 114:128, 1984.

83. McCoy CP: *Characterization of monensin poisoning in the horse*, Masters Thesis, Oklahoma State University, 1982.

84. Mollenhauer HH et al: Ultrastructural observations in ponies after treatment with monensin, *Am J Vet Res* 42:35, 1981.

85. Amend JF et al: Equine monensin toxicosis: some experimental clinicopathologic observations, *Comp Cont Ed* 11:S173, 1980.

86. Matsuoka T: Evaluation of monensin toxicity in the horse, *J Am Vet Med Assoc* 169:1098, 1976.

87. Galitzer SJ et al: Preliminary study on lasalocid toxicosis in cattle, *Vet Hum Toxicol* 24:406, 1982.

88. Van Vleet JF et al: Clinical, clinicopathologic, and pathologic alterations in acute monensin toxicosis in cattle, *Am J Vet Res* 44:2133, 1983.

89. Davidovich A et al: Safety evaluation of lasalocid for growing and finishing steers and heifers, *J Anim Sci* 53(suppl 1):392, 1981 (abstract 651).

90. Van Vleet JF et al: 1985. Effect of pretreatment with selenium-vitamin E on monensin toxicosis in cattle, *Am J Vet Res* 46:2221.

91. Confer AW et al: Light and electron microscopic changes in cardiac and skeletal muscle of sheep with experimental monensin toxicosis, *Vet Pathol* 20:590, 1983.

92. Anderson TD et al: Acute monensin toxicosis in sheep: light and electron microscopic changes, *Am J Vet Res* 45:1142, 1984.

93. Wendt M et al: The effect of treatment with vitamin E or selenium on the course of salminomycin poisoning in swine, *Dtsch Tierarztl Wochenschr* 101(4):141, 1994.

94. Van Vleet JF et al: Clinical, clinicopathologic, and pathologic alterations of monensin toxicosis in swine, *Am J Vet Res* 44:1469, 1983.

95. Hanraha LA et al: Monensin toxicosis in broiler chickens, *Vet Pathol* 18:665, 1981.

96. Shlosberg A et al: Neurotoxic action of lasalocid at high doses, *Vet Rec* 117:394. 1985.

97. Hooper RS: Anticoccidials and turkeys, *Vet Rec* 116:224, 1985.

98. Horrox NE: Salinomycin poisoning in turkeys, *Vet Rec* 114:52, 1984.

99. Dworschak E, Prohaszka L: The effect of improper feeding on the lipid peroxidation of meat animals, *Z Ernahrungswiss* 25(2):96, 1986.

100. Galitzer SJ et al: Pathologic changes associated with experimental lasalocid and monensin toxicosis in cattle, *Am J Vet Res* 47:2624-2626, 1986.

101. Hanrahan LA et al: Monensin toxicosis in broiler chickens, *Vet Pathol* 18:665, 1981.

102. Goras JT, Lacourse WR: Liquid chromatographic determination of sodium salinomycin in feeds, with post-column reaction, *J Assoc Off Anal Chem* 67(4):701, 1984.

103. Hussey RL et al: Liquid chromatographic determination of narasin in feed premixes, *J Assoc Off Anal Chem* 68(3)417, 1985.

104. Lapointe MR, Cohen H: High-speed liquid chromatographic determination of monensin, narasin, and salinomycin in feeds, using post-column derivatization, *J Assoc Off Anal Chem* 71:480, 1988.

105. Martinez EE, Shimoda W: Liquid chromatographic determination of multiresidue fluorescent derivatives of ionophore compounds, monensin, salinomycin, narasin, and lasalocid in beef liver tissue, *J Assoc Off Anal Chem* 69:637, 1986.

106. Newkirk DR, Barnes CJ: Liquid chromatographic determination and gas chromatographic-mass spectrometric confirmation of lasalocid sodium in bovine liver: interlaboratory study, *J Assoc Off Anal Chem* 72:581,1989.

107. Tarbin JA, Shearer G: Improved high-performance liquid chromatographic procedure for the determination of lasalocid in chicken tissues and egg using polymeric and porous graphitic carbon columns, *J Chromatogr* 579:177, 1992.

108. Weiss G, MacDonald A: Methods for determination of ionophore-type antibiotic residues in animal tissues, *J Assoc Off Anal Chem* 68:971, 1985.

109. De Guzman NT, Pressman BC: Cardiovascular effects of the ionophore X-537A, a broad spectrum cation carrier, *Fed Proc* 33:517, 1974.

110. De Guzman NT, Pressman BC: The inotropic effect of the calcium ionophore X-537A in the anesthetized dog, *Circulation* 49:1072, 1974.

111. Whitlock RH: Feed additives and contaminants as a cause of equine disease. *Vet Clin North Am. Equine Pract* 6(2):467, 1990.

Nitrate

1. Worth AJ et al: Nitrite poisoning in cats and dogs fed a commercial pet food, *N Z Vet J*:193, 1997.

2. Johnson JL et al: Post-harvest change in cornstalk nitrate and its relationship to bovine fetal nitrite/nitrate exposure. *Poisonous Plants: Proceedings of the Third International Symposium,* 1992.

3. Bruning-Fann CS, Kaneene JF: The effects of nitrate, nitrite, and N-nitroso compounds on animal health, *Vet Hum Toxicol* 35:237, 1993.

4. Hintz HF, Thompson LJ: Nitrate toxicosis in horses, *Equine Prac* 20:5, 1998.

5. Johnson JL et al: Nitrate exposure in perinatal beef calves, *Proceedings of the 26th Annual Meeting of the American Association of Laboratory Diagnosis,* 1983.

6. van't Klooster ATh et al: On the pathogenesis of abortion in acute nitrite toxicosis of pregnant dairy cows, *Theriogenology* 33:1075, 1990.

7. Burrows GE: Nitrate intoxication, *J Am Vet Med Assoc* 177:82, 1980.

8. Osweiler GD et al: *Clinical and diagnostic veterinary toxicology*, ed 3, Dubuque, Iowa, 1985, Kendall/Hunt.

9. Burrows GE, Tyrl RJ: *Toxic plants of North America*, Ames, Iowa, 2001, Iowa State University Press.

10. Egyed MN, Hanji V: Factors contributing to recent outbreaks of acute nitrate poisoning in farm ruminants, *Isr J Vet Med* 43:50, 1987.

11. Carson TL: Water quality considerations for domestic livestock. *IV Biennial veterinary toxicology workshop, 1978,* Utah State University, Logan, Utah.

12. Ridder WE, Oehme FW: Nitrates as environmental, animal, and human hazard. *Clin Toxicol* 7:145, 1974.

13. Simon J et al: The effect of nitrate or nitrite when placed in the rumens of pregnant dairy cattle. *J Am Vet Med Assoc* 135:311, 1959.

14. Boermans HJ: Diagnosis of nitrate toxicosis in cattle, using biological fluids and a rapid ion chromatographic method, *Am J Vet Res* 51:491, 1990.

15. Johnson JL et al: Evaluation of bovine perinatal nitrate accumulation in western Nebraska. *Vet Hum Toxicol* 36:467, 1994.

16. Harvey JW: In Kaneko JJ, Harvey JW, Bruss ML, eds: *Clinical biochemistry of domestic animals,* 5th ed, San Diego, 1997, Academic Press.

17. Strickland G et al: Nitrate toxicity in livestock. *Bull F-2903,* Oklahoma State University Extension Facts, 1995.

Nonprotein Nitrogen

1. Sniffen CJ et al: A net carbohydrate and protein system for evaluating cattle diets: II. Carbohydrate and protein availability, *J Anim Sci* 70:3562, 1992.

2. Russell JB et al: A net carbohydrate and protein system for evaluating cattle diets: I. Ruminal fermentation, *J Anim Sci* 70:3551, 1992.

3. Osweiler GD et al: *Clinical and diagnostic veterinary toxicology*, ed 3, Dubuque, Iowa, 1985, Kendall/Hunt.

4. Webb DW et al: A comparison of nitrogen metabolism and ammonia toxicity from ammonium acetate and urea in cattle, *J Anim Sci* 35:1263, 1972.

5. Haliburton JC, Morgan SE: Nonprotein nitrogen-induced ammonia toxicosis and ammoniated feed toxicity syndrome, *Vet Clin North Am Food Anim Pract* 5:237, 1989.

6. Kerr LA et al: Ammoniated forage toxicosis in calves, *J Am Vet Med Assoc* 191:551, 1987.

7. Hinz HF et al: Ammonia intoxication resulting from urea ingestion by ponies, *J Am Vet Med Assoc* 157:963, 1970.

8. Davidovich A et al: Ammonia toxicity in cattle: IV. Effects of unprocessed or extrusion-cooked mixtures of grain and urea, biuret or dicyanodiamide and liquid supplements on rumen and blood changes associated with toxicity, *J Anim Sci* 45:1397, 1977.

9. McEvoy TG et al: Dietary excesses of urea influence the viability and metabolism of perimplantation sheep embryos and may affect fetal growth among survivors, *Anim Reprod Sci* 47:71, 1997.

10. Forero O et al: Evaluation of slow release urea for winter supplementation of lactating range cows, *J Anim Sci* 50:532, 1980.

11. Szegedi B, Juhasz B: Pathogenesis of urea poisoning, *Acta Vet Acad Sci Hung* 21:291, 1971.

Sulfur

1. McAllister MM et al: Evaluation of ruminal sulfide concentrations and seasonal outbreaks of polioencephalomalacia in beef cattle in a feedlot, *J Am Vet Med Assoc* 211:1275, 1997.

2. Boila RJ: The sulfate content of water for cattle throughout Manitoba, *Can J Anim Sci* 68:573, 1988.

3. Verdura T, Zamora I: Cerebrocortical necrosis in Cuba in beef cattle fed high levels of molasses, *Rev Cubana Cien Agri* 4:209, 1970.

4. Mella CM et al: Induction of bovine polioencephalomalacia with a feeding system based on molasses and urea, *Can J Comp Med* 40:104, 1976.

5. Dahme VE et al: Zur neuropathologie der jauchegasvergiftung (H$_2$S-vergiftung) beim rind, *Dtsch Tierärztl Wschr* 90:316, 1983.

6. Gould DH: Polioencephalomalacia, *J Anim Sci* 76:309, 1998.

7. Cummings BA et al: Ruminal microbial alterations associated with sulfide generation in steers with dietary sulfate-induced polioencephalomalacia, *Am J Vet Res* 56:1390, 1995.

8. Gould DH et al: High sulfide concentrations in rumen fluid associated with nutritionally induced polioencephalomalacia in calves, *Am J Vet Res* 52:1164, 1991.

9. Bulgin MS et al: Elemental sulfur toxicosis in a flock of sheep, *J Am Vet Med Assoc* 208:1063, 1996.

10. McAllister MM et al: Sulphide-induced polioencephalomalacia in lambs, *J Comp Pathol* 106:267, 1992.

11. Nicholls P: The effect of sulphide on cytochrome aa_3 isosteric and allosteric shifts of the reduced α-peak, *Biochim Biophys Acta* 396:24, 1975.

12. McAllister MM: *Sulfur toxicosis and polioencephalomalacia in ruminants* [Ph.D. dissertation], Colorado State University, Fort Collins, Colo, 1991.

13. Siesjö BK: Cerebral circulation and metabolism, *J Neurosurg* 60:883, 1984.

14. Sager RL et al: Clinical and biochemical alterations in calves with nutritionally induced polioencephalomalacia, *Am J Vet Res* 51:1969, 1990.

15. O'Hara TM et al: Lead poisoning and toxicokinetics in a heifer and fetus treated with CaNa$_2$ EDTA and thiamine, *J Vet Diagn Invest* 7:531, 1995.

16. Raisbeck MF: Is polioencephalomalacia associated with high-sulfate diets? *J Am Vet Med Assoc* 180:1303, 1982.

17. Dickie CW et al: Polioencephalomalacia in range cattle, *J Am Vet Med Assoc* 175:460, 1979.

18. Beke GJ, Hironaka R: Toxicity to beef cattle of sulfur in saline well water: a case study, *Sci Total Environ* 101:281, 1991.

19. Hamlen H et al: Polioencephalomalacia in cattle consuming water with elevated sodium sulfate levels: a herd investigation, *Can Vet J* 34:153, 1993.

20. Gooneratne SR et al: High sulfur related thiamine deficiency in cattle: a field study, *Can Vet J* 30:139, 1989.

21. Jeffrey M et al: Polioencephalomalacia associated with ingestion of ammonium-sulfate by sheep and cattle, *Vet Rec* 134:343, 1994.

22. Low JC et al: Sulphur-induced polioencephalomalacia in lambs, *Vet Rec* 138:327, 1996.

23. Hill FI, Ebbett PC: Polioencephalomalacia in cattle in New Zealand fed chou moellier (*Brassica oleracea*), *N Z Vet J* 45:37, 1997.

24. Khan AA et al: Effects of high dietary sulphur on enzyme activities, selenium concentrations and body weights of cattle, *Can J Vet Res* 51:174, 1987.

25. Rumsey TS: Effects of dietary sulfur addition and Synovex-S ear implants on feedlot steers fed an all-concentrate diet, *J Anim Sci* 46:463, 1978.

26. Weeth HJ, Capps DL: Tolerance of growing cattle for sulfate-water, *J Anim Sci* 34:256, 1972.

27. Suttle NF: The interactions between copper, molybdenum, and sulphur in ruminant nutrition, *Ann Rev Nutr* 11:121, 1991.

28. McLeese JM et al: Evaluation of the quality of ground water supplies used on Saskatchewan swine farms, *Can J Anim Sci* 71:191, 1991.

29. Veenhuizen MF et al: Effect of concentration and source of sulfate on nursery pig performance and health, *J Am Vet Med Assoc* 201:1203, 1992.

30. Corke MJ: An outbreak of sulphur poisoning in horses, *Vet Rec* 109:212, 1981.

31. Jensen R et al: Polioencephalomalacia of cattle and sheep, *J Am Vet Med Assoc* 129:311, 1956.

32. Gould DH et al: In vivo indicators of pathologic ruminal sulfide production in steers with diet-induced polioencephalomalacia, *J Vet Diagn Invest* 9:72, 1997.

Household and Industrial Products

20

ACIDS AND ALKALI

Jill Richardson

Synonyms. Acids are often referred to as corrosives, and alkalis are referred to as caustics.

Sources. Hydrochloric, sulfuric, nitric, phosphoric, and oxalic acids, as well as sodium bisulfate, are used in a wide range of products.[1] Sodium bisulfate forms sulfuric acid when exposed to water. Common sources of acids include toilet bowl cleaners, drain openers, metal cleaners, antirust compounds, gun barrel cleaners, automobile battery fluid, and pool sanitizers.[2] Oxalic acid is used in paint, stain, and varnish removers, rust and ink stain removers, and ceramics. It is also used for general metal and equipment cleaning, wood cleaning, bleaching, and leather tanning.[2]

Alkali ingredients are used in drain openers, oven cleaners, bleaches, industrial cleaners, denture cleaners, bathroom and household cleaners, radiator cleaning agents, hair relaxers, alkaline batteries, electric dishwasher detergents, low-phosphate detergents, some oven cleaner pads, and cement. Ingredient names include lime; potash; caustic soda; potassium or sodium carbonate; calcium, potassium, and sodium oxide or hydroxide; and calcium carbide.

Mechanism of Action. An alkali is defined as a substance that creates hydroxide ions on contact with water.[3] Alkali substances can cause liquefaction necrosis.[3] Lesions are usually deeper and more penetrating with alkalis than with acidic compounds. The ability of alkali compounds to generate caustic injury depends on the concentration, pH, viscosity, amount ingested, and the duration of contact with tissue.[2,3] Serious caustic injury is unlikely with exposures to alkali substances with a pH less than 11.[3] Alkali compounds with a pH of 12 can cause esophageal ulcers, whereas those with a pH of 12.5 or more can cause esophageal perforation.[3] Concentrated forms of alkali can produce transmural necrosis with exposures as short as 1 second.[3]

Acids are corrosives and produce severe burns on contact with tissue. The effect on tissues is a coagulation-type necrosis, which can cause destruction of surface epithelium and submucosa.[2,4,5] Undiluted acids can damage the tissues in the oropharynx and the stomach. Severity of tissue damage is directly related to the concentration. When acids are diluted or have a higher pH, they are irritants. Most cases of exposure to acidic irritants result in mild self-limiting signs of nausea, vomiting, or diarrhea.

Toxicity and Risk Factors. Any species of animal can be affected by an alkali or an acid; however, it is a more common occurrence with companion animals because pets are more likely to be in contact with household cleaners.

Clinical Signs. The severity of the initial symptoms may not correspond to the degree of damage to the gastrointestinal tract. The animal may present with dysphagia, excessive salivation, food refusal, vocalization, bloody vomiting, abdominal pain, polydipsia, or pawing at the mouth. Lesions may be found on the lips, tongue, gums, or esophagus. Ingestion of concentrated acids produces visible lesions of the mucous membranes in the oral cavity. With most acids, damaged tissues are initially gray but soon turn black.[3] However, nitric acid produces a yellow lesion. Irritation to the pharyngeal cavity and laryngeal spasms can also occur. Laryngeal edema could lead to airway obstruction.[1] Swelling may cause dyspnea and asphyxia.[5]

The absence of oral lesions does not rule out the presence of esophageal burns. Because there is immediate pain from acid ingestion, most oral exposures are brief; therefore, esophageal involvement is less likely with exposure to acids than to alkali. Esophageal injuries, such as ulceration, esophagitis, and stricture formation, are more common with alkali agents. Alkali compounds can also cause deeper penetration of esophageal mucosa. The presence of stridor, vomiting, and drooling are frequently related to esophageal injury.[3] Severe burns can also occur in the stomach.[2] The pyloric end of the stomach is usually the most severely affected.

Ingestion of oxalic acids can cause systemic effects in addition to the immediate corrosive effects on the mucous membranes.[2] Oxalic acid binds to calcium, forming a calcium oxide complex, and can result in hypocalcemia and deposition of the complex in the brain and renal tubules.[2] Kidney damage, tetany, seizures, muscle twitching, stupor, and cardiovascular collapse are possible.[2]

Severe dermal burns may occur with dermal contact to concentrated acids. Complications from dermal burns include cellulitis, infection, contractures, and shock.[2] Skin exposure can vary from mild dermatitis to severe ulceration. Dermal contact with alkali may produce pain, redness, irritation, or full thickness burns. Dermal exposures often lead to oral exposures in animals after they groom themselves.

Ocular contact with acid causes corneal ulceration, intense pain, and blepharospasm.[2] Ocular exposure to an alkali can produce severe conjunctival irritation and chemosis, corneal epithelial defects, permanent visual loss, and perforation.[3]

Inhalation of acid vapors, mists, or aerosols may result in dyspnea, pleuritic chest pain, pulmonary edema, hypoxemia, bronchospasm, pneumonitis, tracheobronchitis, and persistent pulmonary function abnormalities.[2]

Treatment. In cases of ingestion, gastric lavage and emesis are contraindicated because these methods increase esophageal exposure to the toxicants.[6] Preferred initial treatment is oral dilution with milk or water.[1,2,5,6] Dilution is most effective if it is performed early.[1] Activated charcoal is ineffective for acids and alkali and is not recommended.[6] Supportive care should be given if diarrhea or vomiting occurs.

For cases of severe stomatitis, pharyngitis, esophagitis, or esophageal ulceration, the animal should be kept strictly NPO, that is, nothing should be given by mouth. Hydration can be maintained with intravenous fluids and a gastrostomy tube may be necessary for nutritional support. Sucralfate slurries can be used for the treatment of oral, esophageal, gastric, and duodenal ulcers.[7] Butorphanol tartrate can be used for pain management. Corticosteroid use is controversial for reduction of inflammation. If used, prednisone can be given at 1 to 2 mg/kg parenterally once daily for 1 to 2 days.[5,7] Additionally, the animal should be monitored for an increase in body temperature or an increase in white blood cell (WBC) count. Broad-spectrum antibiotics are indicated in cases of mucosal damage or secondary infection, or as prophylaxis when using steroids.

For recent ocular exposure to acids or alkali, a minimum of 20 to 30 minutes' irrigation with tepid tap water or physiologic saline is recommended.[1,6] Afterward, the eye should be examined and closely monitored for evidence of corneal ulceration.

After dermal exposure, the animal should be bathed immediately with a mild liquid dish detergent or a non-insecticidal pet shampoo. The animal should be monitored for burns, erythema, swelling, pain, or pruritus. Treatment is symptomatic and may include analgesics, antiinflammatories, and antibiotics.[6]

Prognosis. The prognosis for minor exposures to acids or alkali is good, as long as appropriate care is given to the animal. Animals with esophageal perforations have a poor prognosis unless aggressive care, possibly including surgical intervention, is given. Esophageal strictures are a possible sequela.

Prevention and Control. Animal owners should never allow their pets to have access to the areas in which acids or alkali products are being used or stored.

BATTERIES

Sharon Gwaltney-Brant

Sources. Most small animal battery exposures involve dry cell batteries used in household equipment, watches, and toys. These types of batteries range from 10 mm or smaller disc (button) batteries to rectangular and cylindrical batteries of varying sizes. Alkaline dry cells use potassium hydroxide or sodium hydroxide to generate current.[1] Acidic dry cell batteries contain ammonium chloride and manganese dioxide in an acidic environment. Lithium batteries contain noncorrosive compounds, but can generate alkali as a result of the effects of current on local tissues.[2] Disc, nickel-cadmium, mercuric oxide, and silver batteries are generally of the alkaline type; since 1996, the sale of mercuric oxide–based button batteries has been banned in the United States.[1]

Large animals, particularly cattle, may be exposed to lead acid in automotive batteries that are left in rubbish piles in pastures.

Mechanism of Action. The potential for injury following battery ingestion comes from several sources: acid or alkaline burns from the electrolyte solution or gel within the battery, current-induced tissue necrosis, metal toxicity from battery casings, and gastrointestinal obstruction.[1]

Most household batteries contain alkaline electrolyte solutions or gels that may be released on puncture of the battery casing. Leakage of the alkaline contents onto skin or mucosa results in liquefactive necrosis that may penetrate deep into the local tissues. The contents of lithium- and manganese-containing batteries tend to have the highest potential for severe alkaline tissue injury.[1]

Automotive-type batteries contain sulfuric acid, which, on exposure to tissue, results in coagulative necrosis of tissue. Eschar formation limits the penetration of burns into the tissue and thereby limits the extent of the tissue injury.[3]

In some batteries, notably lithium disc batteries, the electrical current generated between cathode and anode may contact adjacent tissue, resulting in electrolysis of endogenous NaCl and producing NaOH.[2] Accumulation of NaOH may result in extensive alkaline tissue damage in the absence of battery leakage. Disc batteries are a particular concern because even very small batteries may fail to successfully pass from the esophagus into the stomach, leading to severe esophageal burns and possibly perforation; these injuries occur most commonly at the level of the gastroesophageal sphincter. In dogs significant necrosis of esophageal mucosa has been observed after as little as 15 minutes of contact with 3-volt lithium disc batteries.[2] Generation of current may also result in gastric mucosal injury, but the fluid stomach environment and mucous barrier may provide some protection against corrosive injury to the stomach lining.[1]

Casings from batteries may contain a variety of heavy metals, including lead, mercury, zinc, cobalt, and cadmium. In most cases of battery ingestion by a small animal, the transit time of the casing through the gastrointestinal tract is brief enough that significant absorption of metals from the battery casing does not occur.[2] However, there is potential for metal toxicosis (particularly lead and zinc) when the battery casings fail to exit the stomach. In large animals, particularly ruminants, ingestion of lead casing from lead acid batteries is a potential cause of lead intoxication, because the casing is retained in the rumen and gastrointestinal transit times are longer.[4]

Beyond their toxic potential, batteries pose foreign body hazards to animals. Batteries that become lodged as they pass through the digestive tract may result in obstruction or pressure necrosis of adjacent tissue. Choking hazard from smaller alkaline and disc batteries is also a potential risk.

Toxicity and Risk Factors. Pets may be exposed from batteries that are dropped or left around or that happen to fall out of equipment or toys as they are being chewed on by the animal. Cats may be particularly attracted to disc batteries and may ingest them in the process of playing with them. Livestock, especially cattle, may be exposed to old lead acid batteries left in junk piles in poorly managed pastures or from farm equipment left in pastures or barns.

Clinical Signs. Clinical signs may occur within a few hours of exposure. In cases of alkaline battery exposure, signs of oral injury may occur within 2 hours, but can take up to 12 hours for the full extent of injury to become apparent.[3] Acute signs may include depression, hypersalivation, oral inflammation or ulceration, smacking of lips or flicking of the tongue, dysphagia, vomiting (with or without blood), anorexia, abdominal pain, or melena. Significant hyperthermia (>104° F) may accompany oral inflammation. The presence of respiratory stridor may suggest that pharyngeal or esophageal ulceration has occurred; the absence of oral burns does not preclude the development of esophageal burns. Esophageal perforation may result in leakage of ingesta into the pleural cavity, causing pleuritis with dyspnea and fever. Acute dyspnea caused by foreign body airway obstruction by disc batteries may occur. Inhalation of corrosive material may lead to coughing, dyspnea, and moist lung sounds. Vomiting, tenesmus, or obstipation may result from gastrointestinal obstruction from the battery casing.

Dysphagia and regurgitation from esophageal stricture formation may occur during the healing phase in cases of esophageal burns.[1]

Clinical Pathology. Because battery ingestion results in local tissue injury rather than systemic toxicosis, no specific laboratory abnormalities are expected. In extensive soft tissue injury, elevations in the WBC count indicative of inflammation are expected.

Lesions. Gross lesions include oral, pharyngeal, and esophageal ulceration and necrosis. In severe cases esoph-

ageal perforation with hemorrhage and adjacent tissue injury may be present. Perforation of the thoracic esophagus may result in suppurative pleuritis. The formation of esophageal strictures during healing may result in regurgitation, megaesophagus, and aspiration pneumonia. Gastric or intestinal ulceration and perforation are also possible, especially with lithium disc batteries,[5] although esophageal injury is more common.

Respiratory tract corrosive injury caused by inhalation of caustic battery components may be manifested as edema and ulceration of the larynx, trachea, and lower airways. In significant inhalational exposure, pulmonary edema and pneumonitis may occur.

Diagnostic Testing. Radiography is recommended in cases of exposure of small animals to dry cell batteries to determine whether the casing has been ingested and, in the case of disc batteries, whether the battery has become lodged in the esophagus.[2]

Endoscopy of the oropharynx, esophagus, and stomach is recommended when significant exposure to corrosive components is suspected. Because it may take several hours for the full extent of the chemical burns to become apparent, endoscopic evaluation should be delayed at least 12 hours after initial exposure.[1]

Treatment. For recent exposures, dilution with water or milk assists in removing alkaline or acidic products from the oral and esophageal mucosa. In the case of lithium disc batteries, serial administration of tap water (20-ml boluses every 15 minutes) decreases the severity and delays the development of current-induced tissue injury.[5] Skin that has been contacted by battery contents should be bathed copiously in tap water. These measures can be instituted at home in asymptomatic animals before transport to the veterinary hospital.

On presentation animals should be evaluated for the presence of oral or pharyngeal irritation or ulceration. The presence of gray-black residue on the teeth suggests that the animal has punctured the battery and exposed the contents. Radiography to determine the location and appearance of any ingested batteries should be performed. Although deformities in battery casings suggest that leakage of contents may have occurred, the lack of casing deformity on radiography does not guarantee that the casing has not been compromised. Disc batteries lodged in the esophagus should be removed immediately to minimize esophageal burns; ideally, this should be performed using endoscopy.[2]

Whether to remove a battery in the stomach depends on several factors, including the size of the animal, the size of the battery, and evidence that the battery has been punctured.[1] Batteries that are small relative to the size of the animal may readily pass uneventfully through the gastrointestinal tract and be eliminated via the stools. Stools should be examined to ensure that the battery has passed; failure to detect the battery in the stool within 3 days should warrant additional radiography to verify the location of the battery. Batteries that have not passed through the pylorus within 48 hours are unlikely to do so and may require endoscopic or surgical removal.[1] If the battery is suspected to have been punctured, removal via endoscopy is not recommended, because leakage from the battery during extraction may result in esophageal damage.

Treatment of oral or esophageal burns caused by acid or alkaline battery contents depends on the severity of injury, but should include antibiotics to prevent infection, maintenance of adequate nutrition and hydration, and general supportive care.[1] Sucralfate may be used as a general gastrointestinal protectant. As needed, pain medication and antiinflammatories may be used. For severe oral and esophageal lesions, placement of a gastrostomy tube facilitates nutritional support while the mucosa heals. The use of corticosteroids in cases of esophageal burns is controversial; although corticosteroids do help decrease inflammation and minimize the development of scar tissue and thereby stricture formation, they also delay wound healing and increase risk of infection.[1]

Respiratory or dermal injury from exposure to corrosive battery contents should be treated symptomatically.

Prognosis.   The prognosis for animals ingesting batteries depends on the degree of tissue damage that occurs. Most ingestions of intact batteries result in uneventful passage of the batteries out in the stool. Mild to moderate oral ulceration usually heals rapidly and carries a good prognosis. Severe oral burns carry the risk of infection and significant sloughing of oral tissues. Because the esophagus heals poorly and is prone to stricture formation, significant esophageal injury has a more guarded prognosis. Perforation of the esophagus or stomach may result in pleuritis or peritonitis, either of which may be life threatening.

Prevention and Control.   Keeping batteries and battery-containing equipment out of the range of pets is the best method of prevention. For large animal exposures, maintaining clean pastures free of junk piles and old vehicles prevents exposures to automotive batteries.

BLEACHES

Jill Richardson

Synonyms.   Synonyms include bleach, bleaching powder, whitener, Clorox, and chlorox.[1]

Sources.   Bleaches are found in liquid and granular preparations. Most household bleaches contain less than 5% sodium hypochlorite, but granular bleaches can have higher concentrations.[1-3] Powdered chlorine bleaches usually contain calcium hypochlorite, trichloroisocyanuric acid, or dichlorodimethyhydantoin.[1] Commercial bleaches can contain 50% or more calcium hypochlorite.[1] Commercial bleaches may also contain other bleaching agents such as sodium peroxide, sodium perborate, and sodium carbonate.[1] Nonchlorine bleach or colorfast bleaches may contain sodium peroxide, sodium perborate, or enzymatic detergent.[2]

Mechanism of Action.   Bleaches range from being irritating to being corrosive depending on the concentration and the duration of exposure.[1,2,4-6] Household bleaches are usually mild to moderate in toxicity.[1] Bleaches with a pH of 11 to 12 can be corrosive.[1] Solid form bleaches have greater potential for toxicosis because they are concentrated.[2] Sodium peroxide decomposes in the gastrointestinal tract, releases oxygen, and may cause mild gastritis.[1] Sodium perborate decomposes to peroxide and borate. Sodium hypochlorite when combined with an acid or ammonia may produce chlorine and chloramine gas, which can cause mucous membrane and respiratory tract irritation.[1-3]

Toxicity and Risk Factors.   Any species of animal can be affected by bleaches; however, it is a more common occurrence with companion animals because house pets are more likely to be in contact with household items, such as cleaning agents.

Clinical Signs.   The most common clinical signs seen with bleach ingestion include hypersalivation, vomiting or retching, lethargy, and inappetence. Oral ulceration, severe depression, pawing at the mouth, and dysphagia may also be seen with exposures to corrosive formulations. Alkaline bleaches with a pH of 11 to 12 can produce partial-thickness chemical burns.

Dermal exposure to bleach can result in skin irritation and fur bleaching. Eye irritation, lacrimation, blepharospasm, and eyelid edema can occur with exposure to chlorine gas or direct ocular exposure.[1] Ocular exposures to alkaline bleaches can result in corneal damage and ulceration.[1,2,4,6] Inhalation of chloramine gas can result in coughing, choking, and dyspnea, whereas long-term or concentrated inhalation can result in chemical pneumonitis, pulmonary edema, and respiratory failure.[1]

Clinical Pathology.   Hypernatremia and hyperchloremia are possible with large ingestions of hypochlorite bleaches.[1] Metabolic acidosis can occur from a large ingestion or long-term inhalation.[1]

Treatment.   After ingestion of alkaline bleach, gastric lavage and emesis are *not* recommended because of possible corrosive effects. Preferred initial treatment would be oral dilution with milk or water. Dilution is most effective if it is performed early. Activated charcoal is ineffective for caustic agents.[1,3,6] Symptomatic treatment for gastric upset is recommended. Protracted vomiting may require measures to maintain fluid and electrolyte balance. With exposures to bleaches with pH greater than 11, the patient should be monitored for corrosive injury to the mouth, pharynx, and esophagus.

For cases of severe stomatitis, pharyngitis, esophagitis, or esophageal ulceration, hydration can be maintained with intravenous fluids. A gastrostomy tube may be necessary for nutritional support. Sucralfate slurries can be used for the treatment of oral, esophageal, gastric, and duodenal ulcers. Butorphanol tartrate can be used for pain management. Corticosteroid use is controversial for reduction of inflammation. Prednisone can be used at 1 to 2 mg/kg parenterally once daily for 1 to 2 days.[7] The animal should be monitored for an increase in body temperature or an increase in WBC count. Broad-spectrum antibiotics are indicated in cases of mucosal damage and secondary infection or as prophylaxis when using steroids.

After dermal exposure the animal should be bathed immediately with a mild liquid dish detergent or a non-insecticidal pet shampoo. The animal should be monitored for erythema, swelling, pain, and pruritus. Treatment is symptomatic and may include analgesics, antiinflammatories, and antibiotics.

For recent ocular exposure to bleach, a minimum of 20 to 30 minutes' irrigation with tepid tap water or physiologic saline is recommended. Afterward, the eye should be examined for evidence of corneal ulceration. For any product that is identified as corrosive to the eye, an ophthalmologist should be consulted as soon as possible for a thorough eye examination.[3]

Prognosis. The prognosis for minor exposures to household bleaches is good, as long as appropriate care is given to the animal. Animals with exposure to corrosive bleaches resulting in esophageal perforations have a poor prognosis unless aggressive care, possibly including surgical intervention, is given. Esophageal strictures are a possible sequela.

BORIC ACID

Sherry Welch

Sources. Sodium borate, sodium biborate, sodium pyoborate, and sodium tetraborate (in borax cleaners) contain 21% boron by weight. A teaspoon of boric acid crystals contains approximately 2.2 to 4.4 g of boric acid. Sodium borate solution (Dobell's solution) contains 1.5 g of sodium borate, 1.5 g of sodium bicarbonate, and 0.3 ml of liquefied phenol. Boric anhydride, boron oxide, boron trioxide, boric oxide, boron sesquioxide, borax, tincal, and tinkal are 33% boron by weight, sodium metaborate is 16.44% boron, and magnesium perborate is 14% boron. Saturated solutions of boric acid contain 5.55% boron.[1]

Boric acid (H_3BO_3) is prepared by treating sodium borate (borax) with sulfuric acid. Although it is poorly soluble in water at room temperature (l g dissolving in 18 g of water), it dissolves readily in hot water, alcohol, and glycerine. Boric acid in solution is only slightly acidic and acts as a nonirritating, slightly astringent antiseptic, mild enough to be used in eyewash.[2]

Generally, boric acid has a wide variety of uses, including medical, household, and industrial uses. Borates have been used in pharmaceutical preparations including medicated powders, skin lotions, mouthwash, toothpaste (sodium perborate, consisting of sodium borate and hydrogen peroxide), topical astringents, and eyewash solutions. Boric acid and borax are used at concentrations of up to 5% in oral hygiene products in Europe and elsewhere. The effectiveness

of borates as antibacterial and antifungal agents has been questioned, making dermatologic uses in the United States limited.[3,4]

Household uses for boric acid have included its use as a food preservative, water softener, and buffer. Borates have been used as a home remedy for diaper rash and oral discomfort in infants. A mixture of boric acid and honey, in particular, has been applied to pacifiers of irritable infants, resulting in severe toxicity and death from these practices. Boric acid is widely used for control of roaches, ants, and flies, with many formulations containing greater than 90% boric acid. It is available commercially, as well as in homemade mixtures of 100% boric acid with flour or sugar. Accidental ingestion of boric acid–containing bait traps and boric acid powders left out for these purposes is a common occurrence in pets, especially dogs.[3]

Industrial uses of borates or boron-containing compounds include heat-resistant glass, glass fibers, glazes for pottery, enamels, fire-resistant materials and agents, pigments, paints, catalysts, gliding baths, photographic agents, insecticides, and herbicides. Borates are also used in the manufacture of paper and paperboard. Other uses include artificially aging and preserving wood, cleaning compounds, soldering metals, and curing and preserving animal skins.

Toxicokinetics. Absorption of boric acid occurs easily through abraded or excoriated skin. Absorption through intact skin is negligible. Ingestion results in rapid and complete absorption of boric acid from the gastrointestinal tract. Distribution then occurs throughout body water, but with highest concentrations in brain, liver, and kidneys. Most ingested boric acid is excreted unchanged by the kidneys. Greater than 50% of the oral dose is gone within 24 hours, and greater than 90% is excreted within 96 hours of ingestion. Various half-lives have been reported ranging from 5 to 21 hours.[5] Boron has been detected in urine up to 23 days after exposure.[4]

Mechanism of Action. The exact mechanism of action of boric acid is not known, but it is generally considered to be cytotoxic to cells.[4,6] The toxic effects of boric acid depend on the concentration in the exposed organ. Boric acid is freely soluble in body water and can be found in high concentrations in the kidney and, less commonly, in the brain and liver, making these organs predisposed to toxic effects.[4]

Toxicity and Risk Factors. Poisoning has followed ingestion, parenteral injection, enemas, and lavage of cavities. Toxicosis has been produced by excessive topical use for surgical wounds, burns, ulcers, and diaper dermatitis. Fatalities have resulted from accidental administration of boric acid to infants.[1]

In the rat the LD_{50}s of boric acid range from 2 to 4.98 g/kg. The sodium salts are slightly less toxic in animals. There were no deaths or serious systemic effects found in dogs given 1.54 to 6.51 g/kg borax or 1 to 3.09 g/kg of boric acid orally. Most dogs vomited, however. A 2-year chronic test demonstrated that boric acid at 350 ppm could be tolerated in the diets of both dogs and rats. In a 90-day subchronic study boric acid at 525 ppm in feed caused no adverse reaction.[4]

In humans the fatal dose in five infants was 4.5 to 14 g; however, as little as 1 g has been fatal. Systemic poisoning in humans has resulted from the ingestion of as little as 1.2 g/kg of boric acid. Infants have survived ingestions of 1.95 to 20 g. Fatalities have been reported in adults after use of 15 to 30 g.[1] Chronic toxicosis occurred after ingestion of 4 to 5 g of boric acid per day for 3 to 4 weeks, or 6 to 20 g of borax daily for several months. This is equivalent to 2.12 g of boron per day.[1]

Clinical Signs.   With ingestion of boric acid, the severity of clinical signs depends on the amount ingested, the concentration of the agent, and the age and general health of the exposed animal. Young or geriatric animals generally are more susceptible to toxic effects than are adult animals. In a single acute exposure ingestion of toxic levels of boric acid most commonly causes hypersalivation, vomiting, retching, depression, anorexia, diarrhea, and abdominal pain. The vomit and stools may be blue-green in color or may contain blood. Despite these gastrointestinal effects, boric acid is not caustic.[4] In humans acute skin changes have developed after boric acid ingestion or application of a boric acid powder. This may result in erythema, desquamation in 1 to 2 days, and exfoliation resulting in "boiled lobster" syndrome.[1] If a sufficiently high level is ingested, weakness, ataxia, tremors, focal or generalized seizures, oliguria or anuria, renal tubular nephrosis, and, rarely, hepatoxicosis may occur. Seizures may be followed by metabolic acidosis, depression, coma, and death.[1]

Chronic ingestion can cause anorexia, weight loss, vomiting, diarrhea or loose stools, rashes, alopecia, anemia, and death.[4] Renal toxicosis includes oliguria, anuria, and renal tubular necrosis.[4] Death may be caused by cyanosis, hypotension, shock, or severe central nervous system (CNS) depression.[4]

Animal studies have demonstrated that borax and boric acid at very high levels may lead to growth suppression and decreased efficiency of food utilization in rats. Testicular degeneration has been noted in both rats and dogs at very high boron levels, and rats were sterile. Boric acid is a teratogen in chick embryos.[5]

Clinical Pathology.   Clinical pathology parameters may indicate a toxemia, microcytic hypochromic anemia, hypernatremia, hyperchloremia, metabolic acidosis, occasionally hyperkalemia, and possible hepatotoxicosis. Albuminuria, hematuria, proteinuria, and epithelial casts may be noted on urinalysis.[1]

Lesions.   Autopsy findings in human patients who die as a result of boric acid poisoning note significant involvement of several organ systems (skin, gastrointestinal tract, kidneys, liver, and brain). In individuals with skin eruptions pathologic specimens are consistent with an exfoliative dermatitis. The gastrointestinal tract demonstrates inflammatory changes with congestion, edema, and mucosal exfoliation. Renal changes are somewhat variable, ranging from gross pallor to cloudy swelling and tubular degeneration. The CNS is a target organ, demonstrates congestion and edema of the brain, and has in some studies been noted to be the organ with the highest concentration of boric acid in some intoxicated patients. The liver, despite being the organ with the second highest concentration of boric acid, rarely demonstrates clinical manifestations of boric acid toxicosis. Pathologic findings consist of fatty change and congestion, with rare findings of intracytoplasmic inclusion bodies in pancreatic acinar cells.[5]

Diagnostic Testing.   The diagnosis of boric acid toxicosis is usually based on history of ingestion and clinical signs. Boric acid can be detected in urine, cerebral spinal fluid, blood, plasma, and tissues, although concentrations associated with stages of toxicosis have not been well established in animals.[4] Specific urine tests (one drop of the patient's urine is acidified with HCl and applied to turmeric paper; the paper may turn brownish-red if boric acid is present) are unreliable.[1]

In humans serum and urine borate levels reflect the fact that exposure has occurred, but they do not correlate well with the clinical state. In humans signs of toxicosis generally occur when blood levels exceed 20 to 150 μg/ml; however, in a test series with a median age of 2 years, blood borate concentrations as high as 340 μg/ml were not associated with significant toxicosis.[1]

Treatment.   The treatment recommendations depend on the amount of boric acid ingested and the severity of the clinical signs. If a potentially toxic dose has been ingested (400 mg/kg in humans)[1], hospitalization for observation, decontamination, and symptomatic and supportive care is recommended.

Emesis should be induced, unless the patient is already vomiting, is experiencing seizures, is in a coma, or lacks a gag reflex. Gastric lavage is indicated if any of these conditions are present, and should only be performed after endotracheal intubation. Activated charcoal is usually not recommended because of its poor absorption of boric acid. It has been shown experimentally in rats that, in order for activated charcoal to be effective, one would need to administer 5 to 10 times the usual recommended dose, making it impractical clinically.[4] In humans it has been used when the patient was brought in within a few hours after ingestion, but its value remains controversial.[1] Supportive care for vomiting animals includes intravenous fluids (replacement of losses, plus maintenance with isotonic fluids). Gastrointestinal protectants and antiemetics should be administered parenterally during the vomiting phase. Once the vomiting is under control, oral gastrointestinal protectants can be given. Baseline serum chemistries, electrolytes, acid-base status, and urine specific gravity should be determined, with monitoring every 24 hours until the animal has recovered. For acute renal failure, treatment should include intravenous 0.9% saline twice maintenance for a minimum of 48 hours, or until the blood urea nitrogen (BUN), creatinine, and urine specific gravity values return to normal. Sodium bicarbonate should be added to the fluids if the animal is acidotic. Diazepam may be used to control seizures.

If dermal or ocular exposure has occurred, thorough flushing of the affected area is indicated. Dermal lesions may require the application of a topical steroid preparation and prophylactic broad-spectrum antibiotics. Use of ophthalmic ointments containing corticosteroids should be avoided unless the integrity of the cornea is assured.

Prognosis. Unless the amount ingested is large, acute exposures to boric acid in healthy animals usually result in only mild to moderate gastrointestinal signs, and the prognosis is good in most cases. The chance of a good prognosis decreases with chronic exposure or if the amount ingested acutely is high enough to cause severe signs, such as renal, liver, or CNS toxicosis.

Prevention and Control. Boric acid–containing products used in the household should be placed out of reach of pets. When boric acid is used for insect control, it is oftentimes mixed with foods or food-grade additives that may attract some animals, especially dogs. Physical placement of these types of insecticides should be done with care. Chronic or excessive use of topical agents containing boric acid should be avoided, especially if dermal lesions are present, because absorption occurs easily through abraded or excoriated skin, thus increasing the risk of toxicosis.

DETERGENTS

Jill Richardson

Synonyms. Detergents are nonsoap surfactants in combination with inorganic ingredients such as phosphates, silicates, or carbonates. Detergents are classified according to their charge in solution: nonionic, anionic, or cationic.

Sources. Anionic and nonionic detergents are found in shampoos, dishwashing detergents, laundry detergents, and electric dishwashing detergents. Cationic detergents, such as benzalkonium chloride and benzethonium chloride, can be found in fabric softeners, some potpourri oils, hair mousse, conditioners, germicides, disinfectants, and sanitizers.

Mechanism of Action. The mechanism responsible for the systemic effects of cationic detergents is not known. It is hypothesized that these compounds cause ganglionic blocking effects and a curare-like action with the paralysis of neuromuscular junctions of striated muscles.

Toxicity and Risk Factors. Any species of animal can be affected by a detergent; however, it is a more common occurrence with companion animals because pets are more likely to be in contact with household items.

Anionic and ionic detergents are considered irritants and have a low toxicity.[1-3] Cationic detergents are rapidly absorbed and may produce severe local and systemic toxicosis. Cationic concentrations between 1% and 7.5% damage mucous membranes, whereas solutions containing con-centrations greater than 7.5% are corrosive.[1-3] However, oral ulcerations, stomatitis, and pharyngitis can be seen in the cat at concentrations of 2% or less.[4]

Clinical Signs. Nausea, vomiting, and diarrhea are the most common clinical effects seen with ingestion of anionic or nonionic detergents. Persistent gastric upset may result in dehydration and electrolyte abnormalities. Mild eye irritation is possible. Low phosphate detergents (e.g., electric dishwasher detergents) are generally more alkaline and ingestion may result in oral and esophageal burns and should be treated accordingly.

The principal clinical signs from cationic detergents are hypersalivation and vomiting with possible hematemesis, muscular weakness and fasciculations, CNS and respiratory depression, seizures, collapse, and coma. Diarrhea, dermal necrosis, dermatitis, pulmonary edema, hypotension, and metabolic acidosis have also been reported.[1,4] If ingested, solutions of quaternary ammonium compounds may result in corrosive burns of the mouth, pharynx, and esophagus. Eye exposure may cause effects ranging from mild discomfort to very serious corneal damage. Dermal exposure to cationic detergents can result in erythema, edema, intense pain, and ulceration. Hyperthermia and pulmonary edema have been reported.[1,4]

Treatment. After ingestion of detergents, gastric lavage and emesis are *not* recommended because of possible corrosive effects.[4] Instead, oral dilution with milk or water is preferred.[4,5] Dilution is most effective if it is performed early. Activated charcoal is ineffective. Additionally, passing a stomach tube could penetrate damaged esophageal tissue, and charcoal can make visualization of oral and esophageal burns difficult.

Most ingestions of nonionic or anionic detergents are generally self-limiting, requiring only dilution with milk or water. Ingestions of cationic detergents are typically more severe and require more aggressive treatment. For cases of severe stomatitis, pharyngitis, esophagitis, or esophageal ulceration, hydration can be maintained with intravenous fluids. A gastrotomy tube may be necessary for nutritional support. Sucralfate slurries can be used for the treatment of oral, esophageal, gastric, and duodenal ulcers.[4,5] Pain management, such as the use of butorphanol tartrate, may be necessary.[4,5] Corticosteroid use is controversial for reduction of inflammation.[4] Prednisone can be used at 1 to 2 mg/kg parenterally once daily for 1 to 2 days.[4,6] Additionally, the animal should be monitored for an increase in body temperature or an increase in WBC count. Broad-spectrum antibiotics are indicated in cases of mucosal damage, secondary infection, or as prophylaxis when using steroids.[4]

With recent ocular exposure, a minimum of 20 to 30 minutes' irrigation with tepid tap water or physiologic saline is recommended.[1,5] Afterward, the eye should be examined and closely monitored for evidence of corneal ulceration.

After dermal exposure to cationic detergents, the animal should be bathed immediately with a mild liquid dish detergent or a noninsecticidal pet shampoo. The animal should be monitored for burns, erythema, swelling, pain, or pruritus. Treatment for dermal damage is symptomatic and may include analgesics, antiinflammatories, and antibiotics.[5]

Prognosis. The prognosis for most exposures to anionic and ionic detergents is good, as long as supportive care is given to the animal. Exposures to cationic detergents typically require more treatment, but can have a favorable prognosis if prompt and appropriate care is given. Animals with esophageal perforations have a poor prognosis unless aggressive care, possibly including surgical intervention, is given.

Prevention and Control. Animal owners should never allow their pets to have access to the areas where detergents are being used or stored.

DIPYRIDYL HERBICIDES

Fred Oehme and John A. Pickrell

The dipyridyl (bipyridyl) herbicides, paraquat (1,1'-dimethyl-4,4'bipyridylium dichloride; methyl viologen) and diquat (1,1'-ethylene-4,4'bipyridylium dibromide) desiccate plants. Although these toxicants may be absorbed through the percutaneous, respiratory, or digestive routes, only paraquat concentrates in and primarily affects lung tissue. Paraquat is one of the most specific pulmonary toxicants known. A high mortality rate is encountered in paraquat poisoning cases. Alternatively, diquat is less toxic and not concentrated by the lung, and the liver is the primary target organ.[1,2]

PARAQUAT

Sources. Paraquat is one of the most efficient herbicides and often the herbicide of choice to control flourishing vegetation. However, it is one of the most specific pulmonary toxicants known, and a high mortality rate is encountered in poisoning cases. Paraquat has been restricted in the markets of the United States and many other countries; however, more than 130 countries still use paraquat. In developing countries 98% of the workers can obtain paraquat.[1] Because of its widespread distribution and high toxicity, paraquat is considered extremely hazardous.

Toxicokinetics. Paraquat is poorly absorbed (about 5% to 10%) from the intestinal tract.[1] However, it is broken down so slowly that about 50% remains in the digestive tract

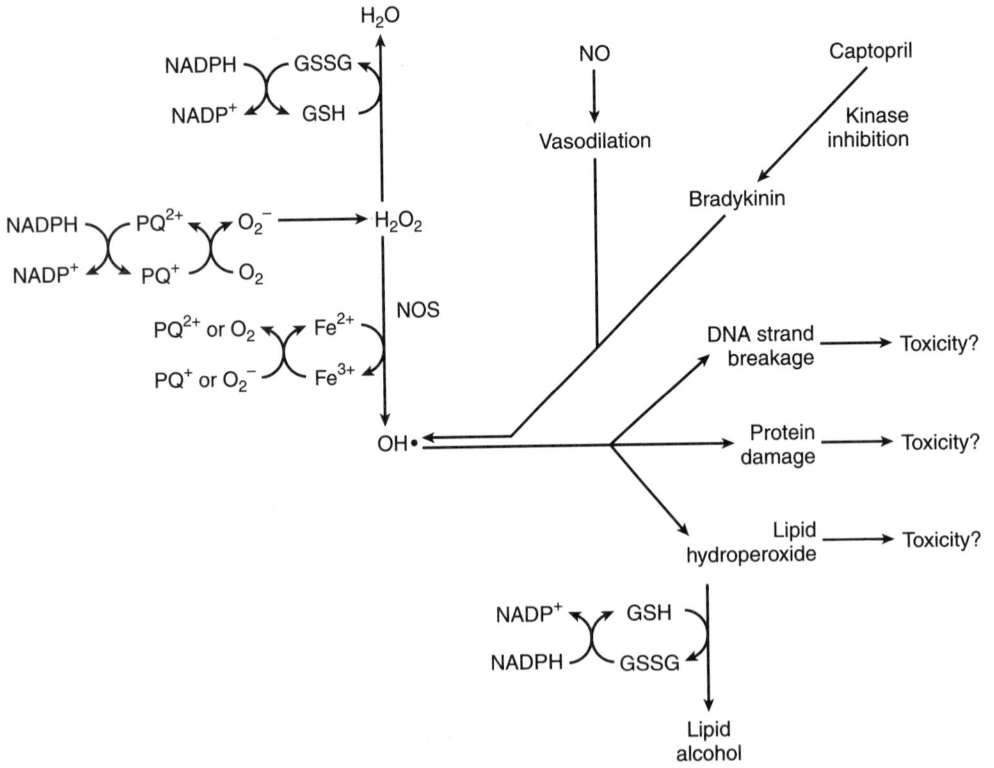

Fig. 20-1 The mechanism of paraquat's (PQ) toxicity is shown. NADPH (reduced nicotine adenine dinucleotide phosphate) oxidation to NADP$^+$ is linked to PQ reduction. PQ reoxidation is linked to reduction of oxygen to produce hydrogen peroxide (H_2O_2). H_2O_2 detoxication is driven by reduced glutathione (GSH) oxidation to oxidized glutathione (GSSG). This is regenerated by linking it to an oxidation of NADPH to NADP$^+$. H_2O_2 can be further oxidized to a hydroxyl radical (OH·) by the ferrous ion being oxidized to the ferric ion, linked to a reduction of either PQ or oxygen (O_2). Nitric oxide synthetase (NOS) is used to create the superoxide radical (O_2^-) which is converted to OH·, potentiating PQ toxicity and depleting the system of needed nitric oxide (NO). The OH· damages tissue, participating in DNA strand breakage, protein damage, and lipid hydroperoxide formation. NO opposes the action of OH· by producing vasodilation. Likewise, kininase inhibition of captopril, which prolongs the action of bradykinin, also opposes the OH· free radical. Finally, lipid hydroperoxide can be reduced to an aldehyde by oxidation of reduced GSH. GSSG is regenerated to reduced GSH by linking it to the oxidation of NADPH.

32 hours after administration. About 45% of the absorbed dose is excreted in the urine by 48 hours after ingestion. Some paraquat is detected in the urine for 21 days after ingestion. Emulsifiers and cosorbents may enhance absorption and toxicity. Intestinal microflora may metabolize less than 30% of the ingestate. Elevated concentrations of paraquat in renal tissue indicate the route of paraquat excretion.[1] The excretion rate of paraquat is greater than the rate of glomerular filtration and is concentration dependent and saturable, indicating secretion by an active transport system.[3]

Mechanism of Action. Paraquat can form free radicals, and tissue necrosis is associated with the same mechanisms of superoxide-induced peroxidation as observed with diquat.[4] In addition, it has special affinity for and concentrates in the lung as a result of a diamine-polyamine concentrator system in alveolar epithelial cells.[4] Paraquat is excreted through the kidney.[1,5]

The initiation of pulmonary injury by paraquat (Fig. 20-1) begins with cyclic reduction-oxidation (redox) reactions. Paraquat undergoes repeated redox cycling, which amplifies production of a toxic reactive oxygen species as well as reduction of reduced nicotine adenine dinucleotide phosphate (NADPH) and other reducing substances, producing a superoxide radical (O_2^-).[6] The O_2^- is converted to hydrogen peroxide (H_2O_2) by superoxide dismutase. Both O_2^- and H_2O_2 can attack polyunsaturated lipids and perpetuate the pulmonary injury.[1]

Nitric oxide (NO) synthetase (NOS) enhances paraquat toxicity by generating superoxide at the expense of NO in several in vitro and cellular models.[7] Neuronal, endothelial, and macrophage NOS activity needed in normal lung tissue are blocked by paraquat. Paraquat-induced endothelial cell toxicity is blocked by inhibitors of NOS that prevent NADPH, but is not attenuated by those that do not.[7] Clinical improvement was seen from NO given late in paraquat toxicosis, suggesting a sparing role of NO in this process.[8] Finally, after undergoing a single electron reduction in tissues, the resultant free radical is readily oxidized by molecular oxygen to the parent compound, and it is excreted unchanged in urine.[1] Paraquat is excreted by an active transport system.[3]

Toxicity and Risk Factors. Paraquat is absorbed by soil, becoming biologically unavailable so that it is of little toxic consequence to animals.[9] However, ingestion of commercial paraquat concentrates before their use or before they have become inactivated by soil is nearly always fatal after a course of 3 to 4 weeks.[1] In animals paraquat shows moderate acute toxicity, with its LD_{50} ranging from 22 to 262 mg/kg.[1] Because about 5% to 10% is absorbed, the polyamine extractor, which increases pulmonary concentrations inordinately,[4,5] is important to the pulmonary toxicity of paraquat. It has been used as a malicious poison.[5]

Clinical Signs. Paraquat is an irritant and a vesicant and thus can cause considerable local toxicosis (erythema, blistering, irritation, blistering of skin, and corneal irritation) from topical exposure, such as splashing at time of application. In uncomplicated cases, full recovery is possible.[9]

In acute poisoning from ingestion, the disease typically occurs in three phases. The initial phase reflects the caustic action of paraquat with the development of pain in the gastrointestinal tract. Pain is followed by vomiting and aphagia. The second phase, renal failure accompanied by hepatocellular necrosis, develops by the second or third day. The renal tubulopathy often resolves uneventfully by the time of death. The third phase is delayed development of pulmonary fibrosis and is responsible for the poor and usually fatal prognosis.[9]

In subacute or chronic poisoning low doses of paraquat allow hyperplasia of type II alveolar epithelial cells and healing by fibrosis. In such cases, cyanosis develops rapidly when the animal is exercised, reflecting the increasing mismatch of ventilation with perfusion, the increasing alveolar-arterial oxygen gradient, and desaturation of hemoglobin with oxygen. Radiographic changes may not reflect the extent of the clinical changes because the extent of mismatch of ventilation with perfusion cannot be seen. In the final stages of fatal paraquat poisoning, decerebration occurs during ventilation with an inspired oxygen fraction of 100% and PAo_2 decreasing to less than 30 mm Hg (torr).[9]

Clinical Pathology. No specific clinical pathology changes are noted with paraquat poisoning.

Lesions. Acutely, alveolar epithelial cells undergo apoptosis or necrosis, leaving a completely denuded basement membrane followed by pulmonary edema, functional impairment, ventilation-perfusion mismatch, and death. Subacutely or chronically, low doses of paraquat can allow hyperplasia of type II alveolar epithelial cells instead of their death. Healing is often by fibrosis.[9]

Diagnostic Testing. A history of consumption of fresh product or association with spraying in an enclosed space is typical.[10] Specific chemical determinations can be made for paraquat in urine, plasma, or lung. If plasma is evaluated paraquat can be measured for up to 30 hours.[6,9] After 30 hours lung tissue contains the highest concentration of paraquat.[9]

Treatment. Treatment for paraquat intoxication should begin quickly.[9] Most of the treatment approaches described apply to human patients and require validation in companion animals.

Although paraquat has no specific antidote captopril, a human antihypertensive and kininase inhibitor given 1 hour or less after exposure to paraquat, reduced lipid peroxidation in rats. It balanced the activities of superoxide dismutase and glutathione peroxidase, thus reducing the development of lung fibrosis. Prolonging kinin action supported the beneficial activity of vasodilation. A limitation to the use of captopril is that it must be given within a short time of exposure.[11]

Gastrointestinal decontamination, via gastric emesis followed by gastric lavage and activated charcoal, is recommended for all cases of acute paraquat poisoning.[9] Time is a factor because energy-dependent lung accumulation of paraquat[4,5] begins as soon as peak plasma paraquat concentrations are achieved. Gastric lavage lowered plasma levels of paraquat in the cat, although therapeutic benefit was not demonstrated.[12] Charcoal is the preferred adsorbent because it more effectively reduces the severity and fatality of paraquat intoxication than does either Fuller's earth or bentonite.

Forced diuresis cannot accelerate paraquat excretion, but it can maintain adequate renal perfusion, which is advantageous to patient survival. Peritoneal dialysis provides no therapeutic advantage because it removes little paraquat. In contrast, hemodialysis can clear up to 150 ml plasma/min.[9,12] Extracorporeal hemoperfusion using a Hemocol cartridge is also effective (113 to 156 ml/min) even when plasma paraquat was only 0.2 ml plasma/L. Survival of dogs exposed to paraquat improves if dogs undergo hemoperfusion for 4 hours at 12 hours after exposure.[12]

Supportive care includes protection of the airway, maintenance of circulation, frequent monitoring of vital signs and blood gases, prompt and timely treatment of secondary infections, adequate pain management, prevention and treatment of renal failure, replacement of blood losses, and treatment of cardiac complications and neurologic signs.[9]

Prognosis. The prognosis for paraquat is extremely guarded in companion animal practice, especially when treatment is delayed. The presence of significant paraquat in plasma or urine (in the first 24 hours) extrapolated from the nomogram in humans is suggestive of a poor prognosis.[13] In animal patients the presence of frank gastric and esophageal ulcers indicates a grave prognosis. The early development of renal failure and concurrent acid-base disturbances heralds a poor outlook. The ability of an animal to excrete paraquat depends mostly on normal or nearly normal renal function.

Prevention and Control. Client education, following all product restrictions, is essential. In the United States paraquat can only be used by a licensed person.

DIQUAT

Sources. Diquat (Reglone) is a rapidly acting contact herbicide used as a desiccant for the control of aquatic weeds and to destroy potato halums before harvesting.[3]

Toxicokinetics. Diquat is poorly absorbed. About 6% of an oral dose is excreted in the urine, whereas 90% to 98% of a subcutaneous dose is excreted in the urine.[1,3]

Mechanism of Action. Diquat can form free radicals, and tissue necrosis is associated with the same mechanisms of superoxide-induced peroxidation as observed with paraquat.[1,3] However, unlike paraquat, it has no special affinity for the lung and it does not appear to respond to the same mechanism that concentrates paraquat in the lung. Thus, diquat is not taken up and concentrated in the lung, but rather by the gastrointestinal tract, liver, and kidney.[1,3] Its desiccant qualities cause large losses of water into the lumen of the gastrointestinal tract.[14]

The initiation of hepatic injury by diquat (in Fischer 344 rats) has been more closely associated with iron chelate–catalyzed oxidations than with depletion of thiols or with thiol s-thiolations.[15] Experimentally, iron chelators (desferox-amine mesylate) provide protection from the toxic reaction, whereas iron salts worsen it.

In addition, the formation of dinitrophenylhydrazine (DNPH)-reactive protein carbonyls may be useful biomarkers of critical mechanisms of injury. These DNPH-reactive protein carbonyls require an oxidant and hydrogen peroxide. Catalase protects in vitro.[16] Thus, diquat enters redox cycling and only then begins to involve glutathione, probably as an adaptation.

Toxicity and Risk Factors. Following high-dose acute exposure or chronic exposure to diquat, major target organs are the gastrointestinal tract, liver, and kidney. Unlike paraquat, diquat has no special affinity for the lung and does not concentrate in the lung.[1] The risk of toxic exposure to cattle is minimal. An expected application rate in a cattle pasture is 320 g/acre and the minimum toxic dose is 5 mg/kg/day for 8 days. The expected application rate on a sheep pasture is about 5 times that of cattle, because the minimum toxic dose is also about 5 times that of cattle, but is documented for 3 days.[5] Because about 6% is absorbed, cattle would have to graze a much larger fraction of an acre than is usual in grazing to become poisoned.[17,18]

The no observed effect level (NOEL) for rats is 25 mg/kg. The LD$_{50}$ is lowest in fish (21 mg/L) and highest in partridges (295 mg/kg). The LD$_{50}$ is 187 mg/kg for dogs and 37 mg/kg for cattle.[5] Experimental intratracheal administration of very high levels of diquat led to the development of respiratory difficulties and pneumotoxicity. However, inhalation exposure to large concentrations of diquat is rare, and the lung neither takes up nor concentrates diquat.[19]

Clinical Signs. With minimal toxic concentrations diquat can produce signs at 8 days in cattle and 3 days in sheep.[17] At higher exposure concentrations signs appear more quickly. Gastrointestinal symptoms, acute renal failure, hepatic damage, and respiratory difficulties have been reported.

The clinical signs of diquat in animals primarily involve the digestive tract. Animals drinking from old diquat containers show anorexia, gastrointestinal distention, and severe loss of water into the lumen of the gastrointestinal tract. Signs of renal impairment, CNS excitement, and convulsions occur in severely affected animals. Lung lesions are uncommon.[14]

Clinical Pathology. No specific clinical pathology changes are noted for diquat. Because it is a desiccant that causes gastrointestinal toxicosis, changes indicating dehydration and electrolyte imbalances may be evident.[14] When exposure concentrations are sufficiently high to elicit liver damage, alanine aminotransferase (ALT) is increased in serum.[15]

Lesions. Animals receiving sufficiently high diquat exposures develop gastritis, hepatic lesions, and occasionally renal failure.[15,17]

Diagnostic Testing. History of a diquat herbicide exposure is usually the most helpful diagnostic aid. Although specific chemical determinations exist for diquat,[20,21] they are usually not available in veterinary diagnostic laboratories.

Treatment. Because of the very low diquat absorption from the gastrointestinal tract, oral administration of adsorbants in large quantities and cathartics is advised.[14] Bentonite (Fuller's earth) is preferred, but charcoal suffices.[14] In conjunction, supportive therapy (rehydration and correction of electrolyte imbalance) and administration of vitamin E and selenium can be helpful if diquat doses are high enough to produce pathologic liver problems. Excretion can be accelerated with forced diuresis induced by mannitol infusion and furosemide administration.[14]

Prognosis. Animals typically must consume diquat directly rather than from sprayed vegetation to receive the minimum toxic dose. However, such animals have a good prognosis for recovery in 1 to 2 weeks with treatment.

Prevention and Control. Little danger exists of even minimal intoxication if the labeled herbicide applications are followed.[14,17]

ESSENTIAL OILS

Charlotte Means

Sources. Essential oils give plants a characteristic odor and are found in all parts of the plant. The volatile oils are a mixture of terpenes (complex hydrocarbons) and other chemicals obtained through a distillation process. The oils are frequently diluted to an essence, which is the concentrated fragrance used in products such as perfume. Medicinally, the essential oil is often diluted in a carrier oil, such as safflower oil. Essential oils should always be diluted before using therapeutically. They are formed into pills, powders, and lozenges and may be mixed into tinctures, teas, and syrups.

The essential oils most commonly used in veterinary medicine are melaleuca, pennyroyal, D-limonene, and linalool. They are used for treating flea infestations, hot spots, and other dermatologic conditions. Shampoos, dips, and ointments often contain essential oils. Melaleuca oil has been marketed as a spot-on flea product, similar to products containing fipronil or imidocloprid. Occasionally, an essential oil such as wormwood may be used as an anthelminthic.[1,2]

Melaleuca oil, also known as tea tree oil, comes from *Melaleuca alternifolia*. Pennyroyal oil is obtained from *Mentha pulegium*. D-Limonene and linalool come from citrus fruits such as oranges and lemons. *Eucalyptus globulus* and *Mentha piperita* are the plants from which eucalyptus oil and menthol are derived. Wormwood, also known as absinthe, comes from *Artemisia absinthium*. Citronella is obtained from *Cymbopogum nardus*. Cinnamon oil comes from the bark of various *Cinnamomum* spp.[3,4]

Toxicokinetics. Essential oils are rapidly absorbed both orally and dermally. The oils are primarily metabolized in the liver by glucuronide and glycine conjugates. The metabolites are excreted in the urine within 48 to 72 hours of exposure.

About 10% of essential oils are excreted in the feces. Repeated exposures to essential oils can cause induction of the hepatic enzyme systems cytochrome P-450 and UPD-glycuronyl transferase systems.[2,3]

Mechanism of Action. The exact mechanism of action is unknown.

Toxicity and Risk Factors. All species can be affected. The acute oral LD$_{50}$ for the major essential oils ranges from 2 to 5 g/kg body weight. However, significant variations exist. Thujone, one of the active ingredients of wormwood, has a subcutaneous (SQ) LD$_{50}$ of 134 mg/kg. If a product is mixed with an organic solvent such as alcohol, increased absorption and toxicity can occur. Surfactants may increase permeability and allow increased absorption.

Animals with preexisting hepatic disease may be at greater risk for development of toxicosis. Some references suggest that cats are more sensitive to the effects of essential oils than are dogs.[2,4,5]

Clinical Signs. The most common clinical signs seen in dogs and cats after dermal exposure include ataxia, weakness, muscle tremors, depression, and behavioral abnormalities. Severe hypothermia and collapse may occur. These signs can occur almost immediately, although signs generally appear within 2 to 8 hours. Transient paralysis has occurred in small breed dogs when melaleuca oil has been applied down the back.

Scrotal dermatitis has developed in cats after being dipped in D-limonene shampoos. Liver failure has been associated with pennyroyal and melaleuca oils.

Oral ingestions can cause vomiting, diarrhea, and CNS depression. Seizures are possible from a large dose. Essential oils can cause aspiration pneumonia if inhaled. Grooming behavior may cause increased toxicity from dermal exposures. In both dermal and oral exposures death is possible.[2,5]

Clinical Pathology. No specific clinical pathology occurs. Hepatotoxicosis is expected to increase liver enzymes. Aspiration pneumonia can cause an increased white blood cell count.

Lesions. No specific lesions occur.

Diagnostic Testing. Gas chromatography–mass spectroscopy (GC-MS) can identify essential oils and metabolites in urine.[1,2,5]

Treatment. Bathing with a mild dish soap is important to remove any residue from the skin and coat. In cases of large oral exposures or heavy grooming, activated charcoal can be used to adsorb the terpenes and limit absorption. Inducing emesis is contraindicated.

No specific antidote exists. Body temperature regulation is critical. Intravenous fluids aid correction of hypotension as well as increase renal elimination of the product. Serum electrolytes should be monitored and corrected as needed. Cardiac and respiratory function should be monitored. Seizures and tremors may be treated with diazepam (0.5 to

1 mg/kg to effect) as needed. If an aspiration pneumonia develops, oxygen and a broad-spectrum antibiotic may be necessary. Hepatic damage usually resolves with good supportive care and the elimination of the product from the environment. N-Acetylcysteine has been used experimentally in pennyroyal toxicosis in humans. Although all patients responded well, it is unknown whether N-acetylcysteine had any bearing on the outcome because all patients received aggressive supportive care as well. N-Acetylcysteine given intraperitoneally (IP) did not help survival rates in rats dosed with lethal quantities of pennyroyal oil. N-Acyetylcysteine has a loading dose of 140 mg/kg and a maintenance dose of 70 mg/kg.[1,2,5]

Prognosis.   Most animals exposed to essential oils have a good prognosis with appropriate treatment. Underlying disease may worsen the prognosis. Many animals require only mild home treatment and observation. In mild exposures signs generally resolve within a few hours. For large exposures signs may resolve over 2 to 3 days with appropriate treatment.

Prevention and Control.   Animal owners often assume that natural products, or products derived from natural sources, are "safe" and cannot harm an animal. Thus, product directions may not be followed or too much product may be given. Clients should be counseled that adverse effects are possible even when a product is derived from a natural source.

ETHYLENE GLYCOL

Rosalind Dalefield

Synonyms.   Ethylene glycol is also known as 1,2-dihydroxy-ethane. Ethylene glycol poisoning is often called "antifreeze poisoning," although antifreeze solutions may be principally composed of methanol or propylene glycol instead. Antifreeze may be called coolant, summer coolant, or radiator coolant.

Sources.   Besides antifreeze, ethylene glycol is found in hydraulic brake and transmission fluids, airplane deicers and antiicers,[1] detergents, lacquers, polishes,[2] cosmetics, and pharmaceuticals.[3] It is also used as an industrial humectant and as a solvent in paints and plastics.[4]

Pure ethylene glycol is a colorless, odorless, sweet-tasting liquid with a boiling point of 197.2° C and a freezing point of −12.3° C. It is slightly viscous and has a density of 1.113. It is miscible in all proportions of alcohol and water.

Toxicokinetics.   Absorption of ethylene glycol is rapid from the gastrointestinal tract after ingestion, from the lungs after inhalation, and from subcutaneous tissues after injection. Metabolism, which occurs primarily in the liver and kidneys, commences within 2 to 4 hours of exposure with most of the ethylene glycol and its metabolites excreted within 24 to 48 hours.[1]

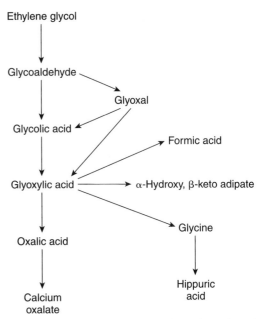

Fig. 20-2 Pathways of ethylene glycol metabolism. The pathway by which the toxicologically significant metabolites are generated is shown vertically.

Metabolism of ethylene glycol is summarized in Figure 20-2. The first step is conversion to glycoaldehyde, which is catalyzed by alcohol dehydrogenase. Glycoaldehyde is then metabolized by aldehyde dehydrogenase to glycolic acid, followed by glyoxylic acid. A minor pathway of glycoaldehyde metabolism is via glyoxal, which is then metabolized to glycolic acid or glyoxylic acid. Glyoxylic acid is metabolized to a number of compounds, of which the major compound, and the most toxicologically significant, is oxalic acid. Other metabolites of glyoxylic acid are formic acid, glycine, and α-hydroxy, β-keto adipate.[1] Excretion of the parent compound and most metabolites is renal, although formic acid is expired as carbon dioxide.

Mechanism of Action.   The central nervous signs of stage I of ethylene glycol toxicosis are principally attributable to the parent compound, which is an alcohol, and to aldehydes. However, high glycolate concentrations may cause clinical CNS effects, and other contributory mechanisms may include cerebral edema and calcium oxalate deposition in cerebral blood vessels.[1]

Because ethylene glycol is a small (molecular weight 62 daltons), water-soluble molecule, it readily causes an increase in serum osmolality. Polydipsia and polyuria that first develop within 1 to 3 hours of ethylene glycol ingestion in the dog may be due to this increasing serum osmolality stimulating thirst, to an osmotic diuretic effect of ethylene glycol, or both. It is also possible that ethylene glycol, like ethanol, inhibits release of antidiuretic hormone.[5]

Stage II of ethylene glycol toxicosis has been characterized as the cardiopulmonary[1] or the acidotic stage.[6] Acidosis is attributable to the acidic metabolites, particularly glycolic acid.[7] Cardiac function may be further compromised by hypocalcemia, which develops as calcium is sequestered in calcium oxalate crystals.

The signs of stage III are those of renal toxicity. This stage is attributed in part to the formation of calcium oxalate crystals in the kidneys and in part to the toxic effects of glycolic acid and glyoxylic acid. These metabolites cause an elevated anion gap and an increase in the serum osmolal gap across cells, which results in renal edema. This edema compromises intrarenal blood flow and promotes renal failure.

A further stage of ethylene glycol toxicosis has been described in humans but not, to date, in animals. This is a delayed neuropathy stage and may be due to the formation of calcium oxalate crystals in the brain and around the cranial nerves, or to a secondary pyridoxine deficiency. Pyridoxine is a cofactor in ethylene glycol detoxification, promoting the metabolism of glyoxylate to glycine.[1]

Salivation and vomiting early in the course of toxicosis may be due to ethylene glycol, which is a gastric irritant and produces nausea, whereas in the later stages of toxicosis, they are more likely caused by uremia and consequent oral ulceration.[8] Increased osmolal gap in ethylene glycol toxicosis is due to the parent compound; metabolites do not contribute to it.[7] Acidosis is exacerbated by the accumulation of lactic acid, which occurs because enzymatic oxidation of ethylene glycol increases the cytoplasmic-reduced nicotinamide-adenine dinucleotide to nicotinamide adenine dinucleotide (NADH:NAD) ratio, and metabolism of lactic acid is catalyzed by NAD-dependent dehydrogenases.[5] Blood phosphorus levels may be elevated as a result of uncoupling of oxidative phosphorylation[1] or the inclusion of phosphate-containing rust inhibitor in antifreeze,[5] but because it occurs even in dogs without azotemia, it is not solely caused by decreased glomerular filtration rate.[9] Hypoglycemia, an inconsistent sign, is believed to be due to inhibition of glycolysis and the Kreb's cycle by aldehydes.[8]

Ethylene glycol is an upper respiratory tract irritant and a minor skin irritant in humans, but does not appear to be a skin sensitizer. Pulmonary irritation from inhaled ethylene glycol has been observed in animals. Slight hepatic toxicity has been reported in several species, and ethylene glycol has been shown to affect hepatic mitochondria, reducing respiration rates and uncoupling oxidative phosphorylation. Ethylene glycol is a reproductive toxicant in mice but not in rats. It has been suggested that oxalic acid may block passage of sperm to the epididymis by inducing the formation of spermatoceles in the efferent ducts and caput epididymis. Several studies have demonstrated that ethylene glycol is a teratogen in laboratory animals. Defects include external and visceral malformations as well as skeletal abnormalities in skull, sternebrae, ribs, and vertebrae. Exencephaly, low-set ears, cleft palate, and ventricular septal defects have also been observed.[1]

Toxicity and Risk Factors. Cases of ethylene glycol toxicosis occur throughout the year with a moderate increase between March and May. Because most exposures occur around the home, this may be because automobile owners are likely to drain their radiators and change the antifreeze in the spring. Most veterinary cases of ethylene glycol toxicosis involve dogs, followed by cats. In both species males and females are at equal risk but intact animals are more often poisoned than are spayed or neutered animals.[10]

An oral dose of 4.4 ml ethylene glycol/kg is lethal in dogs if untreated,[11] whereas the minimum lethal oral dose (MLD) of ethylene glycol in the cat is 1 g/kg, or 0.9 ml/kg.[1] The unusual sensitivity of cats to ethylene glycol is due to their high baseline production of oxalic acid.[1]

An oral dose of 2 ml/kg is sufficient to produce toxicosis in a preruminant calf, but oral doses of 5 to 10 ml/kg are required in ruminating cattle.[12] Toxicosis has also been recognized in swine[13] and a pygmy goat,[14] but the doses ingested were unknown. The lethal dose of ethylene glycol in chickens is 6.7 ml/kg,[15] but may be as low as 2.3 ml/kg in ducks.[16]

Reported MLDs in rats range from 3.8 to 11 g/kg, and LD$_{50}$s from 4 to 8.79 g/kg. LD$_{50}$s reported for mice range from 8.4 to 15.4 g/kg, and those for guinea pigs from 6.61 to 8.2 g/kg. A lethal dose in humans is estimated to be 1.4 ml/kg, or roughly 1.6 g/kg.[1]

Clinical Signs. Although the clinical signs of ethylene glycol toxicosis are classically divided into stages, these stages may overlap, one stage may predominate and eclipse the signs of another, and one or more stages may be clinically inapparent.[17] In veterinary practice it is not unusual for the owner to miss the earlier stages and present the animal only when renal failure has developed.

Stage I begins between 1 and 3 hours after ethylene glycol ingestion. Typical signs in the dog are those of moderate depression, marked polydipsia, and progressive ataxia, which includes knuckling over and stumbling.[5] The dog is inebriated and may become belligerent. Gastric irritation may cause vomiting.

During stage II the polydipsia subsides as the ethylene glycol is metabolized, but the metabolites cause severe acidosis. This stage typically occurs 4 to 6 hours after the first stage in the dog. Clinical signs include tachypnea, vomiting, hypothermia, miosis, and profound depression. The animal may become comatose.[6] Both tachycardia and bradycardia have been reported.[10] Muscle fasciculations may develop.[8]

Stage III of ethylene glycol toxicosis in the dog is that of oliguric renal failure. Clinical signs resulting from uremia may include lethargy, vomiting, oral ulceration, and convulsions.[8]

Anterior uveitis and vitreal hemorrhage have been observed in dogs with ethylene glycol toxicosis. In one case report the anterior uveitis appeared to be temporally associated with azotemia. The dog also exhibited blepharospasm, miosis, enophthalmos, and a unilateral slowed direct pupillary light reflex.[18]

Clinical signs in the cat are essentially the same as those described for the dog. Incoordination first develops in the pelvic limbs, about 1 hour after ingestion.[19]

The first sign of ethylene glycol toxicosis in cattle is a staggering, ataxic gait, which coincides with an increase in plasma osmolality. Other clinical signs observed in cattle include tachypnea, paraparesis progressing to recumbency, initial bradycardia and later tachycardia, hemoglobinuria, epistaxis, and dyspnea.[12]

Clinical signs described in swine include depression, weakness, and ataxia particularly affecting the hindlimbs. Changes noticed in the hindlimbs include knuckling, ataxia, a crouching stance, and pronounced muscle tremors. There is a progressive loss of muscle tone and reflexes, and the pig goes down in sternal recumbency. Ascites, hydrothorax, and weak, muffled heart sounds may also be apparent.[13]

A pygmy goat with ethylene glycol toxicosis exhibited ataxia, polydipsia, constipation, and corneal clouding. Hind-limb ataxia became progressively worse over 4 days, depression and hypersalivation developed, and the goat became recumbent and had tonic-clonic seizures. Other findings included moderate scleral congestion, loss of menace response, and vertical nystagmus. Ruminal motility was decreased, but the feces were described as watery.[14]

Chickens with ethylene glycol toxicosis may exhibit listlessness, ataxia, ruffled feathers, dyspnea, and watery droppings. They adopt a characteristic recumbent posture with drooping wings, closed eyes, and the head resting on the floor with the beak used as a prop. When picked up, they move very little and fluid may drain from their beak.[15] Physical examination may reveal cyanosis of the comb and a crop distended with feed, but the pupils are normal.[20] Signs observed in a probable case of ethylene glycol toxicosis in geese included lethargy and trembling, progressing to recumbency with eyes closed, and flaccidity of the neck and wings.[15]

The stages of toxicosis in humans are similar to those in animals, with the addition of a fourth stage. Stage IV consists of neurologic signs, which appear several days after ingestion and may last for several months. Cranial nerve VII is commonly involved and may be evident as loss of facial expression, loss of the ability to drink through a straw, and difficulty swallowing. Damage to cranial nerves IX and X has also been detected.[21]

Clinical Pathology.
The parent molecule, while present, causes increased serum osmolality, whereas the accumulation of acidic metabolites causes severe metabolic acidosis with a marked increase in the anion gap. In ethylene glycol toxicosis, the anion gap is typically 40 to 50 mEq/L, compared with a normal gap of about 10 to 12 mEq/L. Blood pH is typically less than 7.3.[6] Blood phosphorus levels are elevated but blood calcium is lowered.[1] Hyperglycemia, decreased blood bicarbonate, neutrophilia, and lymphopenia are characteristic.[8] BUN, creatinine, and serum potassium levels are elevated as renal failure develops.[14] Intravascular hemolysis, resulting in anemia and hemoglobinuria, has been observed in cattle.[12]

Oxalate crystalluria generally becomes evident 6 to 8 hours after ingestion of ethylene glycol. Calcium oxalate crystals are birefringent when viewed with polarizing filters. Calcium oxalate dihydrate crystals are dipyramidal octahedrons, sometimes described as "envelope-shaped," whereas calcium oxalate monohydrate crystals are needle-shaped, spindle-shaped, or prism-shaped.[7] Dihydrate crystals are almost always found in human cases of ethylene glycol toxicosis, but are found in only a minority of cases in dogs and cats. Monohydrate crystals are more usual in these species, and hippurate crystals may also be present. Hippurate crystals are similar to monohydrate crystals and are intensely birefringent, so they are virtually indistinguishable by light microscopy.[8]

Hyposthenuria is typical; other findings include proteinuria, glycosuria, and hematuria.[9]

Lesions.
Grossly, the kidneys of dogs that have died of ethylene glycol toxicosis are pale and firm, and may have pale streaks, particularly at the corticomedullary junction.[6,22] Other gross lesions include pulmonary edema with hyperemia and hyperemia of the gastric or intestinal mucosa.[1,22]

The most distinctive and diagnostic histologic lesions of ethylene glycol toxicosis are in the kidneys. Pale-yellow, intensely birefringent calcium crystals are found in and around proximal and distal convoluted tubules. Secondary changes may include multifocal degeneration, atrophy, and, depending on duration, regeneration of tubules. There is inflammatory cell infiltration, and, in advanced cases, there may be severe diffuse interstitial fibrosis of the renal cortex and mineralization of tubular basement membrane.

The glomeruli may show changes such as atrophy, adhesions between capillary tufts and Bowman's capsule, and swelling and hyperplasia of parietal epithelial cells.[22]

Inflammatory changes in the lungs are nonspecific. Mild hepatic fatty change has been reported in dogs subchronically exposed to ethylene glycol aerosol.[1]

The lesions described in cats are essentially the same as those observed in dogs. In acute poisoning there may be frank hemorrhage in the stomach and small intestines of cats. Oral ulcerations are also reported[19] and may be secondary to uremia.

The kidneys of a calf that died 3 to 4 days after ingesting ethylene glycol were green and multicystic. Numerous birefringent crystals were found in the tubules of cortex and medulla. The kidneys also contained foci of fibrosis and lymphocyte infiltration. Tubular epithelium was often absent, although glomeruli were generally normal. Mild-to-moderate periportal lymphocytic infiltration was found in the liver. Of cattle experimentally poisoned with ethylene glycol, some were found on necropsy to have swollen black kidneys with perirenal edema and others had tan, slightly granular kidneys but no perirenal edema. Numerous calcium oxalate crystals were found in the kidneys of these animals, particularly in the cortex. Calcium oxalate crystals were also found in the walls of vessels and adjacent parenchyma of the cerebrum and cerebellum, in the transitional epithelium of the renal pelvices, ureters, and urinary bladder, and in the submucosal glands of the bronchi.[12]

Gross lesions found in swine include edema of the abdominal wall, 250 to 450 ml of clear, straw-colored ascitic fluid, extensive clear, gelatinous perirenal edema, and edema of terminal colon, bladder ligaments, and mesometrium. Kidneys are pale brown with scattered surface petechiae and ecchymoses, and may have hemorrhagic streaks when cut. The heart is dilated and flaccid, pulmonary edema may be marked and includes both interlobular and alveolar edema, and clear, straw-colored fluid is also found in the thoracic cavity.

Histologic renal lesions in pigs are similar to those in other species, including numerous birefringent crystals and necrotic sloughing tubular epithelium. The glomeruli may be hyperemic and the glomerular space may be dilated.[13]

A pygmy goat that died of ethylene glycol toxicosis had swollen, finely granular kidneys that bulged when cut. Other lesions included bloodstained contents of the urinary bladder, diffuse pulmonary edema, and mucosal hyperemia of the distal esophagus. Calcium oxalate crystals were abundant in the renal cortex. Other histologic lesions in the kidneys included swollen epithelial cells with clear cytoplasmic vacuoles, necrotic tubular epithelial cells, and proteinaceous casts and sloughed cells in tubules.[14]

Abundant calcium oxalate crystals are also found in the renal tissue of poultry. Heterophil infiltration of collecting ducts and interstitium occurs.[15] Calcium oxalate crystals may also be present in duodenum and walls of cerebral blood vessels in chickens.[20]

Ethylene glycol also causes oxalate nephropathy in laboratory animals. In addition, ethylene glycol toxicosis may cause focal necrosis of the liver in rats, mice, and guinea pigs. Hyaline degeneration of hepatocytes has been described in mice.[1]

Diagnostic Testing.   In treatment of ethylene glycol toxicosis, time is of the essence. The early signs are relatively nonspecific and may be absent, or missed entirely, and by the time the characteristic crystals appear in urine some 6 to 8 hours after ethylene glycol ingestion, the window of greatest opportunity for successful treatment is closed.

Increased anion and osmolal gaps are highly suggestive of ethylene glycol toxicosis, but these may also occur in a variety of other conditions, such as diabetic ketoacidosis and chronic renal failure. Furthermore, neither of these gaps is universally present at all times in all cases of ethylene glycol toxicosis. The osmolal gap corrects itself as the parent compound is excreted or metabolized, and the anion gap may be within reference range if the patient is presented promptly.[7]

Many antifreeze preparations contain sodium fluorescein, added to help mechanics locate small radiator leaks. Examination of urine with a Woods lamp may therefore be useful in the early diagnosis of ethylene glycol toxicosis. In humans sodium fluorescein is excreted for up to 6 hours after ingestion.[2] However, absence of fluorescence may mean no more than that the ethylene glycol ingested did not contain sodium fluorescein.

Laboratory assay of ethylene glycol may be performed by GC or enzymatic assay, but generally there is not enough time to wait for the results if the patient is to be treated successfully. Ethylene glycol may also be detected in the urine by thin-layer chromatography (TLC).[24]

A colorimetric test kit is marketed for rapid confirmation of the presence of ethylene glycol in dog serum or blood. This kit is not sensitive enough for use in cats. The kit is not specific for ethylene glycol and produces a positive result with propylene glycol and glycerol, which are ingredients found in some medications used for treatment. Therefore, sample collection for testing should be performed before treatment. The kit is most useful for samples collected 30 minutes to 12 hours after ingestion.

The kit is available from PRN Pharmacal, Inc., 5830 McAllister Avenue, P.O. Box 10297, Pensacola, FL 32524; Telephone: (904) 476-9462, 1-800-874-9764.

Glycolic acid is considerably more persistent than ethylene glycol in serum. It may be present for up to 60 hours after ingestion[6] and may be assayed by high-performance liquid chromatography (HPLC). Glycolic acid assay may also be used to evaluate the effectiveness of treatment.[3]

The usefulness of ultrasonography as a diagnostic and prognostic aid in ethylene glycol toxicosis has been explored in dogs and cats.[25,26] Renal cortical echogenicity increases within 4 hours of ethylene glycol toxicosis to a level surpassing that of the liver and approaching or equalling that of the spleen, but this early change is not pathognomonic of ethylene glycol toxicosis. However, the "halo sign," a combination of marked, equal increase in cortical and medullary echogenicity with hypoechoic areas in the corticomedullary and central medullary regions, appears reasonably unique to ethylene glycol toxicosis, having been reported previously only in primary hyperoxaluria in humans.[25] Detection of ultrasonographic changes in ethylene glycol toxicosis warrants a guarded-to-poor prognosis, whereas detection of the "halo sign," which develops concurrently with anuria, warrants a grave prognosis.[26]

After death, the specimen of choice is kidney. The renal histopathology is usually considered diagnostic on its own, but the chemical nature of birefringent crystals in the kidney can be confirmed if frozen kidney is submitted as well as fixed kidney. A urine sample for glycolic acid may also be helpful.

The rumen appears to act as a reservoir for ethylene glycol. Ethylene glycol was detected in ruminal content 4 days after the onset of clinical signs in a pygmy goat. The parent molecule would not normally still be present in a monogastric. Ruminal content may be useful for postmortem diagnosis in ruminants. Glycolic acid was found in both urine and ocular fluid of the same animal. Ocular fluid, which is more stable after death than many other body fluids, may therefore be a useful postmortem specimen.[14]

Treatment.   Early commencement of detoxification markedly improves outcome. Activated charcoal should be given within the first 4 hours if possible. Repeated doses of activated charcoal may be needed in ruminants to decontaminate the rumen.[14] Early and aggressive hemodialysis, which removes ethylene glycol and metabolites including glycolic acid, is recommended in human cases but is not feasible for many veterinary practices. Activated charcoal hemoperfusion, although not sufficient therapy on its own, reduces serum ethylene glycol levels significantly and may be of benefit if used in conjunction with other therapy.[27]

If an early case of ethylene glycol toxicosis is suspected, intravenous fluid therapy should be started, the animal catheterized, and urine production monitored. Fluid diuresis has the dual benefits of accelerating urinary excretion and maintaining renal throughput. Animals in early ethylene glycol toxicosis often have marked polydipsia and should be given water ad libitum. If oliguria or anuria is already present, renal flow should be established with saline before administering fluids that contain potassium.

The traditional antidote for ethylene glycol toxicosis is intravenous 20% ethanol, titrated so that the animal is maintained in a profound stupor for up to 72 hours. Guidelines from which the dose is adjusted are, for dogs, 5.5 ml every 4 hours for five treatments, then every 6 hours for four treatments, and, for cats, 5 ml/kg every 6 hours for five treatments, then every 8 hours for four treatments.[6] Ethanol competes with ethylene glycol for the active site of alcohol dehydrogenase, and alcohol dehydrogenase has a much higher affinity for ethanol than for ethylene glycol. If the alcohol dehydrogenase activity is saturated by ethanol, then ethylene glycol can be excreted as the relatively nontoxic parent compound. However, ethanol treatment has significant disadvantages. It is labor intensive, causes severe CNS depression with risk of respiratory center depression, and exacerbates the osmotic diuresis and plasma hyperosmolality already likely to be present.

An alternative antidote that is safe, effective, and has far fewer side effects is 4-methylpyrazole (4-MP, fomepizole), which was approved by the Food and Drug Administration in November 1996 and became commercially available early in 1997. 4-MP is a specific inhibitor of alcohol dehydrogenase, which is widely used in canine and human cases of ethylene glycol toxicosis, and which has been credited with recent improvements in the survival rate of dogs.[10] Because 4-methylpyrazole does not cause adverse effects, it may be safely given to dogs before ethylene glycol ingestion is confirmed.[9] However, 4-MP is not particularly effective in the cat, so ethanol remains the recommended antidote for cats.[28] 4-Methylpyrazole is readily removed by hemodialysis. Ethanol and 4-MP must never be used together or fatal ethanol toxicosis may result.

Supportive treatment, particularly fluid therapy, is extremely important in ethylene glycol toxicosis. Acidosis is typically severe and should be corrected with intravenous bicarbonate. Renal flow must be established and maintained. Peritoneal dialysis may be required to support renal function until the kidney tubules recover, and peritoneal dialysis also assists in the removal of ethylene glycol and metabolites. Corticosteroids may help control pulmonary edema. If low blood calcium is causing significant problems, 0.25 ml/kg calcium borogluconate may be given daily in a 10% solution.[6]

Administration of pyridoxine and thiamine in doses of 100 mg/day has been recommended in human cases of ethylene glycol toxicosis to promote the conversion of glyoxylic acid to relatively innocuous substances[2] such as glycine and α-hydroxy, β-keto adipate.

The convalescent patient should be given a diet appropriate for an animal with compromised renal function.[6]

Prognosis. Prognosis varies considerably depending on how soon after exposure treatment is instituted. Dogs treated with 4-MP within 8 hours of ethylene glycol ingestion have a good prognosis. However, the prognosis deteriorates rapidly as renal toxicosis develops, and if renal toxicosis is allowed to progress until azotemia is apparent, usually between 24 and 48 hours after ingestion, the prognosis is poor.[9]

Prevention and Control. Owner education, to prevent exposure of animals to ethylene glycol, is extremely important. Animals should not have access to radiator contents or other sources of ethylene glycol. Ethylene glycol spilled from leaking radiators should be promptly adsorbed with bentonite-based kitty litter, which is then carefully disposed of, after which the site of the spill should be washed with copious water. The use of propylene glycol–based antifreeze should be encouraged.

FERTILIZERS

Jay C. Albretsen

Sources. Hundreds of fertilizer products are available with many different manufacturers and distributors. Fertilizers are used for gardening, lawn care, and agricultural purposes.

Fertilizer products generally contain varying amounts of nitrogen, phosphorus, and potassium compounds. Many products list the concentration of these ingredients in the name of the fertilizer, or near the name of the product. For example, a lawn fertilizer may state in the composition: N-P-K (29-3-4). This represents the amounts of nitrogen (29%), phosphorus (3%), and potassium (4%) in the fertilizer. Some nitrogen-containing fertilizers are high in ammonium nitrate. Other fertilizers contain small amounts of minerals such as iron, copper, boron, cobalt, manganese, molybdenum, and zinc. In addition, many fertilizers contain other products such as cocoa bean hulls, herbicides, insecticides, and fungicides.

Toxicokinetics. Because fertilizers are usually a combination of ingredients, there are several toxic principles possible. The major toxic components of fertilizers are nitrogen, phosphorus, and potassium compounds. In general, these ingredients are poorly absorbed and most of the signs are related to gastrointestinal irritation.[1]

Toxicity and Risk Factors. Fertilizers are generally of low toxicity.[1,2] The acute oral LD_{50} in rats is about 5 g fertilizer per kilogram body weight.[1] Other ingredients in the fertilizers may be more toxic, particularly insecticides (e.g., disulfoton), iron (>1%), or calcium cyanamide fertilizers.[1-4] Fertilizers that contain bone meal or blood meal are more palatable to carnivores. Dogs have been known to engorge themselves with fertilizers that contain bone or blood.

Fertilizers high in nitrates are a greater risk to ruminants because of the rapid conversion of nitrates to nitrites by ruminal microorganisms. Nitrate toxicosis can occur in horses but is apparently a rare occurrence.[5] Urea present in several fertilizers is also more of a risk to ruminants than to monogastrics. Urea is more easily converted to ammonia because of the microorganisms in the rumen.[1]

Clinical Signs. The effects of oral fertilizer ingestion depend on the ingredients in the product. Often no clinical signs develop with small ingestions of fertilizers.[2] Fertilizers that contain high percentages of phosphorus and potassium compounds cause primarily gastrointestinal irritation. These signs usually develop within 2 to 10 hours after ingestion. Vomiting, diarrhea, salivation, and lethargy are the most common effects. These signs usually resolve in 12 to 24 hours.[1,2] Other infrequently reported signs are tremors, urticarial rash formation, pruritus, stiffness, and muzzle swelling in dogs.[2,4] Fertilizer ingestions rarely cause death.[1,2,4,6] Dogs that engorge on bone meal or blood meal can develop severe gastroenteritis or pancreatitis.

Fertilizers that contain nitrates as the primary nitrogen source can cause methemoglobinemia, primarily in ruminants. Ammonium salts and urea in fertilizers primarily cause gastrointestinal irritation in monogastrics. However, urea can produce systemic ammonia toxicosis in ruminants. Iron-containing fertilizers may also cause gastrointestinal irritation. However, iron toxicosis is possible if the fertilizer contains more than 1% iron.[1,4] Refer to the appropriate sections in this book to obtain additional information about iron, nitrate, urea, ammonia, insecticide, or herbicide poisoning.

Fertilizers that contain calcium cyanamide can cause skin irritation and ulceration. If the calcium cyanamide is ingested, it may also cause ataxia, rapid breathing, pulmonary edema, hypotension, and shock.[1]

Lesions. Besides gastroenteritis, no specific lesions are caused by fertilizer ingestion, unless other ingredients are present.

Treatment. If the fertilizer ingestion has been recent, emetics such as hydrogen peroxide (1 to 5 ml/kg body weight per os [PO]) or another appropriate emetic is indicated in animals that can vomit. Activated charcoal (1 to 4 g/kg body weight PO) and a cathartic (magnesium sulfate at a dose of 250 mg/kg body weight PO, or 70% sorbitol at 3 ml/kg body weight PO) can be beneficial.[1,2,7,8] Vomiting should not be induced in a symptomatic animal. Often, once the fertilizers have been vomited, the gastrointestinal irritation resolves and no further treatment is necessary. Fluid therapy should be considered in animals that are dehydrated or in shock. Other supportive and symptomatic care is indicated when it becomes necessary.[2] Treating iron, urea, nitrate, insecticide, or herbicide toxicoses are explained in specific sections of this book.

Prognosis. In general, animals showing clinical signs following fertilizer ingestion have a good prognosis and often recover without treatment. Those fertilizers containing nitrates, insecticides, herbicides, urea, iron, and ammonia may result in more serious clinical signs.

Prevention and Control. Ensure that pets are not near while the products are being used, giving the products time to dry or work themselves into the ground before animals have access to the areas. Some fertilizers are palatable to dogs such as blood meal and bone meal. Keep fertilizers and animal feeds in separate locations to prevent mistaken identity.

GASES

Thomas L. Carson

Gases are substances that exist in the vapor state in the normal range of environmental temperatures. When present in high enough concentrations, some of the gases associated with animal housing or production may result in death of animals or adversely affect animal health and performance

(Table 20-1). Toxic gases are of a special concern in closed animal housing where they may be generated from the decomposition of urine and feces, respiratory excretion, or the operation of carbon fuel–burning heaters. The most important gases released from the decomposition of urine and feces in anaerobic under-floor waste pits, in deep litter, or in manure packs are ammonia, carbon dioxide, methane, and hydrogen sulfide. Other toxic gases may be associated with the fermentation of ensiled forages or industrial air pollution.

Natural diffusion and breezes tend to dilute and dissipate air pollutants produced out of doors. However, when these gases are produced inside animal confinement facilities, dissipation and dilution depend directly on the ventilation system of the building. Even at relatively low ventilation rates used during colder weather, concentrations of ammonia and hydrogen sulfide, the two most potentially dangerous gases associated with manure decomposition, usually remain below toxic levels. However, electrical outages, accidents, poor design, and improper operation may result in insufficient ventilation and allow the concentration of poisonous gases to reach toxic levels. In addition to removing potentially toxic gases, ventilation systems also remove heat and moisture from closed animal facilities. Consequently, the buildup of heat and resulting hyperthermia is the most common cause of massive death losses of swine and poultry in confinement facilities or insulated transport trucks after a complete stoppage of mechanical ventilation systems caused by storms, electrical malfunction, or other causes.

Concentrations of toxic gases are usually expressed as parts of the gas per million parts of air (ppm) by volume. Sometimes concentrations are expressed as weight of gas per unit volume of air, for example, as micrograms of the gas per cubic meter of air.

AMMONIA

Sources. Ammonia (NH_3) is the toxic air pollutant most frequently found in high concentrations in animal facilities. Ammonia production is especially common where excrement can decompose on a solid floor.

Toxicity and Risk Factors. Ammonia has a characteristic pungent odor that humans can detect at approximately 10 ppm or even lower. Even though the concentration of ammonia in enclosed animal facilities usually remains below 30 ppm even with low ventilation rates, it may frequently reach 50 ppm or even higher during long periods of normal facility operation. At concentrations usually found in livestock facilities (<100 ppm), the primary impact of aerial ammonia is as an irritant of the eye and respiratory membranes, and as a chronic stressor that can affect the course of infectious disease as well as directly influence the growth of healthy young animals.[1-3]

From the results of a series of experiments conducted at the Illinois Agricultural Experiment Station, the conclusion can be drawn that ammonia in the air can affect the course of infectious disease as well directly influence the growth of healthy young pigs. The rate of gain in young pigs was re-

TABLE 20-1 **Characteristics of Toxic Gases Associated with Animal Production**

Agent	Color, Odor, Weight*	Effect and Prominent Symptoms	Dangerous Working Conditions	Prevention or Precautionary Measures
Ammonia (NH_3)	Sharp, pungent, lighter than air, 0.77 g/L, colorless	Stressor; irritation of respiratory tract; laryngospasm, death at high concentrations	Poor ventilation; decomposition of animal waste; anhydrous ammonia exposure	Adequate ventilation (open doors and windows); turn fans on 10-15 minutes before entering area; wear self-contained breathing apparatus
Carbon dioxide (CO_2)	Odorless, heavier than air, 1.98 g/L, colorless	Trouble breathing, headaches, drowsiness, and asphyxiation	Poor ventilation, combustion engine exhaust and ventilation failure	Adequate ventilation (open doors and windows); turn fans on 10-15 minutes before entering pit; wear self-contained breathing apparatus
Hydrogen sulfide (H_2S)	Rotten egg smell, heavier than air, 1.54 g/L colorless	Irritation of eyes and nose, headache, dizziness, nausea, unconsciousness, and death	Agitation of manure pit; poor ventilation; decomposition of animal waste; pits, enclosed tanks	Adequate ventilation (open doors and windows); turn fans on 10-15 minutes before entering pit; wear self-contained breathing apparatus
Methane (CH_4)	Odorless, lighter than air, 0.72 g/L, colorless	Mild asphyxiant, primarily explosion hazard	Poor ventilation; decomposition of animal waste	Adequate ventilation; no smoking or other ignition sources in area
Carbon monoxide (CO)	Odorless, lighter than air, 1.25 g/L, colorless	Headaches, drowsiness, asphyxiation	Unvented heaters and engines with poor ventilation	Adequate ventilation; adjust, clean and vent heaters
Nitrogen dioxide (NO_2)	Yellowish brown gas, bleach-like smell, heavier than air, 2.03 g/L	Initial irritation of eyes and mucousmembrane; silo filler's disease, shortness of breath, fever and death	Greatest danger during first 48 hours after filling silo; danger exists up to 10 days after filling	Stay away from silo during first 48 hours after filling—after this, if entry is necessary run blower for 20 minutes prior to entry; open all chute doors down to level of silage; wear self-contained breathing apparatus

*The density of dry air at 0° C and 760 mm Hg is 1.29 g/L.

duced by 12% during exposure to aerial ammonia at 50 ppm and by 30% at 100 or 150 ppm.[4] Aerial ammonia at 50 or 75 ppm reduced the healthy young pig's ability to clear bacteria from its lungs.[5] At 50 or 100 ppm, aerial ammonia exacerbated nasal-turbinate shrinkage in young pigs infected with *Bordetella bronchiseptica*, but did not add to the infection-induced reduction in the pigs' growth rate.[6] Ascarid infection reduced young pigs' rate of gain by 28%, and aerial ammonia at 100 ppm by 32% in another study. In this case, however, effects of the infection and the ammonia when imposed on the pigs at the same time were additive.[7] In a study of 28 swine farms in Sweden, a higher incidence of arthritis, porcine stress syndrome lesions, and abscesses had a positive correlation with levels of aerial ammonia in the facilities.[8]

It has recently been recommended that the maximum long-term ammonia exposure limit for swine should be less than 20 ppm because both pathologic data and immunologic data suggest that exposure to ammonia concentrations of 10 to 15 ppm reduce resistance to infection.[9,10] British workers used operant-conditioning techniques, giving pigs

the choice between ambient ammonia levels of 0, 10, 20, and 40 ppm, to demonstrate that pigs have an aversion to atmospheres containing even relatively low levels of ammonia.[11]

In poultry, on the other hand, ammonia is considered the most harmful gas in broiler-chicken housing.[12] Ambient ammonia levels of 50 ppm for prolonged periods irritate respiratory airways and predispose chickens to respiratory infections with the added risk of secondary infections; development of lesions of keratoconjunctivitis of the eye is associated with ambient ammonia levels of 60 ppm.[13] Affected birds close their eyes much of the time, become relatively listless, and reduce feed intake. A reduced rate of bacterial clearance from the lungs was measured in turkeys exposed to 40 ppm aerial ammonia.[14] Excessive mucus production, matted cilia, and deterioration of normal mucociliary apparatus was found in turkeys exposed to ammonia concentrations as low as 10 ppm for 7 weeks.[15]

Clinical Signs. Ammonia is highly soluble in water and reacts with the moist mucous membranes of the eye and

BOX 20-1	CLINICAL EFFECTS OF AERIAL AMMONIA

AMMONIA CONCENTRATION (ppm)	EFFECT
5-10	Very slight to detectable pungent odor
20-25	Easily detected odor; eyes may burn
6-35	Levels often found in swine confinement facilities
50	Reduced pulmonary bacterial clearance
	Growth rate and feed intake of swine reduced 10%
100	Very strong odor
	Eye and respiratory irritation, lacrimation, salivation
	Increased severity of *Bordetella rhinitis* in swine
	Additive growth depressant with *Ascaris suum* in swine
400	Immediate throat irritation
1700	Laryngospasm and coughing
2500	Fatal if greater than 30-minute exposure
5000	Rapidly fatal with acute exposure

respiratory passages. Consequently, excessive tearing, shallow breathing, and clear or purulent nasal discharge are common symptoms of aerial ammonia toxicosis. The effects of increasing concentrations of aerial ammonia are summarized in Box 20-1.

Lesions. No consistent gross or microscopic structural changes tend to be associated with uncomplicated aerial ammonia toxicosis in mammals. When lesions are found, they tend to be minor and confined only to the upper respiratory passages where ammonia has acted as an irritant from the nose to the lungs. This irritation may lead to increased secretion of mucus by the respiratory epithelium, bronchiolar constriction, and hyperplasia of the bronchiolar and alveolar epithelium.

Diagnostic Testing. A diagnosis of aerial ammonia exposure is primarily based on the history and field observation. Laboratory analysis is of limited value in cases of inhalation exposures.

Prevention and Control. Maintenance of adequate ventilation and good sanitary procedures generally alleviate the problems associated with ammonia from animal waste in confined spaces.

ANHYDROUS AMMONIA

Sources. In contrast to the moderate stressor levels of ammonia from animal waste, extremely high and potentially lethal concentrations of ammonia are associated with exposure to anhydrous ammonia gas (gas-NH_3). Although sometimes used as a refrigerant, anhydrous ammonia is most often used as an agricultural fertilizer nitrogen source, by which it presents a unique risk of exposure to both animals and humans because of its use on farms and because it is stored, transported, and applied under high pressure. Poisoning with anhydrous ammonia is generally associated with gas release from broken hoses, failure of valves, and human error in operating the transport or application equipment.

Mechanism of Action. A large release of anhydrous ammonia forms a white vapor cloud that may linger for several hours depending on atmospheric conditions. Once released, anhydrous ammonia rapidly seeks and combines with water to form caustic ammonium hydroxide.

Clinical Signs. The moisture-rich membranes of the cornea, mouth, and respiratory tract of exposed animals are especially susceptible to damage from the resulting strong alkali burns. Acute death from apnea, laryngospasm, and accumulation of fluid in the lungs can occur within a matter of minutes with anhydrous ammonia concentrations more than 5000 ppm. Animals surviving an exposure frequently are blinded by corneal damage, slough epithelium and exude fluid throughout the respiratory tract, and may not regain full productive status. Secondary bacterial invasion of pulmonary tissues is a common outcome and generally affords a guarded prognosis.

Diagnostic Testing. A diagnosis of anhydrous ammonia poisoning is based on history of exposure, clinical signs of sudden death or severe respiratory distress, and lesions of epithelial damage to the eye, skin, mucous membranes, and respiratory tract.[16,17]

Treatment. Treatment is often futile and consists of supportive care and antibiotic therapy to control secondary bacterial pathogens. Humane destruction of clinically affected but surviving animals may be warranted.

CARBON DIOXIDE

Sources. Carbon dioxide is a colorless, odorless gas present in the atmosphere at 300 ppm. It is produced by animals themselves as an end product of energy metabolism and by improperly vented, although properly adjusted, fuel burning heaters. It is also the gas produced in the greatest quantity by decomposing manure. Even so, its concentration in closed animal facilities rarely approaches levels that endanger animal health.[2]

Clinical Signs. Carbon dioxide at 50,000 ppm (5%) is well tolerated by animals, producing only an increase in rate and depth of respiration. In the unlikely event that carbon dioxide, which is heavier than air, collects in a low part of a facility, animals may exhibit anxiety followed by staggering, coma, and finally death as the concentration exceeds 400,000 ppm.

Diagnostic Testing. Diagnosis is usually based on the clinical history, clinical signs, and lack of other obvious causes. Blood P_{CO_2} can be measured if suitable equipment is available, but samples must be protected from exposure to the air for even brief periods of time.

Treatment.   Treatment is simply to provide fresh air. If the respiratory mechanisms are still intact, the body is able to rapidly eliminate the excess CO_2.

Prognosis.   Chronic neurologic damage may result depending on the severity and duration of apnea.

METHANE

Sources.   Methane (CH_4), which is lighter than air, colorless, and odorless, is a product of microbial degradation of carbonaceous materials, but is not a poisonous gas. Methane is also a natural by-product of rumen microflora in cattle, goats, sheep, and other ruminant animals.

Mechanism of Action.   Methane is biologically inert and produces effects on animals only by displacing oxygen in a given atmosphere, thereby producing asphyxiation. Under ordinary pressures, a concentration of 87% to 90% methane is required before irregularities of respiration and eventually respiratory arrest due to anoxia are produced. It has been reported that rabbits breathed a mixture of 1 part oxygen and 4 parts methane for extended periods of time without showing ill effects.[18]

The chief danger inherent in methane is its explosive hazard as concentrations of 5% to 15% by volume in air are reached. Its flammability and explosiveness, rather than toxic effects on living organisms, constitute the major impact of this gas on animal agriculture. Explosions attributed to methane set off by an electrical spark have destroyed buildings.

HYDROGEN SULFIDE

Sources.   Hydrogen sulfide (H_2S) is a potentially lethal gas produced by anaerobic bacterial decomposition of protein and other sulfur-containing organic matter. This colorless gas has the distinctive odor of rotten eggs, is heavier than air, and may accumulate in manure pits, holding tanks, and other low areas in a facility.[19]

The source of hydrogen sulfide that presents the greatest hazard to livestock and other animals is liquid manure holding pits. Consequently, most cases of animal death loss from hydrogen sulfide involve swine, but poultry and cattle can also be affected.[20] Most of the continuously produced hydrogen sulfide is retained within the liquid of the pit. In fact, the concentration of hydrogen sulfide usually found in closed, undisturbed animal facilities (less than 10 ppm) is not detrimental. However, when the waste slurry is agitated to resuspend solids before being pumped from the pit, it rapidly releases much of the hydrogen sulfide that may have been retained. This release of gas on agitation may produce concentrations of hydrogen sulfide up to 1000 ppm or higher within the facility, especially at lower levels closer to the floor.[1,21]

In addition to animal waste, hydrogen sulfide is also associated with natural gas and crude oil production, and some coal deposits. Hydrogen sulfide may also be found as a by-product, waste material, or reactant associated with industrial applications.

Mechanism of Action.   Hydrogen sulfide is an irritant gas. Its direct action on tissues induces local inflammation of the mucous membranes of the eye and respiratory tract. When inhaled, hydrogen sulfide exerts its irritant action more or less uniformly throughout the respiratory tract, although the deeper pulmonary tissues suffer the greatest damage, which often appears as pulmonary edema.

At higher levels hydrogen sulfide can also be readily absorbed through the lung and produce fatal systemic intoxication.[2] At concentrations in air exceeding 500 ppm, hydrogen sulfide must be considered a serious imminent threat to life. Between 500 and 1000 ppm hydrogen sulfide produces permanent effects on the nervous system. Although a number of organs and tissues, including the heart and skeletal muscles, respond, this action is most significantly expressed through its effect on the chemoreceptors of the carotid body. This stimulation results in excessively rapid breathing (hyperpnea), which quickly leads to depletion of the carbon dioxide content of the blood (acapnia). This, in turn, gives way to a period of respiratory inactivity (apnea). If depletion has not progressed too far, carbon dioxide may reaccumulate until spontaneous respiration is reestablished. If spontaneous recovery does not occur and artificial respiration is not immediately provided, death from asphyxia is the inevitable conclusion. At concentrations greater than 2000 ppm, breathing becomes paralyzed after a breath or two. Generalized convulsions frequently begin at this point.

At these higher levels hydrogen sulfide exerts a direct paralyzing effect on the respiratory center that is not related to the carbon dioxide content of the blood.

Toxicity and Risk Factors.   Acute hydrogen sulfide poisoning is directly responsible for more deaths in closed animal facilities than any other gas. Several human deaths are recorded each year from hydrogen sulfide accidents associated with animal and industrial facilities. Humans can detect the typical "rotten egg" odor of hydrogen sulfide at very low concentrations (0.025 ppm) in air. Acute exposures to these low concentrations have little or no importance to human health and thus the detection of odor can be a safe and useful warning signal of its presence. However, at higher concentrations (greater than 200 ppm), hydrogen sulfide presents a distinct hazard as it exerts a paralyzing effect on the olfactory sensory apparatus, effectively blocking the detection of the warning odor.

Differences between mammalian species' susceptibility to toxic concentrations of hydrogen sulfide are small, as demonstrated by the following reported acutely toxic levels of hydrogen sulfide: goat, 900 ppm; guinea pig, 750 ppm; dog, 600 ppm; rat, 500 ppm.[22] However, chickens were found to be less sensitive to hydrogen sulfide than mammals, with exposures of 4000 ppm not resulting in immediate death.[23]

Early experiments examining various levels of acute hydrogen sulfide gas exposure in pigs reported the following associated clinical effects: 50 to 100 ppm, nothing significant;

250 ppm, distress; 500 to 700 ppm, semicomatose; 1000 ppm, intermittent spasms, cyanosis, unconsciousness, convulsions, death.[24] At low levels of hydrogen sulfide exposure, no effect was measured on rate of body weight gain or respiratory tract structure in young pigs breathing air containing 8.5 ppm hydrogen sulfide for 17 days.[25]

Clinical Signs. The clinical and pathologic effects of acute hydrogen sulfide exposure are similar for most species of animals. The clinical effects of increasing concentrations of hydrogen sulfide are presented in Box 20-2.

Diagnostic Testing. Diagnosis of hydrogen sulfide poisoning is most often based on a history of acute death, manure pit agitation, and typical clinical signs and lesions.

Treatment. Breathing is usually never reestablished spontaneously following hydrogen sulfide–induced paralysis of respiration. However, because the heart continues to beat several minutes after respiration has ceased, death from asphyxia can be prevented if artificial respiration is begun immediately and is continued until the hydrogen sulfide concentration in the blood decreases as a result of pulmonary excretion of the gas. Usually after several minutes, normal respiration is reestablished. Victims of acute hydrogen sulfide poisoning who recover usually do so promptly and completely.

Prevention and Control. Management is the most important part of preventing animal deaths from hydrogen sulfide. When manure stored in a pit beneath a building is agitated, the animals should be moved out of the building if possible. When relocation of the animals is not possible, other steps should be taken to protect the animals during agitation. When manure agitation is begun in mechanically ventilated buildings, the fans should be turned up to full capacity, even during the winter. Manure pits in naturally ventilated buildings should not be agitated unless there is a brisk breeze blowing.

When agitation is started, the animals should be watched closely and the pump should be turned off as soon as any clinical signs occur. The critical area of the building is where the pump breaks the liquid surface of the pit. If any animals are affected, they should *not* be immediately rescued, because the rescuer may quickly become a victim of hydrogen sulfide poisoning. The building should not be entered until accumulated toxic gases have escaped. Even if the pit has been emptied, it still may contain little oxygen or high concentrations of hydrogen sulfide.

CARBON MONOXIDE

Sources. Carbon monoxide (CO) is an odorless, colorless, poisonous gas that is a by-product of incomplete combustion of hydrocarbon fuels. One of the primary sources of carbon monoxide is the exhaust of gasoline-burning internal-combustion engines, which may contain up to 9% carbon monoxide. Ambient background levels of CO are 0.02 ppm in fresh air, 13 ppm in metropolitan city streets, and 40 ppm in areas with high vehicular traffic. Lethal concentrations of carbon monoxide may accumulate within 10 minutes if an automobile engine is left running in a closed garage. Animals and people in enclosed cargo areas of vehicles with faulty exhaust systems have been poisoned with carbon monoxide.

High levels of carbon monoxide may frequently be produced when improperly adjusted or improperly vented gas water heaters, space heaters, or furnaces are operated in tight and often poorly ventilated spaces such as basements, farrowing houses, or lambing sheds. In many of these cases producers have greatly reduced ventilation in these heated areas to reduce heat loss and save money. In some instances, fresh air vents were completely covered or flue pipes or chimneys were blocked with bird nests.

Fires are also an important source of exposure, with the concentration of carbon monoxide inside a burning building reaching as high as 10%. Consequently, carbon monoxide poisoning should be suspected in any animal rescued from a fire.

A small amount of carbon monoxide arises from catabolized heme and is endogenously produced in mammals. One mole of carbon monoxide is formed for each mole of heme degraded.[26]

Mechanism of Action. Carbon monoxide is rapidly absorbed through the lungs and acts by competing with oxygen for binding sites on a variety of proteins, including hemoglobin, with which most of the compound is associated in the body. The affinity of hemoglobin for carbon monoxide is about 250 times greater than that for oxygen. When the heme group binds with carbon monoxide, forming carboxyhemoglobin (COHb), the oxygen carrying capacity of the molecule is severely reduced. The degree of carboxyhemoglobin formation is a function of both the concentration of carbon monoxide in the inspired air and the length of exposure time. The higher the level of carbon monoxide the shorter the exposure time necessary to reach 25% to 30% carboxyhemoglobin, a level which is generally associated with onset of clinical effects. In addition, the oxygen dissociation curve is shifted to the left, meaning that the release of oxygen from hemoglobin to tissues is also impaired. Therefore, systemic tissue hypoxia is the consequence of carbon monoxide toxicosis.[27]

BOX 20-2	CLINICAL EFFECT OF INCREASING CONCENTRATIONS OF HYDROGEN SULFIDE IN AIR	
AMMONIA CONCENTRATION OF H_2S (ppm)	**CLINICAL EFFECT**
0.1-0.2	Threshold for odor
3-5	Offensive odor
10	Threshold limit value
50-100	Eye and respiratory irritation
150-250	Olfactory paralysis
300-500	Pulmonary edema
500-1000	Strong nervous system stimulation; apnea
1000-2000	Immediate collapse with respiratory paralysis

BOX 20-3	CLINICAL EFFECT ASSOCIATED WITH INCREASING BLOOD CARBOXYHEMOGLOBIN	
CONCENTRATION OF CARBOXYHEMOGLOBIN IN BLOOD (%)	**CLINICAL EFFECT***	
<1-3	Normal	
6-8	Decreased ability to maintain attention	
10-20	Headache, fatigue, irritability	
20-30	Weakness, dizziness, mild symptoms, fetal hypoxia, stillbirth in swine	
30-60	Increased heart and respiratory rate, confusion, EEG changes, coma	
>60	Usually fatal	

*These are general guidelines because carboxyhemoglobin values may not correlate well with clinical severity, particularly if samples were obtained after oxygen therapy was initiated.

Toxicity and Risk Factors.   Lethal doses of carbon monoxide reported for animals can vary greatly depending primarily on the level of the gas and the exposure time; however, age, metabolic rate, physical activity, and pulmonary and cardiac function also have an impact. In most studies most animals died after carboxyhemoglobin reached a 60% level (Box 20-3). In decreasing order of carbon monoxide susceptibility are the canary, mouse, rat, chicken, cat, dog, pigeon, guinea pig, and rabbit. In general, carbon monoxide levels of 4000 to 5000 ppm in the air are lethal to animals and humans within a few minutes.[28]

Clinical Signs.   The clinical signs of carbon monoxide poisoning reflect the hypoxia of tissues with a high oxygen demand, primarily the brain, heart, and skeletal muscle.

Exposure to relatively high concentrations of carbon monoxide results in acute poisoning and includes a progression of clinical effects including drowsiness, lethargy, weakness, deafness (in dogs and cats), incoordination, and reduced heart excitability. As the concentration of carboxyhemoglobin increases, some animals may show a cherry-red color to skin and mucous membranes. As the animal becomes more severely affected, dyspnea, coma, terminal clonic spasms, and acute death may be observed.

Pregnant animals may abort as carbon monoxide crosses the placenta and produces fetal hypoxia. High concentrations of carbon monoxide (>250 ppm) in swine farrowing houses may increase the number of stillborn piglets.[29,30]

Long-term exposure to lower levels of carbon monoxide may result in chronic poisoning, which is manifested by low exercise tolerance, disturbance of postural and position reflexes and gait, and changes in the electrocardiograph (ECG) consistent with anoxia and necrosis of single heart muscle fibers.

Lesions.   The physical changes and lesions associated with carbon monoxide toxicosis may be minimal. The blood of animals with a high carboxyhemoglobin concentration becomes bright cherry-red in color and often produces a pink coloration of the tissues and nonpigmented skin. The bright red color can also be observed in the tissues of stillborn piglets expelled subsequent to carbon monoxide poisoning.

The physiologic and pathologic changes observed in carbon monoxide–poisoned animals are thought to be the direct results of hypoxia. Changes in the ECG are consistent with necrosis of single heart muscle fibers. Histologic changes in the brain appear as necrosis in the cortex and white matter of the cerebral hemispheres, the globus pallidus, and the brain stem. Also reported are edema and hemorrhage in the brain and necrosis in Ammon's horn of the hippocampus. Demyelination has also been reported.[31]

The brain lesions may result in permanent damage and may be manifested as deafness in dogs and cats. Respiratory alkalosis occurs from hyperventilation caused by a metabolic acidosis, but there is no evidence of CO_2 retention. At postmortem the bronchi are dilated and major blood vessels may be distended.

Diagnostic Testing.   A diagnosis of carbon monoxide toxicosis should be suspected in animals with clinical signs of acute death or hypoxia and when the history suggests exposure to a source of carbon monoxide such as unvented or faulty fuel-burning heaters or automobile exhaust in an area with poor ventilation. Features of the clinical history generally associated with stillbirths in swine include (1) the use of unvented or improperly vented gas space heaters, (2) inadequate or nonexistent ventilation, (3) a high percentage of near-term sows delivering dead piglets within a few hours of being moved into an artificially heated farrowing facility, (4) clinically normal appearance of sows, although the whole litter is born dead, and (5) negative laboratory examination for the detection of infectious causes of abortion.[32]

Suspicion of high levels of carbon monoxide can be verified by measuring the carbon monoxide level in the suspect environment. Sometimes re-creation of the specific heating or ventilation conditions may be required to identify the source of carbon monoxide, and utility officials or heating contractors should be contacted for assistance in this activity.

Measuring the level of carboxyhemoglobin in a whole blood sample of the affected animal may also help confirm carbon monoxide exposure. Elevated carboxyhemoglobin concentration in the blood-tinged fetal thoracic fluid may be used as an aid in confirming carbon monoxide–induced stillbirth in swine.[33] Carboxyhemoglobin in whole blood is relatively stable for several days if refrigerated and can often be measured at veterinary diagnostic laboratories or nearby human hospitals. Interpretation of carboxyhemoglobin values should take into account when the blood sample was collected, because once carbon monoxide exposure has ceased and the animal is treated with oxygen or exposed to fresh air, the carboxyhemoglobin level is likely to return to normal in as little as 3 hours.[34]

Treatment.   The main goal in treatment of the carbon monoxide–poisoned patient is to restore adequate oxygen supply to the brain and heart. The patient should be moved to an area of fresh air to stop further carbon monoxide exposure. A patent airway should be established and maintained, and artificial respiration should be provided if necessary. Patients breathing hyperbaric or 100% oxygen recover more quickly. A significant response to therapy should be observed within 1 to 4 hours.

Prognosis. The prognosis of animals poisoned with carbon monoxide depends on the degree of cellular hypoxia and resulting cellular damage. Recovering animals should have cardiac, pulmonary, and neurologic function monitored for 2 weeks, and physical activity should be minimized for 2 to 4 weeks. In some cases, irritability, personality changes, disorientation, gait disturbance, or other neurologic signs may appear within a few days to as long as 6 weeks after apparent recovery, and are attributed to neuronal anoxia during acute carbon monoxide poisoning.

Prevention and Control. Carbon monoxide poisoning may be prevented by maintaining properly functioning heaters, exhaust systems, and adequate ventilation. Inexpensive carbon monoxide detectors are commercially available and should be considered for use in the home or other enclosed spaces in which carbon monoxide might accumulate. Automobile engines and other sources of carbon monoxide should never be used in or near enclosed spaces.

Veterinarians should also keep in mind that household pets may be affected earlier and more severely than humans in the same environment.[35] Therefore, animals with evidence of carbon monoxide exposure may be indicators of human risk. It is important to establish the source of carbon monoxide so that corrective measures can be taken. Heating system professionals or utility officials should be contacted for assistance in these cases.

NITROGEN DIOXIDE

Synonyms. Nitrogen dioxide is primarily responsible for the pulmonary condition known as "silo fillers" disease in man.

Sources. Nitrogen dioxide, a poisonous gas with a yellow or yellow-brown color and a bleachlike smell, is heavier than air. The most important agriculture source of this gas is from the fermentation process of ensiled forages. Most nitrogen dioxide forms during the first 2 weeks after silage has been harvested and stored in the silo. Highest concentrations of this gas normally are reached during the first 48 hours after filling the silo and may reach levels as high as 1500 ppm. Because it is heavier than air, nitrogen dioxide forms layers on top of the silage within the silo and settles down the chute. It may concentrate in enclosed spaces at the bottom of the chute and move into an adjoining building, possibly exposing animals in the feeding area.[1,36]

Mechanism of Action. Nitrogen dioxide exerts it effect by combining with water in the air or exposed tissues to form corrosive nitric acid. However, because of its relatively low solubility in water, nitrogen dioxide may pass through the upper respiratory tract with little effect but then produce considerable permanent damage in the lungs where the duration of contact and the moisture are greater. The clinical impact of nitrogen dioxide exposure is a function of both concentration of the gas and the length of exposure. Increasing levels of nitrogen dioxide have a direct effect on pulmonary function.

Toxicity and Risk Factors. Concentrations in the 4 to 5 ppm range for a 10-minute exposure period have their maximum effect of increasing expiratory flow resistance some 30 minutes after the exposure ceases. Rats, mice, guinea pigs, rabbits, and dogs have a mortality threshold of between 40 and 50 ppm of nitrogen dioxide for a 1-hour exposure. Once the threshold concentration is exceeded, the death rate for animals increases as exposure period or the concentration is increased. In general, brief exposures to high concentrations of nitrogen dioxide are much more toxic than exposures to low concentrations for longer periods.

Clinical Signs. Humans are able to detect nitrogen dioxide at levels of 0.1 to 0.2 ppm in the air, although detection may vary with relative humidity and individual sensitivity. Breathing air containing a few parts per million of this gas can cause coughing, choking, tightness in the chest, and nausea. Breathing higher concentrations (>200 ppm) can result in immediate death. Inhalation of nonlethal concentrations of this gas may lead to chronic bronchitis or emphysema.

Lesions. The extent of pathologic change in the lung corresponds to the exposure dosage. Acute exposures to nitrogen dioxide with concentrations of 2 to 3 ppm, which are close to ambient levels, have not resulted in an increase in morphologic abnormalities in dogs or rodents nor have these exposures affected cellular structure. At higher concentrations, ultrastructural scanning electron microscopic studies have revealed loss of cilia, swelling, disruption of type I alveolar cells, fibrin deposition on basement membranes, and an influx of macrophages.

Pulmonary congestion, edema, and emphysema are found at necropsy in animals that have died of nitrogen dioxide poisoning.[37]

Diagnostic Testing. Diagnosis of nitrogen dioxide poisoning is based on a history of exposure and the presence of respiratory clinical signs and pulmonary tissue changes. Although conditions in the field may change rapidly, handheld air testing devices are commercially available and may be useful to help document ambient nitrogen dioxide concentrations.

Treatment. Treatment of nitrogen dioxide poisoning should include the administration of oxygen and artificial respiration. Corticosteroids may be used to relieve pulmonary edema, and broad-spectrum antibiotics may be useful in preventing bronchopneumonia. However, no specific treatment is available for nitrogen dioxide poisoning.

Prognosis. The prognosis should be guarded because even animals given fresh air immediately after exposure may die in a few hours to several days later.[38]

GLYPHOSATE HERBICIDES

Sherry Welch

Synonyms.   Glyphosate is an acid, but is often used in salt form, most commonly the isopropylamine salt. It may also be available in acidic or trimethylsulfonium salt forms. Other synonyms include glyphosate-isopropylammonium, glyphosate sesquiodium, and glyphosate-trimesium. Roundup is a commonly used herbicidal product that contains glyphosate.

Sources.   Glyphosate (N-phosphonomethyl) glycine is a nonselective, nonresidual, postemergence herbicide that is effective on deep-rooted species. It is a systemic herbicide used for control of a great variety of annual, biennial, and perennial grasses, sedges, broad-leaved weeds, and woody shrubs. It is also used on a wide variety of crops, as well as for preharvest desiccation of cotton, cereals, peas, and beans. Other uses are for destruction of rye sown to prevent wind erosion of the soil, control of suckers on fruit trees, and aquatic weed control.[1]

It is generally distributed as aqueous solutions, water-soluble concentrates, and powders.[2] There are a variety of products available commercially that contain glyphosate in either the diluted or concentrated form.

Toxicokinetics.   Glyphosate is poorly absorbed dermally and orally, and is largely excreted unchanged by mammals. In human dermal studies, absorption of glyphosate was less than 2%. In rats fed glyphosate for 3 weeks, only minute amounts were found in tissues 10 days after treatment. Cows, chickens, and pigs fed small amounts of glyphosate had undetectable levels (<0.05 ppm) in tissue and fat. Levels in milk and eggs were also undetectable (<0.025 ppm).[2]

Glyphosate appears to undergo minimal metabolism, if any. Results from animal studies (10 mg/kg PO in rats) indicate that essentially no toxic metabolites are produced. Only parent compound was present and it did not persist in the body.[3]

Mechanism of Action.   In plants, glyphosate moves through the plant and is absorbed into the root, inhibiting the enzyme 5-enolpyruvylshikimate-3-phosphate (EPSP) synthetase, which produces EPSP from shikimate-3-phosphate and phosphoenolpyruvate in the shikimic acid pathway of the plant. EPSP inhibition leads to depletion of the aromatic amino acids tryptophan, tyrosine, and phenylalanine, all needed for protein synthesis or for biosynthetic pathways leading to growth.[4] Its low toxicity in animals is attributed to the fact that animals do not possess the EPSP synthetase enzyme or this biochemical pathway.

Glyphosate is representative of a broad class of compounds known as phosphonic acids, which contain a direct carbon-to-phosphorus (C-P) bond. Although the C-P bond is stable, many bacteria, even enteric bacteria such as *Escherichia coli,* have the ability to enzymatically cleave the bond to liberate inorganic phosphate.[5] This inorganic phosphate,

however, has no cholinesterase inhibitory activity.[3] It has been postulated that the mechanism of toxicity in humans and animals is related to uncoupling of mitochondrial oxidative phosphorylation, although this has not been conclusively proven.[3]

Toxicity and Risk Factors.   Glyphosate has a wide margin of safety, with a reported acute LD_{50} of 5600 mg/kg in the rat. The toxicity of the technical grade acid (glyphosate) and the formulated product are nearly the same. Glyphosate is slightly toxic to wild birds. The dietary LD_{50} in both mallards and bobwhite quail is greater than 4500 ppm. Technical grade glyphosate is practically nontoxic to fish and may be slightly toxic to aquatic invertebrates. Some formulations, however, may be more toxic to aquatic species because of differences in salts and the parent acid or of the surfactants used in the formulation.

Typically, animals at risk are those exposed to freshly treated vegetation, to overspray, or to the product directly from the container. The clinical signs associated with exposure to glyphosate-containing products are attributable to the irritating effects of the anionic surfactants (polyoxyethyleneamines) rather than the glyphosate itself. Ingestion of plants treated with a glyphosate herbicide after the product has dried is not expected to cause a serious problem. However, some herbicides can increase the palatability of some plants, increasing the risk of ingesting potentially toxic plants.[6]

Clinical Signs.   Clinical signs expected after exposure to glyphosate herbicides include hypersalivation, vomiting, diarrhea, anorexia, and lethargy. The clinical signs are primarily due to the surfactants in the product, with the severity depending on the amount ingested. In healthy animals with no underlying disease processes, these signs are usually mild and self-limiting, with a duration of 2 to 24 hours.

Lesions.   Some microscopic liver and kidney changes, but no observable differences in function or toxic effects, have been seen after lifetime administration of glyphosate to test animals.[2]

Treatment.   For dermal exposure the animal should be bathed with either liquid dishwashing detergent or noninsecticidal shampoo. If ingestion occurs and the animal is asymptomatic, small amounts of water (or milk in small animals) can be given to dilute the ingested product as much as possible. Treatment is symptomatic and supportive if signs occur. If vomiting occurs, keeping the patient NPO for a minimum of 2 to 3 hours is oftentimes all that is necessary. For persistent vomiting, especially if the patient weighs less than 10 pounds, intravenous fluids to prevent dehydration and electrolyte imbalances is recommended. Ingestion of large amounts of the super-concentrated products may result in more extreme irritation, thus gastrointestinal protectants may be indicated.

Prognosis.   Overall, exposure to glyphosate herbicides carries a good prognosis because of their wide safety margin.

Prognosis generally depends on the amount of product ingested, severity of signs, and overall health of the animal involved. In most cases, the signs are mild and self-limiting, with no long-term sequelae expected.

Prevention and Control. Problems can be avoided by following label instructions with regard to dilution and drying time before animal exposures, as well as keeping containers out of the range of animals. Following manufacturer recommendations with regard to grazing restrictions, as well as meat and milk withdrawal times, is important in the prevention of toxicosis with any herbicide.

NAPHTHALENE

Karyn Bischoff

Naphthalene is most commonly associated with mothballs, even though it has several other uses. Twelve million pounds of naphthalene moth repellants were produced in 1989. However, other substances are becoming more commonly used in mothballs.[1]

Currently, paradichlorobenzene, which is less toxic than naphthalene, is used in mothballs more frequently than naphthalene.[2] Naphthalene mothballs are approximately twice as toxic as paradichlorobenzene mothballs.[3] Clinical signs of paradichlorobenzene exposure are associated with the gastrointestinal tract.[4]

Differentiating between types of mothballs can be difficult if the packaging is not available. Both types of mothballs look much the same, although paradichlorobenzene mothballs may appear more oily.[5] Naphthalene and paradichlorobenzene mothballs both sink in water; however, naphthalene mothballs float in saturated salt water (add 3 heaping tablespoons of salt to 4 ounces of tepid water; mix well) and paradichlorobenzene do not.[2-4] Camphor is used in mothballs in some countries, but, unlike the other two types, camphor mothballs float in fresh water.[2]

Synonyms. Synonyms for naphthalene include tar camphor, white tar, and albocarbon.[1,2,6] Naphthalene mothballs may be labeled "old fashioned mothballs."[4]

Sources. Naphthalene is a dry-appearing, white, solid crystalline material found in mothballs, moth flakes, urinal disks, and toilet bowl and diaper pail deodorant blocks.[1,2,7-9] Naphthalene is a bicyclic aromatic hydrocarbon with the chemical formula $C_{10}H_8$ and molecular weight of 128. This substance has a characteristic "mothball" odor, which can be detected at levels as low as 84 ppb.[1,7] It has various industrial uses and has been used as a soil fumigant.[7-9]

Historically, naphthalene has been used in medicine as an antiseptic, an expectorant, and a treatment for gastrointestinal and dermal disorders.[1] Physicians and veterinarians used to use the compound as an anthelminthic, and veterinarians have used it in insecticide dusting powders.[1,2,6]

Toxicokinetics. Naphthalene is moderately lipophilic.[1] Oral doses are rapidly absorbed, although mothballs may take several days to dissolve and be absorbed in the gastrointestinal tract.[1] When ingested with fatty material, absorption may be enhanced.[1,2] Similarly, dermal absorption may be enhanced in the presence of lipid-containing lotions and ointments.[1,2] In an experiment involving rats, 50% of a dermal dose was absorbed within 2.1 hours.[1] Dermal exposure is usually associated with concomitant inhalation exposure.[1] Naphthalene uptake is rapid in the lungs.[2]

Naphthalene is believed to enter the placental blood supply in humans, causing clinical signs in the neonate.[7,10] The material is also excreted in the milk of humans and cattle and the eggs of poultry.[1] The half-life of naphthalene in guinea pig blood is 10.4 hours and decay is biphasic in other tissues.[1] Low levels of naphthalene were detected in the adipose tissue of experimental swine 72 hours after exposure.[1]

Thus far, at least 21 naphthalene metabolites have been detected in humans and experimental animals.[1] These metabolites are generally less lipophilic than the parent compound.[1] Metabolism occurs via microsomal P-450 enzymes, usually in the liver.[1,2] A primary metabolite is 1-naphthol, and further metabolism of this product results in the production of naphthoquinones, which may be responsible for some of the toxic effects associated with naphthalene.[11] Naphthalene metabolites are usually conjugated to other compounds, frequently gluathione, glucuronide, or sulfate, as the final step in detoxification.[1,11]

The kidney excretes naphthalene and its metabolites.[1] Rats exposed to naphthalene excrete 77% to 93% of the dose in the urine and 6% to 7% in feces.[1] Less than 1% of a dermal dose was excreted in the lungs of experimental rats.[1]

Mechanism of Action. Naphthalene-induced hemolytic anemia is associated with glucose-6-phosphodiesterase deficiency in humans, although it has also occurred in humans with normal glucose-6-phosphodiesterase activity. A metabolite of naphthalene oxidizes hemoglobin to methemoglobin, causing Heinz body formation and erythrocyte lysis.[1] Naphthalene may also deplete cellular glutathione, thus decreasing the ability of the cell to counteract oxidative damage.[1]

Gastrointestinal, dermal, and some ocular effects are caused by the irritant properties of naphthalene.[1] Cataract formation has been reported in experimental animals after oral exposure to naphthalene.[1,8,9] A metabolite of naphthalene alters cellular metabolism in the lens and produces free radical damage.[1,8,9,12]

Pulmonary toxicosis from inhalation and intraperitoneal injection of naphthalene has been reported, but there are species differences in susceptibility, and mice appear to be the most susceptible.[1] Naphthalene is metabolized in the pulmonary Clara cells to a reactive intermediate, which causes cellular damage.[1,13]

Toxicity and Risk Factors. Acute hemolytic anemia in dogs has been reported at 411 mg/kg (about 2.7 g naphthalene/mothball).[3] Hemolytic anemia developed in one dog given one dose of 1525 mg/kg naphthalene in food and in another dog given 1841 mg/kg in food over 7 days.[1]

Clinical Signs.   The most common clinical signs of naphthalene toxicosis in humans and dogs involve the digestive system.[5] Gastrointestinal signs have been seen in humans following both ingestion and inhalation exposure.[1] Vomiting, diarrhea, abdominal pain, and anorexia are commonly encountered.[1,2,5,7,10] Gastrointestinal bleeding has been reported in humans.[1]

Hemolysis may occur in dogs, and pale mucous membranes, anorexia, icterus, collapse, and unconsciousness were reported in a dog with possible naphthalene-induced hemolysis.[5] Respiratory effects, hematuria, and renal damage have been reported in human cases of naphthalene-induced hemolytic anemia.[1,2,7] Hemolytic anemia has been reported in neonates of women who ingested mothballs during pregnancy.[1,10]

Clinical Pathology.   The findings in the case of possible naphthalene-induced hemolysis in a dog include decreased packed cell volume (PCV) and the presence of Heinz bodies.[5] Clinical pathology findings in humans include erythrocyte fragmentation, schistosomes, and methemoglobinemia.[2]

Diagnostic Testing.   A presumptive diagnosis of naphthalene toxicosis may be based on a history of exposure along with appropriate clinical signs.[10] The smell of naphthalene can usually be detected on the dog's breath after consumption. Urine may be submitted to a diagnostic laboratory for isolation of naphthalene and metabolites using TLC or HPLC and identification using GC-MS.[1,2]

Treatment.   Treatment for oral exposure to naphthalene should include inducing emesis and possibly gastric lavage if the exposure occurred within 2 hours of presentation.[1,2] Activated charcoal and a saline cathartic may then be given to decrease absorption of the compound.[1]

Hemolysis in a dog was treated with oxygen and fluid therapy.[5] Physicians have treated naphthalene-induced hemolysis in humans with blood transfusions and bicarbonate to produce alkaline diuresis.[1] Methylene blue has been used to reverse methemoglobinemia.[2] Vitamin E succinate has been used in laboratory animals to decrease oxidative damage in the eye.[8,9]

Dermal exposure is treated by washing affected surfaces with soap and water and avoiding contact with oily substances such as lotions to prevent naphthalene absorption.[1,2] Ocular exposure requires irrigation with isotonic saline or water for 15 or more minutes.[1,2] Animals exposed to naphthalene fumes should be moved to fresh air.[1]

PHENOLS

Tina Wismer

Synonyms.   Phenol is also known as carbolic acid, phenic acid, phenylic acid, phenyl hydroxide, hydroxybenzene, and oxybenzene.

Sources.   Phenol can be manmade, but it is also found naturally in some foods, in human and animal wastes, and in decomposing organic material. It is a hydrolyzed form of benzene and can be further metabolized to other substances. Phenol historically was obtained by distillation of petroleum and by fractional distillation of coal tar. Phenol can be synthesized by fusing sodium benzenesulfonate with sodium hydroxide, by heating monochlorobenzene and aqueous sodium hydroxide under high pressure conditions, or by cumene hydroperoxidation, which yields acetone as a by-product (most common method in the United States).[1-3] Phenol ranks in the top 50 production volumes for chemicals produced in the United States. It is a colorless-to-white crystalline solid when pure; however, the commercial product, which contains some water, is a liquid.[1,4] It has a distinct disinfectant odor that is sweet and tarry.

Phenol is used primarily in the manufacture of phenolic resins, bisphenol A (epoxy precursor), caprolactam (nylon precursor), alkyl phenols (nonionic detergents), and other chemicals and drugs. Phenol is also used as a dye and indicator, a medical and veterinary antiseptic, a disinfectant (in solution or mixed with slaked lime), a reagent in chemical analysis, and a preservative for pharmaceuticals.[2,4]

Phenols have been in use since the 1800s for their antiseptic and local anesthetic properties and are still widely available for medical and home use. Dilute phenol solutions (0.1% to 4.5%) are found in sore-throat lozenges, throat sprays, gargles, gels, ointments, and lotions. Phenol is included in most of these as a local anesthetic for treating pruritus, stings, burns, bites, and sore throats. Some of the skin and mouthwash preparations are also labeled for antiseptic use.[5]

Physicians have found many uses for phenol in the clinical setting. Phenol destroys the outer layers of skin and small amounts of concentrated phenol solutions are sometimes used as a chemical peel to remove warts, skin blemishes, and wrinkles.[2] Phenol is also used for nail bed cauterization by podiatrists. Small amounts of phenol diluted in water have also been injected into nerve tissue to lessen pain.

Toxicokinetics.   Phenol is readily absorbed after inhalation or after oral or dermal exposure.[6-11] Phenol quickly enters the bloodstream and is widely distributed throughout the body.[11-13] Peak tissue concentrations are achieved in most tissues within 1 hour after oral ingestion, with the highest concentrations found in the liver. The gastrointestinal tract, lung, liver, and kidney are the major sites of phenol metabolization.[14-16]

The toxic effects of phenol exposure are due to a combination of effects of the parent compound and its metabolites. The primary pathway for phenol metabolization is conjugation by sulfotransferases and glucuronyltransferases forming phenylsulfate and phenylglucuronide, respectively. Because phenol and its major metabolites compete for the same P-450 and conjugation enzymes, these metabolic reactions are saturable. If the conjugation systems are saturated, phenol can be oxidized to hydroquinone and pyrocatechol.[17] Quinol and catechol are then conjugated or further oxidized to trihydroxybenzene. The conjugation pathways form less toxic metabolites than do the oxidation systems.[6,18]

Although mammals all process phenol to the same metabolites, the ratio of the metabolites varies among species. The glucuronidation pathway predominates in new world monkeys, guinea pigs, swine, and fruit bats and leads to higher amounts of phenylsulfate. Sulfation is the major phenol conjugation pathway for old world monkeys, prosimians, humans, and rats; therefore, larger amounts of phenylglucuronide are formed.[6,19] Cats have extremely low activities of phenol glucuronyltransferase and metabolize phenol to phenyl sulfate nearly exclusively.[6,8,18] Experiments in cats also suggest that hydroquinone formation is an important step in phenol poisoning.[6,10,18]

The amount of phenol and the route of exposure can also influence the route of metabolism.[19] In mice phenyl sulfate is the major urinary metabolite for low doses of phenol; however, as the dose increases, phenol sulfation decreases and glucuronidation of both phenol and hydroquinone increases. This suggests that the sulfation pathway becomes saturated.[10] The sulfate conjugation process in mice also saturates at a lower concentration in males than in females.[10] When phenol is given intravenously, bypassing the initial intestinal sulfate conjugation process, the oxidative pathway becomes more prominent.

A small fraction of phenol may be excreted by the lungs, imparting an aromatic odor to the breath, but phenol and its metabolites are predominantly excreted in the urine.[6-13] Renal excretion varies from 24 to 72 hours in different species.

Mechanism of Action. In dilute solutions, phenol is an irritant, and tissue damage and inflammation may be seen at the site of absorption. In concentrations of 5% or more, phenol rapidly denatures all proteins with which it comes into contact.[13] Although the exact mechanism of multiorgan toxicity is unknown, phenol has been shown to mimic the blocking effect of lidocaine on cardiac sodium channels but has little effect on sodium channels in skeletal muscle.[20] Circulatory depression is thought to be primarily due to a direct toxic effect on the myocardium but central vasomotor depression is also seen.[21] Both phenol and its glucuronide conjugate have CNS effects presumed to be responsible for the excitability of the cortex and the involuntary tremors observed in early phenol poisoning.[22] The CNS stimulation may also be related to the increased acetylcholine release at the neuromuscular junctions.[13] Phenol stimulates respiration by an unknown mechanism, and, if sustained, results in respiratory alkalosis.

Toxicity and Risk Factors. Phenol toxicosis produces identical symptoms in all animal species. All animals develop phenol toxicosis at about the same magnitude, except cats, which are more sensitive because of their limited glucuronide transferase activity.[23,24] The oral LD_{50} in rats, dogs, mice, rabbits, and monkeys is approximately 300 to 500 mg/kg, whereas the minimum oral lethal dose in cats is only 80 mg/kg.[25,26]

An oral dose of 40 mg/kg of phenol per day caused dyspnea, rales, and birth defects when given to pregnant rats on gestation days 6 to 19.[27] A single oral dose of 120 mg/kg of phenol in water given to rats caused mild to severe whole body tremors and decreased motor activity; when the dose was increased to 207 mg/kg, tremors of the muscles around the eyes followed by convulsions and coma were described.[13,28] Finally, when an oral dose of 300 mg/kg of phenol was given to rats, loss of coordination and convulsions preceded death.[26]

Mortality associated with dermal exposure to phenol is greatly influenced by the surface area exposed as well as the concentration of the applied solution. The dilution of phenol in water enhances the dermal absorption; so phenol-water solutions are better absorbed and have greater toxicity than phenol alone.[26,29] Dermal exposure is also potentially more toxic than oral exposure because of the large capacity of the intestines and the liver to conjugate phenol (no first-pass effect following dermal exposure).

The dermal LD_{50} of undiluted phenol was reported to be 669.4 mg/kg in rats and 850 mg/kg in rabbits.[29,30] Among pigs treated with a single dose of 500 mg/kg of undiluted phenol on 35% to 40% of the total body surface (about 1136 cm²; 0.44 mg/cm²/kg), lethargy, dyspnea, cyanosis, convulsions, and coma were observed, and 2 of 3 died within 90 minutes after exposure.[31] Skin discoloration occurred after 20 to 30 minutes of exposure and severe skin necrosis occurred after 8 hours in the remaining pig.[31] Cardiac arrhythmias have been noted in rabbits treated with 2 ml of a 50% phenol solution on a 15 cm² area (23.8 mg/cm²/kg).[32]

Concentration of aerosolized phenol and duration of exposure greatly influence mortality rates. Female rats exposed to 234 ppm phenol delivered in an aerosol demonstrated no neurologic effects at 1 hour, a slight loss of coordination and muscle spasms at 4 hours, and whole body tremors leading to a severe loss of coordination by 8 hours.[30] All animals were normal 24 hours after exposure. No deaths were reported in rhesus monkeys, rats, or mice exposed to 5 ppm phenol continuously for 90 days.[33]

Clinical Signs. Phenol is caustic, and dermal application causes intense pain and blanching of the area and can result in blisters and severe burns. Dermal application of phenol can also cause mydriasis, incoordination, salivation, and nasal discharge within 5 minutes of exposure. Large doses can lead to muscle tremors, convulsions, coma, and death.[31] Dilute phenol solutions on large portions of the body (greater than 25% of the body surface) can also result in death. Other effects following dermal exposure to phenol include liver damage, diarrhea, dark urine, and hemolytic anemia.

Ocular exposure to phenol results in conjunctivitis, epithelial ulceration, and stromal opacity, which may lead to vision loss.[34] Aerosolized phenol can also cause ocular irritation, which usually resolves in 24 hours. Exposure to aerosolized phenol causes respiratory irritation characterized by coughing and reflex apnea.[30,35] In animals exposure to high repeated concentrations of phenol in air for several days produced muscle tremors and loss of coordination. Exposure to high, aerosolized concentrations of phenol for several weeks resulted in paralysis and severe injury to the heart, kidneys, liver, and lungs, followed by death in some cases.

Concentrated phenol is extremely corrosive and, if ingested, may cause oral and esophageal burns. Esophageal stricture formation has been reported but is uncommon.[17] Laryngeal edema as a result of aspiration has also been recognized. Oral phenol exposure in animals causes panting, profuse vomiting (in those species that can vomit), diarrhea, salivation, apprehension, and ataxia, which may progress to gastric ulcers, muscle fasciculations, and methemoglobinemia. Other systemic signs may include CNS stimulation or depression, tremors, seizures, extremity weakness, lethargy, coma, supraventricular and ventricular dysrhythmias, hypotension, pulmonary edema, and severe metabolic acidosis.[22,36] Hepatic and renal damage may occur within 12 to 24 hours.[37]

Clinical Pathology.   Because phenol affects many organ systems, a variety of clinical pathology abnormalities can be noted. Abnormalities in the complete blood count include anemia, neutrophils with basophilic cytoplasms and Dohle bodies, and thrombocytopenia. The anemia appears to be dose related because higher doses led to lower hematocrits.[38,39] Phenols have also been implicated as causing methemoglobinemia and Heinz body hemolytic anemia.[40,41]

Blood chemistry abnormalities are primarily liver related. The enzymes lactate dehydrogenase, aspartate aminotransferase (AST), ALT, glutamate dehydrogenase, alkaline phosphatase, and bilirubin are all commonly elevated after exposure.[42,43] Serum levels of magnesium, potassium, and creatine phosphokinase have also been found to be elevated.[42]

Urinalysis abnormalities include green or black color, albuminuria, hematuria, and the presence of casts.[23] Hemoglobinuria and hematin casts have been reported in the renal tubules of rats treated dermally with a nonlethal dose of phenol.[29]

Lesions.   Dermal application of phenol solutions as dilute as 1% can result in skin necrosis.[17] Other dermal changes include edema, hyperemia of superficial dermal vessels, and dense perivascular infiltration of lymphocytes and neutrophils.[44]

Oral ingestion of phenol causes epiglottal edema and ulceration, hyperemia of the esophageal and gastric mucosa, and multifocal areas of gastric erosion with lymphoid cell infiltration and focal cryptal epithelial metaplasia.[38] Renal tubular necrosis, protein casts, and papillary hemorrhage have been reported with oral ingestion of phenol (224 mg/kg) in rats.[26]

Necrosis or atrophy of the spleen and thymus along with unspecified microscopic changes in the adrenal glands have been reported in rats given a single gavage dose of 224 mg/kg phenol in water.[43] A 30% to 60% decrease in the ratio of polychromatic to normochromatic erythrocytes was observed in the bone marrow of pregnant mice treated by gavage with a single dose of 265 mg/kg phenol in water on gestation day 13.[45]

Aerosolized phenol can cause extensive damage to the respiratory tract. Inflammation, cellular infiltration, pneumonia, bronchitis, endothelial hyperplasia, and capillary thrombosis have all been reported in animals exposed to phenol by inhalation.[26] Aerosolized phenol can also cause myocardial injury characterized by myocardial inflammation,

degeneration, necrosis, interstitial fibrosis, and lymphocyte infiltration.[26] Renal proximal tubule and glomerular injury along with hepatic centrilobular degeneration and necrosis have been reported in guinea pigs and rabbits after chronic inhalation of phenol (26 to 52 ppm phenol for 41 days for guinea pigs and 88 days for rabbits).[26,43]

Diagnostic Testing.   Measurement of phenol requires special laboratory equipment and techniques that are not routinely available in most hospitals or clinics. History of exposure to phenol along with its disinfectant odor are usually all that is needed for diagnosis; however, there are multiple analytical methods used to detect phenol in the body. The presence of phenols may be nonspecifically detected through the use of 10% ferric chloride reagent, or phenols can be specifically determined by using HPLC, polystyrene divinylbenzene resin-based reversed-phase column,[46] NMP urinalysis,[47] or GC-MS.[48]

Because of the short half-life of phenol, testing can only detect exposures that have occurred within 1 to 2 days. Urine is the most often tested substance; however, phenol concentrations can be determined in the blood, stomach contents, and organs. Normal urine can test positive for phenol because it is a metabolite of proteins. Testing can be used to determine whether the urine has a higher than normal concentration of phenol, suggesting recent exposure to phenol or to a substance that is converted to phenol in the body (e.g., benzene).

Treatment.   Treatment of phenol poisoning is controversial, but general management includes decontamination of the body surfaces, removal of ingested phenol, and supportive therapy. Treatment should take place in a well-ventilated area while gloved, gowned, and masked.

With an ocular exposure, the eyes should be flushed with water or saline for at least 30 minutes. If any symptoms persist after 30 minutes of irrigation, ophthalmologic consultation is needed. Inhalation exposure necessitates removal of the patient from the environment and supportive treatment for signs of respiratory distress.

Literature review of dermal decontamination yields many contradictory recommendations. Although several references list polyethylene glycol 300 or 400 as being the most efficacious agent for dermal decontamination,[17,29,44] most veterinarians in the clinical setting do not have this item available. Before washing any contaminated areas of skin, liquefied or solid phenol should first be removed by blotting with an absorbent material. Decontamination with liquid dishwashing detergent and copious amounts of water until phenol can no longer be smelled on the animal is recommended. Using less copious amounts of water only dilutes the phenol and expands the area of exposure, resulting in greater morbidity.[17] For small dermal exposures (<5% body surface area), isopropyl alcohol may be used.[44] If any areas of necrosis are noted after bathing, sodium bicarbonate (0.5%) dressings and further wound management is recommended.

Removal of large amounts of ingested phenol is best accomplished by careful gastric lavage using tap water or normal saline. An endotracheal tube should be placed to reduce the chance of aspiration. Small ingestions may be treated with egg white or milk dilution. Emesis is contraindicated because phenol has corrosive effects and there is potential for rapid CNS depression and seizures. Administration of activated charcoal, which retards phenol absorption, is indicated.

Management of systemic toxicosis is symptomatic and supportive. In all symptomatic exposures, patients should undergo cardiac monitoring and close neurologic observation. Forced diuresis decreases plasma concentrations of phenol and reduces the cardiac effects, but patients must be carefully monitored for development of pulmonary edema. Lidocaine may be used to treat ventricular dysrhythmias. Intravenous administration of sodium bicarbonate may rapidly reverse CNS depression in the presence of metabolic acidosis.[49] *N*-Acetylcysteine may prevent renal and hepatic damage. If methemoglobinemia is present, methylene blue or ascorbic acid may be tried. Ascorbic acid is the drug of choice in cats.[37] Pain control is an important factor in the symptomatic animal.

Prognosis.   Because phenol is rapidly absorbed, if signs of toxicosis do not develop within 2 to 4 hours, the exposure is probably not toxic. Because phenol is also quickly metabolized and excreted, the most critical phase of toxicosis is usually complete in 24 hours. Prognosis depends on the dose and the resulting clinical signs.

Prevention and Control.   All phenol-containing products should be kept away from domestic animals.

PINE OIL

Tina Wismer

Synonyms.   Pine oil is also called arizole, oleum abietis, unipine, and yarmor.

Sources.   Pine oil is the product of pine trees and is composed primarily of terpene alcohols. Terpenes are aliphatic, cyclic hydrocarbons derived from plants rather than petroleum (crude oil) distillates.[1] Pine oil is a component of many household cleaners and disinfectants. Pine-scented formulations contain small amounts of pine oil and therefore have minimal toxicity compared with pure pine oil.

Toxicokinetics.   Pine oil is a mixture of highly lipophilic unsaturated cyclic hydrocarbons that is one fifth as toxic as turpentine in animals.[2] The major component of pine oil is α-terpineol but borneol and other terpene ethers are present along with monoterpenes (α-pinene, carene, β-pinene, and limonene).[3] Adding ingredients that increase pine oil viscosity reduces the aspiration potential.

Oral and dermal absorption of pine oil is considered to be poor.[2] Absorption has been demonstrated vaginally, rectally, and via the uterus.[4,5] Vaginal and uterine absorption may occur if pine oil is used as an abortifacient and rectal absorption has occurred when pine oil is used in enemas.

Metabolization of pine oil is by the epoxide pathway. Pine oil is oxidized in the liver by cytochrome P-450, conjugated principally with glucuronic acid, and then excreted by the kidney into the urine.[6] The volume of distribution is large, with the highest concentrations found in the brain, lungs, and kidneys. High concentrations of pine oil are demonstrable in lung tissue, lending a characteristic pine odor to the breath.[7] Twice the amount of α-terpineol was found in the lungs as in the blood or kidney after an intravenous injection in the horse.[3] α-Terpineol is excreted as the glucuronide and disappears from the urine in a short time.[6] Horses have no α-terpineol in their plasma within 2 hours, and none in any other tissues at 24 hours.[3]

Mechanism of Action.   Pine oils are directly irritating to the mucous membranes, producing erythema of the oropharynx, mouth, and skin. Pulmonary toxicosis may be caused by either aspiration during ingestion or emesis, or chemical pneumonitis resulting from absorption of pine oil from the gastrointestinal tract with subsequent deposition in the lung.[7] The monoterpenes contained in pine oil have spasmolytic, bactericidal, and CNS effects.

Toxicity and Risk Factors.   Because of poor dermal absorption, the dermal LD_{50} in the rabbit is 5 g/kg,[8] whereas the oral LD_{50} for small animals (dogs, cats) is 1 to 2.5 ml/kg.[9] However, much smaller doses can result in severe toxicosis.[10]

Cats are deficient in certain types of glucuronyl transferase activity, including that required for terpene excretion, making cats more susceptible than other species to pine oil toxicoses.[11] In one cat that ingested about 100 ml of Pinesol, containing 20% pine oil and 10.9% isopropanol, severe depression, ataxia, and unresponsive pupils developed, and the cat died. Autopsy revealed pulmonary edema, acute centrilobular hepatic necrosis, and total renal cortical necrosis.[11]

In horses the primary site of toxicosis is the lungs, and the main cause of death is pulmonary edema.[3] Mild segmental degeneration of renal tubular cells has also been noted in the horse.[3]

Clinical Signs.   Dermal exposure to pine oil may cause some erythema, whereas ocular exposure results in severe irritation with blepharospasm, lacrimation, conjunctivitis, and photosensitivity.[10]

Ingestion of pine oil may cause oral and pharyngeal irritation, vomiting, CNS depression, tachycardia, nephritis, and fever.[10] Less commonly seen signs include aspiration pneumonitis, diarrhea, hypotension, bradycardia, respiratory depression, ataxia, coma, renal failure, and myoglobinuria following large ingestions.

Lesions.   Mild segmental degeneration of some renal epithelial tubular cells has been seen in horses and cats.[3,11] Cats with pine oil toxicosis have also been found to have pulmonary edema, acute centrilobular hepatic necrosis, and total renal cortical necrosis.[9,11]

Diagnostic Testing.   The odor of pine oil is the best diagnostic tool, and pine oil can be detected on the breath even if given rectally.[5] The α-terpineol found in pine oil can be identified by GC, but levels are not clinically useful. No therapeutic or toxic levels have been established for either pine oil or α-terpineol.[12]

Treatment.   Animals with dermal exposures to pine oil should be bathed with water and a mild liquid dishwashing detergent. Dilution with milk, egg whites, or water is recommended following ingestion of pine oil disinfectants.[13] Emesis is contraindicated at home and significant exposures should be transferred to a medical facility for lavage.

It is not known whether activated charcoal adsorbs pine oil. Because of the unknown benefit and potential risk of aspiration, the use of activated charcoal is not recommended. A baseline chest x-ray study should be obtained after significant ingestions or in patients with signs of aspiration. There is no specific antidote for pine oil; treatment is symptomatic and supportive. Acid-base status and renal function should be monitored, and fluid and electrolyte balances should be maintained. The patient should be observed for a minimum of 24 hours.

Prognosis.   Serious complications are unlikely to develop in patients who are either asymptomatic or who have only mild gastrointestinal or CNS symptoms after 6 hours.

Prevention and Control.   All pine oil products should be kept away from domestic animals.

PROPYLENE GLYCOL

Rosalind Dalefield

Synonyms.   Propylene glycol (PG) is also known as 1,2-propanediol.[1]

Sources.   Propylene glycol is widely used as a solvent, humectant, plasticizer, bacteriostat, and fungistat in pharmaceuticals, cosmetics, and food. It is also used in coolants and deicing solutions,[2] and is used instead of ethylene glycol in "environmentally safe" automotive antifreeze.

Propylene glycol is often used in semimoist pet food, in which it forms an economical source of metabolizable energy. Propylene glycol is also used therapeutically as a source of energy for ruminants with ketosis and is therefore likely to be present in large animal practices. It closely resembles mineral oil and there have been a small number of cases in which veterinarians have inadvertently given horses propylene glycol instead of mineral oil.[3-5]

Propylene glycol is a colorless, odorless, slightly viscous liquid. It is essentially tasteless. It has a boiling point of 189° C, a freezing point of –60° C, and a density of 1.036. It is miscible in alcohol and water.[2] It is synthetically prepared from propylene or glycerol.[6]

Toxicokinetics.   Propylene glycol is rapidly absorbed from the gastrointestinal tract, via inhalation, and following subcutaneous injection. Metabolism occurs in the liver and

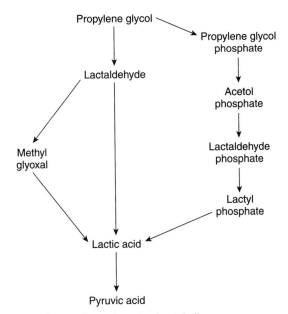

Fig. 20-3 Pathways of propylene glycol metabolism.

kidneys, and metabolites can be detected within 2 to 4 hours of exposure. Excretion is largely completed within 24 to 48 hours.[2]

About one third of ingested propylene glycol is not metabolized, but is excreted renally as the parent compound.[1] Pathways of propylene glycol metabolism are shown in Figure 20-3. Propylene glycol is metabolized by alcohol dehydrogenase to lactaldehyde. Lactaldehyde may be converted directly to lactic acid by aldehyde dehydrogenase, or it may be converted to methyl glyoxal by alcohol dehydrogenase. Methyl glyoxal is converted to lactic acid by glyoxalase.[6]

Propylene glycol may also be metabolized to lactic acid by addition of a phosphate group and conversion that progresses through propylene glycol phosphate, acetol phosphate, lactaldehyde phosphate, and lactyl phosphate to lactic acid.[2]

Both L-lactic acid and D-lactic acid are produced by propylene glycol metabolism.[6] Lactic acid is converted to pyruvic acid. Both lactic acid and pyruvic acid are normal constituents of the citric acid cycle, but at high concentrations may cause lactic acidosis.

Mechanism of Action.   Propylene glycol acts as an osmotic diuretic,[1] and has a narcotic effect on the brain approximately one third that of a similar dose of ethanol. Excessive D-lactic acid accumulates in the brain and may cause encephalopathy.[6]

The mechanism by which propylene glycol induces Heinz body anemia in cats is unknown. Heinz body formation cannot be replicated in vitro by incubating feline erythrocytes with propylene glycol, which suggests that a metabolite may be responsible. Aldehydes react with proteins, but cats treated with propylene glycol show no evidence of aldehyde-hemoglobin adducts.[7] Cats are particularly susceptible to hemoglobin oxidation because they have eight reactive sulfhydryl groups on the hemoglobin molecule; some authors believe that propylene glycol or a metabolite may have oxidant properties,[8] but others reject this mechanism.[7] Feline hemoglobin molecules also dissociate readily from tetramers to dimers, relative to those of other species,[7] and induction of changes in the tertiary structure of hemoglobin by a propylene glycol metabolite has been proposed as a mechanism.[2] Heinz bodies develop in the erythrocytes of cats with diabetes mellitus, and propylene glycol may mimic that process, in that it is metabolized as a carbohydrate substitute.[7]

The mechanism by which anemia develops is also uncertain in cats. In contrast to that of other species, the feline spleen has large pores in pulp venules that allow erythrocytes to pass through without deforming, and thus erythrocytes with Heinz bodies are not sequestered in the spleens of cats as they are in other species.[8] Nevertheless, a dose-dependent reduction in erythrocyte survival in cats with propylene glycol–induced Heinz bodies has been demonstrated.[1,9]

Toxicity and Risk Factors

Dogs. Chronic administration to dogs causes no pathologic effects in kidneys, liver,[2] bone marrow, or spleen.[10] Mild changes in hematologic and serologic parameters, but no overt clinical signs of toxicosis, occur in dogs fed propylene glycol at 5 g/kg/day, or 20% of the diet. A dietary propylene glycol level of 2 g/kg/day, or 8% of the diet, is below threshold for any discernible effect in the dog.[10] A lowest observed adverse effect level of 5000 mg/kg/day has been identified in dogs, the observed effect being increased urinary output.[2]

Cows. Cattle can become intoxicated if overdosed with propylene glycol during treatment for ketosis. The toxic dose 50 (TD_{50}) of propylene glycol in adult cows was calculated as 2.6 g/kg in one study.[11]

Cats. Besides the unique properties of feline hemoglobin, cats may be particularly susceptible to propylene glycol toxicosis because of their limited capacity for glucuronidation. The propylene glycol–glucuronide conjugate makes up a substantial fraction of the propylene glycol in urine in other species. Cats may therefore have limited excretion capacity for propylene glycol compared with other species, resulting in higher circulating levels relative to dose.[2]

Commercial semimoist cat foods may contain between 3% and 13% propylene glycol. A concentration of dietary propylene glycol that has no effect on feline hematology has not yet been reported.[9] Propylene glycol levels as low as 5% of the diet caused increased Heinz bodies numbers in kittens,[12] and dietary propylene glycol of 6% caused increased Heinz body numbers and a slight increase in reticulocytes in adult cats.[9]

Cats with increased food intake, such as lactating queens and growing kittens, are at particular risk from dietary propylene glycol,[1] as are cats exposed to exogenous oxidants such as acetaminophen. Other high-risk individuals are cats with diseases that cause depressed erythropoiesis and cats with diseases that predispose to Heinz body formation, such as diabetes mellitus and hyperthyroidism.[8]

Horses. Iatrogenic propylene glycol toxicosis in horses is a rare event, but has occurred when mistaken for mineral oil during treatment for colic[4,5] or in horses undergoing elective surgery.[3] Three horses of unspecified weight survived oral administration with 1.89 to 3.79 L (0.5 to 1.0 gal) propylene glycol, but a horse weighing 454 kg (1000 lb) died after being given 2 gallons (16.7 ml/kg) of propylene glycol. No treatment was attempted.[3] A stallion that received 7.6 ml/kg died despite treatment attempts,[4] but two mares survived with treatment after receiving doses of 6 ml/kg and 6.25 ml/kg.[3,5]

Clinical Signs

Cows. Ataxia developed in cattle within 2 to 4 hours of ingestion, but the ataxia resolved within 24 hours. Depression and temporary recumbency also occurred.[11]

Cats. Cats fed 8 g/kg of propylene glycol, or 41% dietary propylene glycol, exhibited moderate polyuria and polydipsia and moderate neurologic signs, which included decreased activity, depression, and mild to moderate ataxia.[6] Cats on a diet containing propylene glycol are more susceptible to cyanosis in response to acetaminophen.[8]

Horses. Signs of pain, including salivation and sweating, may become evident within 10 to 15 minutes of accidental oral administration of propylene glycol in the horse. Other signs that may become apparent early in the course of toxicosis are ataxia and circling in the stall.[4] Depression may be apparent within 2 hours.[5] Ataxia is severe and, in the absence of treatment, persistent. At a high dose (16.7 ml/kg), one horse became recumbent within 3 hours. The rapid, shallow breathing characteristic of metabolic acidosis is present, and cyanosis may be evident.[4]

A strong, unpleasant odor, affecting both the horse and its feces, and described in one report as being similar to that of garlic,[5] is characteristic. In one case in which a mare was given 6 ml/kg propylene glycol, this odor was evident 2 hours after the administration,[5] whereas in another case in which a stallion was given 7.6 ml/kg, the odor was not noticed until the next day. The mare survived the toxicosis but the abnormal odor persisted for more than a week.[5]

Clinical Pathology

Cows. Serum and CSF hyperosmolality and an elevated osmolal gap developed in cattle.[11]

Cats. Chronic feeding of dietary propylene glycol (6% to 12% of diet) to adult cats is associated with decreased red blood cell count, increased Heinz bodies, an increase in reticulocytes, and a reduction in erythrocyte survival time. However, no change in bone marrow myeloid to erythroid (M:E) ratio or bone marrow cellularity occurs. Both mean cell hemoglobin concentration and mean cell hemoglobin are elevated, but this may be an artifact of increased sample turbidity caused by Heinz bodies.[9] Propylene glycol at 12% of diet on a dry weight basis, equal to a daily dose of 1.6 g/kg, is sufficient to cause an increased anion gap in cats. This is positively correlated with elevated levels of D-lactate but not L-lactate. At 8 g/kg, or 41% dietary propylene glycol, the bone marrow becomes hypercellular and the M:E ratio is altered by an increase in early erythroid precursors and in erythroblasts.[1]

Horses.   There is very little documented information on clinical pathology of propylene glycol toxicosis in the horse. A mare given propylene glycol instead of mineral oil had a blood pH of 7.32.[5] As in ethylene glycol toxicosis, the parent compound might be expected to cause an increased osmolal gap. Lactic acidosis may also be expected.

Lesions

Cats.   Gross lesions of chronic propylene glycol ingestion in cats may include splenic nodularity and mottling of the liver.[9]

Histologic lesions include hepatocyte vacuolation, which tends to be periportal. The vacuoles stain positively for glycogen with periodic acid–Schiff. After 5 weeks on 12% dietary propylene glycol, iron pigment is slightly increased in liver and spleen. After 3 weeks on 41% dietary propylene glycol, there is a marked increase in iron in both liver and spleen, hemosiderin-laden macrophages are apparent in the liver, and scattered foci of hematopoiesis are observed in the spleen.[1]

Segmental nephritis has been reported in a minority of cats fed 12% propylene glycol for 16 weeks, but it has not been established that propylene glycol causes this lesion.[9]

Horses.   One horse had a dilated stomach that was filled with feed although he had not eaten for 3 days. There was moderate sloughing of the gastric mucosa, and moderate to severe inflammation throughout the intestines and large colon. Ecchymotic hemorrhages were observed on the serosal surface of the small intestine. Renal congestion and cerebral edema were evident grossly, whereas on histologic examination degenerative changes were discovered in hepatocytes.[3]

Diagnostic Testing.   Propylene glycol may be identified and measured in serum, urine, and postmortem fluids by GC with flame ionization.[4]

Treatment.   Generally, cats with propylene glycol–induced Heinz body anemia recover with supportive care.

Three horses recovered within 3 days without treatment after oral doses of 0.5 to 1 gallon of propylene glycol.[3] A mare given 6 ml/kg propylene glycol survived after gastric lavage followed by activated charcoal, then intravenous sodium bicarbonate (0.6 mEq/kg), dexamethasone (0.12 mg/kg), and vitamin C (2.5 mg/kg). Lactated Ringer's solution was continued intravenously at 8 ml/kg/hr, with vitamin B complex supplementation. The mare was also given 1 L of isotonic sodium bicarbonate every 2 hours for the next 10 hours and a repeat dose of vitamin C every 4 hours over the next 12 hours.[5]

Prognosis.   Prognosis for cats with propylene glycol–induced Heinz body anemia is excellent, although it may take 6 to 8 weeks for the anemia to resolve.[12]

Prognosis in horses depends on dose and how quickly the toxicosis is identified and treated. Of seven horses described in the literature, five survived and two died.[3-5]

Prevention and Control.   Cat foods containing propylene glycol may be unsuitable for cats with diseases that cause Heinz bodies or anemia. Cats ingesting diets containing propylene glycol are at particular risk from oxidant insult such as acetaminophen toxicosis. Breeders may prefer to avoid propylene glycole–containing diets for nursing queens and growing kittens.

Propylene glycol is similar to mineral oil in appearance and viscosity. When the two substances are stored in the same area in a veterinary practice, clear labeling is imperative.[4] The University of Minnesota veterinary school uses green food coloring to dye propylene glycol to prevent iatrogenic toxicosis.[5]

TURPENTINE

Tina Wismer

Synonyms.   Turpentine in its various forms may be called gum spirits, gum turpentine, turpentine oil, rectified oil of turpentine, turpentine steam distilled, wood turpentine, and spirits of turpentine.

Sources.   Turpentine is a terpene, which is an aliphatic, cyclic hydrocarbon derived from plants rather than petroleum (crude oil) distillates.[1] Distilled or wood turpentine is the most crude form and is produced by destructive distillation of pine brush, stumps, and sawdust. Distilled or wood turpentine also contains methyl alcohol, formaldehyde, phenols, and pyridine. This is the form used in solvents and paint thinners. Further treatment with sodium hydroxide and water produces rectified turpentine oil. Rectified turpentine oil consisting almost entirely of pinenes (pure turpentine oil) is intended for internal use. Turpentine is in the medium range of viscosity for hydrocarbons.

Turpentine is a distillate from pine trees and is commonly used as a solvent for paints, varnishes, pigments, oils, resins, waxes, and polishes.[2,3] Turpentine has also been used as a fragrance and flavoring in candy, chewing gum, perfume, and deodorizers.

Turpentine has been used in veterinary medicine topically as a rubefacient and counterirritant for treating sprains, muscle pains, and swollen udders. It has also been given internally as an antiseptic, carminative, expectorant, anthelmintic, abortifacient, and treatment for bloat.[2,3]

Toxicokinetics.   Turpentine is easily absorbed through the gastrointestinal tract and lungs, and may also be absorbed dermally at a slower rate.[4] Turpentine is widely distributed in the body with the highest concentrations found in the liver, spleen, kidneys, and brain.[5] The details of turpentine metabolism are unknown, but elimination of turpentine and its metabolites is primarily by the kidneys.

Mechanism of Action. The toxic effect of turpentine on skin is thought to be caused by the dissolution of lipids and resultant cell membrane injury. The proposed mechanism of respiratory toxicosis is that turpentine dissolves the lipids in surfactant, resulting in alveolar collapse and anoxia. The absence of CNS lesions plus the presence of lung pathology may suggest that anoxia also contributes to the development of CNS signs.[6] The exact mechanism of toxicosis is unknown, but it appears that vomiting and diarrhea in small animals are due to gastrointestinal irritation.

Toxicity and Risk Factors. Terpenes produce more CNS and gastrointestinal symptoms than do the aliphatic hydrocarbons. Ingestions of turpentine exceeding 2 ml/kg in humans are considered potentially toxic, and as little as 15 ml in a 2-year-old child has been fatal.[4] The volatile components of turpentine (α-pinene, β-pinene, δ-3-carene) are significant pulmonary aspiration hazards.[7]

The LD_{50} for the rat (oral) is 5760 mg/kg and for the mouse (intravenously) is 1180 mg/kg.[8] The minimum lethal dermal exposure dose in the rabbit is 5010 mg/kg.[8]

Clinical Signs. Turpentine is an irritant, CNS depressant, and aspiration hazard.[2] If applied topically, turpentine can produce mild to severe dermatitis, erythema, burns, blisters, skin necrosis, and limb edema.[9,10] Turpentine is also an eye irritant, and ocular exposure can cause conjunctivitis, eyelid edema, and blepharospasm.

In general, the most severe clinical effects produced by hydrocarbon exposures are related to aspiration pneumonia.[11,12] Because of the lower volatility and higher viscosity of the terpenes, the risk of aspiration is somewhat less than that with the more volatile hydrocarbons, such as gasoline and kerosene. Respiratory signs can include coughing, fever, dyspnea, and cyanosis. Respiratory tract irritation, if severe, can progress to pulmonary edema. Death is usually due to respiratory failure. Radiographic changes associated with hydrocarbon aspiration in dogs are similar to those observed with other forms of aspiration pneumonia.

Systemic evidence of toxicosis has been reported in topically exposed humans and must be considered in animals following heavy dermal exposure.[10] Systemic toxicosis of turpentine primarily results in abdominal pain, vomiting, diarrhea, tachycardia, weakness, ataxia, somnolence, agitation, or coma. Seizures appear to be uncommon.[13] When systemic toxicosis occurs, it usually develops within 2 to 3 hours of the exposure. Gastrointestinal and CNS symptoms generally resolve within 12 hours in moderately severe exposures.[6] Animals that remain asymptomatic for 6 to 12 hours are unlikely to develop clinical signs.

Clinical Pathology. No specific clinical pathology abnormalities are seen with turpentine exposure. However, decreased oxygen saturation and secondary leukocytosis may be seen with aspiration.

Lesions. No specific histopathologic findings are apparent in turpentine exposure. Nonspecific lesions of inflammation (dermal and gastrointestinal) can be seen. If aspiration has occurred, lung tissue has intraalveolar edema, hemorrhage, and increased numbers of intraalveolar cells (mainly mononuclear).

Diagnostic Testing. Turpentine can be positively identified by using GC or a screening test on serum.[14,15] However, the distinctive odor of turpentine along with history and physical examination are usually all that is needed for diagnosis.

Treatment. Treatment of dermal turpentine exposure consists of bathing the animal with copious amounts of water and a mild liquid dishwashing detergent. The skin should be medicated to control drying, cracking, secondary self-trauma, and infection. With ophthalmic exposures, the eyes should be irrigated with water for at least 15 minutes. A corneal stain should be performed after irrigation to check for ulceration.

Treatment for oral turpentine exposure is controversial.[16] Treatment is largely determined by the time and amount of ingestion, evidence of aspiration, and the patient's level of consciousness. In alert animals with large ingestions, emesis may be induced because of the potential for systemic effects. This should be done only under veterinary supervision for the high aspiration potential and quick onset of signs. Gastric lavage may also be used with large ingestions.

Activated charcoal adsorbs turpentine in vitro and should be considered in patients with large ingestions, and should probably be preceded by intubation with a cuffed endotracheal tube.[7,11] Animals without the ability to vomit should be given activated charcoal. Oils are not recommended for animals exposed to hydrocarbons.[16]

For symptomatic animals, oxygen, cage rest, and assisted ventilation may be needed. Corticosteroids have not been shown to be of benefit.[17] If any seizure activity is present, Valium or barbiturates may be used for control. Symptomatic animals should be monitored for at least 12 hours after exposure.

Prognosis. Serious complications are unlikely to develop in animals that are either asymptomatic or that have only mild gastointestinal or CNS symptoms after 6 hours.

Prevention and Control. All turpentine products should be kept out of range of animals.

REFERENCES

Acids and Alkali

1. Coppock RW: The toxicology of detergents, bleaches, antiseptics, and disinfectants in small animals, *Vet Human Toxicol* 30(5):463, 1988.
2. Poisindex® editorial staff: Acid (toxicologic managements). In Rumack BH et al, editors: *Poisindex® system*, vol 100, Englewood, Colo, Micromedex, expires June 2000.

3. Poisindex® editorial staff: Corrosive-alkaline (toxicologic managements). In Rumack BH et al, editors: *Poisindex® system,* vol 100, Englewood, Colo, Micromedex, expires June 2000.
4. Kore A et al: Toxicology of household cleaning products and disinfectants, *Vet Clin North Am Small Anim Pract* 20(2):525, 1990.
5. Ellenhorn M: Household products. In *Medical toxicology*, New York, 1988, Elsevier.
6. Beasley Val et al: Management of toxicoses, *Vet Clin North Am Small Anim Pract* 20(2):307,1990.
7. Plumb DC: *Veterinary drug handbook*, ed 3, Ames, Iowa, 1999, Iowa State University Press.

Batteries

1. Litovitz T: In Haddad LM et al, editors: *Clinical management of poisoning and drug overdose*, ed 3, Philadelphia, 1998, WB Saunders.
2. Tanaka J et al: Esophageal electrochemical burns due to button type lithium batteries in dogs, *Vet Hum Toxicol* 40:193, 1998.
3. Kore A et al: Toxicology of household cleaning products and disinfectants, *Vet Clin North Am Small Anim Pract* 20:525, 1990.
4. Baker JC: Lead poisoning in cattle, *Vet Clin North Am Food Anim Pract* 3:137, 1987.
5. Tanaka J et al: Effects of tap water on esophageal burns in dogs from button lithium batteries, *Vet Hum Toxicol* 41:279, 1999.

Bleaches

1. Poisindex® editorial staff: Bleaches: hypochlorites and related substances (toxicologic managements). In Rumack et al, editors: *Poisindex® system,* vol 100, Engelwood, Colo, Micromedex, expires September 2001.
2. Khan SA: *Toxicology of common household cleaning products in small animals*. Presented at the 98th Annual Fall Conference and Short Course for Veterinarians, University of Illinois, Champaign, Illinois. October 12-13, 1995.
3. McGuigan MA: Bleach, soaps, detergents, and other corrosives. In *Clinical management of poisoning and drug overdose*, ed 3, Philadelphia, 1998, WB Saunders.
4. Coppock RW: The toxicology of detergents, bleaches, antiseptics, and disinfectants in small animals, *Vet Human Toxicol* 30(5):463, 1988.
5. Ellenhorn M: Household products. In *Medical toxicology*, New York, 1988, Elsevier.
6. Kore A et al: Toxicology of household cleaning products and disinfectants. *Vet Clin North Am Small Anim Pract* 20(2):525, 1990.
7. Plumb DC: *Veterinary drug handbook*, ed 3, Ames, Iowa, 1999, Iowa State University Press.

Boric Acid

1. Ellenhorn MJ: *Ellenhorn's medical toxicology*, ed 2, Baltimore, 1997, Williams & Wilkins.
2. Boric acid, Microsoft® Encarta® Online, Encyclopedia 2000, *http://encarta.msn.com*© 1997-2000 Microsoft Corporation.
3. Poisindex® editorial staff: Boric acid (toxicologic managements). In Rumack BH et al, editors: *Poisindex® system,* vol 100, Englewood, Colo, Micromedex, expires March 2001.
4. Kiesche-Nesselrodt A, Hooser SB: Boric acid. *Vet Clin North Am Small Anim Pract* 20:369,1990.
5. Haddad LM et al: Baby powder, borates, and camphor. Borates. In Young-Jin S, Pinkert H, editors: *Clinical management of poisoning and drug overdose*, ed 3, Philadelphia, 1998, WB Saunders.
6. Beasley VR et al: *A systems affected approach to toxicology,* Urbana, Ill, 1999, University of Illinois.

Detergents

1. Poisindex® editorial staff: Detergents and soaps-anionic and nonionic (toxicologic managements). In Rumack BH et al, editors: *Poisindex® system,* vol 100, Englewood, Colo, 1999, Micromedex.

2. Kore A et al: Toxicology of household cleaning products and disinfectants, *Vet Clin North Am Small Anim Pract* 20(2):525, 1990.
3. Ellenhorn M: Household products. In *Medical toxicology*, New York, 1988, Elsevier.
4. Richardson JA: Potpourri hazards in cats, *Vet Med* 94:12, 1999.
5. Beasley V et al: Management of toxicoses, *Vet Clin North Am Small Animal Pract* 20(2):307, 1990.
6. Plumb DC: *Veterinary drug handbook*, ed 3, Ames, Iowa, 1999, Iowa State University Press.

Dipyridyl Herbicides

1. Klaassen CD: *Casarett and Doull's toxicology,* ed 6, New York, 2001, McGraw-Hill.
2. Hughes WW: *Essentials of environmental toxicology*, Washington, DC, 1996, Taylor and Francis.
3. Klaassen CD, Amdur MO, Doull J: *Casarett and Doull's toxicology*, ed 5, New York, 1996, McGraw-Hill.
4. Chen N, Bowles MR, Pond SM: Prevention of paraquat toxicity in suspensions of alveolar type II cells by paraquat specific antibodies, *Hum Exp Toxicol* 13:551, 1994.
5. Chan BS, Scale JP, Duggin GG: The mechanism of excretion in paraquat in rats. *Toxicol Lett* 90:1, 1997.
6. Bischoff K et al: Malicious paraquat poisoning in Oklahoma dogs, *Vet Hum Toxicol* 40:151, 1998.
7. Day BJ et al: A mechanism of paraquat toxicity involving nitric oxide synthetase, *Proc Natl Acad Sci* 96:12760, 1999.
8. Koppel C et al: Inhaled nitric oxide in advanced paraquat intoxication, *J Toxicol Clin Toxicol* 32, 205, 1994.
9. Oehme FW, Mannala S: In Peterson ME, Talcott PA, editors: *Small animal toxicology,* Philadelphia, 2000, WB Saunders.
10. Kishimoto T et al: [Lethal paraquat poisoning caused by spraying in a vinyl greenhouse of causing pulmonary fibrosis with a hepatorenal dysfunction] [article in Japanese], *Nihon Kokyuki Gakkai Zasshi* 36:347, 1998.
11. Candan F, Alagozlu H: Captopril inhibits the pulmonary toxicity of paraquat in rats, *Hum Exp Toxicol* 20:637, 2001.
12. Bisumth C: Treatment of paraquat poisoning. In Bismuth C, Hall A, editors: *Paraquat poisoning,* New York, 1995, Marcel Dekker.
13. Pond MS: Manifestations and management of paraquat poisoning, *Med J Aust* 152:256, 1990.
14. Aiello S, editor: *The Merck veterinary manual*, Whitehouse Station, NJ, 1998, Merck and Co.
15. Gupta S et al: Sex differences in diquat-induced hepatic necrosis and DNA fragmentation in Fischer 344 rats, *Toxicol Sci* 54:203, 2000.
16. Sandy MS et al: Cytotoxicity of the redox cycling compound diquat in isolated hepatocytes: involvement of hydrogen peroxide and transition metals, *Arch Biochem Biophys* 15:29, 1987.
17. Howard JL, editor: *Current veterinary therapy: food animal practice 3*, Philadelphia, 1993, WB Saunders.
18. Osweiler GD: *Toxicology,* Philadelphia, 1996, Williams & Wilkins.
19. Manabe J, Ogata T: The toxic effect of diquat on the lung after intratracheal administration, *Toxicol Lett* 30:7, 1986.
20. Itagaki T, Lai SJ, Binder SR: A rapid monitoring method of paraquat in diquat in serum and urine using ion-pairing bare-silica stationary phase HPLC following a single acidification step of sample pretreatment, *J Liq Chromatog Rel Technol* 20:3339, 1997.
21. Minakata K et al: A new diquat derivative appropriate for colorimetric measurements of biological materials in the presence of paraquat, *Int J Legal Med* 114:1, 2000.

Essential Oils

1. Woolf A: Essential oil poisoning, *Clin Toxicol* 37(6): 721, 1999.
2. Villar D et al: Toxicity of melaleuca oil and related essential oils applied topically on dogs and cats, *Vet Human Toxicol* 36(2):139, 1994.
3. Poisindex® editorial staff: Essential oils. In Toll LL, Hurlbut KM, editors: *Poisindex® system,* Englewood, Colo, Micromedex, expires 2000.

4. DerMardosian A, editor: *The review of natural products*, St Louis, 1996, Facts and Comparisons Publishing Group.
5. Bischoff K, Fesswork G: Australian tea tree *(Melaleuca alternifolia)* oil poisoning in three purebred cats, *J Vet Diagn Invest* 10:208, 1998.

Ethylene Glycol

1. LaKind JS et al: A review of the comparative mammalian toxicity of ethylene glycol and propylene glycol, *Crit Rev Toxicol* 29(4):331, 1999.
2. Church AS, Witting MD: Laboratory testing in ethanol, methanol, ethylene glycol and isopropanol toxicities, *J Emerg Med* 15(5):687, 1997.
3. Hewlett TP, McMartin KE: Ethylene glycol poisoning. The value of glycolic acid determinations for diagnosis and treatment, *Clin Toxicol* 24(5):389, 1986.
4. Marshall DA, Doty RL: Taste responses of dogs to ethylene glycol, propylene glycol, and ethylene glycol-based antifreeze, *J Am Vet Med Assoc* 197(12):1599, 1990.
5. Grauer GF et al: Early clinicopathologic findings in dogs ingesting ethylene glycol, *Am J Vet Res* 45(11):2299, 1984.
6. Osweiler GD: *Toxicology*, Media, Penn, 1996, Williams & Wilkins.
7. Eder A: Ethylene glycol poisoning: toxicokinetic and analytical factors affecting laboratory diagnosis, *Clin Chem* 44(1):168, 1998.
8. Thrall MA et al: Clinicopathologic findings in dogs and cats with ethylene glycol intoxication, *J Am Vet Med Assoc* 184(1):39, 1984.
9. Connally HE et al: Safety and efficacy of 4-methylpyrazole for treatment of suspected or confirmed ethylene glycol intoxication in dogs: 107 cases (1983-1995), *J Am Vet Med Assoc* 209(11):1880, 1996.
10. Khan SA et al: Ethylene glycol exposures managed by the ASPCA National Animal Poison Control Center from July 1995 to December 1997, *Vet Human Toxicol* 41(6):403, 1999.
11. Beckett SD, Shields RP: Treatment of acute ethylene glycol (antifreeze) toxicosis in the dog, *J Am Vet Med Assoc* 158(4):472, 1971.
12. Crowell WA et al: Ethylene glycol toxicosis in cattle, *Cornell Vet* 69:272, 1979.
13. Osweiler GD, Eness PG: Ethylene glycol poisoning in swine, *J Am Vet Med Assoc* 160(5):746, 1972.
14. Boermans HJ et al: Ethylene glycol toxicosis in a Pygmy goat, *J Am Vet Med Assoc* 193(6):694, 1988.
15. Riddell C et al: Ethylene glycol poisoning in poultry, *J Am Vet Med Assoc* 150(12):1531, 1967.
16. Stowe CM et al: Ethylene glycol intoxication in ducks, *Avian Dis* 25:538, 1981.
17. Raisbeck MF: Common small animal intoxications II. In *Proceedings 318, Clinical Toxicology*, PGFVS, Univ. Sydney, 1998.
18. Fox LE et al: Reversal of ethylene glycol-induced nephrotoxicosis in a dog, *J Am Vet Med Assoc* 191(11):1433, 1987.
19. Penumarthy L, Oehme FW: Treatment of ethylene glycol toxicosis in cats, *Am J Vet Res* 36(2):209, 1975.
20. Hutchison TWS, Dykeman JC. Presumptive ethylene glycol poisoning in chickens, *Can Vet J* 38:647, 1997.
21. Spillane L: Multiple cranial nerve deficits after ethylene glycol poisoning, *Ann Emerg Med* 20:208-220, 1991.
22. DiBartola SP et al: Hemodialysis of a dog with acute renal failure, *J Am Vet Med Assoc* 186(12)1323, 1985.
23. Anderson B: Facial-auditory nerve oxalosis (Letter), *Am J Med* 88:87, 1990.
24. Maylin GA: A simple method for detecting ethylene glycol in urine by thin layer chromatography, *Cornell Vet* 70(2):202, 1980.
25. Adams WH et al: Early renal ultrasonographic findings in dogs with experimentally induced ethylene glycol nephrosis, *Am J Vet Res* 50(8):1370, 1989.
26. Adams WH et al: Ultrasonographic findings in dogs and cats with oxalate nephrosis attributed to ethylene glycol intoxication: 15 cases (1984-1988), *J Am Vet Med Assoc* 199(4):492, 1991.
27. Adaudi AO, Oehme FW: An activated charcoal hemoperfusion system for the treatment of barbital or ethylene glycol poisoning in dogs, *Clin Toxicol* 18(9):1105 1981.
28. Dial SM et al: Comparison of ethanol and 4-methylpyrazole as treatments for ethylene glycol intoxication in cats, *Am J Vet Res* 55(12):1771, 1994.
29. Marshall DA, Doty RL: Taste responses of dogs to ethylene glycol, propylene glycol, and ethylene glycol-based antifreeze, *J Am Vet Med Assoc* 197(12):1599, 1990.
30. Harry P et al: Ethylene glycol poisoning in a child treated with 4-methyl-pyrazole, *Pediatrics* 102(3):E31, 1998.

Fertilizers

1. Osweiler GD et al: *Clinical and diagnostic veterinary toxicology*, ed 3, Dubuque, Iowa, 1985, Kendal Hunt.
2. Campbell A, Chapman M: *Handbook of poisoning in dogs and cats*, London, 2000, Blackwell Science.
3. Gerken DF: In Bonagura JD, editor: *Kirk's current therapy XII*, Philadelphia, 1995, WB Saunders.
4. Yeary RA: Oral intubation of dogs with combinations of fertilizer, herbicide, and insecticide chemicals commonly used on lawns, *Am J Vet Res* 45:288, 1984.
5. Schmitz DG: In Reed SM, Bayly WM, editors: *Equine internal medicine*, Philadelphia, 1998, WB Saunders.
6. Haddad LM et al: *Clinical management of poisoning and drug overdose*, ed 3, Philadelphia, 1998, WB Saunders.
7. Dorman DC: In Bonagura JD, editor: *Current veterinary therapy XII*, Philadelphia, 1995, WB Saunders.
8. Leveille-Webste CR: In Morgan RV: *Handbook of small animal practice*, ed 3, Philadelphia, 1997, WB Saunders.

Gases

1. Lillie RJ: Air pollutants affecting the performance of domestic animals. A literature review. *Agriculture Handbook No. 380*, Washington, D.C., 1972, U.S. Department of Agriculture.
2. Curtis SE: *Environmental management in animal agriculture*, Ames, Iowa, 1983, Iowa State University Press.
3. National Research Council (Committee on Medical and Biologic Effects of Environmental Pollutants, Subcommittee on Ammonia): *Ammonia*, Baltimore, 1979, University Park Press.
4. Drummond JG et al: Effects of aerial ammonia on growth and health of young pigs, *J Anim Sci* 50:1085, 1980.
5. Drummond JG et al: Effects of atmospheric ammonia on pulmonary bacterial clearance in the young pig, *Am J Vet Res* 39:211, 1978.
6. Drummond JG et al: Effects of atmospheric ammonia on young pigs experimentally infected with *Bordetella bronchiseptica*, *Am J Vet Res* 42:963, 1981.
7. Drummond JG et al: Effects of atmospheric ammonia on young pigs experimentally infected with *Ascaris suum*, *Am J Vet Res* 42:969, 1981.
8. Donham KJ: Association of environmental air contaminants with disease and productivity in swine, *Am J Vet Res* 52:1723, 1991.
9. Hamilton TD et al: The synergistic role of gaseous ammonia in the aetiology of *Pasteurella multocida* induced atrophic rhinitis in swine, *J Clin Microbiol* 43:2185, 1996.
10. Urbain B et al: Quantitative assessment of aerial ammonia toxicity to the nasal mucosa by the use of the nasal gavage method in pigs, *Am J Vet Res* 55:1335, 1994.
11. Jones JB et al: Behavioral responses of pigs to atmospheric ammonia. In Bottcher RW, Hoff SK, editors: *Livestock environment V*, vol II, , St. Joseph, Mich, 1997, American Society of Agricultural Engineers.
12. Carlile FS: Ammonia in poultry houses: a literature review, *World Poultry Science* 40:99, 1984.
13. Hauser RH, Folsch DW: Methods for measuring atmospheric ammonia in poultry houses: review and approved practices, *J Vet Med* 35:579, 1988.
14. Nagaraja KV et al: Effect of ammonia on the quantitative clearance of *E. coli* from the lungs, air sacs, and livers of turkeys aerosol vaccinated against *E. coli*, *Am J Vet Res* 45:392, 1984.
15. Nagaraja KV: Scanning electron microscope studies of adverse effects of ammonia on tracheal tissues of turkeys, *Am J Vet Res* 44:1530, 1983.

16. Carson TL et al: *Anhydrous ammonia fertilizer poisoning in cattle: peracute death loss and sequelae.* Abstracts of 39th Annual Meeting of the American Association of Veterinary Laboratory Diagnosticians, Little Rock, Ark, October 12-18, 1996.

17. Morgan SE: Ammonia pipeline rupture: risk assessment to cattle, *Vet Human Toxicol* 39(3):159, 1997.

18. U.S. Public Health Service: Toxicity and potential dangers of aliphatic and aromatic hydrocarbons. Public health bulletin no. 255, Washington, D.C., 1940, U.S. Government Printing Office.

19. National Research Council (Committee on Medical and Biological Effects of Environmental Pollutants, subcommittee on Hydrogen Sulfide): *Hydrogen sulfide*, Baltimore, University Park Press, 1979.

20. Hoover SB et al: *Acute pit gas (hydrogen sulfide) poisoning in confined cattle.* Abstracts of 41st Annual Meeting of the American Association of Veterinary Laboratory Diagnosticians, Minneapolis, Minn, October 3-9, 1998.

21. Donham KJ: The concentration of swine production: effects on swine health, productivity, human health, and the environment, *Vet Clin North Am Food Anim Pract* 16(3):559, 2000.

22. Sayers RR et al: *Hydrogen sulfide as an industrial poison.* U.S. Bureau of Mines, Department of the Interior. Reports of Investigations, Serial no. 2491, Washington, DC, U.S. Department of the Interior, 1923.

23. Klenz RD, Fedde MR: Hydrogen sulfide: effects on avian respiratory control and intrapulmonary carbon dioxide receptors, *Respir Physiol* 32(3):355, 1978.

24. O'Donoghue JG: Hydrogen sulfide poisoning in swine, *Can J Compar Med Vet Sci* 25:217, 1961.

25. Curtis SE et al: Effects of aerial ammonia, hydrogen sulfide, and swine: house dust on rate of gain and respiratory tract structure in swine, *J Anim Sci* 41:735, 1975.

26. Landaw SA: Kinetic aspects of endogenous carbon monoxide production in experimental animals, *Ann N Y Acad Sci* 174:32, 1970.

27. Coburn RF: Biological effects of carbon monoxide, *Ann N Y Acad Sci* 174:369, 1970.

28. Bingham E et al: *Patty's toxicol*, vol. II, ed 5, New York, 2001, John Wiley & Sons.

29. Carson TL, Donham KJ: Carbon monoxide abortion in Iowa swine, *Am Assn Vet Lab Diagn* 21:179, 1978.

30. Dominick MA, Carson TL: Effects of carbon monoxide exposure on pregnant sows and their fetuses, *Am J Vet Res* 44:35, 1983.

31. National Research Council (Committee on Medical and Biologic Effects of Environmental Pollutants, subcommittee on Carbon Monoxide): *Carbon monoxide*, Washington, DC, 1977, National Academy of Sciences.

32. Carson TL: Carbon monoxide-induced stillbirth. In Kirkbride CA, editor: *Laboratory of livestock abortion*, 3rd ed, Ames, Iowa, 1990, State University Press.

33. Carson TL, Dominick MA: Diagnosis and experimental reproduction of carbon monoxide induced fetal death in swine, *Am Assn Vet Lab Diagn* 25:403, 1982.

34. Donham KJ et al: Carboxyhemoglobin values in swine relative to carbon monoxide exposure: guidelines for monitoring animal and human health hazards in swine-confinement buildings, *Am J Vet Res* 43:813, 1982.

35. Ilano AL, Raffin TA: Management of carbon monoxide poisoning, *Chest* 97:165, 1990.

36. National Research Council (Committee on Medical and Biologic Effects of Environmental Pollutants, subcommittee on Nitrogen Oxides): *Nitrogen oxides*, Wahington, DC, 1977, National Academy of Sciences.

37. Cutlip RC: Experimental nitrogen dioxide poisoning in cattle, *Pathol Vet* 3:474, 1966.

38. Beasley VR et al: *A systems approach to veterinary toxicology*, Urbana, Ill, 1994, University of Illinois.

Glyphosate Herbicides

1. Spectrum Laboratories: Chemical fact sheet case number 1071836, *http://www.speclab.com/compound/c1071836.htm*

2. EXTOXNET PIP-Glyphosate: *http://ace.orst.edu/cgi-bin/fms/0l/pips/glyphosa. htm.*

3. Poisindex® editorial staff: In Rumack BH et al, editors: *Poisindex® system*, vol 107, Englewood, Colo, Micromedex, expires March 2001.

4. Ahrens W: *Herbicide handbook*, ed 7, Champaign, Ill, 1974, Weed Science Society of America.

5. Wiersema R et al: Glyphosate degradation pathway: *htpp://umbbd.ahc. umn.edu/gly/gly_map.html.*

6. Beasley VR et al: Phenoxy herbicides. In *A systems approach to veterinary toxicology*, Urbana, Ill, 1999, University of Illinois.

Naphthalene

1. U.S. Department of Health and Human Services: *Toxicological profile for naphthalene (update)*, Springfield, Va, 1995, US Department of Commerce National Technical Information Service.

2. Leikin JB, Pacoucek FP: *Poisoning and toxicology compendium*, Hudson, Ohio, 1997, Lexicomp.

3. Beasley et al: *A systems affected approach to veterinary toxicology*, Urbana, Ill, 1994, University of Illinois.

4. Winkler JV et al: Mothball differentiation: naphthalene from paradichlorobenzene, *Ann Emerg Med* 14:30, 1984.

5. Desnoyers M, Hébert P: Heinz body anemia in a dog following possible naphthalene ingestion, *Vet Clin Pathol* 24:124, 1995.

6. Budavari S: *The Merck index*, ed 12, Whitehouse Station, N.J., 1996, Merck.

7. Agency for Toxic Substances and Disease Registry: *ATSDR public health statement, naphthalene*, Springfield, Va, 1990.

8. Bagchi M et al: Naphthalene-induced oxidative stress and DNA damage in cultured macrophage J774A.1 cells, *Free Rad Biol Med* 25:137, 1998.

9. Bagchi D et al: Induction of oxidative stress and DNA damage by chronic administration of naphthalene to rats, *Res Commun Mol Pathol Pharmacol* 101:249, 1998.

10. Anziulewicz J et al: Transplacental naphthalene poisoning, *Am J Obstet Gynecol* 78:519, 1957.

11. Witschi HR, Last JA: In Klaasen CD, editor: *Casarett and Doull's toxicology*, ed 5, New York, 1996, McGraw-Hill.

12. Potts AM: In Klaasen CD: *Casarett and Doull's toxicology*, ed 5, New York, 1996, McGraw-Hill.

13. Honda T et al: Alkylnaphthalene XI. Pulmonary toxicity of naphthalene, 2-methylnaphthalene, and isopropylnaphthalenes in mice, *Chem Pharm Bull* 38:3130, 1990.

Phenols

1. Lewis RJ: *Hawley's Condensed Chemical Dictionary*, ed 12, New York, 1993, Van Nostrand Reinhold.

2. Budavari S, editor: *The Merck index*, ed 12, Whitehouse Station, N.J., 1996, Merck.

3. USITC: *Synthetic organic chemicals, United States production and sales, 1986*, Washington, D.C., 1987, U.S. Government Printing Office Publication no. 2009.

4. Sittig M: *Handbook of toxic and hazardous chemicals and carcinogens*, ed 3, Park Ridge, N.J., 1991, Noyes Publications.

5. Goodman LS, Gilman AG: *The pharmacological basis of therapeutics*, ed 7, New York, 1985, Macmillan.

6. Capel ID, French MR, Millburn P et al: Fate of [^{14}C]-phenol in various species, *Xenobiotica* 2:25, 1972.

7. Edwards VT, Hones BC, Hutson DH: A comparison of the metabolic fate of phenol, phenyl glucoside and phenyl 6-O-malonyl-glucoside in the rat, *Xenobiotica* 16:801, 1986.

8. French MR, Bababunmi EA, Golding RR et al: The conjugation of phenol, benzoic acid, 1-naphthylacetic acid and sulfadimethoxine in the lion, civet, and genet, *FEBS Lett* 46:134, 1974.

9. Kao J, Bridges JW, Faulkner JK: Metabolism of [^{14}C] phenol by sheep, pig, rat, *Xenobiotica* 9:141, 1979.

10. Kenyon EM, Seeley ME, Janszen D et al: Dose-, route-, and sex-dependent urinary excretion of phenol metabolites in B6C3F₁ mice, *J Toxicol Environ Health* 44:219, 1995.

11. Hughes MF, Hall LL: Disposition of phenol in rat after oral, dermal, intravenous, and intratracheal administration, *Xenobiotica* 25:873, 1995.

12. Deichmann WB: Phenol studies. V. The distribution, detoxification, and excretion of phenol in the mammalian body, *Arch Biochem* 3:345, 1944.

13. Liao TF, Oehme FW: Tissue distribution and plasma protein binding of [¹⁴C] phenol in rats, *Toxicol Appl Pharmacol* 57:220, 1981.

14. Cassidy MK, Houston JB: *In vivo* capacity of hepatic and extra hepatic enzymes to conjugate phenol, *Drug Metab Disp* 12:619, 1984.

15. Powell GM, Miller JJ, Olavesen AH et al: Liver as major organ of phenol detoxification, *Nature* (London) 252:234, 1974.

16. Quebbemann AJ, Anders MW: Renal tubular conjugation and excretion of phenol and p-nitrophenol in the chicken: differing mechanisms of renal transfer, *J Pharmacol Exp Ther* 184:695, 1973.

17. Horch R, Spilker G, Start GB: Phenol burns and intoxications, *Burns* 20:45, 1994.

18. Miller JJ, Powell GM, Olavesen AH et al: The toxicity of dimethoxyphenol and related compounds in the cat, *Toxicol Appl Pharmacol* 3:47, 1976.

19. Mehta R, Hirom PC, Millburn P: The influence of dose on the pattern of conjugation of phenol and 1-naphthol in nonhuman primates, *Xenobiotica* 8:445, 1978.

20. Zamponi GW: Arrhythmias during phenol therapies: a specific action on cardiac sodium channels? *Circulation* 89:914, 1994.

21. Botta SA, Straith RE, Goodwin HH: Cardiac arrhythmias in phenol face peeling: a suggested protocol for prevention, *Aesth Plast Surg* 12:115, 1988.

22. Soares ER, Tift JP: Phenol poisoning: three fatal cases, *J Forensic Sci* 27:729, 1982.

23. Dorman DC, Clark JO: Common household chemical hazard. In Bonagura JD, editor: *Kirk's current veterinary therapy XIII small animal practice*, Philadelphia, 2000, WB Saunders.

24. Deichmann WB, Keplinger ML: Phenols and phenolic compounds. In Patty FA, editor: *Industrial hygiene and toxicology*, vol II, *Toxicology*, ed 2, New York, 1962, Interscience Publishers.

25. RTECS®: *Registry of toxic effects of chemical substances. National Institute for Occupational Safety and Health, Cincinnati, OH* (CD-ROM Version), Englewood, Colo, 1999, Micromedex.

26. Deichmann WB, Witherup S: Phenol studies: VI. The acute and comparative toxicity of phenol and o-, m-, and p-cresols for experimental animals, *J Pharmacol Exp Ther* 80:233, 1944.

27. Narotsky MG, Kavlock RJ: A multidisciplinary approach to toxicological screening: II. Developmental toxicity, *J Toxicol Environ Health* 45:145, 1995.

28. Moser VC, Cheek BM, MacPhail RC: A multidisciplinary approach to toxicological screening: III. Neurobehavioral toxicity, *J Toxicol Environ Health* 45:173, 1995.

29. Conning DM, Hayes MJ: The dermal toxicity of phenol: an investigation of the most effective first-aid measures, *Br J Ind Med* 27:155, 1970.

30. Flickinger CW: The benzenediols: catechol, resorcinol and hydroquinone— a review of the industrial toxicology and current industrial exposure limits, *Am Ind Hyg Assoc J* 37:596, 1976.

31. Pullin TG, Pinkerton MN, Johnston RV et al: Decontamination of the skin of swine following phenol exposure: a comparison of the relative efficacy of water versus polyethylene glycol/industrial methylated spirits, *Toxicol Appl Pharmacol* 43:199, 1978.

32. Wexler MR, Halon DA, Teitelbaum A et al: The prevention of cardiac arrhythmias produced in an animal model by the topical application of a phenol preparation in common use for face peeling, *Plast Reconstr Surg* 73:595, 1984.

33. Sandage C: *Tolerance criteria for continuous inhalation exposure to toxic material: I. Effects on animals of 90-day exposure to phenol, CCl₄ and a mixture of indole, skatole, H₂S and methyl mercaptan*, Wright-Patterson Air Force Base, Ohio, 1961, U.S. Air Force Systems Command, Aeronautical Systems Division, ASD technical report 61-519 (I).

34. Murphy JC, Osterberg RE, Seabaugh VM et al: Ocular irritancy responses to various pHs of acids and bases with and without irrigation, *Toxicology* 23:281, 1982.

35. DeCeaurriz JC, Micillion JC, Bonnet P et al: Sensory irritation caused by various industrial airborne chemicals, *Toxicol Lett* (Amst) 9:137, 1981.

36. Spiller HA, Quadrani, KDA, Cleveland P: A five year evaluation of acute exposures to phenol disinfectant (26%), *J Toxicol Clin Toxicol* 31:307, 1993.

37. Coppock RW, Mostrom MS, Lillie LE: The toxicology of detergents, bleaches, antiseptics and disinfectants in small animals, *Vet Human Toxicol* 30:463, 1988.

38. Gieger TL, Correa SS, Taboada J et al: Phenol poisoning in three dogs, *J Am Anim Hosp Assoc* 36:317, 2000.

39. Hsieh G-C, Sharma RP, Parker RDR et al: Immunological and neuro-biochemical alterations induced by repeated oral exposure of phenol in mice, *Eur J Pharmacol* 228:107, 1992.

40. Fertman MH, Fertman MB: Toxic anemias and Heinz bodies, *Medicine* 34:131, 1955.

41. Smith RP, Olson MV: Drug-induced methemoglobinemia, *Semin Hematol* 10:253, 1973.

42. Dalin NM, Kristoffersson R: Physiological effects of a sublethal concentration of inhaled phenol on the rat, *Ann Zool Fenn* 11:93, 1974.

43. Berman E, Schlicht M, Moser VC et al: A multidisciplinary approach to toxicological screening: I. Systemic toxicity, *J Toxicol Environ Health* 45:127, 1995.

44. Hunter DM, Timerding BL, Lenonard RB et al: Effects of isopropyl alcohol, ethanol, and polyethylene glycol/industrial methylated spirits in the treatment of acute phenol burns, *Ann Emerg Med* 21:1303, 1992.

45. Ciranni R, Barale R, Marrazzini A et al: Benzene and the genotoxicity of its metabolites: I. Transplacental activity in mouse fetuses and in their dams, *Mutat Res* 208:61, 1988.

46. Nieminer E, Heikkile P: Simultaneous determination of phenol, cresols, and xylenols in workplace air using a polystyrene-divinylbenzene column and electrochemical detection, *J Chromatogr* 360:271, 1986.

47. Foxall PJD, Bending MR, Gartland KPR et al: Acute renal failure following accidental cutaneous absorption of phenol: application of NMR urinalysis to monitor disease process, *Human Toxicol* 9:491, 1989.

48. Tanaka T, Kasai K, Kita T et al: Distribution of phenol in a fatal poisoning case determined by gas chromatography/mass spectrometry, *J Forensic Sci* 43:1086, 1998.

49. Bennett IL, James DF, Golden A: Severe acidosis due to phenol poisoning, *Ann Intern Med* 32:324, 1950.

Pine Oil

1. Trammel HL, Dorman DC, Beasley VR et al: *Ninth annual report of the Illinois Animal Poison Information Center*, Dubuque, Iowa, 1989, Kendall Hunt.

2. Koppel C, Tenczer J, Tennesmann U et al: Acute poisoning with pine oil: metabolism of monoterpenes, *Arch Toxicol* 49:73, 1981.

3. Tobin T, Swerczek TW, Blake JW: Pine oil toxicity in the horse: drug detection residues and pathological changes, *Res Commun Chem Pathol Pharmacol* 15:291, 1976.

4. Gornel DL, Goldman R: Acute renal failure following hexal-induced abortion, *JAMA* 203:146, 1968.

5. Tauscher JW, Polich JJ: Treatment of pine oil poisoning by exchange transfusion, *J Pediatr* 55:511, 1959.

6. Hill RM, Barer J, Hill LL et al: An investigation of recurrent pine oil poisoning in an infant by the use of gas chromatographic-mass spectrometric methods, *J Pediatr* 87:115, 1975.

7. Brook MP, McCarron MM, Mueller JA: Pine oil cleaner ingestion, *Ann Emerg Med* 18:391, 1989.

8. RTECS®: *Registry of Toxic Effects of Chemical Substances. National Institute for Occupational Safety and Health, Cincinnati, OH* (CD-ROM Version), Englewood, Colo, 1999, Micromedex.

9. Dorman, DC, Clark, JO: Common household chemical hazard. In Bonagura JD, editor: *Kirk's current veterinary therapy XIII small animal practice,* Philadelphia, 2000, WB Saunders.
10. Coppock RW, Mostrom MS, Lillie LE: The toxicology of detergents, bleaches, antiseptics, and disinfectants in small animals, *Vet Human Toxicol* 30:463, 1988.
11. Rousseaux CG, Smith RA, Nicholson S: Acute Pine-Sol toxicity in a domestic cat, *Vet Human Toxicol* 28:316, 1986.
12. McGuigan MA: Turpentine, *Clin Toxicol Rev* 8:1, 1985.
13. Kore AM, Kiesche-Nesselrodt A: Toxicology of household cleaning products and disinfectants, *Vet Clin North Am Small Anim Pract* 20(2):533, 1990.

Propylene Glycol

1. Christopher MM et al: Contribution of propylene glycol-induced Heinz body formation to anemia in cats, *J Am Vet Med Assoc* 194(8):1045, 1989.
2. LaKind JS et al: A review of the comparative mammalian toxicity of ethylene glycol and propylene glycol, *Crit Rev Toxicol* 29(4):331, 1999.
3. Myers VS, Usenik EA: Propylene glycol intoxication of horses, *J Am Vet Med Assoc* 155(12):1841, 1969.
4. Dorman DC, Haschek WM: Fatal propylene glycol toxicosis in a horse, *J Am Vet Med Assoc* 198(9):1643-1644, 1991.
5. McClanahan S et al: Propylene glycol toxicosis in a mare, *Vet Human Toxicol* 40(5):294, 1998.
6. Christopher MM et al: Propylene glycol ingestion causes D-lactic acidosis, *Lab Invest* 62(1):114, 1990.
7. Christopher MM et al: Erythrocyte pathology and mechanisms of Heinz body-mediated hemolysis in cats, *Vet Pathol* 27:299, 1990.
8. Weiss DJ et al: Effects of propylene glycol-containing diets on acetaminophen-induced methemoglobinemia in cats, *J Am Vet Med Assoc* 196(11):1816, 1990.
9. Bauer MC et al: Hematologic alterations in adult cats fed 6 or 12% propylene glycol, *Am J Vet Res* 53(1):69, 1991.
10. Weil CS et al: Results of feeding propylene glycol in the diet to dogs for two years, *Food Cosmet Toxicol* 9:479, 1971.
11. Pintchuk PA et al: Propylene glycol toxicity in adult dairy cows, *J Vet Int Med* 7:150, 1993.
12. Hickman MA et al: Effect of diet on Heinz body formation in kittens, *J Vet Res* 50(3):475, 1990.

Turpentine

1. Trammel HL, Dorman DC, Beasley VR et al: *Ninth annual report of the Illinois Animal Poison Information Center,* Dubuque, Iowa, 1989, Kendall Hunt.
2. Gosselin RE, Smith RP, Hodge HC, editors: *Clinical toxicology of commercial products,* ed 5, Baltimore, 1984, Williams & Wilkins.
3. Windholz M, editor: *The Merck index, ed 11,* Rahway, NJ, 1989, Merck.
4. McGuigan MA: Turpentine, *Clin Toxicol Rev* 8:1, 1985.
5. Sperling F: *In vivo* and *in vitro* toxicology of turpentines, *Clin Toxicol* 2:21, 1969.
6. Jakobson I, Wahlberg JE, Holmberg B et al: Uptake via the blood and elimination of 10 organic solvents following epicutaneous exposure of anesthetized guinea pigs, *Toxicol Appl Pharmacol* 63:181, 1982.
7. Dice WH, Ward G, Kelley J et al: Pulmonary toxicity following gastrointestinal ingestion of kerosene, *Ann Emerg Med* 11:138, 1982.
8. RTECS®: *Registry of Toxic Effects of Chemical Substances. National Institute for Occupational Safety and Health, Cincinnati, OH* (CD-ROM Version), Englewood, Colo, 1999, Micromedex.
9. Ervin ME: Petroleum distillates and turpentine. In Haddad LM, Winchester JF, editors: *Clinical management of poisoning and drug overdose,* Philadelphia, 1983, WB Saunders.
10. Steele RW, Conklin RH, Mark HM: Corticosteroids and antibiotics for the treatment of fulminate hydrocarbon aspiration, *JAMA* 219:1434, 1972.
11. Decker WJ, Corby DG, Hilburn RE et al: Adsorption of solvents to activated charcoal, polymers, and mineral sorbents, *Vet Hum Toxicol* 23:44, 1981.
12. Edwards WC, Niles GA: Dermatitis induced by diesel fuel on dairy cows, *Vet Med Small Anim Clin* 76:873, 1981.
13. Jacobziner H, Raybin HW: Turpentine poisoning, *Arch Pediatr* 78:357, 1961.
14. NIOSH: *Pocket guide to chemical hazards. National Institute for Occupational Safety and Health, Cincinnati, OH* (CD-ROM Version). Englewood, Colo, 2000, Micromedex, (expires April 30, 2000).
15. Kaye S: *Handbook of emergency toxicology,* ed 3. Springfield, Ill, 1973, Thomas.
16. Dorman DC: Petroleum distillates and turpentine, *Vet Clin North Am Small Anim Pract* 20(2):505, 1990.
17. Coppock RW, Mostrom MS, Lillie LE: The toxicology of detergents, bleaches, antiseptics, and disinfectants in small animals, *Vet Human Toxicol* 30:463, 1988.

21

Insecticides and Molluscicides

AMITRAZ

Sharon Gwaltney-Brant

Synonyms. Amitraz has a chemical name of *N'*-(2,4-dimethylphenyl)-*N*-[[(2,4-dimethylphenyl)imino]methyl]-*N*-methylmethanimidamide. Common names for amitraz include amitraze, triazid, and azaform.[1] Trade names of products containing amitraz include BAAM, Ectodex, Mitaban, Preventic, Point-Guard, Taktic, and Triatox.

Sources. Amitraz is a synthetic formamidine acaricide that is labeled for topical use to control ticks, mites, and lice on cattle, pigs, and dogs. The use of amitraz on horses is contraindicated because there are potentially life-threatening complications.[2] For livestock use amitraz is available as a pour-on product and as a dip. For dogs amitraz formulations include dips, shampoos, and tick collars. Although amitraz has been used on cats,[3] it is not approved for such use. Amitraz is also used as an agricultural pesticide for crops, particularly fruit trees. Commercial solutions may contain up to 75% xylene or other solvents, which may contribute to toxicity.

Toxicokinetics. Amitraz has rapid oral absorption in most species. Ingested amitraz is rapidly metabolized in the stomach to at least six metabolites, several of which are active.[1] Peak blood levels occur in 3 hours after oral exposure in dogs. Amitraz metabolites are excreted primarily through the urine over 48 hours, although some fecal excretion occurs.[1] Dermal absorption is relatively low (13.8% in rats), although toxicosis in dogs dipped in amitraz has been reported.[4]

Mechanism of Action. The toxic effects of amitraz are primarily due to α_2-adrenergic agonist activity in the central nervous system (CNS), resulting in sedation.[1] Amitraz also inhibits monoamine oxidase and has weak antiserotonin activity, contributing to CNS depression. Amitraz also has some peripheral α_1- and α_2-adrenergic activity. The bradycardia induced by amitraz is thought to be due to alteration of autonomic function rather than to a direct effect on the heart.[1] Amitraz-induced mydriasis is due to stimulation of postsynaptic α_2 receptors.[1] Amitraz decreases intestinal motility by inhibiting smooth muscle contractility; in horses and ponies a reduction in colonic blood flow has also been associated with administration of amitraz.[1] Amitraz-induced hyperglycemia is thought to be due in part to α_2-adrenergic–mediated suppression of insulin release.[5,6] Amitraz is a weak inhibitor of platelet aggregation and has antipyretic and antiinflammatory activities.[1] Amitraz has no effect on serum acetylcholinesterase activity.[7]

Toxicity and Risk Factors. Amitraz is classified by the Environmental Protection Agency (EPA) as slightly toxic to mammals if ingested orally.[8] Oral and dermal lethal dose 50s (LD_{50}) for several species are listed in Table 21-1. In a 2-year chronic toxicity study in dogs ingestion of 0.25 mg/kg/day was determined to be the no observed effect level (NOEL), whereas dosages of 1 mg/kg/day resulted in CNS depression, ataxia, vomiting, transient bradycardia, hyperglycemia, and hypothermia.[8] Rats fed 50 mg/kg/day had slight decreases in food and water intake, but no other significant clinical abnormalities.[8]

Horses and ponies appear to be particularly susceptible to intestinal stasis induced by amitraz, and fatal ileus has resulted from the use of amitraz on these animals.[1,2,9] This sensitivity may be related to species-related differences in

TABLE 21-1 Acute LD_{50} Values for Amitraz

Species (route)	LD_{50} (mg/kg)
Rat (oral)	523
(dermal)	1600
Mouse (oral)	>1600
Rabbit (oral)	>100
(dermal)	>200
Dog (oral)	100
Pig (oral)	>100
Baboon (oral)	100
Guinea pig (oral)	400

From Knowles CO: In Hayes WJ, Laws ER: *Handbook of pesticide toxicology*, vol 3, San Diego, 1991, Academic Press.

distribution and elimination of amitraz metabolites,[10] or sensitivity of equines to decreases in colonic blood flow caused by amitraz.[1]

Improper mixing of amitraz concentrates before application on livestock or inappropriate use of amitraz products on equines are common causes of amitraz toxicosis in large animals, although transient depression anorexia and ataxia sometimes occur at recommended levels.[1] Amitraz toxicosis has developed in dogs dipped in amitraz solutions at recommended levels.[4] Additionally, ingestion of amitraz collars is a potential cause of toxicosis in dogs.[11] Less commonly, pets or livestock may be exposed through aerial spraying of crops, accidental spills resulting in water or food contamination, and malicious poisonings.

Clinical Signs.   Because many formulations of amitraz include xylene as a carrier, some of the signs resulting from exposure to amitraz compounds may be secondary to xylene toxicosis.[12] Signs of amitraz toxicosis generally begin within 2 to 4 hours of dermal or oral exposure, although in some cases onset of signs is delayed up to 12 hours.[2,13] Clinical signs that have been associated with amitraz toxicosis in dogs and cats include vomiting, depression, disorientation, ataxia, ileus, bradycardia, hypertension or hypotension, hypothermia, coma, and seizures.[14] In ruminants, salivation, depression, anorexia, ataxia, disorientation, tremors, decreased milk production, and coma have been reported.[14] Horses display similar neurologic signs; furthermore, they are particularly prone to the development of ileus, with resulting large intestinal impaction and severe colic.[2,9]

Death resulting from amitraz toxicosis is usually due to profound bradycardia, CNS depression leading to respiratory depression, or, especially in equines, complications of ileus (e.g., intestinal impaction with subsequent vascular compromise, shock, and sepsis).[1,9,13]

Clinical Pathology.   Hyperglycemia has been reported in several species in relation to exposure to amitraz.[1,6,13] Alterations of serum alkaline phosphatase, albumin-globulin ratios, serum potassium, and alanine aminotransferase have been reported in rats in long-term amitraz feeding trials,[1] but similar alterations have not commonly been associated with acute amitraz toxicosis in domestic animals.

Lesions.   In most species few gross or histopathologic lesions are expected in cases of amitraz toxicosis. In equines large intestinal impaction may be seen at necropsy. Long-term feeding studies in dogs and rats revealed only mild and nonspecific histopathologic alterations in the liver and adrenal gland.[1]

Diagnostic Testing.   Amitraz can be detected in stomach contents, urine, feces, and tissues of animals using gas chromatography (GC)-mass spectrometry.[14] In addition, the amitraz metabolite 4-amino-3-methylbenzoic acid has been detected in the urine of humans, although the availability of such testing is not known.[1]

Treatment.   The aims of treatment are to stabilize the patient, prevent further exposure, and provide supportive care. Yohimbine[6,15] and atipamezole[13] have been used in several species to successfully reverse the bradycardia, CNS depression, and hyperglycemia caused by amitraz toxicosis. Atropine is contraindicated in the treatment of amitraz-induced bradycardia, because it can potentiate both hypertension and ileus.[16] Seizures generally respond to diazepam; a barbiturate may be used if diazepam is ineffective, although this compounds any CNS and cardiovascular depression.

Once the animal is stable, dermal exposures can be decontaminated by bathing the animal with a mild detergent and water; because hypothermia is common in amitraz toxicosis, appropriate measures should be taken to keep the animal warm during and after bathing. When mild signs have developed after appropriate topical use of amitraz, no further treatment is usually necessary and signs should subside within 24 to 72 hours.[14]

Emesis may be induced early in oral amitraz exposures; because of the risk of aspiration, emesis is contraindicated in symptomatic animals or in cases of ingestion of formulations containing high percentages of xylene or other volatile solvents. The decision to use activated charcoal in the face of potential amitraz-induced ileus must be made with care. Activated charcoal adsorbs amitraz, but if ileus develops before the charcoal has passed, the amitraz may eventually be released from the charcoal and be available for absorption. In addition, if intestinal surgery becomes necessary, activated charcoal in the gastrointestinal tract may complicate matters. Saline cathartics are recommended whether or not activated charcoal is used.[14] Surgery to remove ingested amitraz collar pieces may be required.

General supportive care includes maintenance of normal body temperature, intravenous (IV) fluid therapy for cardiovascular support, and maintenance of normal gastrointestinal motility.

Prognosis.   With prompt and appropriate treatment, the prognosis in most cases of amitraz toxicosis is good.[13] The prognosis for comatose, seizuring, or moribund animals, or for equines exhibiting evidence of ileus must be considered guarded.

Prevention and Control.   Proper mixing and administration of amitraz per label directions minimize the risk of toxicosis. Amitraz collars should be fitted properly and any excess collar length should be cut off to minimize the risk of the collar being chewed or ingested.

ANTICHOLINESTERASE INSECTICIDES

Gavin L. Meerdink

Synonyms.   Besides the widespread use of anticholinesterases for insect control, some have been developed for chemical warfare and are referred to as "nerve gases."

Sources.   Organophosphorus (OP) and carbamate insecticides have been in common use in agriculture, gardens, and homes since the 1970s. Not all of these are cholinesterase inhibitors; some formulations are used as herbicides or fungicides. Insecticides can be in spray, powder, or granule form.

Aerial spraying can be circumstantially associated with animal illness. Spray dispersion is a function of droplet size and wind velocity. Amounts hazardous to animal health are not likely to be distributed long distances by this method. Most OP insecticides (except dichlorvos) have comparatively low volatility.[1]

Other potential sources can come from medications. Certain members of this class of compounds are used as therapeutic agents, such as deworming products for animals. Some that cross the blood-brain barrier have been proposed for the treatment of Alzheimer's disease. [2]

Toxicokinetics. Most of the agents are absorbed readily by any route. The rate is influenced by lipid solubility and formulation. The agents undergo oxidation and hydrolysis by esterases, namely carboxylesterases and paraoxonases, that are found in the plasma and liver.[2] A variety of conjugation reactions follow primary metabolic processes. Excretion is via urine and feces. Most OPs are excreted as hydrolysis products in the urine.[1,2] The rate of metabolism and excretion may be reduced by the inhibition of esters by the insecticide.[3]

Many of the OPs, specifically the phosphorothioate and phosphorodithioate compounds, contain a sulfur attached by double bond to the phosphorus. The sulfur is exchanged for oxygen by cytochrome P-450 metabolism in the hepatocyte. This "lethal synthesis," oxygen for sulfur substitution, accounts for the full potential efficacy as an insecticide.[1,2]

Mechanism of Action. Acetylcholine transfers impulses at cholinergic nerve synapses and at neuromuscular junctions. Acetylcholine is catabolized (in 0.1 msec) by acetylcholinesterase, or other cholinesterases (ChE), to acetic acid and choline. OP and carbamate insecticides produce their toxic effects by binding with ChE enzymes, thereby inhibiting the catabolism of the acetylcholine. Poisoning is caused by overstimulation of the end organ as a result of the accumulation of acetylcholine. Death results primarily from respiratory failure, often with a cardiovascular component.[1-3]

Like acetylcholine, OP and carbamate insecticides share a structural compatibility with acetylcholinesterase and other ChE and readily bind to at least one of three sites of the ChE enzymes. The more structurally suited relative to binding, the higher the affinity and the more effective the insecticide is in producing the anticholinergic effect. OPs in general have higher affinity for the enzyme sites than do the carbamates. Therefore, OPs are often referred to as "irreversible" inhibitors and carbamates as "reversible" inhibitors of ChE because they can spontaneously dislodge from the enzyme. This distinction is not absolute and cannot be used as a strict separation of the two insecticide groups.[2,4] The stability of the OP-ChE enzyme bond is enhanced through "aging," which is caused by the loss of one of the alkyl groups.[2]

Toxicity and Risk Factors. Errors in use, mixing, or storage of unused materials are common reasons for animal

exposures that result in poisoning. Given the high toxicity of several of these agents, animals have been poisoned by licking empty bags. The color or odor of some insecticides may aid in identification by owners but does not seem to deter ingestion by animals.

Although these two groups of insecticides include some of the most toxic products ever marketed (e.g., LD_{50} of less than 1 mg/kg body weight), the range of toxicity is wide. Consideration of the formula concentration or conditions of use is likely a more important factor for the clinician in deciding the likelihood of poisoning. Listings of toxicities for these insecticides can be found in product data sheets and other publications (e.g., *Farm Chemicals Handbook*[5]). Young animals are poisoned by a lower dose of these agents because of immature development of the hydrolyzing enzyme systems.

Repeated exposure, as might occur with grazing of contaminated pastures or frequent spraying, can be a clinical concern. Most agents from these two groups are metabolized rapidly and excreted within a few days, whereas ChE regeneration requires approximately 2 weeks. Thus, the additive enzyme inhibition is clinically more significant than accumulation of the insecticide in the body.

When a pour-on product containing chlorpyrifos was found to produce unexpected effects in dairy bulls, the label was changed to restrict its use on dairy breeds of any age and bulls of any breed older than 8 months of age. Cholinesterase depression was demonstrated in blood and brain tissues. Heavier, aggressive, older bulls were reported to be more sensitive to chlorpyrifos. This was associated with higher circulating testosterone concentrations.[6]

Clinical Signs. Clinical signs from an excess of these agents result from the overstimulation of the cholinergic nervous system, skeletal muscles, and, to a lesser degree, the CNS. Clinical signs of acute poisoning can occur within 30 minutes, usually within 6 hours, and certainly within 12 hours after exposure. Dermal exposure can result in signs of intoxication within a few hours but may be delayed a few days depending on the rate of absorption.

The duration from the onset of clinical signs to death may be a few minutes to several hours. Sudden collapse and apparent suffocation, occasionally with epistaxis, has been observed from large oral doses. Lesser doses or repeated exposures can result in anorexia, lethargy, and diarrhea of several days' duration.

The progression of clinical signs with acute poisoning often begins with an appearance of apprehension or uneasiness. Evidence of abdominal discomfort with a tucked posture and foot stomping or kicking might be observed. Salivation and lacrimation become more copious and can be accompanied by frequent urination and defecation (collectively known as the *SLUD signs*). Initial fine muscle tremors become more generalized and pronounced, leading to stiffened, jerky movements with ataxia. Dyspnea from increased bronchial secretions and presumably bronchoconstriction becomes pronounced. Convulsive seizures may occur before coma, respiratory depression, and death. Clonic seizures are more often observed in small animals than in ruminants.

The term *intermediate syndrome* has been applied to clinical signs of apparent muscular weakness that occur several days after exposure and that are accompanied by persistent low blood ChE activity. OPs with high lipid solubility and prolonged metabolism from system (cardiovascular, hepatic, or renal) impairment are thought to be involved.[7] A common example is a syndrome in cats that exhibit anorexia, profound weakness, and depression following exposure to chlorpyrifos.

A *delayed neuropathy syndrome* referred to as "Ginger Jake" paralysis arose during the days of prohibition when Jamaican ginger extract contaminated with triorthocresyl phosphate (TOCP) was consumed in place of alcohol. Triarylphosphates, of which TOCP is an example, and certain fluorine-containing alkylorganophosphorus compounds are capable of inducing delayed neurotoxicosis. At least 1 week to approximately 1 month after ingestion of the toxic agent, evidence of sensation deficits or pain leads to weakness and ataxia. Eventually, paralysis changes from flaccid to spastic. Any recovery is slow and usually incomplete. Toxicity is not related to inhibition of ChEs, but another esterase, referred to as a neurotoxic esterase, is inhibited. Systemic effects appear limited to the nervous system and include axon and myelin sheath lesions.[1,2]

Clinical Pathology. Although results are inconsistent, decreased serum potassium and increased serum magnesium have been reported with poisoning.[8] Consistent changes in clinical pathologic parameters do not occur and likely are related to secondary tissue and metabolic changes.

Lesions. Pulmonary edema often is evident at necropsy. Severity varies and is not useful as a diagnostic determinant. Salivation, tracheal fluid, diarrhea, and other signs of cholinergic stimulation might be observed.

Diagnostic Testing. Confirmation of OP or carbamate insecticide poisoning includes (1) detection of the insecticide in ingesta or tissues, (2) demonstration of the adverse biological effect, that is, ChE inhibition, and (3) clinical signs and history consistent with this poisoning.

Specimens for diagnostic submission from the clinical patient should include whole blood for ChE activity determination and vomitus, urine, and suspect material for identification of the agent. Postmortem samples should also contain brain, eyes (retina), liver, and stomach contents. These samples should be submitted chilled (eyes, in particular, should not be frozen to prevent destruction of the retina). An entire brain or hemisphere should be submitted because ChE activity is associated with nuclei and is not homogeneous throughout the tissue. Sections of appropriate tissues for histology should also be saved in 10% formalin for thorough diagnostic investigation.

Treatment. Poisoning by these agents progresses rapidly; treatment must be instituted as soon as possible. Artificial respiration may be successful in maintaining the animal while waiting for the return of sufficient muscular activity. Respiratory failure is the principal cause of death from these insecticides.

Atropine blocks the effects of the excess acetylcholine at the neuromuscular junction. It can control the muscarinic signs, but not the nicotinic signs. Therapeutic response is expected from a dose of 0.25 to 1 mg/kg of atropine. To shorten the response time, about one fourth of the dose can be administered intravenously. The dose should be adjusted by assessing the degree of atropinization, that is, secretion production and heart rate.

Because relapses are common, repeated atropine administration may be necessary to control the return of clinical signs (usually every 2 to 4 hours). The response to atropine becomes less apparent with each successive treatment.

Dosages must be monitored judiciously to prevent overtreatment, especially when treatment is prolonged. Horses are particularly prone to develop ileus from atropine, so no more than a total dose of 65 mg is advised for the average horse.

Activated charcoal is given orally to bind insecticide in the alimentary tract to prevent absorption. This addition to the treatment regimen is beneficial, particularly for ruminants with their large rumen stores, and should be administered as soon as the animal's condition is stabilized.

Oximes, such as pralidoxime Cl, dissociate the insecticide-ChE bond and attach to the insecticide, which allows for reactivation of the ChE enzyme. Because the bond between OPs (but not carbamates) and ChE becomes stronger with time, the efficacy of oximes is better within 24 hours after exposure. The affinity between ChE and carbamates is less than that for OPs; therefore, oximes are not recommended for carbamate insecticide poisoning.[2] Excessive doses of the oximes are contraindicated because these drugs have the molecular capability to inhibit ChE themselves.

Animals with dermal exposure should be washed as quickly as possible with soap and water to prevent further absorption. Other therapeutic measures include diazepam (Valium, Roche Laboratories, Nutley, N.J.), which has been used in addition to atropine or the atropine-oxime combination, and appears to prevent some central effects of accumulated acetylcholine and the bradycardia produced by anticholinergics.[9] Diphenhydramine (Benadryl, Park, Davis & Co., Morris Plains, N.J.) can block effects of nicotine receptor overstimulation and prevent paralysis in dogs.[10]

Drugs that interfere with ChE activity such as morphine, physostigmine, phenothiazine tranquilizers, pyridostigmine, neostigmine, and succinylcholine are contraindicated.[11]

Prognosis. If the dose of anticholinesterase insecticide is not overwhelming and the animal responds to treatment, the prognosis is favorable.

DIETHYLTOLUAMIDE

David Dorman

Synonyms. Diethyltoluamide (DEET) is the common name for *N,N*-diethyl-m-toluamide, a multipurpose insect repellent registered for direct application to human skin, clothing, and household pets. The most commonly used insect repellent is the meta-substituted isomer (*N,N*-diethyl-m-toluamide; *m*-DEET). The *ortho*- and *para*-isomers are also highly repellent but are less effective than *m*-DEET. Additional synonyms for DEET include detamide, diethylbenzemide, diethyl toluamide, m-delphene, and metadelphene, and it is also known by the acronyms DET, DETA, and M-DET.

DEET-based insect repellents are widely used. It is the active ingredient in products such as Autan (Bayer AG, Kansas City, Mo.), Cutters (Cutter Laboratories, Berkeley, Calif.), and Deep Woods Off (S.C. Johnson Wax, Inc., Racine, Wis.).

Sources. DEET-based insect repellents contain from 5% to 100% DEET and are formulated as solutions, gels, sticks, aerosol sprays, and impregnated towelettes. DEET-based repellents may contain ethanol or isopropyl alcohol as solvent carriers, whereas other products contain DEET in a microencapsulated form. A number of products with DEET have veterinary application. For example, a combination insecticide and repellent product (Hartz Blockade), composed of 9% DEET and 0.09% fenvalerate, was developed for the control of fleas and other ectoparasites on dogs and cats; however, this product has been recently discontinued.

Toxicokinetics. A number of experimental studies using in vivo and in vitro approaches have evaluated the dermal absorption of DEET.[2] These experiments have shown that DEET is well absorbed from intact skin and is rapidly distributed to most tissues including the brain and the fetus. Peak plasma concentrations are observed in dogs within 1 to 2 hours after dermal application.[1]

Plasma clearance of DEET is considered rapid (half-life of hours). Accumulation and persistence of DEET in the skin and dermis of topically exposed individuals, however, may occur and can contribute to delays in whole-body elimination. The primary route of excretion of DEET is urinary, with enterohepatic elimination playing a more minor role. The metabolism of DEET by most veterinary species is incompletely understood. Hippuric and m-toluric acid have been identified in the urine of rats and rabbits exposed to a DEET aerosol. Urinary excretion of glucuronide metabolites of DEET has also been demonstrated. Whether cats could be more sensitive to DEET-based products because of their lack of ability to glucuronidate certain exogenous compounds remains unknown at this time.

Mechanism of Action. Despite its widespread use the toxicologic mechanisms of action of DEET have not been fully characterized.

Toxicity and Risk Factors. The toxicity of DEET has been reviewed.[2-4] The toxicity of *m*-DEET is low, with an oral LD_{50} of 1.8 to 2.7 g/kg body weight in the rat. The *ortho* (o-DEET) isomer is somewhat more toxic (oral rat LD_{50} of 1.2 g/kg) and the *para* (p-DEET) isomer is slightly less toxic (oral rat LD_{50} of 2.3 g/kg) than *m*-DEET. The dermal toxicity of DEET is also considered low because a single application of 2 to 4 g/kg to rabbits produced no signs of systemic toxicity. Age (neonates are more sensitive) and gender (females are more sensitive) are known risk factors in rodents and possibly humans and pets.

Clinical Signs. Reports of DEET toxicosis in the human and veterinary literature are limited. Animals topically exposed to DEET have developed dermal and ocular reactions. Repeated dermal application of products containing 15% or more DEET to horses can result in hypersteatosis.[5] Profuse sweating, irritation, and exfoliation have also been observed in horses after repeated dermal application of a solution containing at least 50% DEET.[6] Instillation of DEET into the eyes of rabbits produced mild to moderate edema of the nictitating membrane, lacrimation, conjunctivitis, and corneal injury.

Neurotoxicity has been attributed to excessive DEET exposure in children and adult humans following prolonged external use or appreciable ingestion.[4] Human exposure to DEET has been associated with generalized seizures and a toxic encephalopathy that is characterized by lethargy, ataxia, behavioral changes, abnormal movements, seizures, and coma. Neurotoxicity has also been associated with subchronic exposure of dogs to DEET. Dogs that were given 100 or 300 mg DEET/kg/day for 13 weeks displayed tremors, hyperactivity, and occasionally vomiting.[7] Clinical signs observed in dogs and cats with suspected acute DEET toxicosis may include vomiting, tremors, excitation, ataxia, and seizures.[3]

Clinical Pathology. Cerebral spinal fluid abnormalities (increased cell count, protein, and glucose concentrations) have been reported in DEET-poisoned human patients.

Lesions. Dermal effects including erythema, desquamation, and scarring have been observed in rabbits following repeated dermal exposure to DEET. Kidney, liver, and testes hypertrophy have also been observed in rodents following repeated DEET exposure. Spongiform myelinopathy has been observed in rats following administration of near-lethal doses of DEET.[8]

Diagnostic Testing. Diagnosis of DEET toxicosis in animals is based on excessive exposure to a DEET-based repellent and the development of appropriate clinical signs. Confirmation of exposure by analysis of urine, skin, blood, stomach contents, and vitreous for DEET and its metabolites can be performed by some laboratories, but concentrations associated with toxicosis have not been established.[9]

Treatment. Therapy is primarily directed at decontamination of the gastrointestinal tract and skin. With a recent ingestion and when the animal is asymptomatic, an emetic may be administered. When vomiting has ceased, administration of activated charcoal and saline cathartic is indicated. In cases of dermal exposure, bathing with a mild detergent shampoo is recommended. Animals should be monitored for the development of seizures, and when seizures occur, diazepam or phenobarbital can be given to abolish seizure activity.

Prognosis. Most animals with mild DEET poisoning recover completely within several days.

Prevention and Control. The most effective means of preventing DEET toxicosis is to restrict access of animals to this repellent. Products approved for veterinary use should only be applied to animals. The use of products containing less than 50% DEET decreases the likelihood of excessive dermal exposure.

METALDEHYDE

Patricia A. Talcott

Synonyms.   Slug bait, snail bait, and molluscicide are commonly used names for products that contain metaldehyde. "Shake and bake" syndrome is a common name for the disease that is produced in domestic animals that ingest metaldehyde.

Sources.   Metaldehyde is a tetramer made of acetaldehyde molecules arranged in an eight-member ring.[1] Formulations include pelleted bait, granules, liquids, or wettable powder. Most molluscicides sold within the United States contain less than 5% metaldehyde. Some producers dye the bait blue or green, and some countries and states require that certain formulations be designed so that they are unattractive to nontarget species. Some feed ingredients added to these baits, such as molasses, apples, rice, soybeans, and oats, have made the baits more likely to be palatable to species other than slugs and snails.

Metaldehyde has also been used in several countries as canned or pelletized solid fuel for camping stoves and lamps, as well as being marketed as a color flame tablet for party goods.

Toxicokinetics.   Metaldehyde is poorly soluble in water and is insoluble in fat. It is unclear whether toxicity is due to metaldehyde or to its breakdown product, acetaldehyde. A case involving a human patient showed that metaldehyde, in part, had been absorbed intact from the gastrointestinal tract and was excreted unchanged in the urine.[2] Oral toxicity studies in rats, challenged with 400 mg metaldehyde/kg body weight, showed only metaldehyde residues in serum collected 30 minutes after ingestion.[3] Acetaldehyde was not detected in any of the animals. Additional data to support metaldehyde as the direct toxicant were seen in rats. Tardieu et al[4] reported that rats pretreated with the phenobarbital-DDD P-450 inducer were protected against the toxic effect of metaldehyde. Acetaldehyde administration did not produce any clinical signs of illness. Other studies, however, have suggested that acetaldehyde is the form that is absorbed by the gastrointestinal tract and is responsible for the toxic effects observed in poisoned animals.

Mechanism of Action.   The exact mechanism of action is unclear. Brain concentrations of noradrenaline, 5-hydroxytryptamine, and 5-hydroxyindoleacetic acid were significantly reduced in metaldehyde-poisoned mice.[5] Other studies in metaldehyde-poisoned mice showed a significant decrease in gamma aminobutyric acid (GABA) concentrations in the brain, which appeared to be directly related to survival.[6]

Toxicity and Risk Factors.   Metaldehyde is toxic to all known animals, and reports of poisoning have been documented in dogs, cats, birds, horses, rats, mice, sheep, swine, goats, and cattle. However, dogs are the species most frequently poisoned. Most cases of confirmed poisonings occur in the coastal areas of the United States where the slug and snail populations are high. Poisoning in animals is most likely a result of oral ingestion of the bait; inhalation or topical exposures are not likely routes of poisoning.

The reported acute oral LD_{50} for metaldehyde in rats is 283 mg/kg body weight. Acute oral LD_{50} values for dogs and cats have been reported as being 210 to 600 mg/kg and 207 mg/kg, respectively.[7,8] An exposure dose of 200 mg/kg body weight was lethal to adult cattle; even less was lethal in calves.[9] A dose of 300 mg/kg body weight was estimated to be a lethal dose in sheep.[10] A 100-mg/kg body weight dose was lethal in a colt.[11] Other cases in equine patients have reported lethal doses ranging from 60 mg/kg body weight to 360 mg/kg body weight.[1] The minimum lethal dose reported for chickens is 500 mg/kg and for ducks it is 300 mg/kg.[12] Secondary poisoning has not been commonly reported; it would seem to be only a risk to birds that may be attracted to poisoned slugs and snails.

Clinical Signs.   Acute exposures to metaldehyde are most common. Chronic exposures have not been documented. Signs of poisoning in dogs generally begin to occur within 1 to 2 hours of ingestion. Initial signs may include salivation, restlessness, anxiety, panting, vomiting, and ataxia. Eventually, tremors, hyperthermia and continuous convulsions may be observed. Uncontrolled hyperthermia may lead to disseminated intravascular coagulation and multiple organ failure. Temporary blindness has been infrequently reported in poisoned dogs. Clinical signs can last up to 5 days, but most generally abate over a period of 12 to 72 hours with appropriate and aggressive treatment. Heightened sensitivity to loud noises, light, and touch is often seen in metaldehyde-poisoned patients.

Cats and other species appear to be infrequently poisoned by metaldehyde. Metaldehyde-poisoned ducks and chickens display hyperexcitability, tremors, rigidity, spasm, and dyspnea.[12] Signs of poisoning in cattle, sheep, horses, and goats are similar to those in dogs and include such changes as salivation, ataxia, tremors, dyspnea, hyperpnea, colic, nystagmus, and convulsions. Loss of the menace reflex and blindness have been reported in cattle, as have exaggerated responses to external stimuli.[1]

Clinical Pathology.   No specific clinical pathologic changes are associated with metaldehyde poisoning. Hemoconcentration (elevated packed cell volume and total protein) may be observed in animals showing moderate to severe signs. Changes associated with renal or hepatic disease infrequently are reported and are most likely a result of persistent and uncontrolled elevations in body temperature. A mild metabolic acidosis may be present.

Lesions.   No reported consistent and pathognomonic gross or histologic lesions occur in metaldehyde-poisoned animals. Gross lesions described include generalized renal, hepatic, gastrointestinal, and pulmonary congestion; petechial and ecchymotic hemorrhages scattered throughout the body; subendothelial and subepicardial hemorrhages; and mild enteritis. A few swollen axons in the medulla and mild hepatic degeneration are a few of the histologic changes reported.[1]

Diagnostic Testing. Metaldehyde-poisoned patients are not prone to vomiting, so the *best* samples to confirm exposure are gastrointestinal contents (i.e., vomitus, gastric lavage washings, feces). However, metaldehyde can also be found in serum, plasma, and urine, but the concentrations are relatively low compared to gastrointestinal samples. All samples for metaldehyde testing should be submitted frozen to the laboratory.

Treatment. Treatment aims to decontaminate, to control muscle tremors and seizure activity, and to provide adequate cardiovascular and respiratory support.

Aggressive and effective decontamination of the asymptomatic or moderately symptomatic patient greatly enhances the survival rate. Emetics such as apomorphine (dog: 0.04 mg/kg IV, 0.25 mg/kg conjunctiva; cat: 0.04 mg/kg IV) or 3% hydrogen peroxide (dog, cat: 1 ml/lb PO, not to exceed 50 ml in the dog or 10 ml in the cat; may be repeated) should be administered to the asymptomatic patient. Additional decontamination procedures should include gastric lavage and rectal enemas. Gastric lavage should be performed on lightly sedated animals with a cuffed endotracheal tube in place. The lavage may be followed by oral administration of an activated charcoal or sorbitol slurry. It is not known how well metaldehyde binds to activated charcoal, so its use in all cases is questionable. Rectal enemas have been used to resolve the hyperthermia, along with monitoring the progress of the metaldehyde through the gastrointestinal tract.[13,14]

A variety of sedatives and anesthetics, including diazepam, diazepam and ketamine, phenobarbital, pentobarbital, methocarbamol, and gas anesthesia, have been used effectively in controlling metaldehyde-induced tremors or convulsions. Diazepam is probably the most commonly used drug, and dosages in dogs and cats range from 0.5 to 5 mg/kg and from 0.5 to 1 mg/kg IV, respectively, to effect. The sedated effect may be short-lived, so repeat administration may be necessary. A constant-rate infusion may be necessary. Methocarbamol, at a dose of 55 to 220 mg/kg IV in dogs and cats (administer half rapidly, then wait until the animal relaxes and then continue to administer) has also been shown to be effective. Phenobarbital (3 to 30 mg/kg IV to effect) or pentobarbital (5 to 15 mg/kg IV to effect) can also be used.

IV fluid therapy (lactated Ringer's solution, 0.9% saline, saline with dextrose), at a rate of 50 to 80 mg/kg/hr may be necessary in the initial treatment to combat hemoconcentration and control hyperthermia. Metabolic acidosis can be treated with bicarbonate, but is often corrected after cessation of tremors or seizures and fluid therapy. Pulse rate, quality, and rhythm, along with capillary refill time and mucous membrane color, should be monitored continuously to assess changes in the cardiovascular system. Continuously

monitoring to prevent aspiration of vomitus is critical. Placing the patient in a warm, comfortable, quiet environment lessens the patient's anxiety.

Poisoning in livestock and horses is a challenge because it is difficult to treat acutely seizing patients in the field. Asymptomatic patients should be given oral activated charcoal (2 g/kg body weight), possibly followed by mineral oil. Diazepam (cattle: 0.5 to 1.5 mg/kg IV or intramuscularly; horses: 25 to 50 mg IV; foals: 0.05 to 0.4 mg/kg IV), along with phenobarbital (cattle, horses: 1 to 10 mg/kg IV to effect), and pentobarbital (cattle: 30 mg/kg IV to effect) can be used to control tremors or seizures. Xylazine combined with acepromazine has been used in horses. IV fluid therapy and a warm, quiet environment are useful.

Prognosis. The overall prognosis is good when the patient is aggressively decontaminated and provided quality symptomatic and supportive care. Renal and hepatic changes have been reported rarely in poisoned patients and are generally seen several days after the initial signs develop. No long-term sequelae are expected.

Prevention and Control. Using the bait according to label instructions should greatly reduce exposures to nontarget species. Some less toxic alternatives to control slug and snail populations include diatomaceous earth, beer, crushed rock, coconut oil soap, copper tape, cocoa mulch, and iron phosphate.

NOVEL INSECTICIDES

Tina Wismer

Several new types of insecticides have been introduced into the market in the past few years. They do not fall into the categories that have historically been used in the literature and so are listed separately here.

FIPRONIL

Synonyms. Fipronil is a phenylpyrazole insecticide. It may also be referred to by its generic name 5-amino-1-[2,6-dichloro-4-(trifluoromethyl) phenyl]-4-[(1R,S)-(trifluoromethyl) sulfinyl]-1H-pyrazole-3-carbonitrile. Common trade names include Combat, Frontline, Regent, Maxforce, Termidor, Icon, and Chipco.[1]

Sources. Fipronil is approved for flea and tick control on dogs and cats; home ant, roach, and termite control; pest control on food crops; and turf insect control on golf courses and lawns. Fipronil is available in various forms and comes as a spot-on (9.7% to 9.8%), spray (0.29%), bait (0.01% to 0.05%), gel (0.01%), granular product (0.1% to 1.5%), spray concentrate (40%), and wettable granular product (80%).

Toxicokinetics. Fipronil is lipid soluble but does not readily penetrate skin. Microscopic examination of the skin after topical administration revealed that fipronil is widely distributed in the stratum corneum, viable epidermis, and pilosebaceous units.[2] Fipronil is found on the hair shafts but is not detected in the dermis and adipose tissue, suggesting that it is absorbed and accumulates in the sebaceous glands, from which it is slowly released via follicular ducts.[2] Fipronil can still be detected 56 days after topical application.[2]

Fipronil has slow oral absorption and after ingestion it can be detected in the gastrointestinal tract, liver, adrenals, and abdominal fat.[3] Fipronil is metabolized in the liver into several compounds and is excreted in both the feces and urine.[3]

Mechanism of Action.   Fipronil is a GABA agonist. GABA is an inhibitory neurotransmitter in both invertebrates and vertebrates, and it normally stops transmission of impulses. Fipronil works by binding to the GABA receptors and blocking chloride passage.[4] This causes excitation of the nervous system. The neurotoxicity of fipronil is selective, because the shape of GABA receptors in mammals is different from that in insects; therefore, it is much less toxic in mammals.

Toxicity and Risk Factors.   Fipronil has a wide safety margin. Fipronil has no known interactions with commonly used biologics, pharmaceuticals, or ectoparasites.[5] In dermal toxicity studies, the application of a 0.29% spray to dogs and cats at a dose five times higher than the recommended dose for 6 months did not cause any clinical, biochemical, hematologic, or cutaneous abnormalities.[6] A few skin hypersensitivity reactions have been reported with dermal applications. Fipronil, used off-label, has been reported to cause seizures in rabbits.

In rats an acute oral overdose of technical fipronil of 5 mg/kg led to decreased hind leg splay, and 50 mg/kg caused tremors and seizures.[3,7] In chronic feeding studies no signs were seen in female dogs fed 0.5 mg/kg/day for 13 weeks or in male dogs fed 2 mg/kg/day for 13 weeks.[3,8] Feeding studies in mice did not find any evidence of carcinogenicity and studies in dogs exposed to fipronil also showed no effect on T_4 or thyroid-stimulating hormone levels.[9] Fipronil is virtually nontoxic to waterfowl and earthworms, but is highly toxic to shrimp, oysters, fish, bees, and upland game birds.[8,10,11]

Clinical Signs.   The most commonly reported adverse effect to dermal application of fipronil is a dermal hypersensitivity reaction. Redness, irritation, and alopecia at the application site, along with hiding and other behavior changes are the most commonly reported signs. Some of these reactions are most likely due to the inert carriers rather than the active ingredient present in the product. Dermal hypersensitivity reactions can start within hours of application and last up to 1 to 2 days. (American Society for the Prevention of Cruelty to Animals Animal Poison Control Center [ASPCA APCC], unpublished data, 1998–present.)

Taste reactions to the spray or spot-on are common; salivation and vomiting are commonly seen. Ataxia, tremors, and seizures are rare and are seen only with large ingestions or with dermal application to rabbits.

Diagnostic Testing.   With known or suspected oral exposures, plasma or serum may be tested. Samples may be chilled or frozen; both the manufacturer, Merial, Inc., and Pacific Toxicology Laboratories in Woodland Hills, California (818-598-3110) perform the test.

Treatment.   For dermal hypersensitivity reactions fipronil is easily removed by bathing in the first 48 hours after application.[2] Liquid dishwashing detergent or a follicle-flushing shampoo are recommended. Some animals may need topical or systemic antihistamines or steroids to reduce inflammation and itching. If the area has been abraded, antibiotics may be needed.

Activated charcoal may be given once at 1 to 2 g/kg with large oral exposures. A large oral exposure may be seen with ingestion of the spray concentrate or granular product. Licking or oral ingestion of the spray product or spot-on is not considered to be a large oral exposure. If the animal is seizuring, Valium or phenobarbital may be given. Fluids and other supportive care should be given as needed.

Prognosis.   Prognosis is good for most exposures; however, the prognosis is guarded for seizuring rabbits.

IMIDACLOPRID

Synonyms.   Imidacloprid is a chloronicotinyl nitroguanide insecticide found in a variety of commercial insecticides. In may also be called by its chemical name 1-(6-chloro-3-pyridylmethyl)-*N*-nitroimidazolidin-2-ylideneamine or 1-[(6-chloro-3-pyridinyl)methyl]-*N*-nitro-2-imidazolidinimine. Common trade names include Admire, Advantage, Bayer Advanced, Condifor, Gaucho, Marathon, Merit, Premier, Premise, and Provado.[1]

Sources.   Imidacloprid is used for crop, fruit, and vegetable pest control, termite control, and flea control on dogs and cats. Imidacloprid-based insecticide formulations are available as a dustable powder, granular product, seed dressing (flowable slurry concentrate), soluble concentrate, suspension concentrate, wettable powder (75%), and spot-on (9.1%).[12]

Toxicokinetics.   With a dermal exposure to imidacloprid, there is minimal to no systemic absorption. Imidacloprid is lipophilic and resides in the fatty layer of the skin. Imidacloprid is quickly and almost completely absorbed from the gastrointestinal tract. It is broken down in the liver to the active metabolite 6-chloronicotinic acid. This compound may be conjugated with glycine and eliminated, or it may be reduced to guanidine.[13] Imidacloprid is eliminated via urine and feces. In rats 96% of the parent compound is excreted within 48 hours.[13]

Mechanism of Action.   Imidacloprid works by interfering with the transmission of stimuli in the insect nervous system. Imidacloprid mimics the action of acetylcholine, but it is not degraded by the enzyme acetylcholinesterase. Imidacloprid binds to the acetylcholine receptor on the postsynaptic portion of nerve cells.[14,15] This results in persistent activation preventing transmission of impulses and leading to an accumulation of acetylcholine. The acetylcholine accumulation results in hyperexcitation, convulsions, paralysis, and death of the insect. It has been recently hypothesized that there are two binding sites with different affinities for imidacloprid and that imidacloprid has both agonistic and antagonistic effects on the nicotinic acetylcholine receptor channels.[16]

Toxicity and Risk Factors. Imidacloprid has a wide safety margin. It has low toxicity in mammals because there is a higher concentration of nicotinic acetylcholine receptors in insect nervous tissue than in that of mammals. In addition, imidacloprid has a higher affinity for insect receptors than for vertebrate receptors.[15,17] The 24-hour dermal LD_{50} in rats is more than 5000 mg/kg.[13] Topical application of imidacloprid on dogs and cats at a dose of 50 mg/kg caused no adverse effects.[18] The acute oral LD_{50} of technical-grade imidacloprid is 450 mg/kg and 131 mg/kg in rats and mice, respectively.[12,13] A 1-year feeding study in dogs fed up to 2500 ppm resulted in an NOEL of 1250 ppm (41 mg/kg). Adverse effects at the higher dose included increased cholesterol levels and elevated liver cytochrome P-450 levels.[19]

Imidacloprid is considered safe for use during pregnancy and is considered to be of minimal carcinogenic risk. Imidacloprid is categorized by the EPA as a "group E" carcinogen (evidence of noncarcinogenicity for humans). There were no carcinogenic effects in a 2-year study in rats fed up to 1800 ppm imidacloprid.[20]

Imidacloprid is highly toxic to bees if used as a foliar application, especially during flowering, but it is not considered a hazard when used as a seed treatment.[13] Products containing imidacloprid may be highly toxic to aquatic invertebrates, toxic to upland game birds, and of moderately low toxicity to fish.[12,13]

Clinical Signs. Acute oral ingestions can cause salivation or vomiting. Dermal hypersensitivity reactions (redness, pruritus, alopecia) have been reported. Although rare and only seen at extremely high doses, signs of imidacloprid toxicosis are expected to be similar to nicotinic signs (lethargy, salivation, vomiting, tremors, diarrhea, ataxia, muscle weakness).[21]

Diagnostic Testing. Two methods are used to detect imidacloprid and 6-chloronicotinic acid residues: high-performance liquid chromatography (HPLC) with ultraviolet (UV) detection and enzyme-linked immunosorbent assay.[22,23]

Treatment. For dermal hypersensitivity reactions, imidacloprid can be removed by bathing with a liquid dishwashing detergent or a follicle-flushing shampoo. Antihistamines or steroids may be needed in extreme cases. Oral exposures to imidacloprid should be diluted with milk or water. The animal should be given nothing by mouth if vomiting.

Prognosis. Prognosis is good for most exposures.

HYDRAMETHYLNON

Synonyms. Hydramethylnon is a trifluoromethyl amino-hydrazone insecticide. It may be found listed on product labels as 5,5-dimethylperhydropyrimidin-2-one 4-trifluoromethyl-alpha-(4-trifluoromethylstyryl)-cinnamylidenehydrazone or tetrahydro-5,5-dimethyl-2(1H)-pyrimidinone (3-[4-(trifluoromethyl)phenyl]-1-(2-[4-(trifluoromethyl)phenyl]-ethenyl)-2-propenylidene)hydrazone.[13] Common trade names include Amdro, Maxforce, Combat Blatex, Cyaforce, Cyclon, Impact, Matox, Pyramdron, Seige, and Wipeout.[1]

Sources. Hydramethylnon is used in baits, both indoor and outdoor, to control fire ants, leafcutter ants, harvester ants, big-headed ants, and cockroaches. Hydramethylnon is also available in granules or as a gel.[12]

Toxicokinetics. Hydramethylnon is poorly absorbed by mammals after an oral dose, and greater than 95% is excreted unchanged in the feces.[24] Rats given hydramethylnon orally eliminate 72% of the dose in 24 hours and 92% in 9 days.[25] There were no residues detectable in the milk or tissues of goats fed 0.2 ppm daily for 8 days or in the milk or tissue of cows fed 0.05 ppm for 21 consecutive days.[13,26]

Mechanism of Action. Hydramethylnon works by uncoupling oxidative phosphorylation. It inhibits the electron transport system in the mitochondria. Inhibition of the electron transport system blocks the production of adenosine triphosphate (ATP) and causes a decrease in oxygen consumption by the mitochondria. Disruption of energy metabolism and the subsequent loss of ATP results in a slowly developing toxicosis, with the insect developing lethargy, paralysis, and death.

Toxicity and Risk Factors. The dermal LD_{50} of hydramethylnon in rabbits and rats is greater than 5000 mg/kg, and the oral LD_{50} in rats is reported to be 1100 to 1300 mg/kg.[12,13] In a 26-week feeding study in male and female dogs doses of 3 mg/kg/day resulted in increased liver weights and increased liver-to-body weight ratios. No other biochemical or histopathologic abnormalities were noted.[27] Oral hydramethylnon doses of 6 mg/kg/day for 90 days in dogs caused decreased food consumption, decreased body weight gain, and testicular atrophy.[27,28] Chronic studies in several animal species have shown the testis as a target organ. In an 18-month cancer assay oral hydramethylnon given at 3.8 mg/kg/day was associated with renal amyloidosis.[28]

Hydramethylnon has a large margin of safety when used according to label directions. Grazing animals fed 10 times the recommended field application amount did not develop any problems. Calves fed Amdro (0.5% to 1% hydramethylnon) at 113.5 g/day for 50 days showed no significant difference when compared with control calves for the following parameters: neutrophil and basophil counts, plasma protein and serum Ig concentrations, antibody formation and titers to *Brucella* challenge, physical examination, and necropsy examination.[29] Hydramethylnon did appear to selectively affect production of eosinophils and immunocompetent T and B cells in Holstein calves in the same study.[29]

Leukopenia and eosinopenia have also been reported in ponies fed Amdro-treated grits (1/100th to 1/150th the calculated LD_{50}) for 30 days.[30] A possible effect on the immune system of horses fed Amdro has been suggested.[30] Amdro-fed animals had an increased severity of an upper respiratory disease (strangles), and foals born to mares that had been fed Amdro while pregnant had an increased incidence of diarrhea and upper respiratory infections when compared with control subjects.[30]

Hydramethylnon is nontoxic to honey bees and birds but is highly toxic to fish.[26] Hydramethylnon is often found in grain-based baits and may attract rodents and domestic animals.

Clinical Signs.   The most commonly seen clinical signs are vomiting and gagging after oral ingestion.

Diagnostic Testing.   Hydramethylnon residues can be detected by using chromatography or mass spectrometry.[31] Any tissue, blood, milk, or feed may be tested for the presence of hydramethylnon.

Treatment.   Emesis would be necessary only if large amounts were ingested. Signs are usually mild and self-limiting.

Prognosis.   The prognosis is good for most exposures.

SULFLURAMID

Synonyms.   Sulfluramid is a fluorinated sulfonamide. This unique polyfluorinated insecticide may also be called perfluorooctanesulfonamide, *N*-ethylperfluorooctane sulfonamide, or *N*-ethyl-1,1,2,2,3,3,4,4,5,5,6,6,7,7,8,8,8-heptadecafluro-1-octanesulfonamide. Common trade names include Advance, Firstline, FlourGuard, and RaidMax.[1]

Sources.   Sulfluramid is found in roach and ant bait stations.

Toxicokinetics.   Sulfluramid is highly lipid soluble, and the highest tissue concentrations of sulfluramid after oral ingestion in the rat are found in the liver, kidneys, and adrenal glands; however, no tissue accumulation occurred in rats during a 56-day feeding trial.[32,33] Sulfluramid is de-ethylated by cytochrome P-450 to form perfluorooctane sulfonamide, also called desethylsulfluramid.[32] The rat eliminates 80% of sulfluramid within 72 hours, but desethylsulfluramid is excreted over 10.8 days.[32,33] The routes of excretion in the rat after oral ingestion are 56% via respiratory system, 25% via feces, and 8% in the urine.[32]

Mechanism of Action.   The de-ethylated metabolite of sulfluramid (deselthylsulfluramid) is a potent uncoupler of mitochondrial respiration. The disruption of energy metabolism and the subsequent loss of ATP result in a slowly developing toxicosis, and the effects of sulfluramid include inactivity, paralysis, and death. Insects may take 24 to 48 hours to die.

Toxicity and Risk Factors.   Sulfluramid appears to be safe in dogs and cats. The acute oral LD_{50} in the rat is 500 mg/kg

and the dermal LD_{50} in the rabbit is greater than 2000 mg/kg.[34] Sheep given 5 mg/kg IV or 400 mg/kg intraruminally experienced no adverse effects.[35] When the sheep were given 15 mg/kg IV, they experienced lethargy and dyspnea.[35] Long-term oral doses of sulfluramid in the rat (75 mg/kg of food/56 days) caused a decrease in body weight gain and "large doses" administered to laboratory animals caused diarrhea.[33,34] Preliminary studies in dogs suggested that ingestion of high doses for prolonged periods of time may arrest spermatogenesis.[36] Sulfluramid is slightly toxic to fish and aquatic arthropods and moderately to highly toxic to birds.[34]

Clinical Signs.   The most commonly seen clinical sign with sulfluramid ingestion is vomiting (ASPCA APCC, unpublished data, 1998–2000). Signs are self-limiting and occur within 2 hours after ingestion.

Treatment.   Treatment is rarely needed; signs are usually mild and self-limiting.

Prognosis.   Prognosis is good for most exposures.

ORGANOCHLORINE INSECTICIDES

Steve Ensley

Synonyms.   The chlorinated hydrocarbons of significance to animals include the diphenyl aliphatic compounds, the aryl hydrocarbons, and the cyclodiene insecticides.[1] The diphenyl aliphatics include dichlorodiphenyltrichloroethane (DDT), methoxychlor, perthane, and dicofol. Aryl hydrocarbons include lindane, mirex, kepone, and paradichlorobenzene.[2] The important cyclodiene insecticides are aldrin, dieldrin, endrin, chlordane, heptachlor, and toxaphene (Fig. 21-1). Most of these compounds are banned in the United States, but limited use of lindane and methoxychlor continues. DDT was banned in the United States in 1972.[3]

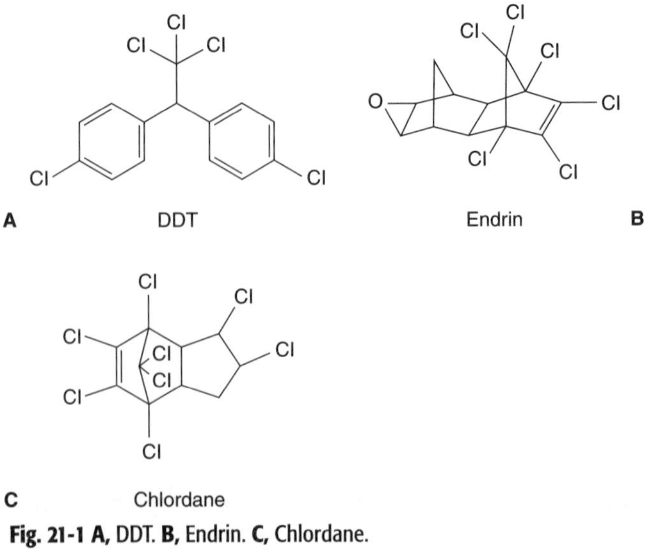

Fig. 21-1 A, DDT. **B,** Endrin. **C,** Chlordane.

Sources. Chlorinated hydrocarbons were heavily used in pest control and agriculture from the 1950s through the early 1970s. Acute contamination of food and water is currently unlikely but the organochlorine insecticides already in the environment are slowly degraded and may persist. The possibility that food and the environment are contaminated with organochlorines is decreasing slowly as contaminated areas are biodegraded and continuing sources are not available.[2]

Toxicokinetics. The organochlorines can be absorbed orally and topically. These compounds are lipid soluble, which makes absorption rapid.[4] Organochlorines are not highly volatile, so inhalation is not a normal route of absorption. Distribution is to the liver, kidney, brain, and any adipose tissue. Acute toxicosis caused by organochlorines is of concern, but bioaccumulation is equally important. The chlorinated hydrocarbons are highly lipid soluble and persist in the environment.[5] These two properties favor bioaccumulation upward in the food chain from environment to animals and humans.

Methoxychlor is rapidly eliminated by dechlorination and oxidation compared to DDT. The diphenyl aliphatics such as DDT are dechlorinated by mixed function oxidases (MFO). Aryl hydrocarbons, like paradichlorobenzene, are rapidly absorbed and undergo glucuronidation and sulfation. The cyclodiene insecticides, such as endrin, are rapidly converted to epoxides by MFOs.[2] Organochlorine metabolites may be more toxic than the parent compound.

The major excretory route of organochlorines is from bile into the digestive tract. Enterohepatic recycling can occur. Metabolites are released slowly from lipid depot storage. The half-life of some diphenyl aliphatics, such as DDT and the cyclodienes, may range from days to weeks. Elimination can sometimes be explained by a two-compartment model, wherein the first phase is rapid elimination and the second is prolonged.

Mechanism of Action. DDT-type organochlorine insecticides affect the peripheral nerves and brain by slowing Na^+ influx and inhibiting K^+ outflow.[2] This results in excess intracellular K^+ in the neuron, which partially depolarizes the cell. The threshold for another action potential is decreased, resulting in increased firing of the neuron.

Mirex, in addition to decreasing action potentials, may inhibit the postsynaptic binding of GABA. The cyclodiene organochlorine insecticides act by competitive inhibition of the binding of GABA at its receptor, causing stimulation of the neuron.

Toxicity and Risk Factors. Cats are the most sensitive species to organochlorines.[3] The LD_{50} for endrin in cats is 3 to 6 mg/kg. The cyclodiene organochlorine insecticides cause more seizure activity and have a lower LD_{50} than the DDT-type insecticides.

The oral LD_{50} for DDT in rats is 113 to 2500 mg/kg, whereas the IV LD_{50} is 47 mg/kg.[3] In humans toxic signs from oral exposure to organochlorines can be observed at 10 mg/kg. The LD_{50} for oral exposure to aryl hydrocarbons, such as paradichlorobenzene, is 3.2, 2.5, and 2.8 g/kg in the mouse, rat, and rabbit, respectively.[3]

Clinical Signs. Acute toxicosis is characterized by abnormalities of the nervous system. Salivation, nausea, and vomiting are early signs of toxicosis. Agitation, apprehension, hyperexcitability, incoordination, nervousness, and tremors are early signs related to the effects on the nervous system.

More advanced signs of organochlorine toxicosis include intermittent clonic-tonic seizures, epileptiform seizures with opisthotonus, paddling, and clamping of the jaw. The seizures may persist for 2 to 3 days. The excessive muscle activity can result in hyperthermia. Between seizures animals may remain normal to depressed. Affected cattle may walk backward, chew or lick excessively, or have abnormal postures.

Birds affected by organochlorine toxicosis can have apparent blindness, disorientation, abnormal postures, depression, and sudden death.[2] Organochlorine insecticides have been associated with eggshell thinning in raptors and can have estrogenic effects in birds that interfere with reproduction.

Clinical Pathology. Clinical chemistry and hematology are usually not helpful in reaching a diagnosis of organochlorine toxicosis. Dogs may experience liver damage from excessive exposure to organochlorines.

Lesions. Usually no lesions are associated with organochlorine toxicosis. Nonspecific lesions that may be observed in all species are trauma from seizures or pale musculature from seizures. Nonspecific lesions observed in dogs include liver necrosis or hemorrhage of the adrenal gland. Large doses may cause centrilobular necrosis of the liver, whereas smaller doses may cause liver enlargement. Liver enlargement can be due to enzyme induction of cytochrome P-450s. Porphyria can be observed with exposure to polychlorinated biphenyls.[6]

Diagnostic Testing. GC is the analytic method used to determine the presence of organochlorines.[6] Acute cases of organochlorine exposure result in insecticide in the blood, liver, or brain. Milk fat or adipose tissue from biopsy samples can be used to confirm chronic exposure. Tissue concentrations of organochlorines are poorly correlated with the severity of signs or survival.

An important detail when submitting tissues for analysis is to avoid contamination from plastic containers; tissues should be packaged in clean glass containers or wrapped in aluminum foil.

Treatment. No specific antidotes for organochlorine insecticides are available. Detoxification is the most essential component of therapy for organochlorine toxicosis. If dermal exposure has occurred, the animal should be washed with water and soap or detergent. The hair of heavily contaminated long-haired animals should be clipped. Personnel treating animals should exercise caution and wear gloves, aprons, or raincoats because these compounds are readily absorbed through the skin.

For oral exposure to organochlorines, activated charcoal (1 to 2 g/kg) should be administered orally.[2] An alternative but less effective treatment is mineral oil. Mineral oil solubilizes the insecticide but does not adsorb it. Approximate oral dose of mineral oil is 2 to 6 ml in cats, 5 to 15 ml in dogs, and 1 to 3 liters in large animals. Adsorbents or nonabsorbable oils are most effective when given within 4 hours of ingestion of the pesticide.

General supportive care includes the use of antiseizure medications such as diazepam, phenobarbital, or pentobarbital.[6] To minimize trauma animals need to be placed in a warm and comfortable area.

Animals recovering from organochlorine insecticide exposure may have to be monitored long term because organochlorines can persist in the body for months or years. The source of the exposure must be identified to eliminate exposure.

One decontamination strategy is to reduce feed intake so that the animal loses body fat, thereby reducing the residue in adipose tissue. Lactating animals rapidly eliminate organochlorine residues because of losses in milk fat. Large animals can be fed activated charcoal (500 to 1000 g/day) to reduce enterohepatic recycling.[2]

Prognosis.   Prognosis depends on the dose of organochlorine and how quickly detoxification occurs.

Prevention and Control.   Preventing exposure by properly disposing of these compounds and their containers is the key to minimizing the impact of organochlorines. State or local authorities can be contacted for assistance in disposing of contaminated animals, soil, or materials.

The EPA and state public health authorities regulate potential human exposure to organochlorines. Slow elimination and high lipid solubility favor the accumulation of unacceptable residues in the edible tissue of food animals. The immediate sale or consumption of products from animals that have recovered from toxicosis is not recommended. All potentially exposed food animals should be evaluated to determine whether residues exist.

PYRETHRINS AND PYRETHROIDS

Petra A. Volmer

Sources.   The marked toxicity of some traditional insecticides to nontarget organisms has led to the demand for, and development of, newer and safer products. Ideal insecticides have great efficacy and selectivity against insect pests with nominal environmental persistence and minimal mammalian toxicity. Pyrethrin-based insecticides were replaced by the cheaper and more stable OP and organochlorine insecticides after World War II.[1] However, in the 1970s they reemerged as a move away from these pesticide groups that had raised concerns about environmental contamination and mammalian toxicity.[1] Pyrethrin and pyrethroid insecticides currently make up more than 25% of the world insecticide market.[2]

Pyrethrins and pyrethroid insecticides are effective against a variety of insect pests on pets, livestock, and other animals, and are readily available for home, farm, and garden use. They are currently marketed as sprays, dusts, dips, shampoos, spot-ons, gels, foggers, ear tags, pour-ons, back rubbers, and face rubbers. Most ready-to-use (RTU) formulations are at concentrations of 2% or less; however, concentrated products are available as high as 40% as wettable powders (WP), granulars (G), soluble powders (SP), and emulsifiable concentrates (EC). The presence of one of these abbreviations in the product name indicates its formulation.

One product of note is the popular spot-on permethrin flea products for dogs, which are available over-the-counter at 45% to 65% concentrations. These products are extremely toxic to cats.[3,4] Most permethrin premise sprays and pet flea sprays contain low concentrations of permethrin (<2%) and do not pose a hazard to cats.

Pyrethrin and pyrethroid products may have one of several carriers, including water, alcohol (usually isopropyl), or a hydrocarbon. Aerosol spray formulations usually contain a halocarbon propellant that may pose a hazard to birds.

Pyrethrum occurs naturally in the flowers of *Chrysanthemum cinerariaefolium* and *Chrysanthemum cineum*. Harvested flowers are dried and powdered, or the oils are extracted with solvents. Pyrethrum is a mixture of six active insecticidal compounds termed *pyrethrins*. Pyrethrins are readily degraded by UV light, acids, or alkalis. Pyrethrins are esters consisting of an acid and alcohol moiety. Sequential replacement of the acid, the alcohol, or both has resulted in synthetic analogues of the original pyrethrin esters that are collectively known as pyrethroids. Pyrethroids tend to have more potent insecticidal properties, tend to be more toxic, and are more stable in the environment than naturally occurring pyrethrins. The absence or presence of a cyano group in the alpha position of the chemical structure of pyrethroids differentiates type I pyrethroids from type II pyrethroids. Addition of the alpha-cyano group increases insecticidal potency.[1] Table 21-2 lists pyrethrins and some commonly encountered pyrethroids.

Synergists are compounds that when combined with an insecticide enhance its toxicity, but have minimal toxicity alone at the dosages used. Synergists are often added to pyrethrin and pyrethroid insecticide products to inhibit mixed function oxidase and esterase enzymes of insects, hindering detoxification of the insecticide and prolonging its action. Inhibition of mixed function oxidase enzymes may, however,

TABLE 21-2 Pyrethrins and Some Commonly Encountered Pyrethroids

Pyrethrins (Compounds in Natural Pyrethrum Extract)	Type I Pyrethroids (Synthetic Pyrethrins that Do Not Contain a Cyano Group)	Type II Pyrethroids (Synthetic Pyrethrins that Do Contain an Alpha-cyano Group)
Pyrethrin I	Allethrin	Cyfluthrin
Pyrethrin II	Bifenthrin	Cyhalothrin
Cinerin I	Permethrin	Cypermethrin
Cinerin II	Phenothrin	Deltamethrin
Jasmolin I	Resmethrin	Genvalerate
Jasmolin II	Sumithrin	Flumethrin
	Tefluthrin	Fluvalinate
	Tetramethrin	Tralomethrin

enhance mammalian toxicity.[1] Commonly used synergists include piperonyl butoxide, N-octylbicycloheptene dicarboximide (MGK 264), sesamolin, sesamex, sesamin, sulfoxide, propynyl ethers, and tropital.

Toxicokinetics. The toxicokinetics of this class vary with the individual compound and data are often limited. This discussion provides a general overview of the insecticide class; refer to relevant literature for information specific to a particular pyrethrin or pyrethroid. Although most pyrethrin and pyrethroid products are applied dermally, the natural grooming behavior of most animals results in oral and possibly inhalational exposures.

Pyrethrin and pyrethroids are incompletely absorbed after oral exposure, with approximately 40% to 60% of an ingested dose being absorbed. The amount absorbed dermally is less (<2%), and the rate of absorption is much slower than the oral route of exposure. Pyrethroids may be stored in the skin and slowly released into the systemic circulation. Inhalation results in rapid absorption of pyrethrins and pyrethroids.[5]

Pyrethroids are lipophilic in nature and are expected to distribute to tissues with a high lipid content, such as fat, and central and peripheral nervous tissues. They are also widely distributed to many other tissues, including liver, kidney, and milk.[5]

Pyrethrins and pyrethroids are rapidly hydrolyzed in the gastrointestinal tract and may bind to components in the ingesta. Once absorbed, many tissue types are involved in the metabolism of pyrethrins and pyrethroids by nonspecific esterases and microsomal mixed-function oxidases. Metabolism of the pyrethroids involves hydrolysis of the central ester bond, oxidation of several sites, and reactions with glycine, sulfate, glucuronide, or glucoside conjugates to produce water-soluble metabolites that are readily excreted. Cleavage of the ester bond results in substantial reduction in toxicity, and the presence of the alpha-cyano group decreases the rate of hydrolytic cleavage of the ester bond. Disruption of the ester bond in type II pyrethroids results in release of cyanide, which is rapidly converted to thiocyanate.[5]

Pyrethroids exhibit first order elimination kinetics, with the majority eliminated from the body in the first 12 to 48 hours. The primary routes of excretion are urine and feces as a mix of parent compound and metabolites.[5]

Mechanism of Action. Pyrethroids appear to bind to the membrane lipid phase of nerve cells near the sodium channel. Activation and deactivation occur much more slowly than in normal, unmodified sodium channels. In other words, pyrethrins and pyrethroids slow the opening and closing of neural sodium channels. The duration of sodium tail currents is much longer for type II pyrethroids than for type I. The result is that repetitive discharges predominate in type I pyrethroids, and membrane depolarization predominates in type II pyrethroids.[6] Paresthesia is thought to result from direct action of pyrethroids on sensory nerve endings, causing repetitive firing of these fibers.[5] Less than 1% of sodium channels must be modified by pyrethroids to produce neurologic signs.[7] High concentrations of type II pyrethroids may also act on GABA-gated chloride channels.[8]

The decreased sensitivity of mammals to this class of compounds compared to insects is due to several factors. Pyrethroids are more potent on the sodium channel at low temperature than at high temperature. This enhances toxicity to insect pests whose ambient temperature is around 25° C compared with mammalians at 37° C.[6] Independent of temperature influences, mammalian sodium channels are at least 1000 times less sensitive to pyrethroids than their insect counterparts.[2] Mammalian sodium channels recover much more quickly from depolarization than do insect sodium channels, and, because of their body size, mammals are much more likely to detoxify pyrethroids before they reach their target site than are insects.[6]

Toxicity and Risk Factors. Animals that are weak and debilitated from a large flea burden or other condition are at increased risk.

Most pyrethroid products for agricultural use (except livestock and premise use) are restricted-use pesticides (RUPs) because of their possible adverse effects on aquatic organisms.[9] Fish are highly sensitive to pyrethrin and pyrethroid products, and contamination of lakes, streams, ponds, or other aqueous habitats should be avoided. Homeowners with aquaria should turn off the tank pump when using pyrethrin- or pyrethroid-based foggers or other products in the home where the aerosol can be drawn into the air intake. The tank and air intake should be covered during application and the home should be well ventilated before uncovering and starting the pump.

The sensitivity of many exotic species, including lagomorphs and reptiles, is not well established, and use on or around these animals should be with caution. Most avian species are thought to be tolerant of pyrethrins and pyrethroids,[9] but carriers or propellants in spray formulations may pose a respiratory hazard to birds. Toxicity studies in birds may not address exotic species and caution should be exercised.

Clinical Signs. All animals may exhibit paresthesia following application of a pyrethrin or pyrethroid product. Of the domestic species routinely exposed to this class of compounds, cats account for most reports of adverse reactions. Cats may exhibit mild, self-limiting signs of hypersalivation and paresthesia after a pyrethrin-based topical spray. Other signs include hypersalivation, paw shaking, ear twitching, flicking of the tail, and twitching of the skin on the back. Some cats exhibit an unusual walk, holding a rear leg out to the side, or the cat hides and becomes reluctant to move. Onset of signs is from minutes to 2 to 3 hours, and signs usually resolve by 24 to 48 hours. The signs may be attributed to the disagreeable taste of the product or to a tingling sensation on the skin or oral mucous membranes (paresthesia).

Following dermal exposure to a pyrethrin or pyrethroid product some dogs (usually small breeds or young animals) may develop a paresthesia-like syndrome. These animals may act uncomfortable, lick or chew at their skin, roll on the floor, or rub their backs. Cattle may exhibit a paresthesia-like syndrome after application of a pyrethroid pour-on product. Cattle may become restless and act uncomfortable, twitch the skin on their backs, and attempt to rub their backs.

Cutaneous exposure of permethrin-containing spot-on products produces pronounced seizure activity in most cats. These products are highly concentrated (45% to 65% in 1- or 2-ml vials) and are labeled for use only in dogs. Close physical contact of a cat with a dog recently treated with a permethrin spot-on product may also result in convulsions in the cat. Within 12 to 18 hours cats exhibit agitation and tremors and can be seizuring by 18 to 20 hours. The convulsions induced by permethrin in cats may be difficult to control. Untreated cats may die within 24 hours. Similar clinical signs may occur in cats after exposure to phenothrin spot-on products labeled for cats. In most cases signs are milder and of shorter duration than those encountered following a permethrin exposure.

Fish are highly sensitive to this class of compounds and may die upon exposure.

Clinical Pathology.   No specific clinical pathologic findings are expected following exposure to pyrethrin- or pyrethroid-containing products.

Lesions.   In general, pyrethrins and pyrethroids are not expected to produce any gross pathologic or histologic lesions. Cats exhibiting severe or prolonged muscle stimulation (e.g., tremors or seizures) following inappropriate application of a permethrin-containing product may exhibit lesions characteristic of trauma, hypoxia, or hyperthermia.

Diagnostic Testing.   Results of analytic testing for pyrethroids depend on the pyrethroid involved. Results may be disappointing because of the insufficient method sensitivity in tissues at the normal level of use. Consultation with a veterinary toxicologist at a diagnostic laboratory is recommended.

Treatment.   Bathing with a mild liquid dish detergent or a keratolytic shampoo is effective in removing most topically applied formulations. Warm water alone does not remove most carriers. The clinician should avoid the use of insecticidal shampoos (often containing pyrethrin or a pyrethroid, a carbamate, or a citrus oil, tea tree oil, or other compound) that may exacerbate or complicate the clinical course. Animals should be thoroughly rinsed, well dried, and kept warm. Large animals may require the use of a garden hose and scrub brush in addition to a liquid dish detergent. Power washers are not recommended for cattle or other large animals because they may result in dermal trauma. Once the pyrethrin-based product has been removed, clinical signs associated with dermal application should resolve over 8 to 24 hours.

Hypersalivation, frothing, smacking the lips, and other unusual behavior following oral exposures to pyrethrin or pyrethroid products can be managed by offering the animal a palatable treat. Signs are thought to occur as a result of either the disagreeable taste of the product or the unusual oral tingling sensation produced by the pyrethrin or pyrethroid itself. Management by dilution or by offering a tasty flavor is sufficient to resolve the clinical effects after oral exposure.

Cats exposed to a permethrin spot-on intended for canines should be treated as medical emergencies because of their profound sensitivity to these products. If application was recent and the cat is not exhibiting clinical signs, the animal should be bathed immediately. If tremoring or seizuring have already developed, control can be achieved with the skeletal muscle relaxant methocarbamol (55 to 220 mg/kg IV). One third to one half the dose is administered as a bolus (not exceeding 2 ml/min), the cat begins to relax while the drug administration is paused, and then the remainder is given to effect. If the tremors recur, methocarbamol can be repeated to a maximum daily dose of 330 mg/kg. Refractory seizures may require a combination of diazepam and methocarbamol. Complete cessation of tremors may not occur after initial treatment with methocarbamol.[3,4] Diazepam alone may be effective for very mild tremors but is ineffective for severe neuromuscular activity. Alternatively, a barbiturate such as phenobarbital or pentobarbital can be given to effect; however, cats may develop severe CNS depression without adequate reduction of peripheral tremors. Gas anesthesia with isoflurane or intravenous propofol at a constant-rate infusion has also been used with variable success.

Once stabilized cats should be bathed as previously described. Activated charcoal is not likely to be of benefit unless a large ingestion has occurred. Supportive care should include IV fluids, blood glucose monitoring and correction, and thermoregulation. Hyperthermia from excess muscle activity can rapidly progress to hypothermia once treatment is initiated. Hypothermia can prolong recovery. IV fluids may act to reduce body temperature and are indicated for the prevention of myoglobinuric-induced renal failure after prolonged, extreme seizure activity. Some cases, especially very young or very old cats, may become profoundly hypoglycemic during the course of the intense muscle activity. Correction with intravenous dextrose is recommended. Most cats fully recover and can be released to the owners in 24 to 72 hours. Permanent sequelae are unlikely unless the animal experienced trauma, extreme hyperthermia, or hypoxia during the seizure activity. Atropine is not indicated for the treatment of pyrethrin or pyrethroid toxicoses and should not be administered.[3,4] No antidotes or direct antagonists are currently available.

Prognosis.   Animals exposed to most pyrethrins and pyrethroids are expected to have an excellent prognosis. Cats exposed to a concentrated permethrin-containing product may have a guarded prognosis if treatment is delayed and severe signs have already developed. Cats treated immediately and aggressively have a favorable prognosis.

Prevention and Control.   Cat owners should be cautioned about the extra-label use of dog products on cats. Keep cats away from dogs that have been recently treated with a permethrin-containing spot-on product. The importance of adhering to label dilution and application instructions should be stressed.

REFERENCES

Amitraz

1. Knowles CO: In Hayes WJ, Laws ER, editors: *Handbook of pesticide toxicology*, vol 3, San Diego, 1991, Academic Press.

2. Roberts MC, Argenzio A: Effects of amitraz, several opiate derivatives and anticholinergic agents on intestinal transit in ponies, *Equine Vet J* 18:256, 1986.

3. Cowan LA, Campbell, K: Generalized demodicosis in a cat responsive to amitraz, *J Am Vet Med Assoc* 192:1442, 1988.

4. Paradis M: New approaches to the treatment of canine demodicosis, *Vet Clin North Am Small Anim Pract* 29:1425, 1999.

5. Hsu WH, Schaffer DD: Effects of topical application of amitraz on plasma glucose and insulin concentrations in dogs, *Am J Vet Res* 49:130, 1988.

6. Smith BE et al: Amitraz-induced glucose intolerance in rats: antagonism by yohimbine but not by prazosin, *Arch Toxicol* 64:680, 1990.

7. al-Qarawi AA et al: Effects of amitraz given by different routes on rats, *Vet Human Toxicol* 41:355, 1999.

8. Pesticide information profile for amitraz, EXTOXNET, 1995, Oregon State University, *http://ace.orst.edu/info/extoxnet/*.

9. Roberts MC, Argenzio A: Amitraz induced large intestinal impaction in the horse, *Aust Vet J* 55:553, 1979.

10. Pass MA, Mogg TD: Pharmacokinetics and metabolism of amitraz in ponies and sheep, *J Vet Pharmacol Ther* 18:210, 1995.

11. Grossman MR: Amitraz toxicosis associated with ingestion of an acaricide collar in a dog, *J Am Vet Med Assoc* 203:55, 1993.

12. Turnbull G.J: Animal studies on the treatment of poisoning by amitraz (a formamidine pesticide) and xylene, *Human Toxicol* 2:579, 1983.

13. Hugnet C et al: Toxicity and kinetics of amitraz in dogs, *Am J Vet Res* 57:1506, 1996.

14. Osweiler GD: *Toxicology,* Philadelphia, 1996, Williams & Wilkins.

15. Hsu WH et al: Effect of yohimbine on amitraz-induced CNS depression and bradycardia in dogs, *J Toxicol Environ Health* 18:423, 1986.

16. Hsu WH et al: Effect of amitraz on heart rate and aortic blood pressure in conscious dogs: influence of atropine, prazosin, tolazoline, and yohimbine, *Toxicol Appl Pharmacol* 84:418, 1986.

Anticholinesterase Insecticides

1. World Health Organization: Organophosphorus insecticides: a general introduction, Environmental Health Criteria, No. 63, Albany, N.Y., 1986.

2. Taylor P: Anticholinesterase agents. In Hardman JG, Limbird LL, Gillman AG, editors: *Goodman and Gilman's the pharmacological basis of therapeutics,* ed 10, New York, 2001, McGraw-Hill.

3. DuBois KP: The toxicity of organophosphorus compounds to mammals, *Bull WHO* 44:233, 1971.

4. Andersen RA et al: Inhibition of acetylcholinesterase from different species by organophosphorus compounds, carbamates and methylsulphonyl-fluoride, *Gen Pharmacol* 8:331, 1977.

5. *Farm chemicals handbook 2002,* vol 88, Willoughby, Ohio, 2001, Meister Publishing.

6. Lein DH et al: Chlorpyrifos (Dursban 44) toxicity in dairy bulls, *Cornell Vet* 72(suppl 9):1, 1982.

7. DeBleecker JL: The intermediate syndrome in organophosphate poisoning: an overview of experimental and clinical observations, *J Toxicol Clin Toxicol* 33(6):683, 1995.

8. Silvestri R, Himes JA, Edds GT: Repeated oral-administration of coumaphos in sheep: effects on erythrocyte acetylcholinesterase and other constituents, *Am J Vet Res* 36(3):283, 1975.

9. Johnson DD, Wilcox WC: Studies on the mechanism of the protective and antidotal actions of diazepam in organophosphate poisoning, *Eur J Pharmacol* 34:127, 1975.

10. Clemmons RM et al: Correction of organophosphate-induced neuro-muscular blockade by diphenhydramine, *Am J Vet Res* 45(10):2167, 1984.

11. Carson TL: Organophosphate and carbamate insecticide poisoning. In Kirk RW, editor: *Current vet therapy VIII,* Philadelphia, 1983, WB Saunders.

Diethyltoluamide

1. Qiu H et al: Pharmacokinetics of insect repellent *N,N*-diethyl-m-toluamide in beagle dogs following intravenous and topical routes of administration, *J Pharm Sci* 86:514, 1997.

2. Robbins PJ, Cherniack MG. Review of the biodistribution and toxicity of the insect repellent N,N-diethyl-m-toluamide (DEET), *J Toxicol Environ Health* 18:503, 1986.

3. Dorman DC: Diethyltoluamide (DEET) insect repellent toxicosis, *Vet Clin North Am Small Anim Pract* 20:387, 1990.

4. Osimitz TG, Murphy JV: Neurological effects associated with use of the insect repellent N,N-diethyl-m-toluamide, *J Toxicol Clin Toxicol* 35:435, 1997.

5. Palmer JS: Toxicologic effects of aerosols of N,N-diethyl-m-toluamide (DEET) applied on skin of horses, *Am J Vet Res* 30:1929, 1969.

6. Blume RR et al: Tests of aerosols of DEET for protection of livestock from biting flies, *J Econ Entomol* 64:1193, 1971.

7. Keplinger ML et al: Subacute oral and dermal toxicity of DEET (N, N-diethyl-m-toluamide). *Fed Proc Fed Am Soc Exp Biol* 20: 432, 1961.

8. Verschoyle RD et al: A comparison of the acute toxicity, neuropathology, and electrophysiology of N,N-diethyl-m-toluamide and N,N-dimethyl-2,2-diphenylacetamide in rats, *Fundam Appl Toxicol* 18:79, 1992.

9. Dorman DC et al: Fenvalerate/N,N-diethyl-m-toluamide (DEET) toxicosis in two cats, *J Am Vet Med Assoc* 196:100, 1990.

Metaldehyde

1. Booze TF, Oehme FW: Metaldehyde toxicity: a review, *Vet Hum Toxicol* 27(1):11, 1985.

2. Keller KH et al: Acetaldehyde analysis in severe metaldehyde poisoning, *Vet Hum Toxicol* 33:374, 1991.

3. Shintani S et al: Adsorption effects of activated charcoal on metaldehyde toxicity in rats, *Vet Hum Toxicol* 41(1):15, 1999.

4. Tardieu D et al: Phenobarbital-type P-450 inducers protect rats against metaldehyde toxicity, *Vet Hum Toxicol* 38(6):454, 1996.

5. Homeida AM, Cooke RG: Pharmacological aspects of metaldehyde poisoning in mice, *J Vet Pharmacol Ther* 5(1):77, 1982.

6. Homeida AM, Cooke RG: Anti-convulsant activity of diazepam and clonidine on metaldehyde-induced seizures in mice: effects on brain-amino butyric acid concentrations and monoamine oxidase activity, *J Vet Pharmacol Ther* 5:187, 1982.

7. Von Burg R, Stout T: Toxicology update, *J Applied Toxicol* 11(5):377, 1991.

8. Hatch E: In Booth NH, McDonald LE, editors: *Veterinary pharmacology and therapeutics,* Ames, Iowa, 1988, Iowa State University Press.

9. Stubbings DP: Three cases of metaldehyde poisoning in cattle, *Vet Rec* 98:356, 1976.

10. Egyed MN, Brisk YL: Metaldehyde poisoning in farm animals, *Vet Rec* 78:753, 1966.

11. Harris WF: Metaldehyde poisoning in three horses, *Mod Vet Pract* 56(5):336, 1975.

12. Delak M, Marzan B: Toxicity of metaldehyde to poultry, *Vet Archiv* 28:95, 1958.

13. Firth AM: Treatment of snail bait toxicity in dogs: literature review, *Vet Emerg Crit Care* 2(1):25, 1992.

14. Firth AM: Treatment of snail bait toxicity in dogs: retrospective study of 56 cases, *Vet Emerg Crit Care* 2(1):31, 1992.

Novel Insecticides

1. Thomson WT: *Agricultural chemicals,* book I: Insecticides, acaricides and ovicides, 14th rev, Fresno, Calif, 1998, Thomson Publications.

2. Weil A, Cochet P, Birckel P: *Skin and hair distribution of 14C-fipronil by microautoradiography following topical administration to the beagle dogs.* In Proceedings of the 42nd Annual Meeting of the American Association of Veterinary Parasitologists, Reno, Nev, 1997.

3. U.S. Environmental Protection Agency: *New pesticide fact sheet,* EPA-737-F-96-005, Washington, DC, 1996, Office of Prevention, Pesticides and Toxic Substances.

4. Cole LM, Nicholson RA, Casida JE: Action of phenylpyrazole insecticides at the GABA-gated chloride channel, *Pesticide Biochem Physiol* 46:47, 1993.

5. Rhone Merieux, Inc. Frontline® product information, Athens, Ga, 1997.

6. Consalvi PJ, Arnaud JP, Jeannin P et al: *Safety of a 0.29% w/w fipronil solution (Frontline® Spray) in dogs and cats. Results of a pharmacovigilance survey one year after launch*. In Proceedings of the 41st Annual Meeting of the American Association of Veterinary Parasitologists, Louisville, Ky, 1996.

7. Gill MW, Wagner CL, Driscoll CD: MB 46030: Single exposure peroral (gavage) neurotoxicity study in Sprague Dawley rats. Union Carbide Bushy Run Research Centre, Laboratory Project ID 91N0099, 27 April 1993.

8. Rhone-Poulenc: *Fipronil worldwide technical bulletin,* Research Triangle Park, N.C., 1996.

9. Keister EM: Pharmaceutical Group of North America, Rhone Merieux, letter to practitioners, 1996.

10. Hamon N, Shaw R, Yang H: Worldwide development of fipronil insecticide. In Herzog GA, Hardee DA (chairs), Ottens RJ, Ireland CS, Nelms JV, editors: *Proceedings Beltwide Cotton Conferences US,* vol. 2, Jan 9-12 1996, Nashville, Tenn, Cotton insect research and control conference, NCC, Memphis, Tenn.

11. Lahr J, Badji A, Ndour KB, Diallo AO: Acute toxicity tests with *Streptocephalus sudanicus* (Branchipoda, Anostraca) and *Anisops sardeus* (Hemiptera, Notonectidae) using insecticides for desert locust control. In Everts JW, Mbaye D, Barry O, Mullie W, editors: *Environmental side-effects of locust and grasshopper control,* vol 3, LOCUSTOX Project—GCP/SEN/041/NET, FAO, Dakar, Senegal, 1998.

12. Meister RT, editor: *Farm chemicals handbook,* vol. 82, Willoughby, Ohio, 1996, Meister Publishing.

13. Kidd H, James DR, editors: *The agrochemicals handbook*, ed 3, Cambridge, UK, 1991, Royal Society of Chemistry Information Services (as updated).

14. Bai D, Lummis SCR, Leicht W et al: Actions of imidacloprid and a related nitromethylene on cholinergic receptors of an identified insect motor neuron, *Pesticide Sci* 33:197, 1991.

15. Lui MY, Cassida JE: High affinity of [3H] imidacloprid in the insect acetylcholine receptor, *Pesticide Biochem Physiol* 46:40, 1993.

16. Nagata K, Song JH, Shono T et al: Modulation of the neuronal nicotinic acetylcholine receptor channel by the nitromethylene heterocycle imidacloprid, *J Pharmacol Exp Ther* 285:731, 1998.

17 Werner G, Hopkins T, Shmidl JA et al: Imidacloprid, a novel compound of the chloronicotinyl group with an outstanding insecticidal activity in the on-animal treatment of pests, *Pharmacol Res* 31:S126, 1995.

18. Griffin L, Hopkins TJ: Imidacloprid: Safety of a new insecticidal compound in dogs and cats. *Compend Contin Educ Pract Vet* 19(suppl):17, 1997.

19. Imidacloprid; pesticide tolerances. July 5, 1995. *Fed Reg* 60(128): 34943.

20. U.S. Environmental Protection Agency: *Imidacloprid; pesticide tolerance and raw agricultural commodities,* 40 CFR Part 180 Section 472, Washington, D.C., 1995.

21. Doull J, Klassen CD, Amdur MO, editors: *Cassarett and Doull's toxicology. The basic science of poisons,* ed 4, Elmsford, N.Y., 1991, Pergamon Press.

22. Placke FJ, Weber E: Method of determining imidacloprid residues in plant materials, *Pflanzenschutz-Nachrichten Bayer* 46(2):109, 1993.

23. Li K, Li QX: Development of an enzyme-linked immunosorbent assay for the insecticide imidacloprid, *J Agri Food Chem* 48(8):3378, 2000.

24. Cyanamid Agricultural Division: *Technical data sheet. Amdro fire ant insecticide (hydramethylnon),* Wayne, N.J., 1986, American Cyanamid Co.

25. American Cyanamid Co: *Technical data sheet. Maxforce (hydramethylnon),* Wayne, N.J., 1988, American Cyanamid Co.

26. U.S. National Library of Medicine: *Hazardous substances databank,* Bethesda, Md, 1995, U.S. National Library of Medicine.

27. U.S. Environmental Protection Agency: *Characteristics of hazardous waste,* 40 CFR 261.2-261.24, Washington, D.C., 1996, U.S. Environmental Protection Agency.

28. U.S. Environmental Protection Agency: Integrated Risk Information System Database, Washington, D.C., 1995.

29. Evans DL, Jacobsen KL, Miller DM: Hematologic and immunologic responses of Holstein calves to a fire ant toxicant, *Am J Vet Res* 1984;45:1023.

30. Miller DM, Caudle AB, Crowell-Davis S: *Effects of consumption of a fire ant toxicant on horses,* American Association of Veterinary Diagnosticians 27th Annual Proceeding, 1984.

31. Stout SJ, Steller WA, Tondreau RE et al: Residue methodology for AMDRO fire ant insecticide (AC 217,300) in pasture grass and crops, *J Assoc Off Anal Chem* 68:71, 1985.

32. Manning RO, Bruckner JV, Mispagel ME, Bowen JM: Metabolism and disposition of sulfluramid, a unique polyfluorinated insecticide, in the rat, *Drug Metab Dispos* 19(1):205, 1991.

33. Grossman MR, Mispagel ME, Bowen JM: Distribution and tissue elimination in rats during and after prolonged dietary exposure to a highly fluorinated sulfonamide pesticide, *J Agric Food Chem* 40(12):2505, 1992.

34. U.S. Environmental Protection Agency: *Pesticide fact sheet #205 (sulfluramid),* Washington, D.C., 1989, U.S. Environmental Protection Agency.

35. Vitayavirasuk B, Bowen JM: Pharmacokinetics of sulfluramid and its metabolite desethylsulfuramid after intravenous and intraruminal administration to sheep, *Pesticide Science,* 55(7):719, 1999.

36. FMC Corporation: *Material safety data sheet. FluorGuard Ant Bait Station insecticide (sulfluramid),* Philadelphia, 1998, FMC Corporation.

Organochlorine Insecticides

1. Buck WB, Osweiler GD, Van Gelder GA: *Clinical and diagnostic veterinary toxicology,* ed 2, Dubuque, Iowa, 1976, Kendall/Hunt Publishing.

2. Osweiler GD: *Toxicology,* Media, Pa, 1996, Williams & Wilkins.

3. Beasley VR, Dorman DC, Fikes FD, Diana SG: *A systems approach to veterinary toxicology,* Champagne, Ill, 1994, University of Illinois.

4. Lorgue G, Lechenet J, Riviere A: *Clinical veterinary toxicology,* Cambridge, Mass, 1996, Blackwell Science.

5. Klaassen CD, editor: *Klaassen Casarett & Doull's toxicology: the basic science of poisons,* ed 5, New York, 1996, McGraw-Hill.

6. Murphy M: *A field guide to common animal poisons,* Ames, Iowa, 1996, Iowa State University Press.

Pyrethrins and Pyrethroids

1. Valentine WM: Pyrethrin and pyrethroid insecticides. *Vet Clin North Am Small Anim Pract* 20(2):375, 1998.

2. Vais H et al: The molecular interactions of pyrethroid insecticides with insect and mammalian sodium channels, *Pest Manag Sci* 57:877, 2001.

3. Volmer PA et al: Warning against use of some permethrin products in cats, *J Am Vet Med Assoc* 213(6):800, 1998.

4. Volmer PA et al: Permethrin spot-on products can be toxic in cats, *Vet Med* 93(12):1039, 1998.

5. Agency for Toxic Substances and Disease Registry (2001): *Toxicological profile for pyrethrins and pyrethroids: draft for public comment,* Washington, D.C., 2001, U.S. Department of Health and Human Services, Public Health Service.

6. Narahashi T: In Soria B, Cena V: *Ion channel pharmacology,* New York, 1998, Oxford University Press.

7. Narahashi T: Neuroreceptors and ion channels as the basis for drug action: past, present, and future, *J Pharm Exp Ther* 294:1, 2000.

8. Ecobichon DJ: In Klaassen CD: *Casarett and Doull's toxicology: the basic science of poisons,* ed 6, New York, 2001, McGraw-Hill.

9. EXTOXNET 1996. *http://ace.orst.edu/info/extoxnet/pips/permethr.htm.*

22

Metals and Minerals

ARSENIC

Steve Ensley

Sources. The commercial forms of arsenic include inorganic and organic arsenic.[1-3] Inorganic arsenic was formerly used as arsenic trioxide, a herbicide and insecticide.[4] Arsenic trioxide is used as a source for other arsenicals. Pentavalent (arsenate, H_3AsO_4) and trivalent (arsenite, H_3AsO_3) forms of inorganic arsenic are used as sodium, potassium, and calcium salts for baits.[5] Paris green (copper acetoarsenite) and lead arsenate have been used as insecticides.[6] Trivalent forms of inorganic arsenic, such as monosodium methanearsonate (MSMA) and disodium methanearsonate (DSMA), are used as herbicides.[2]

Organic forms of arsenic are also present as pentavalent and trivalent forms. Pentavalent arsenicals have been used as feed additives for food animals. The most common feed additives containing arsenic are arsenilic acid, sodium arsanilate, and 3-nitro, 4-hydroxyphenylarsonic acid (3-nitro). Renewed interest in arsenic feed additives has occurred because there are concerns about use of antimicrobials as growth promotants in food animals. Thiacetarsamide, an organic arsenical, has been used for heartworm therapy in dogs.

Sources of arsenic poisoning include areas around mining or smelting sites. Normally soils contain low concentrations of elemental arsenic; however, mine tailings, smoke, fumes, and dust may contaminate soils near mining or smelting sites. The ores arsenopyrite and loellingite are smelted to produce elemental arsenic and arsenic trioxide. Arsenic in the environment is usually present in the pentavalent form and may be methylated by microorganisms.

Exposure to arsenic by animals can result from accidental exposure to old pesticides such as lead arsenate and arsenic trioxide that have been improperly discarded or stored. Wood products treated with arsenic compounds such as copper, chromium, and arsenic (CCA) can cause toxicosis when they are burned and generate ashes.[2] Some ant baits contain sodium or potassium arsenate, which can be consumed by small animals.[5]

An additional source of arsenic exposure can be arsine. Arsine (ASH_3) is the hydride gas of arsenic. Arsine is an industrial gas or gaseous product of the charging of storage batteries.

Arsenic in drinking water has recently come under scrutiny by the Environmental Protection Agency because of the potential of carcinogenicity in humans. Drinking water can become contaminated in abandoned mining areas or contain elevated concentrations (>5 ppb) of dissolved arsenic that is present naturally in the aquifer. Concentrations of arsenic from 10 to 50 ppb in drinking water have not been documented to cause pathologic problems in animals.

Toxicokinetics. The solubility of the formulation, route of exposure, rate of absorption, rate of metabolism and excretion, and acceptability of the formulation to animals influence the toxicity of arsenic. Soluble arsenicals are readily absorbed from the gastrointestinal tract and through the skin.[1] The kidneys may reduce a small portion of orally absorbed pentavalent arsenicals to the more toxic trivalent form. This may explain the nephrotoxicity that can be observed. In vivo methylation of inorganic arsenicals is an important detoxification mechanism and large amounts of methylated arsenic compounds are excreted.[2]

Most pentavalent arsenicals are excreted in the feces and trivalent arsenicals are readily excreted into the intestine via the bile.[2] Excretion of arsenicals is rapid in domestic animals and nearly complete within a few days.

Mechanism of Action. Trivalent arsenicals inhibit cellular respiration. Trivalent arsenicals bind to sulfhydryl compounds, especially lipoic acid and α-ketooxidases. Lipoic acid, a tissue respiratory enzyme cofactor, plays an important role in the tricarboxylic acid (TCA) cycle. Tissues with high oxidative energy requirements such as actively dividing cells of the intestinal epithelium, epidermis, kidney, liver, skin, and lung are most affected. Trivalent arsenic also affects capillary integrity by an unknown mechanism. The capillary system of the gastrointestinal tract is most affected. Capillary dilatation is followed by transudation of plasma into the gastrointestinal tract, resulting in submucosal congestion and edema.

Pentavalent inorganic arsenicals appear to substitute for phosphate in oxidative phosphorylation. Uncoupling of oxidative phosphorylation produces a cellular energy deficit. Unlike other compounds that uncouple oxidative phosphorylation, elevated body temperatures are not characteristic of pentavalent arsenic poisoning.

The hydride gas of arsenic, ASH_3, can combine with hemoglobin and be oxidized to a hemolytic metabolite.

Toxicity and Risk Factors. Cats are the species most susceptible to arsenic, followed by horses, cattle, sheep, swine, and birds. Subacute toxicosis can occur at lower doses received over several days. Chronic toxicosis from inorganic arsenicals is generally not observed in animals.

The ability of the inorganic arsenicals to cause toxicosis depends on valence. Trivalent forms are 10 times more toxic than pentavalent forms.[5] The trivalent forms have varying degrees of toxicity. For most species a lethal single dose of sodium arsenite ranges from 1 to 25 mg/kg body weight. The single lethal dose of arsenic trioxide is 3 to 10 times less than sodium arsenite. The oral lethal dose 50 (LD_{50}) in rats for sodium arsenite is 42 mg/kg and for arsenic trioxide is 385 mg/kg. A chronic lethal dose of sodium arsenite is 0.2 to 0.5 mg/kg/day for several months.[7]

Cattle that ingested MSMA died after five daily doses of 10 mg/kg body weight and six daily doses of DSMA at 25 mg/kg body weight.[2] Sheep that ingested MSMA died after six daily doses of 50 mg/kg body weight and six daily doses of DMSA at 25 mg/kg body weight.[2] Cattle and sheep experience toxicosis when exposed to 8 to 10 daily doses of the herbicide cacodylic acid (dimethyl arsenic acid) at 25 mg/kg body weight. The oral LD_{50} for cacodylic acid in rats is 644 to 830 mg/kg.

Organic arsenical feed additives that are fed too long or at overdoses have caused arsenic toxicosis in swine and poultry. Organic arsenicals produce toxicosis in swine diets at 500 ppm arsanilic acid or 250 ppm 3-nitro, 4-hydroxyphenylarsonic acid for 7 to 10 days.[5] Poultry are affected by dietary exposure at approximately twice the dose that affects swine.

Therapeutic use of thiacetarsamide as a heartworm treatment in dogs has resulted in arsenic toxicosis.

Clinical Signs. Arsenic compounds cause severe effects in the gastrointestinal system.[3] Organic or inorganic trivalent arsenicals cause acute or peracute poisoning. It is common to have high morbidity and mortality rates over 2 to 3 days with peracute and acute episodes of inorganic arsenic poisoning.[2] Vomiting, intense abdominal pain, weakness, staggering, ataxia, recumbency, and weak, rapid pulse with signs of shock are common. Rapid onset of watery diarrhea or rumen and gastrointestinal atony may occur. Subacute poisoning occurs when affected animals survive acute arsenic poisoning and live 3 days or longer.[5] Watery diarrhea can continue in subacute poisonings. Damage to the kidneys can result in oliguria and proteinuria that can follow the initial toxicosis. The resulting dehydration, acidosis, and azotemia may cause death.

Chronic poisoning is rarely seen in domestic animals but has been observed frequently in humans.

Organic pentavalent arsenical feed additives (usually in swine) can cause signs within 2 to 4 days of an overdose. Clinical signs include ataxia, incoordination, torticollis, and blindness. Affected animals assume a dog-sitting position and eventually become paralyzed in lateral recumbency. Appetites remain normal and affected animals are cognizant, except for some with blindness.

Clinical Pathology. Clinical pathology findings are not specific for arsenic poisoning, but increased hematocrit, increased blood urea nitrogen (BUN), proteinuria, increased urine specific gravity, and urinary casts have been reported as a result of renal damage.

Lesions. Gross lesions include generalized or localized redness of the gastric, abomasal, or intestinal mucosa. Gastrointestinal irritation characterized by mucosal congestion, prominent submucosal edema, epithelial necrosis, and massive accumulation of fluids in a dilated atonic intestine is frequently observed with arsenic poisoning. In some cases the necrosis in the gastrointestinal system progresses to perforation. In subacute cases, pale, swollen kidneys, pale, yellow liver, and petechial hemorrhages of the intestinal serosa and mucosa can be seen. Microscopic lesions include intestinal capillary dilatation, submucosal congestion and edema, intestinal epithelial necrosis, renal tubular necrosis, and hepatic fatty degeneration.[2]

Organic arsenicals target the nervous system. Microscopic lesions of arsenilic acid poisoning include mild edema of the white matter in the brain and spinal cord, and a few shrunken and degenerate neurons in the medulla. With arsenilic acid toxicosis, extensive wallerian degeneration can occur in the optic and peripheral nerves. 3-Nitro toxicosis can cause wallerian degeneration in the dorsal proprioceptive and spinocerebellar tracts of the cervical cord, and in the posterior cord there is damage to the lateral and ventral funiculi.[3]

Diagnostic Testing. Increased arsenic in urine, vomitus, feces, liver, and kidney can be found in acute poisonings. During chronic poisoning inorganic arsenic accumulates in the epidermis and hair, persisting for weeks to months after exposure. Suspected baits, feed, plants, or soil can be analyzed for arsenic content.

Organic pentavalent arsenicals accumulate in nervous tissue and may persist at elevated levels for several weeks after an acute poisoning.

Treatment. Early intervention, including gastrointestinal detoxification and supportive therapy, is essential. Emergency and supportive care include correction of shock, acidosis, and dehydration. A blood transfusion may be necessary. Emetics, cathartic agents, or gastric lavage may be used if ingestion is recent.

Dimercaprol (British anti-Lewisite, or BAL) is the classic antidote for arsenic, but it is relatively ineffective unless given before the onset of clinical signs. The dose of BAL is 6 mg/kg every 8 hours for 3 to 5 days. Renal function needs to be monitored when using BAL.[5] Thioctic acid (50 mg/kg every 8 hours at two to three injection sites) is more effective than dimercaprol for arsenic-poisoned cattle; however, it is not available in a commercial dosage form and it is not currently approved for use in food animals.[5]

Mesodimercaptosuccinic acid and dimercaptosuccinic acid (Succimer, DMSA) are water soluble analogues of dimercaprol. Succimer is currently the preferred chelator and is available in the United States. Dimercaptosuccinic acid (DMSA) Succimer is effective for increasing excretion of arsenicals (10 mg/kg three times per day [tid] orally for 10 days).[6]

Convalescent animals need to receive bland diets containing reduced amounts of high-quality protein. Vitamin supplementation is recommended.

Prognosis. The mortality rate is high among animals acutely poisoned with inorganic arsenicals. Animals poisoned with pentavalent organic arsenicals can experience a high morbidity rate, but with good nursing care a low mortality rate. Recovery may require 2 to 4 weeks.

Prevention and Control. Animal exposure to inorganic arsenic as pesticides and herbicides is less frequent than in the past because safer compounds are usually used. Knowing where mining and smelting sites are and avoidance of these sites is important. Not allowing animals access to burn piles of CCA-treated wood is also advisable. When using organic arsenicals in swine feed, one must be aware that not all arsenicals are used at the same dose.

COPPER

Robert B. Moeller, Jr.

Synonyms. Enzootic icterus of sheep in South Africa is believed to be chronic copper poisoning.[1]

Source. Numerous sources of copper are available in the animal's environment. The interaction of copper, molybdenum, and sulfate are critical in the absorption of copper (particularly ruminants) and needs to be evaluated in the diet. Because molybdenum and sulfate bind with copper to form insoluble copper sulfide, deficiencies of molybdenum in the diet can result in excessive copper absorption by the gut and increased hepatocellular copper storage.[2]

The feeding of calf or horse rations (which commonly contain high levels of copper) to sheep is often the source of excessive copper in the diet. Poultry and swine rations should also be avoided. The feeding of monensin in a high copper ration to young animals can also increase intestinal absorption of copper, which can result in toxic copper levels in the animal.[3]

Certain fungicides used in orchards contain copper salts and can result in excessive accumulations in the plants and soil. Copper-containing algicides used in ponds and water tanks can cause increased copper concentrations in the animal. Footbaths containing copper salts ($CuSO_4$) are also potential sources of excess copper. The drainage of copper-containing footbaths into waste collection ponds and the spreading of the copper-contaminated water onto fields can also cause increased copper levels in forage harvested from those fields.

Toxicokinetics. Copper is primarily absorbed in the stomach, duodenum, jejunum, and ileum in monogastric animals. The large intestine is also important for copper absorption in ruminants (particularly sheep) with the rest absorbed in the lower small intestine. Copper is actively transported through the enterocytes into the bloodstream, where it loosely binds to albumin, ceruloplasmin, and the protein transcuprein. Once absorbed into the bloodstream, copper is then distributed to the liver, kidney, and brain, where it is stored. Most of the copper is picked up, stored, and metabolized by the liver. Hepatocytes pick up the copper and store it in the lysosomes and then incorporate it into ceruloplasmin (an α_2-globulin), which stores the copper into a stable electron state for use by the body.[1,4-7]

Although most tissues use copper, elevated levels are often first detected in the liver. When copper levels in the liver reach suspected toxic levels, liver necrosis can occur. Copper is then released into the bloodstream, resulting in erythrolysis, hemoglobinuria, and elevated copper in the serum. This excessive copper is absorbed by the kidneys, causing elevated renal copper levels. Excessive copper is also stored in the bone marrow and brain but at much lower levels than in the kidney.[2-4]

Small amounts of copper are excreted in the urine. Most copper is excreted as insoluble copper complexes from the bile.[2,3, 6] Some of the copper secreted in the bile is reabsorbed via the intestines but most is removed from the body in the feces. In sheep copper is excreted in the urine at 1 µg/kg body weight. Young animals may excrete much more copper in the urine. Biliary excretion of copper is more pronounced with greater than 3 µg/kg body weight per day.[6] The bioavailability of copper is limited to the amount of molybdenum and sulfur ingested. This is particularly true in ruminants. In the rumen molybdenum and sulfur form thiomolybdate, which reacts with copper to form insoluble copper complexes. These insoluble complexes result in decreased absorption of copper in the intestine. Copper/molybdenum ratios of 6:1 to 10:1 are recommended for most ruminant diets to prevent excessive copper accumulation in the liver. Sulfur levels greater than 0.35% can reduce copper absorption. Iron and zinc can also act as antagonists to copper and limit the absorption of copper from the gut.[3,8]

Mechanism of Action. Copper exerts its toxic action primarily on the liver because there are excessive accumulations of copper in the hepatic lysosomes. The excessive copper causes damage to the cell membranes and death of the hepatocytes. Copper is then released into the bloodstream. As long as the liver is able to reabsorb the copper and keep up with the hepatocellular loss, the animal is able to compensate for the hepatic damage. Once the animal is stressed or ingests hepatotoxic substances, such as pyrrolizidine alkaloids (which inhibit cell replication), hepatic compensation is lost and hepatocellular necrosis results. Because the new immature hepatocytes that are forming in the liver lack the ability to rapidly absorb and clear the excess serum copper, large amounts of free copper are released into the circulation. Once in the circulation, the copper damages the membrane of red blood cells, causing the release of hemoglobin by intravascular hemolysis. With the lysis of red blood cells, the animal becomes anoxic causing more compromise to the liver and resulting in additional centrilobular necrosis and copper release. Excessive free copper then accumulates in the kidneys.

Toxicity and Risk Factors.   Sheep are sensitive to copper, whereas cattle, horses, swine, chicken, turkeys, and dogs are relatively resistant to excessive accumulations of copper.

Thirty parts per million copper in the diet of sheep can be toxic (normal dietary levels 10 to 20 ppm), whereas cattle can handle up to 50 ppm (normal 10 to 25 ppm) in the ration. Again the amount of molybdenum in the ration plays an important role in how much of the copper is taken up by the body and stored in the liver.[3] In most ruminants the accumulation of more than 250 ppm copper in the liver is considered toxic. However, in cattle it is rare to see hepatocellular necrosis at these concentrations. Sheep, on the other hand, can have prominent liver necrosis at these concentrations.

Swine and horses are relatively resistant to copper toxicosis. In the horse dietary copper levels greater than 50 ppm are required to cause gastric upset and death when fed for several weeks. Four hundred parts per million total dietary copper can cause depressed growth rates and decreased feed consumption in growing pigs. Levels greater than 500 ppm fed to pregnant sows can cause copper toxicosis in nursing piglets and the fetus. However, feeding copper at 250 ppm has little or no ill effects on pigs. Turkeys can tolerate up to 500 ppm copper, whereas chickens can tolerate more than 300 to 500 ppm.[3,9]

Dogs are fairly resistant to copper. In the dog copper levels greater than 350 to 400 ppm are a concern and are considered toxic. However, the Bedlington terriers, West Highland white terriers, and Skye terriers have an inherited autosomal recessive trait resulting in accumulation of copper in the hepatocytes caused by decreased copper biliary excretion. These breeds commonly have liver concentrations of more than 2000 ppm without significant liver damage.[3,10,11] However, the defect results in toxic accumulations of copper up to 10,000 ppm in the liver.[10-12]

Clinical Signs.   Sheep rarely show clinical signs until the animal is stressed, resulting in a massive liver necrosis and copper release. The released copper then causes intravascular hemolysis of red blood cells, resulting in hemoglobinuria, icterus, anoxia, and death. Urine is dark red (port wine) as a result of the presence of hemoglobin in the urine.[13-15] Usually only one or two animals in the group die at any one time, while the remainder of the flock appears clinically normal. However, once a stressor affects the flock again, several more animals may die. Copper toxicosis in cattle appears similar to that noted in sheep.

In swine copper toxicosis is characterized by anorexia, depression, poor weight gain, icterus, hemoglobinuria, and bloody feces.[9] Young swine are more likely to develop clinical toxicosis than are adults.

In the dog chronic copper toxicosis is seen primarily in the Bedlington and West Highland white terrier breeds. Often animals do not show clinical signs of toxicosis with copper levels at 2000 ppm. However, as copper levels increase, a chronic active hepatitis with slow hepatocellular death and loss develops in affected animals. This eventually results in micronodular and macronodular hepatocellular regeneration in the liver. A hemolytic crisis or hemoglobinuria never develops from a massive release of copper by the liver. Affected dogs usually present with weight loss and anorexia. Later in the disease, ascites sometimes develops, and in some dogs, central nervous system (CNS) signs develop as a result of the inability of the liver to detoxify toxic products from the bloodstream. Liver enzymes are often elevated, but icterus is uncommon.[10-12,16]

Clinical Pathology.   Often clinical signs of copper toxicosis develop acutely and the animals die before clinical parameters are noted. Because these animals have hepatocellular damage, surviving animals may have elevated liver enzymes (aspartate aminotransferase, sorbitol dehydrogenase, alkaline phosphate, and gamma-glutamyltransferase).[13]

Bedlington and West Highland white terriers develop a chronic progressive disease with resulting elevated hepatic enzymes (alkaline aminotransferase and alkaline phosphatase).

Lesions.   In sheep copper toxicosis is usually considered a chronic problem because of the slow buildup of copper in the liver followed by the quick release of copper from the hepatocytes. The lesions of copper toxicosis are hemoglobinuria (from intravascular hemolysis), dark red or bluish-black kidneys (sometimes referred to as gunmetal blue kidneys), and a swollen, friable liver. Histologically, the livers in affected sheep usually show fibrosis of the portal areas, some bile duct duplication, lymphocytic inflammation, and centrilobular coagulative necrosis.

The ingestion of large amounts of copper sulfate or the injection of excess copper compounds can result in acute copper deaths. Affected animals often present dead with icterus, hemoglobinuria, and large, swollen, friable livers. Hemoglobinuria and centrilobular necrosis of the hepatocytes are commonly found in acute copper toxicosis. Because the abomasum or stomach is irritated by the ingestion of copper sulfate, hemorrhage and edema of the abomasal or stomach mucosa may also be noted. Intestinal contents and feces may have a faint blue-green color.

In Bedlington and West Highland white terriers a chronic active hepatitis develops, characterized by markedly elevated levels of copper in the hepatocytes and slow progressive hepatocellular damage. The animals often have pale brown nodular livers with abundant fibrosis. Histologically, the livers are swollen and often contain abundant brownish yellow pigment. Kupffer cells contain abundant hemosiderin and copper pigments. Scattered necrosis of hepatocytes is evident with minimal inflammation. Fibrosis is primarily portal, but can be variable depending on the progression of the disease in the animal. In time micronodular and macronodular regeneration of the liver develop, resulting in the variable sized nodules seen on the capsular surface.

Diagnostic Testing. Serum copper levels can be difficult to interpret. Even though excessive copper is being accumulated in the liver, the serum copper levels often remain normal until hepatocellular necrosis occurs. This elevation may be transient and quickly returns to normal values as a result of renal and hepatic reabsorption if the damage is mild.[3] However, once hepatic compensation is lost, the copper is released from the liver into the bloodstream and a toxic amount of copper is detectable in the serum.

At necropsy it is best to test both the liver and kidney for copper. In many cases the liver releases enough stored copper so that a nontoxic level of copper remains in the hepatic tissues. However, in these cases the released copper will have accumulated in the kidneys, resulting in markedly elevated levels of copper in the kidneys.

In some breeds of dogs particularly the Doberman pinscher, elevated copper levels are caused by chronic active hepatitis with bile stasis, probably because of biliary obstruction and poor release of copper, not because of an inherited trait.[17]

In the Bedlington terrier a DNA microsatellite marker for inherited copper toxicosis is useful in the determination of animals at risk of developing excessive copper accumulation.[18] Liver biopsies also detect excessive copper accumulation.

Treatment. In ruminants with acute copper toxicosis, treatment is often unsuccessful. Ammonium molybdate (50 to 500 mg PO once a day [SID]) and sodium thiosulfate (300 to 1,000 mg PO SID) for 3 weeks should begin to reduce liver copper levels within 4 days of initiation of treatment. Ammonium tetrathiomolybdate (on alternate days for 3 treatments) significantly reduces liver copper levels within 6 days.

D-Penicillamine (10 to 15 mg/kg PO twice daily [bid]) chelates copper and promotes urinary excretion in dogs with copper hepatopathy. 2,3,2-Tetramine is a more potent chelator, but is not available commercially.

Prevention and Control. In ruminants dietary amounts of copper can be regulated by the amount of molybdenum and sulfur in the diet. Ensuring that the copper/molybdenum ratio is 6:1 to 10:1 in the diet greatly assists in decreasing the chances of elevated hepatic copper. In addition, sulfur levels greater than 0.35% assist in lowering copper availability. (Caution: Increased sulfur can lead to thiamine deficiency and polioencephalomalacia.) The addition of zinc to the diet can also decrease copper absorption.[3,8,9]

Water containing excessive copper (copper sulfate in the water to prevent algae formation) should be avoided. Pasturing animals on old orchards where copper-containing pesticides have been used should also be avoided. Sheep should not be fed calf or equine rations.

In Bedlington and West Highland white terriers the problem is not the intake of excess copper, but the increased retention of copper in the hepatocytes. Consequently, the prevention of copper absorption in the stomach and intestine assists in decreasing copper levels. The addition of zinc to the diets of affected dogs can help in forming a mucosal copper block, which ties up copper in the enterocytes and does not allow it to be transported into the enterocytes.[9-11,18]

FLUORIDE

Gary Osweiler

Synonyms. Fluoride is the commonly used term for the monovalent anion of fluorine. As a highly reactive element, fluorine rarely occurs uncombined in nature. Hydrogen fluoride (HF) may be formed in the atmosphere where fluorine gas is generated.[1] HF is a strong acid that is highly reactive with tissues. Synonyms related to fluoride generally are related to sources of fluoride as they occur in nature. These are discussed later.

Sources. Fluorine is present in many sites and forms throughout the world. Soils contain fluorides, generally present as calcium fluoride (CaF_2), which is poorly absorbed by plants. Natural sources include volcanic ash, rock phosphate deposits (RP), iron and aluminum ores, deep wells, geothermal waters, and animal bones. Some of the rock phosphates are used as phosphorus supplements for livestock. If they are fluoride-bearing rocks above regulated levels, they must be defluorinated for use as feed supplements. Water sources of fluorides vary widely across North America. Some geothermal waters in the western United States can contain high levels of fluoride, and sufficient fluorides occur in some deep wells to cause dental mottling or even chronic fluorosis after long-term consumption.[2-4] Other regions of the world with high fluoride concentrations in water include Africa, Argentina, Australia, and India. Local health departments and state departments of natural resources are good sources to learn of specific water fluoride concentrations in the United States. Alfalfa hays from different regions in the United States vary from 0.8 to 36.5 ppm (mean 3.6 ppm) on a dry basis.[5] Pastures in England and Canada appear to range from 7 to 16 ppm.[6,7]

Industrial sources of fluorides may occur during iron and aluminum refining, when fluorides are released from the ore.[5] Fluorine combines with water and particulates in air, eventually settling on vegetation consumed by livestock. Rainfall reduces contamination, and plant levels may decrease when plants lose a large portion of leaves. Gaseous fluoride is also retained in grass and can serve as a fluoride source.[8] Airborne exposure from direct inhalation does not contribute significantly to total fluoride exposure for livestock. When it occurs, contamination is related to the prevailing winds, and fluorides physically contaminate forages near such plants. Current environmental regulations in the United States and other developed countries have largely reduced this threat of contamination.

Sources and exposure to small animals are relatively rare. Sodium fluoride has been used as an insecticide and anthelmintic in the past, but has largely been replaced by safer products with more specific target pests. Other forms of fluorine important in toxicology in the past have included sodium fluoroacetate (compound 1080), formerly used as a rodenticide in the United States, and sodium fluorosilicate.[9] These highly toxic and dangerous rodenticides have been banned from use in the United States, but they may be available in other countries and are occasionally imported illegally.

Exposure to fluorides for large animals, including ruminants and horses, is commonly by use of poorly defluorinated rock phosphate supplements or by forages contaminated with industrial pollutants, dusts, or volcanic ash.[2,10] Rock phosphate supplements used for livestock in the United States must be defluorinated or have a phosphorus/fluorine (P:F) ratio of more than 100:1. At this ratio and higher, the amount of phosphate added to animal rations does not contribute a detrimental amount of fluorides.[2] Products with generally high P:F ratios include defluorinated phosphate, phosphoric acid and sodium phosphate, feed grade diammonium phosphate, and bone meal. Sources with P:F ratios less than 100 include fertilizer grade monoammonium and diammonium phosphate, Curacao rock phosphate, colloidal (soft) phosphate, triple superphosphate, and fluoride rock phosphate. Veterinarians should be aware that attempts to reduce costs in rations could result in adding unapproved sources of phosphate that could promote fluorosis.

Toxicokinetics.   Sodium fluoride is highly available orally and is readily absorbed. It is estimated to be 2 to 5 times more available than common environmental and dietary forms of fluoride (e.g., bone meal, aluminum ore, calcium fluoride, and rock phosphate).[2,10]

Fluorides absorbed from the intestinal tract are transported mainly in the plasma and accumulate most readily in bone. Of the soft tissues, kidney contains the greatest concentrations of fluorides. Approximately half of absorbed fluoride is excreted primarily in the urine by glomerular filtration. Fluoride accumulates in bone with both duration and rate of fluoride intake. If fluoride intake stops, bone fluorides are depleted slowly over a period of months to years. Normal bone fluoride concentrations in cattle are 1000 to 1500 $\mu g/g$. Excessive fluoride concentration in blood of pregnant animals appears to increase neonatal blood concentrations. However, neonatal concentrations appear from twofold to tenfold lower than that in the dam. Fluoride concentrations in milk increase in conjunction with increased plasma fluoride, but specific quantitative relationships appear not to be established.[2]

Mechanism of Action.   The best known and documented effects of fluorides in animals are effects on the teeth and skeletal system.[11,12] Fluorides replace hydroxyapatite in the crystalline structure of bone, resulting in delayed and altered mineralization. Most affected are the matrices supporting formation of enamel, dentine, cementum, and bone. Teeth are affected during development, causing damage to ameloblasts and odontoblasts, and matrix laid down by damaged ameloblasts and odontoblasts fails to accept minerals normally.[13] Structural changes in teeth occur only prior to eruption. Erupted teeth with already formed enamel and dentine are not affected. In fully formed teeth ameloblasts lose their ability to repair enamel, but odontoblasts can produce secondary dentine to accommodate partially for fluorotic damage. Both erupting incisors and molars are affected. These teeth are weaker than normal teeth and wear

rapidly, resulting in excessive pitting and dental wear. Oxidation of organic material in damaged portions of fluorotic teeth causes brown or black discoloration, mainly in the pitted areas.[11,13]

Skeletal fluorosis interferes with formation by osteoblasts of adequate matrix and mineralization. In addition, the substitution of fluoride ion for the hydroxy ion in hydroxyapatite changes the hydroxyapatite crystalline structure and lattice. In skeletal fluorosis there is dysfunction of normal sequences of osteogenesis, acceleration of bone remodeling, production of abnormal bone (exostosis, sclerosis), and in some cases, accelerated resorption. Abnormal and excessive bone remodeling leads to subperiosteal hyperostosis with thickened and irregular surface of long bones.[11,13]

Toxicity and Risk Factors.   Fluoride is present in dietary ingredients and the environment, so a low level of fluoride intake occurs normally throughout life. Several factors may interact to change the toxicity of fluoride in individual animals or herds.[9] Each should be considered as part of the evaluation of fluoride toxicosis. These interacting factors are discussed briefly.

Daily dosage or dietary concentration of fluoride. Fluoride is cumulative during constant or increasing dosage. Chronic fluorosis occurs after prolonged ingestion and results in toxic concentrations in the target tissues, primarily bone and developing teeth. For chronic fluorosis, the National Research Council has established dietary fluoride tolerances for various production animals and horses (Box 22-1).[14,15]

Total exposure time. Because fluorides are cumulative when dietary intake is stable or increasing, exposure time is a major factor in development of dental fluorosis or osteofluorosis.[2] Tolerance levels are based on expected productive lifetime of an animal. Thus dairy cattle with a long productive lifetime and skeletal stresses related to calcium metabolism are considered at highest risk. Long exposure times (2 to 5 years) put animals at higher risk for any given fluoride concentration.

Availability of fluoride in the source ingested. Some tolerance figures have been determined using sodium fluoride (NaF), whereas actual sources of dietary fluoride are likely less available.[2] Thus the established tolerances provide a margin of safety by design as well as by comparative

BOX 22-1	DIETARY FLUORIDE TOLERANCE FOR CHRONIC FLUOROSIS	
ANIMAL	**NRC DIETARY TOLERANCE (ppm)**	
Dairy or beef heifer	30-40	
Adult dairy cattle	40	
Adult beef cattle	40-50	
Finishing cattle	100	
Feeder lambs	150	
Breeding ewes	60	
Horses	40-60	
Swine	50	
Turkeys	150	
Chickens	200	

availability to the NaF standard. Tolerances are determined assuming constant exposure. Intermittent exposures to levels above the tolerances may result in increased severity of bone and tooth lesions. This effect occurs even when the annual average is within tolerances, which is similar to clinical conditions.[16]

Age and species of animal exposed. Box 22-1 shows differences in tolerance among species, as well as between types of animal within species. Furthermore, younger animals are considered at greater risk because of active bone and tooth formation, which increase the opportunity for damage from excessive fluoride. Although not a food animal, mink are considered among the most fluoride resistant of animals where chronic toxicity data are available.[17]

Nutritional factors. Nutritional interrelationships are difficult to interpret. Generally a calcium-deficient diet increases the accumulation and possibly the toxic effects of fluoride, for example, in swine and poultry.[18,19] Increased dietary fat in poultry may also enhance fluoride effects.[20]

Clinical Signs. *Acute fluoride toxicosis* occurs when high doses of a soluble form of fluoride are ingested. The most common source is sodium fluoride. Clinical signs occur between 30 minutes to 1 hour after ingestion. Characteristic acute signs include excitement, seizures, urinary incontinence, defecation, vomiting, weakness, excessive salivation, depression, cardiac failure, and death. Differential diagnosis includes poisoning by metals or metalloids (e.g., arsenic), organophosphate toxicosis, zinc phosphide toxicosis in dogs, and sodium fluoroacetate toxicosis in dogs.[9] The last is a fluorinated organic compound that is no longer readily available in the United States. Because most sources of acute fluoride poisoning are not readily available, acute toxicosis is expected infrequently.

The potentially most important form of fluoride toxicosis is chronic fluorosis of livestock, including horses.[21] Wild herbivores could also be affected if the source is airborne contamination of vegetation. Most documented clinical signs involve the skeletal system and teeth as a result of structural and remodeling changes in those tissues.[9]

Dental fluorosis affects only animals in which active tooth formation is occurring. Teeth already erupted are not susceptible to fluorotic lesions.

Defects in enamel and dentine formation produce mottled and pitted teeth with enamel hypoplasia. The pitted areas become stained with oxidized material, showing brown or black discoloration. As fluoride exposure increases, affected teeth show excessive wear that may abrade incisors and molars as far as the crown of the tooth. Exposure of the pulp cavity and nerves causes dental pain.[22] This lesion leads to difficult mastication, periodic decrease in feed intake, slow growth, and poor performance secondary to reduced feed intake. A characteristic observation in cattle is that they lap water, presumably to lessen the pain of cold water on damaged teeth. Examination of molars and premolars also reveals enamel hypoplasia and excessive dental wear.

Skeletal effects of hyperostosis, enlargement, and roughening of multiple bones are cardinal lesions of fluorosis. These are bilateral and occur initially on the medial surfaces of the proximal one third of the metatarsal bones. As severity

of fluorosis progresses, mandible, metacarpals, and ribs become involved. Periosteal hyperostosis leads to spurring and bridging near joints, leading to intermittent lameness.[12,22] Lameness leads to abnormally reduced hoof wear with elongated toes, especially of the rear legs. Intermittent lameness is typical of chronic fluorosis. In addition, arched back and generalized stiffness may be present periodically. On a herd basis, some animals are likely involved at any one period in time. Visual evidence of hyperostosis may be difficult to detect early in the course of fluorosis. Palpation of metatarsals, ribs, and mandible may assist detection of early skeletal lesions before they are grossly visible.

Animals with chronic fluorosis have dry hair coat and dry, roughened skin. Weight loss and decreased milk production progress as fluorosis becomes more severe and prolonged.[23] Although chronic fluorosis does not directly affect reproduction, severe lameness or dental wear may curtail reproduction because of poor locomotion and malnutrition. Inadequate feed intake caused by dental pain or poor mastication, as well as general physiologic decline, is the likely cause of reduced milk production.[21] Economic losses are due primarily to unthriftiness and low productivity from secondary effects in the skeleton and teeth. One exception is that dairy cattle rations exceeding 150 ppm fluoride for 1 month were associated with signs of reduced grain intake and slightly reduced milk production not attributed to dental fluorosis or osteofluorosis.[16]

Clinical Pathology. Relatively few specific clinical pathology changes occur from acute or chronic fluorosis. Acute toxicosis is likely to cause laboratory changes consistent with dehydration and electrolyte imbalance, as well as renal tubular damage and possible acute leukocyte stress response. For chronic fluorosis in livestock, routine laboratory analysis could reflect severe malnutrition (hypoglycemia, hypoproteinemia), hypothyroidism, anemia, and eosinophilia in cattle clinically diagnosed with moderate fluorosis.[24] Cattle with fluorosis in the Darmous area of Morocco had increased serum potassium, urea, gamma

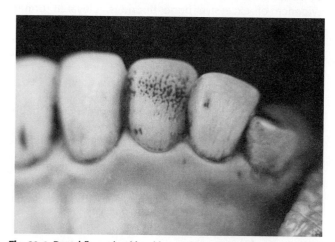

Fig. 22-1 Dental fluorosis with evidence of intermittent fluoride ingestion. Enamel hypoplasia with pitting and staining of enamel is evident in the second incisor. The fourth incisor demonstrates excessive wear resulting from enamel hypoplasia and defective dentin formation.

globulins, lactate dehydrogenase, alkaline phosphatase, and aspartate aminotransferase, whereas calcium, total proteins, and albumin were reduced.[25]

Lesions.   Based on similar eruption times, there is positive correlation between dental fluorosis of some incisors and the abrasion of specific molars and premolars as follows[26]:

Incisor Number	Molar Number
1st	2nd molar
2nd	3rd molar
3rd	2nd premolar

Examination of incisors is a convenient indicator of overall enamel quality in fluorotic cattle.[11,27] Fluorotic enamel is hypomineralized and coronal cementum is hyperplastic. Fluorotic teeth have disrupted subsurface pigment bands, hypoplastic pits, puckered incremental lines, and periodic radiolucent regions.[14] Mild internal structural lesions can best be viewed using lighting from behind the teeth in a moderately darkened area (Fig. 22-1).

When examining bones grossly, the medial aspects of the proximal one third of the metatarsals are affected first with thickening and roughness from periosteal hyperostosis. Similar changes are in metacarpals, mandible, and ribs. Skeletal articular surfaces are not affected.

Microscopic changes of fluorosis include periosteal hyperostosis and thickened cortex, irregular or intermittent mineralization, zones of immature bone, endosteal surface reabsorption, and excessive osteoid tissue. Dysfunctional bone remodeling results in abnormal size and shape of the concentric haversian system of compact bone with evidence of abnormal development of osteoblasts and osteoclasts.[11,13]

Acute fluoride poisoning causes severe gastroenteritis and possible nonspecific renal tubular damage. These changes are expected in animals consuming toxic amounts of sodium fluoride or other fluorinated compounds on an acute basis.

Diagnostic Testing.   Confirmation of a clinical diagnosis is based primarily on knowledge of exposure to fluorides, dental lesions, skeletal fluorosis, intermittent lameness, and evidence of excessive bone fluorides. Elevated urinary concentration of fluorine indicates relatively recent exposure (1 to 3 weeks) or evidence of continuing release from fluorotic bone at 15 to 20 ppm in urine compared with 2 to 6 ppm in normal animals.[9] Radiographic detection of teeth and skeletal changes and microscopic examination of affected bone are helpful adjunct procedures for diagnosis.

Histopathologic and radiographic examination of bones detects bone lesions and tentatively confirms osteofluorosis.[14,26] Biopsy or rib or coccygeal vertebrae is used to obtain samples for skeletal fluoride analysis.[23] Samples at necropsy can include metatarsal, metacarpal, rib, pelvis, and mandible.[11,28] Interpretation of bone assays depends on knowing the normal and abnormal values for different individual bones. Cancellous bone generally contains more fluoride than cortical bone. Results are reported either as ppm of dry fat-free bone or as ppm of bone ash. Normal values for cattle are 400 to 1200 ppm (dry fat-free basis); fluorotic animals contain skeletal fluoride concentrations of 3000 to 5000 ppm (dry fat-free basis). Bone ash values are approximately one third higher than dry fat-free values.[29]

Feed, forages, minerals, and water consumed by fluorotic animals should be analyzed, and other nutritional aspects of the ration (e.g., calcium and phosphorus) should be reviewed.

Treatment.   No specific antidote for either acute or chronic fluoride toxicosis is available. Symptomatic therapy for chronic osteoarthritis, limiting grazing, providing easily masticated feeds, and artificial insemination of valuable breeding animals may help prolong the useful life of livestock. However, for severe fluorosis, economic losses and humane considerations often mandate salvage or euthanasia.

Prognosis.   Prognosis for acute fluoride toxicosis is relatively poor. Soluble fluorides are acute toxicants and the outcome is most related to dose received. Without an effective antidote, provision of prompt gastroenteric detoxification and appropriate supportive therapy for gastroenteritis and renal damage are the major options.

For mild chronic fluorosis prognosis may be relatively good. Mild dental and skeletal changes may be tolerated for many years if ration and grazing are adjusted accordingly. However, fluorosis resulting in excessive dental abrasion or intermittent lameness causes economic damage and is largely insensitive to resolution.

Prevention and Control.   For chronic fluorosis, aluminum sulfate, aluminum chloride, calcium aluminate, and calcium carbonate (1% of dietary intake) reduce the absorption of fluorides in the diet.[30] Substitution of low-fluoride ingredients in a portion of the diet reduces total fluoride intake. Using grains to replace some contaminated forages reduces total fluoride intake because grain crops accumulate little fluoride.

Because fluorosis causes chronic and permanent changes, prevention is the best approach. Producers should understand the sources and quality of their minerals, especially phosphate sources. Low-cost phosphate products not designed for animal rations should never be used in rations. Local health departments and state departments of natural resources can provide information on water fluoride concentrations. One should investigate the possibility of airborne pollution if smelters, refractories, or fertilizer plants are in the environment. Direct analysis of forages is a cost-effective way to confirm airborne fluoride pollution. Early detection of dental lesions in animals exposed before incisor eruption is a good biological indicator of recent toxic levels of fluorosis. A combination of these factors should provide adequate protection from chronic fluorosis.

IODINE

Sandra E. Morgan

Synonyms.   Elemental iodine is classified as a rare element that occurs in soil. Iodide is any binary compound of iodine. Because iodine is an essential element, it is a generally recognized as safe (GRAS) food ingredient for humans and animals.[1] Iodine toxicosis is also known as iodism or iodinism.

Sources. The primary sources of iodine are seaweed and a nitrate-bearing rock known as Chilean Caliche. Other sources are water and a mineral known as "marshite," which contains cuprous iodide. The iodine content of feed depends on the iodine available in the soil. Plant uptake depends on species and soil levels. Pasture levels of up to 1500 ppb iodine have been recorded, but normal grass contains 60 to 140 ppb and normal clover contains 160 to 180 ppb. The Rocky Mountains, Great Lakes, and much of the northeast regions of the United States are considered iodine-deficient areas. Iodine is usually added as part of the mineral mix to feeds and to various products for its antimicrobial action.[1]

Besides being a required element, iodine has therapeutic properties. An organic iodide, ethylene diamine dihydriodide (EDDI), and calcium iodate are widely used as feed additives for livestock and poultry. EDDI has been used to prevent and treat foot rot in cattle (questionable effectiveness) using amounts much higher than dietary requirements. It also has an expectorant action, which stimulates the vagus nerves in the gastrointestinal tract. Iodine salts such as potassium and sodium iodine have been used to treat soft tissue lumpy jaw and foot rot.[2]

Many compounds containing iodine have been used in human and veterinary medicine because of its germicidal activity and low tissue toxicity. Iodophores (povidone-iodine) are water-soluble combinations of iodine with detergents, wetting agents, and other carriers. They are widely used as skin disinfectants before surgery because of their antimicrobial properties. They do not sting or stain and are effective against bacteria, viruses, and fungi, but less so against spores. Iodophore solutions retain good bacterial activity at pH less than 4 even in the presence of organic matter. They are used as teat dips to control mastitis, dairy sanitizers, and general antiseptics for dermal and mucosal infections.

Iodine tincture contains 2% iodine with 2.4% potassium iodide (KI) dissolved in 50% ethanol and is used as a skin disinfectant. Strong iodine tincture contains 7% iodine and 5% KI dissolved in 85% ethanol and is more potent and irritating than tincture of iodine. Iodine solution contains 2% iodine and 2.4% KI dissolved in aqueous solution and is used as a nonirritant antiseptic on abrasions and wounds. Strong iodine solution contains 5% iodine and 10% KI dissolved in aqueous solution.[3]

Most of the *Brassica* spp. (turnips, rape, kale, cabbage), some of the crucifers, and soybeans are goitrogenic, but cooking, heating, or processing destroys the goitrogenic substance. Iodine uptake by the thyroid may be inhibited by diets high in nitrate.[4]

Toxicokinetics. Iodine is readily absorbed from the gastrointestinal tract and freely distributed into the extracellular fluid and glandular secretions. It concentrates in the lacrimal, salivary, and tracheobronchial glands, but the highest degree of concentration is in the thyroid gland (50 times the corresponding plasma level). Iodine metab-

olism essentially consists of the synthesis and degradation of the thyroid hormones and the reuse or excretion of the iodine released. Iodine can be removed from amino acids by the salivary glands and recycled through the gastrointestinal tract. Iodine is excreted primarily in the urine with smaller amounts present in sweat and feces.

The biologic half-life of iodine for most animals is between 6 and 10 hours. Iodine accumulates in the body and leads to iodinism if it is used long term at high levels. Once iodine exposure is discontinued after iodine toxicosis occurs, the blood levels decrease rapidly to near baseline levels within a few days.

Mechanism of Action. Iodine is an essential component of the thyroid hormones thyroxine (T_4) and triiodothyronine (T_3), which regulate the rate of energy metabolism in the body. The thyroid gland traps iodine for iodinization of the amino acids thyroxine, thyronine, 3,5,3-triiodothyropyruvic acid, and 3-monoiodotyrosine. The quantity of heat liberated and the rate of energy exchange are elevated in hyperthyroidism and reduced to below normal in hypothyroidism. Iodine-containing thyroid hormones are essential for growth in all young mammals and birds.[1]

Toxicity and Risk Factors. In cattle 300 to 500 mg/day of EDDI is toxic to stressed cattle. The incidence of bovine respiratory disease is increased when 1 mg/kg body weight of EDDI per day is fed for 5 weeks. Weight gain is reduced in calves if more than 7.5 mg/kg body weight of iodine per day is fed, and levels greater than 2 g/day of iodine as EDDI are toxic to fetuses.

The maximum amount of EDDI that lactating dairy cattle can be fed is 25 to 30 mg/head per day without exceeding 500 µg/L of iodine in milk. The upper safe limit in milk replacer is 10 ppm. Milk replacer with EDDI up to 100 to 200 ppm has reduced protein digestibility and caused toxic signs in calves.[5]

Goiter and weakness in foals were observed in animals at a thoroughbred farm that had added dried seaweed to their ration. The dietary iodine levels were 38 to 432 mg/mare per day. No goiter was found in animals on a control farm that received 6.3 to 7 mg/mare per day.[4]

Clinical Signs. In general clinical signs of iodinism include lacrimation, salivation, increased respiratory secretions, nonproductive cough, dry, scaly skin, reduced appetite, tachycardia, abortion, and infertility. Furthermore, chronic toxicosis results in goiter and decreased cell-mediated and humeral immune response. Cardiomyopathy has been reported in cats.[3]

Clinical Pathology. Thyroid function can be evaluated by testing for T_4 and T_3.

Lesions. Gross lesions of iodine toxicosis include dry, flaky skin, especially around the head, neck, and back. The thyroid gland is usually grossly enlarged to almost twice the normal size and is soft and dark red. The tissue around the thyroid may be edematous, flabby, or thickened.[3] Excessive lacrimation, as well as excess serous to mucopurulent discharge in nasal and tracheal mucosa with congestion of conjunctiva and upper respiratory mucosa, is seen. Histopathologic changes in the trachea are squamous metaplasia, loss of cilia, necrotic areas, and disruption of mucosa with neutrophilic and lymphocytic infiltration. Bronchopneumonia occurs in various stages. The thyroid gland has flat columnar epithelium with excessive pale or granular colloid.[1]

Diagnostic Testing.   Iodine levels have been tested in feed, serum, milk, liver, muscle, thyroid, eggs, and hair. Reference values of various tissues for cattle, dogs, goats, horses, llamas, mink, pigs, poultry, rabbits, and sheep are well documented.[5]

Treatment.   The best treatment for iodine toxicosis is removal of the source of iodine because it is rapidly mobilized and excreted from the tissues.

Prognosis.   The prognosis for iodism depends on the age and species of animal, pregnancy status, and duration and severity of clinical symptoms. Many of the clinical signs are reversible if complications such as pneumonia have not developed.

IRON

Jay C. Albretsen

Synonyms.   Iron is available orally in many different forms. These iron salts contain various percentages of elemental iron. Box 22-2 lists several iron salts and the percentage of elemental iron in each. The injectable forms of iron include iron dextran, iron dextrin, iron sorbitol, and ferric ammonium citrate. Several chelated forms of iron exist and are almost as effective for treating iron deficiencies as are some of the other salts, but are only considered to be about one fourth as toxic.[1-3]

BOX 22-2	IRON SALTS AND THE PERCENTAGE OF ELEMENTAL IRON	
FORM OF IRON		**% ELEMENTAL IRON**
Ferric hydroxide		63
Ferrous carbonate (anhydrous)		48
Ferric phosphate		37
Ferrous sulfate (anhydrous)		37
Ferric chloride		34
Ferrous fumarate		33
Ferric pyrophosphate		30
Ferrous lactate		24
Ferrous sulfate (hydrate)		20
Peptonized iron		17
Ferroglycine sulfate		16
Ferric ammonium citrate		15
Ferrous gluconate		12
Ferrocholinate		12

Data from references 1, 2.

Sources.   Iron is an essential metal and the most abundant trace mineral in the body.[1,2] Products that contain iron include iron supplements (both injectable and oral forms), multivitamins, and iron in other dietary supplements and foods. Most of these products are available over-the-counter and thus large quantities can be consumed. Iron can also be found in fertilizers and is present in soil. [1-3] It is a common practice to supplement young piglets with iron sometime within the first week after they are born. Although the piglets can be supplemented orally, most pigs are given injectable forms of iron supplementation.[3]

Iron toxicosis is usually the result of injecting excessive amounts of iron in baby pigs or the ingestion of large amounts of iron-containing products in other animals. Occasionally, some animals may eat large enough amounts of iron-containing fertilizers to be at risk for an iron toxicosis.[1-3]

Toxicokinetics.   Iron is absorbed from the intestines in a two-step process. First, ferrous iron ions are absorbed from the intestinal lumen into the mucosal cells.[1,2,4] The iron must be in an ionized state for absorption.[1,2,4] Ferrous forms are better absorbed than ferric forms of iron, although both can be absorbed as long as they are ionized.[2] Because iron must be ionized to be absorbed, metallic iron and iron oxide (rust) are not generally of concern when they are ingested.[1,2] Most iron absorption occurs in the duodenum and upper jejunum.[2,4] A high-sugar diet increases iron absorption, and phosphates reduce iron absorption.[3] Iron absorption requires an energy-dependent carrier. A transferrin-like protein facilitates this energy-dependent carrier mechanism and the entry of iron into the mucosal cells. This step is considered the rate-limiting factor in iron absorption.[1-4] However, in acute overdoses iron seems to be absorbed in a passive, concentration-dependent fashion similar to how most other metals are absorbed.[2] In addition, iron seems to be absorbed well along all parts of the intestinal tract in cases of iron overdoses.[1,2,4,5]

The second step in iron absorption is the transfer of iron to ferritin or into circulation bound to transferrin proteins. Transferrin is an α_1-globulin produced in the liver.[1,2] Complexed with transferrin, iron is distributed to other iron storage locations in the body.

About 70% of the iron in the body is found in hemoglobin and about 5% to 10% is found in myoglobin. Iron is in the ferrous (Fe^{2+}) form when bound to normal hemoglobin and myoglobin.[1-3] Most of the remaining iron found in the body is in the ferric (Fe^{3+}) form and is stored in hemosiderin, ferritin, and transferrin. The remaining iron in the body is used in iron-containing enzymes such as peroxidase, catalase, and cytochrome C. Most iron is stored in the liver, spleen, and bone marrow.[1,2,4]

A unique feature of iron metabolism is the almost complete absence of any iron excretion. Any iron lost from hemoglobin degradation is rapidly bound to transferrin and transported to the bone marrow for the resynthesis of hemoglobin.[2] Consequently, very little iron is lost in the urine and feces. In addition, iron loss is not significantly increased even after iron overdose.[2,4] Most iron loss is through the exfoliation of gastrointestinal mucosal cells and through menstrual blood loss.[4] Even though from 2% to 15% of the iron ingested is absorbed, only about 0.01% of the iron body burden is eliminated every day. The amount of iron eliminated varies from 0.5 to 2 mg/day.[1,4]

Mechanism of Action. Acute iron toxicosis has both a direct corrosive effect on the gastrointestinal tract and causes cellular damage as a result of the presence of unbound iron in the circulation.[2] Large doses of iron may break down the rate-limiting absorption step and allow excessive iron to enter the body. When iron-binding proteins become saturated, free iron ions are allowed into the general circulation.[2-5] Free iron penetrates the cells of the liver, heart, and brain. At the cellular level, free iron causes increased lipid peroxidation with resulting membrane damage to mitochondria, microsomes, and other cellular organelles.[1]

Iron exerts its most profound effects on the cardiovascular system. The result of excessive iron on the cardiovascular system is fatty necrosis of the myocardium, postarteriolar dilation, increased capillary permeability, and reduced cardiac output.[2] The stimulation of serotonin and histamine release by free iron does occur, as does systemic metabolic acidosis caused by an accumulation of lactic acid. All of these mechanisms lead to shock. Elevated iron also interferes with clotting mechanisms, augmenting hemorrhagic processes.[1-3]

Metabolic acidosis is caused by iron toxicosis from several mechanisms. First, lactic acidosis results from hypovolemia and hypotension. Iron disrupts oxidative phosphorylation by interfering in the electron transport chain. Thus, anaerobic metabolism is promoted. As ferrous (2+) iron is converted to ferric (3+) iron, hydrogen ions are released, adding to the metabolic acidosis. Free iron ions also inhibit the Krebs cycle and cause an accumulation of organic acids.[4]

Toxicity and Risk Factors. Because no mechanism for the excretion of iron exists, the toxicity depends on the amount of iron already present in the body. Consequently, some animals can develop clinical signs of iron toxicosis even when given doses that cause no problems in other animals.[3] Iron is most toxic when given intravenously. Intramuscular injections are less toxic, and iron given orally is the least toxic, probably because the amount of iron absorbed orally is not 100% of the dose ingested.[3] All animals are potentially susceptible to iron toxicosis.

In most cases it is best to determine the amount of elemental iron ingested to more accurately figure toxic doses (see Box 22-2). Humans between 12 and 24 months of age who ingest 1 to 10 g of iron are considered to have eaten a lethal amount of iron.[4] In dogs ingesting less than 20 mg/kg of elemental iron is considered to be nontoxic. Between 20 and 60 mg/kg of elemental iron when ingested can cause mild clinical signs. When the amount of elemental iron ingested is greater than 60 mg/kg, serious signs of iron toxicosis can develop in dogs.[2] In all animals oral doses between 100 and 200 mg/kg are potentially lethal.[2,3]

Clinical Signs. Excessive iron in the body affects several organs and body systems. Iron has direct corrosive effect on the gastrointestinal mucosa.[1,4] As a result vomiting, hema-

temesis, melena, and even gastrointestinal ulceration can occur.[1,2,4] The greatest mucosal damage occurs on an empty stomach. In humans acute iron overdoses have led to gastric scarring and resulted in pyloric stenosis.[4]

Iron overdoses can cause several cardiovascular abnormalities. Free iron and ferritin are potent vasodilators and cause hypotension and hypovolemia. Iron also injures blood vessels, increasing capillary membrane permeability and exacerbating the hypovolemia and hypotension.[2,4] Fatty degeneration of myocardial cells occurs when excess iron is absorbed into these cells. Ultimately, this degeneration leads to a cardiomyopathy.[4]

The liver accumulates free iron in the Kupffer cells and hepatocytes. The iron localizes in mitochondria and damages several cell organelles.[4] Eventually, hypoglycemia, hyperammonemia, coagulation defects, and hepatic encephalopathy occur.[2,4] Acute hepatic failure is a rare occurrence in humans except after massive overdoses.[4,5] Free iron inhibits the thrombin-induced conversion of fibrinogen to fibrin. Excessive iron also causes metabolic acidosis and thrombocytopenia.[4]

Finally, iron toxicosis results in several CNS signs. Often these signs are secondary to other problems caused by iron. For example, metabolic acidosis and hepatotoxicosis can lead to other signs, such as lethargy and hepatic encephalopathy. Iron can also cause cerebral edema.[4] Other CNS signs that occur are coma, seizures, and tremors.[1,2,4]

Iron toxicosis is clinically manifested in four different phases. The first stage occurs between 0 and 6 hours after the iron overdose. It is characterized primarily by gastrointestinal effects such as vomiting, diarrhea, and gastrointestinal bleeding.[2-5] Most animals with a mild to moderate iron toxicosis do not progress beyond this stage.[4] The second stage occurs 6 to 24 hours after the iron overdose. This is referred to as a latent period or a period of apparent clinical recovery. In severe cases of iron toxicosis, this recovery period is transient and soon progresses to the third stage.[2] The third stage of iron toxicosis occurs about 12 to 96 hours after clinical signs develop. The clinical signs include lethargy, a recurrence of gastrointestinal signs, metabolic acidosis, shock, hypotension, tachycardia, cardiovascular collapse, coagulation deficits, and hepatic necrosis. Death can occur.[2,4,5]

The fourth stage occurs 2 to 6 weeks after the iron overdose in animals that developed gastrointestinal ulcerations.[2,4] As the ulcerations heal, scarring occurs and strictures may develop. Even animals that do not show signs other than gastrointestinal irritation in the first phase of iron toxicosis are at risk of stricture development.[2]

Two syndromes can develop in pigs given iron injections. The first is a peracute syndrome that occurs within a few minutes to hours after the injection. It resembles an anaphylactic reaction and is characterized by sudden death.[3] The second is similar to the iron toxicosis signs previously listed and is characterized by lethargy, coma, and death.[3]

Clinical Pathology. Iron overdoses cause dehydration, hypovolemia, anemia, hypoglycemia, hyperammonemia, and evidence of hepatic necrosis (e.g., elevated alanine aminotransferase and aspartate aminotransferase).[2,4] In addition, iron toxicosis causes coagulation disturbances of thrombo-cytopenia, hypoprothrombinemia, and impaired clotting factor synthesis.[4] The presence of hyperglycemia and leuko-cytosis often indicates a serum iron level of greater than 30 µg/dl.[2]

Lesions.   Oral ingestion of large amounts of iron causes gastroenteritis, gastric ulceration, and edema. Iron does cause hepatic damage, which is evident histopathologically by the presence of cloudy, swollen hepatocytes, portal iron deposition, fatty metamorphosis, and massive periportal necrosis.[2-4] In addition, iron injections cause yellowish-brown discoloration and edema of the tissue around the injection site. Nearby lymph nodes and the kidneys may have a dark color following iron injections.[3]

Diagnostic Testing.   Serum iron levels are the best method to confirm iron poisoning. It is also beneficial to test the total iron-binding capacity (TIBC). Because normal serum iron and normal TIBC can vary from animal to animal, it is best to measure both values. When serum iron exceeds the TIBC, severe systemic effects can be expected.[2] Normal serum iron-binding capacity is usually about 25% to 30% saturated.[2]

Because iron undergoes multicompartmental kinetics, serum iron concentrations can change dramatically during the first few hours after ingestion. Consequently, it is best to test serum iron concentrations 4 to 6 hours after the iron is consumed.[2] Earlier sample collection may be beneficial if massive doses of iron have been ingested. Radiographs of the abdomen can be useful to identify a mass of tablets or metallic foreign bodies.[2] Radiographs help confirm exposure and may help determine the quantity of iron ingested.[4]

Treatment.   Animals that have recently ingested large doses of iron benefit from gastrointestinal decontamination. In animals that can vomit, emesis may be induced with 3% hydrogen peroxide (1 to 5 ml/kg PO), apomorphine, or another appropriate emetic.[6] Gastric lavage can be performed on anesthetized animals. A cuffed endotracheal tube should be used.[2] Activated charcoal does not bind iron effectively. It has been suggested that iron can be precipitated to a nonabsorbable form in the digestive tract using sodium phosphate, sodium bicarbonate, or magnesium hydroxide. However, the clinical significance of this therapy is questionable.[2,3,5]

The restoration of fluid, electrolyte, and acid-base balance is essential for the successful treatment of iron toxicosis. Fluids are also needed to prevent hypovolemic shock. The amount of fluids to be given should be based on the animal's maintenance and replacement needs.[2] Electrolytes should be monitored and abnormalities corrected. Gastrointestinal protectants such as sucralfate, cimetidine, misoprostol, or other inhibitors of gastric acid secretion are helpful.[2,7]

Chelation therapy is indicated in animals at risk of showing signs of severe iron toxicosis. Deferoxamine (Desferal , Ciba) is the chelator with the highest affinity for iron in the body. Calcium ethylene diamine tetraacetate (EDTA) has also been used but has not been shown to reduce mortality in acute iron poisoning. The recommended dose of deferoxamine is 40 mg/kg intramuscularly every 4 to 8 hours. Deferoxamine can be given as a continuous infusion at the rate of 15 mg/kg/hr. Chelation should continue until the serum iron levels decrease below 300 µg/dl or below the TIBC. Often, iron toxicosis requires 2 to 3 days of chelation therapy.[2-4]

All treated animals should be monitored for 4 to 6 weeks for evidence of gastrointestinal obstruction.[2] Peracute iron poisoning following iron injections is often untreatable.[3]

Prognosis.   Once signs have developed, the prognosis is guarded. If serum iron exceeds the TIBC and a chelator (deferoxamine) is unavailable, the prognosis is poor.

Prevention and Control.   All medications, multivitamins, and iron supplements should be kept out of reach of animals. Animals should be kept away from recently fertilized areas and fertilizers should be kept away from animal feeds.

LEAD

Sharon Gwaltney-Brant

Synonyms.   Lead is a heavy metal with the chemical symbol Pb. Lead toxicosis, particularly chronic toxicosis, is sometimes referred to as *plumbism.*

Sources.   Lead is ubiquitous in the environment, and it is used in a large variety of products. Most lead is present as inorganic compounds such as metallic lead or lead salts; organic lead sources (organoleads) include tetramethyl and tetraethyl lead found in leaded petroleum products. Sources of exposure for animals include lead weights (e.g., fishing sinkers, curtain weights), lead-based paints (artist's paints, some agricultural or outdoor paints), lead solders, wire shielding, old metal tubes (especially artist's paints), automotive batteries, leaded gasolines or oils, plumbing caulks, old leaded pipes, linoleum, lead-containing toys, computer equipment, roofing felt, window putty, improperly glazed pottery, lead arsenate pesticides, lead shot for guns, wine cork covers, and contamination of pastures near smelters.[1] The U.S. Congress enacted legislation in 1977 requiring that residential paints contain no more than 0.06% (600 ppm) lead.[1] Even so, lead may still be present in large amounts in agricultural or industrial paints: a thumbnail-sized flake of leaded paint may contain 50 to 200 mg of lead.[2] Further legislation restricting the use of leaded gasolines and oils has resulted in significant reductions in environmental contamination, especially in urban areas.[2]

Toxicokinetics.   Absorption of lead depends on the physical form (metallic, salt, organic) and the route of exposure. In general, metallic lead is less readily absorbed than lead salts, and organolead compounds are better absorbed than the salts. Dermal exposure to organolead compounds can result in toxicosis, but metallic and inorganic salts have virtually no dermal absorption.[2,3] Lead fumes or fine particles of less than 0.5 μm are readily absorbed in the lungs, whereas larger particles may be coughed up and swallowed, resulting in oral exposure. Ingested lead requires ionization within the gastrointestinal tract, primarily in the acidic environment of the stomach, in order to be appreciably absorbed.[3] For this reason, lead embedded in soft tissues (as in lead shot) is poorly absorbed and generally is not considered a significant lead source; however, in areas of active inflammation or in joint cavities, enzymatic activity may allow embedded lead to become ionized and thereby more readily absorbed.[2]

More than 90% of absorbed lead is bound to red blood cells, with small amounts bound to albumin and even lesser amounts present in the plasma as free lead; the unbound lead is distributed widely throughout various tissues.[3] The highest concentrations of lead occur within the bone, teeth, liver, lung, kidney, brain, and spleen.[2] Bone serves as a long-term storage depot for lead, and enhanced bone remodeling may result in the release of stored bone, precipitating toxicosis long after the original lead exposure.[2] Precipitation of lead salts in bone may result in the appearance of "lead lines" on radiographs of long bones.[2] Especially in the young, lead crosses the blood-brain barrier where it concentrates in the gray matter of the CNS. Unbound lead crosses the placenta and may pass into the milk of lactating animals; alterations in calcium metabolism in pregnant and lactating animals may result in significant lead being mobilized from maternal bone and transferred to the offspring.[2] In cattle passage of lead into milk increases exponentially with increasing blood lead levels.[4]

Most ingested lead is excreted in the feces without being absorbed. Absorbed lead is filtered across the glomeruli and tends to accumulate in the renal tubular epithelium. Sloughing of renal tubular epithelium results in slow elimination of lead; chelation therapy can greatly enhance the urinary excretion of lead. In addition to urinary excretion of lead, some species have significant biliary excretion of absorbed lead,[2] and secretions from the pancreas may serve as another means of elimination of lead from the body.[3] The half-life of lead in the body tends to be multiphasic because lead is redistributed from storage depots in the body, such as the CNS or bone. Intravenously administered lead has a triphasic half-life in dogs of 12 days, 184 days, and 4591 days,[2] whereas the half-life of lead in blood of cattle is reported to be 9 days.[4]

Mechanism of Action. Lead has multiple effects on biochemical mechanisms within the body, including binding of cellular and enzymatic sulfhydryl groups, competition with calcium ions, inhibition of membrane-associated enzymes, and alteration of vitamin D metabolism. Lead binds sulfhydryl groups, resulting in inactivation of enzymes involved in heme synthesis, such as δ-aminolevulinic acid dehydratase (ALAD) and ferrochelatase, and causing red blood cell abnormalities.[2] Inhibition of heme synthesis is also thought to be responsible for some of the neurologic effects of lead poisoning; for example, heme depletion may result in inhibition of cytochrome P-450, which in turn results in inhibition of tryptophan pyrrolase, increased plasma tryptophan levels, elevations in brain serotonin levels, and,

ultimately, aberrant neurotransmission of serotonergic pathways.[2] Increased serum ALAD levels may themselves be neurotoxic by interfering with γ-aminobutyric acid (GABA) transmission.[2] Lead competes with calcium ions, resulting in substitution for calcium in bone, alteration of nerve and muscle transmission, and displacement of calcium from calcium-binding proteins such as calmodulin. Damage to membrane-associated enzymes such as sodium-potassium pumps results in red blood cell fragility and renal tubular injury.

Derangements of calcium absorption and metabolism result from interference with vitamin D metabolism. Lead may also alter zinc-dependent enzyme processes and interfere with GABA production or activity in the CNS.[5]

Toxicity and Risk Factors. Lead toxicosis has been reported in mammals, birds, and reptiles.[2,6,7] Relative to other livestock, swine, goats, and chickens are considered to be fairly resistant to the effects of lead.[8] Toxic doses of lead have been determined experimentally for a variety of species (Table 22-1), but it is often difficult to extrapolate these doses to "natural" exposures in which amounts of lead ingested are rarely known.

Young animals absorb lead far more readily than do adults, with up to 50% of ingested lead being absorbed in the young.[2] Lead absorption can also be enhanced in calcium-, zinc-, iron-, or vitamin D–deficient animals.[2] Conversely, zinc or calcium supplementation may decrease the absorption of lead from the gastrointestinal tract.[2,4] Lead may interfere with the absorption of selenium from the gastrointestinal tract in ruminants, resulting in selenium deficiency.[4] Co-ingestion of lead and cadmium may increase the severity of clinical signs of lead poisoning.[2]

Cattle are most commonly exposed to lead through ingestion of discarded automotive batteries, farm machinery grease or oil, roofing felt or lead-based agricultural paints, and caulks or putties.[5] Horses and sheep are most commonly exposed by grazing on pastures contaminated by airborne emissions from nearby smelters.[5] Other potential sources of lead exposure for livestock include water from lead-lined pipes, leaded drinking or feeding utensils, and lead arsenate

TABLE 22-1 **Acute and Chronic Toxic Doses of Lead**

Species	Acute Toxic Dose (mg/kg)	Chronic Cumulative Toxic Dose (mg/kg/day)
Cattle		
Calves	400-600	
Adult	600-800	1-7
Dogs	191-1000	1.8-2.6
Horses	500-750	2.4-7
Ducks	18 pellets of no. 6 shot	2
Geese	5 pellets of no. 4 shot 25 pellets of no. 6 shot	n/a

Data from references 2, 16, 22.

pesticides (although arsenic toxicosis is the more common consequence).[5] Exposure of household pets to lead occurs through ingestion of lead paints in old houses, leaded artist's paints, linoleum, and lead-containing toys, weights, and ornaments.[5] Pets may ingest lead-based paint that may flake off in older houses, or they may be exposed to paint residues in sawdust during remodeling projects. Younger pets may be at increased risk to exposure to lead-containing items because of their increased tendency to play with and potentially swallow these items.[9] Lead toxicosis in waterfowl occurs primarily from ingestion of spent lead shot,[7] although regulations requiring the use of steel shot in hunting waterfowl have decreased environmental contamination with leaded shot.[2] Lead toxicosis has developed in raptors that have ingested wild fowl with lead shot embedded in the muscles.[7] Other nondomestic species may be occasionally exposed through ingestion of lead in discarded items such as batteries and lead sinkers, or by grazing contaminated pastures.

Clinical Signs.   Clinical signs of lead toxicosis vary with species (Table 22-2). Peracute death is possible in any species exposed to very high levels of lead fumes.[2] Ruminants tend to display evidence of central nervous dysfunction, whereas equines tend to display signs of peripheral neuropathy.[4] Dogs and cats show neurologic and gastrointestinal signs.[9] Psittacines display nonspecific gastrointestinal, neurologic, renal, and hematologic dysfunction.[10] Lead toxicosis in waterfowl and raptors manifests as chronic wasting and peripheral nerve dysfunction.[7]

Ruminants with lead toxicosis may show initial depression followed by hyperesthesia, muscle tremors or fasciculations (especially about the head), ataxia, blindness, seizures, dementia or aggression, head pressing, tenesmus, bloat, diarrhea, and death.[4,5] Chronic toxicosis resembles the acute syndrome, but the signs tend to develop over a longer period of time and are not as severe.[5] Arterial hypertension and electrocardiographic abnormalities have been reported in cattle within 30 days of exposure to lead.[4] Because lead can

TABLE 22-2 **Clinical Signs Associated with Lead Toxicosis in Animals**

Species	Clinical Signs	Differential Diagnoses
Ruminants		
Acute	Depression followed by hyperesthesia, muscle tremors or fasciculations (especially about the head), ataxia, blindness, seizures, dementia, aggression, head pressing, tenesmus, bloat, diarrhea, death	Rabies, thromboembolic meningoencephalitis, polioencephalomalacia, listeriosis, nervous coccidiosis, ammoniated forage toxicosis, hepatic encephalopathy
Chronic	Similar to acute but signs take longer to develop and may be of lesser severity; arterial hypertension	
Horses		
Acute	Uncommon; seizures, death	Rabies, other viral encephalitides, hepatic encephalopathy, leukoencephalomalacia, *Centaurea* toxicosis
Chronic	Depression, weight loss, dysphagia, dysphonia, "roaring" laryngeal paralysis, facial nerve deficits, gastrointestinal signs (rare), aspiration pneumonia, seizures, death	
Dogs, cats		
Acute	Anorexia, behavior changes, ataxia, tremors, seizures	Rabies, canine distemper virus, other viral encephalitides, toxoplasmosis, hepatic encephalopathy, idiopathic epilepsy, a variety of gastrointestinal disorders
Chronic	Abdominal discomfort, vomiting, diarrhea, anorexia, lethargy, weight loss, anemia, behavior changes, intermittent seizures, megaesophagus (cats; uncommon)	
Psittacines		
Acute	Rare; seizures, death	Proventricular dilatation syndrome, psittacine beak and feather disease, viral or bacterial encephalitides, hepatic encephalopathy
Chronic	Depression, behavior disorders, anorexia, regurgitation, diarrhea, polyuria, weakness, hemoglobinuria (hemolytic anemia), seizures	
Waterfowl		
Acute	Peracute death	Starvation, botulism, infectious disease
Chronic	Anorexia, depression, emaciation, muscle atrophy, weakness, dysphonia, coma, death	Starvation, botulism, infectious disease
Raptors	Weakness, depression, limb paralysis, dyspnea, seizures	

Data from references 3-5, 7, 9-11.

decrease the absorption of selenium, selenium deficiency, manifested as white muscle disease, may accompany lead toxicosis.[4] Differential diagnoses of lead toxicosis in ruminants include rabies, thromboembolic meningoencephalitis, polioencephalomalacia, listeriosis, nervous coccidiosis, ammoniated forage toxicosis, and hepatic encephalopathy.

In horses lead poisoning is most often a chronic illness, with acute toxicosis being uncommonly seen. The syndrome in horses is characterized by dysfunction of peripheral motor nerves, with relative sparing of sensory nerve function.[8] Horses with lead poisoning may show weight loss, depression, ataxia, dysphagia, dysphonia, "roaring," laryngeal paralysis, facial nerve deficits, seizures, and death.[3-5] Gastrointestinal signs are occasionally present but are not a prominent feature in most cases.[3] Aspiration pneumonia secondary to dysphagia may occur.[3] Differential diagnoses of lead poisoning in horses include rabies or other encephalitides, hepatic encephalopathy, and *Centaurea* toxicosis.

In dogs and cats acute lead toxicosis is most commonly manifested as anorexia, behavior changes, ataxia, muscle tremors, and seizures.[9] Chronic lead poisoning in dogs and cats is sometimes overlooked, because the signs can be insidious in onset and subtle in nature, mimicking a variety of other ailments. Chronic toxicosis in dogs or cats include abdominal discomfort, vomiting, diarrhea, anorexia, lethargy, weight loss, anemia, behavior changes, and intermittent seizures.[9] Megaesophagus has been reported as an uncommon manifestation in cats, and cats may be more prone to lead-induced seizures.[9] Differential diagnoses include rabies and other viral encephalitides (e.g., canine distemper virus), toxoplasmosis, hepatic encephalopathy, idiopathic epilepsy, and a variety of gastrointestinal disorders.

Psittacines rarely develop acute lead toxicosis, which is manifested by seizures and death. Chronic lead toxicosis is more common and is characterized by depression, behavior disorders, anorexia, weakness, regurgitation, greenish-black diarrhea, polyuria, hemoglobinuria, and seizures.[10,11] Differential diagnoses include proventricular dilatation syndrome, psittacine beak and feather disease, viral or bacterial encephalitides, and hepatic disease.

Waterfowl may die acutely from lead poisoning, or chronic disease may be characterized by anorexia, depression, emaciation, coma, muscle atrophy, weakness, and dysphonia.[7] Rule-outs include starvation, botulism, and infectious disease.

Weakness, depression, limb paralysis, dyspnea, and seizures develop in raptors.[7] Differentials include starvation and infectious disease.

Clinical Pathology. Although a variety of hematologic abnormalities have been reported with lead toxicosis, none should be considered pathognomonic for lead toxicosis, nor should the absence of any significant clinical pathology alterations be considered sufficient to rule out lead poisoning as a potential diagnosis in animals exhibiting consistent clinical signs. Hematologic alterations are more commonly encountered in subchronic or chronic toxicosis; serum chemistry alterations, particularly elevations in serum kidney parameters, may be seen in acute cases or during chelation therapy.[12]

Lead-induced alteration of heme metabolism and other erythrocyte functions results in shortened erythrocyte lifespan and decreased erythrocyte replacement, both of which contribute to the anemia that may be seen with chronic lead toxicosis. Depending on species and stage of toxicosis, the anemia may range from microcytic hypochromic to normocytic normochromic.[2-4] Initially, the anemia is regenerative, but in severe, chronic cases a nonregenerative anemia may be present.[2] Basophilic stippling, long considered a hallmark of lead poisoning, must be evaluated with care. Ruminants may normally have a small percentage of stippled erythrocytes; erythrocytic parasites (e.g., *Hemobartonella felis* in cats) may be misidentified as basophilic stippling.[8] Basophilic stippling may be of more diagnostic value in dogs and horses than in other species[13]; however, basophilic stippling may be found in dogs with other diseases.[9] The presence of large numbers of nucleated red blood cells (5 to 40 per 100 white blood cells) without evidence of severe anemia has been reported to be highly suggestive of lead toxicosis in small animals.[9] Increased erythrocyte fragility may result in alterations such as anisocytosis, poikilocytosis, polychromasia, echinocytosis, and target cells. Other hematologic abnormalities include a mature leukocytosis and decreased myeloid/erythroid ratio in the bone marrow.[2]

Hematologic abnormalities reported in birds include heterophilia, hyperchromic and regenerative anemia, and red blood cell vacuolation.[10]

Lesions. In animals dying of acute lead toxicosis, gross lesions may be minimal and generally consist of nonspecific degenerative changes in the nervous system and kidneys. Even in chronic cases of lead toxicosis, lesions may be subtle and not consistently found, although emaciation and muscle wasting is not uncommon. Occasionally, the lead source may be found within the gastrointestinal tract on necropsy.[8] Ruminants with chronic lead toxicosis may have laminar cortical necrosis within the cerebrum, which may sometimes be detected grossly by flattening or yellowing of cortical gyri. Histopathologically, the lesion of lead toxicosis consists of laminar cortical cerebral necrosis with swelling of cerebral and cerebellar capillary endothelium. The lesion of laminar cortical necrosis is not pathognomonic for lead toxicosis, in that similar lesions are seen in sulfur-induced polioencephalomalacia of ruminants, salt toxicosis in swine, and cyanide toxicosis in several species.[8] Cerebral edema, vascular congestion of meningeal vessels, and astrogliosis in the Purkinje and molecular layers of the cerebellum have also been reported.[8] There may be degeneration and necrosis of renal tubular epithelium that may be accompanied by a high number of mitotic figures (regeneration), a lesion reported to be more common in young calves.[8]

Lead toxicosis in horses generally is not associated with consistent gross lesions, although aspiration pneumonia, emaciation, and weight loss are expected in chronic cases.[4] The histopathologic lesions of lead toxicosis in horses have not been well described, but are thought to be similar to the peripheral neuropathy reported in lead-intoxicated humans, in which segmental degeneration of axons and myelin in the distal motor fibers are reported.[8]

In dogs and cats few gross lesions are reported, although, in some cases, lead objects may be found in the gastrointestinal tract. Histopathologically, edema of the white matter of the brain and spinal cord, myelin degeneration within the cerebellum and cerebrum, and spongiosis of deep cerebral structures have been reported.[8] Degenerative changes may be seen in the liver and kidney of dogs with chronic lead toxicosis. Intranuclear inclusion bodies may be found in the renal tubular epithelium and, rarely, the hepatocytes of dogs with chronic toxicosis. Even though the presence of these inclusions is highly suggestive of lead toxicosis, their absence does not rule out lead as a potential cause. Inclusions may be rarely found in other species.[8]

Waterfowl and other wildlife that have died of lead toxicosis are generally emaciated, with extensive muscle wasting possible; in birds, lead shot may be present in the gizzard.[7] Atrophy of breast muscles in birds may result in a "razor keel" appearance.[7] Pale streaks may be seen within the myocardium, corresponding to patchy areas of myocardial necrosis associated with fibrinoid necrosis of arterioles.[7] Other histopathologic lesions reported in waterfowl include hepatocellular necrosis, renal tubular necrosis (with or without intranuclear inclusions similar to those in dogs), brain edema, myelin degeneration of peripheral nerves, and patchy necrosis of gizzard muscles.[7]

Diagnostic Testing. Determination of blood lead levels is a major step in confirming a presumptive diagnosis of lead toxicosis in the living patient. Lead analysis is readily available and affordable, and can be performed in a timely manner. Because more than 90% of circulating lead is bound to erythrocytes, whole blood is required for lead analysis. Although most laboratories run lead levels on EDTA, citrated, or heparinized blood, it is often beneficial to contact the facility before collecting the blood to ensure that the appropriate sample is obtained, because EDTA may interfere with some analytic methods.[9] Because of the widespread distribution of lead within different compartments of the body, blood lead levels in chronically intoxicated animals may not be appreciably high; for the same reason, it is important to remember that blood lead levels are not necessarily reflective of the total body burden of lead nor do they necessarily correlate with the severity of clinical signs.[2] Additionally, reported blood lead levels may vary depending on the individual laboratory and the analytic method. Accordingly, blood lead levels should be interpreted in light of existing clinical signs and history of exposure.

In most species blood lead levels greater than 0.3 to 0.35 ppm (30 to 35 µg/dl) suggest significant lead exposure and, in the presence of appropriate clinical signs, support the finding of lead toxicosis.[3,4,9] Blood lead levels greater than 0.6 ppm (60 µg/dl) are diagnostic for lead toxicosis.[9] In birds levels greater than 0.2 ppm (20 µg/dl) are suggestive and levels greater than 0.5 ppm are diagnostic of lead toxicosis.[14]

When blood lead levels are equivocal, a urinary Ca-EDTA postchelation test may be performed.[15] Measurement of lead in a 24-hour urine sample is performed, then Ca-EDTA is administered, followed by another 24-hour urine lead level evaluation. An increase in urine lead excretion that is greater than 10 times the prechelation value is indicative of lead toxicosis, whereas postchelation levels less than 10 times the prechelation level are not supportive of a diagnosis of lead toxicosis.[15] Because of cost and logistics, this test is not practical for livestock and is generally limited to small animals.

Other confirmatory laboratory tests available for the live patient include measurement of erythrocyte ALAD activity, erythrocyte porphyrin assay, urinary ALA levels, and zinc protoporphyrin levels. Normal values for these tests in domestic and wild animals are generally not widely available, except erythrocyte ALAD activity, erythrocyte porphyrin, and urinary ALA levels in cattle. Erythrocyte ALAD activity levels less than 50 and 100 nmol porphobilinogen/ml erythrocyte/hr in adult cattle and calves, respectively, are considered indicative of lead toxicosis.[16] Reference ranges for erythrocyte porphyrin levels in normal cattle are 113 to 142.8 ± 32.4 µg/dl, and levels of more than 2000 µg/dl have been reported in asymptomatic, chronically exposed cattle.[4] Urinary ALA levels in lead-poisoned cattle generally exceed 500 µg/dl.[4] In waterfowl blood protoporphyrin levels of greater than 40 µg/dl are considered diagnostic of lead poisoning.[7]

Radiography may be used to detect the presence of lead within the gastrointestinal tract or in other parts of the body. The absence of lead densities within the gastrointestinal tract does not necessarily rule out the possibility of lead toxicity. Lead paint, especially in fine particulate form, may not show up on radiography.[9] Radiography may also be used to detect lead lines within the epiphyseal plate of long bones, although this lesion is rarely seen in domestic animals.[9]

Postmortem diagnosis of lead toxicosis is generally accomplished through a combination of analysis of history, necropsy findings, histopathologic lesions, and toxicologic analysis of tissues. In suspect cases liver or kidney should be submitted for lead analysis; most diagnostic laboratories can run heavy metal analysis. In general, levels greater than 10 ppm wet weight should be considered diagnostic for lead.[4] Toxic levels of lead for a variety of species are listed in Table 22-3. Hair and fecal analysis for lead are considered of minimal diagnostic value in animals.[4,9]

Treatment. Management of lead toxicosis in animals consists of (1) stabilization of severe clinical signs, (2) elimination of lead from the gastrointestinal tract, (3) chelation

TABLE 22-3 **Toxic Levels of Lead in Tissues (ppm, wet weight)**

Species	Liver	Kidney
Bovine	5-300	5-700
Canine	5-10	50-200
Equine (chronic)	4-50	4-140
Equine (acute)	10-500	20-200
Poultry	18-90	20-150
Rabbits	>10	>10
Ovine	10-100	5-200
Canada geese	>5	60-1600
Ducks-swans	>6-8	8-55
Bald eagles	>10	n/a

Data from references 7, 16.

therapy, (4) general supportive care, and (5) elimination of the lead source from the animal's environment. Failure to address all of these parameters may result in exacerbation or recurrence of clinical signs in affected animals.

Seizuring animals should be managed with anticonvulsants such as diazepam or barbiturates. Poor response to anticonvulsant therapy or progression of severe CNS signs may require treatment for cerebral edema (e.g., mannitol, diuretics). Fluid and electrolyte abnormalities should be corrected as needed.

Decontamination of the gastrointestinal tract is extremely important in the management of lead toxicosis, because chelating agents may actually enhance gastrointestinal absorption of lead.[4,9,12] Physical removal of relatively large lead objects via rumenotomy or gastrotomy may be necessary, although in dogs and cats with recent ingestions induction of emesis may assist in the removal of small to moderately sized lead objects. Activated charcoal binds poorly to lead and is therefore not generally recommended.[13] Cathartics, enemas, or whole bowel irrigation may be used to assist in emptying the gastrointestinal tract of lead. Sulfate-containing cathartics, such as magnesium or sodium sulfate, may help precipitate lead as lead sulfate in the gastrointestinal tract and impede absorption.[9]

The goal of chelation therapy is to bind lead into a soluble complex (chelate) that is then excreted in the urine. Because most chelators, as well as lead itself, have some degree of nephrotoxicity, careful monitoring of renal parameters and maintenance of adequate hydration during chelation therapy are essential. The chelation agents used most commonly in domestic animals are Ca-EDTA (calcium disodium ethylene diamine tetraacetate), D-penicillamine (Cuprimine), and succimer DMSA (Chemet).

Ca-EDTA has been used as the lead chelator of choice for several decades, and despite the recent development of what many consider to be superior chelators, it is still widely used in veterinary medicine, especially in large animals. Sodium EDTA should not be used for chelation, because it can bind serum calcium and cause hypocalcemia.[17] Ca-EDTA must be given parenterally. Ca-EDTA effectively removes lead from osseous tissues, which can result in increases in blood lead levels during chelation, with subsequent worsening of clinical signs. For this reason Ca-EDTA therapy is sometimes administered in conjunction with BAL because BAL removes lead from parenchymatous tissues (particularly the brain) and may help prevent exacerbation of signs during Ca-EDTA therapy.[13] Ca-EDTA is nephrotoxic, so close monitoring of renal values is important during chelation therapy. Other adverse effects include vomiting, anorexia, diarrhea, depression, and pain on subcutaneous or intramuscular injection. Additionally, Ca-EDTA may bind dietary essential minerals such as zinc, copper, iron, and calcium.[17]

Recommended doses for horses and ruminants are 73 mg Ca-EDTA/kg divided twice daily to three times daily for 3 to 5 days, administered by slow intravenous infusion.[3] If signs are still present, an additional 5-day treatment may be administered after a 2-day "rest." An alternative regimen is 110 mg/kg intravenously twice daily for 2 days, followed by a 2-day "rest," then 2 more days of treatment.[3,4] For dogs, the dose is 100 mg/kg/day for 2 to 5 days with each dose divided into four portions, diluted to a final concentration of 10 mg Ca-EDTA/ml of 5% dextrose, and administered at different subcutaneous sites. The total daily dose should not exceed 2 g of Ca-EDTA per dog to avoid risk of nephrotoxicosis.[9] Clinical improvement is expected within 24 to 48 hours. If further treatment is required after the initial 5 days of therapy, a 5-day rest is recommended between treatment series. Supplementation with dietary zinc minimizes the gastrointestinal side effects of Ca-EDTA.[9] The recommended dose for cats is 27.5 mg/kg in 15 ml of 5% dextrose subcutaneously every 6 hours for 5 days.[9] Ca-EDTA should be used with caution in cats to reduce risk of nephrotoxicity.[18] In psittacines the dose of Ca-EDTA is 35 to 40 mg/kg intramuscularly twice daily for 5 days, with a 5- to 7-day rest if further therapy is needed.[10] Waterfowl and raptors have been successfully treated with Ca-EDTA at 35 to 50 mg/kg intravenously every 12 hours (duration of therapy not mentioned),[7] whereas in a 9.8-kg snapping turtle 20 mg Ca-EDTA given intramuscularly 3 times over 4 weeks was used to successfully treat lead toxicosis (initial blood lead level 3.6 ppm).[6]

BAL is sometimes used in conjunction with Ca-EDTA, especially when severe CNS signs are present. BAL adsorbs lead from erythrocytes and increases both urinary and biliary excretion of lead.[9] BAL can be nephrotoxic and painful on injection, and its use is contraindicated in animals with hepatic dysfunction.[19] Renal toxicity reportedly can be reduced by alkalinization of the urine.[19] Vomiting, tachycardia, hypertension, mercaptan odor to breath, and seizures are reported as side effects of BAL therapy. The reported doses for BAL are 3 to 6 mg/kg intramuscularly 3 to 4 times daily[13] or 2 to 5 mg/kg intramuscularly every 4 hours for 2 days, then every 8 hours for 1 day, then every 12 hours.[19] The dose for caged birds is 2.5 mg/kg intramuscularly every 4 hours for 2 days, then every 12 hours.[10]

Penicillamine has the advantage of being an oral medication, eliminating the painful intramuscular injections of Ca-EDTA. As with Ca-EDTA penicillamine enhances gastrointestinal absorption of lead, so chelation must not be initiated until all lead has been removed from the gastrointestinal tract. Penicillamine also binds dietary copper, iron, and zinc. Penicillamine chelates may be nephrotoxic, so adequate hydration during treatment is important. Side effects of penicillamine include vomiting, fever, lymphadenopathy, hypersensitivity reactions, and blood dyscrasias, with vomiting being the most common side effect by far. Dividing the daily dose or administration of diphenhydramine 30 minutes before penicillamine treatment may decrease the incidence of gastrointestinal side effects. Reported doses of penicillamine in dogs are 30 to 110 mg/kg/day PO divided every 6 hours for 7 days followed by 7 days of rest; the regimen may be repeated as needed. The dose for cats is 125 mg/cat PO (not per kg) every 12 hours for 5 days.[18] The dose for caged birds is 55 mg/kg PO every 12 hours for 1 to 2 weeks and repeated as needed after 3 to 5 days of rest.[10]

Succimer is a structural analogue to BAL that has several advantages over Ca-EDTA and penicillamine. Succimer is administered orally or rectally; the latter route is advantageous in vomiting animals. Unlike Ca-EDTA and penicillamine, succimer is less likely to cause nephrotoxicosis and less likely to bind essential minerals such as zinc, copper, calcium, and iron.[17] And, unlike Ca-EDTA and penicillamine, succimer does not enhance lead absorption from the gastrointestinal tract[17]; indeed, succimer has been shown to reduce gastrointestinal absorption of lead in rats.[20] Succimer also reportedly has a lower incidence of gastrointestinal side effects.[17] The reported dose for dogs is 10 mg/kg PO or PR three times daily for 10 days and the dose can be repeated as needed.[17] In caged birds the dose is 25 to 35 mg/kg PO every 12 hours for 5 days a week for 3 to 5 weeks.[10]

General supportive care for lead-intoxicated animals includes maintaining adequate hydration and nutrition (hand-feeding or force-feeding may be required in severe cases), symptomatic care for vomiting or diarrhea, and management of aspiration pneumonia (horses).[3,9] In ruminants the use of thiamine at 250 to 1000 mg every 12 hours for 5 days has been reported as a useful adjunct to Ca-EDTA therapy and may aid in resolution of CNS signs.[4]

As animals are being treated for lead toxicosis, attempts should be made to identify and remove the source of lead from the animal's environment so that reexposure does not occur.

Prognosis. In animals with mild to moderate signs, early diagnosis and appropriate therapy generally yield a favorable prognosis as long as the lead source can be identified and removed from the animal's environment. Domestic animals with severe CNS signs have a more guarded prognosis. Wildlife are frequently not diagnosed with lead toxicosis until signs are severe, making the prognosis for lead toxicosis in wildlife guarded to poor, even with appropriate therapy.[7]

Prevention and Control. Prevention of exposure to lead in large animals includes proper pasture management, for example, removal of trash and machinery, avoiding the use of lead-based paints on fencing or buildings to which livestock may be exposed, and analysis of lead levels in soil and forage in areas subject to environmental contamination, such as pastures near lead smelters. Contaminated pastures containing soil lead levels exceeding 175 ppm should be mowed, and contaminated forage baled and removed (forage from contaminated pastures may contain more than 300 ppm of lead).[4] Stubble and native grasses should be plowed under or burned (the ashes retain lead). The application of agricultural lime to contaminated pastures increases soil calcium levels and decreases availability of lead.[4] Similarly, adding alfalfa to the diet of herbivores increases the dietary calcium content and may reduce the gastrointestinal absorption of lead.[3]

In pets prevention of household exposures includes removal of lead objects and careful elimination of sources of old lead-based paints (dusts from remodeling projects can be a significant source of lead for pets). When the source of lead cannot be immediately determined, analysis of water and soil may be required to rule out these as potential lead sources.

Because of their relative sensitivity to lead, family pets may serve as sentinel animals that can alert pet owners to the potential for human exposure to lead in the household.[21] Veterinarians diagnosing lead poisoning in household pets should feel obliged to warn the pet owners of the potential for human exposure and direct the owners, especially those with young children, to their physicians or local public health officials for more information. Additional information on human exposures to lead may be found at the Agency for Toxic Substances and Disease Registry website: *http://www.atsdr.cdc.gov/toxprofiles/phs13.html.*

MERCURY

Steve Ensley

Sources. Many forms of mercury can cause a toxicosis in animals.[1] A common source of exposure in dogs is inorganic elemental mercury found in glass thermometers.[2] However, elemental mercury is poorly absorbed from the gastrointestinal tract and so is not considered a health hazard when ingested. Sources that can cause toxicosis include the inorganic mercurial salts such as mercuric (divalent) and mercurous (monovalent) salts, which are used as preservatives and fixatives.[3] Organic alkyl mercurials, such as methyl mercury and ethyl mercury, are used as fungicides.[4] Aryl mercurials, such as phenyl mercuric acetate, are used in antimildew paints and are sources of mercury.

Both acute and chronic mercury poisoning of animals are rare because of the limited availability of toxic amounts of mercury. When mercury poisoning does occur in domestic animals, it is most often related to the accidental consumption of obsolete mercurial products.

Toxicokinetics. The form of mercury found in thermometers may be volatilized to mercury vapor, which is lipid soluble and can be absorbed by inhalation. Ingested elemental mercury and inorganic mercurial salts are absorbed very slowly from the gastrointestinal tract.[1] Organic methyl and ethyl mercury compounds are lipophilic and readily absorbed by the gastrointestinal tract.[1]

Inorganic mercurial salts are transported in erythrocytes and plasma. They accumulate in the renal cortex and localize in the lysosomes. Alkyl organic mercury compounds accumulate in the brain. All forms of mercury can cross the placenta and accumulate in the fetus.[1]

Elemental mercury can be oxidized to divalent mercury by catalases in tissue. Aryl mercurials are rapidly metabolized to inorganic salts. Alkyl mercurials are slowly metabolized to divalent mercury.

Inorganic mercury is excreted primarily in urine. Organic mercurials are excreted mainly in bile and feces.

Mechanism of Action. Inorganic mercurial salts cause direct tissue necrosis and renal tubular necrosis. The mercuric ion binds covalently with sulfur and inhibits sulfhydryl-containing enzymes in microsomes and mitochondria.[4] Mercurial salts may also bind to proteins as mercaptides. Organic alkyl mercurials interfere with metabolic activity and prevent synthesis of essential proteins, leading to cellular degeneration and necrosis. Organic alkyl mercurials target the brain.

Toxicity and Risk Factors.   Toxicity varies among different species and with different forms of mercury. Chronic methyl mercury toxicosis can result from dosages of 0.2 to 5 mg/kg body weight.[1] The kidneys contain the greatest concentrations of mercury following exposure to inorganic salts of mercury and mercury vapor (thermometers). Organic mercury has an increased tendency to accumulate in the brain.

Clinical Signs.   Clinical signs resulting from ingestion of toxic doses of elemental mercury can involve damage to the kidneys. Signs from exposure to toxic doses of mercuric salts include stomatitis, pharyngitis, vomiting, diarrhea, dehydration, and shock. Death may occur within hours of ingestion of mercurial salts. In animals surviving acute toxicosis, oliguria and azotemia can follow.[1]

Clinical signs from alkyl mercurial toxicosis develop slowly over 7 to 21 days. Erythema of the skin, conjunctivitis, lacrimation, and stomatitis are early clinical signs. Intermediate signs include depression, ataxia, incoordination, paresis, and blindness. Dermatitis, pustules, and epithelial ulcers increase during the course of the disease. Anemia can result because of the hematuria and melena. Advanced signs of alkyl mercury toxicosis include proprioceptive defects, abnormal postures, complete blindness, total anorexia, paralysis, slowed respiration, coma, and death. The mortality rate among affected animals is high.

Clinical Pathology.   No specific clinical pathologic abnormalities associated with mercury toxicosis are found.

Lesions.   Lesions resulting from mercury toxicosis include gastrointestinal lesions, gastric ulcers, necrotic enteritis, and colitis. Renal lesions include pale, swollen kidneys with tubular necrosis. Alkyl mercurials cause microscopic brain damage, including fibrinoid degeneration of the media of leptomeningeal arteries.[5] Degeneration of the Purkinje network in the heart is a frequent observation in cattle. Fibrosis and mineralization of the Purkinje network can be a result of the degeneration.[5] In swine extensive degeneration and demyelination of peripheral nerves can occur.

Organomercurials selectively damage the granular cells of the cerebellum in all species. Cerebellar hypoplasia can be observed in kittens born to queens exposed to mercury before and during gestation.

Diagnostic Testing.   In acute exposure, concentrations of mercury in the blood or urine may be elevated. Concentrations of mercury may be elevated in the kidney, liver, and brain during acute and chronic exposure. The best diagnostic samples are tissues, but blood or urine can be analyzed for mercury concentration in acute exposures.

Treatment.   Ingestion of mercury thermometers is a minimal risk because elemental mercury is so poorly absorbed via the gastrointestinal tract. Dogs can be given a high-fiber diet for 2 to 3 days to aid passage of ingested glass.

In acute exposure to elemental mercury or mercuric salts, egg white or activated charcoal may be administered to bind ingested mercury. Oral sodium thiosulfate (0.5 to 1 g/kg body weight) also binds mercury.[1] A saline cathartic or sorbitol increases clearance from the intestinal tract. Oral penicillamine (15 to 50 mg/kg body weight daily) may be administered after the intestine is cleared of mercury.[4] DMSA (succimer) is effective for increasing urinary excretion of inorganic mercurials (10 mg/kg PO three times per day for 10 days).[6] Supplemental selenium and vitamin E are somewhat protective against mercury toxicosis.

Irreversible, substantive damage has already occurred in most cases of alkyl mercurial toxicosis by the time the toxicosis is apparent, and treatment can be futile.

Prognosis.   Exposure to mercurials can have lasting, severe consequences in the fetus. The potential for recovery from the neurologic effects of mercurials is better in acute poisonings than in prolonged exposure. In general, neurotoxicosis from exposure to mercurials is irreversible.

Prevention and Control.   Preventing consumption of obsolete mercurial products is the best method of control. Alkyl mercurials can accumulate in edible organs and musculature; therefore, mercury-intoxicated animals should never be used for food.[7] Cases of human exposure to mercury by consuming pork from poisoned swine have been reported. Mercury contamination in commercial fish is a continuing concern and the Food and Drug Administration (FDA) is addressing these concerns. The FDA has set an action level of 1 ppm methylmercury, which is the form of mercury found in fish and other seafood.

MOLYBDENUM

Robert Coppock and Margita M. Dziwenka

Sources.   In its natural form, molybdenum (Mo) does not exist in the elemental state and is found with copper, lead, and tungsten (wolfram) ores. The predominant form of Mo in soil and ground water is the molybdate anion (MoO_4^{2-}).[1] Mineralization of lakes can result in high concentrations of Mo in sediments. Fossil fuels contain Mo, and the Mo is released during combustion. Fly ash residual from burning fossil fuels can be high in Mo.[2] The use of Mo in catalytic applications can result in Mo being lost from the catalitic bed into the atmosphere. Other atmospheric sources are deposition on forage from Mo emissions from aluminum smelting, steel alloy factories, and factories processing ores containing Mo. Depending on input waste streams, sewage sludge can contain high concentrations of Mo. Mo, as well as lead and cadmium, is used in pipe thread-dope, and cattle can be exposed to this substance in oil and gas field operations, and petroleum transmission pipelines.

Toxicokinetics.   Sulfate shares a common transport system with Mo in the intestine and kidney. Mo is eliminated in the bile of cattle and in the urine of laboratory animals. Care must be taken in making cross species extrapolation on the toxicokinetics of Mo, especially between ruminant and monogastric species. Ruminants fed high-dietary Mo excrete Mo in milk.

Mechanism of Action.   Mo is required for metalloenzymes including xanthine oxidase, xanthine dehydrogenase, aldehyde oxidase, and sulfite oxidase. In blood Mo binds with α-macroglobulin in the membranes of erythrocytes, where it enhances the resistance of the membranes to rupture.[3,4] Because of its requirement in metalloenzymes, Mo is an essential nutrient for essentially all animals.

Mo has a three-way interaction with copper and sulfur.[5] Ruminants are more sensitive than nonruminant species to the toxicity of Mo, and this difference is generally attributed to sulfur metabolism in the rumen. Dietary sulfur is converted to sulfide in the rumen, which decreases the absorption of copper. Increasing Mo in the diet increases the rate that microorganisms in the rumen convert the dietary sulfur to sulfide. The thiomolybdates are absorbed and alter the postabsorptive metabolism of Mo. The dithiomolybdates and trithiomolybdates are radially absorbed from the rumen, but the total significance of this is not known.[6]

Increasing dietary Mo and sulfur increases the amount of trichloroacetic acid insoluble Mo-copper protein complex found in plasma. This occurs in both sheep and cattle, and TCA solubility is a measure of available copper present in plasma. However, clinical signs of copper deficiency can be observed even though plasma and liver copper levels are within normal range. Mo may also alter zinc metabolism in cattle.[7]

The desired ratio of copper to Mo is 4:1 to 10:1.[8] The major factor that can result in the calculated copper to Mo ratio being inadequate is dietary sulfur. Increasing sulfur content in the diet, including sulfur in forage, increases the toxicity of Mo. A dietary sulfur/Mo ratio of 100:1 may be considered safe, as long as neither Mo nor sulfur is present in excess.

Toxicity and Risk Factors.   Ruminants are the most susceptible species. Of the ruminant species cattle are the most sensitive and mule deer are the most resistant.[9] Toxicosis has been reported in horses, swine, and rabbits. Some authors have listed horses as being resistant to the effect of Mo on copper metabolism, but recent reports document that horses are susceptible.

Balancing the trace nutrients in rations, especially the Mo/Cu ratio, is the single most important factor in preventing dietary-linked Mo intoxication. Cattle on a high-sulfur diet, including sulfur in the forage and water, are also at a greater risk. Diets high in sulfur decrease the absorption of copper and increase the susceptibility of cattle to Mo. Diets high in Mo may also decrease the absorption of zinc.[10]

The uptake of Mo from soil by plants is a direct soil-to-plant concentration relationship. Factors affecting this relationship include the concentration of Mo in soil, the mineral composition of the soil, soil water, concentration of exchangeable ions, and soil pH.[11,12] Plants growing on humus soils generally are higher in Mo than plants growing on mineral soils, and the disease condition in animals on organic soils is referred to as "teart." Geologic and sediment origins of soil are important for the concentrations of Mo that

may be found. Changes in cultural and fertilization practices in soil management can increase the Mo available for absorption by plants. Increasing the pH of soils generally decreases the absorption of copper and increases the absorption of Mo. Amending soils with sewage sludge and industrial emissions can be a source of environmental Mo.[13] Concentrations of 231 ppm Mo have been reported in plants growing on Mo-rich soils. Forage growing on soils with Mo levels greater than 10 ppm should be suspect.

The desired dietary ratio of copper to Mo is 4:1 to 10:1.[14] Forages containing less than 3 mg Mo/kg of dry matter are generally considered safe, and forages that contain 3 to 10 mg Mo/kg dry matter are considered to be dangerous in terms of inducing copper deficiency. However, the amount of sulfur and copper in the diet can alter the safe levels of dietary Mo. Reports on the dietary levels of Mo required to induce secondary copper deficiency in cattle are varied.[15,16]

Exposure to 6.2 ppm Mo in forage for 5 to 12 months caused epiphyseal dystrophy in 5- to 12-month-old calves, and 25.6 ppm Mo in pasture for 23 days caused death. Cattle on diets adequate for copper and amended with 100 ppm Mo developed signs of secondary copper deficiency within 18 days and deaths occurred after 11 months. Continual grazing of forage contaminated with Mo caused illness and death in cattle within approximately 2 weeks.[17] Increasing dietary concentrations of Mo influence lactation in beef cows, and growth and fertility in heifers.[18-20] In general, cattle feeds should contain less than 5 ppm Mo, sheep diets less than 3.5 to 4 ppm Mo, horse diets less than 100 ppm Mo, swine diets less than 1000 ppm Mo, and poultry diets 10 ppm Mo.[21] The level of Mo in drinking water for cattle should be less than 0.06 ppm.

Clinical Signs.   A summary of clinical signs of Mo intoxication is given in Box 22-3. In cattle, the most common clinical sign is chronic diarrhea. Copper deficiency causes abnormalities in connective tissue formation in bone. Abnormal bone growth and parostosis are observed. An increase of copper in the TCA insoluble fraction of plasma is an early indicator of Mo and sulfur interaction.[22]

Mo poisoning has been observed in horses grazing in a pasture that had been amended with fly ash containing high levels of Mo. In addition to copper deficiency abortions were observed in pregnant mares.

A field incident of acute Mo poisoning in a feedlot was carefully described and monitored.[23] A total of 831 head of feeder cattle were fed a ration that had sodium molybdate (Na_2MoO_4) containing 39% Mo substituted for sodium bicarbonate. The contaminated finished diet was estimated to contain 7400 ppm Mo, and the finished ration was provided ad libitum with an intended daily consumption of 10 kg of feed/head. Actual daily consumption was estimated to be 1.3 kg/head over a 5-day period. The estimated 5-day average oral intake was 9.6 g Mo per head per day or 31 mg/kg body weight Mo per head per day. Anorexia occurred by exposure day 6. Clinical signs included anorexia, posterior ataxia progressing to ataxia of the pectoral limbs, recumbency, streaming epiphora and ptyalism, dry crusty exudate of the nose, foamy mucoid diarrhea, and protrusion of the membrane nictitans. The animals drank water but feed

BOX 22-3	CLINICAL SIGNS OF Mo INTOXICATION

CLINICAL SIGN	SPECIES
Reduced gain in body mass or loss of body mass	Chicks and turkey poults Cattle Sheep Rabbit Guinea pig
Anemia	Chicks Cattle Sheep Rat
Diarrhea	Cattle Sheep Rat
Decreased milk production	Cattle
Achromotrichia	Cattle Sheep Guinea pig
Alopecia	Cattle Rabbit
Deformity of limbs, periosteosis, lameness, abnormal epiphyseal plate	Cattle Sheep Rat Rabbit Guinea pig
Muscular degeneration	Cattle
Central nervous signs (swayback in lambs)	Sheep Cattle
Abortions	Horses

refusal was evident. The problem was identified and alternative feed was provided. As the syndrome progressed, diarrhea and weight loss persisted. On day 13 additional supplementation with copper was provided to give a daily oral intake of 0.5 g copper per head per day. Over a 90-day interval 90 of 831 steers died, and most deaths occurred within 30 days after the initial exposure.

Clinical Pathology. Clinicopathologic findings in cattle that consumed a diet containing approximately 7400 ppm Mo as sodium molybdate were an increase in aspartate aminotransferase, gamma-glutamyltransferase, glutamate dehydrogenase, creatine kinase, BUN, creatinine, total bilirubin, and calcium. As the disease progressed, BUN decreased. Other authors have reported that sorbitol dehydrogenase is elevated in sheep receiving daily injections of Mo.[24]

Lesions. Animals do not present gross or histopathologic lesions characteristic of Mo-induced copper deficiency that are specifically diagnostic. The most common observation is an emaciated carcass. Lesions of periosteosis and abnormal epiphyseal plate growth may be observed, but must be differentiated from a primary copper deficiency.

Lesions observed at necropsy in cattle that were fed a diet containing approximately 7400 ppm sodium molybdate included swollen and friable livers and pale, swollen kidneys with perirenal edema. Histopathology revealed hydropic hepatocellular degermation progressing to periacinar necrosis and hemorrhage. In some animals hepatocytes were only observed in the periportal areas. Histopathology of the kidney ranged from hydropic degeneration of the kidney to marked necrosis of the proximal and distal tubular cells. Limited regeneration was observed 4 days after exposure ceased.

Two sheep were administered daily doses of 35 mg Na_2MoO_4/kg body weight (sheep 1) and 33.9 mg Na_2MoO_4/kg body weight (sheep 2). Sheep 1 received two 35-mg/kg doses and was euthanized at 48 hours; sheep 2 received three doses and was euthanized at 60 hours. Sheep 1 was anorectic at 48 hours, and sheep 2 was anorectic at 60 hours. Necropsy findings included diffuse subcutaneous petechiae and tan discoloration of the liver with multiple 3- to 5-mm subcapsular ecchymosis. The kidneys were mottled and had areas of pallor on the capsular surface. Histopathology revealed diffuse hemorrhagic hepatic necrosis with a thin rim of hepatocytes in the periportal areas. There was diffuse hydropic degeneration to necrosis of the renal convoluted tubular cells. Lesions were not observed in the gastrointestinal tract, heart, spleen, or lung. Plasma levels of Mo at 48 hours were 48 and 51 ppm for sheep 1 and 2, respectively. For sheep 1, the liver and kidney concentrations of Mo were 26 ppm (wet weight) and 50 ppm, respectively. For sheep 2, the liver concentration was 96 ppm and kidney concentration was 180 ppm.

Rats were exposed to inhaled molybdenum trioxide (MoO_3) at exposure levels of 0, 10, 30, and 100 mg/m³ for 6 hours per day, 5 days a week for 2 years.[25] Lesions observed in the exposed rats were chronic inflammatory lesions located at the peribronchiolar and subpleural sites. The giant cells and macrophages contained cholesterol clefts. Metaplasia of the alveoli consisted of ciliated cuboidal and columnar cells. Hyaline degeneration was observed at level II of the nasal respiratory epithelium, and at levels II and III of the respiratory epithelium. Male rats had an increased occurrence of alveolar and bronchiolar adenomas compared with the control rats.

Diagnostic Testing. Mo toxicosis caused by excess dietary intake of Mo is diagnosed based on clinical signs and the concentration of Mo in blood, liver, and kidney. Blood levels that result in Mo intoxication vary with the dietary intake of copper and sulfur.

The most common finding with Mo intoxication is high concentrations of Mo in the liver and low concentrations of copper. When the diet is high in sulfur and Mo, the concentration of copper in the liver may not decrease, but clinical signs of Mo intoxication are observed.

Treatment.   The diet should be assayed for Mo, copper, and sulfur, and copper should be added to the diet to give a 4:1 to 10:1 copper-to-Mo ratio. Because dietary sulfur can alter the predictive ratio, additional copper may be necessary. The sulfur-to-Mo ratio should be less than 100:1, and neither sulfur nor Mo should be in excess. Mineral supplements for cattle grazing forages high in Mo can induce copper poisoning in sheep. Copper sulfate can be added to cattle drinking water.[26] Cattle can be injected with copper, but most preparations are highly irritating and may produce sterile abscesses.

SELENIUM

Stan W. Casteel and Dennis J. Blodgett

Sources.   Selenium-containing compounds are of considerable interest in veterinary medicine for several reasons:

They have biological importance as an essential dietary constituent.[1]
Domestic livestock that ingest seleniferous plants may become intoxicated with selenium.[2]
Intoxication results from excess selenium supplementation of livestock rations.[3-5]
Domestic livestock and companion animals may become intoxicated with selenium after parenteral overdose.[6,7]
Selenium may produce toxic effects in wild aquatic birds exposed to excess environmental concentrations.[8,9]

Selenium occurs in the earth's crust mainly as selenites, selenates, and selenides in association with sulfide minerals.[1] The selenium concentration of soils varies from 0.005 to 1200 ppm. Selenium-deficient soils contain from 0.005 to 2 ppm. Selenium, with chemical properties similar to sulfur, can exist in nature in one of several oxidation states including selenate (SeO_4^{-2}), selenite (SeO_3^{-2}), elemental selenium (Se^o), and selenide (Se^{-2}). The availability of selenium for uptake by vegetation depends on soil conditions. Consequently, the bioavailability and concentration of selenium in soil dictate whether vegetation grown under such conditions has low, moderate, or even toxic levels of selenium. In well-aerated soils with a pH greater than 7.5, selenium is present as water-soluble selenate, which is readily absorbed by plants. However, insoluble ferric selenite predominates in acid soils and plant uptake is limited.[10]

Soils in many parts of the world, including North America, contain high concentrations of selenium. Seleniferous soils and plants containing excess selenium exist in parts of western Canada, Montana, the Dakotas, Nebraska, Wyoming, Colorado, Kansas, Oklahoma, Arizona, New Mexico, Utah, Nevada, and Idaho. Seleniferous regions are characterized by low rainfall, which facilitates the persistence and availability of water-soluble forms of selenium in the soil. Obligate indicator plants, requiring high concentrations of bioavailable selenium for growth, include species of *Astragalus, Oonopsis, Stanleya,* and *Xylorrhiza.* These plants may accumulate several thousand ppm water-soluble selenium on a dry weight basis, giving them acute toxic potential. However, poor palatability restricts consumption to livestock raised under sparse range conditions. Facultative indicator plants of the genera *Atriplex, Machaeranthera,* and *Sideranthus* may accumulate (but do not require) up to 100 ppm selenium. In addition, various grasses and crops may accumulate from 1 to 25 ppm water-insoluble selenium when grown on seleniferous soils. The differences in selenium accumulation by these three groups are rather indistinct. Grasses are by far the most important group from the standpoint of the sheer numbers of livestock affected. Consumption of these grass species for long periods may induce chronic selenium toxicosis.

Toxic concentrations of selenium can occur through the redistribution and concentration of water-soluble compounds leached from soil into irrigation drainage water. Selenium concentrations in agricultural drainage water entering Kesterson Reservoir in California ranged from 140 to 1400 ppb during 1983 to 1985.[11] Normal selenium concentrations in water average no more than 2 ppb. In alkaline aquatic systems, such as that supplying Kesterson Reservoir, water-soluble selenate is the predominant chemical species present and is readily assimilated by aquatic plant life.

Commercial selenium is obtained primarily as a byproduct of copper refining, with a 1982 world production estimate of 1340 tons.[12] Selenium has several industrial applications, including use in the production of low-voltage rectifiers and other electronic equipment, as a decolorizing agent in glass manufacturing, and as a vulcanizing agent in rubber production. Seleniferous compounds also are used in dandruff shampoos, gun bluing, and for supplementation of livestock. In 1987 the FDA-permitted concentration of supplementary selenium was increased from 0.1 or 0.2 ppm to 0.3 ppm in complete feed for finishing swine (except in feeds for weanling swine, which already was approved at 0.3 ppm), poultry, sheep, and cattle. Selenium may be added to feed supplements for limit-feeding at a level not to exceed 3 mg/head per day in beef cattle or 0.7 mg/head per day in sheep. In addition, selenium can be included in free-choice salt-mineral mixtures for beef cattle at a maximum concentration of 120 ppm if intake does not exceed 3 mg/head per day or at a maximum concentration of 90 ppm for sheep if intake does not exceed 0.7 mg/head per day.

Toxicokinetics.   The duodenum is the primary site of selenium absorption, with little or no absorption occurring from the rumen or abomasum. About 40% of orally administered selenium is absorbed by cattle, depending on the chemical form and other dietary factors. The relatively low selenium absorption in ruminants may be related to a reduction of selenite to insoluble, poorly absorbed forms in the rumen. Most water-soluble selenium compounds are effectively absorbed by the gastrointestinal tract of rats. More than 90% of oral selenite and 80% of selenomethionine or selenocysteine are effectively absorbed by rats, whereas elemental selenium and selenium sulfide are poorly absorbed. Presumably, other monogastrics have a similar absorption efficiency. Selenium may be eliminated in the urine, feces, and expired air; however, most dietary excesses are excreted in the urine.

Mechanism of Action. Physiologic and toxic doses of selenium probably are metabolized via the same pathway.[13,14] The reduction pathway begins with the nonenzymatic oxidation of 4 moles of glutathione for every mole of selenite that is reduced. Intermediate metabolites in the reductive pathway include selenoglutathione (GSSeSG), selenopersulfide (GSSeH), and hydrogen selenide (H_2Se).[14] Hydrogen selenide finally is then either methylated for excretion or incorporated into selenoenzymes. The metabolic pathway can generate superoxide, hydrogen peroxide, and oxyradicals.[15] The catalytic specie responsible is believed to be the metabolic selenide (RSe^-) anion. Selenium compounds that react most with thiols (e.g., glutathione) are more toxic in vitro and in vivo. There is also a good correlation between toxicity and carcinostatic activity of the different selenium compounds.

Porcine focal symmetrical poliomyelomalacia (PFSP) results from an induced deficiency of nicotinamide[16] as well as from selenium intoxication, suggesting the involvement of oxidative metabolic failure in the pathogenesis of the lesion. The most severe lesions of PFSP consistently are found in the cervical and lumbosacral intumescences. The metabolic demands of a large concentration of neuronal elements may partially account for the unique vulnerability of these spinal cord regions. Neurotransmitter interactions also play a significant role in neurodegenerative mechanisms.[17] In addition, the presence and relative densities of the different neurotransmitter receptors at various locations in the CNS suggest a basis for selective neuronal vulnerability.

The precise mechanism of embryotoxicity of excess selenium in aquatic birds has not been established. Studies have shown that selenite inhibits cellular DNA and RNA synthesis in vitro.[18,19] Certainly this would have a dramatic effect on rapidly dividing embryonic cells. The enzymes responsible for this synthesis, DNA and RNA polymerases, are inhibited only by selenite in the presence of sulfhydryl compounds.[20] Endogenous cellular sulfhydryl compounds, other than glutathione, are involved in the inhibition of RNA synthesis by selenite.[21] Selenomethionine is more embryotoxic than sodium selenite, partly because of its greater accumulation in the egg.[22] Accumulation of selenium in mallard eggs was approximately 10 times greater for groups fed a dietary concentration of 10 ppm selenomethionine versus sodium selenite. Another study demonstrated a similar trend in chicken eggs, with accumulation of selenium from selenomethionine being significantly greater than that from sodium selenite.[23] Excess selenium as selenite, but not selenate, promotes lipid peroxidation in mammals[24] and increases organic solvent-soluble lipofuscin pigments in the liver, as well as glutathione peroxidase activity.[25] Similar evidence of increased lipid peroxidation and glutathione peroxidase activity was found in aquatic birds collected from Kesterson Reservoir.[8] Lipid peroxidation could be a consequence of the production of free radicals during selenium metabolism.

Toxicity and Risk Factors. In general, the oral minimum toxic dose of selenium ranges from 1 to 5 mg/kg body weight for most animals. The toxicity and bioavailability of inorganic selenium is related to the solubility of the various oxidation states of the particular chemical species. Water-soluble selenate and selenite salts are the two most toxic commonly encountered compounds. All animals are susceptible to selenium toxicosis, with the most common occurrence in cattle, sheep, and horses ingesting plants grown on seleniferous soils. Organic and inorganic forms of selenium account for poisoning in range animals exposed to seleniferous plants. Intoxication also occurs in swine when excess inorganic selenium is added to complete rations and in other livestock and companion animals exposed to excessive parenteral sources.

Acute selenium intoxication occurs with parenteral and oral overdose of supplements. Iatrogenic selenosis occurred in a Chihuahua found dead 1 hour after an intramuscular injection of 1.5 ml of a vitamin E and selenium mixture.[7] The aqueous and oil phases of this mixture had separated and failure to agitate the bottle resulted in the preferential withdrawal of the more dense aqueous phase. Subsequent analysis of the aqueous phase revealed more than 5 mg of selenium/ml of solution. The calculated dose of 2.5 mg selenium/kg body weight exceeded the minimum lethal dose by intramuscular injection in dogs of 2 mg/kg.[26]

The oral dose of sodium selenite required to induce a lesion-specific form of subchronic selenium intoxication unique to swine has been established in male weaner pigs.[27] Encapsulated sodium selenite at doses of 1.4, 2.6, and 4.2 mg/kg of body weight was administered orally on a daily basis. Porcine focal symmetrical poliomyelomalacia was induced in all groups 3 to 20 days after treatment initiation with the time-to-onset occurring in a dose-dependent fashion. The consistent manner in which this lesion was reproduced in this controlled dosing study implies that feed refusal has complicated previous experiments in which selenium was incorporated into the diet for ad libitum consumption.

Subchronic intoxication was induced in pigs fed high-selenium diets for 9 weeks by mixing either *Astragalus praelongus* (31.6 ppm Se in complete feed), *A. bisulcatus* (31.7 ppm Se in complete feed), or sodium selenate (26.6 ppm Se in complete feed) with a commercial ration.[2] A complicating factor in this experiment was the presence of swainsonine in the *Astragalus* species. Clinical signs and lesions in the CNS consistent with subchronic selenosis were induced in all groups of pigs. In a 5-week pig performance study, it was determined that the concentration of sodium selenite required to cause a reduction in growth rate and feed intake was between 4 and 8 ppm selenium when feeding 20% protein in corn-soybean meal diets.[28] Feed refusal was a significant factor affecting weight gain in pigs fed diets containing 16 or 20 ppm selenium.

Severe lesions and congenital malformations have been identified in aquatic birds and embryos from Kesterson Reservoir in Merced County, California.[8] Mean concentrations of selenium in livers and kidneys were elevated tenfold above those from a control site (94 and 97 ppm dry weight versus 8 and 12 ppm dry weight). Subsurface agricultural drainage water feeding the reservoir contained an average of 300 ppb selenium. Mean selenium concentrations in aquatic plants, invertebrates, and fish from the reservoir were 12 to 130 times (22 to 175 ppm dry weight) those found at a control site not receiving agricultural drainage water.[11] Diets containing 10 ppm selenomethionine or 25 ppm sodium selenite fed to mallard ducks caused a 40% to 44% reduction in egg hatchability.[9] Selenomethionine was more embryotoxic and teratogenic than sodium selenite, inducing stunted growth and a 13.1% incidence of malformations versus a 4% malformation rate for the sodium salt.

Clinical Signs. *Acute intoxication* usually manifests as depression, weakness, dyspnea, and a garlicky odor to the breath caused by a volatile methylated metabolite of selenium. Acute poisoning reported in calves given sodium selenite intramuscularly at 2 mg/kg body weight manifested itself as depression and inability to rise 3 to 6 hours later.[6] Calves became dyspneic and died within 12 hours of injection. Acute toxicosis was reported in young pigs fed a ration contaminated with 300 ppm sodium selenite for 3 days.[29] Clinical intoxication commenced with anorexia and depression 24 to 48 hours after consumption of the contaminated feed. Hindlimb ataxia, dog-sitting posture, and sternal recumbency were observed. The most severely affected pigs were seen in lateral recumbency in a state of generalized flaccid paralysis. Pigs in lateral recumbency became dyspneic, cyanotic, and died of respiratory failure within 1 to 2 hours. Forty-two of 256 pigs died or required euthanasia 3 to 8 days after initial exposure to the contaminated feed.

Subchronic intoxication in pigs exposed to complete rations containing 9.7 to 27 ppm selenium for 45 days is manifest as a CNS disorder characterized by initial hindlimb ataxia progressing to posterior paralysis, then tetraparesis to paralysis.[5] Affected pigs remain alert and attempt to walk while dragging their hindlimbs. Hoof separation at the coronary band also occurs. Toxicosis was induced in pigs fed selenium-accumulating *Astragalus* spp. and sodium selenate.[2] Clinical signs and lesions consistent with *subchronic-chronic* selenium intoxication developed in all groups of pigs. These findings are consistent with previous feeding trials in pigs using selenium accumulator *Astragalus* spp.[30] These trials demonstrated that the selenium concentration of the diet was primarily responsible for the clinical intoxication associated with spinal cord lesions of symmetric poliomyelomalacia.

Chronic intoxication, sometimes referred to as "alkali disease," results from the chronic consumption of seleniferous grasses and crops, including small grains containing 5 to 15 ppm protein-bound, water-insoluble selenium.[31] This syndrome occurs in cattle, horses, sheep, pigs, and poultry and is characterized by lameness, hoof overgrowth, and hoof deformation. In horses horizontal cracks in the hoof wall develop (Fig. 22-2). Hair loss and discoloration also occur. Hair from the mane and tail of horses breaks off and creates a "bobtail" appearance.

"Blind staggers," another alleged form of chronic selenosis, occurs when cattle graze certain plants, such as members of the *Astragalus* genus, known to accumulate high concentrations of water-soluble seleniferous compounds. Blind staggers usually affects cattle and occasionally sheep; it is characterized by blindness, aimless wandering, and inability to eat or drink before death. However, this

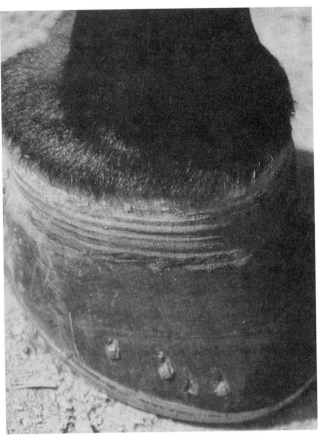

Fig. 22-2 Horizontal rings in the hoof wall, below the coronary band, of a horse with chronic selenium toxicosis. (Photo courtesy of Dr. Frank D. Galey.)

syndrome has not been reproduced by the feeding of selenium-containing compounds and it is questionable whether it has been reproduced by feeding seleniferous forages.[31] Blind staggers is a condition in cattle of questionable etiology in which selenium has little or no involvement.[32] Blind staggers is more likely a syndrome with multiple etiologies including polioencephalomalacia from excessive sulfate ingestion and locoism from ingestion of some *Astragalus* spp.

Pathology. Although the precise physiologic dysfunction occurring in peracute selenium poisoning has not been determined, the lesions induced are consistent with cardiac failure, loss of microvascular integrity, or both. The clinical, biochemical, and pathologic findings all implicate the heart as the major target organ. Gross pathologic findings in sheep include diffuse edema, congestion and focal hemorrhages in the lungs, edema of abdominal viscera, and patchy congestion with occasional hemorrhages in the intestinal mucosa.[33,34] Excessive straw-colored fluid may be found in the thoracic or peritoneal cavities. Histopathologic changes in the heart are of a severe degenerative nature in lethally intoxicated sheep. Other findings in experimentally poisoned sheep include degenerative to necrotic changes in liver, kidney, pancreas, and skeletal muscle, especially the diaphragm.

In acutely poisoned sheep it was shown that the heart has an affinity for selenium, especially following lethal intoxication.[33] Histochemical studies in acutely intoxicated sheep have demonstrated the accumulation of selenium in the cardiac conduction system.[34]

Pulmonary edema was prominent in acute selenosis in a dog as was congestion of the liver and other abdominal organs.[7] Lambs poisoned with sodium selenate used to spike an oral anthelmintic died 5 to 29 hours later; study showed gross lesions of subcutaneous hemorrhage, marked pulmonary edema with hydrothorax, and extensive destruction of renal cortices.[35] Lambs poisoned by parenteral selenium had similar gross lesions.[36] The primary microscopic lesions consisted of necrosis, mineralization, and fragmentation of cardiac myofibers.

Porcine focal symmetrical poliomyelomalacia was induced in pigs 3 to 20 days after initiation of daily oral administration of encapsulated sodium selenite.[27] Spinal cord lesions were confined to the ventral horns of the cervical and lumbosacral intumescences. Lesions varied in severity in a dose- and time-dependent fashion. Lesions of the brain and spinal cord consisted of neuronal chromatolysis, microcavitation of the neuropil, neuronal cytoplasmic vacuolation, perineuronal vacuolation, endothelial proliferation, and swollen axons.

Severe gross and microscopic lesions were found in adult aquatic birds and embryos collected from Kesterson Reservoir in 1984.[8] Adult birds were emaciated, had subacute to chronic hepatic lesions, and excess fluid and fibrin in the peritoneal cavity. Typical liver lesions consisted of moderate focal necrosis, fibrosis, and bile duct hyperplasia. Scattered regenerative nodules also were seen. A variety of malformations were seen in embryos including anophthalmia, microphthalmia, abnormal beaks, amelia, micromelia, ectrodactyly, and hydrocephaly.

Diagnostic Testing. When selenium toxicosis is suspected, it is important to determine the source and the exposure level. Chronic intake of diets containing more than 5 ppm selenium salts induces signs of chronic intoxication. More severe intoxication, with a more rapid onset, is expected with exposure to higher dietary concentrations.

Definitive diagnosis of selenium intoxication is based on compatible clinical signs, lesions, and, most important, chemical analysis of selected tissues and body fluids. Antemortem samples for chemical analysis include blood and urine. High concentrations of selenium in blood and urine reflect recent exposure to excessive dietary or parenteral sources.

Suitable postmortem samples include liver, kidney, and spleen collected and frozen at necropsy. Adequate whole blood selenium concentrations in most species range from 0.08 to 0.35 ppm. Blood concentrations may reach 25 ppm in acute intoxication, whereas 1 to 4 ppm is the likely concentration seen in chronic conditions. Liver and kidney contain the highest selenium concentration in acute and chronic poisoning. Acute cases usually have selenium levels greater than 4 ppm, whereas chronic cases may have 10 to 20 ppm, depending on the time of last exposure. Blood and tissue selenium concentrations are harder to interpret when several days elapse between the last exposure and sample collection.

Peracute selenium intoxication in a Chihuahua found dead 1 hour after an intramuscular injection of a vitamin E and selenium mixture resulted in liver and kidney concentrations of 12.9 and 12.1 ppm wet weight.[7] For comparison, the corresponding dry weight concentrations would be more than 3 times wet weight. Normal liver and kidney selenium concentration in dogs is approximately 1 ppm wet weight. Lambs orally exposed to a lethal concentration of sodium selenate and dying 5 to 29 hours later had liver and kidney concentrations ranging from 3.6 to 9.3 ppm and 1.4 to 2.8 ppm wet weight, respectively.[35]

Subchronic intoxication induced in pigs fed high-selenium diets for 9 weeks (by mixing *A. praelongus* [31.6 ppm Se in the complete ration], *A. bisulcatus* [31.7 ppm], or sodium selenate [26.6 ppm] with a commercial ration) resulted in group mean blood concentrations of 4.2, 3.9, and 3 ppm, respectively.[2] The within-experiment control group had a mean blood selenium concentration of 0.2 ppm. Urine selenium concentrations averaged 9.3, 8.1, and 9.9 ppm, respectively, compared with the experimental control group value of 0.09 ppm. Liver, kidney, and spleen concentrations in principal groups were greater than 22, 24, and 11 ppm dry weight, respectively, compared with the experimental control group averages of 1.8, 5.5, and 1.5 ppm dry weight.

The potential utility of glutathione peroxidase activity for the assessment of selenium status appears limited to selenium-deficient and adequate states. Glutathione peroxidase activity in humans exposed to excessive selenium in drinking water (0.19 to 0.5 ppm versus normal 0.01 ppm) did not show the increased activity seen with supplementation of selenium-deficient subjects.[37] Mice exposed to 4 to 8 ppm selenium in drinking water for 25 weeks had reduced glutathione peroxidase activity in liver homogenates.[38]

Acute selenosis must be differentiated from selenium deficiency and intoxication by ionophores, Japanese yew, gossypol, organophosphates, and carbamates. Infectious agents resembling acute selenosis include pasteurellosis, anthrax, infectious necrotic hepatitis, and enterotoxemia. Subchronic selenosis in swine must be differentiated from organic arsenical toxicosis, water deprivation, calcium-phosphorus imbalances, vitamin B deficiencies, copper deficiency, and pigweed toxicosis. Infectious diseases resembling subchronic selenosis in swine include pseudorabies and edema disease. Chronic selenosis may be confused with freezing of the feet, ergotism, fescue foot, fluorosis, thallium intoxication, and laminitis.

Treatment. Management of acute selenium intoxication is primarily supportive. Cardiopulmonary monitoring is necessary, together with intravenous fluids, supplemental oxygen, and ventilation as needed. An untested treatment is parenteral vitamin E administration.[25] This could potentially help in an acute selenium toxicosis based on the hypothesis of free radical formation with selenium toxicosis. Accelerating the excretion of selenium by adding arsenic-containing compounds may be helpful in chronic intoxication of some species. Feeding rations containing 50 to 100 ppm arsanilic acid is beneficial for calves and pigs. Elimination of the source and provision of selenium-deficient rations is always indicated.

SODIUM

Gene Niles

Synonyms. Hypernatremia, salt poisoning, water intoxication,[1] sodium toxicosis, sodium chloride intoxication, and sodium chloride poisoning are all names given for the disease caused by excess sodium.

Sources. Salt poisoning can occur from ingesting too much sodium (direct toxicosis) or from water deprivation (indirect toxicosis).

Direct sodium ion toxicosis. Direct sodium ion toxicosis is caused by excess sodium intake in either feed or water.[2,3] This syndrome is also called *acute sodium ion toxicosis* because illness develops within 24 to 48 hours of over-consumption of sodium salts.[4-6] Sodium salts composed of sulfate, propionate, acetate, carbonate, sulfonamide, and chloride can cause toxicosis.[2]

Direct sodium ion toxicity frequently occurs from ingesting salt water such as brine from oil field waste.[2,7] These cases often occur during the winter when fresh water sources are frozen. Ground water with naturally high mineral content is a source of toxicosis also.[2-5,8] Saline water that is safe for use during the winter can become a source of toxicosis during extremely hot summer months because of increased consumption and total salt intake.[5] Saline water poses a greater risk to livestock than high sodium levels in feed because the animal cannot drink additional water to dilute the sodium intake.[5] Domestic animals prefer clean, fresh water and generally drink brine or salt water only when fresh water is not available.[4]

One-half percent to 1% salt is added to most livestock rations to fulfill their nutrient requirement for sodium chloride.[1-3] When plentiful, potable water is available, domestic animals can tolerate feeds containing much higher salt levels.[1,2-4,9] Ruminant protein and mineral supplements commonly contain levels of sodium chloride significantly higher than 1%.[2-4] This is done to control intake when these supplements are fed ad libitum.[2-4] These feeds can pose risks to animals that are not properly acclimated to them or are "salt or mineral starved," leading to overconsumption driven by existing mineral or salt deficiencies.[3,9]

Sodium ion toxicosis has developed in bottle-fed calves given only milk substitutes containing high salt levels without access to supplemental water.[1,2,9] The inappropriate use of oral and intravenous fluids with high salt levels in the treatment of calf diarrhea is also a source of sodium ion toxicosis.[10,11]

Using brine or whey in the production of wet mash increases the incidence of sodium ion toxicosis in poultry.[5]

The occurrence of direct sodium ion toxicosis involving dogs or cats is rare, but the ingestion of a high-salt compound caused the death of a dog whose serum sodium concentration was 211 mEq/L at the time of death.[5,12,13] Ingestion of rock salt by dogs generally produces illness involving the gastrointestinal system.[5]

Indirect sodium ion toxicosis. Indirect, or chronic, sodium ion toxicosis generally results from restricted water intake and develops over a period of 4 to 7 days.[2-4,6] Indirect toxicosis is the most common type of sodium ion toxicosis occurring in domestic livestock and generally results from water deprivation.[6,10]

Reasons for water deprivation are numerous, including frozen water sources, overcrowding, unpalatable water because of natural mineral content or added medication, mechanical failure of automatic watering systems, and neglect.

Toxicokinetics. *Osmolality* is the concentration of ions in a solution. Water is the solvent in extracellular fluid (ECF), and sodium with its associated anions is the primary ion affecting the ECF osmolality.[6] Osmoreceptors are specialized neurons in the hypothalamus that monitor the osmolality of the ECF and react to minute increases by stimulating thirst and signaling the release of antidiuretic hormone (ADH) from the posterior pituitary gland.[6] Increased water consumption and increased water retention by the kidneys due to the effect of ADH are the responses that rapidly restore normal osmolality.[6] This mechanism is extremely effective as long as osmolar changes are gradual and ample potable water is available.[6]

Hypernatremia occurs when the sodium content of the ECF increases in relation to its free water content or free water is lost from the ECF without a compensatory decrease in sodium, as can occur with restricted water intake or third space problems.[6,10,14] Third space problems occur when free water is lost into body cavities or the gastrointestinal tract from the development of osmotic gradients that draw fluid into these spaces.[6] Sodium's strong affinity for water causes an influx of water into areas of high sodium concentration.

Although the rate of sodium elimination or retention is the major factor influencing the ECF volume, this does not affect the osmolality of the ECF because water and sodium move proportionally within the kidney.[6]

Mechanism of Action. The ingestion of excess salt has an irritating effect on mucosal surfaces.[5] If the mucosal irritation is not severe, clinical signs include anorexia, vomiting, and diarrhea.[5] When excess salt intake leads to severe gastro-enteritis, electrolyte imbalances, and severe dehydration with losses of body water greater than 10%, acute death can occur.[2-5] If the animal survives the acute insult, in addition to the loss of free body water into the gastrointestinal tract, the blood sodium levels rapidly increase as the sodium is readily absorbed and distributed throughout the body.[5] As hyper-natremia develops, serum sodium levels increase above normal (135 to 155 mEq/L) and sodium passively diffuses into the cerebrospinal fluid (CSF), also increasing its sodium content above normal (135 to 150 mEq/L).[1,2,5,9]

Hypernatremia is *acute* when the serum sodium level goes above 160 mEq/L within 24 to 48 hours.[1,2,6,10] During an acute hypernatremic insult the animal's protective mechanism to maintain cell integrity responds by rapidly concentrating sodium, potassium, and chloride within the neurons of the brain to equalize the osmotic pressures and prevent intracellular fluid loss.[6,10,14] The increase in intra-cellular electrolytes occurs within 3 hours.[6] If the acute insult is quickly resolved without damage to the neurons of the brain, the levels of these electrolytes decline as the CSF sodium levels decline.[10] When this defense mechanism fails, the brain cells shrink from dehydration, tearing blood vessels that lead to hemorrhage, brain infarcts, and cerebral edema.[6]

As brain sodium levels elevate, glycolysis decreases with a corresponding decrease in available energy for normal brain function.[1-7,9] Although sodium passively enters the CSF, it is actively transported out of the CSF into the serum.[1-7,10,13,14] Because an energy deficit develops, sodium becomes trapped in the brain and CSF.[1-7,10,13,14] If access to unlimited water is allowed at this stage and rehydration occurs, blood sodium levels decline and an osmotic gradient is established between the blood and CSF sodium levels. This gradient results in an influx of fluid into the CSF with resultant brain swelling, producing clinical signs and lesions associated with cerebral edema.

When hypernatremia develops over 4 to 7 days, it is *chronic* and involves changes in intercellular osmolality resulting from increased organic osmoles as well as electrolytes.[6,10,14] Organic solutes are called *idaiogenic osmoles* and are composed of taurine, myo-insolitol, glycerophosphoryl-choline, betaine, glutamate, glutamine, and phosphocreatine.[6,10,11,14] These organic osmoles constitute 60% of the increase in intracellular solutes.[10] Idaiogenic osmoles increase to maximum levels within 48 to 72 hours and a similar amount of time is required for their decline as a hypernatremic crisis is resolved.[10] Most cases of sodium ion toxicosis in domestic animals involve increases of intracellular idaiogenic osmoles.[6,10]

The occurrence of water intoxication in bottle-fed calves occurs as a result of their acclimation to high sodium, producing a hyperosmolar state with elevated serum, ECF, CSF, and brain sodium levels. Illness follows when the brain sodium content reaches a level greater than that for which the animal can compensate or when unlimited access to fresh water is allowed. When allowed free access to water, the rapid absorption of water reduces the serum sodium level, thus initiating the disease process.[6,9,10]

Toxicity and Risk Factors. The acute oral lethal dose of salt for swine, horses, and cattle is 2.2 g/kg, whereas it is 4 g/kg and 6 g/kg for dogs and sheep, respectively.[4,5] The toxic dose for poultry is 1.6 g/kg and 0.75 to 3 g/kg is the estimated lethal dose of sodium chloride for humans.[13,15]

Acute salt poisoning can occur in ruminants that have been without salt for an extended period of time (salt starved).[2,4,16] Salt-starved cattle have experienced acute death as a result of severe gastroenteritis after consuming from 1 to 3 kg of salt, even though fresh water was readily available.

Toxicosis has developed in poultry consuming wet mash containing 2% salt because of increased feed consumption as compared to when fed dry feed.[5]

Swine and poultry are the most sensitive to water restriction, with cattle being the next most susceptible species.[5] Lactation increases susceptibility of both sows and cows because of the increased water requirements necessary for milk production. High-producing, early lactation cows are most susceptible.[1,4]

Pregnant mares that underwent 3 weeks of increasing water restriction starting at 72% of normal consumption the first week and decreasing to 58% of normal intake by the last week did not exhibit any life- or pregnancy-threatening effects.[17] In another group of horses feed and water were withheld for 72 hours without ill effect and 62% of their weight loss during the 3-day trial was regained within 1 hour when allowed free access to water.[18]

Sheep are relatively resistant to sodium ion toxicosis, although toxicosis does occur.[5,16]

Clinical Signs. In swine early clinical signs of sodium ion toxicosis are generally unnoticed but include restlessness, thirst, pruritus, constipation, and vomiting.[1-5] These signs progress to aimless wandering, blindness, head pressing, and circling, which is usually characterized by pivoting on one front foot.[1-5,14] Muscle twitches starting at the snout and then spreading to the head occur.[2,4,14] As the tremors progress, pigs back up and assume a dog-sitting position before falling over in lateral recumbency with clonic-tonic seizures and opisthotonos followed by death.[2,4,5] Allowing rapid rehydration increases the number of clinical cases with CNS involvement.[1] Death of 50% or more of affected animals is common.[1,2,5]

In ruminants severe gastroenteritis causes weakness, dehydration, and death within 24 hours when the toxicosis is due to excessive salt intake.[5] Exaggerated goose-stepping motion of the front legs and dragging the rear legs with knuckling of the fetlock is a common sequela of direct toxicosis.[2,9] Signs characteristic of polioencephalomalacia are common when water-deprived cattle are allowed free access to fresh, clean water or are moved into pastures containing water with high salinity. These signs include belligerence or depression, bruxism, circling, cortical blindness, and head pressing. As with swine, fine muscle fasciculations start at the head and progress to clonic-tonic seizures, leading to opisthotonos, paddling, and death. Similar clinical signs can occur in feedlot lambs.[16]

Clinical signs that occur in poultry are depression, weakness, thirst, dyspnea, fluid discharge from the beak, ascites, limb paralysis, diarrhea, and sudden death.[1,2,5,15] In laying hens decreased feed efficiency as well as reduced egg production and egg weight occur. Wet droppings that stain the eggs and cause hock and breast lesions are also common.[15]

Salt poisoning in dogs is rare and generally not life threatening.[5,12,19] Clinical signs generally limited to the gastrointestinal system include vomiting and diarrhea.[5] Vomiting, polyuria, polydipsia, and fine muscle tremors that progressed to continuous clonic-tonic seizures at 36 hours after ingestion of a high-salt compound occurred in a dog that died of hypernatremia.[13]

Clinical Pathology. Measurement of serum and CSF sodium levels is used in the diagnosis of sodium ion toxicosis in all species. Normal reference range values for serum sodium in adult domestic animals range from 135 to 155 mEq/L and normal CSF sodium levels range from 135 to 150 mEq/L.[1,5,9] Serum sodium levels greater than 160 mEq/L confirm hypernatremia.[1,2,6,10] When animals suspected to have sodium ion toxicosis have normal serum sodium levels, it is important to compare serum values with CSF sodium values.[3,4,9] It is common for the sodium level in serum to decline rapidly after gain of free water from either oral or intravenous fluid administration while the CSF sodium levels remain elevated.[6,10]

Elevated serum chloride values in conjunction with hypernatremia aid in the diagnosis of acute toxicosis of sodium chloride.[4,20] Normal serum chloride ranges from 90 to 105 mEq/L.

Eosinopenia can be an early finding in pigs but usually disappears by 48 to 72 hours after the onset of illness.[4,5]

Lesions. Gross lesions associated with the gastrointestinal tract in both large and small animals include inflammation and pinpoint ulcerations containing clotted blood.[1-3] Cerebral and leptomeningeal congestion and edema may be seen.[4] Degeneration and edema of skeletal muscle with anasarca, pulmonary edema, and hydropericardium can occur in swine and ruminants.[2,4,15] Ascites, enlarged hearts, subcutaneous edema, and glomerulosclerosis can occur in poultry.[2,15]

In swine microscopic lesions consisting of eosinophilic meningoencephalitis with eosinophilic perivascular cuffing are observed with acute death.[1-5] This lesion disappears after approximately 48 hours of illness and the eosinophils are replaced with mononuclear cells. Eosinophilic cuffing also can occur in poultry but is not seen in other species.[20]

Polioencephalomalacia with neuronal degeneration occurs in swine and cattle.[1-4,9] Although lesions rarely are noted in sheep, cerebral edema with laminar necrosis has occurred in lambs.[16]

Pulmonary edema and hemorrhage of the gastric mucosa were detected in a dog that died of hypernatremia. Microscopic lesions of renal and liver necrosis were noted along with diffuse vacuolation of the white matter of the brain. Neuronal necrosis was not observed in this dog.[13]

Diagnostic Testing. Brain sodium levels of 1600 and 1800 ppm are considered the upper normal limits for cattle and swine, respectively.[21] Brain sodium levels greater than these values support a diagnosis of sodium toxicosis with values commonly greater than 2000 ppm.[5,20]

Analysis of sodium levels in postmortem eye fluid can aid in a diagnosis of sodium ion toxicosis because sodium has been demonstrated to remain stable in ocular fluid after death.[1,20,22-25] Postmortem autolysis of up to 48 hours' duration does not significantly alter the sodium content of either aqueous humor or vitreous humor.[22] The sodium content of aqueous humor versus vitreous humor is not significantly different when analyzed either fresh or 24 hours postmortem.[22] Vitreous humor sodium levels are 95% of serum levels.[23] Aqueous humor sodium levels of 172 mEq/L and 218 mEq/L were detected in two cows whose brain sodium levels of 3185 mEq/L and 4250 mEq/L confirmed salt toxicosis.[20] Sodium levels in eight cows that died acutely of other causes ranged from 129 mEq/L to 156 mEq/L.[20]

Normal canine brain sodium levels are less than 1840 ppm.[13]

Treatment. The water deficit must be replaced slowly so that iatrogenic cerebral edema does not occur. When sodium level is lowered too rapidly, water follows a concentration gradient and moves into neurons. Ideally, hypernatremia should be corrected over a 48- to 72-hour period. On a herd basis or when sodium cannot be monitored, water intake should be limited to 0.5% of body weight at 60-minute intervals until rehydration is established.[1]

When dealing with sodium ion toxicosis in individual animals, evaluation of the serum sodium level is essential when developing a treatment protocol to correct hypernatremia. The following formula is used to calculate the deficit:

Free water deficit (L) = 0.6 × body weight (kg) × ([current serum sodium concentration/reference range serum sodium concentration] − 1).[10,13]

Serum sodium levels should be reduced by no more than 0.3 to 0.5 mEq/hour.[6] The administration of hypertonic saline solutions instead of isotonic solutions is recommended to reduce the incidence of iatrogenic cerebral edema.[6,10,14] The sodium content of both parenteral and oral fluids should closely match the serum sodium level to prevent the development of osmotic gradients that promote movement of free water into the CSF with subsequent edema.[6,10,14] Physiologic saline (0.9% saline) contains 154 mEq/L sodium. Because serum sodium values in clinical cases of sodium ion toxicosis are generally greater than 160 mEq/L, additional sodium must be added.[6,10,14] When the serum sodium level is unknown but hypernatremia is highly suspected, the initial intravenous fluid should contain 170 mEq/L of sodium. This level should be decreased as clinical signs improve.

The calculated difference between the actual serum sodium values and the base fluid can be made up by adding the necessary quantity of saline from either 5%, 7%, or 23.4% saline, which contain 0.85, 1.19, or 4 mEq/mL sodium, respectively.[6,10] Using the example of an animal with a serum sodium level of 185 mEq/L, the difference in sodium content between the serum concentration and physiologic saline is 31 mEq/L. The addition of 8 ml of 23.4% saline increases the total sodium level to 186 mEq/1.008 L, or 184.5 mEq/L.

Serum sodium levels decrease as excess sodium is eliminated by the kidney; therefore, serum sodium levels should be monitored frequently to allow appropriate adjustments of the sodium level in the intravenous fluids. Also, absorption of water from oral electrolyte solutions, milk replacers, or drinking water can lead to excess free water with rapid decreases in serum sodium.[10] Table salt, which contains 17 mEq/g sodium, can be added to oral fluid sources in appropriate amounts, depending on the sodium content of the fluid source.[10]

When hypernatremia occurs in conjunction with hypoglycemia or acidosis, which are common with protracted diarrhea, the base fluid should be 1.3% sodium bicarbonate (156 mEq/L sodium), to which additional glucose and sodium can be added.[6,10] Glucose in 50% solution should be used instead of 2.5% or 5% glucose to keep from adding unnecessary free water to the solution.[6,10] When 100 ml of 50% glucose is added to 1 L of 1.3% sodium bicarbonate, the resulting solution contains 4.5% glucose and 141.8 mEq/L sodium. Additional sodium can be added to this mixture to increase the sodium content appropriately.

Worsening CNS signs and the development of fine tremors of the facial muscles generally indicate the occurrence of cerebral edema.[6] Mannitol 25% at a dose of 1 to 2 g/kg administered intravenously over 20 to 30 minutes can be used to treat cerebral edema.[6,10] The use of mannitol is contra-indicated if brain hemorrhage is suspected.[6,10] Mannitol also facilitates the elimination of sodium and chloride; therefore, these electrolytes need to be monitored closely.[6] Mannitol may be repeated at 4- to 6-hour intervals for up to 24 hours. Glycerin is a less expensive alternative to mannitol therapy. Glycerin (1 ml/kg) should be diluted with an equal volume of water and administered orally.[6] Dexamethasone at a dosage of 0.44 to 2 mg/kg given intravenously aids in relieving brain swelling.[14,26] Dimethyl sulfoxide administered as a 2% solution intravenously is effective in reducing brain swelling.[14] Diazepam can be administered to control seizures at a dose of 0.5 to 1.5 mg/kg.[10,13,26]

Prognosis. The prognosis for any animal with sodium ion toxicosis should be guarded at best because 50% or more of affected animals die.[1,2,5]

Prevention and Control. The prevention of sodium ion toxicosis relies primarily on the provision of unlimited potable water because livestock and other domestic animals that possess normal thirst-regulating mechanisms can withstand high dietary salt intake.[2,3,9] Livestock water should not contain more than 5000 ppm total salt, although most species can tolerate levels up to twice this amount.[2-4] Salt- and mineral-starved ruminants should have salt gradually reintroduced into their diet to allow reacclimation and prevent overconsumption leading to salt toxicosis.

ZINC

Margita M. Dziwenka and Robert Coppock

Synonyms. Synonyms of zinc are galvanize, blue powder, Asarco L 15, merrillite, and jasad.

Sources. Zinc is an essential nutrient, but when present in excess it can be toxic. Oral exposures account for most zinc intoxications. Toxicity and deficiencies generally are the result of marginal deficiencies, excesses, or interactions with other minerals and can be difficult to diagnose.[1] Because of its electron configuration zinc has a valance of 2. Many metals with a +2 valance interact with zinc. As an essential nutrient, zinc is required for metalloenzymes such as aminopeptidases, alkaline phosphatase, carboxypeptidases, superoxide dismutase, and thymidine kinase.[2,3]

The following list outlines a variety of potential sources of zinc that can lead to toxicosis in domestic animals.

- Nuts from collapsible transport cages can contain zinc.[4,5]
- Some topical ointments contain zinc oxide.
- United States pennies minted after 1982 contain 98% zinc.[6,7]
- Zinc is released from galvanized surfaces, especially if the medium in the container is acid, such as sour milk.[8] In one report it is suggested that a possible source is galvanized pipes and equipment used to deliver feed and milk to pigs.[9]

- Zinc chromate is used as a paste in joining electric cables.
- Fumes from galvanizing factories and foundries may be toxic.
- Forage and soil in pastures near industrial plants can be contaminated.
- Zinc-based paints can contain 50% to 55% zinc.
- Zinc dust is an industrial hazard for guard dogs.
- Careless use of zinc sulfate as a prophylactic and treatment for diseases such as fungi poisoning and ovine foot rot can result in toxicosis.
- Caged and aviary birds may be exposed to zinc oxide, which is produced in the galvanization process used to prevent rusting of wire in cages.[10]
- Other sources include galvanized mesh, nails, containers, dishes, staples, fertilizers, and zinc shampoos,[11] as well as items such as washers, nuts, and snaps.[12]
- Errors can occur in formulation of diets.

Toxicokinetics. Normal zinc metabolism is not completely understood, but the small intestine is the primary site of zinc absorption with the proximal portion being the key site. Absorption is a two-step process consisting of intestinal mucosal uptake and transport to the blood. Transport to the blood occurs rapidly, but is considered the rate-limiting step. Approximately 67% of plasma zinc is bound by van der Waals forces and the remainder is chemically protein bound.[13] The zinc moves to the liver via the portal system where approximately 30% to 40% is extracted and is then released back into the bloodstream. Once it is absorbed, transfer to biologically active tissues such as the liver is rapid and indicates a rapid accumulation and turnover rate in these tissues. Other tissues such as muscle and bone have a slower accumulation and turnover rate and peak concentrations may occur weeks later.

The amount of zinc absorbed is influenced by a variety of factors such as dietary zinc concentrations, age, growth rate, and protein source in the diet as well as the mineral composition of the diet. The interrelationship of zinc with other nutrients plays an important role in zinc metabolism. In monogastric animals nutritional factors such as cadmium, calcium, magnesium, phosphorus, and copper all influence zinc absorption and metabolism.[14] The source of protein in the diet also affects zinc availability. When diets of plant protein origin such as soybean meal are fed to monogastric animals, the requirement for zinc increases as a result of decreased zinc availability and absorption. The reduced absorption seen with plant protein sources is partially due to the phytic acid content of the diet. This effect of phytic acid on zinc metabolism is not evident in ruminants. The exact mechanism of this difference has not been well established. High dietary calcium, especially in the presence of plant protein, reduces the zinc absorption in swine and poultry. The effects of dietary calcium levels on zinc absorption in ruminants, however, are not well established. Cadmium is an important zinc antagonist and causes decreased zinc absorption and affects tissue zinc metabolism in both monogastric and ruminant animals. The relationship between copper and zinc is complex, but copper interferes with zinc absorption and zinc with copper absorption, which may be due to a competition for the same protein-binding sites in the duodenum.

Dietary zinc levels influence the percentage of zinc absorbed from the diet. In a diet that contains excessive zinc, the percentage of zinc absorbed decreases but the total quantity absorbed increases. The reverse holds true for diets that are deficient in zinc.

Zinc is excreted in the feces via the bile, intestinal mucosal secretions, and pancreatic fluid.[15] Fecal zinc excretion increases as dietary zinc levels increase, whereas urinary zinc excretion is generally unaffected by dietary zinc levels. These findings show that homeostatic regulation of zinc concentration in the body takes place in the intestinal tract. Chelated zinc is excreted via the bile and urine. Therefore, tissue levels of zinc are regulated at the level of gastrointestinal absorption, plasma transport, cellular zinc stores, and rate of excretion.[16]

The mechanism of zinc toxicity and its effect on the horse are poorly understood. It has been postulated that the development of osteochondrosis lesions may be related to a copper-deficient state induced by exposure to high zinc and cadmium levels in pasture foliage.[17]

The toxicokinetics of zinc in sheep has not been well established. Sheep have more tightly controlled zinc levels. Adult ruminants, unlike preruminants, reduce zinc absorption and increase fecal excretion of zinc when dietary excesses occur.[18]

Zinc toxicosis in birds can lead to pancreatic injury and lesions in the proventriculus.[19] The exact mechanism of the pancreatic injury is not completely understood. One experimental toxicity study suggests that the injury may be caused by zinc acting directly on the pancreas.[20] This same study also suggests that accelerated and increased normal processes of cell production and desquamation account for the proventricular lesions seen in zinc toxicosis.

Mechanism of Action. The mechanism by which zinc toxicosis causes hemolysis in dogs has not been established. Some possible explanations include inhibition of specific red blood cell enzymes, direct damage to the erythrocytic membrane, and increased susceptibility of the erythrocyte to oxidative damage by other endogenous or xenobiotic agents. Morphologic features of the erythrocytes seen with zinc poisoning have similarities to the erythrocytes seen in dogs with chronic lead poisoning. Therefore, it has been suggested that the same mechanism that causes erythrocyte mechanical fragility and anemia in lead toxicosis may also be responsible for the anemia seen in zinc toxicosis.

The gastrointestinal signs seen in pigs with acute zinc poisonings are likely due to the direct caustic or corrosive properties of certain zinc salts. With chronic exposure to zinc the zinc interacts competitively for absorption with iron, copper, and calcium.[21] These interactions play a significant role in the development of clinical signs seen with chronic zinc exposure.[22]

Excess zinc has been implicated in the formation of osteochondrosis lesions in horses, but the mechanism of action that causes these lesions has not been well established.[23] Evidence suggests that interference with collagen metabolism may be due to interactions between zinc and copper.

The exact mechanism of action of zinc toxicosis in ruminants is unknown, but induced copper or iron deficiency is possibly caused by inhibition of intestinal absorption of these elements.

This may be especially important if dietary levels of copper and iron are marginal for the minimal requirements. This interference results in anemia in nonruminants but not in ruminants, which seem to be more resistant to this effect. Evidence suggests that high dietary zinc intake is antagonistic for copper, iron, and calcium metabolism.

Another effect of zinc toxicosis is the development of lesions in the pancreatic ducts. The exact mechanism for the development of these pancreatic lesions is not known but may be related to the fact that zinc is excreted in high concentrations from the pancreas through the duct system after high daily doses of zinc are administrated. In one report it was hypothesized that the high concentration of zinc in pancreatic secretions may be cytotoxic and thus cause the injury. It has been suggested that the distinct lobular pattern of the pancreatic injury may be caused by blockage of the pancreatic duct, causing subsequent injury to specific lobules drained by a particular blocked duct.

Toxicity and Risk Factors. The toxic dose of zinc for most species has not been established. Zinc may undergo many complex interactions, which often leads to differing toxic levels being reported in the literature (Table 22-4).

Canine and feline. The toxic dose of zinc has not been established. The most likely cause of zinc toxicosis in dogs is ingestion of items made of zinc. Because foreign body ingestion is typically associated with younger animals, they

TABLE 22-4 **Dietary Zinc Levels Associated with Toxicity**

Species	Level of Zinc in Diet/Daily Intake Associated with Toxicosis
Canine and feline	Not available
Porcine	500 ppm feed 2000 ppm feed
Equine	3600 ppm for foal 90 mg Zn/kg body weight/day intake
Ovine	900 to 1000 ppm feed 50 mg Zn/kg body weight/day Acute toxicity: 240 mg Zn/kg body weight/day Pregnant: 10 to 20 mg Zn/kg body weight/day
Bovine	900 to 1000 ppm feed 1700 ppm in diet 900 ppm in diet 2000 ppm diet dry matter
Poultry	10,000 ppm feed 794 to 2000 ppm feed 4000 to 6000 ppm feed 20,000 ppm feed

Data from references 18, 22, 24, 28, 30, 32, 34, 35.

are more likely to develop zinc toxicosis than are mature animals.

Porcine. Pigs, when compared with other species, appear to have a high tolerance for dietary zinc. A diet containing 500 ppm zinc had very little effect on growth or reproductive performance in pigs; however, abnormal articular cartilage was noted, especially on the distal humerus. Pigs fed a diet high (>2000 mg zinc/kg diet) in zinc with associated copper deficiency showed clinical signs including lethargy, unthriftiness, anorexia, and subcutaneous hematomas over the limb joints and the aural pinnae. The Agricultural Research Council lists the toxic level in pig feed as 2 g zinc/kg dry matter.[24]

The dietary level that causes toxicosis depends on formulation of the diet. For example, low levels of calcium in a swill-based diet enhance the potential for toxicity from high dietary zinc. For pigs fed a diet marginal in copper, even low dietary levels of zinc dramatically reduce liver copper levels. High levels of calcium and copper reduce the availability of zinc, and low levels of dietary calcium increase the risk for zinc intoxication.

Equine. Immature horses generally are more at risk for zinc toxicosis than are older animals. In one experiment, the growth rates in foals decreased after the intake exceeded 90 mg zinc/kg body weight per day. This approximates 3600 ppm zinc in the feed on a dry matter basis.[35]

Ovine. Toxicosis is usually associated with feeding errors, contamination of pasture soil and forage with zinc, and access to substances containing zinc.[25-27] Toxicosis has been reported when dietary concentrations exceed 900 to 1000 mg/kg.[28] Clinical signs of toxicosis appear at a dietary intake around 50 mg/kg body weight zinc per day, and acute toxicosis occurs at a dietary intake of 240 mg/kg body weight zinc per day. A discrepancy exists in the literature as to what dietary level of zinc is necessary to cause increased plasma and tissue zinc levels; these differences may be due to conditions of exposure such as diet composition, age, breed, sex, and pregnancy status of the animals. Pregnant ewes are more sensitive to excessive dietary zinc levels than are nonpregnant animals, and dietary levels can cause clinical signs at 10 to 20 mg/kg body weight zinc per/day.

Bovine. Toxic doses of zinc in cattle are not completely defined; however, water levels of 6 to 8 ppm zinc can lead to constipation in cattle. Experimental zinc poisoning at a rate of 1 g/kg body weight caused a reduction in weight gain and feed efficiency. At levels of 1.5 to 1.7 g/kg body weight zinc a reduction in feed consumption was shown.[8] Growing cattle generally are less tolerant of high dietary zinc levels than are older cattle. When dietary levels are high, young cattle absorb more zinc than do old cattle. Preruminant calves cannot tolerate 700 ppm zinc in milk replacer.[29] The control mechanism for maintaining tissue zinc concentrations is less effective in controlling the zinc levels when there is a high dietary intake than when there is a low dietary intake. Under some conditions calves can tolerate diets containing zinc concentrations as high as 600 ppm. However, dietary level of 900 ppm has caused a reduction in feed consumption, pica, diarrhea, and weight loss. Other factors contributing to zinc toxicosis in cattle include bioavailability of zinc complexes, amount of dietary fiber, amount and duration of zinc feeding,

mixing of feed or exposure to contaminated feed, and concurrent disease.

Avian. The literature has various reports on the level of zinc required in the diet to cause clinical signs in birds. The dietary levels range from 794 to 2000 ppm.[30] When chickens were fed a diet containing 25,000 ppm, consumption decreased dramatically. Laying hens fed a diet containing 4000 to 6000 ppm had decreased egg production. Single-comb white Leghorn pullets fed a diet containing 20,000 ppm zinc for 5 days showed a significant reduction in egg production, but removal of the zinc from the diet reversed the effect on egg production.[31] The fertility and hatchability of the eggs from these pullets were also significantly decreased for 14 to 28 days after the zinc supplement was removed. The feed consumption and body weights were also significantly reduced in these pullets. In young chicks zinc dietary levels as low as 6000 ppm zinc can adversely affect body weight.[32] Poultry diets have factors that affect the bioavailability of dietary zinc.[33] An example is phytate in corn-soy–based diets, which decreases the bioavailability of zinc.

The dose of zinc that causes intoxication in caged birds is not well known. Psittacines are at high risk of zinc toxicosis because they naturally chew objects in their surroundings. Factors that cause differences in dose response are species susceptibility, health status, age, and degree of exposure.

Clinical Signs

Bovine. Ruminants, especially young or pregnant, appear to be more susceptible to zinc toxicity. It has been suggested that this increased susceptibility may be due to the adverse effects of zinc on the rumen microorganisms.[34] In acute poisoning of cattle a light green–colored diarrhea and a drastic reduction in milk yield are seen. Severe cases show somnolence, and in severe zinc poisoning paresis may be observed. In calves fed milk replacer containing 700 ppm zinc for 3 weeks, there was a marked reduction in nitrogen digestibility. This reduction in digestibility can be related to a reduction in weight gains experienced by these calves.[29] Other clinical signs noted in nonruminating calves fed milk replacer containing high levels of zinc included general listlessness, marked polyuria, and yellow-green diarrhea. Very high levels of zinc in the diet (1700 mg zinc/kg diet) cause the symptoms described previously with the addition of a depraved appetite, which can be characterized by excessive salt consumption and wood chewing.

Canine and feline. The initial clinical signs of zinc toxicosis observed in dogs are often consistent with gastrointestinal disease. These include vomiting and diarrhea and possibly inappetence. On initial examination they may appear depressed, icteric with pale mucous membranes, tachycardiac, and have a hemoglobinemia and hemoglobinuria.

Porcine. Clinical signs in pigs generally associated with zinc toxicosis include reduced weight gain, reduced litter size and piglet weaning weight, arthritis, and lameness. Pigs chronically fed excessive zinc appeared unthrifty, anorexic, and had a rough hair coat, eventually becoming lame.

Equine. Initial symptoms of chronic zinc toxicosis in the horse may include an unthrifty appearance and a tendency to lie in complete lateral recumbency with reluctance to rise.[35] When taken to exercise, the animals are stiff and reluctant to move faster than a walk or step over curbs. An arched back stance is often noted. Chronic zinc poisoning causes a nonspecific degenerative arthritis, especially at the distal end of the tibia, which is accompanied by effusion and obvious enlargement of the hock joint. Aspirated joint fluid may contain slightly increased numbers of inflammatory cells. The aspirate may include macrophages containing engulfed erythrocytes, free erythrocytes, and neutrophils. Signs observed in experimentally induced zinc poisoning were pharyngeal and laryngeal paralysis, as well as stiffness and lameness resulting from swelling of the epiphyses of the long bones. The skeletal problems differentiate zinc from lead poisoning.

Ovine. In mild cases of zinc toxicosis inappetence and gradual weight loss may be the only signs observed. Sheep with more severe toxicosis may have diarrhea, dehydration, subcutaneous edema, rapid weight loss, weakness, and often death. Excessive dietary zinc can induce a copper deficiency in the ewe and cause a severe copper deficiency in the fetus or neonate. High dietary zinc-induced copper deficiency in both the ewe and fetus can be prevented by copper supplementation, but copper supplementation does not alleviate the effects of the excessive zinc on the appetite of the ewe or the viability of the fetus. Excessive dietary zinc can have a severe effect on the viability of lambs. Suckling lambs exposed to high zinc concentrations via zinc-supplemented milk diets accumulate large amounts of zinc in their kidneys. This accumulation leads to severe renal damage.[36] Therefore, one explanation for the reduced viability may be that the high zinc tissue levels are toxic to the fetus, especially to the kidneys. Another possible explanation is that the decreased feed intake and subsequent reduced feed intake of the ewes lead to the decreased viability of the lambs.

Avian. Reduction in feed consumption, decreased body weight, and decreased egg production are all clinical signs associated with zinc toxicosis in the hen.

Caged and aviary birds often present in good condition with a history of sudden onset of depression, inappetence, and fluffed feathers.[10] Other clinical signs that are often noted include polydipsia, polyuria, vomiting, diarrhea, weight loss, cyanosis, and seizures. Hematuria, crop stasis, and vomiting may also be seen. A common history is that birds have just been introduced to a new cage or aviary and the wire has a fine white powdery coat or flakes of metal attached to it.

Clinical Pathology

Canine and feline. Severe intravascular hemolysis is the most prominent clinicopathologic feature seen in acute zinc poisoning in dogs. A regenerative (often severe) hemolytic anemia, leukocytosis, and neutrophilia are present. Red blood cell morphology may include anisocytosis, polychromasia, target cells, basophilic stippling, nucleated red blood cells, or Heinz bodies. Leukocytosis, consisting of a neutrophilia with a left shift, a monocytosis, and lymphopenia may also be seen. Platelet counts are often normal or slightly decreased. Clinical chemistry changes include a hyperproteinemia, azotemia, increased serum alkaline phosphatase, and bilirubinemia.

Hemoglobinuria is often noted on initial urinalysis. Subsequent urinalysis may reveal bilirubinuria, casts, and persistent hemoglobinuria.[37]

Porcine. The literature does not contain much information on the clinicopathologic effects of zinc toxicosis in pigs. In one report anemia developed in 5 of 6 pigs with zinc toxicosis and associated copper deficiency.[22] Clinicopathologic evidence of hepatocellular and pancreatic acinar damage may also be observed.

Equine. Zinc toxicosis in the horse does not have the same effect in the blood that is seen in the dog or pig. Therefore, clinical pathology results are not indicative of zinc poisoning.

Ovine. The clinicopathologic features of zinc toxicosis in sheep have not been well established. Possible changes may include anemia and neutrophilia. Sheep that survive an acute poisoning may develop clinicopathologic evidence of a severe, fibrosing pancreatitis.[38]

Bovine. The clinicopathologic features of zinc toxicosis in cattle have not been well established. The changes may be the result of other complicating factors such as dehydration and secondary bacterial infection. Possible alterations noted may include neutrophilia, circulating immature erythrocytes, hypernatremia, hyperglycemia, azotemia, elevated lactic dehydrogenase, gamma-glutamyl transferase, and sorbitol dehydrogenase.

Avian. High levels of dietary zinc adversely affect exocrine pancreatic function in the chick without affecting the endocrine function. This effect on the exocrine pancreas is noted as decreased activity of several pancreatic digestive enzymes. Blood analysis is of questionable use because blood uric acid levels are not a reliable measure for detecting early renal damage in birds.

Lesions

Canine and feline. Gross pathology findings are usually nonspecific and may include icterus, splenomegaly, a nodular pancreas, and large, diffusely red-brown kidneys with multiple hemorrhagic foci on cut surface.[39] Hepatomegaly may be seen and the liver may contain disseminated pale intralobular foci. Histopathologic lesions support simultaneous severe cellular injury to multiple organ systems. These include hepatic hemosiderosis with vacuolar degeneration, hepatocellular necrosis, hemoglobinuric nephrosis, pancreatic necrosis of the acinar cells, gastrointestinal hyperemia and serositis, and pulmonary edema and alveolar mineralization. In one reported case renal failure was associated with tubular degeneration and necrosis. The changes were most prominent in the proximal convoluted tubules, which is typical of heavy metal toxicosis. The severity of the lesions seen in the pancreas may be time-dependent and can include necrotic duct epithelium, interstitial fibrosis, and inflammatory infiltrates.

Porcine. Pathology observed with zinc poisoning in pigs is central lobular necrosis of the liver, bone changes at the end of the humerus characterized as collapse of the bony structure under the cartilage and lifting of the cartilage, and atrophy of the pancreatic acini with extensive interstitial fibrosis. Hematomas may be observed in the mesentery, cerebral ventricles, lymph nodes and spleen, and failure of the blood to clot. The skeletal musculature and viscera may be pale, the spleen enlarged, and lymph nodes congested, and serosanguinous fluid may be present in most joints. Excessive pericardial fluid and epicardial petechiation with hemorrhagic foci distributed throughout the lungs may be observed. Ulcerative gastritis and hemorrhagic enteritis can occur.

Histopathologic lesions include centrilobular hepatocellular necrosis and glomerulonephritis. Kupffer cells throughout the liver can be laden with hemosiderin. This finding is consistent with internal hemorrhage.

Equine. At necropsy, the most consistent finding associated with zinc toxicosis is severe generalized osteochondrosis in all limb joints. Often the most severe lesions are in the pastern and fetlock joints.[40] The lesions can include rarefaction, separation, and loss of pieces of hyaline cartilage. Thin cortices in the long bones and less dense long bones and in the vertebral trabeculae have also been noted in equine zinc toxicosis. Enlargement of the epiphyseal areas of the long bones in young, growing horses can occur 7 to 21 days before any noticeable clinical signs of pain or lameness.

Ovine. Necropsy lesions associated with severe, acute zinc poisoning include abomasitis and duodenitis in which the mucosa may appear green. Overall body condition is generally observed to be poor at time of necropsy. Subcutaneous edema, ascites, hydrothorax, and hydropericardium may all be present.[41] Upper gastrointestinal lesions include submucosal edema of the rumen and abomasum, ulceration of the abomasal mucosa with increased amounts of mucus secretions in the abomasum, and catarrhal enteritis with a patchy type of congestion of the small intestine. Abomasal lesions typically are located in the fundic and pyloric areas. The pancreas, a target organ, can range in appearance from normal to mottled and pale to markedly atrophic. The kidneys may also be affected and can range from normal to shrunken and pale to swollen, soft, and orange-brown in color. At necropsy the liver often appears normal.

Histopathology of the pancreas shows a distinct lobular distribution of parenchymal lesions with different stages of pathogenesis between lobules. The acinar cells may appear cuboidal, which is likely due to shedding of the apical cytoplasm and the majority of the secretory material into the lumen. Some acinar cells may be flattened and resemble a metaplastic change to ductal cells. Acini lined by these cuboidal or flattened cells can appear to have enlarged lumens. Areas of secretory cellular necrosis can be apparent, as can edema of the interlobular septa and increased interstitial tissue in affected lobules. A severe necrosis and inflammation of the pancreatic ducts may be seen, and ductular lesions may be the first histopathology observed. A neutrophil or lymphocyte exudate may be observed in the intralobular and interlobular ducts. The lesions may be somewhat regenerative. Lesions have not been observed in the islets of Langerhans.

Histopathology can be observed in the liver and kidney. Zinc-induced lesions in the renal corpuscles include thickening or dilation of Bowman's capsule, collapse of glomeruli, adhesions between glomeruli and the capsule, and pro-

teinaceous material in the corpuscles. Tubular lesions include proteinaceous hyaline and cellular casts in some of the convoluted tubules. Focal infiltration of neutrophils or lymphocytes and early fibroplasia of the interstitial tissue may also be noted. In chronically intoxicated animals an occasional narrow band of interstitial scar tissue with lymphocyte infiltration may occur. Hepatic lesions include multifocal pyogranulomas throughout the parenchyma, characterized by necrotic hepatocytes surrounded by aggregates of neutrophils, and occasionally reticuloendothelial cells and lymphocytes.

Histopathology of the abomasum includes superficial to deep ulceration of the mucosa with congestion and neutrophil infiltration of the lamina propria located below the necrotic epithelium. Dilated gastric glands found in multiple areas of the gastric mucosa can contain cells that resemble parietal cells. Other lesions include submucosal edema, diffuse neutrophil and lymphocyte infiltration of the submucosa and lamina propria, and increased secretory granules in chief cells. In chronically intoxicated sheep a proliferation of neck cells in the gastric glands may be observed.

Bovine. Acute zinc poisoning in cattle has produced generalized pulmonary emphysema, pale, flabby myocardium, renal hemorrhages, severe hepatic degeneration, and lesions in the pancreas. Chronic zinc poisoning can lead to lesions in many organs; however, the pancreas appears to be a target organ.

The histopathologic lesions of the pancreas generally are similar to those in sheep with the lesions in cattle being more diffuse with little flattening of acinar cells and marked vacuolation of the apical cytoplasm. Hepatic lesions observed in calves also are similar to those in sheep, but in the bovine there is diffuse infiltration of neutrophils in the parenchyma. Ulceration of the abomasum can occur and the histopathology is similar to that in sheep.

Avian. Distinct necropsy lesions that confirm a diagnosis of zinc toxicosis have not been described for birds. Zinc poisoning of birds can cause the koilin lining of the proventriculus (gizzard) to appear roughened, fissured, and ulcerated. The histopathology of the proventriculus includes epithelial desquamation and cellular infiltration associated with the macroscopic lesions.

Gizzard lesions can be similar to those seen in copper sulfate intoxication in poultry. Changes that may be observed in the pancreas include dilation of acinar lumina, cytoplasmic vacuolation, hyaline globule formation, and occasionally necrosis of the exocrine cells.

Hens fed a diet containing 10,000 ppm zinc oxide for 4 days showed lesions in the gizzard and pancreas. However, no lesions developed in the gizzard and pancreas of hens fed this same diet for 4 days and then a control diet for 28 days.[32] These observations suggest that zinc poisoning in birds is reversible.

Caged and aviary birds that ingest metallic zinc have kidneys that appear pale and swollen, with other internal organs appearing normal. Lesions associated with visceral gout may be seen but this is a variable finding. A significant observation for a diagnosis of zinc intoxication is finding small metallic fragments in the gastrointestinal tract. Histopathology of the pancreas may include necrosis of the acinar cells seen as diffuse degeneration with vacuolation of the parenchyma and loss of zymogen granules in the remaining cells. When the kidney is involved, nephrosis of the proximal tubules has been observed. The tubules appear dilated with flattened, immature epithelium, occasional necrotic cells, and proteinaceous or granular casts; urate tophi may be present.

Diagnostic Testing. High levels of zinc accumulate in the serum, liver, kidney, pancreas, and bone with lesser amounts in other tissues.[42] Testing of the pancreas, kidney, and liver are helpful in making a diagnosis of zinc toxicosis. Tissue samples collected for zinc analysis should be stored frozen until analyzed.

The rubber found in stoppers for syringes and blood tubes is contaminated with zinc and can falsely elevate zinc levels in blood samples collected with them. Therefore, serum should be collected in royal blue–top tubes, which have stoppers made of plastic rather than rubber.

Treatment. In small animals initial treatment involves symptomatic and supportive therapy. This may include intravenous fluids, electrolytes, and blood transfusion if warranted by the severity of the anemia. If abdominal radiographs reveal a metallic foreign body, endoscopic retrieval or surgery is warranted as soon as the patient is stable. Serum zinc concentrations decrease rapidly after removal of the source of zinc. Chelation therapy can be used to accelerate renal excretion. Ca-EDTA diluted in 5% dextrose has been administered at 100 mg/kg divided into four subcutaneous doses per 24 hours. Serum zinc levels are used to determine the length of chelation therapy. Dehydration and nephrotoxic antibiotics should be avoided.

For birds Ca-EDTA is the most common chelating agent used.[35] A dose of 0.029 mg/g body weight is administered three times daily by intramuscular injection until the bird is asymptomatic. This regimen is followed by a dose of 0.057 mg/g body weight administered orally three times per day until all the zinc particles have been removed from the gastrointestinal tract. Other regimens are 10 to 40 mg Ca-EDTA/kg body weight administered intramuscularly twice daily,[41] 55 mg D-penicillamine/kg body weight twice daily for 10 days,[41] or 2.5 mg dimercaprol (BAL)/kg body weight administered intramuscularly every 4 hours for 2 days and then twice daily until the bird is asymptomatic.

In large animals with zinc toxicosis augmented by copper deficiency, supplementation of copper resulted in a rapid and dramatic clinical response. The use of Ca-EDTA therapy may be helpful.

Prognosis. Once clinical signs have appeared, prognosis is dependent on the severity of clinical signs. However, serum zinc levels usually decrease rapidly after the source of zinc is removed from the animal or its environment.

In small animals the outcome depends on the severity of the anemia and the associated organ failure. When surgical intervention is needed to remove foreign bodies, there are two critical postoperative periods: the first is related to the hemolytic crisis and the second occurs 4 to 5 days later as the result of generalized organ failure possibly induced by or secondary to the hemolytic crisis.

Prevention and Control. Preventive measures are limited to preventing access to sources of excess zinc and ensuring that dietary formulations are correct for trace elements.

REFERENCES

Arsenic

1. Buck WB et al: *Clinical and diagnostic veterinary toxicology,* ed 2, Dubuque, Iowa, 1976, Kendall/Hunt Publishing.
2. Beasley VR et al: *A systems approach to veterinary toxicology,* Champagne, Ill, 1994, University of Illinois.
3. Jubb KV et al: *Pathology of domestic animals,* ed 4, New York, 1993, Academic Press.
4. Klaassen CD, editor: *Casarett & Doull's toxicology: the basic science of poisons,* ed 5, New York, 1996, McGraw-Hill.
5. Osweiler GD: *Toxicology,* Media, Penn, 1996, Williams & Wilkins.
6. Murphy M: *A field guide to common animal poisons,* Ames, Iowa, 1996, Iowa State University Press.
7. Lorgue G et al: *Clinical veterinary toxicology,* Cambridge, Mass, 1996, Blackwell Science.

Copper

1. Bath GF: Enzootic icterus: a form of chronic copper poisoning, *J South Afr Vet Assoc* 50:3, 1979.
2. Gooneratne SR et al: Review of copper deficiency and metabolism in ruminants, *Can J Anim Sci* 69:819, 1989.
3. Puls R: *Mineral levels in animal health,* ed 2, Clearbrook, British Columbia, 1994, Sherpa International.
4. Mahmoud OM, Ford EJH: Absorption and excretion of organic compounds of copper by sheep, *J Comp Pathol* 93:551, 1983.
5. Solaiman SG, Maloney MA, Qureshi MA, Davis G, D'Andrea G: Effects of high copper supplements on performance, health, plasma copper and enzymes in goats, *Small Ruminant Res* 41:127, 2001.
6. Suttle NF: The nutritional requirement for copper in animals and man. In Howell JM, Gawthorne JM, editors: *Copper in animals and man,* vol 1, Boca Raton, Fla, CRC Press.
7. Luza SC, Speisky HC: Liver copper storage and transport during development implications for cytotoxicity, *Am J Clin Nutr* 63:812S, 1996.
8. Van Ryssen JBJ: The effectiveness of using supplementary zinc and molybdenum to reduce the copper content in the liver of hypercuprotic sheep, *J South Afr Vet Assoc* 65:59, 1994.
9. Hatch RC, Blue JL, Mahaffey EA, Jain AV, Smalley RE: Chronic copper toxicosis in growing swine, *J Am Vet Med Assoc* 174:616, 1979.
10. Ludwig J, Owen CA Jr, Barham SS, McCall JT, Hardy RM: The liver in the inherited copper disease of Bedlington terriers, *Lab Invest* 43:82, 1980.
11. Haywood S, Rutgers HC, Christian MK: Hepatitis and copper accumulation in Skye terriers, *Vet Pathol* 25:408, 1988.
12. Sternlieb I: Copper toxicosis of the Bedlington terrier, *J Rheumatol* 7:94, 1981.
13. Lewis NJ, Fallah-Rad AH, Connor ML: Copper toxicity in confinement-housed ram lambs, *Can Vet J* 38:496, 1997.
14. Ishmael J, Gopinath C, Howell JM: Experimental chronic copper toxicity in sheep, *Res Vet Sci* 13:22, 1972.
15. Johnson GF, Gilbertson SR, Goldfischer S, Grushoff PS, Sternlieb I: Cytochemical detection of inherited copper toxicosis of Bedlington terriers, *Vet Pathol* 21:57, 1984.
16. Johnson GF, Zawie DA, Gilbertson SR, Sternlieb I: Chronic active hepatitis in Doberman pinschers, *J Am Vet Med Assoc* 180:1438, 1982.

17. Rothuizen J, Ubbink GJ, van Zon P, Teske E, van den Ing TSGAM, Yuzbasiyan-Gurkan V: Diagnostic value of microsatellite DNA marker for copper toxicosis in West-European Bedlington terriers and incidence of the disease, *Anim Genet* 30:190, 1999.
18. Brewer GJ: Wilson disease and canine copper toxicosis, *Am J Clin Nutr* 16:1087S, 1998.

Fluoride

1. Meldrum M: Toxicology of hydrogen fluoride in relation to major accident hazards, *Regul Toxicol Pharmacol* 30:110, 1999.
2. Underwood EJ, Suttle NF: *The mineral nutrition of livestock,* ed 3, New York, 1999, CABI Publishing.
3. Warren JJ, Levy SM: Systemic fluoride. Sources, amounts and effects of ingestion, *Dent Clin North Am* 43:695, 1999.
4. Araya O et al: Evolution of fluoride concentrations in cattle and grass following a volcanic eruption, *Vet Hum Toxicol* 35:437, 1993.
5. Suttie JW: Fluoride content of commercial dairy concentrates and alfalfa forage, *J Agr Food Chem* 17:1350, 1969.
6. Linzon SN: *Phytotoxicology fluoride studies in Ontario,* Ontario Industrial Waste Conference, 1978, p 105.
7. Underwood EJ: *Trace elements in human and animal nutrition,* ed 4, New York, 1977, Academic Press.
8. Bunce HW: Fluoride in air, grass, and cattle, *J Dairy Sci* 68:1706, 1985.
9. Osweiler GD et al: *Clinical and diagnostic veterinary toxicology,* ed 3, Dubuque, Iowa, 1985, Kendall/Hunt.
10. Clay AB, Suttie JW: The availability of fluoride from phosphorus sources. *J Anim Sci* 51(suppl 1):352(abstr), 1980.
11. Greenwood DA et al: *Fluorosis in cattle.* Special Report No. 17, Logan, Utah, 1964, Utah Agricultural Experiment Station.
12. Shupe JL, Alther EW: 1966. The effects of fluorides on livestock, with particular references to cattle. In Smith FA: *Handbook of experimental pharmacology. Pharmacology of fluorides,* vol XX/1, New York, 1966, Springer-Verlag.
13. Shearer TR et al: Bovine dental fluorosis: histologic and physical characteristics, *Am J Vet Res* 39:597, 1978.
14. National Research Council: *Effects of fluorides in animals,* Washington, DC, 1974, National Research Council-National Academy of Sciences.
15. National Research Council: Mineral tolerance of domestic animals, Washington, DC, 1980, National Research Council-National Academy of Sciences.
16. Suttie JW et al: Effects of alternating periods of high- and low-fluoride ingestion on dairy cattle, *J Dairy Sci* 55:790, 1972.
17. Aulerlich RJ et al: Chronic toxicity of dietary fluorine to mink, *J Anim Sci* 65:1759, 1987.
18. Ammerman CB, Henry PR: Dietary considerations when choosing fluoride supplements reviewed, *Feedstuffs* March 21:22, 1983.
19. Forsythe DM et al: Dietary calcium and fluoride interactions in swine: in utero and neonatal effects, *J Nutr* 102:1639, 1972.
20. Bixler D, Muhler JC: Retention of fluoride in soft tissues of chickens receiving different fat diets, *J Nutr* 70:26, 1960.
21. Shupe JL, Olson AE: Clinical aspects of fluorosis in horses, *J Am Vet Med Assoc* 158:167, 1971.
22. Shupe JL: Clinical and pathological effects of fluoride toxicity in animals, *Ciba Foundation Symposium* 2:537, 1971.
23. Suttie JW, Kolstad DL: Effects of dietary fluoride ingestion on ration intake and milk production, *J Dairy Sci* 60:1568, 1977.
24. Hillman D et al: Hypothyroidism and anemia related to fluoride in dairy cattle, *J Dairy Sci* 62:416(abstr), 1979.
25. Kessabi M et al: Serum biochemical effects of fluoride on cattle in the Darmous area, *Vet Hum Toxicol* 25:403, 1983.
26. Shupe JL: Clinicopathologic features of fluoride toxicosis in cattle, *J Anim Sci* 51:756-758, 1980.
27. Shearer TR et al: Microhardness of molar teeth in cattle with fluorosis, *Am J Vet Res* 41:1543, 1980.
28. Suttie JW, Kolstad DL: Sampling of bones for fluoride analysis, *Am J Vet Res* 35:1375, 1974.
29. Suttie JW: Vertebral biopsies in the diagnosis of bovine fluoride toxicosis, *Am J Vet Res* 28:709, 1967.
30. Allcroft R et al: *Fluorosis in cattle. 2. Development and alleviation: experimental studies.* Animal Disease Surveys Report No. 2, Part 2. London, 1965, HMSO.

Iodine

1. Osweiler GD et al: *Clinical and diagnostic veterinary toxicology,* ed 3, Dubuque, Iowa, 1973, Kendall/Hunt.
2. Buchanan-Smith JG: *Nutrient requirements of beef cattle,* ed 7, Washington, DC, 1996, National Academy Press.
3. Aiello SE, editor: *The Merck veterinary manual,* Whitehouse Station, NJ, 1998, Merck.
4. Beasley VR et al: *A systems affected approach to veterinary toxicology,* Urbana, Ill, 1999, Illinois University Press.
5. Puls R: *Mineral levels in animal health,* ed 2, Clearbrook, British Columbia, 1994, Sherpa International.

Iron

1. Goyer RA: In Klaassen CD, editor: *Casarett & Doull's toxicology: the basic science of poisons,* ed 5, New York, 1996, McGraw-Hill.
2. Greentree WF, Hall JO: In Bonagura JD, editor: *Kirk's current therapy XII,* Philadelphia, 1995, WB Saunders.
3. Osweiler GD et al: *Clinical and diagnostic veterinary toxicology,* ed 3, Dubuque, Iowa, 1985, Kendall/Hunt.
4. Hillman RS: In Hardman JG, Limbird LE, editors: *Goodman & Gilman's the pharmacological basis of therapeutics,* ed 9, New York, 1995, McGraw-Hill.
5. Liebelt EL: In Haddad LM et al: *Clinical management of poisoning and drug overdose,* ed 3, Philadelphia, 1998, WB Saunders, pp 757-766.
6. Dorman DC: In Bongura JD, editor: *Current veterinary therapy XII,* Philadelphia, 1995, WB Saunders.
7. Plumb DC: *Veterinary drug handbook,* ed 3, Ames, Iowa, 1999, Iowa State University Press.

Lead

1. Keogh J: In Sullivan J et al: *Hazardous materials toxicology,* Baltimore, 1992, Williams & Wilkins.
2. Abadin H, Llados F: *Toxicological profile for lead,* Washington, D.C., 1999, Department of Health and Human Services, pp. 19-257, http://www.atsdr.cdc.gov/toxprofiles/tp13.html.
3. Schmitz DG: In Reed SM et al, editors: *Equine internal medicine,* Philadelphia, 1998, WB Saunders.
4. George LW: In Smith BP, editor: *Large animal internal medicine,* ed 2, St Louis, 1996, Mosby.
5. Gwaltney-Brant SM: Heavy metals. In Haschek-Hock W et al, editors: *Handbook of toxicologic pathology,* ed 2, San Diego, 2002, Academic Press.
6. Borkowski R: Lead poisoning and intestinal perforations in a snapping turtle *(Chelydra serpentina)* due to fishing gear ingestion, *J Zoo Wildlife Med* 28:109, 1997.
7. Locke LN, Thomas NJ: In Fairbrother A et al, editors: *Noninfectious diseases of wildlife,* Ames, Iowa, 1996, Iowa State University Press.
8. Jubb KVF, Huxtable CR: In Jubb KVF et al, editors: *Pathology of domestic animals,* ed 4, San Diego, 1993, Academic Press.
9. Kowalczyk DF: In Kirk RW, editor: *Current veterinary therapy IX,* Philadelphia, 1986, WB Saunders.
10. LaBonde J: Toxicity in pet avian patients, *Semin Avian Exotic Pet Med* 4:23, 1995.
11. McDonald SE: In Kirk RW, editor: *Current veterinary therapy IX,* Philadelphia, 1986, WB Saunders.

12. Shannon M: In Haddad L et al, editor: *Clinical management of poisonings and drug overdosage,* ed 3, Philadelphia, 1998, WB Saunders.
13. Osweiler GD et al: *Clinical and diagnostic veterinary toxicology,* ed 3, Dubuque, Iowa, 1973, Kendall/Hunt Publishing.
14. LaBonde J: In Bonagura JD, editor: *Current veterinary therapy XII,* Philadelphia, 1995, WB Saunders.
15. Mount ME: In Ettinger SJ, editor: *Textbook of veterinary internal medicine,* ed 3, Philadelphia, 1989, WB Saunders.
16. Puls R: *Mineral levels in animal health,* Clearbrook, British Columbia, 1988, Sherpa International.
17. Ramsey D et al: Use of orally administered succimer (meso-2, 3-dimercaptosuccinic acid) for treatment of lead poisoning in dogs, *J Am Vet Med Assoc* 208:37, 1996.
18. Plumb DC: *Veterinary drug handbook,* ed 3, Ames, Iowa, 1999, Iowa State University Press.
19. Neiger RD: In Peterson ME, Talcott PA, editors: *Small animal toxicology,* Philadelphia, 2001, WB Saunders.
20. Kapoor S et al: Influence of 2,3-dimercaptosuccinic acid on gastrointestinal lead absorption and whole body retention, *Toxicol Appl Pharmacol* 97:525, 1989.
21. Dowsett R, Shannon M: Childhood plumbism identified after lead poisoning in household pets, *N Engl J Med* 331:1661, 1994.
22. Clarkson TW: In Hayes J, Laws E, editors: *Handbook of pesticide toxicology,* vol 2, Ames, Iowa, 1991, Iowa State University Press.

Mercury

1. Osweiler GD: *Toxicology,* Media, Penn, 1996, Williams & Wilkins.
2. Klaassen CD, editor: *Casarett & Doull's toxicology: the basic science of poisons,* ed 5, New York, 1996, McGraw-Hill.
3. Buck WB et al: *Clinical and diagnostic veterinary toxicology,* ed 2, Dubuque, Iowa, 1976, Kendall/Hunt.
4. Beasley VR et al: *A systems approach to veterinary toxicology,* Champagne, Ill, 1994, University of Illinois Press.
5. Jubb KV et al: *Pathology of domestic animals,* ed 4, New York, 1993, Academic Press.
6. Murphy M: *A field guide to common animal poisons,* Ames, Iowa, 1996, Iowa State University Press.
7. Lorgue G et al: *Clinical veterinary toxicology,* Cambridge, Mass, 1996, Blackwell Science.

Molybdenum

1. Barceloux DG: Molybdenum, *Clin Toxicol* 37:231, 1999.
2. Ladefoged O, Sturup S: Copper deficiency in cattle, sheep, and horses caused by excess molybdenum, *Vet Hum Toxicol* 37:63, 1995.
3. Lener J, Bibr B: Effects of molybdenum on the organism (a review), *J Hyg Epidemiol Microbiol Immunol* 28:405, 1984.
4. Lesperance AL et al: Interaction of molybdenum, sulfate and alfalfa in the bovine, *J Anim Sci* 60:791, 1985.
5. Mason J: Molybdenum-copper antagonism in ruminants: a review of biochemical basis, *Irish Vet J* 35:221, 1981.
6. Hynes M et al: Some studies on the metabolism of labelled molybdenum compounds in cattle, *J Inorgan Biochem* 24:279, 1985.
7. Parada R: Zinc deficiency in molybdenum poisoned animals, *Vet Hum Toxicol* 23:16, 1981.
8. Buck WB: Diagnosis of feed-related toxicoses, *J Am Vet Med Assoc* 156:1434, 1970.
9. Ward GM: Molybdenum toxicity and hypocuprosis in ruminants: a review, *J Anim Sci* 46:1078, 1978.
10. National Research Council: *Nutrient requirements of beef cattle,* ed 4, Washington, DC, 1996, National Academy Press.
11. Jarrell WM et al: Molybdenum in the environment, *Residue Rev* 74:1, 1980.
12. Delhaize E et al: In Howell JMcC, Gawthorne JM, editors: *Copper in animals and man,* vol 1, Boca Raton, Fla, 1987, CRC Press.
13. Schalscha EB et al: Lead and molybdenum in soils and forage near an atmospheric source, *J Environ Qual* 16:313, 1987.
14. Buck WB: Diagnosis of feed-related toxicoses, *J Am Vet Med Assoc* 156:1434, 1970.
15. National Academy of Sciences: Copper. In *Mineral tolerances of domestic animals,* Washington, DC, 1980, National Academy Press.
16. National Academy of Sciences: Molybdenum. In *Mineral tolerances of domestic animals,* Washington, DC, 1980, National Academy Press.
17. Sas B: Secondary copper deficiency in cattle caused by molybdenum contamination of fodder; a case history, *Vet Hum Toxicol* 31:29, 1989.
18. Phillippo M et al: The effect of dietary molybdenum and iron on copper status and growth in cattle, *J Agric Sci Camb* 109:315, 1987.
19. Phillippo M et al: The effect of dietary molybdenum and iron on copper status, puberty, fertility and oestrus cycles in cattle, *J Agric Sci Camb* 109:321, 1987.
20. Wittenberg KM et al: Effects of dietary molybdenum on productivity and metabolic parameters of lactating beef cows and their offspring, *Can J Anim Sci* 67:1055, 1987.
21. Puls R: *Mineral levels in animal health: diagnostic data,* Clearwater, British Columbia, 1988, Sherpa.
22. Lamand M et al: Biochemical parameters useful for the diagnosis of mild molybdenosis in sheep, *Ann Res Vet* 11:141-145, 1980.
23. Swan DA et al: Molybdenum poisoning in feedlot cattle, *Aust Vet J* 76:345, 1998.
24. Auza N et al: Hematological and plasma biochemical disturbances in experimental molybdenum toxicosis in sheep, *Vet Hum Toxicol* 31:535, 1989.
25. Chan PC et al: Lung tumor induction by inhalation exposure to molybdenum trioxide in rats and mice, *Toxicol Sci* 45:58, 1998.
26. Farmer PE et al: Copper supplementation of drinking water for cattle grazing molybdenum-rich pastures, *Vet Rec* 111:193, 1982.

Selenium

1. National Research Council Subcommittee on Selenium, Committee on Animal Nutrition, Board on Agriculture, National Research Council: *Selenium in nutrition,* Washington, DC, 1983, National Academy Press.
2. Baker DC et al: Toxicosis in pigs fed selenium-accumulating *Astragalus* plant species or sodium selenate, *Am J Vet Res* 50:1396, 1989.
3. Harrison LH et al: Paralysis in swine due to focal symmetrical poliomalacia: possible selenium toxicosis, *Vet Pathol* 20:265, 1983.
4. Wilson TM et al: Selenium toxicity and porcine focal symmetrical poliomyelomalacia: description of a field outbreak and experimental reproduction, *Can J Comp Med* 47:412, 1983.
5. Casteel SW et al: Selenium toxicosis in swine, *J Am Vet Med Assoc* 186:1084, 1985.
6. MacDonald DW et al: Acute selenium toxicity in neonatal calves, *Can Vet J* 22:279, 1981.
7. Janke BH: Acute selenium toxicosis in a dog, *J Am Vet Med Assoc* 195:1114, 1989.
8. Ohlendorf HM et al: Selenium toxicosis in wild aquatic birds, *J Toxicol Environ Health* 24:67, 1988.
9. Hoffman DJ, Heinz GH: Embryotoxic and teratogenic effects of selenium in the diet of mallards, *J Toxicol Environ Health* 24:477, 1988.
10. Fishbein L: Environmental selenium and its significance, *Fundam Appl Toxicol* 3:411, 1983.
11. Ohlendorf HM et al: Embryonic mortality and abnormalities of aquatic birds: apparent impacts by selenium from irrigation drainwater, *Sci Total Environ* 52:49, 1986.
12. U.S. Bureau of Mines: *Minerals yearbook, 1983,* Washington, DC, 1983, U.S. Bureau of Mines, Department of the Interior.
13. Ganther HE, Hsieh HS: Mechanism for the conversion of selenite to selenides in mammalian tissues. In Hoekstra WG, Suttie JW, Ganther HE, Mertz W, editors: *Trace element metabolism in animals,* ed 2, Baltimore, 1974, University Park Press.
14. Diplock AT: Metabolic aspects of selenium action and toxicity, *CRC Crit Rev Toxicol* 4:271, 1976.

15. Spallholz JE: On the nature of selenium toxicity and carcinostatic activity, *Free Radical Biol Med* 17:45, 1994.

16. O'Sullivan BM, Blakemore WF: Acute nicotinamide deficiency in the pig induced by 6-aminonicotinamide, *Vet Pathol* 17:748, 1980.

17. Mattson MP: Acetylcholine potentiates glutamate-induced neuro-degeneration in cultured hippocampal neurons, *Brain Res* 497:402, 1989.

18. Medina D, Oborn CJ: Selenium inhibition of DNA synthesis in mouse mammary epithelial cell line Yn-4, *Cancer Res* 44:4361, 1984.

19. Frenkel GD: Effects of sodium selenite and selenate on DNA and RNA synthesis *in vitro, Toxicol Lett* 25:219-225, 1985.

20. Frenkel GD et al: Inhibition of RNA and DNA polymerases by the product of the reaction of selenite with sulfhydryl compounds, *Mol Pharmacol* 31:112, 1987.

21. Frenkel GD, Falvey D: Involvement of cellular sulfhydryl compounds in the inhibition of RNA synthesis by selenite, *Biochem Pharmacol* 38:2849-2852, 1989.

22. Heinz GH et al: Reproduction of mallards fed selenium, *Environ Toxicol* 6:42, 1987.

23. Swanson CA et al: Comparative utilization of inorganic and organically-bound forms of selenium by the laying hen, *Fed Proc* 44(5):1510, 1985.

24. Dougherty JL, Hoekstra WG: Stimulation of lipid peroxidation *in vivo* by injected selenite and lack of stimulation by selenate, *Proc Soc Exp Biol Med* 169:209-215, 1982.

25. Csallany AS et al: Effect of selenite, vitamin E, and N,N'-diphenyl-p-phenylenediamine on liver organic solvent-soluble lipofuchsin pigments in mice, *J Nutr* 114:1582, 1984.

26. National Research Council Committee on Medical and Biologic Effects of Environmental Pollutants: *Selenium,* Washington, DC, 1976, National Academy of Sciences.

27. Wilson TM et al: Porcine focal symmetrical poliomyelomalacia: experimental reproduction with oral doses of encapsulated sodium selenite,. *Can J Vet Res* 52:83, 1988.

28. Goehring TB et al: Toxic effects of selenium on growing swine fed corn-soybean meal diets, *J Anim Sci* 59:733, 1984.

29. Hill J et al: An episode of acute selenium toxicity in a commercial piggery, *Aust Vet J* 62:207, 1985.

30. Hartley WJ et al: Pathology of experimental locoweed and selenium poisoning in pigs. In Seawright AA et al, editors: *Plant toxicology, Proceedings of the Australia-U.S.A. Poisonous Plants Symposium, Brisbane, Australia, 1984.* Yeerongpilly, Australia, 1985, Queensland Poisonous Plants Committee.

31. James LF, Panter KE: *Selenium poisoning in livestock.* Presented at the 3rd International Symposium on Poisonous Plants, Logan, Utah, July 1989.

32. O'Toole D et al: Selenium-induced "blind staggers" and related myths. A commentary on the extent of historical livestock losses attributed to selenosis on western U.S. rangelands, *Vet Pathol* 33:104, 1996.

33. Blodgett DJ, Bevill RF: Acute selenium toxicosis in sheep, *Vet Human Toxicol* 29:233, 1987.

34. Smyth JBA et al: Experimental acute selenium intoxication in lambs, *J Comp Pathol* 102:197, 1990.

35. Hopper SA et al: Selenium poisoning in lambs, *Vet Rec* 116:569, 1985.

36. Taylor RF, Mullaney TP: *Selenium toxicosis in neonatal lambs,* Proceedings of the 27th Annual Meeting of the American Association of Veterinary Laboratory Diagnosticians 1984, Fort Worth, Tex, pp 369-378.

37. Valentine JL et al: Human glutathione peroxidase activity in cases of high selenium exposures, *Environ Res* 45:16, 1988.

38. Jacobs M, Forst C: Toxicological effects of sodium selenite in Swiss mice, *J Toxicol Environ Health* 8:587, 1981.

Sodium

1. Osweiler GA: *Toxicology,* Philadelphia, 1998, Williams & Wilkins.

2. Poppenga RH: In Smith RA and Howard JL, editors: *Current Veterinary Therapy 3: Food Animal Practice*, Philadelphia, 1993.

3. Jubb KVF, Kennedy PC, Palmer N: *Pathology of domestic animals*, ed 4, San Diego, 1993, Academic Press.

4. Radostits OM, Gay CC, Blood DC et al: *Veterinary medicine*, ed 9, London, 1999, Saunders.

5. Beasley VR et al: *A systems approach to veterinary toxicology: reference notes for toxicology* VB320, Urbana, Ill, 1998, Illinois University Press.

6. Angelos SM, Van Metre DC: *Veterinary clinics of North America: food animal practice*, Philadelphia, 1999, WB Saunders.

7. McCoy CP, Edwards WC: Sodium ion poisoning in livestock from oil field wastes, *Oklahoma Veterinary Medical Association* 31:1:12, 1979.

8. Thilsted JP et al: *Sodium salt toxicity in beef cows resulting from the consumption of saline water,* Proceedings of the 24th Annual Meeting of the American Association of Veterinary Laboratory Diagnosticians, 1981, St Louis, pp 229-233.

9. Pearson EG, Kallfelz FA: A case of presumptive salt poisoning (water deprivation) in veal calves, *Cornell Vet* 72:142, 1981.

10. Angelos SM et al: Treatment of hypernatremia in an acidotic neonatal calf, *J Am Vet Med Assoc* 214:1364, 1999.

11. Pringle JK, Berthiaume LMM: Hypernatremia in calves, *J Vet Int Med* 2:66, 1988.

12. Marks SL, Taboada J: *Veterinary clinics of North America Small Animal Practice*. Philadelphia, WB Saunders, 28:533, 1998.

13. Kanna C et al: Fatal hypernatremia in a dog from salt ingestion, *J Am Anim Hosp Assoc* 33:113,1997.

14. Banks P et al: High-sodium crystalloid solution for treatment of hyper-natremia in a Vietnamese pot-bellied pig, *J Am Vet Med Assoc* 209:1268, 1996.

15. Puls R: *Mineral levels in animal heath,* Clearbrook, British Columbia, 1994, Sherpa International.

16. Sarratt WK et al: Water deprivation-sodium chloride intoxication in groups of feeder lambs, *J Am Vet Med Assoc* 186:977, 1985.

17. Houpt KA et al: Effect of water restriction on equine behaviour and physiology, *Equine Vet J* 32:341, 2000.

18. Carlson GP et al: Physiologic alterations in the horse produced by food and water deprivation during periods of high environmental temperatures, *Am J Vet Res* 40:982, 1979.

19. Crawford MA et al: Hypernatremia and adipsia in a dog, *J Am Vet Med Assoc* 184:818, 1984.

20. Osweiler GD et al: Water deprivation-sodium ion toxicosis in cattle, *J Vet Diagn Invest* 7:583, 1995.

21. Martin T et al: Evaluation of normal brain sodium levels in cattle, *Vet Hum Toxicol* 28:308, 1986.

22. Hanna PE et al: Postmortem eye fluid analysis in dogs, cats, and cattle as an estimate of antemortem serum chemistry profiles, *Can J Vet Res* 54:487, 1990.

23. McLaughlin PS, McClaughlin BG: Chemical analysis of bovine and porcine vitreous humors: correlation of normal values with serum chemical values and changes with time and temperature, *Am J Vet Res* 48:467, 1987.

24. Lincoln SD, Lane VM: Postmortem magnesium concentration in bovine vitreous humor: comparison with antemortem serum magnesium concentration, *Am J Vet Res* 46:160, 1985.

25. Boermans HJ: Diagnosis of nitrate toxicosis in cattle, using biological fluids and a rapid ion chromatographic method, *Am J Vet Res* 51:491, 1990.

26. Plumb DC: *Veterinary drug handbook*, ed 3, Ames, Iowa, 1999, Iowa State University Press.

Zinc

1. Miller WJ: *Zinc metabolism in farm animals.* Proceedings of a Panel on the use of Nuclear Techniques in Studies of Mineral Metabolism and Disease in Domestic Animals, International Atomic Energy Agency, Vienna, 1971, pp 23-41.

2. Underwood EJ: *Trace elements in human and animal nutrition,* ed 4, New York, 1977, Academic Press.

3. Herrick JB: The role of zinc in nutrition of food-producing animals, *Vet Med Small Anim Clin* 69:85, 1974.

4. Latimer KS et al: Zinc-induced hemolytic anemia caused by ingestion of pennies by a pup, *J Am Vet Med Assoc* 195:77, 1989.

5. Breitschwerdt EB et al: Three cases of acute zinc toxicosis in dogs, *Vet Hum Toxicol* 28:109, 1986.

6. Meurs KM et al: Postsurgical mortality secondary to zinc toxicity in dogs, *Vet Hum Toxicol* 33:579, 1991.

7. `Petersen ME, Talcott PA: *Small animal toxicology*, Philadelphia, 2001, WB Saunders.

8. Radostits OM et al: *Veterinary medicine: a textbook of the diseases of cattle, sheep, pigs, goats and horses*, ed 9, London, 2000, WB Saunders.

9. Grimmett RER et al: Chronic zinc-poisoning of pigs, *N Z J Agricul* April 20, 1937, p 216.

10. Doneley R: Zinc toxicity in caged and aviary birds: "new wire disease," *Aust Vet Practit* 22:6, 1992.

11. Rupley AE: *Manual of avian practice*, Philadelphia, 1997, WB Saunders.

12. Bauck L, LaBonde J: *Avian medicine and surgery*, Philadelphia, 1997, WB Saunders.

13. Ogden L et al: Zinc intoxication in a dog from the ingestion of copper-clad pennies, *Vet Hum Toxicol* 30:577, 1988.

14. Miller WJ: Zinc nutrition of cattle: a review, *J Dairy Sci* 53:1123, 1970.

15. Poulsen HD, Larsen T: Zinc excretion and retention in growing pigs fed increasing levels of zinc oxide, *Livestock Prod Sci* 43:235, 1995.

16. Gabrielson KL et al: Zinc toxicity with pancreatic acinar necrosis in piglets receiving total parenteral nutrition, *Vet Pathol* 33:692, 1996.

17. Miller WJ et al: In Mills CF, editor: *Trace element metabolism in animals*, Proceedings of WAAP/IBP International Symposium, Aberdeen, Scotland, 1969.

18. Graham TW et al: A pathologic and toxicologic evaluation of veal calves fed large amounts of zinc, *Vet Pathol* 25:484, 1988.

19. Samour J: *Avian medicine*, London, 2000, Mosby-Harcourt.

20. Wight PAL et al: Zinc toxicity in the fowl: ultrastructural pathology and relationship to selenium, lead and copper, *Avian Pathol* 15:23, 1986.

21. Reese DE: *Diseases of swine*, ed 8, Iowa, Ames, Iowa, 1999, Iowa State University Press.

22. Pritchard GC et al: Zinc toxicity, copper deficiency and anaemia in swill-fed pigs, *Vet Rec* November 23:545, 1985.

23. Glade MJ: The control of cartilage growth in osteochondrosis: a review, *Equine Vet Sci* 6:175, 1986.

24. Agriculture Research Council: The nutrient requirements of pigs. Technical review by an Agricultural Research Council working party. Farnham Royal, Commonwealth Agriculture Bureau 1981, p 215.

25. Reif JS et al: Chronic exposure of sheep to a zinc smelter in Peru, *Environ Res* 49:40, 1989.

26. Henry PR et al: Effect of high dietary zinc concentration and length of zinc feeding on feed intake and tissue zinc concentration in sheep, *Anim Feed Sci Technol* 66:237, 1997.

27. Dargatz DA et al: Toxicity associated with zinc sulfate footbaths for sheep, *Agri Pract* 7:30, 1986.

28. Campbell JK, Mills CF: The toxicity of zinc to pregnant sheep, *Environ Res* 20:1, 1979.

29. Jenkins KJ, Hidiroglou M: Tolerance of the preruminant calf for excess manganese or zinc in milk replacer, *J Dairy Sc* 74:1047, 1991.

30. Stahl JL et al: Breeding: hen and progeny performance when hens are fed excessive dietary zinc, *Poultry Sci* 69:259, 1990.

31. Palafox AL, Ho-A E: Effect of zinc toxicity in laying white Leghorn pullets and hens, *Poultry Sci* 59:2024, 1980.

32. Dewar WA et al: Toxic effects of high concentrations of zinc oxide in the diet of the chick and laying hen, *Br Poultry Sci* 24:397, 1983.

33. Junxuan L, Combs GF: Effect of excess dietary zinc on pancreatic exocrine function in the chick, *J Nutr* 118:681, 1988.

34. Mertz W: *Trace elements in human and animal nutrition*, ed 4, Orlando, Fla, 1986, Academic Press.

35. Willoughby RA et al: Lead and zinc poisoning and the interaction between Pb and Zn poisoning in the foal, *Can J Comp Med* 36:348, 1972.

36. Davies NT et al: The susceptibility of suckling lambs to zinc toxicity, *Br J Nutr* 38:153, 1977.

37. Torrance AG et al: Zinc-induced hemolytic anemia in a dog, *J Am Vet Med Assoc* 191:443, 1987.

38. Allen JG et al: Zinc toxicity in ruminants, *J Comp Pathol* 93:363, 1983.

39. Luttgen PJ et al: Heinz body hemolytic anemia associated with high plasma zinc concentration in a dog, *J Am Vet Med Assoc* 197:1347, 1990.

40. Gunson DE et al: Environmental zinc and cadmium pollution associated with generalized osteochondrosis, osteoporosis, and nephrocalcinosis in horses, *J Am Vet Med Assoc* 180:295, 1982.

41. Smith BL, Embling PP: Sequential changes in the development of the pancreatic lesion of zinc toxicosis in sheep, *Vet Pathol* 30:242, 1993.

42. Ott EA et al: Zinc toxicity in ruminants. IV. Physiologic changes in tissues of beef cattle, *J Anim Sci* 25:432, 1966.

23

Mycotoxins

AFLATOXINS

Gavin L. Meerdink

Synonyms. "X disease" was the term applied to afla-toxicosis in 1960 when the undiagnosed disease was recognized in British turkeys. The source of the poisoning was found to be related to *Aspergillus flavus,* and *aflatoxin* was thus named. Many cases of fatal hepatitis in dogs during the 1950s were termed "hepatitis X," which was likely aflatoxicosis.

Sources. Aflatoxins comprise more than a dozen related bisfuranocoumarin metabolites produced by *A. flavus, A. parasiticus,* and *A. nomius.* These were formerly attributed to storage problems; however, aflatoxins can also be formed in the field before harvest. Mold growth and toxin production is enhanced by grain moisture greater than 15%, sustained relative humidity greater than 75%, warm temperatures, and sufficient oxygen (greater than 0.5%).[1] *A. flavus* is not known for its ability to invade intact, active plant tissues. The fungus is more appropriately classified as a saprophyte that occurs primarily in damaged or inactive tissues.[2]

Toxin types B_1, B_2, G_1, and G_2 aflatoxins can be produced by strains of *A. parasiticus.* Most strains of *A. flavus* produce only the B aflatoxins. Strains of these two mold species have been identified that produce no aflatoxins. The letter designations relate to their fluorescence in ultraviolet light: blue for B_1 and B_2, and green for G_1 and G_2. M_1 and M_2 are hydroxylation derivatives from animal metabolism of aflatoxin B_1 and B_2 and can be found in tissues, meat, milk, and eggs. P_1 is a urinary metabolite of aflatoxin B_1 from monkeys. Molecular weights vary from 298 to 346, and melting points range from 190° C to approximately 300° C.[3] Aflatoxin B_1 (AB_1) is the most toxic and carcinogenic member of the group, usually the sole analyte of analytic interest, and in highest concentration in naturally occurring cases.

Aflatoxins are most often found in crops with substantive energy content such as corn, peanuts, cottonseed, rice, sweet potatoes, potatoes, wheat, oats, barley, millet, sesame, sorghum, cacao beans, and almonds and other nuts. Other less common sources include soybeans, copra and coconut, safflower, sunflower, palm kernels, cassava, and spices (cayenne pepper, chili powder, dried chili peppers, black pepper, capsicum peppers, nutmeg).[4,5] Concentrations of aflatoxins in shelled corn vary widely from year to year because of the variety of environmental and climate conditions, corn variety, and degree of insect damage. From 1990 to 1992, which were years of unfavorable climate conditions for corn production, approximately 40% of the samples from the Corn Belt were positive for aflatoxin.[6]

Toxicokinetics. Absorption is by passive diffusion from the small intestine, especially the duodenum. Consistent with the low molecular weight and lipophilic properties of aflatoxin B_1, absorption has been found to be rapid and complete. Aflatoxin B_1 is more lipophilic than G_1 and has a higher rate of absorption. The rate of absorption is higher in young animals.[7] AB_1 can reversibly bind to albumin and other proteins in the circulation; an equilibrium is established between bound and unbound. The unbound AB_1 passes from the vessels into the surrounding tissues. The plasma biologic half-lives ($t_{1/2}$) were 36.5, 28.9, and 12.9 for the monkey, rat, and mouse, respectively. AB_1 accumulates more readily in the liver, kidney, bone marrow, and lungs and to a lesser degree in brain, muscle, and body fat. The highest concentration is found in liver. Elimination of the toxin occurs via bile, urine, and feces, and into milk or eggs. Rates of elimination cannot be generalized except that in most species the majority of the toxin is excreted within 24 hours after exposure. Routes and rates depend on the products of biotransformation as well as the impact of any toxin effects on cellular mechanism or other lesions. Aflatoxins do not accumulate in tissues; however, the effects from long repeated or term exposure may leave lasting deleterious effects in tissues.[8,9]

Biotransformation occurs in the liver, kidney, and small intestine. The proportions of aflatoxin converted to metabolites that bind to critical cellular macromolecules determine the extent of toxicity or carcinogenicity. A key transformation for the toxicity of aflatoxin is the activation of AFB_1 to the reactive epoxide intermediate, which is carried out by the P-450 enzyme system. Binding of AB_1-epoxide to various cellular macromolecules is believed to be responsible for cellular injury and death. Once bioactivated, AB_1 can bind to DNA, RNA, and proteins, resulting in reduced synthesis of DNA, nuclear and nucleolar RNA, and protein. In general, transformations result in more polar compounds, which can be conjugated (usually to less toxic compounds) to aid in excretion. Details of aflatoxin biotransformations have been reviewed.[10,11] Aflatoxin M_1 (AM_1) is formed from the hydroxylation of AB_1 by hepatic microsomal enzymes. It is a major excretion product in several species via urine and milk. Data from studies suggest that 3 to 6 days of daily ingestion of AB_1 is required before steady-state excretion of AM_1 in the milk is achieved. AM_1 becomes undetectable 2 to 4 days after withdrawal from the contaminated diet. Excretion of AM_1 in milk varies among animals and between days and milkings. The ratios of the concentration of AB_1 in feed to AM_1 in milk were estimated at 34 to 1600 with an average ratio near 300. The amount of AM_1 excreted was 0% to 4% of the amount of AB_1 ingested with an average amount of about 1%. A linear relationship between AB_1 intake (mg/kg) and AM_1 in milk (μg/L) has been shown with a slope of approximately 0.7.[9] Cows in early lactation tend to convert a larger portion of the AB_1 and excrete a higher percentage of AM_1 than do cows in later lactation on the same feed (and AB_1) intake. This is believed to be related to increased liver metabolism as well as higher production.[12]

Mechanism of Action.   The reactive metabolites, particularly the epoxide of AB_1, bind with cellular components including nucleic acids, subcellular organelles, and regulatory proteins that disrupt normal anabolic and catabolic processes. The results include disruption of organ function, carcinogenesis, immunosuppression, mutagenesis, and teratogenesis.[13]

AB_1 suppresses the cell-mediated immune responses and, to a lesser degree, humoral immunity. AFB_1 apparently suppresses B cell function and components of phagocytic functions.[14] Several factors make interpretation of the published information difficult: the differences between species, inconsistency of research findings, and usage of higher dosages than are found in most field cases.[15] The toxin dose relative to immunosuppression of clinical significance remains obscure.

Aflatoxin detoxification by rumen microbes has been proposed to explain the lower sensitivity of ruminants. However, significant degeneration of toxin by rumen microbes has not been found.[16] To the contrary, sufficient concentrations of aflatoxin in some studies have had deleterious effects on rumen microbial systems related to cellulose digestion, volatile fatty acid digestion, and proteolysis.[17]

Toxicity and Risk Factors.   In naturally occurring cases of aflatoxin exposure, the total dose received by the animals is often difficult to ascertain because the amount ingested and duration is seldom known. The alleged offending feed source is gone and likelihood of disease depends on a number of other factors. Thus, dose-related data from anecdotal evidence and clinical case reports should be scrutinized carefully.

The nutritional plane of the animals and feed quality are important variables in the severity of disease. A few of the more striking modulating effects related to nutrition follow.

Protein.   Low-protein diets enhance hepatotoxicosis and necrosis but might protect against the development of hepatocellular carcinoma.[10] Hepatic lesions can be made more severe by feeding a protein-deficient diet.[18]

Amino acids.   Ducklings, at least, have a profound increase in sensitivity to AB_1 when dietary concentrations of arginine and lysine are increased only slightly. Casein may be protective. A low choline and methionine dietary status is associated with increased hepatocarcinogenesis and shortened time to first tumors.[19]

Vitamins.   Vitamin A and carotene apparently modify the metabolism of AB_1 and consequently decrease toxicity. Repair of AB_1-damaged DNA also may be defective in vitamin A deficiency.[19] Hypersupplementation of vitamin A has no effect on carcinogenesis, although suboptimal vitamin A status is related to increased tumor incidence. Riboflavin deficiency in rats reduced the in vitro activation of AFB_1 (to effect a reduced toxicity).[10]

Antioxidants and selenium.   Antioxidants reduce the toxicity and enhance repair of the nucleic acid and other organelle damage. Whether the experimental administration corrected a deficiency or provided an excess is not clear. AB_1 intoxication is reduced by addition of 1 ppm selenium (0.1 ppm is the recommended level) to the diet.[19]

Nonnutritive compounds.   Cruciferous vegetables (broccoli, brussels sprouts, cabbage) are protective. Increased conjugation of the activated AB_1-epoxide is the suspected mechanism. Organosulfur compounds (found in garlic), capsaicin (active principle of hot chili peppers), and benzoflavones apparently reduce binding of AB_1 to DNA.[10] Methyl group deficiency increases carcinogenesis and preneoplastic changes.[20]

The determinations of lethal dose 50 (LD_{50}) values (lethal dose 50%, or dose required to kill 50% of the sample population) in Box 23-1 for different animal species shed light on their relative susceptibilities, but are unrelated to chronic or carcinogenic parameters. Biotransformation (including activation) pathways of aflatoxin metabolism vary between species, breeds, and sexes, which impacts the dose-response relationships.[21]

The most common question encountered by practicing veterinarians regarding aflatoxins relates to the interpretation of a toxin level found in a contaminated feed. The analysis of the feed for aflatoxin is often prompted by undiagnosed production problems and, perhaps, chronic disease problems—signs that are common with the prolonged ingestion of low-level aflatoxin contaminated feedstuffs. In such a scenario aflatoxicosis can easily be overdiagnosed.

Because of the appearance of AM_1 residues in milk, exposure to aflatoxins is detected when it might have otherwise gone unnoticed. Table 23-1 lists the results of some experimental feeding trials. Hepatic lesions generally develop at dosage levels lower than those that can cause clinical change. When in doubt, blood and serum samples from a representative number of the herd for clinical pathology examinations are advised.

BOX 23-1	COMPARATIVE SINGLE DOSE LD$_{50}$ VALUES FOR AFLATOXIN B$_1$

SPECIES	LD$_{50}$ (mg/kg)
Rabbit	0.3-0.5
Duckling	0.3-0.6
Cat	0.55
Swine	0.62
Dog	1 (ca.)
Guinea pig	1.4-2
Sheep	2
Calf	1.5
Monkey, cynomolgus, M	2.2
Monkey, macaque, F	8
Chicken	6.5-16
Chicken, 21 days	18
Turkey, 15 days	3.2
Mice	9
Mouse, neonate	1.5
Mouse, weanling	7.3
Hamster	10
Hamster, 42 days, F	5.9
Hamster, 30 days, M	12.8
Rats	5.5-18
Catfish, channel	11.5

Data from references 19, 22-24.

The maximum allowable concentration for aflatoxin M$_1$ in milk is 0.50 ppb. Consequently, total dietary concentrations of aflatoxin for dairy animals should not exceed 20 ppb. Violative milk residues can be expected if the total ration exceeds 40 ppb AB$_1$.

Table 23-2 provides a clinical guide to aflatoxin in swine. Acute aflatoxicosis is expected when swine receive oral doses of aflatoxin exceeding 0.2 mg/kg of body weight (equivalent to approximately 5000 to 7000 ppb).[28] Feed contaminations this high are exceedingly rare in naturally occurring cases. Sheep are evidently more tolerant to aflatoxin exposure than are cattle; few reports of chronic aflatoxicosis are documented.

Mice and rats are among the most resistant of animals to the effects of aflatoxins. Mice tolerated diets with approximately 3.6 ppm aflatoxin B$_1$ for at least 3 months with no adverse effects. Age and sex influence the toxicity of aflatoxin in rats. Castration had a sparing effect on mortality when performed before 10 weeks of age but was not beneficial after 10 weeks. Administration of testosterone increased the mortality rate over that in animals not receiving the hormone.[23]

Trout are particularly sensitive to the carcinogenic effects of AB$_1$. A diet concentration of 0.4 ppb can cause liver cancer in less than a year in trout. Hepatomas have been reported also in some species of salmon. A thorough review of aflatoxin in aquatic animals is available.[29]

TABLE 23-1 Clinical Effects in Cattle by Aflatoxin Dose and Time

Type	Exposure Time	Dose* (µg/kg BW)	Equivalent Feed† 3%	Result
Heifers (400 kg)	140 days	12	300‡	No effect on feed intake, average daily gain, feed efficiency, estrus cycles (SGOT increase at high dose)
Cows, lactating	14 days	15	500	No effect on feed intake or production
Steers	133 days	16	533	Decreased intake
Cows, lactating	13 months	20	667	No decrease in intake or milk production; intermittent decreased intake in first-calf heifers
Calves, 5 months	6 weeks	40	1333	Biliary hyperplasia
Calves, 5 months	6 weeks	60	2000	Intake not changed; reduced gain
Calves, 5 months	6 weeks	80	2667	Decreased feed intake in 1 week
Cows, adult	5 days	110	3667	Depressed feed intake in 12 hours; gradual recovery over 14 days
Cows, adult	5 days	330	11,000	Immediate anorexia; slow recovery

Data from references 25, 26.

BW, Body weight.

* Dose of aflatoxin, µg/kg body weight.

† Equivalent feed concentration of aflatoxin if animal consumes 3% of its body weight.

‡ Actual animal dose and feed concentration in this case.

TABLE 23-2 **Clinical Guide to Aflatoxin in Swine**

Category of Pigs	Dietary Level	Clinical Effects
Grow-finish	<100 ppb	No clinical effect; residues in liver
	200-400 ppb	Reduced growth and feed efficiency; possible immunosuppression
	400-800 ppb	Microscopic liver lesions, cholangiohepatitis; increased serum liver enzymes; immunosuppression
	800-1200 ppb	Reduced growth; decreased feed consumption; rough hair coat; icterus; hypoproteinemia
	1200-2000 ppb	Icterus; coagulopathy; depression, anorexia; some deaths
	>2000 ppb	Acute hepatosis and coagulopathy; deaths in 3-10 days
Brood sows	500-750 ppb	No effect on conception; deliver normal piglets that grow slowly because of aflatoxin in milk

Data from reference 27.

Clinical Signs. The aflatoxin dose and duration of exposure determine the time of onset and observed effects. Following high lethal doses anorexia, depression, weakness to prostration, dyspnea, emesis, diarrhea often with blood and mucus, fever followed by subnormal temperature, convulsions (dogs), and epistaxis may be seen. Icterus follows.[30]

Chronic intoxication is more common. The onset is often subtle and the changes (eventually) reflect liver disease. Reduced weight gain with roughed hair coats is generally the first evidence of intoxication noticed. Concurrent with the degree of hepatic damage, the disease might advance to anemia, jaundice, anorexia, and depression.[31] Dogs more often develop gastrointestinal disturbances with occasional hemorrhage and ascites. Poults and ducklings have loss of appetite, appearance of nervous symptoms, and, in young birds, high and rapid mortality. With prolonged feeding ducks are more likely than poultry to develop tumors.[32]

Dairy cows have detectable residues of AM_1 at doses much lower than needed for clinical change, and milk residues precede clinical signs if doses are high. Toxigenic doses in cattle usually first cause reduced feed intake, which is followed by reduced milk production.[26]

AB_1 is a teratogen in hamsters, rats, and some mouse strains.[33] Fetal malformations include anencephaly, growth retardation, ectopia cordis, microcephaly, umbilical hernia, harelip, and severe diffuse hepatic degeneration, necrosis, and hemorrhage.[23]

Clinical Pathology. Hematologic changes are similar among species. Relative changes are represented in Box 23-2 and generally reflect liver pathology.[34,35]

The greatest amount of cellular γ-glutamyltransferase (GGT) is in the brush borders of renal and bile duct epithelia. With this unique specificity and sensitivity, GGT is a prime marker of bile duct epithelial proliferation that is typical of aflatoxicosis.[35] Changes in urinalysis are not specific for aflatoxicosis.

Lesions. High doses causing acute intoxication can result in a tan-colored appearance of the liver surface and parenchyma; hemorrhage into the intestines; and hemorrhages associated with the heart, pericardium, fat, muscle, and subcutaneous tissue.[28] Microscopically, early (3 hours) liver changes following acute poisoning include disorganization of hepatocytes with vacuolization in cytoplasm. This is followed by swelling of cells, centrilobular congestion, necrosis, and

BOX 23-2	**CLINICAL PATHOLOGY CHANGES CAUSED BY AFLATOXINS**		
Hematocrit	+/-	Alkaline phosphatase	++
Hb	+/-	γ-Glutamyltransferase	+++
Leukocytes	+/-	Aspartate aminotransferase	++
BUN	-	Alanine aminotransferase	++
Prothrombin time	+	Sorbitol dehydrogenase	+++
Bilirubin	+		
Icterus index	+		
Total protein	-		
Albumin	-		

leukocyte infiltration. Swelling and necrosis of the renal tubule epithelium have also been reported.[21]

With lower doses and longer duration, a proliferation of reticular fibers and bile duct cells among septal borders can be observed. The cytoplasm of hepatocytes becomes granular and vacuolated or completely absent. Bile duct proliferation and nodules of regenerating liver cells become evident. The rate of development of the changes depends on the dose.[28]

In cases of chronic exposure to toxic levels, there is diffuse fatty change of the liver, and proliferation of bile ducts may accumulate to the extent that lobular architecture is distorted. Mitotic figures might be seen in biliary cells. The accumulation of lipids is centrilobular in mild cases and diffusely involves hepatocytes throughout the lobule in more severe lesions.[23,30,32]

Cutaneous lesions of vesicles filled with serous exudate and epithelial necrosis can occur when aflatoxin is applied to the skin of rabbits.[36]

A number of species develop hepatocellular carcinomas and other neoplasms following multiple exposures to aflatoxins.[23]

Diagnostic Testing. Bioassay procedures using eggs or larvae of tadpoles, salamanders, brine shrimp, and ducklings, among others, have long been replaced by a number of sensitive chemical analytic detection and immunoassay methods. Most diagnostic laboratories offer tests on feedstuffs that can provide sensitivities near 3 ppb for AB_1. Toxin detection in tissues, particularly liver, is possible.

The mere demonstration of an aflatoxigenic fungus or a trace of the toxin in feed components is insufficient proof. Characteristic biological alterations as clinical signs and pathologic changes must be demonstrated. Analytic confirmation of aflatoxins in the material ingested is necessary.[31]

Certain metabolites of *Aspergillus* sp. react under black light (approximately 366 nm) to produce a blue-green color. However, the reactant is not aflatoxin. A positive black light test suggests presence of the mold but does not confirm the presence of aflatoxins.

Treatment. No antidote or specific treatment exists for aflatoxicosis beyond prompt removal from the contaminated source. Optimizing the quality of the diet, with particular attention to protein, vitamins, and trace elements, aids in recovery but does little to ameliorate the damage done. Individual treatment depends on the clinical condition and liver function support.

A number of nutritional supplements have been tested, but results were mixed. Oxytetracycline (10 mg/kg), administered daily, apparently reduces hepatic damage and mortality. Use in combination with steroids is not advised. Activated charcoal is helpful, especially when used soon after exposure. The combination of oxytetracycline and activated charcoal is promising.[37]

The poisoned animals may be immunocompromised, which affects biosecurity and treatment decisions. Vaccinations may have to be repeated.

Prognosis. Recovery may be prolonged, and return to normal production may not be realized. Assessment of liver function and the response following removal of the source aids in developing a prognosis.

Prevention and Control. Procedures to prevent crop damage, such as insect control, can decrease fungal invasion. Handling corn to minimize seed coat damage and drying to 15% or less prevents mold growth and production of additional toxin. Mold retardants, such as propionic acid, can help in storage but do nothing to the toxin that was produced before harvest.

Ammoniation of feeds such as corn and cottonseed is practiced in several areas of the country. This procedure hydrolyzes the lactone ring of AB_1 to various end-products that are less toxic.[38]

Na Ca aluminosilicate, an adsorbent, binds aflatoxin and reduces toxic effects significantly. This has not been found to work on other mycotoxins.[39] Other binding agents such as clay or bentonite have produced mixed, usually disappointing, results.

The U.S. Food and Drug Administration (FDA) has established the following "action levels" as guidelines for acceptable levels of aflatoxin in the specified food and feed (*http://vmcfsan.fda.gov/~lrd/fdaact.html*):

Commodity Action Level (ppb)
Corn and peanut products intended for finishing (i.e., feedlot) beef cattle, 300
Cottonseed meal intended for beef, cattle, swine,

or poultry (regardless of age or breeding status), 300
Corn and peanut products intended for finishing swine of 100 pounds or greater, 200
Corn and peanut products intended for breeding beef cattle, breeding swine, or mature poultry, 100
Animal feeds, except listed above, 20
Milk, 0.5 (aflatoxin M_1)

CITRININ AND OCHRATOXIN

Gavin L. Meerdink

Synonyms. Ochratoxin and citrinin are discussed in the same section because the two produce indistinguishable clinical syndromes, are produced by the same genera of fungi, and have structural similarities.[1]

Poisoning by these agents has been referred to as *porcine mycotoxin nephropathy*. A European syndrome in humans associated with ochratoxin has been termed *Balkan endemic nephropathy*.

Sources. Ochratoxins are a family of compounds with the general structure of a phenylalanine linked by an amide bond to dihydroisocoumarin. Ochratoxin A (OA) contains chlorine, which is not present in ochratoxin B (OB); ochratoxin C is the ethyl ester of OA. OA is the most toxic of the three.[2] A hydroxyl group attached to the isocoumarin moiety is ionizable and must exist in the dissociated form for ochratoxin intoxication.[3] Ochratoxin α (Oα) is the nontoxic product of OA hydrolysis (with loss of phenylalanine group) by microorganisms in the rumen, cecum, and large intestine. The citrinin structure is similar to OA without the phenylalanine and replacement of the Cl with a methyl group.

Ochratoxins and citrinin are produced by *Aspergillus* and *Penicillium* species. Multiple species of both genera have been found to produce ochratoxin; however, *A. ochraceus* (*A. alutaceus*) and *P. verrucosum* are most commonly associated with disease.[4-6]

Citrinin was first isolated from *Penicillium citrinum* and can be produced by a number of *Penicillium* and *Aspergillus* spp., usually in concert with ochratoxins. Citrinin has been isolated from an Australian plant, *Crotalaria crispata*, and can be found with other mycotoxins such as patulin and oxalic acid.[6]

Ochratoxins, often including citrinin, have caused problems from contaminated corn, barley, rye, and wheat; they are also found in oats, soybeans, buckwheat, rice, sorghum, white beans, peanuts, Brazil nuts, surface of hams, red pepper, black pepper, coffee, decaying vegetation, and soil. Citrinin can persist in nature for several months. It has bacteriostatic and bactericidal properties, primarily against gram-positive bacteria.[4,7] Naturally occurring concentrations are usually less than 0.5 ppm, although higher levels of contamination do occur. The amount of the fungal mass does not correlate with the quantity of mycotoxin produced.[2]

Toxicokinetics. OA is absorbed by passive diffusion from the gastrointestinal tract, primarily stomach, in the nonionized (or partially ionized) form rather than the ionized form. The hydroxyl group of OA, of primary importance in its absorption, exists in the nonionized form at a low pH and in the ionized form at a high pH. The proportion of the two forms can be calculated from its pKa value of 7.1. Thus, absorption is enhanced by the acid environment of the stomach. The pH of ingesta also affects absorption; OA is absorbed more readily in cattle and sheep on high concentrate rations (with lower pH) than on forage rations.[2]

OA has a high binding affinity to albumin (more likely smaller molecular-weight protein fractions), which facilitates passive absorption of the nonionized form from the digestive tract and retards OA elimination and contributes to the prolonged half-life of the toxin. The smaller protein carrier enhances passage through the glomerular membrane to enable accumulation of OA in the kidney. The positive association between the binding of OA to plasma protein and the elimination $t_{1/2}$ contributes to the following differences following intravenous injection of OA: the $t_{1/2}$ for quail was 12 hours; rat, 170 hours; pig, 150 hours; monkey, 840 hours. OA is excreted in the bile and reabsorbed in the intestine; this enterohepatic recycling also contributes to its prolonged half-life. The organic anion transport system in the proximal and distal tubules of the kidney actively reabsorbs OA, which adds to the $t_{1/2}$ of the toxin and contributes to its renal concentration.[2]

OB is hydrolyzed (in vitro) by bovine carboxypeptidase A and by various rat tissue extracts much faster than OA. This factor plus the higher acid dissociation constant of the hydroxyl group for OA might account for the lower toxicity of OB. The greater toxicity of OA has also been associated with the ionizable hydroxyl group.[6]

Rumen microbes cleave OA to Oα.[8] Oα is nontoxic because it does not dissociate under physiologic conditions. The same reaction occurs in the lower intestinal tract of nonruminants but is of less protective significance than that which occurs in ruminants. Hydrolysis of OA to Oα does not occur in tissues.[2]

Liver cytochrome P-450 microsomes metabolize OA, in the presence of NADPH, to (4R)- and (4S)-hydroxyochratoxin A. OA is primarily excreted in the urine as Oα and OA. Smaller amounts of the two forms are excreted in the feces. Ruminants generally excrete a larger proportion of Oα.[2] In trout, ochratoxins A and B are thought to be metabolized to their water-soluble dihydroisocoumarin moieties, which are readily excreted.[9]

Generally, OA is a stable compound. About 15% of the toxin in cereals can survive autoclaving, increasing to 35% with higher moisture. In beans, about half of the OA concentration remains after blanching, salting, and heat processing in tomato sauce for 1 hour.[6]

Citrinin is readily absorbed; serum concentrations can be detected within 3 hours after ingestion.[6]

Mechanism of Action.
OA is thought to act by at least three defined mechanisms: (1) inhibition of phenylalanine metabolizing enzymes, (2) promotion of lipid peroxidation, and (3) inhibition of mitochondrial adenosine triphosphate (ATP) production. Other effects appear to be secondary.[2] OA affects DNA, RNA, and protein synthesis, presumably because

of its phenylalanine moiety and inhibition of phenylalanine hydroxylase. Protein and mRNA pools are reduced in kidney cells by 30% to 40%. Renal gluconeogenesis and phosphoenolpyruvate carboxykinase (PEPCK) is inhibited in rats and swine. (The enzyme PEPCK is a key regulator of the gluconeogenic pathway and is regulated by the kidney.) One result is interference with carbohydrate metabolism and glycogen stores or utilization. Lipid peroxidation produces free radicals that have toxic effects in multiple ways. By acting as a competitive inhibitor of carrier proteins, OA inhibits mitochondria respiration, resulting in depletion of intramitochondrial ATP.[2]

The immunosuppression effects may be related to inhibition of peripheral B and T lymphocyte proliferation and interleukin-2 and its receptor production. However, depressed T-independent or T-dependent antigen responses are not seen when OA is administered in the diet. Phenylalanine (which provides some protection against OA intoxication) has been shown to attenuate OA-induced immunosuppression in mice. The complement system is significantly reduced in chickens fed OA, but is unaffected in guinea pigs.[10]

OA has been found to be carcinogenic in some experimental laboratory animals. Carcinogenesis and immunosuppression may be related. Suppression of natural killer cell activity by oral OA appears to be the result of inhibition of endogenous interferon levels. The ability of OA to modulate natural killer cell activity may contribute to its capacity to induce renal and hepatic carcinomas because (1) the dose for tumor induction is similar to that required for immunosuppression, (2) immunosuppression precedes development of detectable tumors, and (3) immune alterations are consistent with those involved in tumor immunity and correlate with changes in resistance to transplantable syngeneic tumor cells. However, most immunodeficiency tumors are lymphomas and leukemias, which do not occur with OA. Furthermore, these three points were determined with high doses that are not encountered naturally.[10]

Citrinin can cause parasympathomimetic activity such as vasodilation bronchoconstriction, and increase in muscular tone (at a high dose, 67 mg/kg body weight).[6]

Toxicity and Risk Factors.
Toxicity is affected by the dissociation constant of the hydroxyl group, which differs accordingly between the four forms. The LD_{50} values for young chicks are OA, 150 μg (3 to 4 mg/kg); OB, 1900 μg; OC, 216 μg; and Oα, not toxic at 1000 μg.[2]

Toxicity varies considerably among species and is influenced by diet, age, sex, route of administration, genetic differences, and the form of ochratoxin. LD_{50} values (mg/kg body weight) are listed in Table 23-3.

Dogs develop no signs of toxicosis at oral doses of 0.1 mg OA/kg body weight (for 21 days). At doses of 0.2 to 0.3 mg/kg body weight, dogs survived 11 to 14 days with anorexia, weight loss, emesis, tenesmus, blood in feces, polydipsia/polyuria, dehydration, and prostration. Oral doses of more than 2 mg/kg body weight can kill dogs within 3 days with severe clinical signs.[7]

Pigs fed diets containing 0.2 to 4 ppm OA developed nephropathy after 4 months. Feed levels less than 0.2 ppm

TABLE 23-3 **LD$_{50}$ Values for Ochratoxin A**

Species	LD$_{50}$ (mg/kg BW)
Swine	1-6
Dogs	0.2
Chickens	3.3-3.9
Cattle, adult	20
Rats, neonate	3.9
Rats, adult	20-30
Mice	46-58
Peking ducklings	3

Data from references 2, 11, 15, 18.
BW, Body weight.

had little effect on daily gain and feed efficiency. Higher dietary levels, more than 5 to 10 ppm OA, result in extrarenal lesions involving liver, intestine, spleen, lymphoid tissue, and leukocytes in pigs.[2] A single lethal oral dose for swine is about 11 mg/kg body weight (similar to that for calves that do not yet have a functional rumen).[12]

Broiler chicks fed diets containing 0.5 to 8 ppm OA had dose-related reductions in weight gains up to 80%. Reductions in laying hens' egg production and feed consumption can occur with OA dietary concentrations of 0.5 ppm for 6 weeks.[11]

Ochratoxicosis has rarely been reported in ruminants, presumably because of the ability of ruminal microorganisms to hydrolyze OA to nontoxic Oα. In young calves, doses of 2 mg/kg body weight have caused some clinical depression, reduced weight gain, and dehydration; however, the signs improved within a month.[2] Adult cattle develop transitory anorexia, diarrhea, difficulty in rising, and loss of milk production following a single oral dose of 13 mg/kg body weight and can recover without further sequelae.

Pregnant cows given 2.5 and 0.25 mg/kg body weight OA orally for 5 days had no clinical evidence of illness and all delivered normal calves.[4] A sheep study suggested that OA does not cause abortion and only trace amounts of the toxin penetrate the ovine placenta.[13]

OA fed to pregnant rats induced fetal death and resorption at 25 mg/kg body weight, but not at 12.5 mg/kg. Teratogenic changes can also occur. A single oral dose of 1 mg OA/kg body weight during gestation produced gross malformations in a mouse and rat fetus. Hamsters fed 50 and 100 ppm OA for 14 days developed depression, decreased feed consumption, and loss of condition.[2,7]

The LD$_{50}$ value 48 hours after exposure to OA administered into the yolk sac is about 17 µg/egg in 5-day-old chicken embryos. (This is approximately 70 times greater than the LD$_{50}$ value for aflatoxin B$_1$.)[14] Following a single oral dose of 16 mg/kg OA, 3-week-old chicks became listless, huddled, and developed diarrhea in 6 hours; at 18 hours they developed a catatonic-like appearance with a loss of righting reflex, followed by intermittent fine tremors of leg and neck muscles with prostration and death at 24 hours.[11] White leghorn pullets (14 weeks of age) fed a diet containing OA up to 4 ppm had dose-related mortalities of up to 35.4% after 6 weeks. Up to 64% of laying hens on these diets died after 6 months.[15]

Japanese quail (*Coturnix coturnix japonica*) fed a diet containing 4 to 16 ppm of pure OA had decreased body weight, emaciation, inactivity, less feathering, and a range of dose-related mortalities up to 90% at 10 days.[15,16]

The LD$_{50}$ of OA in trout by intraperitoneal injection is 4.67 mg/kg body weight. In long-term feeding trials OA fed to rainbow trout in a semipurified diet at levels up to 4 ppm caused no liver or kidney tumors. The immature stage of brine shrimp (*Artemia salina*) has a 90% mortality after 24 hours at OA concentrations of approximately 5.0 µg/ml (at a temperature of 37.5° C).[9]

In cattle, OA is excreted in minute quantities in milk and urine when the oral dose is more than 100 mg OA per day. When 1 g of OA was fed daily for 4 days, the compound was detected in milk on days 3, 4, and 5.[17] Dietary concentrations of at least approximately 60 ppm OA are needed to produce milk residues.[18] Dietary concentrations of less than 0.5 ppm for less than 3 months are not likely to result in violative OA residues in tissues.[19]

Citrinin is less toxic. Six young beagle dogs given oral doses of 2.5 or 5 mg/kg body weight citrinin for 6 weeks appeared clinically normal. Dogs on a diet containing 25 ppm citrinin had an increased blood urea nitrogen (BUN) after 15 days on the feed, decreased urine specific gravity, presence of urine glucose in excess of 0.5%, and necrotic renal epithelial cells in the sediment. Oral doses of 20 mg/kg body weight citrinin resulted in deterioration and death in 5 days. Hamsters fed 250 and 500 ppm diets for 2 weeks had little change in body weight and no clinical signs, and all survived with no gross or histologic changes in kidney, spleen, jejunum, or liver.[7]

Clinical Signs. Acute poisoning with high doses of OA results in gastroenteritis, diarrhea, emesis, tenesmus, depression, anorexia, and dehydration. Elevated body temperature, bilateral purulent conjunctivitis, tonsillitis, polydipsia, polyuria, and bloody feces can also occur from high doses.[2]

The mycotoxin concentrations more often found in field cases with chronic exposure cause a slower onset and often subtle signs related to kidney disease. Water intake and urination frequency is increased. Production parameters (e.g., weight gain, egg production, feed efficiency) decrease. Evidence of exposure might not be noticed antemortem but is discovered at slaughter from the chronic kidney lesions.

Clinical Pathology. Changes with ochratoxin and citrinin poisoning generally reflect renal damage. BUN may not be altered with acute poisoning, but it increases with the progression of lesions and is a characteristic of field cases. Additional clinical pathologic evidence of kidney damage and hepatic injury can be seen depending on the dose, duration of exposure, and degree of tissue damage.[7]

In chickens, reductions of serum total protein and albumin are the most sensitive indicators of ochratoxicosis. Other changes include decreased serum globulin, urea nitrogen, cholesterol, triglycerides, and potassium. Serum uric acid and creatine increase as do the activities for serum phosphatase, GGT, and cholinesterase.[20]

Decreased renal PEPCK activity is a highly sensitive and specific indicator of OA intoxication in pigs, but not for rats.

Renal tubular function changes in swine include decreased transport of *p*-aminohippuric acid (Tm-PAH), a decreased Tm-PAH/inulin clearance, glucosuria, proteinuria, and reduced urine concentration. A dose-related increase in urine albumin and large-molecular-weight proteins, suggestive of glomerular proteinuria, can be seen. Polydipsia, polyuria, and increases in serum creatinine and BUN occur eventually as the renal lesions develop.[2]

Changes in dogs are similar with decreased urine specific gravity, granular casts, and necrotic renal epithelium with acute poisoning. BUN changes are variable early in the disease process.[7]

In a case of suspected citrinin poisoning in feeder steers being fed moldy high-moisture corn, the principal changes included increased serum BUN, plasma protein, and fibrinogen. Serum sodium, potassium, and calcium were decreased.[21]

Lesions.   The morphologic change classically associated with ochratoxin and citrinin poisoning is nephropathy, specifically degeneration of the proximal renal tubules. Variations in lesions and the rate of appearance are determined by dose and duration of exposure.

Dogs administered 0.2 to 3 mg/kg OA had gross lesions of tonsillitis, enlarged lymph nodes, and mucohemorrhagic enteritis of the cecum, colon, and rectum. Histopathologic alterations in the kidneys consisted of necrosis and desquamation of epithelial cells that were more pronounced in the proximal convoluted tubules. Tubules contained eosinophilic granular casts. Necrosis of lymphoid tissues—especially germinal centers—occurred in the spleen, tonsils, thymus, and mesenteric lymph nodes. Hepatic changes consisted of centrilobular necrosis and fatty change.[22] Lesions in pigs that died soon after ingesting 1 or 2 mg/kg body weight OA were similar to those described in the dogs[12] Limited studies suggest that citrinin lesions predominate in the kidney tissues without the extrarenal changes found with OA.[7]

Poultry develop emaciation, dehydration, dry and firm gizzard mucosal surfaces, proventricular mucosal hemorrhages, and visceral gout. The liver, pancreas, and kidney are pale and might contain focal hemorrhages. Acute nephrosis, hepatic vacuolation or necrosis, catarrhal enteritis, suppression of hematopoiesis in bone marrow, and depletion of lymphoid elements from the spleen and bursa of Fabricius are seen microscopically. As the duration of the disease syndrome increases, bile duct proliferation with diffuse vacuolation of hepatocytes can occur (even in the absence of kidney lesions). Ducklings consistently have fatty livers.[15]

Guinea pigs develop ochratoxin and, to a lesser degree, citrinin lesions in proximal and distal convoluted tubules, loops of Henle, and collecting ducts with little change in glomeruli. Hamsters fed diets with 50 or 100 ppm OA for 14 days had lesions limited to the kidneys with dilated tubules in focal areas of the renal cortex. Rabbits develop similar renal proximal convoluted tubule lesions.[7]

Rats fed 9.6 or 24 ppm OA develop enteritis of duodenum and jejunum and pale liver and kidneys. Relative kidney weights increase (at the higher dose), but the absolute weights of liver and kidneys are reduced. Microscopic lesions are similar to those described for dogs. Neoplasia was not noted in rats fed 100 or 300 mg OA for 5 days per week for 53 weeks. Citrinin lesions in rats consist of kidney changes, primarily tubular, as described earlier.[7]

Ultrastructure changes in rats (5 ppm OA for 90 days) include proliferation of smooth endoplasmic reticulum accompanied by residual bodies and thickening of renal tubular basement membrane epithelium. Hepatocytes have hyperplasia of the agranular endoplasmic reticulum with the formation of compact masses of smooth membranes that correspond to the foci of hyaline degeneration observed by light microscopy.[23]

Although not clinically documented in other species, OA is a potent teratogen in mice. Pregnant mice injected intraperitoneally on various gestation days had higher fetal mortality, decreased fetal weights, higher rates of malformations, and skeletal defects (exencephaly, malformations of the face, eyes, digits, and tail).[24]

Diagnostic Testing.   Chemical analytic and immunoassay methods are available for the detection of ochratoxin. Clinicians should contact the analytic laboratory for the optimum sample selections and sensitivity capability. Ochratoxin can be found in feed and often tissues, such as liver and kidney. However, Oα as the metabolite of OA is more likely to be found in milk or urine and is likely the analyte of choice for determination of exposure.[6]

Blood ochratoxin can provide an indication of exposure; levels can relate to intake.[19] One study indicated that as long as the concentration of OA in blood was less than 200 ppb, the risk of nephropathy was minor.[25]

Tissue concentrations depend on time length of ingestion as well as the dose, and can be found in the absence of lesions. Diets containing more than 0.5 ppm for more than 2 weeks can result in kidney and liver residues. Ochratoxin tissue concentrations of 5 to 10 ppb can result from ingestion of feed containing 1 ppm for a month. Residues in eggs are possible following 1 ppm dietary levels for several weeks. Kidney and liver tissues are likely to contain the highest concentration of ochratoxin; the toxin might also be found in muscle and fat tissues.[19]

Tissue ochratoxin residue levels have been legislated in Denmark: 25 ppb OA in kidneys is the maximum allowed. Some relationships between kidney, meat, and blood levels have been established. Blood tests allow preharvest testing; about 4 weeks on uncontaminated feed usually allows for elimination from tissues.[19]

Little data exist regarding the likelihood of finding citrinin in tissues. For diagnostic purposes, feed analyses are recommended.

Treatment.   Agents that slow absorption, such as activated charcoal, may be of value in acute poisoning. Supportive therapy for the kidney disease that results from these toxins depends on the degree of organ damage and the particular physiologic abnormalities that warrant intervention.

Ascorbic acid added to the diet (at 300 ppm) partially ameliorates the negative effects of OA intoxication on egg production and physiology in laying hens.[26]

Prognosis.   Prediction of recovery hinges on the degree of kidney damage. Sufficient testing of plasma and urine parameters along with clearance test procedures can be used to assess functional status. The duration of exposure to the contaminated feed is a large factor.

Blood can provide early indication of exposure to OA. Studies in pigs indicate that as long as the concentration of OA in the blood was less than 200 ppb, the risk of nephropathy is minor.[25] Even with the serum protein binding that somewhat "levels" intake fluctuation, the difficulty with this approach is knowing dose consistency and duration of exposure.

Prevention and Control. The first means of prevention is to employ the feed management practices necessary to prevent growth of the fungi and production of the toxins. Moisture and temperature are critical to mold growth and toxin production. Feedstuffs must be stored at less than 15% moisture to avoid the production of OA. This is particularly important in regions of high humidity.

In areas of higher moisture, procedures such as anaerobic storage (silos or "ag-bags"), sterilization, mold inhibition, or introduction of competitive nontoxigenic microflora should be considered. Electron or γ beam irradiation is effective in destroying the spores of *A. alutaceus* that produce OA. Phosphine (Zn or Al phosphide fumigants) is effective at inhibiting fungal growth. For feeds with pH values of about 4.5 to 6, methyl paraben, K^+ sorbate, or Na^+ propionate can effectively inhibit the production of OA. Ammoniation reduces aflatoxin concentrations and has a similar effect on OA; this technique also inhibits mold growth. Inoculation with a competitive nontoxigenic microbe, such as *Lactobacillus* sp., reduces the concentration of OA in silage.[2]

Feeding the contaminated feedstuff to less sensitive species, such as ruminants, is a viable option. Adequate testing should be done to assure a toxin dose that is not harmful. Because the detoxification in the rumen is enhanced in a higher pH environment, the margin of safety is increased with high roughage (versus concentrate) diets.

Binding agents have not been found to offer practical control for OA contamination. The addition of hydrated Na^+/Ca^+ aluminosilicate (1%) and bentonite (1% and 10%) had no effect on the OA in swine. The addition of activated charcoal at 10% of the diet did reduce the uptake of OA but is not regarded as practical. Cholestyramine is a commercial anion exchange resin that has been shown to sequester bile salts and reduce hypercholesteremia in humans. Rat studies have revealed that cholestyramine (at 0.5% of diet) reduced OA blood concentrations. Further studies are needed to determine efficacy and search for less expensive anion exchange adsorbents.[2]

The coadministration of phenylalanine with OA reduces the OA-associated inhibition of protein synthesis. Injections of phenylalanine prevent OA-induced immunosuppression in mice. However, when added to diets of chicks, OA toxic effects were reduced, but an amino acid imbalance was created. Thus, little or no benefit is obtained by supplementing OA-contaminated diets with phenylalanine. High-protein diets also afford some protection in chicks, presumably because of the increased concentration of phenylalanine in the diet. The cost does not warrant the relatively small benefit.[2]

ERGOT

Tim J. Evans, George E. Rottinghaus, and Stan W. Casteel

Synonyms. Ergotism is an ancient disease, which is also referred to as "ergot" or "ergot poisoning." The term *ergot* has also been used to refer to species of *Claviceps* fungi in general or, more specifically, to refer to the visible fungal growth (sclerotium or ergot body) formed by *Claviceps purpurea* on rye *(Secale cereale).*[1,2] Unless otherwise stated in this chapter, *ergotism* refers to disease syndromes caused by *C. purpurea* or identical conditions associated with other members of the *Claviceps* genus.

Ergotism is associated with a variety of disease syndromes in many animal species, including humans. Terms for these conditions are used interchangeably with "ergotism" in some references. Several syndromes, such as "gangrenous ergotism" (cutaneous ergotism), a "summer slump"–like condition in cattle, and adverse effects on reproduction and lactation in horses may be clinically indistinguishable from "fescue foot," summer slump, and equine fescue toxicosis, respectively. The term *ergot alkaloid toxicosis* may be used to collectively refer to both ergotism and fescue toxicosis. Many aspects of ergotism and fescue toxicosis are similar enough that the reader is directed to the section on Fescue Toxicosis when comparisons between the two syndromes are referred to in this chapter.

Another syndrome referred to as "convulsive ergotism" or "nervous ergotism" may be confused with toxicoses associated with tremorgens, including those produced by *Claviceps paspali.*[1-5] In fact, there remains some debate regarding the nomenclature and the actual incidence of this particular condition.[1-3,6] Further controversy exists regarding the association between ergotism and human diseases and abnormal behavior such as that which occurred in Saint Anthony's fire or Saint Vitus's dance in the Middle Ages, witchcraft in Salem, Massachusetts, in 1692, and the "Peasants' Revolt" during the French Revolution.[1-3,5]

Sources. The sclerotia or ergot bodies of *C. purpurea* represent the mycelia, along with the hardened exudate or "honeydew" containing fungal conidia, which replace the ovarian tissue of the infected grass or cereal grain (Fig. 23-1). Although slightly larger, the dark brown, purple, or black sclerotia mature at the same rate as the grain or grass seeds they replace and fall to the ground to overwinter. The fungal life cycle is completed when sclerotia germinate and produce ascospores, which infect the stigma of grass or cereal grain flowers and allow for the spread of fungal hyphae to the ovarian tissue. Insects can pick up fungal conidia in the moist "honeydew" (before hardening) and infect other grass or grain flowers with *C. purpurea.*[1,2]

Of the cereal grains, rye and triticale, which are cross-pollinators, appear to be the most susceptible to infection by *C. purpurea*, but wheat, barley, and oats can also be ergotized. A wide variety of grasses (Box 23-3) are frequently associated with clinical cases of ergotism.[1,2,7-9] Both endophyte-free and endophyte-infected fescue grass are susceptible to

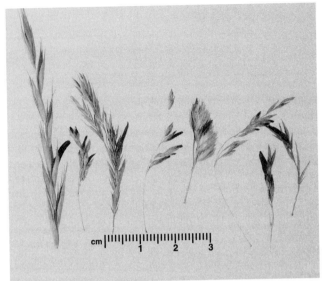

Fig. 23-1 *Claviceps purpurea* sclerotia (ergot bodies) occur in a number of shapes and sizes and vary in appearance with the type of grain or grass from which they originate. (Photo courtesy of Howard Wilson and Don Connor.)

infection by *C. purpurea*, and it is important to take this into consideration when designing feeding trials with fescue seed or when evaluating clinical cases of fescue toxicosis in which concentrations of ergovaline are less than expected. Ergotism is a worldwide problem, with predisposing weather conditions frequently occurring in the northern Great Plains and northwestern regions of the United States. However, ergotism has also been reported throughout the midwestern United States and even on the Atlantic seaboard.[1,4,7,8,10]

The naturally occurring ergot alkaloid, ergonovine (also known as ergometrine or ergobasine), has been used medicinally for its oxytocic effects.[1] Synthesized ergot alkaloids, such as bromocriptine, pergolide, and cabergoline, have a variety of therapeutic applications in human and

BOX 23-3	COMMON GRASSES SUSCEPTIBLE TO *Claviceps purpurea* INFECTION

COMMON NAME	LATIN NAME
Bentgrasses and redtops	*Agrostis* spp
Blue grasses	*Poa* spp
Brome grasses	*Bromus* spp
Canary grasses	*Phalaris* spp
Cocksfoot and orchard grasses	*Dactylis* spp
Fescue grasses	*Festuca* spp
June grasses	Koeleria spp
Love grasses	*Eragrostis* spp
Quack grasses and wheat grasses	*Agropyron* spp
Rye grasses	*Lolium* spp
Timothy grasses	*Phleum* spp
Wild barleys	*Hordeum* spp
Wild oats	*Avena* spp
Wild ryes	*Elymus* spp

Data from references 1, 7, 9.

veterinary medicine, including treatment of Parkinson's disease and prolactin-secreting pituitary adenomas.[11,12] These compounds have also been used for the suppression of lactation and the regulation of the reproductive cycle in dogs and cats and Cushing's-like disease in horses.[13,14] The occurrence of clinical signs related to those of ergotism is a potential side effect of excessive therapeutic or accidental exposure to these and related compounds.

Toxicokinetics.   The broad class of compounds known as the ergot alkaloids encompasses all of the toxic principles responsible for the clinical signs of ergotism.[1-5] Ergot alkaloids are composed primarily of the ergopeptine alkaloids (ergotamine, ergocristine, ergosine, ergocryptine, ergocornine, and ergovaline) and the ergoline alkaloids (lysergic acid, lysergol, lysergic acid amide, and ergonovine). Unlike fescue toxicosis, there is less debate regarding the relative roles of the ergopeptine and ergoline alkaloids in the pathogenesis of ergotism. Most clinical signs of ergotism are attributable to the recognized pathophysiologic effects of ergopeptine alkaloids.[1,2,4,8,9] Ergotamine, ergocristine, ergosine, ergocornine, and ergocryptine are the predominant, physiologically active ergopeptides present in ergot bodies.[4,8] Unless otherwise indicated, the remaining discussion in this chapter focuses on the toxicokinetics and pharmacodynamics of ergopeptine alkaloids in animal species.

In contrast to the toxicokinetics of the ergot alkaloids in endophyte-infected fescue, there is a lack of recent information on the digestion, absorption, metabolism, and excretion of the ergot alkaloids contained in fungal sclerotia. Intestinal absorption of ergopeptine alkaloids has been reported in nonruminants.[15] Research performed in cattle has shown that, although their effects may persist for a period of time, intravenously (IV) administered ergopeptine alkaloids are rapidly cleared from the blood by the liver.[2,16] Because of their larger size, ergopeptine alkaloids undergo primarily biliary excretion, whereas the smaller ergoline alkaloids are generally excreted in urine.[15] Ergot alkaloids are not excreted in the milk of cows consuming the sclerotia of *C. purpurea.*[2]

Mechanisms of Action.   As in fescue toxicosis, the mechanisms of action of the ergopeptine alkaloids involve vasoconstriction associated with D_1 dopaminergic receptor inhibition and partial agonism of α_1-adrenergic and serotonin receptors by ergopeptine alkaloids. In addition, stimulation of D_2-dopamine receptors by ergopeptine alkaloids has been shown to decrease prolactin secretion by lactotropes located in the anterior pituitary. Vasoconstriction and hypoprolactinemia are either directly or indirectly associated with the pathogenesis of many of the clinical abnormalities noted in ergotism.[1,3,5,8-10] The sedative properties of lysergic acid amide may be mediated by a neurotransmitter imbalance in the pituitary and pineal glands involving receptors for norepinephrine, epinephrine, dopamine, serotonin, and melatonin. Uterine contraction associated with the stimulation of α_1-adrenergic receptors by some ergot alkaloids, especially ergonovine, has been proposed to play a role in producing some of the clinical signs of fescue toxicosis.[1-3]

Toxicity and Risk Factors. Ergotism can affect humans and a wide range of animal species consuming sufficient quantities of ergopeptine alkaloids in ergotized grasses or cereal grains.[1-5,8,9] Total ergot alkaloid concentrations in the sclerotia of *C. purpurea* vary considerably and have been reported to range between 2000 and 6000 mg/kg (ppm) or between 0 and almost 10,000 mg/kg (ppm), depending on the reference.[4,8] The relative amounts of the different ergopeptine alkaloids and other ergot alkaloids contained within the sclerotia of *C. purpurea* vary.[1,4,7,8] In addition, there is a wide range of clinical signs related to ergotism and a variety of risk factors that impact the development of clinical signs. As a result of this apparent variability and changes in analytic methods, no real consensus exists in the literature regarding threshold levels of total ergot alkaloids or ergopeptine alkaloids capable of causing ergotism in animals.

Some references have suggested that relatively large doses of ergot alkaloids are necessary to produce clinical disease. Agalactia and reproductive problems in horses have been reported in horses ingesting grain containing 1100 to 2600 mg/kg (ppm) of total ergot alkaloids.[18] Ergotism has been observed in cattle consuming sclerotia with total concentrations of ergot alkaloids reportedly ranging from 1300 mg/kg (ppm) to 3100 mg/kg (ppm). The duration of exposure before onset of disease in these instances appeared to vary from 2 to almost 15 weeks and, surprisingly, was independent of total ergot alkaloid concentration. Total amounts of ergot alkaloids consumed ranged from 3.7 to 8.2 g.[8] Cattle consuming rations with 0.5% ergot bodies have been reported to exhibit a summer slump–like syndrome, and dietary levels of 0.3% to 1% sclerotia have been associated with gangrenous ergotism in cattle.[4,17] Based on the cited ranges of total ergot alkaloid concentrations in sclerotia, these levels of ergot contamination are roughly equivalent to the consumption 6 to 90 ppm of ergot alkaloids in the total ration. However, these extrapolations are only estimates.[4,8] Some references have suggested that consumption of 40 to 60 mg/kg body weight of ergot alkaloids is toxic to animals.[4]

In contrast, exposure to lower concentrations of ergot alkaloids appears to produce clinical signs of ergotism under certain circumstances probably involving a variety of risk factors. Daily doses of ergot alkaloids ranging from 0.3 to 0.6 mg/kg have been associated with ergotism in cattle and sheep.[19] It has been estimated that adult cattle, if allowed to graze selectively, ingest approximately 30 mg of ergot alkaloids daily (daily dose of 0.07 mg/kg body weight) when grazing ergotized ryegrass.[9,19] Several weeks of this level of exposure represent a total dose of approximately 0.5 to 1 g of ergot alkaloids, which is expected to be associated with clinical signs of ergotism. Extensive research has not been done regarding the dietary concentrations of the primary ergopeptine alkaloids in *C. purpurea* sclerotia capable of causing ergotism. It seems logical, however, that threshold ergovaline levels associated with clinical fescue toxicosis (0.2 to 0.8 mg/kg of total ration) could serve as an approximate guideline for threshold levels of total ergopeptine alkaloid concentrations likely to produce ergotism in livestock species. A total concentration of 1.6 mg/kg (ppm) of the five primary ergopeptine alkaloids produced by *C. purpurea*, in

ergotized grass, has been associated with gangrenous ergotism in dairy cattle. Likewise, samples of a processed feed, which was incorporated into equine rations, contained 0.5 to 1.5 mg/kg (ppm) total ergopeptine alkaloids from screenings of ergotized grain, and exposure to these rations decreased lactation in mares exposed during late gestation.[7] It has recently been reported that that 0.01 mg/kg body weight per day of ergopeptine alkaloids administered to dairy cattle for 10 days during summer heat stress resulted in increased body temperature and respiratory rate with marginally decreased feed intake and milk production.[20]

As in fescue toxicosis, there do appear to be species, breed, age, gender, and physiologic state differences in susceptibility to the various clinical signs of ergotism. It has been speculated that ruminal pH values and diets favoring fermentation predispose ruminants to ergotism because of enhanced extraction of ergot alkaloids from sclerotia.[19] Swine and mice are traditionally considered to be more resistant to ergotism than other animals.[2,3,9,19] However, the risk of ergotism in animals is ultimately determined by the likelihood of exposure to a toxic dose of ergopeptine alkaloids. For instance, swine rations are normally based on cereal grains. The relative portions of potentially ergotized grains (e.g., rye, wheat, barley, oats, and triticale versus corn and soybeans) in the diet impact the risk of ergotism in this species. This situation is analogous to the historically enhanced risk of ergotism in socially disadvantaged people consuming inexpensive rye.[1-3] In grazing species, ergotized grain may represent a relatively small portion of the diet; however, ergotized grasses pose a significant risk to these animals. Concurrent exposure to endophyte-infected fescue in grazing animals increases the likelihood of clinical signs common to both ergotism and fescue toxicosis.

Seasonal variations and stages of plant growth affect the levels of ergopeptine alkaloids in ergot sclerotia. Cool, damp weather in the spring delays pollination and favors the germination and growth of *C. purpurea*. The ergopeptine alkaloid content and the size of ergot sclerotia increase as the plant grows. The species of grass affects the size and appearance of the ergot body and the relative concentration of the ergopeptine alkaloids.[1,2,4,8] No-till farming practices, shallow seeding, and failure to rotate crops favor germination of ergot sclerotia. Pasture management allowing access of livestock to infected seed heads increases the chances of ergotism in exposed animals.[2] Ergot bodies are indistinguishable in processed or pelleted cereal grain preparations, and accidental exposure to ergopeptine alkaloids is more likely when these types of feedstuffs predominate in animal diets.[2,4] Because of their decreased density, ergot bodies or their fragments may be partially removed from cereal grains using gravity tables, and consumption of grain screenings greatly increases the risk of exposure to ergopeptine alkaloids.[4]

As in fescue toxicosis, environmental conditions and animal husbandry practices have the potential to lower the minimum ergopeptine alkaloid levels necessary to produce disease. Low and high environmental temperatures predispose susceptible species to gangrenous ergotism and to a hyperthermic, summer slump–like syndrome, respectively.[1,2,4,9,18] Inadequate housing and insufficient water and supervision facilitate the development and progression of ergotism in livestock species.

Clinical Signs. Ergotism generally occurs sporadically after subacute or chronic exposure to ergopeptine alkaloids. Depending on the level of exposure and the species involved, ergotism may be associated with low or relatively high morbidity.[3,9,18] Ergotism occurs in many of the same species as fescue toxicosis, and traditionally ergotism has been divided into the gangrenous, hyperthermic, reproductive, and nervous forms, of which the first three are also associated with fescue toxicosis.[1-3] Gangrenous or cutaneous ergotism, which is identical to fescue foot, and hyperthermia, resembling summer slump, are the predominant clinical presentations of ergotism in cattle.[1-3,9,17,20] As in fescue toxicosis, decreased lactation and subfertility may also be observed in cattle exposed to ergopeptine alkaloids, but the role of these compounds in ruminant abortions remains controversial.[1,4,8,19,20] Because of the differences in grazing behavior and, therefore, reduced exposure, the clinical signs of ergotism in sheep have been reported to be mild compared to those in cattle. Affected sheep exhibit necrosis of the tip of the tongue, excessive salivation, nausea, diarrhea, lameness, and decreased lambing rates.[1,3,22] Milk production is also decreased in sheep exposed to ergot alkaloids in *C. purpurea* sclerotia.[8] "Fat necrosis," which is generally associated with several years of exposure to endophyte-infected fescue in ruminants, is not commonly reported with ergotism.

Agalactia, prolonged gestation, dystocia, abortion, retained placenta, neonatal mortality, and subfertility are generally associated with ergotism, as well as fescue toxicosis, in horses.[1,7,18,23] However, unlike endophyte-infected fescue, in which ergovaline concentrations range from 0.2 to 0.6 mg/kg (ppm), heavily ergotized grasses or cereal grains may contain much larger concentrations of ergopeptine alkaloids (up to 10,000 mg/kg, or 1%), which can cause gangrenous ergotism in horses or even death in cattle and horses.* Although not specifically reported in the literature, laminitis, heat intolerance, and other clinical abnormalities in horses, which have been associated with fescue toxicosis, logically seem possible with sufficient duration and level of exposure to ergopeptine alkaloids in ergot bodies.

Because cereal grains can be infected by *C. purpurea*, the gangrenous, hyperthermic, and reproductive forms of ergotism can also occur in species rarely exposed to endophyte-infected fescue and, therefore, not generally susceptible to fescue toxicosis, including humans. Feed refusal, decreased weight gain, agalactia, shortened gestation, neonatal mortality, abortion, and even some gangrenous lesions have been reported in swine exposed to heavily ergotized cereal grains.† In poultry, comb gangrene, along with poor growth and feathering and necrotic beaks, toes, and toenails is reported with exposure to fungal sclerotia.[2] Rabbits are extremely sensitive to the hyperthermia associated with ergot alkaloids.[1] On the other hand,

rats and mice seem to be more sensitive to the embryocidal and abortifacient effects of ergot alkaloids than other animal species.[1,2,8,19] Similarly, dogs, which like rodents are dependent on prolactin for maintenance of corpora lutea, can be aborted by therapeutic or possibly accidental exposure to ergot alkaloids.[13] The susceptibility of humans to gangrenous ergotism is well documented and may be associated with abnormal cutaneous sensation as well as dry gangrene of the distal extremities.[1-3]

The convulsive or nervous form of ergotism was previously reported to be more common than the other forms of ergotism in carnivora, horses, and sheep.[8] However, the existence of convulsive disease caused by *C. purpurea* is currently considered questionable.[1,2,6] "Convulsive" or "nervous" ergotism may be confused with toxicoses associated with tremorgens, including those produced by *Claviceps paspali*. Alternatively, nervous system abnormalities, such as ataxia and confusion, may actually be produced by the ingestion of ergot alkaloids related to lysergic acid diethylamide (LSD) and may not be related to tremorgenic disease.[1-3]

Clinical Pathology. The clinical pathologic alterations associated with ergot alkaloid exposure have been reviewed in detail in the section on Fescue Toxicosis in this chapter.

Lesions. The gross and microscopic lesions in the distal extremities observed with gangrenous ergotism are indistinguishable from those of fescue foot depicted in the section on Fescue Toxicosis in this chapter.[1,2,4,9] Because of the high concentrations of ergopeptine alkaloids in fungal sclerotia, visceral structures, including the intestines, liver, kidneys, heart, and even the brain may exhibit abnormalities related to the vascular changes occurring with ergotism. Deaths in cattle have been related to gastrointestinal ulceration and perforation.[9] The fetal and placental lesions associated with ergopeptine alkaloid exposure in late gestational mares are identical to those seen in equine fescue toxicosis.[18,23]

Diagnostic Testing. Diagnostic testing for ergotism currently involves detection of *C. purpurea* sclerotia, which may require feed microscopy in ground or milled feeds, and the determination of forage, hay, or processed feed concentrations of ergotamine, ergocristine, ergosine, ergocornine, and ergocryptine concentrations by high-performance liquid chromatography.[24] Analysis for ergovaline should also be performed if the forage or hay contains fescue. The analysis of biologic tissues for the presence of ergot alkaloids or their metabolites has not been developed to the same degree in ergotism as it has in fescue toxicosis. However, the same type of testing, particularly in urine, may be applicable.

Treatment. As in fescue toxicosis, the key to successful treatment of ergotism in animal species is the early recognition of the clinical signs.

Ergotism is rare in human populations but most likely is underdiagnosed in animals. The most logical approach to managing ergotism is the removal of animals from the source of ergopeptine alkaloids. The early signs of ergotism are often reversible, with the cutaneous vascular effects of

---

*References 1, 3, 8, 9, 20, 24.
†References 1, 2, 4, 8, 19, 21.

the ergopeptine alkaloids usually subsiding shortly after removal from ergot-contaminated pastures, hay, grains, or processed feeds.[1,2,4] The treatment of more severe cases of ergotism and its sequelae in cattle, horses, and other animals should follow the therapeutic approaches outlined for fescue toxicosis.

Prognosis. As in fescue toxicosis, the prognosis for recovery from ergotism is dependent on the severity of the clinical signs at the time of removal from ergopeptine alkaloid exposure and the prevention of sequelae such as dystocia in mares.

Prevention and Control. The prevention and control of ergotism (e.g., fescue toxicosis) in animals may be the best approach to this disease. Logically, the keys to prophylaxis are the recognition of the potential for exposure to ergotized grasses or cereal grain and an understanding of the risk factors that may predispose animals to the development of clinical signs of ergotism. This is particularly true for pregnant mares and sows, for which knowledge of breeding dates, confirmed pregnancy diagnoses, and careful monitoring of mammary development are all critical steps in the identification of susceptible individuals and the early recognition of the disease.

Unlike fescue toxicosis, ergotism generally occurs sporadically, and there is usually adequate access to sufficient quantities of nonergotized grasses and cereal grains. Nonetheless, pastures, hays, and grains should be periodically monitored for the presence of *C. purpurea* sclerotia. The analysis of suspect grasses or grains for ergopeptine alkaloid concentrations may be advisable. *C. purpurea* infection of cereal grains can be reduced by the use of clean seed, the rotation of crops, and the deep cultivation of ergot-resistant grains, such as wheat, barley, and oats.[2] The incorporation of grain screenings in animal feeds should be avoided. The U.S. Department of Agriculture has a tolerance level of 0.3% ergot sclerotia in grain, and it has been recommended that ergot body concentrations be kept to less than 0.1% in the grain portion of the diet to reduce the risk of ergotism in animals.[2,4]

In situations involving diagnosed ergotism in mares, the prophylactic approaches outlined for fescue toxicosis may be applicable. In environments that favor the germination and growth of *C. purpurea* or when the risk of the incorporation of ergotized grains in the ration is increased, the use of a variety of binders to prevent the absorption of ergopeptine alkaloids has been advocated. However, as in fescue toxicosis, the in vivo efficacy of these products remains questionable.

FESCUE

Tim J. Evans, George E. Rottinghaus, and Stan W. Casteel

Synonyms. *Fescue toxicosis* or, more specifically, *"tall fescue toxicosis,"* is associated with several disease syndromes in multiple animal species. Fescue toxicosis is observed clinically as fescue foot, summer slump, summer syndrome, summer fescue toxicosis, and fat necrosis or lipomatosis in cattle and other species.[1,2]

Sources. The potentially misleading descriptive term, fescue toxicosis, is derived from the close association between the development of the clinical signs of these syndromes and the ingestion of tall fescue grass (*Festuca arundinacea* Shreber) from pastures or hay.[1-3] Tall fescue grass, especially the extremely vigorous Kentucky 31 cultivar, is a perennial cool season grass growing on more than 35 million acres in predominantly the upper southeastern and lower midwestern regions of the United States.[2,3] It is estimated that in North America tall fescue grass is one of the primary forages for more than 8.5 million cattle and 700,000 horses.[3,4] Unlike other typical pasture grasses, tall fescue is not associated with toxicoses related to nitrate accumulation, cyanogenesis, and photosensitization.[2]

As part of a symbiotic relationship with tall fescue grass, the fungal endophyte, *Neotyphodium coenophialum* (formerly known as *Acremonium coenophialum* and *Epichlöe typhina)*, grows entirely within the intercellular spaces of the leaf sheaths, stems, and caryopses or seeds (highest concentrations) of *F. arundinacea* and possibly other grass species.[1,2,4] It is generally well accepted that tall fescue grass or fungal endophyte interactions play an essential role in the etiology of fescue-associated disease syndromes and the survivability of fescue grass under adverse conditions.[1-4]

Toxicokinetics. Tall fescue, with or without endophyte, contains a multitude of potentially toxic chemical compounds. Pyrrolizidine alkaloids, such as loline, *N*-formyl loline, and *N*-acetyl loline, and the diphenanthrene alkaloids, perloline and perlolidine, have been found in endophyte-free and endophyte-infected tall fescue. However, these potential toxins, along with the vasoactive amine, halostachine, and various other compounds found in fescue, are considered to be relatively minor contributors to the pathogenesis of fescue toxicosis.[1,2] Ergot alkaloids, composed primarily of the ergoline alkaloids (lysergic acid, lysergol, lysergic acid amide, and ergonovine) and the ergopeptine alkaloids (ergovaline, ergosine, ergotamine, ergocristine, ergocryptine, and ergocornine), have been suggested to be the toxic principals responsible for most of the clinical signs associated with fescue toxicosis.[1,2,4-6]

There has been some debate regarding the relative roles of the ergopeptine and ergoline alkaloids in the pathogenesis of fescue toxicosis.[4,6] The more traditional view is that most of the clinical signs of fescue toxicosis are attributable to the recognized pathophysiologic effects of ergopeptine alkaloids, of which ergovaline is the predominant compound in endophyte-infected *Festuca.*[1,2] The injection of the semisynthetic ergopeptine alkaloid, bromocriptine, into late gestational pregnant pony mares simulated fescue toxicosis in these animals.[7] Grass and hay concentrations of ergovaline have been reported to correlate well with development of the clinical signs of fescue toxicosis.[1,2,5,8] In vitro studies with ergovaline have confirmed the ability of this ergopeptine alkaloid to mediate the predominant pathophysiologic effects associated with the clinical signs of fescue toxicosis.[9,10]

Some researchers have suggested that the ergoline alkaloids play a more important role in the pathogenesis of fescue toxicosis than was traditionally thought. Passive immunization of cattle exposed to endophyte-infected tall fescue, with monoclonal antibodies for the lysergic acid moiety common to the ergoline alkaloids (some ergopeptine alkaloid cross reactivity), prevented the suppression of prolactin usually associated with fescue toxicosis.[11] Although attempts to simulate fescue toxicosis in calves with intravenous infusion of ergonovine were unsuccessful, the vasoconstrictive properties of ergonovine and lysergic acid amide have been demonstrated in vitro.[12-14] The results of one study indicated that observed changes in feed intake and reduced weight gain in rats exposed to endophyte-infected fescue were independent of concentrations of ergovaline.[15] In addition, other data suggest that ergoline alkaloids are the primary ergot alkaloids absorbed from the gastrointestinal tract of ruminants.[1,6]

Given the number and diversity of the different ergot alkaloids, it is not surprising that significant data gaps still exist regarding the toxicokinetics of this class of compounds in animal species. The results of ongoing research may eventually elucidate the differences, if any, between the fates of these compounds in ruminant and monogastric species. The results of these studies should also provide additional data regarding the gastrointestinal breakdown, absorption, metabolism, and excretion of the various types of ergot alkaloids.

Intestinal absorption of the ergot alkaloids has been reported in nonruminants.[16] Investigators have speculated that the ruminal breakdown of fescue-associated ergot alkaloids in cattle results in ergoline alkaloid-type compounds.[1,6] The absorption of the ergoline alkaloids was more efficient than the absorption of ergopeptine alkaloids in a recently reported in vitro study, and the absorption of lysergic acid and lysergol were shown to be greater across the ruminal than omasal epithelium.[6] Research performed in cattle has shown that, although the effects of ergot alkaloids may persist for a period of time, IV-administered ergopeptine alkaloids are rapidly cleared from the blood by the liver.[1,17] In another study, urinary ergot alkaloid concentrations began to increase or decrease accordingly within 12 hours of introduction of cattle to or withdrawal of cattle from endophyte-infected fescue pastures.[18] As expected, the metabolism and excretion of ergot alkaloids, at least in nonruminant species, appear most likely to be based on the molecular weight of these compounds. The ergopeptine alkaloids (>450 Da) undergo primarily biliary excretion, whereas the smaller ergoline alkaloids (<350 Da) are generally excreted in the urine.[16,18] Recently, it was found that 90% of the ergot alkaloids, as detected by an enzyme-linked immunosorbent assay (ELISA) for the lysergic acid moiety, were excreted in the urine of steers grazing *Neotyphodium*-infected fescue pastures.[18] Extrapolation of the nonruminant toxicokinetic data to these results suggests that ergoline alkaloids were the products of digestive breakdown or hepatic metabolism in cattle.[6,16,18]

Mechanisms of Action. The pathogeneses of the thermoregulatory and circulatory disturbances, the alterations

in nutrient intake, absorption, and metabolism, the decreased lactation or agalactia, and the impaired reproductive function associated with fescue toxicosis are generally thought to involve ergot alkaloid-mediated interactions with a variety of receptor types. These ergot alkaloid/receptor interactions lead to vasoconstriction, suppression of prolactin secretion, and other physiologic effects.* Vasoconstriction, which is associated with D_1-dopaminergic receptor inhibition and partial agonism of α_1-adrenergic and serotonin receptors by ergot alkaloids, results in hyperthermia from inadequate heat dissipation from the body surface and dry gangrene, necrotic fat, and abortion or altered placental function from impaired circulation to the extremities, abdominal and pelvic fat stores, and the placenta.†

Stimulation of D_2-dopamine receptors by ergopeptine alkaloids, including ergovaline, has been shown to decrease prolactin secretion by lactotropes located in the anterior pituitary.‡ Prolactin is involved in the endocrine regulation of many physiologic processes, including lactogenesis, lipid and carbohydrate metabolism, maintenance of electrolyte balance, immune function, and steroidogenesis. Lactational abnormalities related to hypoprolactinemia are one of the hallmark features of ergot alkaloid exposure in animal species.[1,2,19-22] Prolonged gestation in mares may be related to hypoprolactinemia-induced alterations in uterofetoplacental steroid metabolism or may be mediated by a speculated direct or indirect inhibition of corticotropes in the fetal anterior pituitary by ergot alkaloids.[19]

Decreased feed intake and alterations in gut motility and nutrient absorption may be associated with interactions between ergot alkaloids and D_1, D_2, and other dopaminergic receptor types located within the central or peripheral nervous systems.[19,20] Impaired adaptations to seasonal changes in photoperiod and temperature have also been observed with fescue toxicosis. These effects, as well as the sedative properties of lysergic acid amide, may be mediated by a neurotransmitter imbalance within the pituitary and pineal glands, involving interactions between ergot alkaloids and the receptors for norepinephrine, epinephrine, dopamine, serotonin, and melatonin.[1,21,22] Uterine contraction, associated with the stimulation of α_1-adrenergic receptors by some ergot alkaloids, has also been proposed to play a role in producing some of the clinical signs of fescue toxicosis.[1,20]

Toxicity and Risk Factors. Because of the widespread distribution of dopaminergic, adrenergic, and serotonin receptors within animals, fescue toxicosis can affect a wide range of animal species consuming sufficient quantities of ergot alkaloids in endophyte-infected tall fescue pasture or hay.[1,20] Cattle, sheep, and horses are the domestic species that appear to be most sensitive to the effects of fescue "toxicosis," but various laboratory animal species and wild ruminants have also been shown to be sensitive to the effects of ergovaline and other ergot alkaloids. Ergovaline concentrations in fescue grass generally range between 200

---

*References 1, 2, 4, 7, 9, 10, 12-14, 19-22.
†References 1, 2, 4, 7, 9, 19-22.
‡References 1, 2, 9, 10, 12-15, 19, 21-23.

and 600 μg/kg (200 to 600 ppb), with seed head concentrations generally exceeding 1000 ppb (1 ppm). Levels of ergovaline as low as 200 ppb in the total ration have been associated with the clinical signs of "summer fescue toxicosis" in heat-stressed steers.[1,8] Dietary levels of ergovaline as low as 150 ppb (approximately 6.8 μg of ergovaline/kg of body weight) have been reported with reduced growth rate and lower blood levels of prolactin in lambs.[1,2,24] Fescue foot in cattle and sheep has been produced experimentally with levels of ergovaline in the diet ranging from 400 to 750 ppb in cattle and from 500 to 800 ppb in sheep.[25] Clinical cases of agalactia have been observed in mares ingesting fescue-contaminated hay containing 100 ppb or more ergovaline.[26]

There do appear to be species-, breed-, age-, gender-, and physiologic state–dependent differences in susceptibility to the clinical signs of fescue toxicosis in animals. The absence of placental lactogen production during equine gestation appears to predispose mares to the development of agalactia in cases of fescue toxicosis.[19,21,27] The prolonged gestation, alterations in placental endocrine function, and fetal abnormalities associated with exposure to Neotyphodium-infected tall fescue appear to be unique to mares.[1,2,19,21,27-29] Although exposure to endophyte-infected tall fescue has been implicated in laminitis and hyperthermia in horses, the development of fescue foot, summer slump, and fat necrosis have been described primarily in cattle and other ruminant species.* Breed differences are reported to exist in the susceptibility of cattle to fescue foot and summer slump. Brahman-type cattle are apparently more likely than European breeds to develop gangrene of the extremities associated with fescue foot, whereas cattle breeds of European origin may be more predisposed to ergot alkaloid–related heat stress.[1,2,4] Young animals are obviously more likely than mature animals to have impaired growth associated with exposure to the ergot alkaloids in endophyte-infected fescue, and puberty was delayed in heifers raised entirely on endophyte-infected pasture.[1,21,22] Although ergot alkaloid–induced hypoprolactemia has been associated with reduced libido in rams and decreased gonadal and accessory sex gland weights in rodents, the relative lack of data regarding the adverse effects of fescue toxicosis on male fertility as opposed to female reproductive efficiency implies that gender plays a role in predisposing individual animals to the reproductive clinical effects of fescue toxicosis or, at least, the ease of detection of those clinical effects.[1,22] Male and female ruminants, however, both appear to be susceptible to the adverse effects of ergot alkaloid exposure related to an enhanced intolerance to heat stress.[1,2,4,8,22] Lactation and pregnancy, particularly in mares, appear to be the physiologic states most susceptible to the effects of ergot alkaloid exposure.[1,2,19,27-29]

Seasonal variations, stages of plant growth, and pasture management can affect the levels of ergot alkaloids in endophyte-infected fescue. Reflecting the synergistic nature of fescue-endophyte interactions, endophyte infection rates are generally less than 10% or greater than 80%. Adverse

climatic conditions usually considered stressful to nonfescue grasses are more likely to favor the growth of Neotyphodium-infected fescue, rather than endophyte-free tall fescue.[1,2,4] Reflecting seasonal variations and stage of fescue growth-dependent interactions with Neotyphodium, ergovaline concentrations are highest in the seed heads (followed by the stems with leaf sheaths and leaf blades) in mid- to late June. In addition, peak levels of ergovaline may vary from year to year and appear to increase with nitrogen fertilization.[1,2,8] Low grazing pressure may actually lead to higher ergovaline concentrations in pastures, and infrequent mowing may enhance the chances of ergot alkaloid exposure in grazing animals syndromes.[1,2,22,33,34]

Environmental conditions and animal husbandry practices have the potential to lower the minimum ergot alkaloid levels necessary to produce disease, thereby predisposing animal populations to fescue toxicosis or exacerbating the clinical signs observed with this syndrome. The minimum dietary levels of ergovaline impairing the adaptation of livestock species to hypothermic and hyperthermic environments are dependent on environmental temperature and humidity. The clinical signs of summer slump in cattle and other ruminants are more likely to be induced at ambient temperatures greater than 32° C, especially with high humidity. In contrast, cattle and sheep are predisposed to fescue foot at lower environmental temperatures.* Differences in normal feeding and management practices, reflected in increased levels of exposure, may predispose beef cattle to be impacted more dramatically by fescue toxicosis than are dairy cattle. Additionally, suboptimal animal husbandry practices, such as a lack of ample water and shelter, and inadequate nutrient supplementation, observation, and reproductive management predispose animals to more severe clinical signs and prevent the early recognition of the disease syndromes.[1,2,22,33,34]

Clinical Signs. *Fescue foot*, indistinguishable from the dry gangrene of the extremities associated with ergotism in cattle and sheep, is generally associated with exposure to ergot alkaloids under hypothermic conditions and normally occurs in late fall or winter. Fescue foot has been reported to develop from one to several weeks after introduction to tall fescue hay or pasture and most commonly affects the hind limbs, frequently beginning in the left hind leg. In its early stages, the condition is characterized by swelling and reddening at the coronary band, knuckling of the pastern joint, arching of the back, and shifting of weight from one hind limb to the other. In more severe cases of fescue foot, animals appear unthrifty, with progressive lameness, increased swelling above the hoof, and ischemic necrosis of the hooves, associated phalanges, and possibly other extremities, such as the tips of the ears and tail.† Secondary infections, with bone and joint involvement, may occur in some cases.

Summer slump is probably the most common and economically significant syndrome associated with fescue toxi-

---

*References 1, 2, 4, 21-23, 25, 30-32.

*References 1, 2, 8, 21, 22, 25, 32.
†References 1, 2, 4, 25, 26, 32.

cosis in livestock.[1-4,21,22] Summer slump results from alterations in the thermoregulatory ability and the endocrine milieu of affected animals and is related to reduced cutaneous heat transfer and neurotransmitter and hormonal imbalances.[1,2,4,21,22] In cattle and sheep, this syndrome is characterized by decreased feed intake, weight gain, and growth rate, reductions in milk production, delayed shedding and "bleaching" of the hair coat, immunosuppression, and impaired reproductive function, as indicated by reduced conception and calving rates and delays in the onset of puberty. Clinically affected animals exhibit lethargy, diarrhea, hyperthermia, tachypnea, and alterations in behavior, spending less time grazing and more time standing in the shade or in ponds.[1,2,4,21,22] It has recently been reported that the exacerbated poor performance in beef cattle under the conditions of heat stress, commonly seen with exposure to endophyte-infected fescue, is associated with the disruption of the normal patterns of diurnal core temperature and impaired follicle and corpus luteum development.[35,36]

Fat necrosis has been observed in a variety of ruminant species and is associated with the presence of necrotic fat in the abdominal and pelvic cavities. Fat necrosis, or lipomatosis, requires several grazing seasons of exposure to heavily fertilized endophyte-infected fescue and is probably asymptomatic in many cases. Masses of necrotic fat can frequently be palpated transrectally in affected cattle. Lipomatosis becomes clinically significant if it is associated with gastrointestinal disease, such as chronic bloating and colonic constriction, or if masses of necrotic adipose tissue are obstructing the genitourinary tract, resulting in dystocia or nephrosis and uremia.[1,2,4,23]

Equine fescue toxicosis is most commonly recognized as a disease syndrome of mares during late gestation and early postpartum period. The clinical signs of fescue toxicosis in pregnant mares grazing on endophyte-infected fescue pasture are almost exclusively limited to reproductive function. These signs include agalactia, prolonged gestation, abortion, dystocia, fetal asphyxia, weakness, dysmaturity and mortality, and placental abnormalities, such as premature placental separation, thickening and edema of fetal membranes, and retained placenta.* The signs of impending parturition in pregnant mares, such as the rapid increase in udder development and the commonly observed "waxing" or accumulation of colostrum at the teat orifices, are often minimal in ergot alkaloid-exposed, late gestational mares. These foalings are frequently unexpected and, therefore, unattended.[2,19,33,34] Fetal dysmaturity and increased fetal size associated with maternal exposure to endophyte-infected fescue contribute to the development of dystocias and the subsequent complications in mares and foals. Potentially life-threatening maternal tissue trauma, metritis, septicemia, endotoxemia, and laminitis are frequent sequelae to fescue toxicosis in mares.[33,34] Failure of passive transfer and neonatal septicemia and decreased viability commonly occur in foals from agalactic mares with a history of exposure to *Neotyphodium*-infected fescue pasture or hay. Exposure to endophyte-infected fescue has also been associated with an increased incidence of laminitis and postexercise disturbances in thermoregulation within equine populations. Irregularities in estrous cycles, prolongation of winter anestrus and the vernal transition period, and increased occurrence of early embryonic death have also been reported in mares exposed to *N. coenophialum*.[30,31,33,34]

Clinical Pathology. Several significant variations have been noted in the hemograms, routine serum biochemical profiles, and other blood, plasma, and serum parameters of beef cattle and other ruminants chronically exposed to endophyte-infected fescue pastures. The average number of erythrocytes appears to be increased, whereas the mean corpuscular hemoglobin and volume values and the average number of eosinophils are decreased in exposed cattle. Additionally, cattle grazing *Neotyphodium*-infected tall fescue pastures have decreased serum levels of cholesterol, globulin, and total protein; suppressed activities of alanine aminotransferase (ALT) and alkaline phosphatase (ALP); and increased levels of bilirubin and creatinine in the serum.[37] Serum copper levels in cattle grazing endophyte-infected tall fescue pastures are routinely decreased, reflecting the lower amounts of copper accumulated in fescue infected with *N. coenophialum*.[1,37,38] Although prolactin assays are not routinely done in most veterinary diagnostic laboratories, hypoprolactinemia is a consistent finding and occurs within several days in a dose-dependent fashion in cattle and other ruminants exposed to ergot alkaloids.* Total leukocyte numbers may be increased or decreased in cattle grazing endophyte-infected fescue pastures, and this lack of a consistent pattern may be a reflection of the wide variety of pathophysiologic effects and sequelae, such as infection, inflammation, and stress associated with ergot alkaloid exposure in livestock species.[1,37]

Any significant variations from normal values in the hemograms or routine biochemical profiles of foaling mares exposed to endophyte-infected fescue are most likely reflections of tissue trauma, inflammation, infection, septicemia, endotoxemia, or stress associated with the occurrence of dystocia or retention of fetal membranes. Despite nasogastric intubation with high-quality colostrum, blood IgG levels are frequently decreased in foals whose dams were exposed to endophyte-infected fescue during late pregnancy.[33] Foals of mares with fescue toxicosis may exhibit abnormalities in their hemograms or biochemical profiles if dystocia-related trauma or infection secondary to diagnosed failure of passive transfer has occurred.[1,2,19,33,34] Fescue toxicosis is associated with alterations in circulating levels of several hormones for which assays are available in some diagnostic and research laboratory settings. Exposure of late gestational mares (after day 300 of gestation) to ergot alkaloids consistently results in significant decreases in plasma or serum levels of prolactin, radioimmunoassayable progestins, and relaxin, a sensitive indicator of placental function in the mare.† In conjunction with hypoprolactinemia, the calcium concentrations of the minimal mammary secretions present in agalactic mares

---

*References 1, 2, 7, 19, 21, 33, 34.

*References 1, 2, 4, 21, 22, 24, 37.
†References 1, 2, 7, 19, 21, 27, 28, 33, 34, 39, 40.

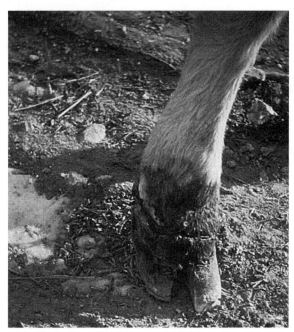

Fig. 23-2 The lower extremity of a cow with fescue foot. The pastern is swollen and contains an area of necrotic tissue. A line of demarcation exists where the deformed hoof is separating from the coronary band.

seem to rarely exceed 50 ppm.[26] Reportedly increased levels of circulating radioimmunoassayable total estrogens in ergot alkaloid–exposed pregnant mares appear to be less consistent clinical pathologic findings.[34,39,40] Plasma levels of radioimmunoassayable progestins, cortisol, and tri-iodothyronine are decreased in the foals of mares grazing endophyte-infected tall fescue pastures.[29,33]

Lesions. In severe cases of fescue foot, there is usually a distinct line of demarcation between necrotic and viable skin and underlying tissues (Fig. 23-2). Ergot alkaloid–induced tissue necrosis and sloughing are associated with vascular changes distinguished microscopically by perivascular edema and hemorrhages, the thickening of blood vessel walls, and vascular fibrosis.[1,2,25,32] In some complicated cases of fescue foot, osteomyelitic changes and lesions consistent with septic arthritis may be present.

Fat necrosis occurs in ruminants chronically exposed to ergot alkaloids and is often evident within the mesentery surrounding the intestines. Necrotic fat appears grossly as hard, caseous, yellowish, or chalky white nodules or masses of adipose tissue. Microscopically, lipomatosis is characterized by focally extensive areas of adipocytes undergoing coagulative necrosis, with occasional foci of macrophages and saponification.[1,4,23]

Prolonged gestation in mares exposed to *Neotyphodium*-infected tall fescue grass or hay is often associated with perinatal mortality. Grossly, these deceased, overmature foals are larger with overgrown hooves, irregular dental eruption, decreased muscle mass, and flexor tendon laxity. Histologically, the thyroid glands from the foals of mares grazing endophyte-infected fescue may exhibit enlarged thyroid

follicles distended with colloid, and other tissues may demonstrate microscopic changes consistent with inflammation, infection, and sepsis secondary to failure of passive transfer.[1,33,34] The fetal membranes from ergot alkaloid–exposed mares are grossly thickened because of edema, and increased cellularity and connective tissue have been reported.[33,41] Dystocia, retention of fetal membranes, and subsequent laminitis have been associated with mortality in ergot alkaloid–exposed mares, and gross and microscopic changes reflect the trauma, inflammation, infection, and sepsis related to these sequelae of fescue toxicosis.[33,34,40]

Diagnostic Testing. Diagnostic testing for fescue toxicosis encompasses detection of *N. coenophialum* in plant tissues or seeds, determination of forage or hay concentrations of ergovaline, or the analysis of biological tissues for the presence of ergot alkaloids or their metabolites. Because endophyte infection of tall fescue is not visibly distinguishable, a variety of analytic techniques have been described for the detection of endophyte in the stems, leaf sheaths, and seeds of tall fescue. Agricultural extension personnel or area agronomists should be consulted before sample collection for such analyses. It is generally recommended that approximately 30 sample-sites/field (5 sample-sites/acre) of forage or seeds or 2 ounces of stored seed should be collected. Forage or seeds from fields should be gathered between May and December. Specifically with regard to forage samples, three stems per sample-site should be cut to fit within a test tube half-filled with water.[34] A variety of staining protocols, including a 0.5% solution of rose bengal in 5% aqueous ethanol, or other procedures, such as ELISA methods or tissue-print immunoblotting techniques, can be used to detect *N. coenophialum* elements in submitted samples.[2,4,33,34]

The advent of genetically modified, nontoxigenic ("friendly"), endophyte-containing tall fescue and the high incidence of endophyte infection in flourishing tall fescue pastures, along with the lack of direct evidence for animal consumption of endophyte-infected tall fescue, limit the diagnostic usefulness of endophyte testing for fescue toxicosis. The determination of ergovaline by ELISA or high-performance liquid chromatography (HPLC), although similarly limited by the lack of evidence confirming ingestion by livestock species, has the advantage over endophyte testing in that an actual toxic principle associated with the development of the clinical signs of fescue toxicosis is detected in forages and seeds.[1,2,8,33] Because the clinical signs of ergotism can be indistinguishable from those of fescue toxicosis and fescue seed heads can be ergotized, analyses for the other ergopeptine alkaloids normally associated with ergot may be advisable to get a more accurate appreciation of the level of total ergopeptine alkaloid exposure. This is particularly important when seeds, forage, or hay containing fescue seed heads is submitted.

As debate exists regarding the role of the various classes of ergot alkaloids in the etiology of fescue toxicosis, it would be argued by some researchers that low ergovaline levels in submitted samples may not necessarily eliminate fescue toxicosis as the cause of suboptimal performance, lameness, reproductive problems, or other disease syndromes in livestock species.* ELISA testing for urinary excretion of ergot alkaloids is approaching commercial availability and has recently been proposed as a sensitive and reliable dose-dependent diagnostic tool for use in cattle with possible exposure to endophyte-infected fescue pastures or hay.[42] Because circulating ergopeptine alkaloids are eliminated almost immediately from the blood and are "masked" from detection, this analytic technique, if performed within 24 to 48 hours of animal removal from suspect pasture or hay, may provide a method of definitively confirming ergot alkaloid exposure in cattle, and, potentially, other livestock species.[1,17,42,43] Ongoing research is attempting to identify the specific compounds in urine detected by this ELISA for the lysergic acid moiety (Hill NS: Personal communication, 2001).

Treatment.   The key to successful treatment of fescue toxicosis in livestock species is the early recognition of the clinical signs. The most logical approach to managing fescue toxicosis, particularly the summer slump syndrome in cattle in its earliest stages, is the removal of animals from the source of endophyte-infected fescue. Likewise, the early signs of fescue foot are often reversible, and the cutaneous vascular effects of the ergot alkaloids have been reported to subside within a week of removal from endophyte-infected fescue pastures. However, the lack of alternative forages and sources of hay in many areas may make withdrawal from endophyte-infected fescue an impractical therapeutic approach.[1,2,4,22] In geographic regions where grasses free of toxigenic *N. coenophialum* are often unavailable, the use of a variety of binders to prevent the absorption of ergot alkaloids has been advocated; however, the in vivo efficacy of these products remains questionable (Rottinghaus GE: Personal communication, 2001).[22]

Nutrient supplementation, primarily in the form of increased dietary energy, protein, amino acids (arginine), and/or trace elements (copper), has been used, with limited success, to ameliorate the effects of ergot alkaloids in cattle. Although the administration of ivermectin and thiamine to ergot alkaloid-exposed beef cattle has been reported to be of some therapeutic benefit to these animals, supplementation with selenium and implantation with progesterone and/or estrogen implants are of questionable value in improving the feed efficiency of beef cattle grazing endophyte-infected fescue.[2,4,13,22,43] Immunomodulation with antibody formation to the lysergic acid moiety has been used experimentally in passive and active immunization schemes to treat or prevent the clinical signs associated with fescue toxicosis and may have practical implications in the future.[2,11,44]

D_2 receptor antagonists, such as metoclopramide and pinquidone, the α_1-adrenergic antagonist, prazosin, and α_1-adrenergic and serotonin receptor blockers, such as phenoxybenzamine, have shown some clinical or experimental efficacy in decreasing the clinical signs of fescue toxicosis in ruminants. The need for individual animal administration, the lack of approval for use in food animal species, potential side effects, and potential drug residue concerns, however, limit the practicality of these therapeutic approaches in most herd situations.[1,22,39] Although its use has been associated with nervousness and hyperexcitability, metoclopramide (15 mg/kg by mouth [PO] 3 times weekly) has been utilized in instances in which treatment or prevention of fescue toxicosis in particularly valuable individual animals not intended for human consumption has been warranted.[2,4,39] The inflammation and secondary infections often seen with fescue foot, as well as the impaired immune function associated with summer slump, may require the appropriate use of antiinflammatory medications or antibiotics in individual animals.

As in other animal species, successful treatment of fescue toxicosis in horses is dependent on the early recognition of the clinical signs and, particularly in the case of pregnant mares, careful preparturturient monitoring and assistance during foaling.[33,34] Because of the severity of the clinical signs, the delay in cessation of clinical effects following termination of exposure, and the failure of some owners to recognize the presence of endophyte-infected fescue pasture or hay, withdrawal of pregnant mares from ergot alkaloid exposure is an often impractical and ineffective therapeutic approach.[1,2,33,34] As in cattle, the in vivo efficacy of ergot alkaloid binders has not been clearly demonstrated in mares[22] (Rottinghaus GE: Personal communication, 2001).

Likewise, the therapeutic or prophylactic benefits of increased dietary energy content, selenium supplementation, and phenothiazine administration to pregnant mares showing signs of fescue toxicosis are doubtful.[2,19,33]

Because of the economic value and emotional attachment associated with horses and the life-threatening nature of the potential complications of ergot alkaloid exposure, a variety of compounds have been proposed for the individual treatment of mares with prolonged gestation or agalactia associated with exposure to endophyte-infected fescue. Domperidone (1.1 mg/kg PO once a day [SID]), sulpiride (3.3 mg/kg PO SID), perphenazine (0.3 to 0.5 mg/kg PO twice daily [BID]), and acepromazine (20 mg/horse intramuscularly [IM] four times a day [QID]), the actions of which are mediated through D_2 receptor antagonism, have all been reportedly used successfully in the treatment of agalactia in ergot alkaloid–exposed mares.* The rauwolfian alkaloid reserpine (2.5 to 5 mg per 450-kg horse SID), through the depletion of brain depots of dopamine, serotonin, and norepinephrine, has also been effective in treatment of agalactia in mares with a history of ergot of alkaloid exposure.[33,34,40,45] Domperidone is effective for the treatment of ergot alkaloid–associated prolonged gestation in mares. Decreased circulating levels of immunoassayable progestins and prolactin, measured in bromocriptine-treated pony mares exhibiting prolonged gestation with agalactia, rapidly increased after the initiation of domperidone therapy. These domperidone-treated pony mares experienced uneventful parturitions with the birth of normal offspring. Although a small number of animals were used experimentally, there were no similar significant alterations in the endocrine parameters of pregnant pony mares treated with reserpine, and these mares experienced dystocia with neonatal mortality of one foal.[40,45]

---

*References 4, 6, 11, 15, 34, 42.

*References 2, 7, 19, 33, 34, 39, 40, 45.

In contrast with domperidone therapy, which does not cross the blood-brain barrier, and sulpiride treatment, in which adverse effects are rare, the use of perphenazine in horses has occasionally been associated with extrapyramidal side effects, such as excitability, hyperesthesia, and increased muscle tone.[19,33,34,39] Diphenhydramine has been used therapeutically for these adverse reactions.[34] Domperidone administration has been associated with excessive dripping of milk and the loss of colostral antibodies, and some horses treated with reserpine have been observed with prolonged sedation, diarrhea, and hypotension.[34,40,45] These adverse effects have been managed successfully by dose adjustment, discontinuation of administration, and, in the case of domperidone, nasogastric intubation of foals with high-quality colostrum to prevent failure of passive transfer. With the therapeutic or prophylactic use of domperidone in pregnant mares, calcium concentrations in mammary secretions increase rapidly after daily administration of domperidone and are no longer useful as predictors of impending parturition.[26] Regarding the medicolegal aspects of treating fescue toxicosis in mares, acepromazine is approved for use in the horse, and domperidone is approaching approval and commercial availability. Perphenazine and reserpine are human pharmacologic agents used for the treatment of psychoses (perphenazine and reserpine) and hypertension (reserpine), and the recognized side effects of these drugs should also be taken into consideration before prescribing their use in clinically affected mares.[34,40]

The severe complications of fescue toxicosis in pregnant mares, including dystocias and neonatal disease, often require intensive therapeutic management. Veterinary intervention in equine dystocias ranges from manual manipulations to cesarean sections. Anesthesia, intravenous fluids, antiinflammatory and antibiotic medications, and prolonged intrauterine therapy are often necessary in these clinical situations. Parturient trauma, fetal membrane retention, and laminitis are additional maternal sequelae to fescue toxicosis, which may require surgical correction or long-term treatment.[33,34,46] Fetal complications from fescue toxicosis, such as dysmaturity and neonatal septicemia related to failure of passive transfer, require intensive nursing care and monitoring, transfusion with plasma, and administration of intravenous fluids, antibiotics, and other medications. Other potential sequelae related to sepsis and neonatal stress may include gastric ulceration, urachal patency and other umbilical abnormalities, joint infections, and pneumonia.[34,47]

Perphenazine has been used with some success to advance seasonal cyclicity in pony mares exposed to bromocriptine.[48] The potential efficacies of domperidone and sulpiride for the stimulation of normal cyclic behavior in anestrous or transitional mares, even in the absence of endophyte-infected fescue, may involve interactions with ambient temperature and may be best demonstrated in warmer environments.[49] Given the critical nature of early foaling dates in intensive breeding management systems, the use of perphenazine, domperidone, or sulpiride may be indicated to treat delayed or irregular cycling related to ergot alkaloid exposure, especially in the southeastern United States. In less intense horse breeding systems or in colder parts of the United States, however, withdrawal of brood mares from endophyte-infected fescue grass or hay or other therapeutic approaches may be the treatments of choice for delayed seasonal cyclicity.

Prognosis. With regard to summer slump, and mild cases of fescue foot and "fat necrosis" in ruminants, complete recovery or, as in the case of fat necrosis, termination of disease progression would be anticipated in most situations. Animals with more severe lameness associated with tissue sloughing, osteomyelitis, or arthritis may need to be salvaged for slaughter. Humane destruction of affected animals may even be necessary in the worst cases of fescue foot. Likewise, animals with severe fat necrosis characterized by large masses of necrotic adipose tissue causing gastrointestinal or genitourinary complications may need to be sold for slaughter or destroyed humanely, depending on the clinical circumstances.[1,2,4]

Regarding early embryonic death, cyclic irregularities, and thermoregulatory disturbances noted in horses exposed to endophyte-infected fescue, complete recovery would be anticipated in most situations. Agalactic mares, which do not develop mastitis, appear to be able to lactate normally following withdrawal from endophyte-infected pastures or hay or after successful therapeutic intervention, and subsequent lactations in these mares appear to be normal. Pony mares treated for prolonged gestation with domperidone responded quickly and without complications.[40,45] The prognoses for future fertility and survival in ergot alkaloid–exposed mares are directly related to the occurrence and severity of dystocia and possible complications, such as parturient trauma, metritis, septicemia and endotoxemia, retention of fetal membranes, and laminitis.[19,33,34] Although a slight delay in normal postpartum cyclicity might be anticipated, ergot alkaloid–exposed pregnant mares that have uncomplicated foalings do not appear to be adversely affected in their ability to produce live foals in the future. Complicated dystocias, on the other hand, often result in impaired fertility and potentially mortality in mares. The prognosis for fetal survival is adversely affected by ergot alkaloid exposure and is dependent, in each individual case, on the degree of fetal dysmaturity, foal immunoglobulin status, the severity of septicemia and related clinical signs that develop in the foal, and the availability of adequate nursing care and veterinary facilities to address the clinical problems.[33,47]

Prevention and Control. The prevention and control of fescue toxicosis in livestock species may be the best approaches to this problem and involve many of the same pasture and hay withdrawal and pharmacologic intervention approaches described under therapy. Logically, the keys to prophylaxis are the recognition of the potential for exposure to endophyte-infected fescue and an understanding of the risk factors, which may predispose animals to the development of clinical signs of fescue toxicosis. This is particularly true for pregnant mares, wherein knowledge of breeding dates, confirmed pregnancy diagnoses, and careful monitoring of mammary development are all critical steps in the identification of susceptible individuals.[33,34]

Livestock management systems will require individual evaluation to determine the best prevention and control measures to implement under specific animal husbandry circumstances. Avoidance of the use of toxigenic *N. coenophialum*-infected tall fescue is the optimal goal for livestock producers, but there are inherent financial, practicality, and efficacy challenges to this prophylactic approach. *N. coenophialum* is killed by 24 months of seed storage or subsequent to treatment with heat or fungicides. Complete pasture renovation and reseeding with this endophyte-free fescue or other grass species following tillage or application of herbicides has been traditionally recommended to livestock producers; however, the practicality of this approach has been limited by the symbiotic nature of tall fescue grass and *Neotyphodium* interactions. Endophyte-free tall fescue is less adaptable to weather extremes and less resistant to plant diseases and insect infestation than fescue infected with *N. coenophialum*. As a result, pastures of this less vigorous fescue grass do not flourish in many of the environments to which endophyte-infected tall fescue has readily adapted. The passage of endophyte-infected seed through the gastrointestinal tract of livestock species for up to 72 hours after removal from affected pastures also increases the difficulty of preventing pasture reseeding with infected seed.[4,22,33,34] Endophyte-infected fescue will never be replaced in many areas, and livestock producers will have to live with the problem unless other means of control are found. Recently the introduction of tall fescue infected with a genetically altered "friendly" endophyte, which reportedly produces lower levels of ergot alkaloids while maintaining fescue vigor, has shown promise in the prevention of the clinical signs of fescue toxicosis in cattle and horses.[50,51] This approach to fescue toxicosis prophylaxis is primarily limited by financial, labor, and time constraints, and the possible reintroduction of fescue grass infected with "unfriendly" endophyte.

Strategic timing of livestock withdrawal from endophyte-infected pasture or hay or alternative pasture management strategies may be easier to accomplish than the complete avoidance of exposure to toxigenic *N. coenophilaum*. In ruminants, ergot alkaloid exposure presents the greatest threat to livestock health and performance under conditions of extreme heat (summer slump) and cold (fescue foot). Switching pastures or sources of hay when these weather conditions are anticipated may be beneficial. Although periods as long as 60 to 90 days of tall fescue withdrawal before anticipated foaling date have been recommended for pregnant mares, desirable results have been achieved by removing pregnant mares from endophyte-infected pastures and preventing exposure to endophyte-infected hay 30 days before the expected foaling date (approximately day 300 of gestation).[2,27,33,34] It may also be advisable to prevent ergot alkaloid exposure to mares before the onset of normal cyclicity and the first 30 days of pregnancy, particularly when foaling dates early in the calendar year are desired or for individual mares with a history of subfertility.[33] When withdrawal from tall fescue is impractical, frequent mowing, heavy grazing pressure, and chemical treatment to prevent or retard seed head development have been recommended as ways to decrease ergot alkaloid concentrations in pastures.[2,22,34] Dilution of fescue pastures with at least 20% palatable legumes such as clovers has also been recommended, and the nitrogen fixation associated with leguminous forages may be a means of decreasing levels of ergot alkaloids.[1,2,22,33] Ammoniation of hay has also been demonstrated to dramatically decrease the effects of exposure to endophyte-infected fescue in cattle.[1,2,4]

Pharmacologic intervention has been used experimentally and clinically, primarily in late gestational mares, to prevent the clinical signs of fescue toxicosis. Medications successfully used for fescue toxicosis prophylaxis beginning at day 300 of gestation include the D_2-dopamine receptor antagonists domperidone (1.1 mg/kg PO SID), sulpiride (3.3 mg/kg PO SID), and perphenazine (0.3 to 0.5 mg/kg PO BID).[7,19,39] Most recently, another D_2 receptor antagonist, fluphenazine (25 mg IM in pony mares on day 320 of gestation) has also been used successfully for the prevention of fescue toxicosis.[28] Domperidone has been used in field cases for the prevention of fescue toxicosis starting 10 to 14 days before the expected foaling date or on approximately day 330 of gestation when mammary development is less than anticipated. Domperidone has been reported experimentally to be more effective than sulpiride and is less likely to be associated with the extrapyramidal signs occasionally seen with the use of perphenazine and fluphenazine.[2,33,34,39]

FUMONISIN

Geoffrey W. Smith and Peter D. Constable

Synonyms. Fumonisin toxicosis is known as equine leukoencephalomalacia (ELEM) and as porcine pulmonary edema (PPE).

Sources. Fumonisins (B_1 and B_2) are a group of naturally occurring mycotoxins produced by the fungus *Fusarium verticillioides* (formerly *F. moniliforme*). Apart from reports of fumonisin B_1 and B_2 in "black oats" feed from Brazil and in New Zealand forage grasses, the only commodities in which fumonisins have been detected so far are corn and corn-based foods. ELEM has long been associated with the consumption of moldy corn and has been reported in many areas of the world. However, cases of ELEM that were directly associated with fumonisin-contaminated feed have been reported in South Africa, the United States, Brazil, Mexico, Hungary, Spain, Egypt, and New Caledonia. Additionally, cases of PPE have been associated with fumonisin-contaminated feeds in the United States, Hungary, and Brazil.

Toxicokinetics. Fumonisins are a group of structurally related compounds with the terminal carboxy group composed of propane-1,2,3-tricarboxylic acid involved in ester formation with the C-14 and C-15 hydroxy groups. The structures of FB_1 and FB_2 have the empirical formulas of $C_{34}H_{59}NO_{15}$ and $C_{34}H_{59}NO_{14}$, respectively, with the only difference being the hydroxyl group present at the C-10 position in FB_1 (Fig. 23-3). Four additional fumonisin metabolites have been isolated (B_3, B_4, A_1, and A_2) but appear to

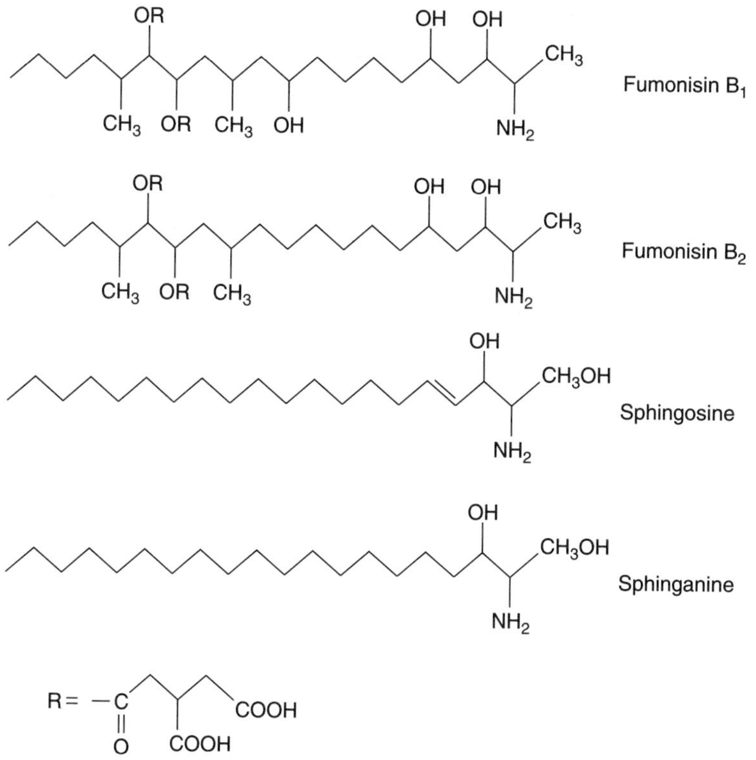

Fig. 23-3 The structure of fumonisin B₁, fumonisin B₂, sphingosine, and sphinganine.

occur in much lower concentrations than FB₁ or FB₂ and are not considered important at this time.

The toxicokinetics of radiolabeled fumonisin B₁ have been examined after intragastric (0.5 mg fumonisin B₁/kg) or IV (0.4 mg fumonisin B₁/kg) administration to bile-cannulated and noncannulated pigs.[1] Fumonisin-derived radioactivity was not detected in the plasma of IV-administered pigs after 180 minutes in the noncannulated group or after 90 minutes in the cannulated group. Urinary excretion began within 3 hours of administration and virtually ended after 8 hours, accounting for only a small amount of administered toxin. Fecal excretion of fumonisin persisted for 48 hours. The excretion in the IV-administered group occurred primarily via the bile, with biliary excretion being greatest during the first 4 hours but persisting for 24 to 36 hours.

Plasma radioactivity in intragastrically administered pigs was first detected 30 to 45 minutes after administration, with maximal activity present between 60 and 90 minutes. As reflected in plasma and elimination data, systemic bioavailability of the dose ranged from 3% to 6%. Excretion of fumonisin occurred primarily via feces, with only trace amounts excreted via urine or bile.

At 72 hours after administration, tissue radioactivity was highest in the liver, kidney, and large intestine in all groups. Intragastrically administered groups had tenfold to twentyfold lower tissue concentrations than did IV-administered groups, and only IV-administered groups had measurable radioactivity in brain, lung, and adrenal tissue. The liver and kidney are therefore the primary organs of fumonisin metabolism and excretion in the pig, and following biliary excretion, enterohepatic circulation prolongs the persistence of fumonisin in the body. Meat residues do not appear to be a major problem associated with fumonisins because they are rapidly eliminated from muscle and only negligible toxin concentrations appear in milk.[2] The toxicokinetics of fumonisin B₁ in horses have not been evaluated.

Mechanism of Action. Fumonisins are structurally related to sphingosine, the major long chain base backbone of cellular sphingolipids (see Fig. 23-3). They are specific inhibitors of sphinganine and sphingosine N-acyltransferase, key enzymes in the de novo sphingolipid biosynthetic pathway (Fig. 23-4). Fumonisins disrupt sphingolipid metabolism, resulting in increased sphinganine and sphingosine, and decreased complex sphingolipids.[3] These elevations in sphinganine and sphingosine concentrations have also been observed in vivo in several species including pigs, horses, and calves.[4-6]

Disruption of sphingolipid metabolism is widely thought to be the primary mechanism of fumonisin toxicity in animals. In pigs, administration of high doses of fumonisin inhibits cardiovascular function, producing acute left-sided heart failure and pulmonary edema within 5 days of exposure.[4,7] The mechanism of cardiotoxicity is believed to be due to a sphingosine-mediated inhibition of the myocardial L-type calcium channels. This calcium channel blockade causes a decrease in cardiac contractility, resulting in left-sided heart failure and pulmonary edema.[8]

Although the mechanism of ELEM is not well understood, a recent study showed that fumonisin administration induced cardiovascular dysfunction in horses. This study reported an association between neurologic signs, increased serum and myocardial sphingosine concentrations, and cardiovascular

Fumonisin Inhibition of Sphingolipid Biosynthesis

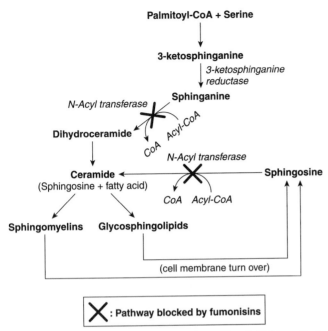

Fig. 23-4 The effect of fumonisin on the sphingolipid biosynthetic pathway.

depression in fumonisin-treated horses,[9] indicating that cardiovascular dysfunction may contribute to the pathophysiology of leukoencephalomalacia in the horse.

Toxicity and Risk Factors.	The primary diseases of veterinary importance associated with fumonisin toxicosis are ELEM and porcine pulmonary edema. The doses associated with toxicity in each species have varied in the literature; however, horses are generally considered to be the most sensitive species to fumonisin.

Horses.	Doses of fumonisin reported from naturally occurring cases of ELEM have varied. One field report calculated that the ingestion of 0.6 to 2.1 mg fumonisin B_1/kg of body weight would induce ELEM in 24 to 28 days.[10] Another study found that leukoencephalomalacia was associated with ingestion of feed containing fumonisin B_1 concentrations greater than 10 ppm and concluded that feed with fumonisin B_1 concentrations greater than 10 ppm was not safe to be fed to horses.[11]

Swine.	Reported fumonisin doses needed to induce pulmonary edema include 100 ppm of fumonisin B_1 and fumonisin B_2 in naturally contaminated corn, 16 mg fumonisin B_1/kg per day as fumonisin containing culture material, and 20 mg fumonisin B_1/kg per day as culture material. Pigs that ingest fumonisin at concentrations high enough to cause pulmonary edema usually die after about 4 days in field cases and after 3 to 6 days of fumonisin exposure experimentally. Pigs that survive chronic exposure to high doses of fumonisin without developing pulmonary edema typically demonstrate hepatic disease with anorexia, weight loss, and generalized icterus.[12,13]

Cattle.	Adult cattle appear relatively resistant to fumonisin. Feeder calves fed a diet containing fumonisin

concentrations up to 148 ppm (μg/g) for 31 days had only mild hepatotoxicity.[14] Although it is tempting to speculate that cattle are able to break down the toxin, fumonisin has been shown to be poorly metabolized by the rumen.[15] Instead it is thought that cattle have an increased tolerance to fumonisin because of differences in the mechanism of action.

In milk-fed calves given purified fumonisin B_1, the kidney was shown to be the primary target organ.[6] This study also showed that sphingosine and sphinganine concentrations did not increase in the serum of treated calves to the same degree that has been shown in pigs and horses.

Poultry.	Research has also indicated that fumonisins can be toxic to chickens with concentrations in the feed as low as 100 mg/kg, causing decreased body weight gain, diarrhea, and hepatotoxicity.[16] There has also been an association between the fungus that produces fumonisin and an acute death sydrome recognized in young chicks (called *spiking mortality syndrome*). It was initially hypothesized that fumonisins were directly cardiotoxic to poultry and were related to this syndrome; however, later research suggested it was moniliformin (another mycotoxin produced by *F. verticillioides*) and not fumonisin.

Clinical Signs.	Clinical signs associated with the development of pulmonary edema consistently develop 3 to 6 days after initial exposure to fumonisins. These include dyspnea and open mouthed breathing, increased respiratory rate, cyanosis of skin and mucous membranes, inactivity, and sudden death.[13] Pigs usually die within a few hours of the onset of definitive respiratory distress.

In horses, several reports have considered ELEM and hepatotoxicosis to be two separate syndromes associated with fumonisin toxicosis in horses, with the terms *classic neurotoxic syndrome* and *hepatic syndrome* being used.[17] However, it appears more likely these are not true "distinct" syndromes but are related to the concentration of fumonisin in the feed, the duration of toxin consumption, and the tolerance of the individual horse to fumonisin. In some outbreaks, horses have died from ELEM, whereas other horses have died from hepatotoxicosis, and occasionally individual horses exhibiting both neurologic and hepatic signs have been described. Reported clinical signs associated with hepatic disease include icterus, mucous membrane petechiae, and swelling of the lips or muzzle. The clinical signs associated with the development of ELEM have been poorly documented; however, they are usually summarized as a sudden onset of one or more of the following: frenzy, aimless circling, head pressing, paresis, ataxia, apparent blindness, depression, and hyperexcitability. Other reported clinical signs associated with fumonisin toxicosis in horses include abdominal breathing, cyanosis, and labored breathing.[18]

Clinical Pathology.	Serum biochemical changes associated with fumonisin toxicosis in horses have been predominantly related to hepatotoxicity. Increased activities of serum enzymes such as ALP, aspartate aminotransferase (AST) and gamma-glutamyl transpeptidase (GGT), and sorbitol dehydrogenase (SDH), and concentrations of total bilirubin, and bile acids have been reported with varying doses of fumonisin. Cerebrospinal fluid findings have only been reported from two affected horses, which had a leuko-cytic pleocytosis and a large increase in protein and myelin basic protein concentrations.[17,19]

In pigs, hepatic toxicosis occurs before the development of pulmonary edema, and alterations are time and dose dependent.[20] Increased activities of serum enzymes such as ALP, AST, and GGT and concentrations of total bilirubin, bile acids, and cholesterol have been reported as early as 1 day after the initiation of fumonisin exposure at doses high enough to induce pulmonary edema.[12,13,20,21] These altera-tions reflect hepatocyte damage as well as altered hepatic function.

Lesions. Gross lesions associated with ELEM include liquefactive necrosis and degeneration of the white matter of one or both cerebral hemispheres (Fig. 23-5). Necrotic areas can vary in size from pinpoint to large. The regions of the brain adjacent to the necrosis are often edematous and large areas of hemorrhage have also been reported, with most lesions being centered around the cerebral vasculature. Gross hepatic changes associated with fumonisin toxicosis in horses include swollen, discolored (yellowish brown) livers with irregular foci or nodules scattered throughout. Histo-logic findings include centrilobular necrosis and fibrosis, portal fibrosis, bile stasis, bile duct proliferation, and fatty disposition of hepatocytes.

Pigs that die in respiratory distress have pulmonary edema characterized grossly by heavy, wet lungs with widened interlobular septa (Fig. 23-6), as well as fluid in the airways and the thoracic cavity. Histologically the major alteration is the presence of clear fluid and markedly dilated lymphatics in connective tissue around vessels, bronchi, subpleurally, and in interlobular septa. Inflammation is not generally ob-served. Hepatic changes in pigs exposed to fumonisins include elevation of liver-associated enzyme activities, altered serum biochemical values, changes in sphingolipid param-eters, and morphologic alterations. Hepatic changes asso-

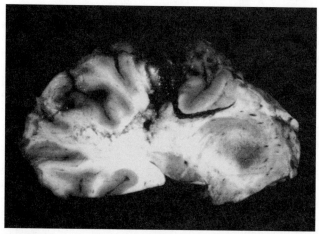

Fig. 23-5 A cross section of a horse's cerebral hemisphere demonstrating liquefactive necrosis of the white matter typical of equine leukoencephalo-malacia.

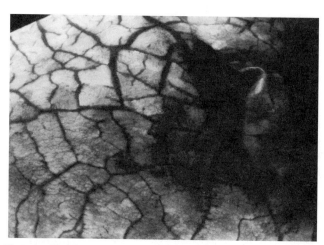

Fig. 23-6 Lung from a pig fed fumonisin-containing culture material at a dose of 20 mg fumonisin B$_1$ per kg of body weight for 4 days. Pulmonary edema is characterized by severe widening of the interlobular septa.

ciated with fumonisin toxicosis in swine include hepatic cord disorganization, cytoplasmic vacuolation, apoptosis, scattered necrosis, and increased cell proliferation. Long-term fumon-isin exposure can result in fibrosis or development of hyper-plastic nodules in the liver and medial hypertrophy of the small pulmonary arteries.

Diagnostic Testing. Fungal culture of feeds has little value in diagnosing fumonisin toxicosis because some corn sam-ples contain very high concentrations of toxin with very low levels of fungus, whereas other samples have heavy growths of *Fusarium* fungus with little to no detectable fumonisin. This is partly because the fungus that produces fumonisin also produces numerous other mycotoxins. Therefore, the definitive diagnosis of fumonisin toxicosis in animals generally requires analyzing feed for the actual toxin. Many diagnostic laboratories across the United States offer assays to detect both fumonisin B$_1$ and B$_2$ in corn and feed sam-ples. The two most commonly used tests for the detection of the toxin are chromatography (HPLC) and ELISA assays. To date, there are no commercially available assays that detect fumonisin in serum or tissues.

Another assay that may be used in the future to diagnose fumonisin toxicosis in animals is the sphinganine to sphingosine ratio (Sa:So ratio). Because of the fumonisin-induced disruption of sphingolipid biosynthesis discussed earlier, the Sa:So ratio increases in the serum and tissues of pigs and horses exposed to fumonisin. It has been suggested that this assay could be used to help diagnose fumonisin toxicosis when feed analysis is not possible. Sphinganine and sphingosine data may soon be available from enough pigs and horses to provide values for normal and affected animals.

Treatment. To date there have been no treatments described for either ELEM or fumonisin-induced PPE. Gen-erally the onset of clinical signs is acute and the progression of disease is rapid for both syndromes. The most important treatment is to identify and remove the source of con-

TABLE 23-4 Recommended Levels for Total Fumonisins in Animal Feeds

Animal	Recommended Maximum Level of Total Fumonisins in Corn to Be Used for Feed (ppm[a])	Recommended Maximum Level of Total Fumonisins in the Ration (ppm[a])
Horse[b]	5	1
Swine	20	10
Ruminants[c]	60	30
Poultry[d]	100	50
Ruminant and poultry breeding stock[e]	30	15
Catfish	20	10
Other animals[f]	10	5

From the United States Food and Drug Administration, Center for Veterinary Medicine.
[a]Total fumonisins = fumonisin B_1 + fumonisin B_2.
[b]Includes donkeys, asses, and zebras.
[c]Cattle, sheep, goats, and other ruminants that are ≥3 months of age and are fed for slaughter.
[d]Turkeys, chickens, ducklings, and other poultry fed for slaughter.
[e]Includes lactating dairy cows, bulls, laying hens, and roosters.
[f]Includes dogs and cats.

taminated feed to prevent other animals from developing toxicosis.

Prevention and Control. Guidelines for the maximum recommended levels of fumonisins in animal feeds have been published by the FDA Center for Veterinary Medicine (Table 23-4). It is important that livestock producers be aware of these guidelines and have their corn periodically tested for mycotoxins. Research has not yet found effective ways of decreasing fumonisin concentrations in corn through processing or feed additives (e.g., binding agents). Corn containing significant levels of fumonisin should be discarded, diluted with corn containing lower concentrations of fumonisin, or fed to a less-sensitive species (e.g., ruminants or poultry intended for slaughter).

OOSPOREIN

Robert Coppock and Margita M. Dziwenka

Synonyms. A synonym for oosporein is chaetomidin.

Sources. The fungi *Oospora colorans*, *Chaetomium trilaterale*, and *C. aureum* and numerous other filamentous fungi have been identified as producers of oosporein.[1] Finished poultry feeds, cereal grains, peanuts, and other feedstuffs and foodstuffs have been identified as favorable substrates.

Toxicokinetics. The chemical structure of oosporein is 3,3′,6,6′-tetrahydroxy-5,5′-dimethyl-2,2′-bi-*p*-benzoquinone.[2] The toxicokinetics of oosporein have not been described.

Mechanism of Action. Oosporein has been identified as a nephrotoxin. The mechanism of action has not been clearly identified. Oosporein has been demonstrated in vitro to inhibit erythrocytic ATPases,[3] but in vitro studies found that oosporein did not inhibit mitochondrial function in rat proximal renal tubular cells.[4] In poultry, uric acid excretion has been found to be impaired, but the clinicopathologic mechanism has not been described. Studies in vivo in poultry suggest that the mitochondria may be a target subcellular organelle.

Toxicity and Risk Factors. Feeding studies in broiler chicks found that the organic acid form was less toxic than the sodium or potassium salt forms of oosporein. The relative order from the most to the least toxic was sodium salt of oosporein (LD_{50} of 4.56 mg/kg body weight) > potassium salt of oosporein (LD_{50} of 5 mg/kg body weight) > oosporein organic acid (LD_{50} of 5.77 mg/kg body weight).[5]

Chickens are susceptible to oosporein.[6] In a feeding trial, day-old male chicks were placed on starter diets amended with oosporein. After 3 weeks, significant depression of body weight was observed in the group receiving dietary levels of 40 μg oosporein/g of feed, but not in the group receiving the diet amended with 20 μg oosporein/g. Birds on a diet amended with 200 μg oosporein/g had a 7% mortality over a 3-week period. Birds on diets with 200 μg/g or more were observed to have both visceral and articular gout. Birds on the high dietary levels were asymptomatic until 24 hours before death.

Turkeys are more resistant to oosporein than are chickens.[7] In a feeding study, 1-day-old male turkey poults were placed on diets containing 0, 500, 1000, and 1500 μg oosporein/g of finished feed. In the second and third weeks, all of the birds had a reduction in body weight. Birds in the group receiving diets amended with 1000 and 1500 μg oosporein/g of feed also consumed less feed. The first mortalities were observed on study day 6 and peaked at study day 7. This probably was due to a reduced intake of oosporein.

Clinical Signs. The sequence of clinical signs in chickens is anorexia, increased water consumption, diarrhea, lethargy, and coma. Birds that die acutely of oosporein toxicosis have visceral gout, especially of the pericardium. The longer the birds live the more tendency there is for gout to be observed in the feet, legs, and head.

Clinical signs observed in turkeys include increased water consumption, listlessness, decreased feed intake, lethargy, ataxia, and death. The macroscopic lesions are similar to those reported for chickens. Visceral and articular urate deposits are observed.

Clinical Pathology. Turkeys on diets amended with oosporein had dose-related increases in serum urea nitrogen, and birds receiving high-dose diets had an increase in serum uric acid. Birds in the high-dose group had a decrease in serum albumin.

Lesions. The renal lesions of oosporein have been reported in chicks.[8] In the acute phase of the toxicosis, macroscopic lesions include enlarged pale kidneys, and white granular urate crystals are observed on the pericardium and peritoneal surfaces. Histopathology demonstrated multifocal proximal tubular necrosis in paracentral locations. The tubular epithelial cells had pyknotic nuclei, karyorrhectic or enlarged clear nuclei, and nuclei containing eosinophilic inclusions. Basophilic casts were present. The interstitium contained multinucleated giant cells. Distal tubules contained hyalin eosinophilic casts. Periodic acid-Schiff–positive granules were observed in the cells of the macula densa.

Ultrastructure histopathology identified gaps in the basement membrane of the proximal tubules. Some of the epithelial cells in the collecting ducts contained myelin bodies.

In the subchronic phase of the toxicosis, the macroscopic pathology was minimal to marked articular and visceral gout, and all the birds had enlarged pale kidneys. Histopathology demonstrated lobules of dilated tubules, enlarged glomeruli, hyperplasia of parietal epithelium, periglomerular fibrosis, and atrophied sclerotic tuff. The proximal tubules were reduced in number and were dilated. The proximal tubular epithelium in some tubules was tall and was intensely eosinophilic and these cells had an increased mitotic index. Anisokaryosis was moderate and nuclear inclusions were observed. Compressed proximal tubules had epithelial cells containing vacuoles. The distal tubules contained hyalin basophilic material and urate crystals. The interstitial space was fibrotic and had polygranulomas around the urate crystals. Ultrastructure histopathology of the proximal tubular epithelium revealed enlarged mitochondria, some being ring-shaped, and some cells with enlarged smooth endoplasmic reticulum. Some epithelial cells had electron dense lysosomes.

Diagnostic Testing. Birds with visceral and articular gout should be suspect for oosporein intoxication. Suspect feed should be submitted to an analytic toxicology laboratory for mycotoxin analysis.

Treatment. Specific treatment for oosporein poisoning does not exist.

Prevention and Control. The best prevention of oosporein intoxication is to store feedstuffs at less than 14% moisture and avoid the use of moisture-damaged ingredients in formulating poultry feeds. Finished feed that has a moldy appearance or smell should not be fed. On a regular schedule, feeders and storage tanks should be emptied and cleaned.

PATULIN

Robert Coppock and Margita M. Dziwenka

Synonyms. Patulin is the name for (2,4-dihydroxy-2H-pyran-3(6H)-ylidene)-, 3,4-lactone.[1] Other names include clairformin, clavacin, clavatin, claviform, claviformin, expansin, expansine, gigantin, mycoin, mycoin c, mycoin C3, mycoine C3, patuline, penatin, penicidin, tercinin, and terinin.

Sources. Patulin is produced by a number of the filamentous fungi (Table 23-5) in a variety of substrates.[2] Patulin is formed from 6-methylsalicyclic acid and the biochemical pathway is magnesium dependent. Other pathways exist,

TABLE 23-5 **Species of *Penicillium* and *Aspergillus* that Have Been Identified with Production of Patulin**

Fungi	Substrate	Comments
Paecilomyces sp (*Byssochlamys nivea*)	Silage	Produces large quantities of patulin
Penicillium urticae *P. patulum*	Silage, stubble residue, apples, cider, chick starter, fruit juices	Uses a low nutrient level substrate Levels of patulin produced may be phytotoxic; can produce g/L quantities of patulin
P. expansum	Apples, pears, fresh and processed foods, cider	Known to produce large quantities of patulin
P. maltum	Malt feed	
P. granulatum	Isolated from corn silage	2.8 g/L in 18 d at 26° C; find 1 to 5 ppm in silage
P. roqueforti	Corn silage substrate	15.9 mg/kg at 4 d; find 1 to 5 ppm in silage
P. vulpinum *P. claviforme*	Foodstuffs and feedstuffs	Produces patulin
Aspergillus clavatus *A. giganteus*	Barley	Peak production at 17° C
A. terreus	Foodstuffs and feedstuffs	Territrems, possible producer of patulin

and patulin can also be formed from acetate, fructose, galactose, maltose, and glucose.

Penicillium expansum growing in apple juice was found to require a narrow pH range of 3.2 to 3.8 for patulin production.[3] Others have found strains of *P. expansum* that can produce patulin in temperatures ranging from 0° C to 25° C.[2] Temperatures for maximal production of patulin were 25° C and 17° C, respectively, for production of patulin in pears and apples. Maximal time for production in apples was 12 to 14 days. The optimum temperature for the production of patulin by *Aspergillus clavatus* growing on barley substrate was 16° C.

Patulin can be produced in fruit juices (especially apple, pear, and grape), fresh fruit, sea buckthorn, processed foods, barley, malt, rice, silage, wheat straw, grass and fruit tree clippings, and soil amended with the roots and bark of fruit trees.[4] Patulin is stable in apple, grape, and pear juices, but it is not stable in orange juice. Rotten apples can contain up to 18 mg/apple, and apple cider has been found to contain 45 mg of patulin/L. The use of rotting pears in the manufacture of juices can result in patulin levels of 300 mg/L. Rotting fruit can be a source of patulin for livestock and poultry. The use of fruit pomace in feedstuffs can be a source of exposure for livestock. However, cereal grains and flour were found to have less than 5% potential for patulin production. Patulin has also been found at concentrations of 1.5 mg/kg in mulch residues after minimum tillage.[5]

Toxicokinetics. Few studies have reported residues of patulin in tissues. In vitro studies have found that blood and liver homogenates inactivate patulin. Rats were given ^{14}C-labeled patulin and 49% of the radiolabel was recovered from the feces, 36% was recovered from the urine, and 2% was recovered in respired air. Studies in chickens given radio-labeled patulin found the radiolabel in eggs. However, the radiolabeled metabolite was not identified. Using in vivo studies, the highest concentration of radiolabel was found in the red blood cells. Penicillic acid has been reported to potentiate the toxicity of patulin in dogs.

The indices of patulin toxicity are summarized in Table 23-6.

Mechanism of Action. Patulin is an unsaturated α, β-lactone and its cytotoxicity is linked to its rapid reaction with SH-groups, and less rapidly with NH_2-groups.[6] Patulin has been found to inhibit protein synthesis by inhibiting amino acid uptake by cells. The cytotoxic effects of patulin were studied in rat hepatocytes and the pathogenesis of cell injury was found to be simultaneous suppression of gap junction–mediated intercellular communications and depletion of intercellular glutathione, production of reactive oxygen species, mitochondrial membrane depolarization, and an increase in intracellular Ca^{2+}. Protein synthesis (in vivo and in vitro) has been found to be inhibited in rat liver by patulin. Maximal in vivo inhibition was observed 5 hours after administration. Patulin inhibits membrane functions including the inhibition of Na^+-K^+ ATPase, thereby increasing Na^+ influx and K^+ efflux from cells. After 4.2 hours of incubation, patulin levels of 1 mM completely reversed the intracellular and extracellular concentrations of K^+ and Na^+. The effects of patulin on Na^+ and K^+ flux were reversible by the addition of dithiothreitol and glutathione. Patulin has been reported to include a dose-dependent inhibition of Na^+-K^+ ATPase activity in mouse brain and kidney tissue. This is postulated to be the mechanism of action for the neurotoxicity of patulin.

Toxicity and Risk Factors. The LD_{50} of IV administered patulin in dogs was estimated to be 10.4 mg/kg body weight. Penicillic acid has been reported to potentiate the toxicity of patulin in dogs.

TABLE 23-6 Indices of Patulin Toxicity

Dose (Route)	Dose Outcome/Species	Comment
17 mg/kg (oral)	LD_{50}/mouse	Pulmonary edema, fatty degeneration of the liver
27.790 mg/kg (oral)	LD_{50}/rat	Behavioral: changes in motor activity (specific assay) Lungs, thorax, or respiration: dyspnea
10 mg/kg (IV)	LD_{50}/dog	Somnolence, hypermotility of gastrointestinal tract, diarrhea, pulmonary edema
31.5 mg/kg (oral)	LD_{50}/hamster	
392 mg/kg (oral)	TDL_0/rat*	14-day interval. Alteration in gastric secretion, gastritis
84 mg/kg (oral)	TDL_0/rat	4-wk interval. Changes in urine composition, weight loss or decreased weight gain, central nervous system toxicity
60 mg/kg (oral)	TDL_0/rat	30-day interval. Enzyme inhibition, induction, or change in blood or tissue levels: phosphates
232 mg/kg (SC)	TDL_0/rat	58-wk interval. Tumors at injection site

Data from reference 12. *IV,* Intravenous administration; *SC,* subcutaneous administration.
*TDL_0, Toxic dose low. The lowest dose of a substance given in a specified period of time and reported to produce any toxic effects.

In a 6-week feeding trial, an Egyptian strain of laying hens was fed a laying mash containing 100 ppb patulin.[7] Eggs were examined by a number of parameters, but only the eggshell thickness, when compared with control hens, was significantly decreased by patulin. Ash content and the concentration of magnesium in the eggshell were not significantly reduced. Eggs from hens on the patulin diet had a cycloid eminence in the middle of the egg. Patulin did not alter the ash content of the tibia. However, the fat content of the liver increased whereas the water and vitamin A content decreased.

In another study, white leghorn cockerels were given 5 to 80 mg (per gavage) in pH 5 buffer.[8] The LD_{50} was determined to be 170 mg/kg body weight. Birds were observed to be listless 1 hour after administration, and birds that survived the first 24 hours were asymptomatic at 72 to 96 hours.

Macaca nemestria were given 5 mg patulin/kg body weight per day for 6 weeks by offering dried fruit amended with patulin before the morning feeding.[9] ALP activity significantly decreased in serum. No other changes in clinicopathology and body weights were observed.

Male and female rats (Wistar) were exposed to 0, 24, 84, or 295 mg patulin/L in drinking water for 4 weeks. Food and water consumption was decreased in the mid- and high-dose groups. In the high-dose group, creatinine clearance was decreased and ulcers were observed in the fundic region of the stomach. In another study, male rats were given patulin by the oral, subcutaneous, and intraperitoneal routes and the 72-hour LD_{50} values were 55, 11 and 10 mg/kg body weight, respectively.

Syrian golden hamsters were given oral, subcutaneous, and intraperitoneal injections of patulin. The LD_{50} was 31.5, 23, and 10 mg/kg body weight, respectively.

Clinical Signs.
A dose of 10 mg/kg body weight produces lethargy, diarrhea, hematemesis, and dyspnea in dogs.

Patulin has been implicated in cattle consuming malted barley.[10] *Penicillium utrice* isolated from the malt was found to produce patulin. Cultures of *P. utrice* were fed to mice and a bull and produced signs of motor nerve paralysis, hyperesthesia, and seizures. It is not known whether penicillic acid was also present. Patulin at 100 and 300 µg/mL concentrations in an in vitro rumen culture was found to depress the growth of rumen bacteria and the production of acetic acid.[11]

Patulin is neurotoxic in rats, resulting in signs that include seizures, tremors, ataxia, stiffness of rear legs, and waggling of the head. The AChE activity in the cerebral hemispheres, cerebellum, and medulla oblongata was significantly lower than in control subjects. Rats administered 25 mg of patulin/kg body weight had seizures before death.

Clinical Pathology.
In hens, blood glucose and ALP may increase.

Clinicopathologic observations in rats are metabolic alkalosis with respiratory compensation, decreased serum Na^+, increased blood glucose, reduction in total plasma protein, and leukocytosis with a neutrophilia.

Lesions.
Cats given an intracardiac dose of 5 mg patulin/kg body weight had immediate clinical signs of salivation and dilation of the pupils. The cats were necropsied 5 days after exposure with findings of pulmonary edema and congestion of the liver.

A dose of 10 mg/kg body weight produces pulmonary edema, pulmonary hemorrhage, and gastrointestinal hemorrhage.

Chicks given 67 mg of patulin (per gavage)/kg body weight developed ascites and watery crop contents within 12 hours after administration. At 16 to 48 hours, hemorrhage was observed in the entire digestive tract.

Histopathology findings in rats include protein and neutrophils in the alveoli. Mice injected with 100 mg patulin/day developed a lymphopenia. Necropsy examination revealed pulmonary edema with the alveoli containing a protein exudate and leukocyte infiltration, along with congestion of the liver. Hyperemia and congestion of the intestine were observed. Rabbits have similar pulmonary lesions as mice.

Patulin given at a dose of 20 mg/kg body weight resulted in lung edema and hemorrhagic foci in rabbits.

Pathologic observations in Syrian golden hamsters were hyperemia, congestion, and ulceration of the gastrointestinal tract. The antimicrobial effects of patulin were thought to have altered the natural flora of the lower intestinal tract and contributed to the observed effects.

Diagnostic Testing.
Patulin intoxication should be in the differential diagnosis for animals with pulmonary edema or central nervous system (CNS) dysfunction. When a history of feeding fruit, especially apples, pears, fruit pumice silage or malt, malt by-products, and wet grains exists, then patulin should be ruled out by diagnostic procedures. Suspect feedstuffs should be submitted chilled or frozen to the analytic toxicology laboratory for patulin analysis. Fungal cultures of suspected feedstuffs and analysis of the culture for patulin production may be helpful in establishing a diagnosis. Patulin may be found in acidic stomach or rumen contents. Because patulin has not been identified in animal tissues or blood, these may not be suitable specimens.

Treatment.
Specific antidotes for patulin intoxication do not exist. Symptomatic and supportive treatment is indicated. Pulmonary edema should be treated aggressively.

Prognosis.
Animals with pulmonary edema and CNS dysfunction can recover.

Prevention and Control.
Prevention of exposure is the best method of controlling patulin poisoning in companion and domestic animals. The high-risk feedstuffs given in decreasing order are rotten apples > apple pumice > fruit pumice > barley and wheat malt > moldy grains > moldy silage.

Patulin is stable at acid pH and is destroyed at alkaline pH. The stability of patulin was tested in phosphate buffer at pH levels of 6, 6.5, 7, 7.5, and 8, using Sorensen's phosphate buffer (25° C). The half-life values ranged from 64 hours for pH 8 to 1310 hours for pH 6. Studies with apple juice found that 50% of added patulin survived heating to 80° C for 10 to

20 minutes. Vitamin B_1 (thiamine), citric acid, and sulfur dioxide (used as a preservative in fruit juices) destroy patulin. Exposure of pomace to ammonia also destroyed patulin. Patulin was degraded in 15 seconds by 20% ozone.

PENITREM A AND ROQUEFORTINE

Birgit Puschner

Synonyms.   Tremorgens, tremorgenic mycotoxins, moldy walnut mycotoxin, moldy dairy product mycotoxin, garbage mycotoxins, and indole alkaloids are names used for these toxins.

Sources.   Mycotoxins are secondary fungal metabolites that may pose a significant risk to animals and humans. Penitrem A and roquefortine are the two most important tremorogenic mycotoxins associated with natural disease outbreaks in small animals. Tremorgenic mycotoxins primarily affect the CNS and are produced by fungi belonging to the genera *Penicillium, Aspergillus,* and *Claviceps.*[1]

Penitrem A is primarily produced by *Penicillium crustosum* and is the most toxic tremorgenic *Penicillium* mycotoxin.[2] It has been isolated from moldy cream cheese,[3] bread,[4] and walnuts.[5] Roquefortine is mainly produced by *P. roqueforti,* but can be produced by many other *Penicillium* spp., including *P. crustosum. P. roqueforti* also produces the mutagenic PR toxin. PR toxin has not been detected as a natural contaminant in foods, but has been produced in *Penicillium* cultures. Roquefortine is typically found in blue cheese and blue cheese products,[6] but can also occur in decaying organic matter such as silage, garbage, and compost.[7] In general, members of the genus *Penicillium* are commonly found in feedstuffs in temperate climates, are microaerophilic, and are acid-tolerant.

Toxicokinetics.   Both penitrem A and roquefortine are readily absorbed following ingestion, and both are excreted primarily through the bile.[8] Therefore, enterohepatic recirculation and continued reabsorption may contribute to the prolonged recovery seen in animals exposed to penitrem A or roquefortine. Penitrem A is excreted unchanged, whereas roquefortine undergoes some transformation during elimination by the biliary route.

Mechanism of Action.   Penitrem A and roquefortine are indole alkaloids (Fig. 23-7), and their lipophilic properties allow crossing of the blood-brain barrier into the CNS. They exert multiple effects on receptors and on neurotransmitter release mechanisms at both central and peripheral levels.[9] The exact mechanism of toxicosis is unknown, but penitrem A may influence presynaptic acetylcholine release,[10] may antagonize the production of glycine in the CNS,[11] or may act as a surrogate of α-aminobutyric acid (GABA).[12] The mechanism of action of roquefortine has not been investigated in detail.

Toxicity and Risk Factors.   In dogs, intraperitoneal administration of purified penitrem A resulted in the onset of acute tremors and death when given at a dose of 0.5 mg/kg.[13] In the same experiment but with a dose of 0.125 mg/kg penitrem A,

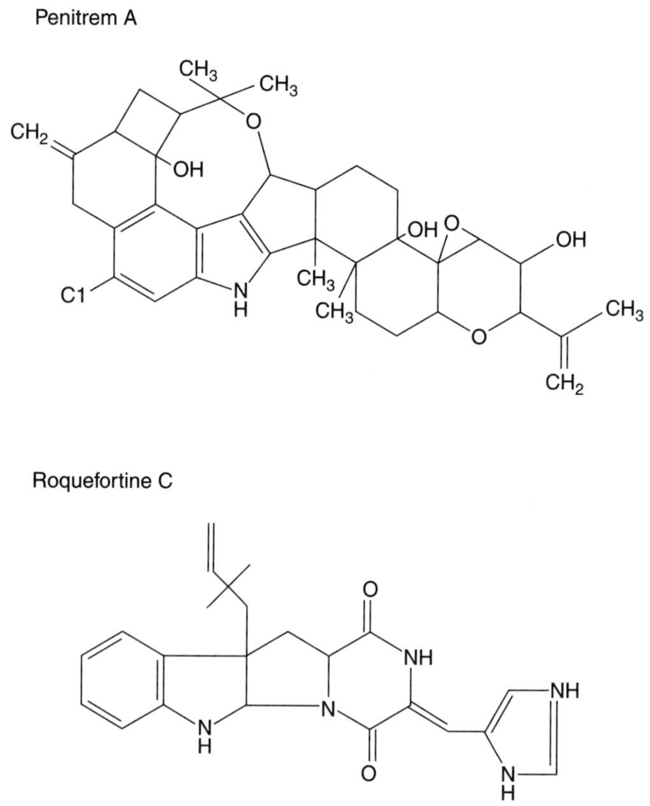

Penitrem A

Roquefortine C

Fig. 23-7 Structures of penitrem A and roquefortine.

dogs developed tremors within 30 minutes but recovered completely. Oral exposure to penitrem A from moldy bread at a concentration of approximately 0.175 mg/kg body weight was sufficient to produce severe muscle tremors in dogs.[4] The oral LD_{50} for penitrem A in mice is 10 mg/kg, whereas the intraperitoneal LD_{50} is 1.1 mg/kg.[14] Roquefortine has an LD_{50} in mice of 20 mg/kg body weight.[15] Oral lethal doses or concentrations resulting in clinical signs of roquefortine toxicosis in dogs and cats are not reported in the literature.

Dogs are more frequently affected by penitrem A and roquefortine toxicosis than are other animals. Their behavior patterns, such as scavenging for food in garbage and other decaying organic matter, increase the risk for exposure to mycotoxins associated with moldy feed.

Clinical Signs.   Clinical signs of penitrem A or roquefortine toxicosis in dogs usually occur within 30 minutes after exposure, but can be delayed for 2 to 3 hours. In the early stage of toxicosis, clinical signs include increased irritability, weakness, muscle tremors, rigidity, hyperactivity, and panting.[4,16] Eventually, the tremors may become more severe, and opisthotonus, seizures, nystagmus, and recumbency with paddling may be observed. In addition, poisoned animals may be sensitive to noise and often develop a body temperature of greater than 40° C. The increased muscle activity may ultimately lead to exhaustion, metabolic changes, rhabdomyolysis, and dehydration. In most cases, vomiting occurs before the onset of neurologic signs.

No confirmed cases of penitrem A or roquefortine mycotoxicosis have been reported in cats.

Clinical Pathology. Any tremor or seizure activity may result in an increased anion gap caused by the accumulation of lactate. In addition, increased muscle activity may result in elevated levels of plasma creatinine phosphokinase, lactic dehydrogenase, and AST. Also, severe fluid loss can cause dehydration. Therefore, the minimum database should include a complete blood count, serum electrolytes, enzyme activities, assessment of serum anion gap, and urinalysis.

Lesions. Gross and histologic examinations usually reveal no specific lesions, unless aspiration pneumonia has occurred during the clinical course. Sometimes, pieces of walnuts may be found in the vomitus or gastrointestinal contents.

Diagnostic Testing. Chromatographic methods have been developed to determine the presence of penitrem A and roquefortine in vomitus, gastric lavage washing, stomach contents, or bile.[16,17] If penitrem A or roquefortine poisoning is suspected, at least 10 g of testing material should be collected, kept frozen in a plastic container, and submitted to a diagnostic laboratory for analysis. Finding of penitrem A or roquefortine in any of the submitted specimens collected from the animal is consistent with exposure to tremorgenic mycotoxins from the environment. If clinical signs are consistent with a tremorgenic mycotoxicosis, a diagnosis is established. If testing is negative for penitrem A and roquefortine, analysis should be considered for other tremor- and seizure-inducing poisons such as strychnine, metaldehyde, bromethalin, zinc phosphide, methylxanthines, mushrooms, certain drugs, organophosphorous and carbamate insecticides, pyrethroids, and chlorinated hydrocarbons. If gastrointestinal contents are unavailable, source material such as moldy walnuts or moldy cheese can be analyzed for the presence of penitrem A and roquefortine.

Treatment. Most essential is the stabilization of vital signs, that is, maintenance of respiration and cardiovascular function, and control of CNS signs and body temperature. After the assessment of vital signs and stabilization of the patient, decontamination procedures should be initiated.

Emesis is recommended in patients that are at no risk for developing aspiration pneumonia. Reliable emetics include apomorphine in dogs at 0.03 mg/kg IV or 0.04 mg/kg IM, and xylazine in cats at 1.1 mg/kg IM or subcutaneously (SQ). Enterogastric lavage is recommended when massive ingestion has occurred or emesis is unproductive, or when the patient is symptomatic. Generally, gastric lavage requires anesthesia (inhalation or short-acting barbiturate), with intubation before initiating the procedure. Administration of activated charcoal is indicated in all cases in which significant toxicant ingestion has occurred. It can be given orally or by gastric tube at 1 to 4 g/kg in 50 to 200 ml of water and can be repeated every 6 to 8 hours. Multiple doses of activated charcoal every 4 to 6 hours for 2 to 3 days may be indicated because penitrem A and roquefortine are subject to enterohepatic recirculation. It is important to keep the patient adequately hydrated when activated charcoal is administered repeatedly.

If an acid-base imbalance has been diagnosed, sodium bicarbonate should be administered. If available, pH and arterial blood gas measurements should be used to guide treatment. Metabolic acidosis is evidenced by a pH of less than 7.2 and a blood bicarbonate concentration of less than 17 mEq/L in dogs and 15 mEq/L in cats. Sodium bicarbonate is administered as follows: mEq of bicarbonate required = $0.3 \times$ body weight (kg) $\times$ (desired total CO_2 mEq/L – measured total CO_2 mEq/L). If blood gas parameters are not known, sodium bicarbonate is given at 0.5 to 1 mEq/kg IV over 1 to 3 hours. An 8.4% solution of sodium bicarbonate contains 1 mEq/L.

In case of seizures, diazepam is a highly effective anticonvulsant but its duration of action is short, ranging from 20 to 60 minutes. It is given at 0.5 to 5 mg/kg IV to either dogs or cats for initial control of convulsions. This dose can be repeated at 10-minute intervals up to three times. If initial diazepam treatment has no effect and tremors or seizures continue, general anesthesia with pentobarbital should be induced.[5,16] The initial recommended dose is 3 to 15 mg/kg IV, slowly given to effect. Pentobarbital is effective within 5 to 10 minutes after administration and the patient should be maintained under general anesthesia for 4 hours, using additional boluses of pentobarbital if required. Alternatively, phenobarbital can be used to treat patients with penitrem A or roquefortine toxicosis. Often, phenobarbital administration is recommended to supplement diazepam, because its onset is about 15 to 30 minutes after administration. Phenobarbital is typically administered IV at 6 mg/kg to effect. It can be repeated every 15 minutes up to a maximum dose of 20 mg/kg in dogs and cats. For muscle relaxation, methocarbamol (150 mg/kg IV, not to exceed 330 mg/kg/day) or guaifenesin (5%, 110 mg/kg IV) can be administered to dogs and cats.

Prognosis. The prognosis is good if the animal receives decontamination treatment soon after exposure. Treatment is then directed toward controlling seizures and correcting metabolic acidosis. Most poisoned animals recover without sequelae within 24 to 48 hours with aggressive treatment. If gastric emptying was not performed, the prognosis is guarded and depends on the amount of penitrem A or roquefortine ingested.

Prevention and Control. Prevention is primarily based on education of animal owners. Pet owners should prevent their dogs from accessing walnut trees and orchards, especially when walnuts are found on the ground and have become colonized by fungi. Pet owners should not feed moldy dairy products to their animals and should keep animals away from garbage, compost, and other decaying organic matter.

PHOMOPSINS

Jeremy Allen

Synonyms. Lupinosis is the name for the disease caused by phomopsin toxicosis. Note, lupinosis is different from lupin or lupine poisoning, which is due to the consumption of quinolizidine alkaloids that may be present in lupin plants.

Sources. Lupinosis is a hepatotoxicosis caused by the ingestion of lupin plants infected by the fungus *Diaporthe toxica* (anamorph *Phomopsis* sp.), which produces the toxic phomopsins under certain environmental conditions. *D. woodii* (anamorph *Phomopsis leptostromiformis)* also infects lupin plants and is able to produce phomopsins, but it is weakly toxicogenic.[1]

Lupinosis has been reported in Germany, the United States, Poland, New Zealand, Australia, the Republic of South Africa, and Spain. However, it is only in Australia, particularly Western Australia, where lupinosis has assumed major importance because this is where lupins are grown extensively as a commercial crop, and after harvest the dead lupin plant is used for fodder.[2]

Virtually all cases of lupinosis result from consumption of the dead lupin stems. This can occur when stock graze on the lupin stubble (remnant of the lupin crop after it has been harvested) or are fed baled lupin stems, late-cut lupin hay, or lupin crop fines (this is small and fine material that is normally passed out of the back of the harvester during harvest). *D. toxica* infection of lupin seed occurs, but it is not a major toxicologic problem.[2]

Phomopsins are also produced by *Phomopsis emicis,*[3] a natural pathogen of the annual winter weed *Emex australis* (double gee). *P. emicis* has a considerable capacity to produce phomopsins in laboratory cultures, but to date no field cases of a lupinosis-like disease have been reported in sheep known to eat this weed.

Toxicokinetics. The phomopsins are a group of low-molecular-weight natural toxins. Phomopsins A and B were isolated in crystalline form more than 20 years ago.[4] Phomopsin A has the chemical formula $C_{36}H_{45}ClN_6O_{12}$ and the molecular weight of 788. It is a linear hexapeptide modified by an ether bridge to form a 13-membered macrocyclic ring.[5] Phomopsin B is the des-chloro analogue of phomopsin A.[6] Phomopsins C, D, and E have been isolated and all are toxic.[7,8]

Knowledge of the distribution of phomopsins within the body is limited to that provided by the detection of lesions in organs of affected animals. The liver is always affected, and functional failure of the liver is the main cause of death in lupinosis,[9] so phomopsins are regarded primarily as hepatotoxins. Other organs directly affected by the phomopsins include the kidneys, adrenal glands, pancreas, hepatic lymph nodes, rumen, and reticulum.

A study involving the inhibition and stimulation of the hepatic microsomal enzymes in rats has indicated that the phomopsins are potent primary toxins that are rapidly metabolized to less toxic metabolites.[10,11] In support of this conclusion is the detection of phomopsin-induced lesions in the rumen and reticulum of intoxicated sheep[10] and the numerous studies of the tubulin-binding capacity of phomopsin A, in which the pure toxin has been used.[12]

Mechanism of Action. Phomopsins are potent cytotoxic and antimitotic agents. They exert these effects through their ability to bind with microtubule subunit proteins (tubulin) and inhibit the formation (polymerization) of the microtubules that are cytoskeletal macromolecules vital to the functioning of cells. Intracellular transport mechanisms and cell division are two processes that require the microtubules. Two distinct binding sites of phomopsin A on tubulin include a high-affinity site and a low-affinity site, and phomopsin A both inhibits the polymerization of tubulin and depolymerizes the polymerized tubulin.[2]

Other mechanisms of action by the phomopsins have been suggested. Phomopsins inhibit complex I of the respiratory chain, resulting in inhibition of uptake of inorganic phosphate and oxygen consumption by mitochondria, so they probably cause impairment of mitochondrial respiration. Changes in the activities of some membrane-associated enzymes and redistribution of Golgi apparatus membranes indicate that cell membranes may be directly affected by these mycotoxins. Phomopsins can also induce chromosomal aberrations, so it has been suggested that they react directly with DNA. They are embryotoxic and carcinogenic in rats. Finally, histochemical and chemical studies have demonstrated considerable disruption of various enzyme systems and metabolic pathways in the liver and kidney of intoxicated mice, rats, and sheep. It is not known whether these latter changes are primary or secondary effects of the phomopsins.[2]

Toxicity and Risk Factors. Lupinosis is recognized primarily as a disease of sheep, but natural outbreaks have also been reported in cattle, goats, donkeys, horses, and pigs. It has been produced experimentally in rabbits, guinea pigs, mice, rats, dogs, ducklings, and chickens.[2]

The toxicity of the phomopsins is affected by the animal species intoxicated, the age and pregnancy state of the affected animal, and the route and pattern of administration of the phomopsins. Sheep are the most susceptible species studied, followed by pigs, rats, and mice in decreasing order of susceptibility. Cattle are less susceptible than sheep, and, although lupinosis is not often seen in horses, they may be highly susceptible because the disease in them is usually acute and fatal. Goats are believed to have intermediate susceptibility between sheep and cattle.[2]

Information on toxic doses of the phomopsins relates only to phomopsin A, the only phomopsin to be isolated in sufficient quantities for toxicity studies. Phomopsin A is twice as toxic as phomopsin B,[9] but the relative toxicity of the other phomopsins is unknown.

The LD_{50} of a single oral dose of phomopsin A to sheep (6 to 9 months old) is 1000 to 1350 µg/kg and for nursing rats (2 weeks old) is 35 mg/kg. Toxicity is considerably greater when the phomopsins are administered intraperitoneally or subcutaneously, with the LD_{50} of a single parenteral dose of phomopsin A to sheep being 10 to 27 µg/kg and to nursing rats being 1.6 mg/kg. The LD_{50} of a single subcutaneous dose of phomopsin A to adult rats (10 weeks old) is approximately 5.5 mg/kg, indicating that older animals are less susceptible. No comparable study has been done with sheep, but once sheep are weaned, not sex, age, or pregnancy affect the toxicity of the phomopsins in laboratory studies. In the field, young sheep (4 to 9 months of age) appear more susceptible than older sheep, but this may be because they are less selective in what they eat. Rats in early pregnancy (days 6 to 10) appear more susceptible than those in later stages of pregnancy (days 11 to 15), and in the field, late pregnant cows appear more susceptible than nonpregnant cattle. However, with cattle this apparent increased susceptibility is associated with the concurrent development of a secondary nutritional ketosis.[9,13,14]

The pattern of administration (or intake) of phomopsins also influences toxicity. For example, 1 of 3 sheep died after a single intraruminal injection of 1000 μg/kg of phomopsin A, whereas 3 of 3 died after receiving either five doses of 200 μg/kg or 20 doses of 50 μg/kg. Multiple smaller doses appear more toxic than a single large dose. However, there is an apparent limit to how small the multiple doses can be for an effect to be seen. It is suggested that the virtual no-effect daily oral dose for sheep is one-eightieth of the LD_{50}.[9,13]

Lupinosis primarily occurs in summer and autumn when livestock graze the dead lupins. Temperature, rainfall, humidity, dew, and cloud cover all probably influence toxin production, but the precise requirements for each are not known. In the laboratory, 25° C is the optimum temperature for toxin production by the fungus in liquid culture. Once lupins develop toxicity they remain toxic for several months, and in some cases, years. In the summer and autumn immediately after the lupins grow, subsequent periods of toxin production are additive. Thus, lupin stubbles are generally least toxic at the start of summer and most toxic at the end of autumn. Decline in the toxicity of stubbles has occasionally been observed, but conditions that lead to breakdown of the phomopsins in the field are unknown. The fungus dies over the subsequent winter, so toxicity does not increase after the first autumn.[14,15]

Clinical Signs. Lupinosis is mainly characterized by severe liver damage, which results in inappetence, loss of condition, lethargy, jaundice, and often death. The course of the disease may be acute, subacute, or chronic depending on the quantity of phomopsins consumed in relation to time. The disease has also been associated with abortion in late pregnant sheep and cattle, death of embryos in early pregnant sheep, up to a 50% reduction in lambing percentage in ewes, reduced wool production and staple strength in sheep, and starvation ketosis in cattle. Photosensitization is uncommon in sheep but is often seen in cattle.[2]

Two secondary complications are common to lupinosis in sheep. The first is hepatoencephalopathy resulting from hyperammonemia. This is often brought on when sheep with lupinosis are fed lupin seeds in an attempt to improve their condition. The lupin seeds contain approximately 30% crude protein and the damaged liver is unable to metabolize the influx of ammonia. Affected sheep stand apart from the rest of the flock, wander in a disorientated manner, and may exhibit repetitive sideways head movements, head pressing, or "star gazing."[14]

The other condition is lupinosis-associated myopathy. This is seen in young sheep (4 to 9 months of age) and is considered to be a nutritional myopathy that cannot be successfully treated or prevented with traditional selenium or vitamin E therapies. This is possibly due to lupinosis interfering with the normal metabolism of selenium and vitamin E.[16] It normally only affects skeletal muscles. Affected sheep move with stiff limbs and, if severely affected, are reluctant to

move; they stand with hunched backs and feet placed closely under the body.[14]

Clinical Pathology. The clinical biochemistry changes in lupinosis are consistent with those expected with any hepatotoxicosis. There is increased activity in plasma enzymes of hepatic origin and increased concentrations of plasma bilirubin. In chronic lupinosis, plasma albumin concentrations decrease and plasma globulin concentrations increase. Plasma concentrations of cholesterol are reduced in acute lupinosis, but increased in chronic lupinosis. Plasma triglyceride concentrations are increased in all forms of lupinosis. If the sheep also have lupinosis-associated myopathy, plasma creatine kinase activities are increased. Plasma concentrations of urea, creatinine, and magnesium are increased and concentrations of sodium and bicarbonate are decreased if there is concurrent nephrosis and degenerative changes in the adrenal cortex.[17]

Sheep may develop an increased packed cell volume (possibly the result of dehydration), leukocytosis, and neutrophilia in acute lupinosis or anemia in chronic lupinosis.[18]

Lesions. Gross pathology varies depending on whether the disease is acute, subacute, or chronic. In acute and uncomplicated subacute lupinosis, there is generalized jaundice and the liver is greatly swollen. It is bright yellow, orange, or cream in color and the cut surface is very greasy. The gall bladder is usually enlarged, and the adrenal glands are swollen and cream-colored. The kidney is usually normal in appearance, but may be golden-brown or pale depending on the degree of hemosiderin or fat deposition that has occurred. Often ascites and edema of connective tissues are found. The cecum is frequently distended with dry, hard fecal material that may contain blood. Petechial hemorrhages may be present in subcutaneous tissues and the epicardium. Evidence of myopathy may be seen as obvious areas of pallor or subtle pale streaking in the skeletal muscles, and occasionally, cardiac muscle.[14]

In chronic lupinosis, jaundice is frequently not a feature. The liver is small, hard, coppery, or tan in color, and often misshapen. The ruminal contents are watery, and the abomasum and small intestine contain very little solid material. The cecum may contain hard, dry, impacted fecal material. Ascites and evidence of muscle wastage may be present.[14]

When sheep are moved on and off lupin stubble, it is not uncommon for them to suffer episodes of subacute lupinosis. In such sheep, the color, size, shape and consistency of the liver can vary considerably.[14]

The characteristic features of the microscopic pathology observed in the liver are individual death of many hepatocytes, predominantly by apoptosis, and arrested and abnormal mitosis affecting variable numbers of hepatocytes. Other changes in hepatocytes include megalocytosis and karyomegaly, variable degrees of fat accumulation, the presence of intranuclear pseudoinclusions, and the presence of intracytoplasmic hyaline globules. Variable degrees and patterns of fibrosis, increased size and number of Kupffer cells, the presence of a golden-brown pigment (lupinoid pigment) in Kupffer cells, and bile duct cell proliferation are other changes seen in the liver.[10]

In cases of fatal, acute lupinosis, parenchymal cells undergoing apoptosis or in arrested mitosis can be seen in the renal cortex, adrenal cortex, pancreas, and epithelium of the rumen and reticulum.[10]

Spongiform change in the white matter of the brain, particularly in the central white substance of the cerebellum, occurs in animals with hepatoencephalopathy.[19] Segmental hyaline degeneration and subsequent regeneration of muscle fibers is found in animals with lupinosis-associated myopathy.[10]

Diagnostic Testing.   Fixed liver, collected by biopsy or at a necropsy, is the sample of choice. The microscopic pathology of lupinosis is reasonably pathognomonic. A sensitive and specific ELISA for the detection of phomopsins in feedstuffs is available.[20]

Treatment.   No specific treatment is available, but an animal that is eating rarely dies of lupinosis. Therefore, the primary aim of any treatment is to stimulate the appetite by removing access to the toxic feed and immediately providing good-quality hay and cereal grains as supplementary feed. Some animals may be more attracted to lucerne hay than a cereal or pasture hay. Spraying the supplementary feed with molasses, butyric acid, aniseed essence, or rumen fluid from healthy livestock may encourage eating. High-protein grains or supplements should not be fed with urea.[14] If the animals are on green pasture, access to shade should be provided.

Additional treatments include a single drench with zinc sulfate (there is a reduction in liver zinc concentrations in sheep with lupinosis) and an injection with vitamin B_{12} (some studies have shown a substantial reduction in liver cobalt concentrations in sheep with lupinosis). For an adult sheep, the suggested dose of zinc is 1 g in a 20 ml solution of zinc sulfate.[14] In valuable animals, any treatment to stimulate rumen movement may be beneficial, including drenching with the rumen contents from healthy livestock.[14]

Prognosis.   Livestock that regain their appetite recover completely.

Prevention and Control.   Planting *Phomopsis*-resistant lupins is the best method of controlling the occurrence of lupinosis. The first *Phomopsis*-resistant lupins were released in Australia in 1989, resulting in a substantial reduction in the occurrence of lupinosis. Studies have indicated that the prevalence of lupinosis on farms has been reduced from 56% to 8% and sheep mortality from 4% to 0.2%, by growing phomopsis-resistant rather than phomopsis-susceptible lupins.[2] Even though most work on phomopsis-resistant lupins has concentrated on *Lupinus angustifolius*, the ultra and Kiev mutant varieties of *L. albus* are also resistant.[2]

Phomopsis-resistant lupins do not completely remove the risk of lupinosis. The following sheep management procedures can further reduce the risk of disease: graze the lupin stubbles immediately after harvest; provide young stock with access to lupin seeds for a few days before placing them on the lupin stubbles; do not stock lupin stubbles at rates greater than 20 sheep/hectare (ha); remove the sheep from the stubbles when the amount of spilt lupin seed falls to 50 kg/ha or less; provide adequate watering points; and regularly observe the flock for lethargic sheep falling behind the flock, which is the first indication that lupinosis is developing.

An experimental vaccine against lupinosis is undergoing refinement and evaluation in field studies. If it proves to be suitable for commercial release, it will be invaluable in situations where livestock have access to *Phomopsis*-susceptible lupins.[21,22]

SLAFRAMINE

Gavin L. Meerdink

Synonyms.   Slaframine has also been referred to as "slobber factor." The syndrome produced has been called slobber syndrome or clover poisoning and, less often, rhizoctonia poisoning.

Sources.   Slaframine is an indolizidine alkaloid synthesized from lysine by the fungus *Rhizoctonia leguminicola*, which infects plants to cause black patch disease.[1] Slaframine production by fungal isolates is consistent, although production is decreased at temperatures greater than 25° C (in vitro).[1]

Black patch disease primarily has been reported in association with clovers (*Trifolium* spp.). Early reports involved red clover; however, cases have occurred with white and alsike clovers. Although black patch disease is usually associated with clovers, it has been found in other legumes such as soybean, kudzu, cowpea, blue lupine, alfalfa, Korean lespedeza, and black medick.[2,3] The pathogen can overwinter on infected plants and survive at least 2 years on infected seed. Black patch is encountered more during summer periods of wet weather and high humidity. The dead, brown, diseased plant parts can be confused with normal maturation of the clover plant. *R. leguminicola* also produces the structurally similar alkaloid swainsonine that is believed responsible for locoism, a nervous system disease.[4]

Toxicokinetics.   Slaframine is absorbed and produces effects rapidly. Slaframine is activated by a hepatic microsomal flavoprotein oxidase to a ketoimine metabolite. This transformation includes the addition of an ester function that is required for parasympathomimetic activity.[4] The slaframine active metabolite may be structurally transitory and readily convert back to the slaframine parent compound. Slaframine seems to have a higher specificity for the gastrointestinal tract, although tissue predilections are not known. However, the active ketoimine form is not likely to cross the blood-brain barrier because of a charged quaternary nitrogen component.[4]

Purified slaframine has a prolonged (6 to 10 hours) stimulatory effect on secretion from salivary glands, pancreas, and other exocrine and endocrine glands. This is longer than signs are usually seen with single doses of naturally contaminated material.[1] The reason for this is not clear, but may relate to its affinity for target receptor or the kinetics of liver activation.[4]

Mechanism of Action.
Slaframine acts as a para-sympathomimetic agent to stimulate exocrine and endocrine glands, particularly salivary glands and the pancreas. It has been classified as a cholinergic agonist.[4] The action of slaframine can be blocked by preadministration of atropine; however, atropine does not reverse the salivary response once initiated.[1]

Salivary secretion can be increased by greater than 50% (as measured in cattle). The effects on pancreatic activity are variable. Some studies with purified slaframine reported increased pancreatic fluid and enzyme secretion in the calf, goat, and sheep.[5] Another study reported only increases in pancreatic trypsin secretion with no changes in pancreatic protein secretion or other digestive enzymes with partially purified slaframine.[6]

Slaframine has no effect on cardiovascular function or blood pressure at dosages stimulatory to exocrine glands, except, possibly, in dogs.[1] Slaframine does not inhibit blood cholinesterase activity.[4]

Slaframine infused into the abomasum (doses of 10, 20, and 30 μg/kg body weight) after once daily feeding resulted in increased rumen volume and pH as well as decreased ruminal volatile fatty acids, ammonia concentrations, and ruminal NDF (neutral detergent fiber) digestion. Rumen dry matter and starch digestion apparently increased with the lowest dosage and decreased at the higher two dosages of slaframine. Abomasal infusion of slaframine alters ingesta passage and the site of digestion of nutrients between the rumen and the lower digestive tract. The highest level shifted the site of digestion to the lower tract, whereas lower dosages enhanced ruminal digestion.[7]

Slaframine has been administered to feeder cattle to assess its value in prevention and control of acidosis associated with high-concentrate diets. Cattle injected with 66 μg slaframine per kg body weight had increased salivary flow (approximately 50% greater). The decrease in rumen pH was reduced with subacute acidosis, but the lactate concentrations were not effectively changed. Slaframine does not have a beneficial effect on acute ruminal acidosis.[8] Daily injections of slaframine dichloride (at 30 and 60 μg slaframine free-base per kg body weight) did increase saliva flow, increase ruminal pH, and increase serum somatotropin. However, insulin-like growth factor was not affected and the higher dose (60 μg/kg) resulted in reduced dry matter intake and weight loss.[9]

Toxicity and Risk Factors.
Though slaframine is a potent pharmacologic agent, few studies have been conducted to measure this lethality. The LD_{50} of slaframine in day-old male broiler chicks is estimated at approximately 81.6 mg/kg body weight.[4]

Cats administered 0.3 g/kg pure slaframine began salivating within 40 minutes; signs were at maximum after 1 hour and returned to normal after about 6 hours.[10] Second doses resulted in reduced response.[1] As noted earlier, cattle given 60 μg/kg body weight daily (by abomasal infusion) had decreased feed intake and reduced body weight.

Clinical Signs.
Signs of intoxication are similar among species. Following ingestion of contaminated forages, animals begin to salivate within 15 minutes (e.g., guinea pigs and small animals) to several hours (e.g., cattle). Species differences in time of onset are apparently not related to sensitivity. Guinea pigs and ruminants seem particularly sensitive to the toxin versus others, such as the rat, that do not salivate at doses that can cause severe reactions to others.[11] A single dose can result in a salivation episode lasting a few hours to a day or two. Although uncommon and related to dose and exposure duration, additional signs can include anorexia, diarrhea, frequent urination, and bloat. Lacrimation occurs periodically, but is rarely intense.[2,12] Decreased milk production can be expected when a significant reaction occurs in milking animals. Joint stiffness, abortion, and death have been reported in isolated cases. Slaframine intoxication has been observed in cattle, sheep, horses, goats, swine, poultry, cats, dogs, guinea pigs, rats, and mice.[1,4]

Dyspnea with open mouth breathing and cyanosis has been reported in sheep, pigs, and guinea pigs. Experimentally, pigs have also been observed to cough, vomit, and walk with stiffened pelvic limbs.[11] Calves had increased pancreatic secretion that continued for 10 hours; bile flow did not change.[10]

Dogs fed nonlethal doses exhibited decreased heart and respiratory rates, and decreased left ventricular and aortal pressure with an accompanying 50% decrease in cardiac output.[13] In guinea pigs, respiration rates decreased from 118 to 36 per minute in a 5-hour induced response, and heart rates declined from an initial 340 to approximately 110 within 40 minutes. Body temperatures declined in guinea pigs from 39° C to 32° C in 2 hours.[10,11] Slaframine administered on day 19 of gestation to pregnant rats caused uterine hemorrhage, abortion, and frequent maternal death; similar effects were observed in pregnant guinea pigs.[10,14]

Lesions.
Because death is rare, lesions from field cases are not well documented. Morphologic change is related to respiratory effects of excess fluid secretions and dyspnea.

Experimentally, gross or microscopic lesions were not observed after a chronic 3-week exposure in guinea pigs to sublethal doses of slaframine.[12] With lethal doses, vascular congestion of the thoracic and abdominal cavities was observed grossly.[2] Microscopically, areas of emphysema, disruption of the alveolar structure, pulmonary edema, congestion of the liver with areas of centrilobular necrosis, and apparent excessive activity of trachea submucosal glands have been described. Death is believed to be due to suffocation from pulmonary edema and or emphysema or, possibly, cardiac arrest.[2]

Diagnostic Testing.
The first assay method was a bioassay procedure based on the salivary response of guinea pigs.[1,11] Chromatographic analytic methods have been developed for detection of the slaframine alkaloid in plant materials. However, detection of metabolites from blood or urine of affected animals has not been sufficiently reliable to be useful in diagnostic testing.

Diagnosis depends on detection of plant lesions, animal clinical signs, recovery following the removal of the offending feedstuff, and detection of the toxin in feedstuffs by chemical analysis.

Treatment. Atropine administered soon after ingestion of a toxic dose of slaframine can reduce the severity of some clinical signs. However, once salivation has become excessive, reversal with atropine is unlikely. Atropine doses approximating 0.3 mg/kg body weight have been efficacious; however, with severe poisoning, doses greater than 2 mg/kg have been needed to prevent death. Antihistamines might also provide some relief of clinical signs.[2,11]

Prognosis. Naturally occurring field outbreaks generally are recognized early in the course of the condition. Early removal from the offending forage conveys rapid resolve of the problem with few aftereffects. With higher doses and longer exposure times, sequelae from dehydration and prolonged cholinergic stimulation can include loss in milk production, intestinal disturbances, and, possibly, abortion. Death is rare.

Prevention and Control. Feasible methods to detoxify or neutralize the effects of consumption of pasture and hay contaminated with this fungus have not been found. Thus, replacement with forages that do not cause problems is necessary. Precautionary test feeding of clover forage to a few animals before general feeding might be useful to avoid larger outbreaks.

SPORIDESMIN

Rosalind Dalefield

Synonyms. Sporidesmin toxicosis is also known as facial eczema and as pithomycotoxicosis.

Sources. The sporidesmins are mycotoxins found in the spores of the saprophytic fungus *Pithomyces chartarum*, formerly known as *Sporidesmium bakeri*. More than 90% of the sporidesmin produced by *P. chartarum* in culture is sporidesmin A. The remainder consists of small amounts of sporidesmins B, C, D, E, F, G, H, and J. The fungus grows on dead plant material, and pasture litter presents an ideal warm, humid microclimate for its proliferation and sporulation. Field cases of disease are restricted to ruminants grazing on improved pastures.[1] Toxicosis has been reported in New Zealand, Australia, Brazil, Uruguay,[2] South Africa,[3] France,[4] and the United States.[5] Only some isolates of *P. chartarum* produce sporidesmin; in one study, sporidesmin was produced by 86% of New Zealand isolates, 67% from Australian isolates, 28% of Uruguayan isolates, and 2% of Brazilian isolates.[2]

Toxicokinetics. Sporidesmin, which is hydrophobic, is rapidly absorbed from the gastrointestinal tract and concentrated in the liver and biliary tract. Sporidesmin has been detected, unchanged, in ovine bile only 10 minutes after

a single oral dose, with maximum concentrations being reached between 2 and 8 hours after administration and excretion largely complete at 24 hours.[6] Enterohepatic cycling may occur but is not thought to significantly increase the severity of lesions.[1]

It appears that at least some sporidesmin undergoes metabolism. Ovine hepatic microsomes have been shown to metabolize sporidesmin in vitro and those from Merinos do so much more efficiently than those of Romneys. Merinos are significantly more resistant to toxicosis in the field than Romneys, which shows a strong correlation with shorter sleeping time in response to pentobarbitone. Furthermore, induction of hepatic mixed function oxidases in sheep by pretreatment with hexachlorobenzene confers protection against sporidesmin toxicosis both by oral administration and in the field.[7]

Sporidesmin and metabolites are excreted predominantly in the bile and to a lesser extent in the urine.[1] Sporidesmin has not been identified in milk, but signs of toxicosis have been reported in calves that had no access to grass but were suckling cows that had clinical signs of sporidesmin toxicosis.[8]

Mechanism of Action. The reduced form of sporidesmin readily undergoes a cyclic reduction/autoxidation reaction in vitro. This reaction, which generates the superoxide radical, is strongly catalyzed by copper.[9] It is thought that the superoxide radical initiates tissue damage in vivo. The protective role of zinc salts in vivo has been attributed to the inhibition by zinc of intestinal absorption of copper in ruminants,[10] or to the reaction between zinc and reduced sporidesmin to form a stable mercaptide, which has been demonstrated in vitro.[11] Zinc also activates superoxide dismutase and may protect against oxidative injury by this mechanism.[1]

On the other hand, sporidesmin induces apoptosis in vitro, which may contribute to its toxicity in vivo. In that study it was found that the complex between zinc salts and the sporidesmin is not strong enough to prevent autoxidation of the mycotoxin but that zinc has a direct inhibitory effect on apoptosis.[12]

Sporidesmin is acutely toxic to bile canalicular membranes, with consequent reduction in bile flow, and causes swelling of hepatic mitochondria.[1] The overall result of the cellular damage is an obstructive cholangitis and hepatitis with hepatogenous photosensitization. Excretion into bile of phylloerythrin, a photodynamic porphyrin pigment derived from microbial breakdown of chlorophyl in the gastrointestinal tract, is impaired. Elevated levels of phylloerythrin in the blood cause a photodermatitis if pale skin is exposed to sunlight for even a few minutes.

Evidence exists that sporidesmin may cause direct capillary injury and vascular exudative reactions[1] and that repeated dermal application may result in a direct dermal hypersensitivity reaction that is independent of solar radiation.[8]

Sporidesmin is a potent clastogen (substance that causes chromosomal breaks) in vitro but not in live mice or sheep.[13,14]

Toxicity and Risk Factors. In the field, sporidesmin toxicosis affects grazing ruminants, although toxicosis has been induced experimentally in some laboratory species. Toxicosis is most likely to occur where there is close grazing of leafy, well-controlled pastures that include dead plant material. Toxicosis is usually associated with perennial ryegrass (*Lolium perenne*) pastures in New Zealand. Sporulation of *P. chartarum* is most abundant between 20° C and 25° C when night minimum grass temperatures exceed 14° C and humidity is close to 100%. High spore counts are most typical of late summer or early autumn after at least 4 mm rain. Spore numbers can increase significantly within 48 hours. Counts of 100,000 or more spores per gram of grass are generally considered dangerous.[15] Repeated small doses of sporidesmin over several days cause greater pathology than one large dose.[16]

Of the ruminants commonly farmed in New Zealand, sheep and fallow deer (*Cervus damadama*) are the most susceptible to sporidesmin toxicosis. Photosensitization of 60% of animals, icterus, and 100% mortality within 24 days have been achieved by giving fallow deer 0.3 mg/kg or more of sporidesmin for 3 days. Toxicosis typical of a serious field outbreak, featuring 50% incidence of photosensitivity and 7% to 15% mortality, has been replicated by orally giving sheep 0.5 to 0.8 mg/kg sporidesmin for 3 days or more. Merino sheep are less susceptible than breeds of English origin. In contrast to fallow deer, giving red deer (*Cervus elaphus*) up to 1.8 mg/kg orally for 3 days produced liver injury in only 25% of animals, without clinical signs.

Toxicosis typical of a serious field outbreak, featuring marked weight loss, photosensitization of 50% of animals, icterus, and some mortalities has been induced in gravid cows with oral doses of 1 mg/kg sporidesmin for 3 days. By contrast, 0.5 mg/kg for 3 days caused largely subclinical illness, whereas 3 mg/kg for 3 days caused 100% mortality within 3 to 5 days in calves.[1] In New Zealand, the incidence of overt toxicosis is higher in dairy cows than in beef cattle. Within dairy herds the incidence is highest in lactating cows, lower in weaner calves, and lowest in replacement heifers.[1] However, a study in Brazil found the highest prevalence in cattle 7 to 12 months old.[17]

Compared with sheep, goats are relatively resistant to sporidesmin toxicosis. Oral administration of sporidesmin has shown that Saanen goats require a dose 2 to 4 times greater than that given to sheep to elicit the same serologic evidence of liver injury, whereas feral goats and feral x Angora goats require 4 to 8 times the sheep dose. In the field, goats may be even more resistant to toxicosis because they prefer to browse rather than graze[7] and therefore are less likely to ingest the spores, which are most numerous on leaf litter.

Oral administration of 3 mg/kg sporidesmin for 3 days caused mild duct lesions and no clinical signs in swine.

Horses are highly resistant to sporidesmin toxicosis.[1] Many of the areas of the North Island of New Zealand where serious outbreaks of sporidesmin toxicosis have occurred in ruminants are also popular areas for horse breeding, but sporidesmin toxicosis has never been reported in a horse. Furthermore, some degree of periportal fibrosis, indicative of mild sporidesmin toxicosis, is present in virtually all livers from adult sheep and cows in the North Island, but similar lesions are not routinely found in equine livers. No record exists in the literature of any attempt to experimentally dose horses with sporidesmin.

Sporidesmin toxicosis has been experimentally induced in a number of laboratory species. A single oral dose of 1.2 mg/kg sporidesmin has caused 50% mortality in rabbits within 14 days. In guinea pigs, 1 to 2 mg/kg for 21 days caused morbidity and 3.5 mg/kg caused 100% mortality within 14 to 21 days. Hepatic and pulmonary lesions with eventual mortalities have been induced with doses of 0.02 mg/day in rats and 0.1 to 0.2 mg/day in mice. Daily doses of 0.5 mg/kg cause 100% mortality within 14 days in week-old chickens.[1]

Clinical Signs. In field cases, the first signs observed in sheep develop 10 to 20 days after ingestion of sporidesmin and are those of dermal photosensitization. Areas exposed to sunlight, particularly the ears, eyelids, face, and lips, develop edema and erythema. Edema often causes the ears to droop. The animal tends to shake its head, scratch or rub the affected areas, and seek shade. Serum exudation from the affected areas results in scabs, while the rubbing causes secondary trauma and bleeding. Necrotic skin may slough from nostrils, lips, and ears. Secondary bacterial infection is commonplace, and flystrike (cutaneous myiasis) may also occur. Photosensitized sheep develop icterus. The urine is deeply colored as a result of bilirubinuria and, in some cases, of hemorrhagic ulcerations in the urinary bladder. Sheep develop urinary cystitis and may exhibit urinary incontinence and urine-staining of the fleece. For every sheep that shows overt photosensitization, there are likely to be many more in the flock that have hepatic lesions without accompanying skin lesions.[4] Subclinical cases may cause decreased growth rates, decreased wool production, and reproductive inefficiency.

The first sign in dairy cattle is often a sudden decrease in milk production. Lesions of dermal photosensitization follow, usually developing 14 to 24 days after exposure. The site of lesions varies depending on the markings of the individual animal, because lesions are generally confined to lightly pigmented or pink skin. Areas with sparse hair cover, such as ears, face, lips, escutcheon, udder, teats, and coronets are particularly vulnerable. Erythema and edema progress to exudation, ulceration, scab formation, and bleeding. Photosensitized cattle develop icterus and bilirubinuria. A small proportion of cattle may develop erythrocyte fragility, massive intravascular hemolysis, hemoglobinuria, and anemia, which may be severe enough to cause them to collapse when stressed.[1] Dark-colored cattle, such as Jersey/Friesian cross cows, which are often dark brown and have white markings only on the belly or udder, may sustain severe hepatic injury yet show little or no dermatitis, because their skin is protected by the presence of melanin.

The incidence of overt toxicosis in farmed red deer is low in the field and is confined to subtle signs of minor liver injury. In contrast, fallow deer develop photosensitization with 7 to 14 days of exposure and exhibit severe distress. Clinical signs include violent shaking of the head and ears, frantic rubbing and licking, restlessness, searching for shade, and intense icterus and bilirubinuria. The animals develop cystitis and frequent urination. Exposure of the tongue to sunlight while licking results in severe inflammation and ulceration of the tongue. Acute mortality is relatively high in this species—more than 50% in some field outbreaks.[1]

Experimental induction of sporidesmin toxicosis in goats results in lesions similar to, although less florid than, those in sheep. Photosensitized goats exhibit lacrimation, periocular edema, and exudation around the eyes, nostrils, mouth, and sometimes the ears. The ears tend to be less edematous and pendulous in affected goats compared to affected sheep.[7]

Rabbits and guinea pigs develop icterus and hepatic failure, whereas signs in mice include icterus, anemia, ascites, and dyspnea resulting from pleural effusion. Rats develop icterus; effusions from the peritoneum or pleura are terminal changes. Rats that survive chronic dosing for more than 4 months develop glaucoma and blindness.[1]

Clinical Pathology.   Cholestasis leads to increases in serum GGT, bilirubin, cholesterol, triacylglycerols, phospholipids, and bile acids. Cytolysis results in elevations of serum AST, ornithine carbamoyltransferase, and glutamate dehydrogenase (GDH). Liver function impairment leads to a decrease in serum albumin, increased prothrombin time, and increased bromosulfophthalein retention. An increase in total serum proteins is caused largely by increases in γ-globulins and, to a lesser degree, increases in γ-globulins. Conflicting reports exist in the literature concerning changes in ALP and ALT; however, ALT is known to be of poor sensitivity as a marker for hepatic damage in sheep.

Elevation of serum GGT is the best criterion for detecting liver pathology as a result of sporidesmin toxicosis in sheep and cattle.[4] Elevations in both conjugated bilirubin and free bilirubin occur. A normocytic, normochromic anemia may be present in subchronic and chronic cases,[18] whereas occasional cattle develop an acute hemolytic anemia.

Urinalysis reveals marked bilirubinuria. Hematuria, inflammatory cells, hemoglobinuria, and secondary bacterial infections may also be present.

Lesions.   Histologically, the skin features ballooning degeneration of epidermal cells, edematous separation at the dermoepidermal junction, and formation of vesicles and pustules. Inflammatory cell infiltration is initially angiocentric. Thrombi are common in dermal blood vessels.[5]

Grossly, the tissues of affected sheep become icteric. In acute toxicosis, the liver is pale and moderately swollen, and it may be mottled. Later it becomes green or yellow-green. The gall bladder is distended and its mucosal surface may be severely ulcerated. The extrahepatic bile ducts are enlarged and may be occluded. Sheep with protracted photosensitization develop adrenal cortical hyperplasia sufficient to more than double the total adrenal weight.[1]

Experimental dosing of sheep has shown that over the first 48 hours, histopathology of the liver is confined to vacuolation of single, scattered hepatocytes. Degenerative changes in the bile duct epithelium become apparent after 48 hours, and cholangitis and pericholangitis become progressively more severe, necrotizing, and obliterative. Both intrahepatic and extrahepatic bile ducts are involved. Edema, necrosis, and granulation tissue with inflammatory infiltrate occur in the peribiliary tissue. Biliary occlusion by inspissated bile and sloughed, necrotic cells is apparent. Hepatocellular vacuolation, particularly of centrilobular hepatocytes, is apparent and bile pigment may be observed in hepatocytes.[1,19] Centrilobular hepatocytes in particular may exhibit glycogen accumulation. Hepatocellular and sinusoidal definition are lost and microabscesses may be present.[19]

In the recovering liver, there is proliferation of bile ducts and periportal fibroplasia, which may be extensive enough to produce fibrous bridges between portal triads.[5] The liver may become grossly misshapen, with areas of atrophy and others of regeneration.[1] Because of streaming of blood in the portal vein, the left lobe typically suffers the most severe atrophy and fibrosis.

Histopathologic findings in bovine livers are similar to those in sheep, although fibrosis tends to be more diffuse and less distinctively periportal. Saccular dilatations commonly occur in the larger intrahepatic bile ducts. Suppurative cystitis and pyelonephritis may be present.

Fallow deer that die early in the course of the disease may have severe pulmonary edema and interstitial emphysema. Lesions of the liver and urinary tract are similar to those in sheep. Other findings in fallow deer include severe inflammation and ulceration of the tongue, and, in some animals, gastric and intestinal ulcerations that may have perforated and led to local or general peritonitis.[1]

Hepatic and urinary tract lesions in goats are similar to those in sheep. Profuse yellow ascitic fluid, dark, swollen kidneys, and pulmonary lesions of emphysema and interlobular edema have also been reported in goats.[7]

Gross lesions in rabbits include gall bladder distention, edema of extrahepatic bile ducts, and firm livers with an accentuated lobular pattern. Hepatic infarcts may be present. Distended, fibrosed intrahepatic bile ducts are sometimes visible from the capsular surface in rabbits. Histopathologic findings in rabbits are generally similar to those in sheep, consisting of acute necrotizing cholangitis and cholecystitis. Heterophils may be found within and around intrahepatic bile ducts. Mild fatty change occurs in hepatocytes and scattered hepatocytes become necrotic. Hepatic arteries may exhibit fibrinoid degeneration in the wall nearest to a necrotic bile duct, and portal venules may contain thrombi attached to the wall nearest to a bile duct. As in sheep, features of recovery are bile ductule proliferation and periportal fibrosis, which may form bridges between triads.[20]

Guinea pigs also suffer hepatobiliary injury. The liver is markedly enlarged. The histopathologic features are similar to those in other species. Wedge-shaped areas of coagulative necrosis may occur in hepatic lobules. Thrombosis of the portal vein is also reported in this species.

Besides severe hepatic and bile duct lesions, rats may also have ascites, pleural effusions, pulmonary edema and, in chronic toxicosis, ocular lesions associated with glaucoma. Mice may exhibit pulmonary edema and bile-stained pleural exudation, in addition to hepatic and hepatobiliary lesions.[1]

Diagnostic Testing.   In New Zealand, diagnosis is usually made on clinical signs and consideration of the season alone. In areas where sporidesmin toxicosis is less frequent, exposure to *P. chartarum* should be confirmed. This is most readily done by pasture spore count.

To detect spores, pastures should be cut at about 1 cm above the soil line to prevent inclusion of soil, trimmed to 6 to 8 cm in length, chopped, and mixed. Fifteen grams of plant material is placed in a plastic bag with 150 ml sterile water containing 0.05% Tween. The bag is squeezed by hand approximately once per second for 1 minute. A 1-ml aliquot is examined using a hemocytometer slide.[21] The spores are distinctive structures, often described as resembling hand grenades. They are 8-20 micrometers wide × 10-30 micrometers long with zero to five (usually three) transverse septa and zero to three (usually two) longitudinal septa.[1] Spore counts in excess of 100,000 spores per gram of pasture are considered dangerous.

In a novel outbreak, it should further be confirmed that the *P. chartarum* is a toxigenic strain. Methods for the culture of *P. chartarum* and assay of sporidesmin are described in the literature.[1,22]

Treatment. Treatment is purely supportive. Photosensitized animals should be housed or provided with deep shade and put out to graze only at night. Animals may develop severe lesions in response to only a few minutes of direct sunlight, and sun block creams cannot be relied on for protection. Secondary bacterial infections should be treated as required. Many animals that show no signs of photosensitization have nevertheless sustained liver injury and should be managed accordingly.

Because clinical signs often do not become apparent for 10 to 14 days after ingestion, it may be too late for detoxification, but administration of zinc salts to prevent further toxicosis may be considered.

Prognosis. Animals may be affected repeatedly; immunity to the disease does not develop.

Prognosis is worse for fallow deer, many of which die early in the course of toxicosis with severe pulmonary edema. Others may succumb to various complications, including peritonitis following perforation of gastrointestinal ulcers.

Some sheep may die of debilitation, stress, extensive superficial lesions, or secondary complications. Most sheep eventually recover fully.

Cattle generally recover from icterus and photosensitization more rapidly than sheep, but general debility may persist for 3 to 4 months. Some cows may die the next spring, having insufficient hepatic reserve to meet the metabolic demands of late pregnancy, parturition, and lactation. This is particularly true of dairy cattle.

Prevention and Control. In the North Island of New Zealand, district advisories on spore counts are routinely broadcast by radio in the summer and early autumn. However, the distribution of spores is not uniform. Hot spots may occur, particularly on ridges, north-facing slopes, and near hedges.[15] Therefore, farmers may choose to purchase or lease a microscope and hemocytometer slide to do their own spore counts, which allows assessment of the problem on a paddock-by-paddock basis. An alternative approach is to use a "spore trap" that is pushed over the pasture like a lawn mower. The trap features beaters, which dislodge the spores from the pasture, and a vacuum system to deposit the spores on a sticky film, which may then be examined under a microscope.

Not all strains of *P. chartarum* are toxigenic and the sporidesmin is less stable than the spores, which may disappear within days, washed off by rain or broken down by sunlight.[1] Therefore, there is considerable interest in the development of a simple, sensitive immunoassay for sporidesmin measurement in the field.[23]

When exposure to pasture with high spore counts is probable, administration of zinc salts provides a cost-effective method of preventing toxicosis in livestock. Zinc salts are not effective if given after the sporidesmin exposure. Animals should receive a daily dose of a zinc salt equivalent to 25 mg/kg zinc. Mixing zinc sulfate in the water is an effective approach in dairy cows, but sheep cannot be relied on to drink water regularly. Both sheep and dairy cattle may be drenched with zinc oxide slurry. Sheep should be drenched at least once a week, which creates practical problems because of the large sizes of sheep flocks and sheep farms in New Zealand and Australia. The zinc oxide slurry may block the drench gun, or zinc oxide may settle out of suspension.

An alternative approach is to add the slurry to a feed, such as chopped maize or hay, to which the sheep have become accustomed and which is spread in the paddock. It is impossible to ensure that all animals receive an effective dose by this method. Zinc toxicosis is unlikely.

The pasture may be sprayed with zinc oxide. This method works well on dairy pasture but there may be considerable loss of zinc oxide between plants on shorter sheep pasture. The cows are confined for 24 hours on a small area that has previously been sprayed with zinc oxide. The spraying rate depends on the anticipated pasture utilization.

Research has been directed at the use of intraruminal bullets that release zinc slowly.[15] Iron is also protective against sporidesmin toxicosis and, although iron salts are too irritating to the gastrointestinal tract to be used alone for this purpose, they may prove to be a useful adjunct to zinc salts.[11]

Spraying with benzimidazole fungicides may prevent fungal growth on pasture. This method is expensive but may be justified for valuable livestock where the topography of the land permits. Fungicides include benomyl at 150 g active ingredient per hectare and thiophanate and thiabendazole, both at 140 g active ingredient per hectare. The fungicide is sprayed using a boom and nozzle. Recommended spray rate is 225 L/ha at 276 kPa from a vehicle traveling at 6.5 km/hour. Usually enough pasture to last 7 days is sprayed at one time. Sprayed pasture may remain safe for up to 6 weeks, but must be sprayed again if, within 3 days of spraying, more than 25 mm of rain falls within a 24-hour period. Pasture that is already high in sporidesmin may be made safe by spraying with benzimidazole fungicide, as long as stock do not graze within 5 days of spraying.[15]

Pasture can be managed to minimize toxicosis.[1] Animals should not be forced to graze close to the ground because this increases the risk of ingesting pasture litter and therefore spores. Alternative fodder, such as crops, may be provided but this is not a popular approach with New Zealand farmers and hill country farms may be nonarable. Hay may be provided as alternative feed. The sporidesmin level declines rapidly on grass under normal methods of hay making and storage. This may be a result of photolysis during outdoor drying, because sporidesmin retains its toxicity in hay dried artificially in a stream of hot air.[24]

It has recently been found that atoxigenic strains of *P. chartarum* can compete with toxigenic strains in the field and that deliberate addition of an atoxigenic strain to pasture can result in up to 80% less sporidesmin 14 weeks later.[20] This method may have practical application.

Practical methods to reduce susceptibility of grazing livestock to sporidesmin toxicosis by mixed function oxidase induction or immunoprophylaxis have not been developed. On the other hand, the heritability of resistance to sporidesmin toxicosis is sufficiently high in both sheep[1,15] and cattle[25] to make selective breeding for resistance promising in the long term. Prospective sires are challenged with a standardized dose of sporidesmin and response is measured by serum GGT assay. Those that show the least and slowest response are selected as sires.[15,25]

No one method of prevention is both absolutely effective and practical, so a combination of several methods is recommended.

STACHYBOTRYOTOXINS

Robert Coppock and Margita M. Dziwenka

Synonyms. Initially the toxins produced by *Stachybotrys* sp. were called stachybotryotoxins.[1] Five of these were identified as macrocyclic trichothecenes. Of these, three were identified as satratoxins F, G, and H, and two were identified as verrucarin J and roridin E. Trichoverrols A and B can also be produced. The compounds generally found in the highest concentration are satratoxins G and H.

Sources. Stachybotryotoxins are produced by filamentous molds generally growing on cellulose-rich substrates. Species of *Stachybotrys* are important producers of the stachybotrys group of toxins. *Stachybotrys* sp. can grow over a wide temperature range (0° C to 40° C), but they require a moisture content of 15% in the substrate and a relative humidity of about 90%.

Roughages, coarse grains, paper, wood, and other cellulose-containing materials, celluloid,[2] and foam materials in buildings can, under moist conditions, provide a suitable substrate for the growth of *Stachybotrys* sp.[3] Indoor environments can become contaminated with spores and hypha, and having direct contact with the fungal contaminated material can expose people and domestic animals. The conidia of *S. atra* made from cultures contain satratoxin H, satratoxin G, and trichoverrols A and B.[4] *S. chartarum* has been found to produce stachybotrys-type mycotoxins in high cellulose greenhouse pots.

Stachybotryotoxicosis in humans is linked to exposure from handling contaminated roughage[5] and from filamentous mold growing on suitable substrates in damp areas of buildings.[6] Dogs can develop contact dermatitis from exposure to bedding including straw contaminated with stachy-

botryotoxins, or being in an environment that has *Stachybotrys* spores in the air. Pigs can develop the disease when contaminated straw is used for bedding or contaminated coarse grains are fed. Poultry can be exposed to stachybotryotoxins from contaminated fiber being used for litter.

Stachybotryotoxicosis has been reported in sheep consuming wheat straw that was baled while having high moisture content.[7] The straw was black spotted and the black spots contained pure cultures of *S. atra*. Mycotoxins isolated were satratoxins G and H. In another incident, forage cubes made from wheat, barley, and rye straw were reported as the cause of stachybotryotoxicosis in sheep, and many of the animals also had a *P. haemolyticum* septicemia.[8]

Toxicokinetics. The toxicokinetics of the stachybotryotoxins have not been well defined.

Mechanism of Action. The macrocyclic trichothecenes are extremely irritating to skin and mucous membranes, and produce necrotizing lesions. They have been identified as potent disrupters of protein synthesis, and they suppress the immune system. They also have been demonstrated to disrupt cellular division; tissues with a high rate of cell division and metabolism are the most susceptible. Target tissues identified include bone marrow, gastrointestinal tract, and lymphoid tissue.

Toxicity and Risk Factors. Spores (10^6) from a mycotoxin-producing strain of *S. atra* were found to contain satratoxin G (0.04 µg), satratoxin H (0.1 µg), stachybotry-lactone (80 µg), and stachybotrylactam (20 µg). Mice (NMRI) were exposed to 10^6 spores of the *S. atra* by intranasal injection.[9] The mice became lethargic after exposure. One mouse died 10 hours after exposure; another mouse was killed in extremis at 24 hours after exposure. Two mice were killed 3 days after exposure and showed decreased body weight.

Clinical Signs. In general, animals have oral lesions, severe contact dermatitis, and signs related to inhalation of an irritating-necrotizing substance.

Humans. Clinical signs from handling contaminated roughage are reported as occurring in stages. The initial stage is a rash located in body areas with high perspiration. A rash under the armpits, in the genital area of both male and females, and on the breasts of females has been reported. A burning sensation occurs in the nose, eyes, and throat with epistaxis sometimes being observed. In the next stage, vesicles develop on the skin. Necrotizing skin lesions sometimes occur. Finally, marked irritation of the upper respiratory tract occurs. Fever, malaise, headache, and fatigue are also concurrent observations.

Pulmonary hemorrhage and hemosiderosis lesions in infants with sudden infant death syndrome in Ohio have suspicious links to stachybotryotoxins.[10] Common to all were water-damaged homes caused by flooding, leaking plumbing, or leaking roofs. Fungal species found to produce stachybotryotoxins in the laboratory have been isolated from some of these homes.[11] Controversy exists as to the links between finding the toxigenic fungi and the syndrome observed in the infants.

Horses. Stachybotrys was first recognized in eastern Europe in 1938 as the cause of death in horses.[12] Clinical signs are ptyalism with erythema and edema of the nose, lips, buccal mucosa, and tongue. Necrotic lesions occur in the oral cavity, which is malodorous. Necrosis and hypertrophy of regional lymph nodes generally follow edema of oral and nasal mucosa. The animal has neutropenia, decreased platelet count, and gastroenteritis with diarrhea. The febrile phase is sometimes accompanied by hemorrhage from the mucous membranes.

Sheep. Two weeks after contaminated wheat straw was introduced into the diet, lambs developed anorexia, ptyalism, lethargy, and weakness. Some animals had dyspnea, foamy and sometimes blood-streaked nasal discharge, diarrhea, wool loss, and pyrexia.

Cattle and bison. Cattle consuming roughage contaminated with toxigenic strains of *Stachybotrys* develop oral lesions similar to those described for sheep and horses.[13] Acute death from stachybotryotoxins can occur in cattle. Because of immune suppression, a variety of infectious type lesions may be observed. *C. perfringens* may be a complication of stachybotryotoxicosis, and this complication may occur in vaccinated animals. Because of partial feed refusal, a chronic form of intoxication was found to be more common in cattle in eastern Europe.

Clinical signs include partial anorexia, ptyalism, diarrhea, serous to purulent discharge from the nostrils, erythema of the nose, scabs appearing on the nose, lips, and tongue, weakness, and ataxia. Necrohalitosis develops from necrotic ulcers on the tongue. Profuse diarrhea sometimes contains shreds of intestinal epithelium. Leukocytosis occurs early, subsequently followed by a panleukopenia. At this stage, cattle are depressed, weak, and prefer to remain in recumbency. Some animals may abort. Hemorrhage is sometimes observed.

Swine. The first clinical sign is a contact dermatitis. The lips and underline are erythematous. Scabby lesions are observed on the nose and around the mouth of piglets and on the nipples and udder of sows. Agalactia has been observed in nursing sows. An acute, serous dermatitis progresses to multifocal areas of skin necrosis. Other signs include ptyalism, emesis, and depression.

Other aspects of stachybotrys in swine have been reported.[14] When present in the diet, it has been suspected of causing abortions in swine. Stachybotryotoxins have also been implicated in interfering with iron metabolism in piglets. This could be an indirect effect due to the role of ferritin as an acute phase protein. The toxicokinetics of stachybotryotoxins being excreted in milk are not known.

Dogs. Dogs given oral extracts from fungal cultures of *S. atra* developed an acute syndrome in 2 to 3 days; the dogs died in 4 to 6 days.[15] Leukocytosis was observed.

Dogs given small doses over longer periods of time developed leukopenia in 5 days, which persisted for 10 to 20 days and was followed by a leukocytosis and then a leukopenia. The dogs also developed a thrombocytosis followed by a thrombocytopenia with the thrombocytopenia following the leukopenia by a few days. Petechiae were observed in the mouth, larynx, and pharynx.

Poultry. Oral administration and feeding studies found that chickens are susceptible to stachybotryotoxins.[15] Necrosis of the tongue and mouth was observed in birds consuming contaminated feed. Contaminated litter resulted in contact dermatitis on the legs and beak. Clinical signs of depression, lethargy, ataxia, and anorexia were the first observed signs. Hematologic findings were leukopenia and thrombocytopenia.

The clinical signs and pathogenesis of stachybotryotoxicosis in turkeys, geese, and ducks are similar to those in the chicken.

Clinical Pathology. Hematologic changes include an acute leukocytosis, followed by a thrombocytopenia, leukopenia, eosinophilia, and hemorrhage.

Lesions. Pathologic findings in horses include erosions in the mouth and esophagus, ulceration of gastric mucosa, swollen intestinal mucous membranes, hemorrhage in muscles and intestinal tract, and lymphoid necrosis. In dogs affected chronically, extensive hemorrhages are found in the subcutaneous tissue, pleura, and diaphragm. In chickens, degenerative lesions were observed in the liver, kidney, and myocardium.

Pathologic findings in sheep include subcutaneous ecchymosis, swollen, dark-red lymph nodes, and petechia to ecchymosis on the diaphragm, mediastinum, pericardium, heart, and membranes of the peritoneal cavity, pleura, and spleen. Mucous membranes of the rumen and abomasum have hemorrhage and erosions, and scattered hemorrhages are observed in the small intestine. The mucous membranes of the throat are swollen and hyperemic, and the tonsils have areas of necrosis. The nasal passages and trachea may contain foamy, reddish mucous. Many of the animals have a *P. haemolyticum* septicemia, and the septicemia is a complication of the mycotoxicosis.

Severity of the lesions in target tissues may vary with route of exposure. Erosions have been observed to occur in the entire gastrointestinal tract after oral exposure. Histopathology reveals necrosis of the enterocytes, especially in the crypt regions. The gut-associated lymphoid tissue areas may have erosions. The bone marrow may be devoid of cellular material or a large number of cells with pyknotic nuclei may be observed. Lympholysis occurs especially in the B-lymphocyte regions of the visceral lymph nodes, peripheral lymph nodes, and spleen. Necrosis of the thymus may also be observed.

Inhalation exposure can result in irritation and necrosis of the respiratory tract. Diffuse hemorrhages may occur as a result of thrombocytopenia. Mice exposed intranasally to spores and dust from mycotoxin-producing strains of *S. atra* were observed to have severe interalveolar and interstitial inflammation and hemorrhagic exudate in the alveoli. The inflammatory exudate contained neutrophils and macrophages. Focal areas of necrosis were observed in the bronchi around the fungal spores. Mice exposed to non–mycotoxin-producing strains had a mild inflammatory reaction, but did not have necrosis occurring around the spores.

Diagnostic Testing. The owner should be questioned regarding the appearance of black spots on roughage and coarse grains, or if buildings used to house the animal could have nooks and crannies that favored the growth of toxigenic fungi. Samples of roughage or bedding can be submitted to a diagnostic laboratory for culturing and other methods of fungal identification. Samples of the feedstuffs and bedding can be analyzed for the toxins. Liver, kidney, rumen, or gastric contents may contain the toxins and should be collected during necropsy. The samples should be frozen and stored at −20° C.

Treatment.   Specific antidotes for stachybotryotoxicosis do not exist. Symptomatic and supportive treatment are indicated. Broad-spectrum antibiotics often are indicated. These animals generally are immune compromised. Therefore, they will not have a good immune response to vaccines, and animals vaccinated during the toxicosis should be revaccinated.

Prognosis.   The prognosis is generally guarded, especially if the animal is leukopenic. Multiple blood samples should be taken to determine whether the animals are leukopenic and thrombocytopenic. In most situations, the problem is not recognized early and the toxicosis is advanced.

Prevention and Control.   The best prevention of stachybotryotoxicosis is to bale roughage and bedding at less than 20% moisture and to keep the bales dry. Roughage or bedding that is observed to have black spots and emit a very irritating dust should not be used. Moisture buildup in animal quarters or water damage from leaking roofs and such can provide a suitable area for the growth of cellulophilic molds. When the molds dry, the spores and hypha can form into dust. These small dust particles are inhaled deep into the respiratory system causing extreme irritation to the respiratory tract and necrotizing lesions.

Occurrences of stachybotryotoxicosis in pet animals that are linked to "sick" building syndrome do not appear to have been reported. However, pets would be susceptible.

TREMORGENIC FORAGES

John A. Pickrell, Fred Oehme, and Shajan A. Mannala

Synonyms.   The disease syndrome caused by these plants is often referred to as "staggers."

Sources.   Sclerotia or endophyte fungi growing on grasses cause toxicosis in the animals that consume them. Table 23-7 lists the forages that have known or suspected mycotoxin tremorgens.[1-5]

Toxicokinetics.   Signs occur within 7 days of grazing.[3,6] Cattle return to normal 3 to 7 days after cessation of the consumption of forage. Residues are not a problem because alkaloids do not accumulate in fat.[1]

Mechanism of Action.   All tremorgens cause presynaptic motor release and prolonged depolarization, facilitating transmission at the motor endplate. These tremorgens are associated with reduced concentrations of inhibitory amino acids, such as GABA or glutamate that lead to responses in the CNS. Finally, these compounds cause vasoconstriction

TABLE 23-7 Tremorgenic Mycotoxins in Forages

Forage	Fungus	Mycotoxin
Perennial rye grass	*Acremonium lolii*	Lolitrem B
Dallis grass and bahia grass	*Claviceps pasapali*	Paspalitrems
Bermuda grass	Unknown	Unknown

in the cerebrum leading to cerebral anoxia, which also supplements the nervous signs.[1]

Toxicity and Risk Factors.   The toxicity is not well defined in domestic animals.

Clinical Signs.   When at rest, animals appear to move and graze normally.[3,6] Only a few minutes of excitement or movement is needed to exaggerate these signs from minimal fine tremors around the head and neck to placement tremors, stiffness, ataxia, hypermetria, seizures, and opisthotonus.[6-8] In a typical episode, animals may stand with their hind legs extended and sway. When forced to run, animals have exaggerated flexure of the forelegs and incoordination that causes them to fall. They remain recumbent for several minutes, gain an upright position, and walk slowly away.[3] The signs usually revert to those at resting in a few minutes. Animals can injure themselves during hypermetria, seizures, or opisthotonus. If animals fall into bodies of water, they may drown.[1-6]

Clinical Pathology.   Abnormalities are not reported.[1,9]

Lesions.   Significant Purkinje cell necrosis (torpedoes) develops, with or without axonal swellings.[4,9] These lesions are not specific for type of tremorgen.[4]

Diagnostic Testing.   Tests to measure tremorgens in body fluids are neither routinely available nor reliably interpreted.[1]

Treatment.   Contaminated forage should be replaced and animals should be kept in a quiet, secure place until they recover. Animals should receive protection from the sun and dehydration. Medications that enhance glycine in the CNS have been used experimentally to reduce clinical signs in mice.[1]

Prognosis.   The prognosis is good. Morbidity is high, but mortality is generally low. Cattle generally return to normal 3 to 7 days after cessation of the consumption of grass.[1]

Prevention and Control.   Animals should be denied access to endophyte-infested grass. Only endophyte-free grass seed should be planted.

TRICHOTHECENE MYCOTOXINS

David Villar and Thomas L. Carson

Synonyms.   Trichothecenes belong to a class of chemicals called *sesquiterpene lactones*, which are characterized by the tetracyclic 12,13-epoxy-trichothec-9-ene skeleton. The compounds that are best known and of greatest concern in domestic animals include deoxynivalenol (vomitoxin or DON), T-2 toxin, diacetoxyscirpenol (DAS), nivalenol, and satratoxin (*Stachybotrys*).

Sources. Trichothecenes are mainly produced by various strains of the *Fusarium* fungi, which infect corn, wheat, barley, and other cereals in the field. The molds require cool, wet weather during the flowering and seed development stage of the infected plant and tend to produce their toxin in late-harvested or overwintered grain. Contamination of grains is therefore associated predominantly with fungal infection in the field rather than during storage and is often associated with periods of excessive rainfall, high humidity, and muddy field conditions that delay the harvesting of the crop.

Toxicokinetics. In general, most trichothecenes are rapidly metabolized and excreted as hydroxylated metabolites in the bile and urine within 2 to 3 days after ingestion. As a consequence, significant residues in edible animal tissues are not a practical problem and have not been found 24 hours after ingestion.[1] Also, because of rapid metabolism and excretion, normal feed intakes quickly resume once the toxin is removed. Metabolism of DON is of particular interest because it explains the marked differences in susceptibility among species to its toxic effects.

In pigs, DON is rapidly and efficiently absorbed, extensively distributed throughout the body but poorly metabolized (detoxified).[2] Little biotransformation occurs in pigs and most is excreted unchanged through the urine within 24 hours.

Unlike in swine, metabolism is a major process of elimination of DON in ruminants. Studies have revealed that both ruminants and poultry are capable of microbial transformation of DON into its metabolite 3α,7α,15-trihydroxy-trichothec-9,12-diene-8-one (DOM-1); therefore, very little DON (<1% to 5%) is bioavailable for absorption.[3,4] Most DON is converted to DOM-1 by the rumen microflora and then excreted through the feces or absorbed and conjugated

with glucuronide in the liver before excretion through the urine.[5] When metabolized to DOM-1, DON loses its cytotoxic activity in vitro[6] and in vivo[7]; therefore, this metabolite is assumed to be biologically inactive. No significant amount of DON or its metabolite DOM-1 is transferred to milk[8]; in fact, only insignificant traces were detected in some studies when cows were given extremely high doses.[5,9]

Mechanism of Action

DON. It appears that DON causes mild to moderate lesions in the mucosa of the stomach and intestines of pigs[10,11] and this may impair the absorption of certain nutrients, which is one of the mechanisms of toxic effects proposed by some authors.[12] It is believed that DON acts via the chemoreceptor zone of the medulla oblongata to induce vomiting rather than involving direct effects on the gastrointestinal tract.[2]

Unlike in rodents, the studies in swine exposed to feed levels of 2 and 5 ppm DON for 6 weeks did not find any immune response inhibition or stimulation in a wide battery of tests.[13] The authors concluded that at levels normally found in suspected contaminated feeds (i.e., <5 to 10 ppm), immunosuppressive effects are most unlikely, although they cannot be excluded. Other authors have concluded that effects on selected immunologic and hematologic parameters are difficult to separate from the impact of a lower feed intake.

DAS and T-2. Both toxins have been classed as potent radiomimetic substances because they affect rapidly dividing cells (i.e., those of the bone marrow, lymph nodes, intestinal mucosa) and thus cause similar lesions to those produced by ionizing radiation.

Toxicity and Risk Factors

DON. DON, also called vomitoxin, is by far the most commonly detected *Fusarium* mycotoxin and the least toxic. There is marked difference in sensitivity among species to DON, which is reflected by the FDA advisory levels: 5 ppm in total diet for cattle and poultry, 1 ppm for swine feed, and

TABLE 23-8 **Toxicity of Trichothecenes in Domestic Animals**

Toxin	Species	Dietary Level	Clinical Effect
Deoxynivalenol (DON, vomitoxin)	Swine (growing-finishing)	1 ppm	No sickness, minimal reduction in feed consumption
		5-10 ppm	25%-50% reduction in feed consumption
		20 ppm	Complete refusal
	Cattle	12 ppm	No effect
	Sheep	16 ppm	No effect
	Poultry	20-40 ppm	No effect
	Horses	~15 ppm	No effect
	Dogs	4 ppm	Reduced food ntake
		8 ppm	Vomiting
T-2 toxin and DAS	Swine (growing-finishing)	1 ppm	No effect
		2 ppm	Decreased feed consumption
		≥4 ppm	Decreased feed consumption; oral/dermal irritation; immunosuppression
		16 ppm	Complete feed refusal; vomiting

2 ppm for all other animal species including finished products for human consumption. The relationship between feed levels of DON and clinical effect for various species is summarized in Table 23-8.

In swine, dose-related studies have shown that feed refusal can be expected when feeds contain more than 1 ppm DON.[14] An almost linear dose-effect relationship exists between the feed concentration of DON and the clinical response in pigs (see Table 23-8).

In dairy cattle, no effect on total feed intake or milk production was observed at levels of 12 ppm dry matter (total daily intake of 104 mg DON/cow).[8] In other studies in which pregnant yearling crossbred beef heifers were fed diets with 3.4 kg of barley averaging 36.8 ppm DON (total daily of 134 mg DON/cow), no effects on feed intake, heifer weight gain, calf birthweight, or blood metabolites were observed (Vern Anderson, personal communication). Similarly, crossbred lambs fed wheat diets containing DON at 15.6 ppm for 28 days did not exhibit changes in feed consumption, weight gain, feed efficiency, or hematologic or serum biochemical variables.[15]

Horses are also relatively resistant to DON; when fed barley containing levels of 36 to 44 ppm DON for 40 days, no evidence of illness or feed refusal was observed.[16]

Occasionally, cases of dogs and cats exposed to contaminated food have occurred. Commercial dry-extruded pet foods may contain large quantities of grain and grain by-products, and because DON is stable at high temperatures and pressure processes, it can contaminate pet foods.[17] In a recent controlled study it was shown that dogs and cats are quite sensitive to DON and exhibit reduced food intake at dietary levels of DON at greater than 4 ppm and greater than 7 ppm, respectively. Vomiting is expected in both species at more than 8 ppm within 2 to 3 hours after feeding.[18]

Chickens and turkeys are tolerant to DON. The authors are unaware of studies in which poultry being fed diets with high levels of DON reported any detrimental effects. When end-of-lay hens were fed diets containing 38 ppm DON (i.e., higher levels than expected from natural contamination) for 4 weeks, no adverse effects occurred with egg production, feed consumption, body weight, or gross pathology.[19] In general, the literature indicates that poultry are relatively insensitive to DON; thus, the possibility has been raised that grains contaminated with DON in field situations may be incorporated into poultry diets without affecting performance.[20]

DAS and T-2. Although much research has been conducted with DAS and T-2 toxin, they rarely occur at toxic concentrations in North American grains and no proven field occurrences could be found in the literature. Both are potent toxins compared to DON and are well known for their effects on the skin. A no-effect level in swine is less than 1 ppm for DAS and T-2 toxin in the ration.

Clinical Signs.   The clinical signs caused by DON are feed refusal, followed by vomiting at higher doses.

DAS and T-2 also can cause decreased feed consumption and vomiting. In swine, oral lesions as well as intestinal necrosis have been reported, together with effects on body weight and feed consumption.[21] Some studies give detail descriptions of the skin lesions at levels greater than 4 ppm after 9 days of the experimental period.[22] Lesions consist of a crusting dermatitis of the snout, buccal commissures behind the ears, and around the prepuce. Even though chickens are assumed to be tolerant to DON, such assumption should not be extended to these more potent trichothecenes. Chickens show a dose-related increase in the extent of mouth lesions and feed refusal starting at levels as low as 1 ppm (Fig. 23-8).[23] In a probable outbreak of T-2 toxicosis in dairy cattle, animals consuming a diet with 2 ppm T-2 or more over a 5-month period developed anorexia, high frequency of abortion, high temperatures, and occasional deaths with extensive hemorrhages on the serosal surfaces of internal organs.[24]

Diagnostic Testing.   Knowledge of the origin of grain and the weather conditions during the growing season may suggest conditions for fungal growth and may alert the practitioner as to the potential presence of mycotoxins. However, the identification of a specific mold organism or the measurement of mold spore counts does not necessarily imply presence of toxins. The recommended method of establishing a diagnosis is by representative sampling and analysis of feed for the specific mycotoxin.

In recent years, analytic techniques for the detection of common mycotoxins have improved and immunoassay test kits are available for screening or quantitation of DON and T-2 toxin as well as for other mycotoxins. These immunoassay tests are generally only accurate for the matrix intended, usually grain, and may give false-positive results on mixed feed or hay samples. When in doubt, other methods are available at veterinary diagnostic laboratories and private testing laboratories to provide more definitive results.

A common fallacy is to associate health herd problems with very low levels of mycotoxins. In these cases, a reexamination of the feed for nutritional composition, of the herd health history, and of the management practices often reveals other causes unrelated to mycotoxins.

Prevention and Control.   In general, these toxins tend to be stable in the environment and resistant to normal food

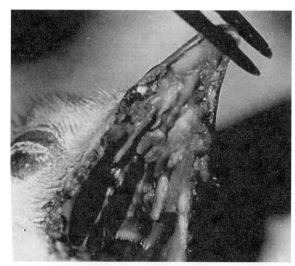

Fig. 23-8 Lesions in the hard palatine region of the oral cavity in a chicken offered feed containing 13.5 ppm T-2 toxin. Notice the ulcerated areas along the margin of the beak. (Courtesy of Dr. Gary Osweiler.)

processing conditions, including sterilization temperatures (120° C) and feed milling processes.[17]

ZEARALENONE

Gavin L. Meerdink

Synonyms. The disease was first described in U.S. swine in the 1920s and termed *vulvovaginitis* when reproduced and found to disappear after removal of the moldy corn. This *Fusarium* toxin was first referred to as F-2 toxin and was later named zearalenone (derived as "zea" from primary host *Zea mays;* "ral" from its resorcylic acid lactone chemical group; and "en" and "one" for a double bond and the ketone moiety in the molecule).[1-3]

Sources. Zearalenone, a resorcylic acid lactone, is a natural metabolite produced by strains of *Fusarium roseum* (or *F. graminearum), F. tricinctum, F. gibbosum, F. oxysporum, and F. moniliforme. F. graminearum* is the conidial stage of *Gibberella zeae.*[4,5] Enzymes responsible for the biosynthesis of zearalenone in crops are apparently induced at low temperature (12° C to 14° C). Optimum production of this mycotoxin is enhanced in most grain sources by higher temperatures (27° C).[6]

Clinical problems are more frequently reported from the temperate zones of northern United States and Canada. Corn is the substrate most frequently reported with problem cases; zearalenone has also been reported from wheat, sorghum, barley, oats, sesame seed, and corn silage. Stored ear-corn has provided a toxin source often in past cases.

Although rarely found in forages, evidence of zearalenone metabolites has been found in the urine of pasture-fed animals in New Zealand. The levels found were similar to those expected from treatment with the anabolic agent zeranol.[7] Zeranol (or α-zearalanol) was first derived from zearalenone by saturation of one double bond and conversion of the aldehyde to an alcohol. This agent is now synthetically produced for use as a growth-promoting implant in beef cattle and sheep (Ralgro).[8]

The toxin is generally stable in the environment; it can survive the heat of pelleting and can remain unaltered in grain for long periods of time. The quantity of toxin cannot be related to the amount of the mold present in the grain source.[5]

Toxicokinetics. Zearalenone is readily absorbed from the gastrointestinal tract. Liver metabolism results in α-zearalenol and its epimer by conversion of the ketone to a hydroxyl group. With the saturation of a double bond, α-zearalanol (zeranol) and α-zearalanol (taleranol) are formed. Zearalenone and its metabolites are conjugated with glucuronides and sulfates; these products can be found in urine and feces. Detectable concentrations in urine or feces are dose dependent and unlikely beyond 1 to 2 weeks after exposure. Enterohepatic recycling is sufficient to extend the half-life of plasma zearalenone and prolong its effects.[3,9]

Less than 1% of a dose of zearalenone in lactating cows is found in milk as free or conjugated forms. Single, one-time doses of up to 6 g of zearalenone to dairy cows resulted in total residues in milk of 16 ppb, which is about 0.01% of the dose.[10] Discrepancies in transmission of residues to cow's milk occur and may be due to dietary effects and differences in rumen protozoa available to metabolize zearalenone.

An in vitro study indicated that rumen microbes can degrade about 38% of the zearalenone to α- and β-zearalenol within 48 hours.[11]

Mechanism of Action. Even though structurally dissimilar, zearalenone functions as a weak estrogen and binds to receptors for estradiol-17β. This complex binds to estradiol sites on DNA and specific RNA synthesis is initiated that promotes signs of estrogenism. Ovarian follicle maturation and ovulation is inhibited by the reduction in plasma follicle stimulating hormone concentrations resulting from increased estrogenic negative feedback on the pituitary.[9,12]

Experimentally, zearalenone and zearalenol have been found to be capable of inducing thymic atrophy and macrophage activation, and of inhibiting mitogen-stimulated lymphocyte proliferation. The toxins have no effect on antibody or delayed type hypersensitivity responses and immunosuppression has not been recognized as an important clinical entity.[13]

Toxicity and Risk Factors. The extent of zearalenone metabolism to its alcohol metabolites is variable among species. Also, species sensitivity to the metabolic products varies, which impacts the dose-response differences among species.

Swine are the most sensitive species. Clinical signs in young gilts can become evident at about 1 ppm zearalenone in the diet; signs become more obvious or severe with higher doses. Infertility becomes evident at diet concentrations of approximately 3 to 5 ppm. Once pregnant, diet concentrations up to 15 ppm do not appear to affect litter development. Concentrations of greater than 20 ppm ingested by sows 7 to 10 days after conception can cause failure of implantation and embryonic death. Removal of zearalenone-contaminated feed at least 2 weeks before insemination generally restores normal reproduction efficiency. Low levels (<5 ppm) fed throughout pregnancy and lactation had no effect on postweaning rebreeding.[8,9,12,14]

Zearalenone, in sufficient concentrations, can reduce testes weights, spermatogenesis, and libido in young boars. The adverse effects generally disappear with removal of the contaminated feed. Mature boars are unaffected by dietary concentrations of at least 60 ppm (up to 200 ppm).[8,12,15] Prolonged feeding at 20 mg/kg body weight caused no testicular changes in rats.[16]

Zearalenone is not a major factor in bovine infertility. In one study, heifers (364 kg average) fed 250 mg zearalenone daily through three estrus cycles did not have lower conception rates. Doses of 500 mg zearalenone per head per day for two estrus cycles had no effect on health parameters or estrus. In order for zearalenone to have adverse effect on the conception rate in dairy cows, the ration must contain at least 50 ppm in the complete feed.[17,18]

Zeranol implants (doses of 36 mg) in young bulls adversely affect scrotal circumference, serving ability, and semen quality. The first two parameters can improve in time, but semen quality does not improve.[19]

Ewes administered zearalenone doses of 12 to 24 mg per head per day (equivalent to 4 to 8 ppm feed concentrations) before mating had a dose-related decline in ovulation rates. Estrus cycle length decreased and duration of estrus increased with increasing dose levels. When ewes were administered similar doses after mating, zearalenone treatment had no effect on pregnancy rate or embryonic loss.[20]

Rats developed linear increases in uterine weight with doses of 20 to 650 μg per rat per day for 7 days.[21]

Poultry are resistant to effects of zearalenone. Broiler chickens and turkey poults fed up to 800 ppm of pure zearalenone had only minor effects that occurred at the higher exposure levels.[8,22,23]

Clinical Signs. Animals develop signs of hyperestrogenism with hyperemia and swelling of the vulva, mammary glands, and uterus, as well as ovarian atrophy. Anabolic properties resulting in increased weight gain and feed efficiency can also be seen.

Swine, especially young gilts, are the most apt to develop signs of intoxication. Swelling of the vulva in gilts as well as edema of the prepuce in boars or barrows is usually the first evidence of adverse effects. With increased severity, a vaginal discharge may be seen and the mucosal irritation may be sufficient to cause straining, resulting in rectal prolapse. Difficulty in micturition can result from the edematous pressure on the urethra. Morbidity is usually high, signs are evident within a few days to 2 weeks depending on the dose and age of the animals. Mortality is essentially nonexistent, except for possible sequelae such as rectal prolapse complications. Removal of the contaminated source usually results in resolution of clinical signs within days; recovery may be a few weeks with higher doses and more severe effects on reproduction.[5,12,24]

Dietary concentrations of zearalenone in excess of 3 ppm fed to nongravid sows early in the estrus cycle can prevent follicular development and promote signs of persistent estrus or nymphomania. Exposure during the middle of the estrus cycle (days 11 to 14) promotes formation and persistence of functional progesterone-secreting corpora lutea that leads to anestrus and pseudopregnancy. High dietary concentrations of zearalenone (>20 ppm) given to pregnant sows 7 to 10 days after conception cause failure of implantation and embryonic death. The effect is not necessarily associated with changes in the serum concentration patterns of luteinizing hormone or follicle-stimulating hormone. Because of its luteotropic effects, zearalenone is not considered an abortifacient in swine.[9,12,14]

Young boars can have signs of preputial swelling, testicular atrophy, enlargement of the mammary glands, decreased libido, and reduced sperm quality. These signs abate and reproductive potential returns to normal.[8,15]

Zearalenone has no adverse effect on appetite or feed consumption. (In fact, the anabolic effects may enhance appetite.) Confusion arises due to the concurrent presence of DON (vomitoxin) that is also produced by *F. roseum* and is often present with zearalenone.[12]

Field case clinical reports in ruminants include signs of estrogenism. However, controlled studies have described little more than evidence of decreased fertility and delayed estrus.[8,12,17,18]

Clinical Pathology. Biochemical alterations associated with chronic zearalenone ingestion are essentially limited to elevated serum progesterone levels with decreased prolactin and luteinizing hormone concentrations.[25]

Lesions. *Vulvovaginitis* is perhaps a misnomer because no primary inflammatory changes occur in the vulva or the vagina as a direct result of zearalenone toxicosis. Inflammation follows from the irritation or eversion. The gross morphologic changes include swelling of the vulva, enlargement of the mammary glands, and increased size and weight of the uterus. Microscopic changes involve edema and hyperplasia of the uterus with thickening of the myometrium and endometrium with, eventually, duct proliferation of the mammary gland and squamous metaplasia of the cervix and vagina. Changes are indistinguishable in immature gilts between zearalenone and other estrogenic substances, namely estradiol.[8,25,26]

Ovaries of prepuberal gilts can appear hypoplastic with numerous small follicles and no evidence of corpora luteal formation. Sows can have considerable secondary follicular development and concurrent follicular atresia. Evidence of ovulation and corpora lutea in the ovarian tissue may be absent. Mammary gland and nipple enlargement is from edema, epithelial hyperplasia, and squamous metaplasia along with an increased mitotic index principally of the mammary ductal tissue.[25,26]

Diagnostic Testing. Bioassay procedures entailing feeding trials on laboratory animals with measurement of uterine change are used to detect estrogenic substances in feedstuffs. The specific detection of zearalenone is routinely performed on feed sources with chemical analytic and immunoassay test procedures by most veterinary diagnostic laboratories.

Analysis of tissues is possible but is seldom a reliable estimate of exposure. Toxin was not detected in muscle, liver, kidney, blood, or milk of dairy cows fed 1.9 ppm zearalenone for 11 weeks before slaughter. After 40 ppm dietary zearalenone for 21 days, less than 6 ppb total residue was detected in milk of cows. Low-level natural exposures have not been found to result in meat or egg residues.[10]

Treatment. Prompt removal from the contaminated feed source generally corrects the problem. Treatment of external genitalia physical damage may be indicated. Anestrus due to retained corpora lutea can be corrected by administration of prostaglandin F2-α.

Clays, bentonites, and other absorbents have not been shown to be of value.

Prognosis. Estrogenic signs usually disappear within about a week after removal of the contaminated feed with no significant aftereffects. With long durations of excessive doses, the infertility effects may require a prolonged period (as much as 3 months) for resolution.[26]

Prevention and Control. Adequate drying (<16% moisture) of the harvested crop to prevent further toxin production is the first means of prevention. Contaminated grain can be fed to a less susceptible species such as feeder cattle. If fed to market hogs, the zearalenone concentration of the source should be accurately determined for risk assessment. DON (vomitoxin), a common cocontaminant with zearalenone, should also be monitored to avoid feed intake problems. Grains from crops with mold infestations should be analyzed, especially if used in breeding herd diets.

REFERENCES

Aflatoxins

1. Diekman MA, Green ML: Mycotoxins and reproduction in domestic livestock, *J Anim Sci* 70:1615, 1992.
2. Sauer DB: Contamination by mycotoxins: when it occurs and how to prevent it. In Wyllie TD, Morehouse LG, editors: *Mycotoxic fungi, mycotoxins, mycotoxicoses; an encyclopedic handbook*, vol 3, New York, 1978, Marcel Dekker.
3. Jones BD: Chemistry of aflatoxin and related compounds. In Wyllie TD, Morehouse LG, editors: *Mycotoxic fungi and chemistry of mycotoxins*, vol 1, New York, 1977, Marcel Dekker.
4. Jones BD: Occurrence in foods and feeds, aflatoxin and related compounds. In Wyllie TD, Morehouse LG, editors: *Mycotoxic fungi, mycotoxins, mycotoxicoses; an encyclopedic handbook*, vol 1, *Mycotoxic fungi and chemistry of mycotoxins*. New York, 1977, Marcel Dekker.
5. Wilson DM, Payne GA: Factors affecting *Aspergillus flavus* group infection and aflatoxin contamination of crops. In Eaton DL, Groopman JD, editors: *The toxicology of aflatoxins; human health, veterinary, and agricultural significance*, New York, 1994, Academic Press.
6. Wood GE: Mycotoxins in foods and feeds in the United States, *J Anim Sci* 70:3941, 1992.
7. Kumagai S: Intestinal absorption and excretion of aflatoxin in rats, *Toxicol Appl Pharmacol* 97:88, 1989.
8. Wyatt RD: Poultry. In Smith JE, Henderson RS, editors: *Mycotoxins and animal feeds*, Boca Raton, Fla, 1991, CRC Press.
9. Hsieh DPH, Wong JJ: Pharmacokinetics and excretion of aflatoxins. In Eaton DL, Groopman. JD, editors: *The toxicology of aflatoxins; human health, veterinary, and agricultural significance*, New York, 1994, Academic Press.
10. Eaton DL et al: Biotransformation of aflatoxins. In Eaton DL, Groopman JD, editors: *The toxicology of aflatoxins; human health, veterinary, and agricultural significance*. New York, 1994, Academic Press.
11. Patterson DSP: Biochemistry and physiology of aflatoxin and related compounds. In Wyllie TD, Morehouse LG, editors: *Mycotoxic fungi, mycotoxins, mycotoxicoses; an encyclopedic handbook*, vol 1, *Mycotoxic fungi and chemistry of mycotoxins*, New York, 1977, Marcel Dekker.
12. van Egmond HP: Aflatoxins in milk. In Eaton DL, Groopman JD, editors: *The toxicology of aflatoxins; human health, veterinary, and agricultural significance*, New York, 1994, Academic Press.
13. Wogan GN et al.: Structure-activity relationship in toxicity and carcinogenicity of aflatoxins and analogs, *Cancer Res* 31:1936, 1971.
14. Pier AC: The influence of mycotoxins on the immune system. In Smith JE, Henderson RS, editors: *Mycotoxins and animal foods*, Boca Raton, Fla, 1991, CRC Press.
15. Miller DM, Wilson DM: Veterinary diseases related to aflatoxins. In Eaton DL, Groopman JD, editors: *The toxicology of aflatoxins; human health, veterinary, and agricultural significance*, New York, 1994, Academic Press.
16. Kiessling KH et al: Metabolism of aflatoxin, ochratoxin, zearalenone, and three trichothecenes by intact rumen fluid, rumen protozoa, and rumen bacteria, *Appl Environ Microbiol* 47(5):1070, 1984.

17. Bodine AB, Mertens DR: Toxicology, metabolism and physiological effects of aflatoxin in the bovine. In Diener UL, et al, editors: *Aflatoxin and Aspergillus flavus in corn*, Auburn, Ala, 1983, Alabama Agriculture Experiment Station, Auburn University.
18. Madhavan TV, Gopalan C: Effect of dietary protein on aflatoxin liver injury in weanling rats, *Arch Pathol* 80:123, 1965.
19. Cullen JM, Newberne PM: Acute hepatotoxicity of aflatoxins. In Eaton DL, Groopman JD, editors: *The toxicology of aflatoxins; human health, veterinary, and agricultural significance*, New York, 1994, Academic Press.
20. Rogers AE: Nutritional modulation of aflatoxin carcinogenesis. In Eaton DL, Groopman. JD, editors: *The toxicology of aflatoxins; human health, veterinary, and agricultural significance*, New York, 1994, Academic Press.
21. Patterson DSP: Toxin-producing fungi and susceptible animal species. In Wyllie TD, Morehouse LG, editors: *Mycotoxic fungi, mycotoxins, mycotoxicoses; an encyclopedic handbook*, vol 1, *Mycotoxic fungi and chemistry of mycotoxins*, New York, 1977, Marcel Dekker.
22. Patterson DSP: Metabolism as a factor in determining the toxic action of the aflatoxins in different animal species, *Food Cosmet Toxicol* 11:287, 1973.
23. Carlton WW, Szczech GM: Mycotoxicoses in laboratory animals. In Wyllie TD, Morehouse LG, editors: *Mycotoxic fungi, mycotoxins, mycotoxicoses; an encyclopedic handbook*, vol 2, *Mycotoxicoses of domestic and laboratory animals, poultry and aquatic invertebrates and vertebrates*, New York, 1978, Marcel Dekker.
24. Lynch GP: Response of calves to a single dose of aflatoxin, *J Anim Sci* 35(1), 651972.
25. Mertens DR: Biological effects of mycotoxins upon rumen function and lactating dairy cows. In *Interaction of mycotoxins in animal production*, Washington, DC, 1979, National Academy of Sciences.
26. Lynch GP et al: Responses of dairy calves to oral doses of aflatoxin, *J Dairy Sci* 54:1688, 1971.
27. Osweiler GD: Mycotoxins. In Straw B et al, editors: *Diseases of swine*, ed 8, Ames, Iowa, 1999, Iowa State University Press.
28. Armbrecht BH: Aflatoxicosis in swine. In Wyllie TD, Morehouse LG, editors: *Mycotoxic fungi, mycotoxins, mycotoxicoses; an encyclopedic handbook*, vol 2, *Mycotoxicoses of domestic and laboratory animals, poultry and aquatic invertebrates and vertebrates*, New York, 1978, Marcel Dekker.
29. Sinnhuber RO, Wales JH: The effects of mycotoxins on aquatic animals. In Wyllie TD, Morehouse LG, editors: *Mycotoxic fungi, mycotoxins, mycotoxicoses; an encyclopedic handbook*, vol 2, *Mycotoxicoses of domestic and laboratory animals, poultry and aquatic invertebrates and vertebrates*, New York, 1978, Marcel Dekker.
30. Newberne PM et al: Acute toxicity of aflatoxin B1 in the dog, *Pathol Vet* 3:331, 1966.
31. Armbrecht BH: Aflatoxicosis in sheep. In Wyllie TD, Morehouse LG, editors: *Mycotoxic fungi, mycotoxins, mycotoxicoses; an encyclopedic handbook*, vol 2, *Mycotoxicoses of domestic and laboratory animals, poultry and aquatic invertebrates and vertebrates*. New York, 1978, Marcel Dekker.
32. Austwick PKC: Aflatoxicosis in poultry. In Wyllie TD, Morehouse LG, editors: *Mycotoxic fungi, mycotoxins, mycotoxicoses; an encyclopedic handbook*, vol 2, *Mycotoxicoses of domestic and laboratory animals, poultry and aquatic invertebrates and vertebrates*. New York, 1978, Marcel Dekker.
33. Terao K, Ohtsubo K: Biological activities of mycotoxins: field and experimental mycotoxicoses. In Smith JE, Henderson RS, editors: *Mycotoxins and animal foods*, Boca Raton, Fla, 1991, CRC Press.
34. Asquity RL: Mycotoxicoses in horses. In Smith JE, Henderson RS, editors: *Mycotoxins and animal foods*, Boca Raton, Fla, 1991, CRC Press.
35. Kramer JW: Clinical enzymology. In Kaneko JJ, editor: *Clinical biochemistry of domestic animals*, ed 4, San Diego, 1989, Academic Press.
36. Joffe AZ, Ungar H: Cutaneous lesions produced by topical application of aflatoxin to rabbit skin, *J Invest Dermatol* 52:504, 1969.
37. Hatch RC: Poisons causing abdominal distress or liver or kidney damage. In Booth NH, McDonald LE, editors: *Veterinary pharmacology and therapeutics*, ed 5, Ames, Iowa, 1982, Iowa State University Press.

38. Park DL et al: Review of the decontamination of aflatoxins by ammoniation: current status and regulations, *J Assoc Official Analyt Chem* 71:685, 1988.
39. Lindemann MD et al: Potential ameliorators of aflatoxicosis in weanling/growing swine, *J Anim Sci* 71:171, 1993.

Citrinin and Ochratoxin

1. Prelusky DB et al: Toxicology of mycotoxins. In Miller JD, Trenholm HL, editors: *Mycotoxins in grain, compounds other than aflatoxin,* St Paul, 1994, Eagan Press.
2. Marquardt RR, Frohlich AA: A review of recent advances in understanding ochratoxicosis, *J Anim Sci* 70:3968, 1992.
3. Chu FS: Studies in ochratoxin, *CRC Crit Rev Toxicol* 2:499, 1974.
4. Ribelin WE: Ochratoxicosis in cattle. In Wyllie TD, Morehouse LG, editors: *Mycotoxic fungi, mycotoxins, mycotoxicoses; an encyclopedic handbook,* vol 2, *Mycotoxicoses of domestic and laboratory animals, poultry and aquatic invertebrates and vertebrates,* New York, 1978, Marcel Dekker.
5. Ciegler A: Bioproduction of ochratoxin A and penicillic acid by members of the *Aspergillus ochraceus* group, *Can J Microbiol* 18:631, 1972.
6. Scott PM: Penicillium mycotoxins. In Wyllie TD, Morehouse LG, editors: *Mycotoxic fungi, mycotoxins, mycotoxicoses; an encyclopedic handbook,* vol 1, *Mycotoxic fungi and chemistry of mycotoxins,* New York, 1977, Marcel Dekker.
7 Carlton WW, Szczech GM: Mycotoxicoses in laboratory animals. In Wyllie TD, Morehouse LG, editors: *Mycotoxic fungi, mycotoxins, mycotoxicoses; an encyclopedic handbook,* vol 2, *Mycotoxicoses of domestic and laboratory animals, poultry and aquatic invertebrates and vertebrates,* New York, 1978, Marcel Dekker.
8. Kiessling KH et al: Metabolism of aflatoxin, ochratoxin, zearalenone and three trichothecenes by intact rumen fluid, rumen protozoa and rumen bacteria, *Applied Environ Microbiol* 47:1070, 1984.
9. Sinnhuber RO, Wales JH: The effects of mycotoxins on aquatic animals. In Wyllie TD, Morehouse LG, editors: *Mycotoxic fungi, mycotoxins, mycotoxicoses; an encyclopedic handbook,* vol 2, *Mycotoxicoses of domestic and laboratory animals, poultry and aquatic invertebrates and vertebrates,* New York, 1978, Marcel Dekker.
10. Pestka JJ, Bondy GS: Immunotoxic effects of mycotoxins. In Miller JD, Trenholm HL, editors: *Mycotoxins in grain, compounds other than aflatoxin,* St Paul, 1994, Eagan Press.
11. Huff WE et al: Ochratoxicosis in the broiler chicken, *Poultry Sci* 53:1585, 1974.
12. Szczech GM et al: Ochratoxin A toxicosis in swine, *Vet Pathol* 10:347, 1973.
13. Munro IC et al: Ochratoxin A: occurrence and toxicity, *J Am Vet Med Assoc* 163(11):1269, 1973.
14. Yamazaki M et al: The toxicity of 5-chloro-8-hydroxy-3, 4-dihydro-3-methyl-isocoumarin-7-carboxylic acid. A hydolyzate of ochratoxin A, *Jpn J Med Sci Biol* 24:245, 1971.
15. Peckman JC: Ochratoxicosis in poultry. In Wyllie TD, Morehouse LG, editors: *Mycotoxic fungi, mycotoxins, mycotoxicoses; an encyclopedic handbook,* vol 2, *Mycotoxicoses of domestic and laboratory animals, poultry and aquatic invertebrates and vertebrates,* New York, 1978, Marcel Dekker.
16. Doster RC et al: Comparative toxicity of ochratoxin A and crude *Aspergillus ochraceus* culture extract in Japanese quail *(Coturnix coturnix japonica),* *Poultry Sci* 52:2351, 1973.
17. Still PE: Mycotoxins as possible causes of abortion in dairy cattle. Ph.D. Thesis, 1973, University of Wisconsin, Madison.
18. Ribelin WE et al: The toxicity of ochratoxin to ruminants, *Can J Comp Med* 42:172, 1978.
19. Prelusky DB: Residues in food products of animal origin. In Miller JD, Trenholm HL, editors: *Mycotoxins in grain, compounds other than aflatoxin,* St Paul, 1994, Eagan Press.
20. Huff WE et al: Progression of ochratoxicosis in broiler chickens, *Poultry Sci* 67:1139, 1988.
21. Lloyd WE et al: *A case of probable citrinin toxicosis in a herd of Iowa feeder cattle,* American Association of Veterinary Laboratory Diagnosticians 21st Annual Proceedings, Buffalo, NY, 1978.
22. Szczech GM et al: Ochratoxicosis in beagle dogs, *Vet Pathol* 10:219, 1973.
23. Theron JJ et al: Acute liver injury in ducklings and rats as a result of ochratoxin poisoning, *J Pathol Bacteriol* 91:521, 1966.
24. Hayes AW et al: Teratogenic effects on ochratoxin A in mice, *Teratology* 9:93, 1973.
25. Mortensen HP et al: Ochratoxin A contaminated barley for sows and piglets. Pig performance and residues in milk and pigs, *Acta Agric Scand* 33:349, 1983.
26. Haazele FM et al: Beneficial effects of dietary ascorbic acid supplement on hens subjected to ochratoxin A toxicosis under normal and high ambient temperatures, *Can J Anim Sci* 73:149, 1993.

Ergot

1. Burrows GE, Tyrl RJ: *Toxic plants of North America,* Ames, Iowa, 2001, Iowa State University Press.
2. Cheeke PR: *Natural toxicants in feeds, forages, and poisonous plants,* ed 2, Danville, Ill, 1998, Interstate Publishers.
3. Hintz HF: Molds, mycotoxins, and mycotoxicosis, *Vet Clin North Am Equine Pract* 6:419, 1990.
4. Carson TL: In Howard JL, Smith RA, editors: *Current veterinary therapy 4: food animal practice,* Philadelphia, 1999, WB Saunders.
5. Bryden WL: In Colegate SM, Dorling PR, editors: *Plant-associated toxins: agricultural, phytochemical, and ecological aspects,* Wallingford, UK, 1994, CAB International.
6. Bourke CA: In Colegate SM, Dorling PR, editors: *Plant-associated toxins: agricultural, phytochemical, and ecological aspects,* Wallingford, UK, 1994, CAB International.
7. Evans TJ: University of Missouri, 2001, unpublished data.
8. Burfening PJ: Ergotism, *J Am Vet Med Assoc* 163:1288, 1973.
9. Coppock RW et al: Cutaneous ergotism in a herd of dairy calves, *J Am Vet Med Assoc* 194:549, 1989.
10. Pier AC et al: Implications of mycotoxins in animal disease, *J Am Vet Med Assoc* 176:719, 1980.
11. Montastruc JL et al: Treatment of Parkinson's disease should begin with a dopamine agonist, *Mov Disord* 15:361, 2001.
12. Philosophe R, Seibel MM: Novel approaches to the management of hyperprolactinemia, *Curr Opin Obstet Gynecol* 3:336, 1991.
13. Feldman EC, Nelson RW: *Canine and feline endocrinology and reproduction,* ed 2, Philadelphia, 1996, WB Saunders.
14. Dybdal N: In Robinson NE, editor: *Current therapy in equine medicine 4,* Philadelphia, 1997, WB Saunders.
15. Eckert H et al: In Berde B, Schild HO, editors: *Ergot alkaloids and related compounds,* Berlin, 1978, Springer-Verlag.
16. Moubarak AS et al: HPLC method for detection of ergotamine, ergosine, and ergine after intravenous injection of a single dose, *J Agric Food Chem* 44:146, 1996.
17. Ross AD et al: Induction of heat stress in beef cattle by feeding ergots of *Claviceps purpurea, Aust Vet J* 66:247, 1989.
18. Riet-Correa F et al: Agalactia, reproductive problems and neonatal mortality in horses associated with ingestion of *Claviceps purpurea, Aust Vet J* 65:192, 1988.
19. Mantle PG: The role of alkaloids in the poisoning of mammals by sclerotia of *Claviceps* spp. *J Stored Prod Res* 5:237, 1969.
20. Al-Tamimi HJ et al: Thermoregulatory response of dairy cows fed ergotized barley during summer heat stress, *J Vet Diagn Invest,* 15(4):355, 2003.
21. Lopez TA et al: Ergotism and photosensitization in swine produced by the combined ingestion of *Claviceps purpurea* sclerotia and *Ammi majus* seeds, *J Vet Diagn Invest* 9:68, 1997.

22. Burfening PJ: Feeding ergot to pregnant ewes, *Theriogenology* 3:193, 1975.

23. Ireland FA et al: Effects of bromocriptine and perphenazine on prolactin and progesterone concentrations in pregnant mares during late gestation, *J Reprod Fertil* 92:179, 1991.

24. Rottinghaus GE et al: An HPLC method for the detection of ergot in ground and pelleted feeds, *J Vet Diagn Invest* 5:242, 1993.

Fescue

1. Cheeke PR: *Natural Toxicants in Feeds, Forages, and Poisonous Plants*, ed 2, Danville, Ill, 1998, Interstate Publishers.

2. Burrows GE, Tyrl RJ: *Toxic plants of North America*, Ames, Iowa, 2001, Iowa State University Press.

3. Hoveland CS: In Joost RE, Quisenberry SS, editors: *Acremonium/grass interactions*, Amsterdam, 1993, Elsevier.

4. Kerr LA, Kelch WJ: In Howard JL, Smith RA, editors: *Current veterinary therapy 4: food animal practice*, Philadelphia, 1999, WB Saunders.

5. Garner GB et al: In Joost RE, Quisenberry SS, editors: *Acremonium/grass interactions*, Amsterdam, 1993, Elsevier.

6. Hill NS et al: Ergot alkaloid transport across ruminant gastric tissues, *J Anim Sci* 79:542, 2001.

7. Ireland FA et al: Effects of bromocriptine and perphenazine on prolactin and progesterone concentrations in pregnant mares during late gestation, *J Reprod Fertil* 92:179, 1991.

8. Rottinghaus GE et al: An HPLC method for quantitating ergovaline in endophyte-infested tall fescue: seasonal variation of ergovaline levels in stems with leaf sheaths, leaf blades, and seed heads, *J Agric Food Chem* 39:112, 1991.

9. Strickland JR et al: Effect of ergovaline, loline, and dopamine antagonists on rat pituitary cell prolactin release *in vitro*, *Am J Vet Res* 55:716, 1994.

10. Schöning C et al: Complex interaction of ergovaline with 5-HT$_{2A}$, %-HT$_{1B/1D}$, and alpha$_1$ receptors in isolated arteries of rat and guinea pig, *J Anim Sci* 79:2202, 2001.

11. Hill NS et al: Antibody binding of circulating ergot alkaloids in cattle grazing tall fescue, *Am J Vet Res* 55:419 1994.

12. Oliver JW et al: Evaluation of a dosing method for studying ergonovine affects in cattle, *Am J Vet Res* 55:173, 1994.

13. Oliver JW et al: Effects of phenothiazine and thiabendazole on bovine dorsal pedal bone contractility induced by ergonovine and serotonin; potential for alleviation of fescue toxicity, *J Vet Pharmacol Ther* 15:247, 1992.

14. Oliver JW et al: Vasoconstriction in bovine vasculature induced by the tall fescue alkaloid lysergamide, *J Anim Sci* 71:2708, 1993.

15. Piper EL et al: In Bacon CW, Hill NS, editors: *Neotyphodium/grass interactions*, New York, 1997, Plenum Press.

16. Eckert H et al: In Berde B, Schild HO, editors: *Ergot alkaloids and related compounds*, Berlin, 1978, Springer-Verlag.

17. Moubarak AS et al: HPLC method for detection of ergotamine, ergosine, and ergine after intravenous injection of a single dose, *J Agric Food Chem* 44:146, 1996.

18. Stuedemann JA et al: Urinary and biliary excretion of ergot alkaloids from steers that grazed endophyte-infected tall fescue, *J Anim Sci* 76:2146, 1998.

19. Cross DL et al: Equine fescue toxicosis; signs and solutions, *J Anim Sci* 73:899, 1995.

20. Berde B, Stürmer E: In Berde B, Schild HO: *Ergot alkaloids and related compounds*, Berlin, 1978, Springer-Verlag.

21. Porter JK, Thompson FN: Effects of fescue toxicosis on reproduction in livestock, *J Anim Sci* 70:1594, 1992.

22. Paterson J et al: The effects of fescue toxicosis on beef cattle productivity, *J Anim Sci* 73:889, 1995.

23. Wolfe BA et al: Abdominal lipomatosis attributed to tall fescue toxicosis in deer, *J Am Vet Med Assoc* 213:1783, 1998.

24. Debessai W et al: Effects of feeding endophyte-infected tall fescue seed on lamb performance and serum prolactin (abstr), *J Anim Sci* 71(suppl 1):200, 1993.

25. Tor-Agbidye J et al: Correlation of endophyte toxins (ergovaline and lolitrem B) with clinical disease: fescue foot and perennial ryegrass staggers, *Vet Human Toxicol* 43:130, 2001.

26. Evans TJ: University of Missouri, 2001, unpublished data.

27. Boosinger TR et al: In Sharp DC, Bazer FW, editors: *Equine reproduction VI*. Ann Arbor, Mich, 1995, Society for the Study of Reproduction, p 61.

28. Ryan PL et al: Systemic relaxin in pregnant pony mares grazed on endophyte-infected fescue: effects of fluphenazine treatment, *Theriogenology* 56:471, 2001.

29. Brendemuehl JP et al: *Equine reproduction VI*, Ann Arbor, Mich, 1995, Society for the Study of Reproduction.

30. Rohrbach BW et al: Aggregate risk study of exposure to endophyte-infected (*Acremonium coenophialum*) tall fescue as a risk factor for laminitis in horses, *Am J Vet Res* 56:22, 1995.

31. Vivrette S et al: Cardiorespiratory and thermoregulatory effects of endophyte-infected fescue in exercising horses, *J Equine Vet Sci* 21:65, 2001.

32. Jensen R et al: Fescue lameness in cattle I. Experimental production of the disease, *Am J Vet Res* 17:196, 1956.

33. Brendemuehl JP: In Robinson NE, editor: *Current therapy in equine medicine 4*, Philadelphia, 1997, WB Saunders.

34. Green EM, Raisbeck MF: In Robinson NE, editor: *Current therapy in equine medicine 4*, Philadelphia, 1997, WB Saunders.

35. Al-Haidary A et al: Thermoregulatory ability of beef heifers following intake of endophyte-infected tall fescue during controlled heat challenge, *J Anim Sci* 79:1780, 2001.

36. Burke JM et al: Interaction of endophyte-infected fescue and heat stress on ovarian function in the beef heifer, *Biol Reprod* 65:260, 2001.

37. Oliver JW et al: Alterations in the hemograms and serum biochemical analytes of steers after prolonged consumption of endophyte-infected tall fescue, *J Anim Sci* 78:1029, 2000.

38. Dennis SB et al: Influence of *Neotyphodium coenophialum* on copper concentration in tall fescue, *J Anim Sci* 76:2687, 1998.

39. Redmond LM et al: Efficacy of domperidone and sulpiride as treatments for fescue toxicosis in horses, *Am J Vet Res* 55:722, 1995.

40. Evans TJ: *The effects of bromocriptine, domperidone, and reserpine on circulating maternal levels of progestins, estrogens, and prolactin in pregnant pony mares*, Master's thesis, University of Missouri, 1996.

41. Loch WE et al: The effects of four levels of endophyte-infected fescue seed in the diet of pregnant pony mares, *J Reprod Fertil Suppl* 35:535, 1987.

42. Hill NS et al: Urinary alkaloid excretion as a diagnostic tool for fescue toxicosis in cattle, *J Vet Diagn Invest* 12:210, 2000.

43. Beconi MG et al: Growth and subsequent feedlot performance of estradiol-implanted vs nonimplanted steers grazing fall accumulated endophyte-infested or low-endophyte tall fescue, *J Anim Sci* 73:1576, 1995.

44. Filipov NM et al: vaccination against ergot alkaloids and the effect of endophyte-infected fescue seed-based diets on rabbits, *J Anim Sci* 76:2456, 1998.

45. Evans TJ et al: A comparison of the relative efficacies of domperidone and reserpine in treating equine "fescue toxicosis," *Proc Am Assoc Equine Pract* 45:207, 1999.

46. Threlfall WR: In Youngquist RS: *Current therapy in large animal theriogenology*, Philadelphia, 1997, WB Saunders.

47. LeBlanc MM: In Youngquist RS: *Current therapy in large animal theriogenology*, Philadelphia, 1997, WB Saunders.

48. Bennett-Wimbush K et al: The effect of perphenazine and bromocriptine on follicular dynamics and endocrine profiles in anestrous mares, *Theriogenology* 49:717, 1998.

49. McCue PM et al: Efficacy of domperidone on induction of ovulation in anestrous and transitional mares, *Proc Am Assoc Equine Pract* 45:217, 1999.

50. Bouton JH et al: In Paul VH, Dapprich PD, editors: *Proceedings of the 4th International Neotyphodium/Grass Interaction Symposium*, Soest, Germany, 2000.

51. Ryan PL et al: Effects of exposing late-term pregnant mares to toxic and non-toxic endophyte-infected tall fescue pastures (abstr), *Biol Reprod* 64(suppl 1):612, 2001.

Fumonisin

1. Prelusky DB et al: Pharmacokinetic fate of ^{14}C-labelled fumonisin B$_1$ in swine, *Nat Toxins* 2:73, 1994.
2. Spotti M et al: Fumonisin B$_1$ carry-over into milk in the isolated perfused bovine udder, *Vet Hum Toxicol* 43:109, 2001.
3. Wang E et al: Inhibition of sphingosine biosynthesis by fumonisins, *J Biol Chem* 266:14486, 1991.
4. Smith GW et al: Purified fumonisin B$_1$ decreases cardiovascular function but does not alter pulmonary capillary permeability in swine, *Toxicol Sci* 56:240, 2000.
5. Goel S et al: Effects of *Fusarium moniliforme* isolates on tissue and serum sphingolipid concentrations in horses, *Vet Hum Toxicol* 38:265, 1996.
6. Mathur S et al: Fumonisin B$_1$ is hepatotoxic and nephrotoxic in milk-fed calves, *Toxicol Sci* 60:385, 2001.
7. Smith GW et al: Sequence of cardiovascular changes leading to pulmonary edema in swine fed culture material containing fumonisin, *Am J Vet Res* 60:1292, 1999.
8. Constable PD et al: Ingestion of fumonisin B$_1$-containing culture material decreases cardiac contractility and mechanical efficiency in swine, *Toxicol Appl Pharmacol* 162:151, 2000.
9. Smith GW et al: Cardiovascular changes associated with intra-venous administration of fumonisin B$_1$ in horses, *Am J Vet Res* 63: 538, 2002.
10. Wilson TM et al: Fumonisin B$_1$ levels associated with an epizootic of equine leukoencephalomalacia, *J Vet Diagn Invest* 2:213, 1990.
11. Ross PF et al: Fumonisin B$_1$ concentrations in feeds from 45 confirmed equine leukoencephalomalacia cases, *J Vet Diagn Invest* 3:238, 1991.
12. Colvin BM et al: Fumonisin toxicosis in swine: clinical and pathologic findings, *J Vet Diagn Invest* 5:232, 1993.
13. Osweiler GD et al: Characterization of an epizootic of pulmonary edema in swine associated with fumonisins in corn screenings, *J Vet Diagn Invest* 4:53, 1992.
14. Osweiler GD et al: Effects of fumonisin-contaminated corn screenings on growth and health of feeder calves, *J Anim Sci* 71:459, 1993.
15. Caloni F et al: *In vitro* metabolism of fumonisin B$_1$ by ruminal microflora, *Vet Res Commun* 24:379, 2000.
16. Ledoux DR et al: Fumonisin toxicity in broiler chicks, *J Vet Diagn Invest* 4:330, 1992.
17. McCue PM: Equine leukoencephalomalacia, *Compend Cont Ed Pract Vet* 11:646, 1989.
18. Ross PF et al: Experimental equine leukoencephalomalacia, toxic hepatosis, and encephalopathy caused by corn naturally contaminated with fumonisins, *J Vet Diagn Invest* 5:69, 1993.
19. Brownie CF, Cullen J: Characterization of experimentally induced equine leukoencephalomalacia (ELEM) in ponies (*Equus caballus*): preliminary report, *Vet Hum Toxicol* 29:34, 1987.
20. Motelin GK et al: Temporal and dose-response features in swine fed corn screenings contaminated with fumonisin mycotoxins, *Mycopathol* 126:27, 1994.
21. Haschek WM et al: Characterization of fumonisin toxicity in orally and intravenously dosed swine, *Mycopathology* 117:83, 1992.

Oosporein

1. Wyatt RD: In Smith JE, Henderson RS, editors: *Mycotoxins and animal foods*, London, 1991, CRC Press.
2. *Registry of Toxic Effects of Chemical Substances* (RTECS on CD-ROM), Bethesda, Md, 2000, National Library of Medicine.
3. Jeffs LB, Khachatourians GG: Toxic properties of *Beauveria* pigments on erythrocyte membranes, *Toxicon* 35:1351, 1997.
4. Aleo MD, Wyatt RD, Schnellmann RG: Mitochondrial dysfunction is an early event in ochratoxin A but not in oosporein toxicity to rat renal proximal tubules, *Toxicol Appl Pharmacol* 107:73, 1991.

5. Manning RO, Wyatt RD: Comparative toxicity of *Chaetomium* contaminated corn and various chemical forms of oosporein in broiler chicks, *Poultry Sci* 63:251, 1984.
6. Pegram RA, Wyatt RD: Avian gout caused by oosporein, a mycotoxin produced by Chaetomium trilaterale. *Poultry Sci* 60:2429, 1981.
7. Pegram RA et al: Oosporein toxicosis in the turkey poult, *Avian Dis* 26:47, 1982.
8. Brown TP et al: Microscopic and ultrastructure renal pathology of oosporein-induced toxicosis in broiler chicks, *Avian Dis* 31:868, 1987.

Patulin

1. Hazardous Substances Data Bank (HSDB on CD-ROM), Bethesda, Md, 2000, National Library of Medicine.
2. Pitt JI, Leistner: In Smith JE, Henderson RS, editors: *Mycotoxins and animal foods*, London, 1991, CRC Press.
3. Moss MO: In Smith JE, Henderson RS, editors: *Mycotoxins and animal foods*, London, 1991, CRC Press.
4. Lillehoj EB et al: In Smith JE, Henderson RS, editors: *Mycotoxins and animal foods*, London, 1991, CRC Press.
5. Reiss J: In Wyllie TD, Morehouse LG, editors: *Mycotoxic fungi, mycotoxins, mycotoxicoses*, vol 3, New York, 1978, Marcel Dekker.
6. Fliege R. Metzler M: Electrophilic properties of patulin. Adduct structures and reaction pathways with 4-bromothiophenol and other model nucleophiles, *Chem Res Toxicol* 13: 363, 2000.
7. Abdelhamid AM, Dorra TM: Study on effects of feeding laying hens on separate mycotoxins (aflatoxins, patulin, or citrinin)-contaminated diets on the egg quality and tissue constituents, *Arch Tierernahr* 40:5, 1990.
8. Lovett J: Patulin toxicosis in poultry, *Poultry Sci* 51:2097, 1972.
9. Garza HC et al: Toxicological study of patulin in monkeys, *J Food Sci* 42:1229.
10. Hawig J, Munro IC: Mycotoxins of possible importance in diseases of Canadian farm animals, *Can Vet J* 16:125, 1975.
11. Escoula L: Patulin production by *Penicillium granulatum* and inhibition of rumen flora, *J Environ Path Toxicol Oncol* 11:109, 1992.
12. Registry of Toxic Effects of Chemical Substances (RTECS on CD-ROM), Bethesda, Md, 2000, National Library of Medicine.

Penitrem A and Roquefortine

1. Cole RJ, Dorner JW: Role of fungal tremorgens in animal disease. In Steyn PS, Vleggar R, editors: *Mycotoxins and phycotoxins*, Amsterdam, 1985, Elsevier.
2. Cole RJ: Fungal tremorgens, *J Food Prot* 44:715, 1981.
3. Richard JL, Arp LH: Natural occurrence of the mycotoxin penitrem A in moldy cream cheese, *Mycopathologica* 67(2):107, 1979.
4. Hocking AD et al: Intoxication by tremorgenic mycotoxin (penitrem A) in a dog, *Aust Vet J* 65(3):82, 1988.
5. Richard JL et al: Moldy walnut toxicosis in a dog, caused by the mycotoxin, penitrem A, *Mycopathologica* 76:55, 1981.
6. Ware GM et al: Determination of roquefortine in blue cheese and blue cheese dressing by high pressure liquid chromatography with ultraviolet and electrochemical detectors, *J Assoc Off Anal Chem* 63(3):637, 1980.
7. Auerbach HE et al: Incidence of *Penicillium roqueforti* and roquefortine C in silages, *J Sci Food Agr* 76:565, 1998.
8. Wilson DM, Payne GA: Factors affecting *Aspergillus flavus* group infection and aflatoxin contamination of crops. In Eaton DL, Groopman JD, editors: *The toxicology of aflatoxins: human health, veterinary and agricultural significance,* San Diego, 1994, Academic Press..
9. Knaus H-G et al: Tremorgenic indole alkaloids potently inhibit smooth muscle high-conductance calcium-activated potassium channels, *Biochemistry* 33:5819, 1994.
10. Wilson BJ et al: Effects of a fungus tremorgenic toxin (penitrem A) on transmission in rat phrenic nerve-diaphragm preparations, *Brain Res* 40(2):540, 1972.
11. Cole RJ, Cox RH: Tremorgen group. In *Handbook of toxic fungal metabolites,* New York, 1981, Academic Press.

12. Selala MI et al: Fungal tremorgens: the mechanism of action of single nitrogen containing toxins—a hypothesis, *Drug Chem Toxicol* 12:237, 1989.

13. Hayes AW et al: Acute toxicity of penitrem A in dogs, *Toxicol Appl Pharmacol* 35(2):311, 1976.

14. Ueno Y, Ueno I: Toxicology and biochemistry of mycotoxins. In Uraguchi K, Yamazaki M, editors: *Toxicology biochemistry and pathology of mycotoxins,* New York, 1978, John Wiley and Sons.

15. Boysen ME et al: Molecular identification of species from the *Penicillium roqueforti* group associated with spoiled animal feed, *Appl Environ Microbiol* 66(4):1523, 2000.

16. Lowes NR et al: Roquefortine in the stomach contents of dogs suspected of strychnine poisoning in Alberta, *Can Vet J* 33:535, 1992.

17. Braselton WE, Rumler PC: MS/MS screen for the tremorgenic mycotoxins roquefortine and penitrem A, *J Vet Diagn Invest* 8:515, 1996.

Phomopsins

1. Williamson PM et al: *Diaporthe toxica* sp. *nov.,* the cause of lupinosis in sheep, *Mycological Research* 98:1364, 1994.

2. Allen JG: In Gladstones JS et al, editors: *Lupins as crop plants: biology, production and utilization,* Oxon, UK, 1998, CAB International.

3. Shivas RG et al: In Colegate SM, Dorling PR, editors: *Plant-associated toxins: agricultural, phytochemical and ecological aspects,* Oxon, UK, 1994, CAB International.

4. Culvenor CCJ et al: Isolation of toxic metabolites of *Phomopsis leptostromiformis* responsible for lupinosis, *Aust J Biol Sci* 30:269, 1977.

5. Culvenor CCJ et al: Structure elucidation and absolute configuration of phomopsin A, a hexapeptide mycotoxin produced by *Phomopsis leptostromiformis, Tetrahedron* 45:2351, 1989.

6. Edgar JA: In Keeler RF, Tu AT, editors: *Handbook of natural toxins,* New York, 1991, Marcel Dekker.

7. Allen JG, Hancock GR: Evidence that phomopsins A and B are not the only toxic metabolites produced by *Phomopsis leptostromiformis, J Appl Toxicol* 9:83, 1989.

8. Cockrum PA et al: In Colegate SM, Dorling PR, editors: *Plant-associated toxins: agricultural, phytochemical and ecological aspects,* Oxon, UK, 1994, CAB International.

9. Peterson JE: *The toxicity of phomopsin,* Proceedings of the Fourth International Lupin Conference, Geraldton, Western Australia, 1986.

10. Allen JG: *Studies of the pathogenesis, toxicology and pathology of lupinosis and associated conditions,* Doctoral thesis, Murdoch University, 1989.

11. Allen JG: In James LF et al, editors: *Poisonous plants: Proceedings of the Third International Symposium,* Ames, Iowa, 1992, Iowa State University Press.

12. Hamel E: Antimitotic natural products and their interactions with tubulin, *Med Res Rev* 16:207, 1996.

13. Peterson JE et al: The toxicity of phomopsin for sheep, *Aust Vet J* 64:293, 1987.

14. Allen JG: Lupinosis, *Vet Clin Toxicol,* Proceedings No. 103, University of Sydney Post-Graduate Committee in Veterinary Science, 1987.

15. Allen JG: *Lupinosis, a review,* Proceedings of the Fourth International Lupin Conference, Geraldton, Western Australia, 1986.

16. Smith GM, Allen JG: Effectiveness of α-tocopherol and selenium supplements in preventing lupinosis-associated myopathy in sheep, *Aust Vet J* 75:341, 1997.

17. Allen JG, Randall AG: The clinical biochemistry of experimentally produced lupinosis in the sheep, *Aust Vet J* 70:283, 1993.

18. Allen JG, Cousins DV: In Garland T, Barr AC: *Toxic plants and other natural toxins,* Oxon, UK, 1998, CAB International.

19. Allen JG, Nottle FK: Spongy transformation of the brain in sheep with lupinosis, *Vet Rec* 104:31, 1979.

20. Than KA et al: In James LF et al: *Poisonous plants: Proceedings of the Third International Symposium,* Ames, Iowa, 1992, Iowa State University Press.

21. Allen JG et al: In Colegate SM, Dorling PR: *Plant-associated toxins: agricultural, phytochemical and ecological aspects,* Oxon, UK, 1994, CAB International.

22. Than KA et al: In Colegate SM, Dorling PR: *Plant-associated toxins: Agricultural, phytochemical and ecological aspects,* Oxon, UK, 1994, CAB International.

Slaframine

1. Aust SD: *Rhizoctonia leguminicola*-slaframine. In Purchase IFH, editor: *Mycotoxins,* Amsterdam, 1974, Elsevier.

2. Smalley EB: Salivary syndrome in cattle. In Wyllie TD, Morehouse LG, editors: *Mycotoxic fungi, mycotoxins, mycotoxicoses,* vol 2, *Mycotoxicoses of domestic and laboratory animals, poultry and aquatic invertebrates and vertebrates,* New York, 1978, Marcel Dekker.

3. Weimer JL: Black patch of soybean and other forage legumes, *Phytopathology* 40:782, 1950.

4. Croom WJ Jr et al: The involvement of slaframine and swainsonine in slobbers syndrome: a review, *J Anim Sci* 73:1499, 1995.

5. Aust SD: Effect of slaframine on exocrine gland function, *Biochem Pharmacol* 19:427, 1970.

6. Walker JA et al: Effects of slaframine and 4-diphenylacetoxy-N-methylpiperidine methiodide (4DAMP) on pancreatic exocrine secretion in the bovine, Can J Physiol Pharmacol 72:39, 1994.

7. Froetschel MA et al: Effects of abomasal slaframine infusion on ruminal digesta passage and digestion in steers, *Can J Anim Sci* 75:157, 1995.

8. Hibbard B et al: The effect of slaframine on salivary output and subacute and acute acidosis in growing beef steers, *J Anim Sci* 73:516, 1995.

9. Hibbard B et al: The effect of daily slaframine injection on salivary score, feed intake, ruminal pH, and circulating concentrations of somatotropin and insulin-like growth factor I, *J Anim Sci* 73:526, 1995.

10. Smalley EB: Chemistry and physiology of slaframine. In Wyllie TD, Morehouse LG, editors: *Mycotoxic fungi, mycotoxins,* vol 1, *Mycotoxic fungi and chemistry of mycotoxins,* New York, 1977, Marcel Dekker.

11. Crump MH et al: Pharmacologic properties of a slobber-inducing mycotoxin from *Rhizoctonia leguminicola, Am J Vet Res* 28:865, 1967.

12. Crump MH: Slaframine (slobber factor) toxicosis, *J Am Vet Med Assoc* 163(11):1300, 1973.

13. Edwards WC, Crump MH: The effect of rhizotoxin on the cardiac system and plasma histamine in the canine, Proceedings of the 49th Conference of Research Workers in Animal Diseases, Chicago, 1968.

14. Carlton WW, Szczech GM: Mycotoxicoses in laboratory animals. In Wyllie TD, Morehouse LG, editors: *Mycotoxic fungi, mycotoxins, mycotoxicoses,* vol 2, *Mycotoxicoses of domestic and laboratory animals, poultry and aquatic invertebrates and vertebrates,* New York, 1978, Marcel Dekker.

Sporidesmin

1. Mortimer PH, Ronaldson JW: In Keeler RF, Tu AT, editors: *Handbook of natural toxins,* vol I, *Plant and fungal toxins,* New York, 1983, Marcel Dekker.

2. Collin RG et al: Sporidesmin production by *Pithomyces chartarum* isolates from Australia, Brazil, New Zealand and Uruguay, *Mycological Res* 102(2):163, 1998.

3. Marasas WFO et al: First report of facial eczema in sheep in South Africa, *J Vet Res* 39(2):107, 1972.

4. Bonnefoi M et al: Clinical biochemistry of sporidesmin natural intoxication (facial eczema) of sheep, *J Clin Chem Clin Biochem* 27:13, 1989.

5. Hansen DE et al: Photosensitisation associated with exposure to *Pithomyces chartarum* in lambs, *J Vet Med Assoc* 204(10):1668, 1994.

6. Mortimer PH, Stanbridge TA: The excretion of sporidesmin given by mouth to sheep, *J Comp Pathol* 78:505, 1968.

7. Smith BL, Embling PP: Facial eczema in goats: the toxicity of sporidesmin in goats and its pathology, *N Z Vet J* 39:18, 1991.

8. Fagliari JJ et al: Intoxicação natural de bovinos pela micotoxina esporidesmina. II. Aspectos clínicos, *Arq Bras Med Vet Zoot* 45(3):275, 1993.

9. Munday R: Studies on the mechanism of toxicity of the mycotoxin, sporidesmin. I. Generation of superoxide radical by sporidesmin, *Chem Biol Interact* 44(3):361, 1982.

10. Munday R: Studies on the mechanism of toxicity of the mycotoxin sporidesmin. IV. Inhibition by copper-chelating agents of the generation of superoxide radical by sporidesmin, *J Appl Toxicol* 5(2):69, 1985.

11. Munday R, Manns E: Protection by iron salts against sporidesmin intoxication in sheep, *N Z Vet J* 37:65, 1989.

12. Waring P et al: Apoptosis induced in macrophages and T blasts by the mycotoxin sporidesmin and protection by Zn2+ salts, *Int J Immunopharmacol* 12(4):445, 1990.

13. Ferguson LR et al: *In vitro* and *in vivo* mutagenicity studies on sporidesmin, the toxin associated with facial eczema in ruminants, *Mutat Res* 268(2):199, 1992.

14. Munday R et al: Mouse micronucleus assays of sporidesmin, the toxin associated with facial eczema in ruminants, *Mutat Res* 302(1):71, 1993.

15. Bruère AN et al: *Veterinary clinical toxicology,* Publication 127, Veterinary Clinical Education, 1990, Massey University, Palmerston North, New Zealand.

16. Wright DE: Toxins produced by fungi, *Ann Rev Microbiol* 22:269-282, 1968.

17. Fagliari JJ et al: Intoxicação natural de bovinos pela micotoxina esporidesmina. I. Aspectos epidemiológicos, *Arq Bras Med Vet Zoot* 45(3):263, 1993.

18. Fagliari JJ et al: Estudo de alguns consituintes sangüíneos de bovinos intoxicados naturalmente pela micotoxina esporidesmina, *Arq Bras Med Vet Zoot* 45(5):457, 1994.

19. Flåøyen A et al: Glycogen accumulation and histological changes in the livers of lambs with alveld and experimental sporidesmin intoxication, *Vet Res Commun* 15:443, 1991.

20. Thompson KG et al: Sporidesmin toxicity in rabbits: biochemical and morphological changes, *J Comp Pathol* 93(2):319, 1983.

21. Fitzgerald JM et al: Biological control of sporidesmin-producing strains of *Pithomyces chartarum* by biocompetitive exclusion, *Lett Appl Microbiol* 26(1):17, 1998.

22. Le Bars et al: Ecotoxinogenesis of *Pithomyces chartarum, Food Addit Contam* 7(suppl.1):PS19, 1990.

23. Collin R et al: Development of immunodiagnostic field tests for the detection of the mycotoxin, sporidesmin A, *Food Agric Immunol* 10(2):91, 1998.

24. Richard JL: Mycotoxin photosensitivity, *J Am Vet Med Assoc* 163(11):1298, 1973.

25. Morris CA et al: Genetics of susceptibility to facial eczema in Friesian and Jersey cattle, *N Z J Agric Res* 41(3):347, 1998.

Stachybotryotoxins

1. Lacey J: In Smith JE, Henderson RS, editors: *Mycotoxins and animal foods,* London, 1991, CRC Press.

2. Croft WA, Jarvis BB, Yaiawara CS: Airborne outbreaks of trichothecene mycotoxicosis, *Atm Environ* 20:549, 4986.

3. Bisset J: Fungi associated with urea-formaldehyde insulation in Canada, *Mycopathology* 99:47, 1987.

4. Sorenson WG, Frazer DG, Jarvis BB, Simpson J, Robinson VA: Trichothecene mycotoxins in aerosolized conidia of *Stachybotrys atra, Appl Microbiol* 53:1370, 1987.

5. Hintikka EL. Human stachybotryotoxicosis. In Wyllie TD, Morehouse LG: *Mycotoxic fungi, mycotoxins, mycotoxicoses,* vol 3, New York, 1978, Marcel Dekker.

6. Trout T, Bernstein J, Martinez K, Biagini R, Wallingford K: Bioaerosol lung damage in a worker with repeated exposure to fungi in a water damaged building, *Environ Health Perspect* 109(6):641, 2001.

7. Hajtos I et al: Stachybotryotoxicosis as a predisposing factor of ovine systemic pasteurellosis, *Acta Veter Hung* 31:181, 1983.

8. Schneider DJ et al: A field outbreak of suspected stachybotryotoxicosis in sheep, *J S Afr Vet Assoc* 50:73, 1979.

9. Nikulin M et al: Experimental lung mycotoxicosis in mice induced by *Stachybotrys atra, Int J Exp Pathol* 77:213, 1996.

10. Update: pulmonary hemorrhage/hemosiderosis among infants: Cleveland, Ohio 1993-1996, *Morb Mortal Wkly Rep* 46:206, 1997.

11. Jarvis BB et al: Study of toxin production by isolates of *Stachybotrys chartarum* and *Memnoniella echinata* isolated during a study of pulmonary hemosiderosis in infants, *Appl Environ Microbiol* 64:3620, 1998.

12. Szathmary CI: In Ueno Y, editor: *Trichothecenes: chemical biological and toxicological aspect,* New York, 1983, Elsevier.

13. Hintikka EL: Stachybotryotoxicosis in cattle and captive animals. In Wyllie TD, Morehouse LG, editors: *Mycotoxic fungi, mycotoxins, mycotoxicoses,* vol 2, New York, 1978, Marcel Dekker.

14. Hintikka EL: Stachybotryotoxicosis in swine. In Wyllie TD, Morehouse LG, editors: *Mycotoxic fungi, mycotoxins, mycotoxicoses,* vol 2, New York, 1978, Marcel Dekker.

15. Hintikka EL: Stachybotryotoxicosis in poultry. In Wyllie TD, Morehouse LG, editors: *Mycotoxic fungi, mycotoxins, mycotoxicoses,* vol 2, New York, 1978, Marcel Dekker.

Tremorgenic Forages

1. Osweiler GD: *The National Veterinary Medical Series Toxicology,* Philadelphia, 1996, Williams & Wilkins.

2. Fischer G et al: Mycotoxins of *Aspergillus fumigatus* in pure culture in native bioaerosols from compost facilities, *Chemosphere* 38:1745, 1999.

3. Galey FD: In Howard JL, Smith RA, editors: *Current veterinary therapy 4, food animal practice,* Philadelphia, 1999, WB Saunders.

4. Summers BA, Cummings JA, de Lahunta A: *Veterinary neuropathology,* St Louis, 1995, Mosby.

5. Braselton WE, Rumler PC: MS/MS screen for the tremorgenic mycotoxins roquefortine and penitrem A, *J Vet Diagn Invest* 8:515, 1996.

6. Galey FD et al: Staggers induced by consumption of ryegrass in cattle and sheep from northern California, *J Am Vet Med Assoc* 199:466, 1991.

7. McLeay LM et al: Tremorgenic mycotoxins paxilline, penitrem and lolitrem B, the non-tremorgenic 31-epilolitrem B and electromyographic activity of the reticulum and rumen of sheep, *Res Vet Sci* 66:119, 1999.

8. Carson TL: In Howard JL, Smith RA, editors: *Current veterinary therapy 4, food animal practice,* Philadelphia, 1999, WB Saunders.

9. Galey FD: Toxic topics: hot items from the small animal case log. Paper presented at the American VMA, New Orleans, La, 1999.

Tricothecene Mycotoxins

1. Coppock RW et al: Preliminary study of the pharmacokinetics and toxicopathy of deoxynivalenol (vomitoxin) in swine, *Am J Vet Res* 46:169,1985.

2 Prelusky DB et al: Pharmacokinetic fate of 14C-labeled deoxynivalenol in swine, *Fund Appl Toxicol* 10:276, 1988.

3. He P et al: Microbial transformation of deoxynivalenol (vomitoxin), *Appl Environ Microbiol* 58:3857, 1992.

4. Prelusky DB: Excretion profiles of the mycotoxin deoxynivalenol, following oral and intravenous administration to sheep, *Fund Appl Toxicol* 6:356, 1986.

5. Côte LM et al: Excretion of deoxynivalenol and its metabolite in milk, urine, and feces of lactating dairy cows, *J Dairy Sci* 69:2416, 1986.

6. Kollarczik B et al: *In vitro* transformation of the Fusarium mycotoxins deoxynivalenol and zearalenone by the normal gut microflora of pigs, *Nat Toxins* 2:105, 1994.

7. He P et al: Microbially detoxified vomitoxin-contaminated corn for young pigs, *J Anim Sci* 71:963, 1993.

8. Charmley E et al: Influence of levels of deoxynivalenol in the diet of dairy cows on feed intake, milk production, and its composition, *J Dairy Sci* 76:3580, 1993.

9. Prelusky DB et al: Nontransmission of deoxynivalenol (vomitoxin) to milk following oral administration to dairy cows, *J Environ Sci Health B* 19:593, 1984.

10. Côte LM et al: Sex-related reduced weight gains in growing swine fed diets containing deoxynivalenol, *J Anim Sci* 61:942, 1985.

11. Trenholm HL et al: Feeding trials with vomitoxin (deoxynivalenol)-contaminated wheat: effects on swine, poultry, and dairy cattle, *J Am Vet Med Assoc* 185:527,1984.

12. Prelusky DB: Effect of intraperitoneal infusion of deoxynivalenol on feed consumption and weight gain in the pig, *Nat Toxins* 5:121, 1997.

13. Øvernes G et al: Effects of diets with graded levels of naturally deoxynivalenol-contamined oats on immune response in growing pigs, *J Vet Med Assoc* 44:539, 1997.

14. Bergsjø B et al: Effects of diets with graded levels of deoxynivalenol on performance in growing pigs, *J Vet Med Assoc* 39:752, 1992.

15. Harvey RB et al: Effects of deoxynivalenol in a wheat ration fed to growing lambs, *Am J Vet Res* 47:1630, 1986.

16. Johnson PJ et al: Effect of feeding deoxynivalenol (vomitoxin)-contaminated barley to horses, *J Vet Diagn Invest* 9:219, 1997.

17. Wolf-Hall CE et al: Stability of deoxynivalenol in heat-treated foods, *J Food Prot* 62:962, 1999.

18. Hughes DM et al: Overt signs of toxicity to dogs and cats of dietary deoxynivalenol, *J Anim Sci* 77:693, 1999.

19. Moran ET et al: Impact of high dietary vomitoxin on yolk yield and embryonic mortality, *Poultry Sci* 66:977, 1987.

20. Kubena LF et al: Effects of feeding deoxynivalenol (DON, vomitoxin)-contaminated wheat to female white leghorn chickens from day old through egg production, *Poultry Sci* 66:1612, 1987.

21. Weaver GA et al: Diacetoxyscirpenol toxicity in pigs, *Res Vet Sci* 31:131, 1981.

22. Rafai P et al: Effect of various levels of T-2 toxin on the clinical status performance and metabolism of growing pigs, *Vet Rec* 136:485, 1995.

23. Brake J et al: Effects of trichothecene mycotoxin diacetoxyscirpenol on feed consumption, body weight, and oral lesions of broiler breeders, *Poultry Sci* 79:856, 2000.

24. Hsu IC et al: Identification of T-2 toxin in moldy corn associated with a lethal toxicosis in dairy cattle, *Appl Microbiol* 24:684, 1972.

Zearalenone

1 McNutt SH et al: Vulvovaginitis in swine, *J Am Vet Med Assoc* 73:484, 1928.

2. Urry WH et al: The structure of zearalenone, *Tetrahedron Lett* 27:3109, 1966.

3. Cheeke PR: *Natural toxicants in feeds, forages and poisonous plants*, ed 2, Danville, Ill, 1998, Interstate Publishers.

4. Ciegler A et al: Mycotoxins: occurrence in the environment. In Shank RC, editor: *Mycotoxins and N-nitroso compounds: environmental risks*, Boca Raton, Fla, 1981, CRC Press.

5. Kurtz HJ, Mirocha CJ: Zearalenone (F-2) induced estrogenic syndrome in swine. In Wyllie TD, Morehouse LG, editors: *Mycotoxic fungi, mycotoxins, mycotoxicoses; an encyclopedic handbook,* vol 2, *Mycotoxicoses of domestic and laboratory animals, poultry and aquatic invertebrates and vertebrates,* New York, 1978, Marcel Dekker.

6. Mirocha CJ et al: F-2 (zearalenone) estrogenic mycotoxin from *Fusarium*. In Kadis S et al, editors: *Microbial toxins*, vol 7, New York, 1971, Academic Press.

7. Erasmuson AF et al: Natural zeranol (a-zearalanol) in the urine of pasture-fed animals, *J Agric Food Chem* 42:2721, 1994.

8. Prelusky DB et al: Toxicology of mycotoxins. In Miller JD, Trenholm HL, editors: *Mycotoxins in grain, compounds other than aflatoxin*, St Paul, 1994, Eagan Press.

9. Osweiler GD: In Osweiler GD, Galey FD, editors: Mycotoxins, contemporary issues of food animal health and productivity, *Vet Clin North Am Food Anim Pract* 16(3):511, 2000.

10. Prelusky DB: Residues in food products of animal origin. In Miller JD, Trenholm HL, editors: *Mycotoxins in grain, compounds other than aflatoxin,* St Paul, 1994, Eagan Press.

11. Kiessling KH et al: Metabolism of aflatoxin, ochratoxin, zearalenone, and three trichothecenes by intact rumen fluid, rumen protozoa, and rumen bacteria, *Appl Environ Microbiol* 47(5):1070, 1984.

12. Diekman MA, Green ML: Mycotoxins and reproduction in domestic livestock, *J Anim Sci* 70:1615, 1992.

13. Pestka JJ, Bondy GS: Immunotoxic effects of mycotoxins. In Miller JD, Trenholm HL, editors: *Mycotoxins in grain, compounds other than aflatoxin,* St Paul, 1994, Eagan Press.

14. Long GG, Diekman MA: Characterization of effects of zearalenone in swine during early pregnancy, *Am J Vet Res* 47(1):184, 1986.

15. Ruhr LP: The effect of the mycotoxin zearalenone on fertility in the boar. PhD thesis. University of Missouri, Columbia, 1979.

16. Milano GD et al: Effects of long-term zearalenone administration on spermatogenesis and serum luteinizing hormone, follicle-stimulating hormone, and prolactin values in male rats, *Am J Vet Res* 56(7):954, 1995.

17. Weaver GA et al: Effect of zearalenone on the fertility of virgin dairy heifers, *Am J Vet Res* 47:1395, 1986.

18. Weaver GA et al: Effect of zearalenone on dairy cows, *Am J Vet Res* 47:1826, 1986.

19. Deschamps JC et al: Effects of zeranol on reproduction in beef bulls: scrotal circumference, serving ability, semen characteristics and pathologic changes of the reproductive organs, *Am J Vet Res* 48(1):137, 1987.

20. Smith JF et al: Reproductive performance of Coopworth ewes following oral doses of zearalenone before and after mating, *J Reprod Fertil* 89:99, 1990.

21. Mirocha CJ et al: Estrogenic metabolite produced by *Fusarium graminearum* in stored corn, *Appl Microbiol* 15:497, 1967.

22. Chi MS et al: Effect of zearalenone on female white leghorn chickens, *Appl Environ Microbiol* 39:1026, 1980.

23. Allen NK et al: Effects of dietary zearalenone on finishing broiler chickens and young turkey poults, *Poultry Sci* 60:124, 1981.

24. Nelson GH et al: *Fusarium* and estrogenism in swine, *J Am Vet Med Assoc* 163(11):1276, 1973.

25. Kurtz HJ et al: Histologic changes in the genital tracts of swine fed estrogenic mycotoxin, *Am J Vet Res* 30:551, 1969.

26. Chang K et al: Effects of the mycotoxin zearalenone on swine reproduction, *Am J Vet Res* 40(9):1260, 1979.

Pharmaceuticals

ANALGESICS

Joseph D. Roder

NONSTEROIDAL ANTIINFLAMMATORY AGENTS

Synonyms. Aspirin and the salicylates are carboxylic acids found in numerous products ranging from aspirin and arthritis creams (methyl salicylate) to Pepto-Bismol. The propionic acids are a class that includes ibuprofen (Advil, Nuprin), ketoprofen (Orudis), carprofen (Rimadyl), and naproxen. The enolic acids include oxyphenbutazone, phenylbutazone, and piroxicam. The acetic acids are represented by etodolac (EtoGesic), sulindac, and indomethacin.

Toxicokinetics. These compounds share a common kinetic profile. They are well absorbed from the stomach and proximal small intestine following oral administration and are highly (>90%) protein bound. Most of these drugs are metabolized to inactive forms and have a low volume of distribution (<0.2 L/kg).

Mechanism of Action. These compounds reduce inflammation by inhibiting the cyclooxygenase (COX) enzyme system. COX mediates the production of cyclic endoperoxides from arachidonic acid to yield prostaglandins. COX1 and COX2, which are encoded by different genes, are two different isoforms of the COX enzyme. Some of the newer nonsteroidal antiinflammatory drugs (NSAIDs) preferentially inhibit COX2 more than COX1.[1] It is thought that the majority of the antiinflammatory, analgesic, and antipyretic actions are due to inhibition of COX2, whereas most of the adverse effects are due to inhibition of COX1.

These enzymes have differences in function and location. COX1 is the constitutive isoform found in almost all tissues.[2] COX1 is produced continuously, is only slightly regulated, and is involved in tissue homeostasis (production of cytoprotective prostaglandins, modulation of blood flow). COX2 is an inducible isoform, is not commonly found in most tissues during basal conditions, and is highly regulated with more enzyme produced in response to infection or cytokines.

Cells that increase production of COX2 in response to infection include macrophages, fibroblasts, chondrocytes, epithelial cells, and endothelial cells.

NSAIDs cause several toxicologic syndromes: gastrointestinal, renal, hepatic, and central nervous system (CNS). Gastrointestinal toxicosis is a complex and multifactorial process resulting from direct drug effects and the inhibition of COX isozymes. The acidic nature of some NSAIDs decreases barrier characteristics of the gastrointestinal mucous layer and uncouple oxidative phosphorylation, further decreasing mucus barrier functions. In vitro, uncoupling of oxidative phosphorylation is not a characteristic of highly specific COX2 inhibitors. Additionally, there is the potential of ion trapping of the acidic NSAIDs resulting in a higher local concentration. Inhibition of prostaglandin production (PGE and PGI) decreases the cytoprotective properties of gastric mucus and increases the hydrogen ion release from the gastric gland via the H+/K+-ATPase.

Nephrotoxicity caused by nonsteroidal antiinflammatory drugs (NSAIDs) relates primarily to inhibition of prostaglandin synthesis and renal blood flow. Inhibiting COX1 production of PGI, PGE, and PGD increases vascular resistance, constricts renal capillary beds, and redistributes blood away from the medulla. The resulting vasoconstriction and medullary ischemia account for renal papillary necrosis. This process is reversible if noted early, in that only a minority of nephrons have loops of Henle extending into the papillae.

Acute intoxication with aspirin or salicylates can cause hyperthermia. The mechanism for this syndrome relates to the ability of the salicylate molecule to uncouple oxidative phosphorylation. Salicylates diminish the proton gradient across mitochondrial membranes by carrying protons from the outside to the inside of this organelle. This prevents the function of adenosine triphosphate (ATP) synthase, which is powered by the proton gradient. Uncoupled, the energy of phosphorylation is dissipated as thermal energy or an elevated body temperature. This promotes anaerobic metabolism with elevations of lactate, pyruvate, and ketones, which contribute to the development of acidosis and an anion gap.

NSAIDs may also produce hepatotoxicosis. In veterinary medicine this syndrome has been more commonly associated with the administration of carprofen (Rimadyl), although many of the NSAIDs can cause liver damage.[3] In humans, hepatotoxicosis is uncommon, with an incidence of less than 0.1%, but with 20 million patients regularly taking NSAIDs, this may result in significant potential for hepatotoxicosis. The mechanism of hepatotoxicity in humans is not well understood but is thought to relate to an idiosyncratic susceptibility by the patient, either by an immune-mediated hypersensitivity or by a metabolic idiosyncrasy with the production of unusual toxic metabolites. A similar mechanism may be responsible for the hepatotoxicity noted in dogs.

Toxicity and Risk Factors.   NSAIDs are prevalent and are found in most households in the United States, thus posing a significant exposure potential to pets. Animals may become poisoned by accidental ingestion (more common in dogs) or inappropriate administration by owners. The long-term use of NSAIDs in the management of orthopedic disease predisposes some animals to the development of toxicosis.

Acute intoxication is more typically noted in small animals and particularly dogs. More long-term (several days to weeks) administration of NSAIDs may result in toxicosis in all species. Cats are more susceptible to salicylate intoxication because of the relatively low capacity of their hepatic glucuronyl transferase system. Gastrointestinal (ulcerogenic) signs are the most common in all species and may occur after normal administration. Flunixin meglumine (2.2 mg/kg) produced lesions of the gastric mucosa within 4 days.[4] Naproxen-induced toxicosis was reported in a dog after a dose of 220 mg.[5] Protein-losing enteropathy has been noted in ponies and horses with phenylbutazone at doses between 8 and 12 mg/kg given over a period of 8 to 10 days.[6]

Older and younger animals are at greater risk for developing gastrointestinal ulcers or nephrotoxicosis. Animals with diminished renal or hepatic function are more likely to develop toxicosis. Dehydration during NSAID therapy predisposes animals to development of nephropathy, especially with phenylbutazone. NSAIDs that are more commonly associated with nephropathy include phenylbutazone, ibuprofen, mefenamic acid, and fenoprofen. Some NSAIDs that carry a manufacturer's notification of potential human fulminant hepatic failure include indomethacin, ibuprofen, naproxen, piroxicam, and mefenamic acid.

Clinical Signs.   In animals acutely poisoned with salicylates, the initial sign is an altered respiratory pattern. The animal may vomit early in the clinical course with signs possibly progressing to depression, hyperthemia, dehydration, and, sometimes, seizure activity. The most common presentation for acute intoxication by other NSAIDs is gastrointestinal distress with signs that include nausea, vomiting, hematemesis, melena, anorexia, and colic. Clinical signs associated with nephrotoxicosis include an acute onset of oliguria. Animals suffering from the hepatotoxic syndrome may present with anorexia, jaundice, hepatic encephalopathy, coagulopathy, or ascites.

Clinical Pathology.   Metabolic acidosis with an elevated anion gap may suggest salicylate intoxication. Decreased serum proteins (albumin) may be noted in phenylbutazone

intoxication resulting from a protein-losing enteropathy.[7] Hypoalbuminemia is also possible with NSAID-induced gastric or intestinal ulcers as well as those that cause nephrotoxicosis. Gastric ulceration can be monitored using packed cell volume (PCV) or fecal occult blood. Increased blood urea nitrogen (BUN) and creatinine suggesting decreased renal function may be noted with NSAID-induced nephrotoxicity. Elevated serum alanine aminotransferase (ALT), aspartate aminotransferase (AST), alkaline phosphatase (ALP), and hyperbilirubinemia are associated with the hepatotoxic syndrome.

Lesions.   Gastrointestinal mucosal lesions include irritation, erosions, hemorrhage, ulceration, edema, and perforation of the stomach, intestines, or colon.[4,7-9] The glandular portion of the gastric mucosa and the right dorsal colon of the horse are most commonly affected by phenylbutazone.[7] In horses, renal lesions associated with phenylbutazone include renal papillary necrosis.[7]

Diagnostic Testing.   Diagnostic evaluation of serum for salicylates and ibuprofen is available in human hospitals. However, knowing the serum concentration for these NSAIDs is not useful in the management of the poisoned patient. Ultrasound may be used in foals and horses to document the presence of renal papillary damage associated with phenylbutazone.[10] Endoscopy can be used to identify gastric ulceration associated with NSAID administration.[8] Occult fecal blood is more correlated to gastric ulceration as compared to PCV or a physical examination when using endoscopy as the gold standard.

Treatment.   No specific antidote is available for NSAID intoxication so the treatment is symptomatic and supportive. Initial decontamination includes emesis, in appropriate species, for a recent ingestion. Activated charcoal and sorbitol cathartic (Toxiban) administration is necessary to adsorb any of the drug remaining in the gastrointestinal tract. Fluid therapy is indicated in the poisoned patient to maintain renal function and urine flow.[11] Urinary alkalinization using sodium bicarbonate may increase the elimination of aspirin. This allows the ionized aspirin molecules to be trapped in the urine. The rationale for this is sound in that many acutely intoxicated animals also have a metabolic acidosis. The patient must be closely monitored during this therapy to ensure that electrolyte abnormalities and overhydration do not develop.[12] Blood transfusions may be necessary if severe anemia develops. If seizures occur, they can generally be controlled with diazepam. Gastrointestinal mucosal protection using sucralfate or cimetidine may prevent further damage to the gastric mucosa. Omeprazole, a proton pump inhibitor, increases the healing of gastric ulcers in humans patients.

Prognosis.   The gastrointestinal lesions are generally reversible; however, perforation of the intestine has a guarded prognosis because of peritonitis. Most of the renal effects of the NSAIDs are reversible by discontinuation of the drug; renal papillary necrosis is a permanent change that may not adversely affect renal function of the horse.

Prevention and Control.   NSAIDs should be used at lower doses in foals than in adult horses.[13] It is necessary to maintain hydration status and electrolyte balance in all animals receiving NSAIDs. The decision to place an animal on long-term NSAID therapy should not be taken lightly. This is especially true with older animals suffering from osteoarthritis that will require continuous therapy. The animal must be routinely monitored (renal and liver function tests) to assess the efficacy of therapy and development of potential toxic effects. Additionally, the animals should be closely observed for any early signs of illness (anorexia or depression) so the veterinarian might be contacted immediately.

ACETAMINOPHEN

Synonyms.   Tylenol, Paracetamol, Anacin-3, Tempra, and many other products contain acetaminophen.

Sources.   Acetaminophen is found in a variety of over-the-counter (OTC) pain relievers as well as in cold, flu, and allergy medications. It represents one of the most common analgesics found in human medications.

Toxicokinetics.   Acetaminophen is rapidly absorbed from the gastrointestinal tract and removed in most species following hepatic metabolism. Acetaminophen is generally conjugated by sulfation or glucuronidation before elimination.[14] Glutathione serves as an intracellular scavenger of reactive metabolites produced by the metabolism of acetaminophen.

Mechanism of Action.   Acetaminophen exerts its toxic effects via the production of toxic metabolites, especially N-acetyl-p-benzoquinonamine. Normally, this is a minor metabolic pathway and toxic metabolites are conjugated and eliminated. In the case of an overdose, the conjugation pathways are outstripped and the reactive metabolite then interacts with glutathione to produce nontoxic metabolites. After glutathione supplies are exhausted, the toxic metabolite binds to sulfhydryl-containing proteins in the liver cell and causes lipid peroxidation, disrupting the cell membrane. These events eventually lead to cell death.

Toxicity and Risk Factors.   Acetaminophen is absolutely contraindicated in the cat. The cat lacks sufficient glucuronyl transferase to adequately metabolize and excrete acetaminophen.[15] A single acetaminophen tablet may cause intoxication in the cat and repeated administration increases the risk of clinical disease.[16] Acetaminophen at doses greater than 60 mg/kg induced methemoglobinemia in cats.[17] Doses of acetaminophen greater than 100 mg/kg induced toxicosis in dogs.[14] Many intoxications occur when owners treat their pets with acetaminophen, not realizing the difference in toxicity for this drug between humans and animals.

Clinical Signs.   Dogs are more likely to have signs related to hepatotoxicosis: nausea, vomiting, depression, and anorexia. The red blood cell of the cat is more susceptible to oxidative injury following depletion of glutathione, so cats are more likely to have signs related to methemoglobin production: cyanosis or dark mucous membranes, dyspnea, and edema of the front paws and face. At high doses of acetaminophen, the dog also develops methemoglobinemia and the cat develops hepatic disease.

Clinical Pathology.   Methemoglobin concentrations will be elevated in cats exhibiting clinical signs. Liver enzymes (ALT, AST) may be elevated, especially in dogs.

Lesions.   The primary lesion noted with acetaminophen intoxication in dogs is a centrilobular hepatic necrosis. Cats exhibit a diffuse hepatic necrosis.[14]

Treatment.   Initial therapy for acute ingestion focuses on prevention of absorption of acetaminophen and administration of the specific antidote. Induction of emesis for recent ingestions may be indicated as long as it does not delay the administration of activated charcoal. Gastric lavage is generally not necessary unless the animal has consumed a very large dose. Administration of activated charcoal (Toxiban) that contains sorbitol decreases absorption of acetaminophen from the gastrointestinal tract. This stage of therapy should be followed immediately with administration of N-acetylcysteine, which serves as a sulfhydryl source that binds reactive toxic metabolites and as a glutathione precursor.[16,18,19] The initial dose is 140 mg/kg orally or intravenously, followed by 70 mg/kg doses every 6 hours for at least 48 hours. Treatment is most effective against toxicosis when started within 8 hours of ingestion. Treatment between 8 and 24 hours after ingestion lowers mortality but offers incomplete protection from hepatotoxicity. An additional component of treatment may be the inclusion of cimetidine or ranitidine, which appears to reduce metabolism of acetaminophen.[20,21]

Prognosis.   The prognosis is guarded in cats presenting with clinical signs.

Prevention and Control.   Client education is paramount to prevent this disease in cats.

ANTICONVULSANTS

Joseph D. Roder

BARBITURATES

Synonyms.   Several classes of barbiturates and related drugs are used in the treatment and prevention of seizures. Phenobarbital (long-acting) and pentobarbital (short-acting) are two of the more commonly used barbiturate agents.

Toxicokinetics.   Phenobarbital exhibits enterohepatic recycling.

Mechanism of Action.   The therapeutic effects of the barbiturates relate to their ability to increase the binding of gamma-aminobutyric acid (GABA), the major inhibitor neurotransmitter of the CNS, to its receptor. This results in a greater influx of chloride into the cell, causing hyperpolarization and decreased excitability. Isolated cases of hepatotoxicosis have been reported secondary to idiosyncratic or hypersensitivity reactions.

Toxicity and Risk Factors.   Hepatotoxicosis has been most often reported in dogs following chronic use.[1-3] Generalized bone marrow suppression has been noted with the use of these agents to control seizures in dogs.[4] This may represent a hypersensitivity or idiosyncratic reaction.

Clinical Signs.   Clinical signs associated with an acute toxicosis include shallow respiration, incoordination, lethargy, coma, loss of reflexes, and dilated pupils. Clinical signs associated with hepatotoxicosis include icterus, depression, and ascites.[1]

Clinical Pathology.   Mild elevations of liver enzymes (lactate dehydrogenase and AST) may be noted in chronic cases. Sulfobromophthalein excretion is generally prolonged; serum bile acids (resting and postprandial) may be elevated. Marked increases in serum ALT, serum ALP, total bilirubin, and sulfobromophthalein retention indicate hepatotoxicosis.[1,2] Additionally, animals may have decreased albumin and increased BUN. Neutropenia, thrombocytopenia, and anemia may also be noted in response to long-term barbiturate therapy.

Lesions.   Dogs receiving long-term phenobarbital therapy may have chronic hepatic fibrosis with nodular regeneration. Infrequently with chronic phenytoin use, toxic hepatitis may develop and lead to liver necrosis and chronic inflammation along with cholangitis.[3]

Diagnostic Testing.   Testing of serum concentrations may be performed; however, serum concentrations are not predictive of the clinical outcome.

Treatment.   A specific antidote is not available. Decontamination includes repeated administration of activated charcoal every 4 to 6 hours. Activated charcoal acts as a "sink" for phenobarbital even when given parenterally.

A saline cathartic is often beneficial because of the reduction of gastrointestinal motility and subsequent constipation that is often noted with barbiturate administration. However, the cathartic should be used judiciously because repeated administration of cathartics can produce uncontrolled diarrhea and dehydration.

Increased elimination of the barbiturates may be achieved by alkalinization of the urine with sodium bicarbonate. The change in the urinary pH ionizes and traps the barbiturate in the urine. When using this method, careful monitoring of the serum electrolytes and respiratory function must be performed.

Symptomatic therapy includes maintenance of a patent airway with intubation and oxygen therapy, if necessary. Hypotension and hypothermia may be treated with warmed intravenous fluids and blankets. Treatment of the hepatotoxic

syndrome includes discontinuation of the drug and symptom management.[1,2]

Prognosis.   The prognosis for an acute overdose that is aggressively managed is good. Many of the dogs that present with hepatotoxicity return to normal hepatic function after removal of the offending barbiturate.[1,2]

Prevention and Control.   The chronic use of barbiturates to control epilepsy in dogs should include regular screening of hepatic and renal function. Additionally, a baseline complete blood count (CBC) should be done before therapy and regularly during treatment to examine for possible bone marrow depression.[4]

BROMIDE

Synonyms.   Bromide intoxication is also known as bromism.

Sources.   Bromide toxicosis is caused by the ingestion of too much potassium or sodium bromide as an adjunct therapy for seizures in patients that do not exhibit good control with barbiturates. Other sources include home permanent solutions, the salts of drugs, and methyl bromide fumigants.

Toxicokinetics.   Bromates are readily absorbed following oral administration and are eliminated by the kidneys. Bromide has a long half-life and can accumulate after subsequent administration. It requires several weeks to months to achieve a steady-state condition with bromide during anticonvulsant therapy. Bromide is also eliminated in the milk and can be transferred across the placenta.

Mechanism of Action.   Bromide substitutes for the chloride ions in plasma, extracellular fluid, and intracellular fluid. Of greatest interest is the replacement of chloride in excitable membranes and the CNS where it may replace up to 30% of the chloride ions. As the concentration of bromide ions increases, there is a generalized membrane depressant effect.[5]

Toxicity and Risk Factors.   All animals are susceptible, but the disease is more commonly noted in dogs. This intoxication may be acute or chronic in nature. Animals with renal dysfunction are at greater risk of developing toxicosis. Also, a recent change in diet in which chloride is lowered (salt-restriction diet) increases the potential for poisoning. Cattle were intoxicated after ingesting hay containing 6800 and 8400 ppm bromide ion.[6]

Clinical Signs.   Animals with bromism have signs of generalized weakness, depression, ataxia, hyporeflexia, or sedation. Animals may initially present with muscle pain or weakness.[5] Often animals that have ingested a large dose acutely have nausea and vomiting, which may limit the dose absorbed.

Clinical Pathology.   The most prominent alteration of the serum chemistry is an increased serum chloride and a decreased anion gap.

Diagnostic Testing.   Serum bromide testing can be performed to confirm intoxication. Serum bromide concentrations greater than 3000 µg/ml are generally above the therapeutic range and may suggest toxicosis.[7]

Treatment.   No specific antidote for bromide intoxication is available. Emesis as the initial step in decontamination therapy may be warranted unless the animal has recently vomited. Activated charcoal does not readily adsorb the inorganic salts of bromide. The key to therapy is increased elimination by providing intravenous 0.9% NaCl. The chloride in the fluids drastically reduces the serum half-life of bromide. As an adjunct therapy, furosemide may be needed to increase diuresis. Additionally any barbiturate or other CNS depressant used to control the animal's seizures should be discontinued or reduced. The animal should be closely monitored because the elimination of bromide may be associated with an onset of seizures. These seizures should be controlled symptomatically with diazepam. Other supportive therapy includes intubation and oxygen therapy if the animal is comatose.

Prognosis.   Mortality resulting from bromide intoxication is uncommon. Animals with normal renal function should be able to adequately eliminate the bromide. The prognosis is good with proper therapy.

Prevention and Control.   The key to prevention is client education concerning the signs of bromide intoxication. The animal can then be given emergency care. The owners need to be compliant and diligent in administering medications.

ANTIDEPRESSANTS

Sharon Gwaltney-Brant

Antidepressants used in human medicine encompass several different classes of drugs, including the tricyclic antidepressants (TCAs), selective serotonin reuptake inhibitors (SSRIs), monoamine oxidase inhibitors (MAOIs), and "atypical" antidepressants. Examples of specific compounds in each class are listed in Box 24-1.

TRICYCLIC ANTIDEPRESSANTS

Synonyms.   The TCAs include amitriptyline, amoxapine, clomipramine, desipramine, dothiepin, doxepin, imipramine, lofepramine, maprotiline, nortriptyline, protriptyline, and trimipramine. In general, TCAs differ from each other in their relative abilities to block neurotransmitter reuptake, in their relative anticholinergic and antihistaminic effects, and in their sedative properties. For example, amoxapine and maprotiline result in less cardiovascular toxicity and more CNS toxicity than the other TCAs in humans.[1]

Toxicokinetics.   TCAs are rapidly and completely absorbed from the gastrointestinal tract following ingestion, with some reaching peak plasma levels as soon as 30 to 60 minutes following ingestion (Table 24-1).[2] Although onset of signs

---

BOX 24-1	CLASSIFICATION OF ANTIDEPRESSANT DRUGS

TRICYCLIC ANTIDEPRESSANTS

Amitriptyline (Elavil)
Amoxapine (Asendin)
Clomipramine (Anafranil, Clomicalm)
Despiramine (Norpramin)
Doxepin (Sinequan, Adapin)
Imipramine (Tofranil)
Maprotiline (Ludiomil)
Nortriptyline (Pamelor)
Protriptyline (Vivactil)
Trimipramine (Surmontil)

MONOAMINE OXIDASE INHIBITORS

Phenelzine (Nardil)
Selegiline* (Anipryl, Eldepryl)
Tranylcypromine (Parnate)

SELECTIVE SEROTONIN REUPTAKE INHIBITORS

Fluoxetine (Prozac)
Fluvoxamine (Luvox)
Nefazodone (Serzone)
Paroxetine (Paxil)
Sertraline (Zoloft)
Trazodone (Desyrel)
Venlafaxine (Effexor)

"ATYPICAL" ANTIDEPRESSANTS

Bupropion (Wellbutrin)

*Selegiline is used to treat cognitive dysfunction in humans and dogs and is not classified as an antidepressant, but it is included here because the toxic effect of overdose would be similar to that of other monoamine oxidase inhibitors.

---

may develop quickly, the anticholinergic effects of TCAs may decrease gastrointestinal motility and delay drug absorption for several hours after ingestion.[1] TCAs are highly protein bound (>85%) and have a large volume of distribution.[1] Distribution into milk has been demonstrated for several TCAs, including amitriptyline and clomipramine.[3]

Hepatic metabolism is the primary mechanism of elimination of TCAs, with little to any excretion of either parent compound or active metabolite through the urine. Prolongation of TCA half-lives may occur as a result of saturation of metabolic pathways or when hepatic metabolic pathways are deficient (e.g., very young, very old, preexisting hepatic disease).[1] Several TCA metabolites are active and may contribute to toxicosis after the first 12 to 24 hours[1]; additionally, enterohepatic recirculation of parent compound or metabolites may prolong signs of toxicosis.[2] Inactive metabolites of TCAs are excreted in the urine.[1]

Mechanism of Action.   The exact mechanism of the antidepressant effects of TCAs is not known, but it is thought to involve both neurotransmitter reuptake blockade and anticholinergic effects.[1] TCAs inhibit reuptake of dopamine, norepinephrine, and serotonin in the CNS, resulting in higher levels of these neurotransmitters within neuronal synapses and thereby potentiating their effects. TCAs also have potent anticholinergic and antihistaminic effects.[1]

In TCA toxicosis, the most life-threatening effects relate to the cardiovascular and central nervous systems.[1] Cardiovascular effects result from direct effects on the myocardium and vasculature and from indirect effects mediated by the

TABLE 24-1 **Veterinary Dosages and Kinetics for Selected Antidepressant Drugs**

Drug	Therapeutic Dosage (Oral)	Peak Plasma* Levels	Half-life*
Tricyclic antidepressants			
Amitriptyline	Dogs: 1-4.4 mg/kg q12-24hr Cats: 0.1-1.5 mg/kg q24hr	2-12 hr	6–8 hr (dog)
Clomipramine	Dogs: 2-3 mg/kg/day Cats: 0.5-1.5 mg/kg q24hr	1.2 hr (dogs) 1 hr	4 hr (dog)
Doxepin	Dogs: 0.5-5.5 mg/kg q12hr	1-2 hr (dogs)	8–24 hr
Imipramine	Dogs: 2.2-4.4 mg/kg q 2-24hr Cats: 2.5-5 mg q12 hr	1-2 hr	18–34 hr
Nortryptiline	Dogs: 1-2 mg/kg q12hr Cats: 0.5-2 mg/kg q12-24hr		16–36 hr
Selective serotonin reuptake inhibitors			
Fluoxetine	Dogs: 1 mg/kg q24hr Cats: 0.5 mg/kg q24hr	4-8 hr	48-72 hr
Paroxetine	Cats: 1 mg/kg q24hr Dogs: 1-3 mg/kg prn	5.2 hr 5.4-8.4 hr	12-21 hr 26 hr
Sertraline	No dose available		
Monamine oxidase inhibitors			
Selegiline	Dogs: 0.5-2 mg/kg q24hr	<30 min (dogs)	1 hr(dogs)
Nefazodone	No dose available	40 min (dogs)	6.8-14.2 hr
Serotonin agonists			
Buspirone (Buspar)	Dogs: 1 mg/kg q24hr or 2.5-10 mg/dog q8-12hr Cats: 0.5-1 mg/kg q12hr or 2.5-7.5 mg/cat	40-90 min	24 hr

Data from references 1-4, 8, 11-14.
*Values listed are from human information unless otherwise specified. For some drugs, the half-life may be increased in cases of overdose caused by saturation of metabolic pathways.

autonomic nervous system. Inhibition of myocardial sodium channels results in myocardial conduction delays, decreased cardiac contractility, and ventricular arrhythmias. Although the overall effect of sodium channel blockade might be expected to be bradycardia, tachycardia is often seen as a result of anticholinergic blockade and inhibition of norepinephrine reuptake.[1] Accordingly, sinus tachycardia is the most common arrhythmia seen in human TCA toxicosis.[1] Vasodilation resulting from vascular alpha-adrenergic blockade and decreased cardiac contractility contributes to the profound hypotension seen in TCA toxicosis.[1] Anticholinergic effects of TCAs contribute to sinus tachycardia, hyperthermia, agitation or hyperactivity, ileus, urinary retention, pupillary dilatation, coma, and perhaps seizures.[1] Blockade of serotonin reuptake may contribute to the signs seen in TCA toxicosis by inducing a serotonin syndrome (see Serotonergic Drugs).

Toxicity and Risk Factors. In general, TCAs have narrow therapeutic windows, with toxic doses being only slightly higher than therapeutic doses in many cases. Lethal doses for animals are not well established; however, TCA doses as low as 15 mg/kg have been reported to be lethal.[2] In dogs, the subcutaneous lethal dose for amitriptyline has been reported to be 50 mg/kg, and the oral lethal dose of clomipramine is 100 mg/kg[2]; serious clinical signs may be seen at doses much lower than these.

Most instances of TCA overdosage in dogs or cats are accidental. Owners may give pets the wrong medication by mistake, or pets may ingest tablets while chewing on bottles or chasing dropped pills. Rarely, human patients feed their medication to their pet to avoid having to take it themselves. Very rare instances of suicide victims wishing to "take their pet with them" have occurred; in these cases, the potential for involvement of multiple drugs must be considered.

Clinical Signs. Clinical signs may begin within 30 minutes of ingestion of TCAs, and death can occur within a few hours if the patient is not given prompt and aggressive treatment.[2] Initial signs generally include ataxia and lethargy, which may be rapidly followed by hypotension, disorientation, hyperactivity, vomiting, tachycardia, mydriasis, dyspnea, urinary retention, ileus, cardiac arrhythmias, acidosis, hyperthermia, coma, seizures, myoclonus, pulmonary edema, and death.[1,2]

Clinical Pathology. Laboratory evaluation may reveal metabolic acidosis.

Lesions. No specific lesions are expected in animals dying of acute TCA toxicosis. In severe or prolonged cases, evidence of damage secondary to prolonged seizuring or hyperthermia includes rhabdomyolysis, disseminated intravascular coagulation (DIC), cerebral edema, renal tubular necrosis, and hepatic necrosis.

Diagnostic Testing. TCAs can be qualitatively detected in the urine or serum by chromatography, although this is not commonly done. Quantitative measurement of TCA levels in serum is not considered to be of much value in managing human TCA overdoses.[1]

Treatment. Treatment for recent TCA ingestions in asymptomatic animals includes decontamination and monitoring. For very recent (less than 15 minutes) ingestions, emesis may be induced, but it should be performed under veterinary supervision because clinical signs may manifest rapidly. For other ingestions, activated charcoal with a cathartic (1 to 2 g/kg orally)[3] may be administered.[2] If the ingestion involved a large amount of drug, gastric lavage might be considered, although in human medicine, there is controversy as to the benefit of lavage, and some clinicians omit this step in favor of administering activated charcoal as rapidly as possible.[1] Certainly the risk of sedation or anesthesia (which may complicate TCA-induced hypotension and acidosis and mask TCA-induced depression) must be considered when deciding whether to perform gastric lavage. Following administration of activated charcoal, the animal should be closely monitored (including electrocardiography) for a minimum of 6 hours for the development of hypotension, hyperthermia, or arrhythmias.[1]

For symptomatic animals, the goals are to stabilize the animal, decontaminate (if not already accomplished), and provide supportive care. Intravenous fluids (Normasol or physiologic saline) are vital in maintaining cardiovascular function and adequate blood pressure. Fluid rates of $1\frac{1}{2}$ to 2 times maintenance rate help counter hypotension and may aid in managing mild arrhythmias.[1]

Tachycardia rarely needs to be directly addressed, in that it generally resolves once other signs are under control; beta-blockers, because of their potential to exacerbate hypotension, are contraindicated.[1] Bradycardia, if present, should not be treated with atropine, because anticholinergic effects may be potentiated. Seizures or myoclonus, if present, generally respond to diazepam, and benzodiazepines are less likely to contribute to cardiovascular abnormalities than are barbiturates.[1]

Blood gas monitoring should be instituted because acidosis is a common effect that can increase the severity and duration of clinical signs.[1] Experimental studies have shown that maintaining a blood pH between 7.5 and 7.55

can reduce cardiotoxicity of TCAs in dogs, and hypertonic sodium bicarbonate is recommended in the treatment of human TCA toxicosis.[1] However, bicarbonate administration should not be instituted unless blood gases can be monitored because iatrogenic alkalosis may result.[2] Hyperventilation improves cardiovascular performance in dogs with experimental TCA toxicosis[1] and might be considered when blood gas monitoring is not available.

Body temperature in symptomatic patients should be monitored at least every 30 minutes, and hyperthermia should be treated as needed, because prolonged hyperthermia may result in serious complications such as DIC and multiorgan failure. Treatment of hyperthermia can be instituted using fans, cool water enemas, and cool intravenous fluids. Animals should be monitored for a minimum of 24 hours after the cessation of clinical signs for the development of complications such as pulmonary edema, coagulation disorders, and pancreatitis.[1]

Prognosis. Animals exhibiting mild to moderate signs should respond well to prompt and aggressive therapy. Severely symptomatic animals, especially those with seizures, hypotension, or arrhythmias that are poorly responsive to therapy, have a guarded prognosis. Animals with preexisting cardiac problems may be at increased risk for severe cardiac dysfunction from TCA toxicosis.

SEROTONERGIC DRUGS

Synonyms. The discovery that drugs that affect CNS levels of serotonin (5-hydroxytryptamine) are useful in the treatment of a variety of human mood disorders has resulted in a growing number of serotonergic drugs being introduced for prescription use. These drugs include the SSRIs and MAOIs, examples of which are listed in Box 24-1. Additionally, two herbal products, Griffonia seed extract (L-5-hydroxytryptophan), a serotonin precursor, and St. John's wort (*Hypericum perforatum*), an MAOI, are available over the counter and are used by some as "alternative" therapies for depression. Selegiline, although not used as an antidepressant, is an MAOI that is used in veterinary medicine for treatment of cognitive dysfunction and Cushing's disease.[3] TCAs also have some serotonergic activity within the CNS.

Toxicokinetics. Like TCAs, SSRIs are well absorbed orally, are highly protein bound, and have wide volumes of distribution and rapid onsets of action (see Table 24-1). In contrast, although MAOIs are well absorbed orally, many have an extensive first pass effect, resulting in low initial bioavailability; bioavailability improves with repeated administration of MAOIs.[4] The serotonin precursor 5-hydroxytryptophan is rapidly absorbed orally and readily crosses the blood-brain barrier into the CNS.[5] Buspirone is likewise well absorbed orally with a rapid onset of action.

SSRIs are metabolized in the liver, and the formation of active metabolites may prolong effects of the drug after the parent compound has been largely cleared from the body (e.g., fluoxetine is converted to norfluoxetine, which peaks 76 hours after fluoxetine administration and has activity that mirrors the parent compound). As with TCAs, half-lives of

SSRIs may increase in cases of overdose because of saturation of metabolic pathways.[2] Metabolites of SSRIs are excreted in urine. MAOIs are rapidly cleared from the blood by hepatic metabolism and excretion of metabolites via the urine, resulting in relatively short half-lives (less than 3 hours).[6] However, the duration of action of MAOIs may be prolonged because of irreversible inactivation of the monoamine oxidase enzyme.[6] Most MAOI metabolites are inactive, but selegiline is metabolized to methamphetamine and amphetamine, which may contribute to its activity.[3]

MAOI metabolites are largely eliminated through the urine. 5-Hydroxytryptophan is excreted via the urine as parent compound, or it can be metabolized in the kidneys to serotonin before excretion.[7] Buspirone is metabolized in the liver to inactive metabolites, and both parent compound and metabolites are excreted in the urine.[8]

Mechanism of Action.   Serotonin (5-hydroxytryptamine) acts as a CNS neurotransmitter, regulator of smooth muscle function in the gastrointestinal tract and cardiovascular system, and promoter of platelet aggregation.[9] Within neurons, some nonneural cells (e.g., enterochromaffin cells of the gastrointestinal tract), and platelets, serotonin is synthesized from tryptophan, an essential amino acid. Tryptophan is converted to 5-hydroxytryptophan by the enzyme tryptophan hydroxylase in a rate-limiting fashion. 5-Hydroxytryptophan is then constitutively converted to serotonin (5-hydroxytryptamine) by L-aromatic amino acid decarboxylase.[9] Within neurons, serotonin is packaged in vesicles and released into the synapse during depolarization.

Serotonin binds to one of several different types of serotonin receptors on the postsynaptic neuron membrane as well as an autoregulatory receptor on the presynaptic neuron; the receptor most important in toxicosis from serotonergic drugs is 5-HT1A.[10] On release from receptors, serotonin is pumped back into the presynaptic membrane, where it is either recycled into secretory vesicles or metabolized to hydroxyindoleacetic acid (the primary metabolite) by monoamine oxidase located on the outer mitochondrial membrane (Fig. 24-1).

Serotonergic drugs affect the activity of serotonin in the CNS through various mechanisms (Box 24-2; see Fig. 24-1): (1) increasing the production of serotonin within the neuron (e.g., 5-hydroxytryptophan), (2) decreasing the breakdown of serotonin within neurons by inhibiting metabolic enzymes (e.g., MAOIs), (3) decreasing the reuptake of serotonin from the synapse, thereby increasing synaptic serotonin levels (e.g., SSRIs), (4) increasing serotonin release (e.g., MAOIs), or (5) acting as serotonin agonists (e.g., buspirone). *Serotonin syndrome* describes the clinical presentation of serotonin excess, characterized by abnormalities of cognitive, behavioral, autonomic nervous system, and neurologic function.[10]

Toxicity and Risk Factors.   Besides accidental overdose of serotonergic drugs, signs of serotonin excess may occasionally develop in humans or animals on therapeutic doses of SSRIs or MAOIs, or when SSRIs are administered too soon after cessation of MAOI therapy (because most MAOIs cause irreversible enzyme inhibition, several weeks may be required for MAO levels to return to normal following cessation of

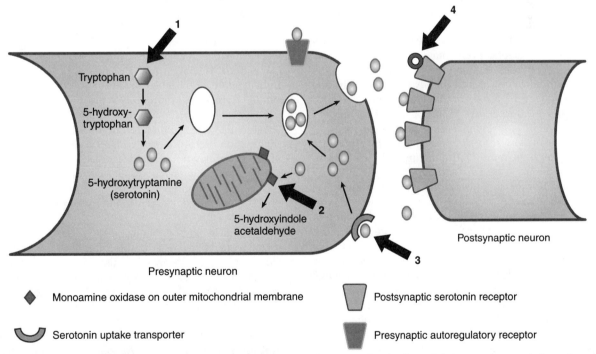

Fig. 24-1 Mechanism of serotonergic drugs. *(1)* Increases in tryptophan or 5-hydroxytryptophan levels result in increased serotonin formation within the presynaptic neuron. *(2)* Monoamine oxidase inhibitors decrease the breakdown of serotonin to 5-hydroxyindole acetaldehyde, resulting in elevated serotonin levels in presynaptic neurons. *(3)* Impairment of serotonin uptake back into the presynaptic neuron by selective serotonin reuptake inhibitors results in elevations of serotonin levels in the synapse. *(4)* Serotonin agonists stimulate postsynaptic serotonin receptors.

BOX 24-2

MECHANISM OF ACTION OF SEROTONERGIC DRUGS

DRUGS THAT ENHANCE SEROTONIN SYNTHESIS

L-Tryptophan
L-5-hydroxytryptophan

DRUGS THAT INCREASE SEROTONIN RELEASE

Amphetamines and amphetamine derivatives
Monoamine oxidase inhibitors
Cocaine

DRUGS THAT INHIBIT SEROTONIN UPTAKE

Selective serotonin reuptake inhibitors
Tricyclic antidepressants
Amphetamines and amphetamine derivatives
Cocaine
Dextromethorphan
Meperidine

DRUGS THAT INHIBIT SEROTONIN METABOLISM

Monoamine oxidase inhibitors

DRUGS THAT ACT AS SEROTONIN AGONISTS

Buspirone
Sumatriptan
Lysergic acid diethylamide (LSD)

MAOI therapy).[6,10] In general, signs developing at therapeutic levels are mild and resolve on cessation of the drug.

Toxic doses of many serotonergic drugs have not been established for domestic animals. In general, low doses of SSRIs (close to therapeutic levels) may be expected to cause mild sedation, whereas higher levels can result in signs consistent with serotonin syndrome.[2,10] In dogs, sertraline causes anorexia at 10 to 20 mg/kg, hypersalivation and muscle tremors at 30 to 50 mg/kg, and death at 80 mg/kg.[2] Paroxetine, fluoxetine, and venlafaxine have been reported to cause depression at 1 mg/kg in dogs; at 10 mg/kg venlafaxine caused tremors in dogs.[2] The minimum lethal dose of fluoxetine is reported to be greater than 100 mg/kg in dogs.[2] Dogs ingesting 10 mg/kg of fluvoxamine have demonstrated depression and tremors.[2]

At therapeutic doses, selegiline is a selective inhibitor of monoamine oxidase B (MAO-B) and is therefore considered to be less likely to cause unwanted side effects, but this selectivity is lost in overdose situations in which selegiline is expected to result in signs similar to those of other MAOIs.[3] Selegiline has caused stereotypic behavior, dehydration, salivation, and panting at 3 and 6 mg/kg in dogs.[3] Tremors have been reported in dogs with 5.5 mg/kg of phenelzine and 2.2 mg/kg of tranylcypromine.[2]

Buspirone has a lethal dose 50 (LD_{50}) in dogs of 586 mg/kg,[3] although significant signs can occur at much lower levels. In one report, the minimum toxic dose in dogs for 5-hydroxytryptophan was 23.6 mg/kg, and the minimum lethal dose was 128 mg/kg.[5]

Clinical Signs.   The toxic effects of serotonergic drugs relate to excess serotonin within the body, and the primary systems affected include the CNS, cardiovascular system, and gastrointestinal tract. At therapeutic doses or low overdoses, signs associated with serotonergic drugs may be limited to mild lethargy, but at higher doses, more severe signs may be seen. The term *serotonin syndrome* describes the clinical manifestation of overstimulation of serotonin receptors.[10] Serotonin syndrome is a potentially life-threatening disorder that has been described in humans, laboratory rodents, and dogs.[1,5] Signs commonly associated with serotonin syndrome in humans include myoclonus, hyperthermia, vomiting and diarrhea, ataxia, agitation, and tremors.[1] Similar signs have been described in dogs ingesting 5-hydroxytryptophan, with the most common signs being seizures (47%), hyperthermia (body temperatures up to 108 °F; 37%), depression (31%), tremors (26%), hyperesthesia (26%), diarrhea (26%), vomiting (26%), and ataxia (21%).[5] Other signs in these dogs included vocalization (19%), transient blindness (16%), death (16%), abdominal pain (16%), hypersalivation (11%), disorientation (11%), tachycardia (5%), weakness (5%), bloat (5%), coma (5%), recumbency (5%), and hyper-reflexia (5%).

Clinical Pathology.   No direct clinical pathologic alterations are expected from patients with serotonin syndrome. However, protracted seizures or hyperthermia may result in rhabdomyolysis, organ damage, or DIC, so clinical laboratory values should be monitored in symptomatic animals.

Lesions.   No specific lesions would be expected from animals ingesting overdoses of serotonergic drugs. Lesions consistent with rhabdomyolysis, DIC, or renal tubular necrosis may be present as secondary changes in severely affected animals.

Diagnostic Testing.   Many of the serotonergic drugs may be detected via chromatography, but levels are not considered to be useful in managing overdose situations.

Treatment.   Because of the potential for rapid onset and progression of clinical signs, decontamination is best done under veterinary supervision. Decontamination should consist of emesis (in asymptomatic animals only) and administration of activated charcoal; the benefits of repeated doses of activated charcoal in serotonergic drug overdose have not been established.[1]

Seizures in dogs generally respond to diazepam[5]; other anticonvulsants such as barbiturates may be considered if diazepam is not effective. The use of phenothiazines in the treatment of serotonin syndrome in humans is controversial as their use has had mixed results.[1] Cyproheptadine, a serotonin antagonist, has been used with success in humans and dogs exhibiting serotonin syndrome[1,5]; the recommended dose in dogs is 1.1 mg/kg orally or per rectum if the oral route is not feasible.[5] As with TCAs, thermoregulation and fluid support are important aspects of managing an animal with serotonin syndrome. Cardiovascular abnormalities generally respond to supportive care and rarely require specific pharmacologic intervention. Although propranolol has some serotonin antagonist activity, its use in serotonin syndrome is rarely indicated.[1] Because the clinical status of animals with serotonin syndrome rapidly changes, it is imperative that affected animals be closely monitored until clinically normal.

Prognosis. Although serotonin syndrome is a potentially life-threatening condition, most animals respond to prompt and aggressive therapy. In dogs with serotonin syndrome resulting from 5-hydroxytryptophan ingestion, the majority of signs resolved within 12 hours of initiation of treatment, and all dogs were clinically normal within 36 hours.[5]

Prevention and Control. All medications should be stored in areas well away from pets. Owners should be advised of the narrow therapeutic window of TCAs that are prescribed for their pets, and they should be made aware of signs of adverse reactions or overdoses in pets that are receiving TCAs or serotonergic drugs. Human and veterinary drugs should be stored separately to avoid accidental mix-up of medication, and pets should be kept out of the area while a human medication is being taken to avoid ingestion of dropped pills by pets. Children should be watched closely while they take their medications to ensure that they are not "slipping" the medication to a pet. Likewise, if medication for one pet is put into food, the pet should be closely observed to be sure that another pet does not "steal" the medication.

ANTIHISTAMINES

Sharon Gwaltney-Brant

Synonyms. *Antihistamine* is a term used to describe drugs that block H_1 receptors for histamine.[1] A large variety of antihistamines encompass several different classes (Box 24-3). Some of the more commonly available first-generation antihistamines used in veterinary and human medicine include brompheniramine (Dimetane), chlorpheniramine (Chlor-Trimeton), clemastine (Tavist), cyproheptadine (Periactin), dimenhydrinate (Dramamine), diphenhydramine (Benadryl), hydroxyzine (Atarax), meclizine (Antivert), promethazine (Phenergan), trimeprazine (Temaril), and tripelennamine (PBZ).[1,2] Second-generation antihistamines lack the sedative properties of first generation antihistamines and include astemizole (Himanal), cetirizine (Zyrtec), fexofenadine (Allegra), loratadine (Claritin), and terfenadine (Seldane). Terfenadine was removed from the market in 1997 in the United States because of the risk of cardiac arrhythmias in humans but may still be in household medicine cabinets. Other drugs such as the TCA amitriptyline (Elavil) may be used for their antihistaminic effects.[2]

Sources. Antihistamines are widely used in human and veterinary medicine for control of allergic disorders, including anaphylaxis, for sedation, for motion sickness and antiemesis, for treatment of laminitis (cattle),[3] and for some mood disorders in humans.[1] Because antihistamines are often formulated along with decongestants that can have serious clinical effects, such as pseudoephedrine, careful questioning is needed to determine the exact product involved in an overdose situation.

Toxicokinetics. Antihistamines are well absorbed orally in monogastric animals, but are poorly absorbed in ruminants.[2] Delayed gut emptying following anticholinergic effects of antihistamine may delay absorption.[4] After ingestion, plasma levels of most antihistamines peak within 2 to 5 hours and onset of action is rapid, often within 30 to 40 minutes.[1] Most antihistamines have a high degree of protein binding (>70%) and a wide volume of distribution.[1] Intravenous injection of antihistamines may result in CNS stimulation or other unwanted effects, whereas similar effects are not commonly seen with intramuscular injection.[2] Most classes of first-generation antihistamines enter the CNS after administration, and the nonsedative properties of second-generation antihistamines (e.g., loratadine, terfenadine) are due in large part to their inability to cross the blood-brain barrier at therapeutic levels. However, in overdose situations, even second-generation antihistamines may enter the CNS and cause CNS effects.[4,5] Virtually all antihistamines undergo metabolism in the liver and metabolites are excreted in the urine; an exception is cetirizine, which is an active metabolite of hydroxyzine that is excreted unchanged in the urine.[1] The metabolism of antihistamines may be delayed in cases of hepatic, and some cases of renal, dysfunction. Half-lives of antihistamines vary with the individual drug; most

---

BOX 24-3	CLASSIFICATION OF ANTIHISTAMINE DRUGS

ALKYLAMINE	Pyrilamine
Brompheniramine	Thenyldiamine
Chlorpheniramine	Tripelennamine
Dexbrompheniramine	
Dexchlorpheniramine	**PHENOTHIAZINE**
Dimethindene	Methdilazine
Pheniramine	Promethazine
Pyrrobutamine	Trimeprazine
Triprolidine	
	PIPERADINE
ETHANOLAMINE	Astemizole
	Levocabastine
Bromodiphenhydramine	Loratadine
Carbinoxamine	Terfenadine
Clemastine	
Dimenhydrinate	**PIPERAZINE**
Diphenhydramine	
Diphenylpyraline	Buclizine
Doxylamine	Cetirizine
Phenyltoloxamine	Chlorcyclizine
	Cyclizine
ETHYLENEDIAMINE	Hydroxyzine
	Meclizine
Antazoline	Niaprazine
Methapyrilene	
Phenyldiamine	

of these drugs have a therapeutic duration of action of 3 to 12 hours.[2]

Mechanism of Action. Three classes of histamine receptors (H_1, H_2, and H_3) have been described, and by convention the term *antihistamine* is used to describe drugs that block H_1 receptors.[1] H_1 receptors are present on a variety of cell types, including capillary endothelium, smooth muscle cells of the gastrointestinal and respiratory tract, peripheral nerves, and neurons of the CNS (particularly within the hypothalamus).[1] Stimulation of histamine receptors leads to increased capillary permeability, bronchoconstriction, large blood vessel dilation, contraction of gastrointestinal smooth muscle, and the classic wheal, flare, pain, and itch of dermal allergic responses. Antihistamines function by binding to H_1 receptors, competitively blocking histamine from the receptors and thereby lowering cell responses to released histamine. Most antihistamine binding to histamine receptors is reversible, but in overdose situations, receptor binding may become irreversible.[5] The effects of H_1 blockade include CNS depression (or occasionally stimulation), inhibition of smooth muscle response to histamine, inhibition of histamine-driven capillary permeability, and modulation of allergic reactions. In humans, the cardiac effects seen with the second-generation H_1 antagonists terfenadine and astemizole are thought to result from impaired metabolism of these antihistamines by hepatic P-450 enzymes, leading to accumulation of unmetabolized product and development of ventricular tachycardia.[1] Many first-generation antihistamines also have pronounced anticholinergic (atropine-like) effects following inhibition of muscarinic receptors, and some H_1 antagonists have local anesthetic effects.[1] Phenothiazine antihistamines have alpha-adrenergic blocking effects.[4] Cyproheptadine, in addition to being an H_1 blocker, also has significant serotonin antagonist activity.[4]

Toxicity and Risk Factors. In animals, although adverse effects such as sedation may occur at therapeutic levels, specific toxic doses for many H_1 antagonists have not been determined. In dogs given a variety of antihistamine products at therapeutic levels, chlorpheniramine maleate most consistently produced side effects.[6] Although preclinical studies on terfenadine showed no clinical effects in dogs fed 30 mg/kg for 2 years, reports of accidental ingestion of terfenadine in dogs indicated that signs of toxicosis could occur at doses of 6.6 mg/kg and greater.[5] Clemastine has an oral LD_{50} in dogs of 175 mg/kg.[7]

Because many H_1 antagonists are metabolized in the liver, animals with hepatic dysfunction may experience prolonged effects from antihistamines. Likewise, animals with renal dysfunction may show prolonged effects from antihistamines or active metabolites that are excreted unchanged in the urine (e.g., cetirizine).

Clinical Signs. The adverse effects of antihistamines include CNS depression, gastrointestinal upset (vomiting and diarrhea), and anticholinergic effects (dry mouth, urinary retention); these effects are features of first generation antihistamines and are rarely seen with second generation H_1 blockers such as loratadine, astemizole, fexofenadine, and terfenadine.[1] Comparisons of major adverse effects between the different antihistamine classes are listed in Table 24-2. Cardiac abnormalities in humans, specifically ventricular tachycardia, have been reported with use of terfenadine and astemizole, and resulted in terfenadine being removed from the U.S. market[1]; similar effects have not been reported in domestic animals. Oral or topical antihistamine use has been associated with induction of drug allergy, resulting in allergic dermatitis, drug fever, and photosensitization.[1] Teratogenic effects from antihistamines of the piperazine class have been reported in experimental animals.[1]

Clinical signs of antihistamine toxicosis may develop rapidly following oral exposure, often within 15 to 30 minutes.[5] Overdose situations may result in exacerbation of adverse effects, although the most significant effects of antihistamine overdose relate to the CNS and anticholinergic effects.[4] In many cases, antihistamines that tend to have CNS depressive effects at therapeutic doses (e.g., diphenhydramine) may instead cause CNS stimulation at higher doses.[2] Human children and young animals may be more prone to developing signs of CNS stimulation, whereas adults may more often become depressed.[5] CNS stimulation may also be seen in animals when antihistamines are administered too rapidly via the intravenous route.[2] Affected animals may become hyperactive, disoriented, anxious, aggressive, and ataxic.[3,5] In severe cases, seizures may develop. Conversely, antihistamine overdose may result in profound CNS depression, coma, respiratory depression, and death.[3] Anticholinergic effects include mentation abnormalities (disorientation, "hallucination," etc.), hyperthermia, tachycardia, cardiac arrhythmias, hypertension or hypotension,

TABLE 24-2 **Adverse Effects of Different Classes of Antihistamines**

Class of H_1 Antagonist	*Reported Adverse Effects at Therapeutic Doses*				
	CNS Depression	CNS Stimulation	GI	Anticholinergic	Cardiac
Ethanolamines	+++	+	+	+++	0
Ethylnediamines	++	+	+++	+	0
Alkylamines	++	+++	++	+	0
Piperazines	+	+	+	+	0
Phenothiazines	++	+	+	+	0
Piperidines	0	0	0	0	+

Data from reference 1. *CNS,* Central nervous system; *GI,* gastrointestinal; *0,* none; +, small; ++, moderate; +++, large.

xerostomia, mydriasis, hypertension, ataxia, seizures, and coma.[4,5]

Clinical Pathology. No specific clinical pathologic abnormalities are expected in antihistamine toxicosis. Animals that have exhibited prolonged or severe signs may develop metabolic acidosis or electrolyte abnormalities, so these parameters should be monitored closely. Baseline values for liver and kidney function should be obtained to detect any previously existing problems that may delay elimination of the drug.

Lesions. No specific necropsy or histopathologic lesions are expected in animals with antihistamine toxicosis. Any lesions are secondary to complications such as rhabdomyolysis and DIC.

Diagnostic Testing. Antihistamines and their metabolites can be measured in serum and urine, and are of most value in verifying exposure. Quantitative values are of little prognostic value.[4]

Treatment. No specific antidotes for antihistamine toxicosis are available. The goals of treatment should be to stabilize the patient, decontaminate, and provide supportive care. Seizures may be managed with benzodiazepines or barbiturates, but care should be taken to avoid a severe "rebound" depression.[4] In humans, the use of physostigmine to treat anticholinergic-mediated seizures is controversial, and its use is usually not recommended because of the risk of potentiating cardiovascular dysfunction or seizures.[4] Comatose animals may require endotracheal intubation to maintain respiratory support. Severe cardiac arrhythmias should be treated as necessary, whereas mild or moderate arrhythmias may respond to intravenous fluid therapy.[4] Atropine is contraindicated in the management of brady-arrhythmias resulting from potentiation of anticholinergic effects. Other methods of stabilization, such as control of hyperthermia, should be instituted as needed.

Activated charcoal with a cathartic may be used in patients once they are stabilized. In asymptomatic animals, emesis may be induced under veterinary supervision, but emesis should be avoided in symptomatic animals because of the potential for aspiration.[4] Some antihistamines undergo enterohepatic recirculation, so multiple doses of activated charcoal may be of benefit in symptomatic animals.[4,5]

Supportive care should include monitoring and correcting abnormalities of cardiac function, acid-base and electrolyte status, blood pressure, and body temperature. Intravenous fluids aid in cardiovascular support and promote adequate renal blood flow and urine production, thus enhancing antihistamine elimination.

Prognosis. Clinical signs of antihistamine toxicosis may persist for up to 72 hours, although most affected animals improve markedly within 24 hours of initiation of treatment.[8] The prognosis for recovery in animals displaying signs of antihistamine toxicosis corresponds to the severity of signs displayed; that is, animals exhibiting mild to moderate signs generally have a good prognosis, whereas the prognosis should be considered guarded in those displaying severe signs (e.g., seizures, coma).

Prevention and Control. All medications should be stored in areas away from pets. Owners should be made aware of signs of adverse reactions or overdoses in pets that are prescribed antihistamines. Human and veterinary drugs should be stored separately to avoid accidental mixup of medication, and pets should be kept out of the area while a human medication is being taken to avoid exposure to dropped pills. If medication for one pet is put into food, the pet should be closely observed to be sure that another pet does not "steal" the medication. Those administering intravenous antihistamines should do so cautiously to avoid CNS stimulation from rapid intravenous infusion; use of alternate administration routes (e.g., intramuscular), when feasible, minimizes this risk.[2]

ANTIMICROBIALS

Joseph D. Roder

SULFONAMIDES

Synonyms. Some of the more common sulfonamides include sulfadimethoxine, sulfadiazine, sulfamethazine, sulfaquinoxaline, sulfathiazole, sulfamerazine, sulfasalazine, and sulfachloropyridazine.

Sources. A wide variety of sulfonamides are used to treat bacterial infections and to prevent coccidiosis. Sulfaquinoxaline is used as an adjunct in some anticoagulant rodenticide products. Additionally, several of the sulfonamides are combined with trimethoprim to produce the potentiated sulfonamides that exhibit a broader antibacterial spectrum.

Toxicokinetics. Most sulfonamides are weak acids and have limited water solubility. Acetylation is a major mechanism of conjugation for sulfonamides in ruminants and pigs. Other species use glucuronidation as a means of conjugating these antibiotics to increase urinary elimination. Elimination of the sulfonamides may occur in the urine, bile, feces, sweat, tears, or milk.

Mechanism of Action. The antimicrobial effects of sulfonamides are due to inhibition of dihydropteroate synthase, a bacterial enzyme required to produce tetrahydrofolate. The mechanism of toxicosis relates to the physiochemical properties of these drugs, their actions on normal bacterial flora, or the ability to elicit hypersensitivity reactions. The development of crystalluria is due to the decreased water solubility of the parent compound or metabolites (especially acetylated metabolites). The parent compound or metabolite becomes less soluble in the glomerular filtrate and precipitate in the renal tubules, causing renal damage. This presentation is less commonly noted since the reformulation of older sulfonamides and awareness have increased.

Coagulopathy is produced by the inhibition of vitamin K epoxide reductase by the sulfonamide or its metabolites. This syndrome is more commonly associated with sulfaquinoxaline.

Aplastic anemia is another syndrome associated with the sulfonamides, especially the potentiated sulfas that are combined with trimethoprim.[1] This syndrome is thought to be caused by the reduction in serum folate resulting from the antibacterial actions of the sulfonamides. The reduced bacterial population of the gastrointestinal tract can no longer produce sufficient folate to maintain the normal replication of the bone marrow progenitor cells.

Keratoconjunctivitis sicca (KCS) has been reported in dogs associated with sulfonamide therapy and is thought to be a hypersensitivity reaction resulting in decreased tear production.[2,3] Other hypersensitivity or idiosyncratic reactions to the sulfonamides are possible and include skin lesions (urticaria, eruptions),[4] hepatic necrosis,[5,6] hemolytic anemia,[7] and hypothyroidism.[8] The production of thyroid tumors following chronic feeding of sulfamethazine to rodents causes some concern. The current therapeutic use of sulfamethazine does not pose a toxicologic risk for thyroid tumors in humans or domestic species.[9]

Toxicity and Risk Factors.   All species are susceptible. Chronic therapy with the sulfonamides increases the risk of developing a toxic syndrome. Younger, dehydrated animals, especially calves, are at greater risk for the formation of crystals in the kidneys. Reports of KCS are more commonly associated with dogs following prolonged therapy.[3] Hepatotoxicity is reported in dogs given 18 to 53 mg/kg of trimethoprim-sulfonamide.[6]

Clinical Signs.   Animals may present with signs of acute renal failure or urinary tract infections, specifically oliguria, anuria, hematuria, or crystalluria. Animals may also exhibit signs of coagulation abnormalities including subcutaneous bruising or prolonged bleeding from wounds. Dogs may exhibit decreased tear production, blepharospasm, corneal ulcers, and increased sensitivity to light as an indication of possible KCS.[3] Clinical signs referable to hepatotoxicity include anorexia, vomiting, and depression.

Clinical Pathology.   A CBC may show leukopenia and thrombocytopenia. A reduced PCV is consistent with hemolytic anemia. Tests of coagulation function may indicate an elevated prothrombin time, partial thromboplastin time, or increased bleeding time. Urinalysis may detect crystalluria and hematuria. Serum chemistry analysis may reveal elevated BUN and creatinine in animals with renal tubular dysfunction associated with sulfonamide precipitation.

Lesions.   The kidneys of animals affected with the renal syndrome are gritty when cut and have crystals.

Diagnostic Testing.   A Schirmer tear test may be performed on dogs to aid in the diagnosis of KCS.[3] Sulfonamide crystals in the kidneys have been detected with ultrasound in humans.

Treatment.   The initial step in therapy is to discontinue the use of the offending agents from all sources, including therapeutic sources, feed, or water. Fluid therapy is indicated in the dehydrated or crystalluric patient. Increased elimination of the sulfonamide may be achieved by alkalinization of the urine with sodium bicarbonate. Animals must be monitored to ensure that overhydration (pulmonary edema) does not occur.

The coagulopathy syndrome responds well to vitamin K_1 therapy for 7 to 10 days. The treatment of KCS may require cyclosporine or pilocarpine to stimulate tear production.[2,3]

Prognosis.   The aplastic anemia is generally reversible after discontinuing the use of the sulfonamide. The coagulopathy syndrome generally responds well to vitamin K therapy. The prognosis for animals with crystalluria depends on the degree of renal damage that occurred before diagnosis and therapy. Animals with KCS may not respond to pharmacologic therapy to restore tear production.

Prevention and Control.   To reduce the likelihood of crystalluria, animals must be well hydrated and offered plenty of fresh water at all times during therapy with sulfonamides. Animals, especially dogs, receiving chronic sulfonamide therapy should have monthly screens for CBC, white blood cells (WBCs), platelets, and coagulation function. Additionally, it may be prudent to monitor the function of the lacrimal gland using a Schirmer tear test. Client education is essential to ensure that the animals are evaluated early after onset of clinical signs.

PENICILLINS

Mechanism of Action.   Penicillin and all of the beta-lactam antibiotics exhibit antimicrobial activity by acting on the cell wall of bacteria. The beta-lactams inhibit the action of transpeptidases (penicillin-binding proteins) that form the bacterial cell wall. The mechanisms of toxicosis relate to hypersensitivity reactions, other immune-mediated reactions, or selective overgrowth of some enteric bacterial species. Anaphylaxis is possible with administration of any of the beta-lactam antibiotics. Immune-mediated hemolytic anemia is more commonly noted in horses given penicillin.[10,11] Penicillin induces bacterial overgrowth in the intestinal tract of guinea pigs with a resulting increase in production and absorption of bacterial exotoxins.[12]

Toxicity and Risk Factors.   Animals with a previous reaction to penicillin have a greater risk for subsequent adverse events. The risk of toxicosis is also greater with venous administration and prior antimicrobial therapy (production of antibodies). The toxic syndromes associated with penicillin may be noted with normal therapeutic doses.

Clinical Signs.   Clinical signs associated with an anaphylactic reaction may include hemorrhagic enterocolitis or respiratory distress. Signs associated with immune-mediated hemolytic anemia include icterus, depression, pale mucous membranes, red-brown urine, splenomegaly, or tachycardia. Procaine toxicosis is most commonly associated with excitement or loss of coordination.[13] Bacterial overgrowth in guinea pigs may result in acute death without other clinical signs.

Clinical Pathology. Hemolytic anemia may be associated with decreased PCV and hemoglobin.

Treatment. The treatment of anaphylaxis should focus on emergency and supportive care. The animal's airway should be maintained and oxygen provided, if necessary. Epinephrine (0.5 to 1 ml of 1:10,000 dilution) may be necessary to maintain the vascular tone. Fluid therapy may be necessary to provide sufficient volume for the cardiovascular system. Immune-mediated hemolytic anemia also requires fluids and possibly transfusion. Fluid therapy should be maintained to prevent hemoglobin-mediated damage to the renal tubules.

Prognosis. Acute anaphylaxis and hemolytic anemia are associated with a guarded prognosis. Positive response to symptomatic and supportive therapy in the early phases of these diseases is encouraging.

Prevention and Control. Consider alternative therapy for animals with previous reaction to penicillin. Penicillin should be used with caution in guinea pigs.

TETRACYCLINES

Synonyms. Oxytetracycline, chlortetracycline, tetracycline, and doxycycline are several types of this antibiotic.

Mechanism of Action. The tetracyclines exert their antimicrobial action by inhibiting the 30s ribosomal unit of bacteria resulting in reduced protein synthesis. The mechanisms of toxicosis do not appear to be related to the antimicrobial action of the drug. One proposed mechanism for the cardiovascular effects is due to a propylene glycol vehicle. It is thought that the propylene glycol induces histamine release leading to cardiovascular collapse.[14] Another proposed mechanism for cardiovascular collapse relates to the ability of tetracycline to chelate calcium[15] in serum acute renal failure. Hepatotoxicity may be noted with tetracycline administration that is due to triglyceride accumulation in the mitochondria of hepatocytes.[16]

Toxicity and Risk Factors. Animals that are dehydrated are at greater risk of toxicosis. Intravenous administration is a risk factor for cardiovascular toxicosis. Cattle given tetracycline dissolved in saline at a dose of 10 mg/kg intravenously over a period of 1 minute collapsed.[15] Dogs receiving 25 mg/kg intravenously for 2 days exhibited renal toxicosis.[14] The risk of enamel hypoplasia and tooth discoloration is greater if the dam is given tetracycline in the later term of pregnancy or early in the neonatal period.

Clinical Signs. Clinical signs associated with tetracycline-induced renal disease include vomiting, diarrhea, dehydration, and oliguria. Signs associated with cardiovascular toxicosis include severe hypotension, decreased heart rate, collapse, and acute death.[14,17]

Clinical Pathology. Urinalysis may reveal proteinuria, increase in tubular casts, and the inability to concentrate urine.[17] Serum chemistries may show elevated urea, creatinine, and hyperphosphatemia.[18,19] Hemoglobinuria may be associated with tetracycline administration. Elevated serum concentrations of hepatic enzymes may be associated with administration of tetracyclines.

Lesions. Renal nephrosis is associated with tetracycline-induced nephrotoxicosis.[19,20]

Treatment. Animals that exhibit cardiovascular collapse may be treated symptomatically with fluids and calcium gluconate. Concurrent intravenous administration of fluids and diuretics (mannitol and furosemide) may prevent renal toxicosis by maintaining normal urine production. Hemodialysis may be necessary if the renal function is severely compromised.[21]

Prognosis. The prognosis is guarded with cardiovascular collapse.

Prevention and Control. Tetracycline that is given intravenously should be diluted in fluids and administered slowly to prevent possible cardiovascular effects. The hydration status must be addressed in animals with decreased renal function.

FLUOROQUINOLONES

Synonyms. The fluoroquinolones are relatively new to veterinary medicine. Members of this group include enrofloxacin (Baytril, difloxacin, ciprofloxacin, and orbifloxacin (Orbax).

Toxicokinetics. The fluoroquinolones exhibit rapid gastrointestinal absorption and a large volume of distribution.[22] These antibiotics are excreted by the kidneys.

Mechanism of Action. The antimicrobial activity of the fluoroquinolones is due to their ability to inhibit the type II topoisomerase of the bacteria.[22] This prevents the coiling and therefore the replication and synthesis of DNA. The mechanism of action for fluoroquinolone-mediated arthropathy may be related to the ability to chelate magnesium. The chelation of magnesium from these critical sites in the articular cartilage may account for the lesions.[23] The mechanism of action that may account for seizures is related to the ability of these antibiotics to act as GABA antagonists and bind to the *N*-methyl-D-aspartate receptor.[24]

Toxicity and Risk Factors. Immature animals of all species are at greatest risk of developing arthropathy. There is some variability between species in this concern. Arthropathy was induced by norfloxacin at 25, 50, and 100 mg/kg/day in young rabbits, dogs, and rats, respectively.[25] Ofloxacin caused articular lesions in immature dogs at 20 mg/kg/day for 8 days.[26] Subhuman primates do not appear to be as susceptible as other mammals to the articular cartilage effects of fluoroquinolones.[25]

Clinical Signs. As a class of antimicrobials, the most common adverse effects are to the gastrointestinal tract (nausea, vomiting, and diarrhea) and CNS (seizures).[22] These toxic syndromes tend to be mild and reversible. The unique aspect of the fluoroquinolones is the clinical picture of a younger animal with lameness and pain of a weight-bearing joint.

Clinical Pathology.   Serum hepatic enzymes may be mildly elevated in response to fluoroquinolone therapy.

Lesions.   Gross lesions of fluoroquinolone-induced arthropathy include erosions or vesicle formation of the articular cartilage. Histopathologic examination of affected tissues indicates necrosis of chondrocytes followed by disruption of extracellular matrix and formation of fissures.[27,28]

Treatment.   The antibiotic should be discontinued at the first sign of toxicosis. Supportive therapy includes fluids to maintain urine production and flow to increase elimination of the fluoroquinolone.

Prognosis.   The gastrointestinal, hepatic, and CNS toxic effects of the fluoroquinolones are generally reversible after discontinuation of therapy.[24] Arthropathy induced by the fluoroquinolones in younger animals carries a more guarded prognosis.

Prevention and Control.   These products should not be used in immature animals. Small dogs should be older than 8 months of age and giant breeds should be older than 18 months of age when using fluoroquinolones.

AMINOGLYCOSIDES

Synonyms.   The more commonly used aminoglycosides in veterinary medicine include gentamicin (Gentocin, Garacin, Gentaglyde, and other generics), kanamycin (Kantrim, Amforol), streptinomycin (Spectam, Adspec, Prospec), amikacin (Amiglyde-V), apramycin (Apralan), neomycin (Biosol, Neomix), and tobramycin (Nebcin).

Toxicokinetics.   As a group, these drugs are highly water soluble and poorly lipid soluble. They are poorly absorbed from the gastrointestinal tract following oral administration, but they exhibit excellent absorption from intramuscular and subcutaneous injections. Elimination occurs by renal processes with little protein binding.

Mechanism of Action.   Aminoglycosides bind to the bacterial 30s ribosomal subunit and inhibit bacterial protein synthesis, which explains the efficacy of these antibiotics on rapidly growing bacteria. The transport of aminoglycosides into cells is concentration dependent and uses a specific carrier. The carrier is energy dependent and transports charged, polar molecules. The carrier uses a transmembrane electrical driving force. Anaerobic bacteria lack aminoglycoside transport mechanisms.

Differences of opinion concern the exact mechanism of action of aminoglycoside-induced nephrotoxicity or ototoxicity. In the mammalian kidney and ear, the aminoglycosides are electrically attracted to the charged phospholipids (phosphatidylinositols). Aminoglycosides accumulate in the proximal

renal tubular epithelial cells and the endolymph of the ear. Aminoglycosides are sequestered in the lysosomes and interact with ribosomes and mitochondria to cause cellular death.[29,30]

Toxicity and Risk Factors.   It is difficult to predict a toxic dose for a particular species because of the complex interaction of drug, disease, and animal factors. In calves, neomycin given at doses greater than 2.25 mg/kg twice daily intramuscularly caused nephrotoxicosis.[31] On the other hand, cats appear to be more sensitive to the vestibular toxic effects of the aminoglycosides.

The risk factors for aminoglycoside-induced toxicosis are age (both old and young), dehydration, compromised renal function, aminoglycoside dose, duration of therapy, hypovolemia, severe sepsis, endotoxemia, concurrent diuretic therapy, or other nephrotoxic agents.[30,32]

Clinical Signs.   Several different clinical syndromes of intoxication are associated with the aminoglycosides. The primary syndromes of clinical interest are nephrotoxicosis and ototoxicosis. Nephrotoxicosis presents as anorexia, vomiting, and depression as a result of acute renal tubular necrosis.

The ototoxicosis involves damage to cranial nerve VIII (vestibulocochlear), which may cause vestibular or auditory dysfunction. Signs of vestibular dysfunction include nystagmus, incoordination, and loss of righting reflex. Signs of auditory dysfunction include permanent damage to the hair cells of the organ of Corti, with an initial loss of the high-frequency auditory function.[29]

Neuromuscular blockade induced by aminoglycosides is expressed as muscular weakness and respiratory arrest, which is more pronounced under general anesthesia.

Clinical Pathology.   Aminoglycoside-induced nephrotoxicosis is marked by elevation in serum creatinine, increased serum urea nitrogen, and decreased osmolality.[31] Urinalysis of animals affected by aminoglycoside-induced nephrotoxicosis reveals granular casts, proteinuria, and low urine specific gravity. In sheep, the concentration of urinary enzymes, gamma-glutamyltransferase, and beta-N-acetyl-glucosaminidase precedes other indicators of renal damage.[33] In dogs, urine gamma-glutamyl transpeptidase (GGT)-to-creatinine ratio increases 3 times above baseline values before azotemia and other abnormalities occur.[34]

Lesions.   Aminoglycoside-induced nephrotoxicosis is characterized by proximal tubular degeneration and necrosis.[31]

Diagnostic Testing.   Therapeutic monitoring of the serum concentrations of several of the aminoglycosides can be used to prevent intoxication. Auditory brain stem response may be beneficial to determine loss of hearing in intoxicated animals.[29]

Treatment.   At the first indication of clinical signs, aminoglycoside therapy should be discontinued. Attention to the hydration of the patient is essential for elimination of the aminoglycoside and the animal should be monitored for renal function. Peritoneal dialysis to remove nitrogenous wastes may be necessary for animals with severe renal injury. The use of a renal vascular vasodilator (misoprostol: 3 µg/kg orally every 8 hours) did not maintain renal function in gentamicin-induced nephrotoxicosis in dogs.[35]

Prognosis. The nephrotoxicosis may be reversible, depending on the severity of damage. The damage to the vestibulocochlear nerve is permanent and irreversible.

Prevention and Control. A greater risk of toxicosis exists in the dehydrated patient. Concurrent administration of calcium (20 mg/kg body weight intravenously every 12 hours) has been shown to prevent the majority of nephrotoxic effects of gentamicin in ponies.[36]

CHLORAMPHENICOL

Synonyms. Chloramphenicol is also known as Tevcocin, Chlorasol, Chloromycetin, Chlora-Tabs, Chloricol, and Anacetin.

Toxicokinetics. The drug is metabolized by the liver and eliminated as a glucuronide conjugate. This may partially explain the increased sensitivity of the cat to potential toxic effects.

Mechanism of Action. Antibacterial activity of chloramphenicol is related to the actions of the drug on peptidyl transferase that is associated with the 50s ribosomal unit. The mammalian and bacterial mitochondria are similar, and chloramphenicol may inhibit the replication of cells in the bone marrow.

Toxicity and Risk Factors. Cats appear to be more sensitive to the hematologic effects of chloramphenicol. Cats that received 100 to 120/mg/kg/day for more than 2 weeks developed bone marrow suppression.[37] Hepatic disease or dysfunction can predispose the animal to intoxication. Chronic chloramphenicol therapy is also a risk factor for developing toxicosis. Some humans develop a life-threatening aplastic anemia in response to chloramphenicol exposure. This is the reason that this drug is not approved for use in food-producing animals.[38]

Clinical Signs. Anorexia, vomiting, and diarrhea are nonspecific signs of intoxication.

Clinical Pathology. A reduction in the packed cell volume is possible, as are alterations in the WBC differential, including neutropenia, lymphocytopenia, and thrombocytopenia.

Lesions. Histopathologic lesions included decreased bone marrow cellularity.

Treatment. The initial step in treatment is to discontinue the use of the drug. No specific antidote exists, and the animal must receive supportive and symptomatic therapy.

Prognosis. Bone marrow depression in cats generally resolves after cessation of therapy.[37]

Prevention and Control. This antibiotic should not be used for more than 2 weeks without monitoring the WBC population in the systemic circulation.

LINCOMYCIN

Synonyms. Lincomycin (Lincocin, Lincomix) is an antimicrobial that has been associated primarily with a severe pseudomembranous colitis. Other antimicrobials that have been implicated in this syndrome include tylosin and tetracycline.[39]

Mechanism of Action. The antibacterial action of lincomycin is the ability of the drug to bind to the 50s ribosomal unit and inhibit protein synthesis. Lincomycin causes a reduction in the microflora of the intestine, allowing the colonization and proliferation of *Clostridium* spp. (*Clostridium difficile, Clostridium spiroforme*). The clostridial organisms then elaborate toxins that result in toxicosis.[40] One such toxin that has been suggested is the *Clostridium perfringens* type E iota toxin.[41]

Toxicity and Risk Factors. Oral administration of these drugs increases the risk of intoxication. The species that are most susceptible to the syndrome are horses, rabbits, guinea pigs, hamsters, and ruminants.[41-43] Guinea pigs and hamsters may develop enteritis following treatment with penicillin, erythromycin, oxytetracycline, and cephalosporins.[44]

Clinical Signs. The clinical syndrome consists of gastrointestinal distress with diarrhea, colic, and death.

Lesions. At necropsy, hemorrhagic colitis with pseudomembranous plaques may be noted. Lesions are found in the colon and ceca. The presence of distended, nonhemorrhagic, fluid-filled ceca in rabbits treated with lincomycin is highly suggestive of this syndrome.

Treatment. The antibiotic must be discontinued and symptomatic treatment for diarrhea including fluid therapy should be initiated.

Prognosis. This syndrome carries a poor prognosis for hamsters and guinea pigs.

Prevention and Control. These antibiotics should be avoided in susceptible species.

TILMICOSIN

Synonyms. Tilmicosin is marketed as Micotil 300 and Pulmotil 90.

Mechanism of Action. The antibiotic effects of tilmicosin result from the drug binding the 50s ribosome of bacteria and reducing protein synthesis. The mechanism of toxicity for tilmicosin relates to the negative inotropic actions of the drug. The negative inotropic actions of tilmicosin are relatively nonspecific.[45,46]

Toxicity and Risk Factors.   Pigs, nonhuman primates, and horses may be most sensitive. Cattle may be poisoned by inappropriate administration. Cattle exhibited clinical signs at a dose of 150 mg/kg (15 times the normal dose). Pigs developed clinical signs following intramuscular injections of 10 mg/kg. Doses of 5 to 10 mg/kg given intravenously caused death in cattle, horses, sheep, and goats.[45]

Clinical Signs.   An overdose of tilmicosin given subcutaneously induced tachycardia in cattle. Nontarget species exhibited tachypnea, vomiting, seizures, ataxia, and acute death.

Treatment.   No specific antidote is available. An animal exhibiting clinical signs should be given symptomatic treatment and be closely monitored for cardiovascular abnormalities. Dobutamine may help improve cardiac function in symptomatic animals.[46]

Prognosis.   Animals surviving the acute episode of an overdose or inappropriate route of administration may survive with minimal residual problems.

Prevention and Control.   Tilmicosin is labeled for use in cattle by subcutaneous injection at a dose of 10 mg/kg. This product should not be used in powered syringes. Human exposures are generally from accidental injection or a scratch from a needle. The dose is generally less than 1 ml in these exposures. These human exposures can be treated symptomatically and pose a limited toxicologic risk.[47]

KETOCONAZOLE

Synonyms.   Ketoconazole is an antifungal agent that is available as a human product called Nizoral.

Toxicokinetics.   The oral absorption of ketoconazole is increased in an acidic environment. Ketoconazole is extensively metabolized in the liver and is eliminated primarily in the bile, but it is also passed in the milk. Ketoconazole is a potent inhibitor of cytochrome P-450 3A4 isozyme system in humans and has been shown to inhibit drug metabolism in animals.

Mechanism of Action.   Ketoconazole inhibits fungal replication by interfering with erosterol synthesis, specifically sterol 14-alpha-demethylase. This enzyme contains a group that is similar to cytochrome P-450. It is thought that ketoconazole may also act directly on the fungal cell membrane. Ketoconazole can inhibit testosterone synthesis. Ketoconazole is a teratogen, which must be considered before beginning therapy.[48] The mechanism of hepatotoxicity is not well understood and does not appear to be immune mediated.[49]

Toxicity and Risk Factors.   Acute toxicity is not common because the oral LD_{50} for a dog is more than 500 mg/kg. Hepatotoxicity is more common in cats than in dogs.[50]

Clinical Signs.   Clinical signs are most commonly associated with gastrointestinal distress: anorexia, weight loss, vomiting, and diarrhea.[51] Hepatotoxicosis has also been reported in cats.[52]

Clinical Pathology.   Animals with hepatotoxicosis may exhibit elevated bilirubin concentrations as well as increased hepatic enzymes.

Lesions.   Evidence of massive centrilobular necrosis[49] and cholestasis may be found in the intoxicated animal.

Treatment.   If an animal exhibits signs of hepatotoxicosis, the drug should be discontinued. No specific antidote exists and the animal must be provided with symptomatic and supportive therapy. If an acute oral ingestion has occurred, oral administration of, or gastric lavage with, sodium bicarbonate may be considered in addition to symptomatic and supportive therapy.

Prognosis.   Mild hepatotoxicosis is generally reversible after termination of the drug.

Prevention and Control.   Nausea and vomiting may be controlled by administering the drug with food or dividing the dose.

AMPHOTERICIN B

Synonyms.   Amphotericin B is an antifungal agent that is available as human products such as Fungizone, Amphotec, Amphotericin B, and AmBisome.

Toxicokinetics.   Amphotericin B is highly bound to serum proteins and is eliminated in the urine and bile. Elimination is often prolonged after cessation of therapy.

Mechanism of Action.   The antifungal actions of amphotericin relate to the drug's ability to inhibit ergosterol synthesis. Ergosterols are components of the cell membrane that are unique to fungal organisms but similar to the sterols found in mammalian membranes. Amphotericin is a potent nephrotoxic agent that acts by causing renal vasoconstriction and a reduction in the glomerular filtration rate. There also may be direct actions of amphotericin on the cell membranes of the renal tubule cells.[53]

Toxicity and Risk Factors.   Clinical toxicosis can occur at therapeutic doses, and cats appear to be more sensitive to nephrotoxicosis, but all species are susceptible. Animals with preexisting renal disease and dehydration may be at greater risk of intoxication.

Clinical Signs.   The clinical syndrome is similar to acute renal failure with signs of depression, anorexia, and vomiting.

Clinical Pathology.   Elevated BUN and creatinine with decreased serum potassium and sodium are commonly found as a result of intoxication.

Lesions. Amphotericin B causes an acute renal tubular necrosis.[53,54]

Treatment. Initial therapy is to discontinue administration of the drug. Aggressive fluid therapy is indicated to prevent further damage to the kidneys. The addition of mannitol may increase the elimination of amphotericin B.[55]

Prognosis. The prognosis depends on the severity of renal damage.

Prevention and Control. Prevention of intoxication starts with calculating the proper dose. This drug should be given intravenously by a slow bolus.[54] Pretreatment evaluation of the BUN, creatinine, total protein, and packed cell volume is necessary to establish the baseline values of these parameters before therapy. Amphotericin B should be discontinued if the BUN and creatinine become elevated during therapy. Intoxication (renal vasoconstriction) may be minimized by saline loading before and after treatment. Liposomal formulations of amphotericin B may reduce the likelihood of toxicosis[56]; however, the additional cost of this drug may not be feasible in veterinary medicine.

GRISEOFULVIN

Synonyms. Griseofulvin is also known as Fulvicin U/F, Grysio, or Grifungal.

Toxicokinetics. Griseofulvin is distributed to many tissues with high concentrations found in the skin, hair, and nails. The drug is metabolized in the liver and excreted in the urine.

Mechanism of Action. The antifungal activity produced by griseofulvin is inhibition of fungal spindle activity leading to distortions of the fungal hyphae. In mammals, griseofulvin exerts its toxic effects by mitotic spindle arrest during metaphase or anaphase.[57] This may account for the teratogenic effects of griseofulvin. The mechanism of the bone marrow suppression is unknown and may be an idiosyncratic reaction.

Toxicity and Risk Factors. Cats, especially kittens, are more sensitive to the teratogenic and hematologic syndromes.[58,59] A cat given 40 mg/kg developed bone marrow suppression.[58] Conversely, eight cats given 110 to 145 mg/kg/day for 11 weeks failed to produce bone marrow depression.[60] Cats given 500 to 1000 mg of griseofulvin orally at weekly intervals exhibited teratogenesis.[61]

Clinical Signs. Anorexia, vomiting, diarrhea, and anemia may be noted in the poisoned animal. Ataxia and fever have been reported in a kitten.[59]

Clinical Pathology. CBC may detect leukopenia[62] and thrombocytopenia, whereas serum chemistry may show increased bilirubin and glucose with decreased sodium and potassium concentrations. Bone marrow cytology may exhibit profound hypoplasia of progenitor cells.[58]

Lesions. The teratogenic effects of griseofulvin produce a myriad of lesions in cats, including exencephaly, hydrocephalus, spina bifida, cleft palate, absence of maxillae, lack of coccygeal vertebrae, atresia ani, cyclopia, and anophthalmia with absence of optic nerves.[61] Microphthalmia, severe brachygnathia, and palate abnormalities were noted in a foal.[63]

Treatment. The initial step is to discontinue the use of the drug. There is no specific antidote, so the animal must receive supportive and symptomatic therapy.

Prognosis. Many of the bone marrow changes revert to normal after removal of the drug.[62] In some cases, the bone marrow suppression may not respond to the removal of the drug or treatment.[58]

Prevention and Control. Griseofulvin should not be used in pregnant animals. The hematologic toxicosis may be an idiosyncratic reaction; therefore, no prevention is possible.

ANTINEOPLASTICS

Joseph D. Roder

ANTIMETABOLITES

Synonyms. The more common antimetabolite antineoplastics are 5-fluorouracil and methotrexate. Fluorouracil (5-FU, Adrucil, Efudex, Fluoroplex, Fluorouracil, Fluorouracil injection) is formulated for intravenous injection and is a 5% topical cream formula. Methotrexate (MTX) is available from several generic manufacturers in an intravenous or tablet formulation.

Toxicokinetics. Fluorouracil is well absorbed following oral administration and is well absorbed from the skin. Methotrexate is well absorbed following oral administration and is widely distributed. Methotrexate has a plasma protein-binding of approximately 50% and is eliminated through the urine.

Mechanism of Action. Fluorouracil is a prodrug that is metabolized to compounds that inhibit thymidylate synthase or RNA function. Methotrexate inhibits the enzyme dihydrofolate reductase as well as other folate-dependent enzymes. Methotrexate reduces the availability of single carbon sources and thereby inhibits the production of purines, DNA, and other cellular proteins. Tissues that have a high rate of cellular metabolism, such as neoplasms, gastrointestinal mucosa, and bone marrow, are most sensitive to the effects of the antimetabolites.[1] Acute nephrotoxicity associated with methotrexate is due to the precipitation of the drug in the renal tubules.

Toxicity and Risk Factors. Dogs and cats may be poisoned following ingestion of the cream formulation of 5-FU used by their owners. Cats are highly sensitive to 5-FU; an overdose may cause acute death from CNS damage. In dogs, fluorouracil can elicit signs of intoxication at 20 mg/kg and death at 43 mg/kg.[2]

Clinical Signs.   Some of the clinical signs often reported in small animals are nausea, vomiting, diarrhea, depression, and ataxia. The stools and vomitus may contain blood.[2] Fluorouracil has been reported to induce cerebellar ataxia in dogs and severe neurotoxic effects in cats.

Clinical Pathology.   These agents decrease the production of leukocytes and platelets. A CBC with differential shows neutropenia and thrombocytopenia with a maximum depression approximately 1 week after administration.

Lesions.   Fluorouracil produces neurologic ultrastructural lesions of vacuolation, myelin lamellar splitting, and separation between the axon and innermost myelin layer.[3]

Treatment.   The initial step in treatment for ingestion of either of these agents is gastrointestinal decontamination. Administration of neomycin orally may reduce the amount of methotrexate absorbed from the gastrointestinal tract. Saline diuresis, possibly alkalinized with sodium bicarbonate, may increase elimination of methotrexate. Leucovorin (folinic acid) is a reduced form of folic acid that can be used as a treatment for methotrexate overdose.[1]

Prognosis.   Cats poisoned with 5-FU and exhibiting clinical signs have a grave prognosis. Dogs that ingest greater than 43 mg/kg of 5-FU have a grave prognosis. Methotrexate-induced neutropenia and thrombocytopenia is generally reversible after discontinuation of therapy.

Prevention and Control.   Owners should be warned of the risks to cats and small dogs posed by the topical fluorouracil creams. The veterinarian may inform the local pharmacist of this risk as well so the owner might be counseled when filling the prescription.

ALKYLATING AGENTS

Synonyms.   The alkylating agents are one of the oldest classes of antineoplastics. These agents are sometimes called the nitrogen mustards from their historical origins as weapons used in World War I. This class is represented by cyclophosphamide (Cytoxan, CTX, CTY, CPM), ifosfamide, melphalan, carmustine (BCNU), chlorambucil, and mechlorethamine. Cyclophosphamide is the most commonly used of these agents and is discussed in the most detail.

Mechanism of Action.   The alkylating agents are considered to be cell cycle nonspecific agents with the greatest effect seen in rapidly dividing cells (gastrointestinal, bone marrow, and hair cells). Cyclophosphamide interferes with normal DNA function by alkylation and cross-linking the strands of DNA, and possibly by protein modification, resulting in potent immunosuppressive activity. Cyclophosphamide must be metabolized in the liver to the active form. Hepatic metabolism of the parent compound produces reactive intermediates that bind nitrogen contained in guanine residues in DNA. This results in improper base pairing and inhibition of DNA replication. The toxic principle for the sterile hemorrhagic cystitis is believed to be acrolein, which is found in high concentrations in the urine and acts on urinary bladder mucosa.[4]

Toxicity and Risk Factors.   Hemorrhagic cystitis is more common in dogs than in cats and may occur at therapeutic doses over a period of time. The lethal dose of cyclophosphamide in the dog is reported to be 40 mg/kg.[4] This drug should be used with caution in animals with renal or hepatic dysfunction.

Clinical Signs.   Hematuria, stranguria, and pollakiuria are a result of the sterile hemorrhagic necrotizing cystitis. Bone marrow suppression is more commonly noted than gastrointestinal effects. Nausea and vomiting are not a common clinical syndrome.

Clinical Pathology.   Sterile hemorrhagic cystitis may be suggested by large numbers of red blood cells in the urine, inability to culture bacterial pathogens in the urine, and clinical signs.[5] Myelosuppression may be noted on a differential count of the WBCs.

Lesions.   Sterile hemorrhagic cystitis causes mucosal ulceration, edema, and necrosis.[5]

Treatment.   The hemorrhagic cystitis can been treated with infusions of dimethyl sulfoxide (DMSO) into the urinary bladder. Patients not responding to this therapy may require surgical intervention to remove necrotic urinary mucosa.[6] Other treatments proposed for the treatment of sterile hemorrhagic cystitis include acetylcysteine to bind the active metabolite and infusion of 1% formalin.[7]

Prognosis.   Myelosuppression is generally reversible after discontinuation of the drug. The cystitis generally only requires discontinuation of cyclophosphamide and treatment.

Prevention and Control.   Concurrent administration of prednisone may decrease the likelihood of the development of cystitis.[7]

MITOTIC INHIBITORS

Synonyms.   The vinca alkaloids vincristine (Oncovin, Vincasar PFS) and vinblastine (Velban) are derived from the periwinkle plant *(Vinca rosea* or *Catharanthus rosea).*

Toxicokinetics.   The vinca alkaloids are well absorbed via the oral route, with variable distribution and hepatic elimination.[8] Compared with vinblastine, vincristine has a longer terminal half-life and greater cellular accumulation, which may explain the higher incidence of neurotoxic effects associated with vincristine.

Mechanism of Action.   The dose-limiting toxic effect of vincristine is neurotoxicity, whereas the dose-limiting toxic effect of vinblastine is myelosuppression. The vinca alkaloids bind to tubulin and inhibit microtubular formation, therefore arresting cell division at metaphase by disrupting the formation of the mitotic spindle.[8]

Toxicity and Risk Factors. Cats are more prone to the neurotoxic effects of the vinca alkaloids.[9]

Clinical Signs. General signs of intoxication include anorexia and vomiting, indicating damage to the gastrointestinal mucosa.

Clinical Pathology. Leukopenia and other indications of myelosuppression are commonly associated with vinca alkaloid treatment and overdose.[10]

Lesions. Histopathology may reveal neuropathy and peripheral nerve degeneration.[11]

Diagnostic Testing. Electrodiagnostic testing of peripheral nerve and muscle function may indicate deficits. Additionally, animals may have a decreased nerve conduction velocity.[12]

Treatment. Discontinuation of therapy is recommended for animals exhibiting signs of peripheral neuropathy. There is not a specific antidote or adjunct therapy for vinca alkaloid intoxication. Depending on the severity of the toxicosis, symptomatic and supportive care should be instituted.

Prognosis. Affected animals may return to normal function with good supportive and nursing care. The healing of the peripheral nerves may require several weeks or months.[12]

Prevention and Control. Animals should be given frequent neurologic examinations during therapy. Owners should be educated to recognize the signs of peripheral neuropathy and to contact the veterinarian if emesis occurs. Accurate administration and weight should help prevent iatrogenic overdose.

ANTIBIOTIC ANTINEOPLASTICS

Synonyms. Examples of anthracyclines include doxorubicin (Adriamycin D), daunorubicin, and idarubicin.

Sources. The anthracycline antineoplastic agents are used to treat a wide variety of tumors. They are isolated from *Streptomyces peucetius* var *caesius.*

Toxicokinetics. Doxorubicin is administered intravenously. Doxorubicin distributes throughout the body tissues and is extensively bound to DNA. Doxorubicin is 75% bound to plasma proteins, extensively metabolized in the liver, and eliminated primarily as glucuronide or hydroxylated conjugates.

Mechanism of Action. Doxorubicin and other anthracyclines act through several different mechanisms. Doxorubicin intercalates between DNA base pairs causing a tertiary structural change that can interfere with strand elongation by inhibiting DNA polymerase. Additionally, this structural change can inhibit RNA polymerase, which affects protein synthesis. Doxorubicin can alter the activity of topoisomerase II, which allows unwinding of the DNA double helix during transcription. Another mechanism of cytotoxicity for doxorubicin involves the formation of complexes with iron or copper. These complexes can cause membrane and mitochondrial damage especially in the presence of oxygen via the formation of free radicals. The free radicals can cause membrane lipid peroxidation, DNA strand damage, and oxidation of purines or pyrimidines.[13]

Toxicity and Risk Factors. Cardiomyopathy is seen following cumulative doses greater than 250 mg/m^2 in dogs.[14] Clinical signs, hematologic changes and death may be seen after one or two doses of 30 mg/m^2 in dogs.[15] Animals with preexisting heart disease or hepatic dysfunction are at greater risk of intoxication.

Clinical Signs. The most common signs of toxicosis are vomiting, diarrhea, colitis, anorexia, and pruritus.[15,16] Acute reactions may occur during or immediately after an infusion period. These reactions are associated with hypotension, tachycardia, and elevated serum histamine.[17] Acute cardiac death may result from this reaction.[14] Cardiomyopathy induced by doxorubicin causes signs consistent with congestive heart failure.

Clinical Pathology. Leukopenia and thrombocytopenia are commonly noted following administration of doxorubicin. Anemia is less commonly noted.

Lesions. Doxorubicin induces a dilated cardiomyopathy in dogs.

Treatment. No specific antidote exists. Treatment of intoxication is primarily supportive and symptomatic. Cardiac monitoring with an electrocardiogram (ECG) may help identify potential cardiac problems.

Prognosis. The development of dilated cardiomyopathy is associated with a guarded prognosis. These animals develop congestive heart failure that may not respond to traditional pharmacotherapy. The hematologic changes are generally reversible.

Prevention and Control. To prevent acute hypersensitivity reactions, dogs may be pretreated with diphenhydramine or dexamethasone. To prevent the cardiomyopathy, one must maintain accurate records of total dose of doxorubicin administered and use iron chelators such as dexrazoxane (Zinecard).[18] Liposomal formulations of doxorubicin may reduce the incidence of cardiomyopathy. The use of antioxidants as an adjunct therapy may help reduce the risk of free radical generation with resulting cardiac damage.

CISPLATIN

Synonyms. Cisplatin is also known as Platinol, Platinol-AQ, *cis*-DDP, CDDP, *cis*-diamminedichloroplatinum.

Sources.   Cisplatin is a platinum-containing therapeutic agent that is used for a wide variety of tumors.

Toxicokinetics.   Cisplatin is given intravenously and exhibits wide distribution and high concentrations in the prostate, liver, and kidney. Most of the drug is eliminated in the urine within 24 hours.

Mechanism of Action.   Cisplatin passively enters the cells where it is activated into an electrophile by replacing two chloride groups with hydroxyl or water. The activated cisplatin then binds primarily at the N-7 positions of guanine and adenine of DNA, RNA, and macromolecules resulting from attractive binding properties of the imidazole ring at this position. Cisplatin binds to DNA and forms intrastrand crosslinks, leading to conformational changes in the tertiary structure and preventing the replication of DNA by DNA polymerase, RNA polymerase, RNA translocation, and other key critical enzymes.[19,20] The nephrotoxic effects of cisplatin relate to the renal elimination of this drug and the reactive metabolites interacting with and binding renal cellular macromolecules. Cisplatin is thought to cause neurotoxicosis by altering the myelin sheath and damaging the Schwann cells of peripheral neurons.

Toxicity and Risk Factors.   Cisplatin is contraindicated in cats. Dehydration during the treatment period predisposes the animal to nephrotoxicosis. Animals with preexisting renal disease are at greater risk for the nephrotoxic effects of cisplatin. Cats given cisplatin at doses greater than 40 mg/m^2 are at risk for developing pulmonary signs.[21]

Clinical Signs.   Intractable nausea and vomiting may be observed in dogs. Vomition is common following administration and may last 24 hours after therapy. Anorexia and hemorrhagic diarrhea were observed in one dog. Anaphylaxis is also possible in dogs. Peripheral neuropathy can be present with ataxia or loss of cutaneous sensation. In cats, cisplatin is associated with severe respiratory distress and death.[21]

Clinical Pathology.   Abnormalities relate to the nephrotoxicity of cisplatin and are typified by azotemia, increased serum creatinine, and electrolyte abnormalities. Bone marrow suppression may result in thrombocytopenia and granulocytopenia.

Lesions.   The nephrotoxicosis primarily affects proximal tubules with lesions of tubular degeneration, loss of brush border, necrosis, and mineralization of tubular epithelial cells. Cats that die following cisplatin intoxication have severe hydrothorax, pulmonary edema, and mediastinal edema. Histopathologic lesions include thickened alveolar septa, congested alveoli with macrophages, neutrophils, and thrombi.[21]

Treatment.   Antiemetic therapy may be initiated before administration of activated charcoal and cathartic. Butorphanol (0.4 mg/kg) proved highly effective in preventing cisplatin-induced vomiting by reducing the proportion of dogs that vomited.[22] Aggressive fluid therapy with normal saline for a minimum of 24 hours after cisplatin ingestion decreases the severity of nephrotoxicosis.[23]

Prognosis.   The prognosis is grave in cats that are exhibiting clinical signs.

Prevention and Control.   Newer, liposomal encapsulated cisplatin formulations appear to have less toxic effects.[24] Maintaining hydration during the treatment period is essential to prevent renal toxic effects.

ANTIPARASITICALS

Joseph D. Roder

PIPERAZINE DERIVATIVES

Synonyms.   Piperazine is a widely used anthelminthic agent that also may be known as Sergeants Worm Away for Dogs and Cats, Wazine, Purina Liquid Dog Wormer, and other names in combination with other agents. Diethylcarbamazine is a derivative of piperazine and is known as Dirocide, Filaricide Capsules, Filaribits, Carbam, Pet-Dec, and other names in combination with other anthelminthics.

Toxicokinetics.   These drugs are rapidly absorbed from the stomach and small intestine and exhibit significant renal elimination. Generally these agents are considered to have a wide margin of safety.

Mechanism of Action.   Piperazine and diethylcarbamazine are GABA agonists.[1] GABA is a major inhibitory neurotransmitter and the stimulation of GABA receptors causes an influx of chloride ions that hyperpolarize the neuronal membrane. This renders the neuronal membrane less excitable and decreases nerve transmission. The mechanism of diethylcarbamazine-induced hypotension involves antigens released from killed heartworm microfilaria. The antigens activate complement and induce immune complex formation, yielding vasoactive mediator release and causing shock. This is not thought to be a classic type I hypersensitivity mediated by histamine in that infusion of microfilarial antigens into healthy dogs can mimic the syndrome.[2]

Toxicity and Risk Factors.   Piperazine may cause neurologic signs following doses between 20 and 110 mg/kg.[1] Diethylcarbamazine may elicit hypotension after normal administration in microfilarial positive dogs.[2]

Clinical Signs.   Piperazine neurotoxicosis in cats and dogs is manifested by muscle tremors, ataxia, depression, incoordination, and ataxia. High doses of piperazine may cause vomiting and diarrhea in addition to neurologic signs.[1] Diethylcarbamazine-induced reactions are characterized by tachycardia, hypovolemia, and hypotension.

Diagnostic Testing. A Knotts test for microfilaria in the systemic circulation may aid in a diagnosis of diethyl-carbamazine-induced shock.

Treatment. Piperazine-induced intoxication requires supportive and symptomatic therapy; no antidote is available. Aggressive fluid therapy, thermoregulation, and possibly oxygen therapy are needed for diethylcarbamazine-induced shock.

Prognosis. Piperazine-induced intoxication is generally mild and transitory. Diethylcarbamazine-induced shock has a rapid onset and death may occur in a few hours. Survival of the animal depends on a rapid diagnosis and aggressive therapy.

Prevention and Control. All animals receiving diethyl-carbamazine should be heartworm and microfilaria negative.

IMIDAZOTHIAZOLES

Synonyms. Representatives of this class of antiparasitic agents include butamisole (Styquin) and levamisole (Levasole, Tramisol, Totalon).

Toxicokinetics. These agents exhibit good oral absorption.

Mechanism of Action. Levamisole has a structural and functional similarity to nicotine. Levamisole acts by producing a sustained depolarization of the nematode muscle membrane and blockade of the neuromuscular junction. Intoxication can result in muscarinic and nicotinic effects.[3]

Toxicity and Risk Factors. Levamisole caused toxicosis following an acute oral dose of 12 mg/kg in dogs.[4] In goats, signs of intoxication were noted with levamisole at doses greater than 35 mg/kg.[5] In pigs, the subcutaneous LD_{50} for levamisole was approximately 40 mg/kg and pretreatment with pyrantel tartrate lowered the lethal dose to 27.5 mg/kg.[6]

Clinical Signs. In sheep and pigs, the most common syndrome of levamisole intoxication produced nausea, vomiting, hypersalivation, frequent urination and defecation, muscle tremors, ataxia, anxiety, convulsions, depression, dyspnea, prostration, and death.[5,6] In dogs, toxicosis elicits vomiting, bradycardia, tachypnea, hypothermia, cerebro-cortical depression, and diarrhea.[3,4]

Lesions. Lesions are not specific to levamisole intoxication but may be related to terminal convulsions. Lesions include cardiac and thalamic hemorrhages, enteritis, hepatic degeneration, necrosis, and splenic congestion.[3]

Treatment. No antidote is available. Supportive and symptomatic therapy are indicated in poisoned patients. Atropine may be beneficial in controlling some of the cholinergic signs.

Prognosis. Animals that survive or can be supported during the acute phase of intoxication have a good chance of complete recovery.

ORGANOPHOSPHOROUS COMPOUNDS

Synonyms. This group is represented by several compounds that include dichlorvos (Atgard, Equigard, Task, Equigel, DDVP), trichlorfon (Combot, Dyrex, Freed), halaxon (Halox), and coumaphos (Asuntol, Baymix, Meldane). These products are provided in a variety of formulations: crumbles, drench, tablets, paste, and powder.

Mechanism of Action. As organophosphorous compounds, these agents all act on acetylcholinesterase. These compounds have a greater affinity for helminth acetyl-cholinesterase than for insect acetylcholinesterase. These agents are nonselective pesticides and can inhibit mammalian acetylcholinesterase.

Toxicity and Risk Factors. Some sheep have a hereditary absence of plasma esterase activity, making them more sensitive to haloxon intoxication than other domestic species. Sheep without the esterase had an oral LD_{50} of greater than 543 mg/kg, whereas presence of the enzyme increased the lethal dose to greater than 11,000 mg/kg.[7,8] The risk of intoxication increased following exposure to environmental or management stressors.

Clinical Signs. The most common clinical presentation of intoxication is a cholinergic syndrome that can include hypersalivation, diarrhea, vomiting, and muscular weakness. Haloxon intoxication in sheep is associated with ataxia or "staggers" marked by limb paresis with knuckling of the fetlocks.[9]

Lesions. After trichlorfon administration to pregnant guinea pigs, the offspring had reduced brain weight, especially of the cerebellum, medulla, thalamus, and hypothalamus.[10] Similar findings were noted in piglets following administration to pregnant sows.[11] Haloxon can produce degeneration of myelinated neurons of the brain stem, spinal cord, and some peripheral nerves in sheep.

Treatment. Gastric decontamination with activated charcoal and a cathartic may be indicated. In severe cases, atropine or oxime therapy may be necessary to control the clinical signs.

Prognosis. Animals surviving the acute intoxication have a good prognosis if they receive prompt supportive care. Sheep with haloxon-induced ataxia have a worse prognosis in that the damage to the peripheral nerves is not reversible.

MACROLIDE ENDECTOCIDES

Synonyms. Representatives of this group include ivermectin (Ivomec, Heartgard, Eqvalan, Zimerctin), abamectin (Avomec), dormectin (Dectomax), milbemycin oxime (Interceptor), and moxidectin (Cydectin, ProHeart, Quest).

Sources. This class of compounds includes fermentation products of fungi from the genus *Streptomyces*.

Toxicokinetics. These compounds are eliminated in the feces with significant biliary excretion. A potential for enterohepatic recycling exists.

Mechanism of Action. This group of drugs includes agonists for the neurotransmitter GABA, a major inhibitory neurotransmitter. In mammals, GABA-containing neurons and receptors are found in the CNS, whereas in arthropods and nematodes, GABA is found primarily in the peripheral nervous system, specifically the neuromuscular junction (NMJ). This is the reason for the large margin of safety of ivermectin-containing products in mammals. The binding of ivermectin to a neuronal membrane increases the release of GABA, which then binds to the GABA receptor-chloride channel complex of postsynaptic neuronal membranes, causing an influx of chloride ions.[12] The influx of chloride ions hyperpolarizes the neuronal membranes, making them less excitatory and decreasing nerve transmission. The hyperpolarization of neuronal membranes (at the NMJ) mediates a flaccid paralysis in arthropods and nematodes.

Toxicity and Risk Factors. Collies and collie-type dogs are at greater risk for developing intoxication compared with other breeds of dogs. The toxicity of ivermectin is 0.1 to 0.2 mg/kg (15 to 30 times the therapeutic dose) in collie-type dogs and 2.5 to 40 mg/kg (greater than 200 times the therapeutic dose) in beagles.[13] The toxicity of milbemycin oxime to collie-type dogs is 10 mg/kg (approximately 20 times the therapeutic dose).[14] In other animals, the risk of ivermectin toxicosis is greater in younger animals (foals younger than 4 months old or kittens). Additionally, animals of small body size (parakeets) can receive a toxic dose of ivermectin from a lack of proper dilution of the product. Chelonians (red-footed and leopard tortoises) appear to be highly sensitive to these compounds.[15]

Clinical Signs. Intoxication is characterized by depression and coma. The clinical signs of poisoning include mydriasis, depression, coma, tremors, ataxia, stupor, emesis, and hypersalivation. Treatment of heartworm-positive dogs with milbemycin may result in a shocklike syndrome with hypotension, pale mucous membranes, weak heart sounds, dyspnea, decreased skin temperature, and increased intestinal peristalsis.[16,17]

Diagnostic Testing. Chemical analysis for ivermectin and related compounds may be performed but is not routine. The method used is either high-pressure liquid chromatography (HPLC) or enzyme-linked immunosorbent assay of liver, fat, gastrointestinal contents, and feces.

Treatment. No specific antidote for ivermectin toxicosis exists. Therapy should focus on gastrointestinal decontamination with activated charcoal and a sorbitol cathartic. Repeated doses of activated charcoal may be needed. Symptomatic and supportive care help most intoxicated animals. Supportive therapy may be prolonged in dogs (days to weeks). Therapy consists of intravenous fluids, padding for the comatose animal, frequent turning of affected animals to prevent pressure sores, and careful monitoring. Physostigmine may be used to induce a transient increase in mental status (reversal of coma) as a diagnostic tool or to allow the animal to eat or drink briefly.[18] Fluids may be necessary for dogs that develop hypotension following milbemycin therapy.

Prognosis. The course of therapy may be prolonged in dogs, but the prognosis is generally good.

Prevention and Control. Attention to proper administration to animals, especially more sensitive breeds, is essential.

DISOPHENOL

Synonyms. Disophenol is also known as D.N.P. This product has been voluntarily withdrawn from the market by the sponsor.

Toxicokinetics. Disophenol is rapidly absorbed from oral or subcutaneous injections. Little of the drug is eliminated in the 24 hours following administration.

Mechanism of Action. This drug uncouples oxidative phosphorylation in the mitochondrial membrane of mammalian cells. Maintenance of a proton gradient across the mitochondrial membrane is essential to the production of ATP. In cases of poisoning, the uncoupling by disophenol allows the energy normally used to convert adenosine diphosphate to ATP to be dissipated as heat.

Toxicity and Risk Factors. Small animals are more commonly intoxicated. The toxicity of disophenol has been experimentally induced with greater than 33 mg/kg.[19] Large, long-haired dogs in a warm environment may be predisposed to intoxication following disophenol administration.

Clinical Signs. The most common signs of intoxication are increased body temperature, respiratory rate, and heart rate. Often, intoxicated animals vomit. Young animals may exhibit reversible opacity of the lens.[20,21]

Clinical Pathology. Poisoned animals may have an increased packed cell volume.

Treatment. The treatment of disophenol intoxication is focused on reducing and controlling the body temperature. Poisoned animals may be treated with antipyretic agents and intravenous fluid administration. To increase the evaporative cooling of a poisoned animal, the fur and skin may be dampened with water and a fan placed over the patient. Additionally, ice baths may be used to increase cooling. Animals should be kept calm in a cool environment.

Prognosis. The prognosis for animals exhibiting clinical signs is guarded. In younger animals, the opacities of the lenses may be reversible.

ARSENICAL ANTHELMINTHICS

Synonyms. The arsenic-containing anthelminthics include thiacetarsamide (Carparsolate) and melarsomine (Immiticide). Thiacetarsamide poses the greater risk of intoxication and as such the following discussion relates primarily to this drug.

Toxicokinetics. Dogs given an intravenous injection of thiacetarsamide (2.2 mg/kg) had an elimination half-life of 43 minutes and a clearance of 200 ml/kg/min.[22] Significant variability in the kinetics of thiacetarsamide may exist between animals. The drug is metabolized in the liver, excreted in the bile, and eliminated via the feces and the urine.

Mechanism of Action. The trivalent arsenic form is the cause of toxicosis. Arsenic interacts with sulfhydryl groups within cells. The binding of trivalent arsenic to sulfhydryl groups of proteins or enzymes can disrupt aerobic metabolism in kidneys, liver, and the gastrointestinal tract. The capillaries of these tissues are more commonly affected. Exposure to either of these arsenic agents results in a loss of pulmonary artery endothelial cells. In vitro studies have shown that thiacetarsamide can decrease nitric oxide–mediated relaxation of the pulmonary artery.[23] Additionally, thiacetarsamide may induce a coagulopathy with increased risk of emboli formation.[24]

Toxicity and Risk Factors. These compounds should not be used in animals with hepatic or renal dysfunction. Hepatic and renal damage may occur when using recommended therapeutic doses of thiacetarsamide. The general therapeutic dose for thiacetarsamide in dogs is 2.2 mg/kg twice daily every 2 days. The safety margin for melarsomine is two to three times the therapeutic dose.[25]

Clinical Signs. A common response to animals treated with thiacetarsamide is vomiting. This is not indicative of intoxication unless other clinical signs are noted. Some of the clinical signs associated with toxicosis include depression, anorexia, icterus, and possibly orange-colored urine.[26] Dogs intoxicated by thiacetarsamide may also have fever and diarrhea. An overdose of melarsomine may cause panting and other signs related to noncardiogenic edema.[27] Dogs may exhibit pain at the injection site associated with melarsomine administration.

Clinical Pathology. Nephrotoxicosis may result in increased tubular casts in the urine. The BUN should be monitored during and after therapy. Hepatotoxicity may occur during thiacetarsamide therapy and may result in increased serum ALT and ALP concentrations. Additionally, increased bilirubin in the serum and urine may be noted as a result of liver damage.[26]

Treatment. Therapy should be immediately discontinued in dogs that exhibit clinical signs of intoxication. The patient should be treated aggressively with fluids. The goal is to maintain urine flow and increase the elimination of thiacetarsamide. The patient should be managed with supportive and symptomatic therapy for signs of renal or liver dysfunction. An intramuscular injection of dimercaprol (BAL in oil) 3 mg/kg may bind excessive arsenic if administered soon after an overdose.[27] If thiacetarsamide is given outside of the vein, the surrounding area may be treated symptomatically with hot packs and topical antiinflammatory agents (DMSO or steroids).

Prognosis. The ultimate prognosis depends on the severity of heartworm disease and the physiologic state of the animal.

Prevention and Control. Before administration of the compound, the patient should be screened using a complete physical examination, CBC, serum chemistry, and urinalysis. Accurate weight should be obtained. During the course of therapy, the patient's baseline renal and hepatic function should be monitored. Careful attention to the administration of these agents in dogs is necessary. An accurate accounting of the total dose is essential in preventing toxicosis.

Thiacetarsamide is formulated as an alkaline product that is irritating to tissues. Placement of an intravenous butterfly catheter for the duration of infusion may reduce the risk of extravascular deposition of thiacetarsamide and the resulting perivascular tissue necrosis.

BRONCHODILATORS

Marcy Rosendale

Three major classes of drugs are used to produce bronchodilation: the beta-receptor agonists, the methylxanthines, and the anticholinergics. The beta-receptor agonist drugs are the most effective bronchodilators of the three classes and are addressed here.[1] The methylxanthines and anticholinergic drugs are covered separately elsewhere.

Synonyms. Beta-agonists are customarily divided into two groups: the nonselective agonists that stimulate both beta-1 and beta-2 receptors, and the selective agonists that are designed to selectively stimulate beta-2 receptors. Isoproterenol is a nonselective beta-agonist that has been used to produce bronchodilation in dogs, cats, and horses. Albuterol and clenbuterol are selective beta-2 agonists that have been used as bronchodilators in dogs and horses, respectively.[2] Other beta-2 agonists found in the human literature include metaproterenol, bitolterol, pirbuterol, terbutaline, and salmeterol.[3] Albuterol overdoses may be encountered more frequently than overdoses of other beta-agonists, with dogs being involved more often than other species. Because the mechanism of action is the same, guidelines for treating albuterol overdoses may be applied to the treatment of other pure beta-agonists.[4]

Albuterol (salbutamol) and albuterol sulfate are available as generic and proprietary preparations. Proprietary preparations include Airet, Proventil, Proventil HFA, Proventil Repetabs, Ventolin, Ventolin Nebules, Ventolin Rotacaps, and Volmax. No veterinary-approved albuterol products are currently marketed.[2]

Sources.   Albuterol and its sulfate salt are available in several forms. Tablets are available in immediate- and extended-release formulations. Some immediate-release tablets have an extended-release core. Albuterol also comes in an oral syrup form, in solutions for nebulization, and in powder and aerosols for inhalation. Chlorofluorocarbons (trichlorofluoromethane and dichlorofluoromethane) or a fluorocarbon (tetrafluoroethane) are propellants used in the aerosol formulations.

Toxicokinetics.   Albuterol is rapidly and well absorbed when ingested or inhaled. Peak plasma concentrations of albuterol following the oral administration of either syrup or immediate-release tablets were seen in humans approximately 2 hours after exposure, with the plasma half-life ranging from 2.7 to 5 hours. Ingestion of the extended-release tablets resulted in peak plasma levels approximately 5 to 7 hours after exposure. Peak plasma levels of inhaled albuterol in humans were found 2 to 5 hours after exposure, with one study finding peak levels 10 minutes after exposure. The elimination half-life for inhaled albuterol in humans was thought to be approximately 3.8 hours in one study, with another study finding a half-life range of 1.7 to 7.1 hours.[5] A study that exposed dogs, rats, and monkeys to aerosolized albuterol powder found peak drug concentrations in all species immediately following exposure.[6]

Albuterol crosses the blood-brain barrier with concentrations in the brain reaching approximately 5% of the plasma concentration. Albuterol is believed to cross the placenta. It has not been determined whether albuterol is distributed in milk.

Albuterol is metabolized in the liver to albuterol 4'-O-sulfate, which has no beta-adrenergic effects. In humans with asthma, approximately 70% of an albuterol dose is excreted in the urine within 24 hours, with 80% to 100% of both albuterol and its metabolites being excreted within 72 hours of exposure. In humans, up to 10% of an albuterol dose may be excreted in the feces.[5]

Mechanism of Action.   Albuterol stimulates beta-2 receptors found on the surface of specific cells. Stimulation causes a conformational change in the receptor, which, in turn, triggers the conversion of ATP into the second messenger cyclic adenosine monophosphate (cAMP). The accumulation of cAMP within cells ultimately leads to the phosphorylation of certain cellular proteins responsible for causing the physiologic responses of the beta-2 adrenergic agonists.[1] In overdoses, the beta-2 agonists lose their specificity, causing adverse effects that are usually associated with the stimulation of both beta-1 and beta-2 receptors.[7] Most adverse effects of the beta-agonists occur as a direct result of the excessive stimulation of these receptors.

Toxicity and Risk Factors.   Animals that have access to human albuterol prescriptions or are being treated for bronchoconstriction with albuterol are potentially at risk for adverse effects. Individuals of any species with preexisting cardiovascular disease are at increased risk of experiencing adverse effects from albuterol use.[8] Dogs may be at risk of developing myocardial necrosis and fibrosis following exposures to albuterol and other bronchodilators.[9] Rodents, humans, and some nonhuman primates are at lesser risk of developing cardiotoxicosis following albuterol exposure.[6] The oral LD_{50} of albuterol in rodents is greater than 2 g/kg.[5]

Even though a toxic dose for albuterol has not been established, adverse effects are possible at therapeutic doses. Oral therapeutic doses of albuterol suggested for companion animals include a dose of 0.05 mg/kg every 8 hours in the dog.[2] Skeletal muscle tremors and restlessness were common signs in dogs given 0.02 mg/kg of albuterol syrup every 12 hours.[10] Between 7.2 and 18 mg of active ingredient is found in albuterol asthma inhalers, depending on the size of the canister.[5] The entire contents are available when dogs bite into the pressurized canister, potentially exposing dogs to large doses of albuterol. In addition, the Freon in some albuterol inhalers is known to sensitize the myocardium to arrhythmogenic effects of beta-agonists, potentially increasing the risk of arrhythmias in those dogs biting into inhalers.[11] In the cat, a dose of 0.02 to 0.05 mg/kg (unspecified route of exposure) up to 4 times per day has been published.[12] Hypokalemia has been seen in cats within 15 minutes of receiving an unspecified dose of albuterol. Baboons developed sinus tachycardia within 30 seconds and hypokalemia within 10 minutes of receiving an intravenous albuterol bolus equivalent to a therapeutic human bronchodilator dose.[13] Given that clinical signs are well documented at therapeutic doses, albuterol should be considered to have a narrow margin of safety, particularly in individuals with preexisting health problems.

Clinical Signs.   Beta-2 receptors are found in many different tissues, the most important of which are smooth muscle (especially bronchial, vascular, gastrointestinal, and uterine), skeletal muscle, the myocardium, and the liver.[8] Stimulation of these receptors causes smooth muscle relaxation, which may result in peripheral vasodilation with subsequent hypotension and reflex tachycardia. Stimulation of beta-2 receptors in the lungs causes bronchodilation, the desired clinical effect. Albuterol has been used in humans to inhibit uterine contractions during premature labor. Stimulation of beta-2 receptors on skeletal muscle cells causes increased contractility and may lead to muscle tremors. Beta-2 receptor stimulation in the heart can cause increases in the heart rate and various arrhythmias, with overdoses in humans also causing precordial pressure or chest pain.[14]

Signs that have been seen in dogs that bite into albuterol inhalers include hyperactivity, depression, tachycardia, premature ventricular contractions, tachypnea, muscle tremors, vomiting, and death.[11] Heart rates of up to 300 beats per minute have been reported in dogs that bite into albuterol inhalers. Some dogs developed prolonged weakness several hours after exposure when tachycardia was not treated.[4] Pulmonary edema, which may be secondary to ruptured chordae tendineae, has been seen in dogs treated with albuterol.[15]

Clinical Pathology.   Hypokalemia, hyperglycemia, increased plasma insulin, hypomagnesemia, and increased free fatty acids have been associated with therapeutic albuterol use in humans. Hypokalemia is secondary to the intracellular movement of potassium, not a net loss of potassium.[16] Hypokalemia has been reported in numerous canine albuterol overdoses. Serum potassium levels as low as 0.9 mmol/L have been reported in some cases in which the tablet formulation was ingested. Hyperglycemia has been associated with albuterol overdoses only rarely in the dog. Hypomagnesemia has not been reported in the dog following albuterol overdoses, presumably because testing for serum magnesium has not been routine.[4]

Lesions.   Albuterol and other beta-agonists have been found to cause cardiovascular lesions in the dog. Six- to 7-month-old beagle dogs treated once daily with aerosolized albuterol powder at 19 to 90 times the clinical dose developed mild fibrosis of the left ventricular papillary muscles of the heart after approximately 14 days of treatment. Some dogs also developed a slight mineralization of the left ventricular papillary muscle. These lesions were not found in the rat or monkey.[6] Albuterol, as well as other beta-agonists, has caused intramural coronary arteriosclerosis in dogs.[9] It is not known whether these lesions exist following one acute overdose of albuterol.

Diagnostic Testing.   Testing for albuterol levels is possible, but not clinically relevant. Albuterol levels are not performed routinely at human hospitals. Albuterol may be measured in plasma by either gas chromatography or HPLC.

Treatment.   Decontamination may not be necessary or advisable in many cases of albuterol overdose. Because of the rapid absorption and onset of clinical signs, emesis should not be attempted in cases of aerosol, syrup, or solution ingestion. In these instances, little, if any, of the drug may be evacuated during emesis. In addition, clinical signs could begin during emesis, increasing the risk of aspiration pneumonitis. Activated charcoal may also be of limited benefit in these cases because of the rapid and complete absorption of the liquid and aerosol formulations. Cases involving the ingestion of large amounts of syrup or solution may warrant the administration of activated charcoal if administered within the first hour after exposure. Decontamination should be considered when albuterol tablets are ingested. Emesis should only be performed within approximately 15 to 30 minutes of ingestion and should not be attempted after the onset of clinical signs. Activated charcoal and a cathartic should be administered within 2 hours of ingestion in cases involving the ingestion of multiple tablets or when extended-release tablets are ingested.

Clinical signs should be treated supportively. Heart rate and rhythm should be monitored for a minimum of 12 hours after exposure. Intravenous fluids may help correct hypotension, if present. Hyperactivity or tremors are not generally severe and usually respond well to diazepam.

Tachycardia and tachyarrhythmias should be treated with intravenous propranolol (a nonspecific beta-blocker) when the heart rate exceeds 160 beats per minute in large dogs or 180 beats per minute in small dogs. The dose range for intravenous propranolol is 0.02 to 0.06 mg/kg, given slowly as needed. Oral propranolol may be given at 0.2 to 1 mg/kg,[2] but is usually less effective and more difficult to administer than via the intravenous route. The more selective beta-1-blocking drugs, such as metoprolol, are not as effective as propranolol in controlling tachycardia. This suggests that excessive beta-2-receptor stimulation is the primary cause of tachycardia in albuterol overdoses. It is possible that propranolol could cause bronchoconstriction, especially in an asthmatic cat. However, propranolol has been used to treat cases of human albuterol overdoses in asthmatics without causing bronchoconstriction.[17]

Propranolol has also been effective in reversing hypokalemia in humans.[18] Serum potassium levels should be monitored and potassium supplemented as needed. If propranolol is administered concurrently with potassium, serum potassium levels should be monitored carefully because potassium eventually shifts back out of the cells, perhaps causing hyperkalemia.

Most dogs are asymptomatic within 12 hours of exposure. Dogs exhibiting arrhythmias may be symptomatic for up to 48 hours. Dogs that do not receive treatment may develop weakness, presumably due to prolonged tachycardia and hypokalemia. Limited activity and supportive care are indicated in these cases.

Prognosis.   The prognosis for healthy individual animals following the acute ingestion of albuterol is good, assuming that prompt, appropriate medical treatment is provided. Overdoses of tablets have the potential for causing more severe signs than those involving the albuterol inhalers, even though the inhalers contain between 80 and 200 doses of albuterol per full canister.[5] Animals with preexisting heart disease have a more guarded prognosis.

Prevention and Control.   Dogs may be especially attracted to the albuterol inhalers.[4] All medications should be kept in a secured location. Owners should be advised to report any adverse reactions their pet may have to therapeutic doses of the beta-agonist bronchodilators.

CARDIOVASCULAR DRUGS

Joseph D. Roder

CARDIAC GLYCOSIDES

Synonyms.   The major therapeutic representatives of this group include digoxin and digitoxin. Commonly, digitalis refers to the entire groups of compounds.

Sources.   The term *digitalis* specifically refers to the mixture of active ingredients contained in the dried leaves of the purple foxglove (*Digitalis purpura*).

Toxicokinetics.   These compounds are well absorbed following oral administration. Digitoxin is highly bound (70%

to 90%) to protein, whereas digoxin exhibits low protein binding (<25%). Both digitoxin and digoxin are metabolized by hepatic enzymes. Digitoxin and digoxin have a narrow therapeutic index. Animals must be dosed for their lean body weight and the dose based on the body surface area.

Mechanism of Action.   These drugs act on the Na^+/K^+-ATPase enzymes of excitable triggers throughout the body. They might inhibit the activity of the enzyme, which results in elevation of the intracellular sodium. The elevated sodium is exchanged for calcium, elevating the intracellular free calcium. This leads to increased calcium-dependent contraction of the cardiac muscle cells. These drugs also decrease the intracellular potassium concentrations that lower the resting membrane potential. This affects the cardiac pacemakers (SA and AV nodes) and allows vagal tone to predominate.

Toxicity and Risk Factors.   Cats are more sensitive than dogs to the toxic effects of digitalis. Male cats have higher serum digoxin concentrations than females.[1]

Clinical Signs.   Animals suffering from digitalis intoxication exhibit gastrointestinal and cardiac signs. The more common gastrointestinal signs include nausea, vomiting, and diarrhea.[1] Animals may also lose body weight over a longer period of time. The cardiac abnormalities are more life threatening in the acute intoxication. Some of the cardiac effects include weakness, decreased beat (sinus bradycardia), heart block, and ventricular tachycardia.[2]

Clinical Pathology.   Hyperkalemia is the most consistent alteration of the serum chemistry.

Diagnostic Testing.   Serum digoxin concentrations may be performed but are not beneficial in managing the poisoned patient.

Treatment.   The treatment of digitalis overdose should be directed at preserving cardiac function. The animal should be monitored with an ECG for any arrhythmias.[2] Decontamination with activated charcoal and sorbitol (Toxiban) should proceed immediately. Emesis may be indicated if ingestion has recently occurred.

The treatment of hyperkalemia is essential for management of the patient. Sodium bicarbonate infusion forces elevated serum potassium back into cells. Glucose and insulin therapy also decreases the serum potassium concentrations by forcing the cation into cells. Serum potassium concentration should be monitored frequently. Sodium polystyrene sulfonate (Kayexalate) has been used to decrease serum potassium. This therapy may require several hours for maximal effectiveness.

Symptomatic therapy consists of establishing a clear airway and providing supplemental oxygen if needed. Bradycardia is treated with atropine. Arrhythmias (ventricular tachycardia) are treated with lidocaine or phenytoin.[3] In human intoxication, Digibind (a Fab portion of digoxin-specific antibodies) is used in refractory or severe intoxication. The cost of therapy is generally beyond practical use in veterinary medicine.

Prognosis.   The outcome is guarded because of cardiac complications.

Prevention and Control.   In the treatment of the elderly veterinary patient, the owner should watch closely for changes in eating and drinking behaviors. Depressed animals should be taken immediately to the veterinarian.

CALCIUM CHANNEL BLOCKING AGENTS

Synonyms.   Representatives of this class of compounds include verapamil, diltiazem, nifedipine, and nimodipine.

Toxicokinetics.   All calcium antagonists are rapidly absorbed from the small intestine. First pass effect is significant with these compounds, which may become saturated in the intoxicated animal, leading to greater drug absorption.

Mechanism of Action.   All calcium antagonists act by preventing the opening of voltage-gated calcium channels (the L type). They slow the influx of calcium into the cell and inhibit the calcium-dependent processes in cardiac cells. The desired therapeutic response is vasodilation (coronary and peripheral), decreased cardiac contractility, and decreased nodal activity and conduction. The result of the conducting system blockade is more noted at the SA and AV nodes because there are no sodium channels in these areas and conduction is dependent on calcium flux.[4]

Toxicity and Risk Factors.   In humans, two to three times the normal dose may cause intoxication. Experimentally, doses greater than 0.7 mg/kg altered hemodynamic parameters in dogs.[4] Cats and small dogs, because of their lower weight, are at greatest risk of intoxication from accidental ingestion of their owners' medications.

Clinical Signs.   Animals presenting with overdose may have depression or loss of consciousness resulting from hypotension and bradycardia.[4,5] Other earlier signs can include nausea, vomiting, and disorientation.

Treatment.   The animal should have a patent airway and oxygen therapy should be given, if needed. Activated charcoal and sorbitol (Toxiban) should be administered if clinical signs are not severe and the danger of aspiration is minimal. Repeated administration of activated charcoal may be beneficial, especially if the cardiac medication is a sustained-release type.

Therapy for hypotension symptoms includes intravenous fluids. Specific antidotal therapy is the administration of calcium (calcium chloride or calcium gluconate). Refractory hypotension should be treated with glucagons[6] or isoproterenol, or with vasopressor therapy (norepinephrine, epinephrine, and dopamine).[4] Alternatively, insulin reverses the hemodynamic alterations induced by calcium channel antagonists.[7] ECG monitoring aids in the diagnosis of any arrhythmias.

Prognosis.   The prognosis is guarded for animals exhibiting severe clinical signs. In humans, the prognosis is correlated to the degree of heart block. Human overdose patients who present with hypotension and no heart block generally respond to fluid therapy. For the veterinary patient, the prognosis depends on coingestion of other drugs, underlying heart disease, age of the animal, and the delay from ingestion to presentation.

Prevention and Control. Pet owners should be reminded of the dangers that their medications pose to their pets.

DECONGESTANTS

Charlotte Means

SYMPATHOMIMETICS

Synonyms. Sympathomimetic decongestants include pseudoephedrine, phenylephrine, and phenylpropanolamine. Some herbal (botanical) products, including ma huang *(Ephedra sinica),* other *Ephedra* species, and *Sida cordifolia,* also contain the sympathomimetic alkaloids ephedrine and pseudoephedrine.

Sources. Various plants produce the alkaloids pseudoephedrine and ephedrine.[1-3]

Pseudoephedrine is formulated in medications to treat cold and allergies as both OTC and prescription products. Pseudoephedrine is found in brand name medications as well as generics. Frequently, pseudoephedrine is combined with a variety of antihistamines such as diphenhydramine and chlorpheniramine, among others. Combination products may also include analgesics such as ibuprofen or acetaminophen. Cough suppressants such as guaifenesin or dextromethorphan may be included in the formulation as well.

Ma huang and *S. cordifolia* are used to treat asthma, colds, and allergies. Most commonly, these herbs are found in weight loss products. Weight loss products often contain caffeine as well, usually derived from guarana, green tea extract, or other naturally occurring caffeine sources. A few trade names include Metabolife, Metabolize and Save, and Dexatrim Natural. Ma huang is also abused in products such as Herbal Ecstasy, advertised as a legal form of the street drug "ecstasy."

Phenylephrine is most commonly found in nasal sprays. Some hemorrhoidal creams and ointments also contain phenylephrine for its vasoconstrictive properties.

Phenylpropanolamine (PPA) was most commonly used as a weight loss aid, as well as a decongestant in cold and allergy medications, both OTC and prescription. Like pseudoephedrine, PPA was combined with a variety of antihistamines, analgesics, and cough suppressants. PPA has been withdrawn from the market because some individuals suffered strokes while taking the medication. It is still available for use in veterinary medicine by drug compounding or in products that are for veterinary use only.

Toxicokinetics. Sympathomimetics are well absorbed orally. Onset of action for most formulations is rapid, frequently less than 1 hour.[1,2] The onset of action is often slower if extended-release or botanical products are ingested. Regardless of formulation, signs are expected by 8 hours after ingestion.[3]

Sympathomimetics are presumed to cross into the cerebrospinal fluid, can be excreted into breast milk, and may cross the placenta. Sympathomimetics are partially metabolized in the liver. Elimination is through the urine. About 55% to 75% of the drug is excreted as unchanged drug. The urine pH partially determines the rate of excretion; acidic urine accelerates elimination. The serum half-life ranges between 2 and 21 hours for pseudoephedrine (depending on urine pH).[2,4] PPA has a half-life of about 3 to 4 hours.[5]

Mechanism of Action. Sympathomimetics stimulate alpha- and beta-adrenergic receptors. This response causes the release of endogenous catecholamines in the brain and heart, resulting in peripheral vasoconstriction and cardiac stimulation. Increased blood pressure, tachycardia, mydriasis, ataxia, and restlessness result. The decongestant activity occurs from a combination of vasoconstriction and bronchodilation.[1,2,4]

Toxicity and Risk Factors. A therapeutic dose of pseudoephedrine to treat urethral sphincter hypotonus resulting in urinary incontinence in dogs is usually given at 1 to 2 mg/kg every 12 hours.[6] PPA is given at 1.1 mg/kg in dogs. Cats are typically given a 75-mg sustained-release capsule orally once daily. Topical 0.25% and 2.5% solutions of phenylephrine are used to diagnose Horner's syndrome.[5]

Clinical signs of pseudoephedrine toxicosis have been seen at 5 to 6 mg/kg (with both pharmaceutical and botanical preparations) and deaths may occur at 10 to 12 mg/kg.[1] Toxicity can be enhanced when ephedrine or pseudoephedrine is combined with other drugs. For example, when ma huang and guarana are consumed, signs are seen at 4.4 mg/kg of guarana (caffeine) and 1.3 mg/kg of ma huang (ephedrine). Death in dogs has occurred at 19.1 mg/kg guarana (caffeine) and 5.8 mg/kg ma huang (ephedrine).[3]

Increased risk of toxicosis exists if preexisting disease is present. In particular, diabetes, hypothyroidism or hyperthyroidism, cardiac disease and hypertension, seizure disorders, renal disease, gastric ulcers, and glaucoma increase the risk of adverse effects. Many drug interactions are possible, especially with digoxin, halothane, MAOIs, and methylxanthines.[1,3,4]

Dogs, ferrets, and potbelly pigs are more at risk because of their inquisitive natures and willingness to eat nonfood items. These types of drugs are frequently placed in areas for easy access, such as coffee tables, night stands, and purses. Powdered drinks and nutrition bars are often attractive and dogs willingly consume large quantities.

Clinical Signs. Initial signs usually include restlessness, agitation, and pacing. Some animals vocalize. Dogs may exhibit hallucinogenic behavior, such as staring and snapping at invisible objects. Mydriasis, tachycardia, and hypertension are usually present. Neurologic signs such as muscle tremors, seizures, and head bobbing may occur. Death is usually due to cardiovascular collapse.[1,3]

Hyperthermia (temperature >104° F) frequently occurs as a result of excess muscular activity. If untreated, DIC or rhabdomyolysis may develop. Rhabdomyolysis can cause myoglobinuria and result in acute renal failure.[1,3]

Clinical Pathology.   Hyperglycemia and hyperinsulinemia can be caused by sympathomimetics. Hyperinsulinemia often results in hypokalemia caused by a shifting of potassium from extracellular to intracellular spaces.[2]

Lesions.   No specific lesions occur.

Diagnostic Testing.   Diagnosis is generally based on exposure history and appropriate clinical signs. Pseudoephedrine can be detected in the urine and plasma.

Treatment.   Decontamination is important in early exposures. Emesis should be induced in asymptomatic animals when the exposure is less than 30 minutes. Activated charcoal and a cathartic are effective in preventing absorption of the drug.

Tremors, seizures, hyperactivity, and agitation should be controlled by acepromazine (0.05 to 1 mg/kg intravenously, intramuscularly, or subcutaneously), chlorpromazine (0.5 to 1 mg/kg intravenously or intramuscularly), or a barbiturate such as phenobarbital (3 mg/kg intravenously to effect).[5] When acepromazine or chlorpromazine is used, the low end of the dosage range is started and increased as necessary. Benzodiazepines, such as diazepam, are not recommended because the dissociative effects of benzodiazepines may be exaggerated in sympathomimetic overdose. A dog may become more agitated after administration of diazepam.[1,3]

Cardiac function and blood pressure should be monitored. Propranolol (0.02 to 0.06 mg/kg slowly intravenously)[3] can control tachycardia and often stabilizes hypokalemia. Intravenous fluids should be administered and the animal monitored. Pulmonary edema is possible if pulmonary hypertension occurs, but this is rare. Baseline CBC and chemistry values should be obtained. Clinical signs may last for 24 to 72 hours.[1,3]

In humans, urinary acidification enhances pseudoephedrine elimination. Whether urinary acidification benefits dogs is unknown. Acidification can be accomplished with ammonium chloride (50 mg/kg orally four times per day) or ascorbic acid (20 to 30 mg/kg intramuscularly or intravenously every 8 hours).[5] When acidifying urine, the animal's acid-base status must be monitored.

Prognosis.   Most animals respond favorably to treatment. Some clinical signs can indicate a poor prognosis. These signs include uncontrollable seizures, the development of DIC or myoglobinuria, or head bobbing.[7]

Prevention and Control.   Clients should be advised to keep all medications in areas where animals do not have access.

IMIDAZOLINES

Synonyms.   Imidazoline decongestants are commonly found in nasal sprays and eyedrops. Active ingredients include naphazoline, oxymetazoline, tetrahydrozoline, and xylometazoline. Drugs with a similar mechanism of action include clonidine, which is used to treat hypertension and attention deficit disorder. Brimonidine is used topically to treat glaucoma or intraocular hypertension.[4]

Some brands of nasal sprays include Privine nasal spray, Allerest, Dristan Long Acting Spray, Sinarest, and Sinex. Eyedrops include Murine Plus, Soothe Eyedrops, and Clear Eyes.

Sources.   Imidazoline decongestants work as topical vasoconstrictives. Nasal sprays provide relief of congestion due to colds, allergies, and sinusitis. Eyedrops relieve redness associated with conjunctival inflammation. These products are available at discount, grocery, and drug stores. They are available OTC and include a wide variety of name brand and generic products. Ocular decongestants are not recommended for use in veterinary medicine.[8]

Toxicokinetics.   Imidazoline decongestants are sympathomimetic agents that affect alpha-adrenergic receptors. Imidazolines are rapidly absorbed after oral ingestion and some absorption occurs from the nasal mucosa as well. Topical effects can be seen within 10 minutes and can last up to 6 hours. Systemic effects, after an ingestion, occur between 30 minutes and 4 hours. Specific information on the distribution and excretion of all imidazoline decongestants is not known; however, clonidine is metabolized in the liver and about half of an oral dose is excreted unchanged in the urine. The half-life of the parent compound in humans is 2 to 4 hours.[2,4,9]

Mechanism of Action.   Imidazolines interact with alpha-2-adrenoceptors. When imidazolines bind to central receptors, norepinephrine release is inhibited, resulting in decreased sympathetic effects. Hypotension, bradycardia, and sedation occur. Peripherally, agonist activity at postsynaptic alpha-2-adrenergic receptors causes vasoconstriction and hypertension. In oral overdoses, central effects usually predominate and drive the clinical syndrome.[4,9]

Toxicity.   Imidazolines have a narrow margin of safety. The oral LD_{50} of oxymetazoline in mice is 10 mg/kg, whereas the oral LD_{50} of xylometazoline is 215 mg/kg and of tetrahydrozaline is 335 mg/kg.[2] Preexisting disease, especially cardiac or renal disease, can cause increased clinical effects. Drug interactions occur with sympathomimetic drugs, MAOIs, other alpha-2 adrenergics, digitalis, calcium channel blockers, phenothiazines, and hypoglycemic agents.[4,9]

Clinical Signs.   Most dogs present with vomiting, weakness, collapse, and bradycardia. Poor capillary refill time may be present. Hypotension is common but hypertension can occur as well. Drowsiness or coma can occur. Some dogs are hyperactive and develop muscle tremors. Dogs should be observed for at least 4 hours after ingestion. Signs can persist for 24 to 36 hours.[7]

Clinical Pathology. Although no specific clinical pathology is expected, electrolytes should be monitored in symptomatic animals.

Lesions. No specific lesions are expected.

Treatment. Because of the rapidity with which clinical signs occur, emesis usually is not practical. Activated charcoal can be given to an asymptomatic animal.[9]

All animals should be monitored closely, including monitoring heart rate and rhythm. A continuous ECG should be considered in affected animals. A baseline CBC and chemistry panel can be obtained. Intravenous fluids should be given. Atropine can be given at a preanesthetic dose (0.01 to 0.02 mg/kg intravenously as needed) for bradycardia. Blood pressure must be monitored. In human medicine, naloxone (0.4 mg/kg intravenously) is used to reverse effects. However, in cases of severe respiratory depression, intubation and ventilation may be indicated.[2,9] Yohimbine, as an alpha-2-antagonist, is effective at reversing clinical signs, especially sedation and bradycardia.[7] Yohimbine is dosed at 0.1 mg/kg intravenously.[5]

Prognosis. With appropriate treatment, prognosis is generally good. Monitoring is important to provide optimal treatment.

Prevention and Control. Clients should be discouraged from keeping medications in baggies and in objects, like a purse, that may be placed on the floor within easy reach of a pet.

DIABETES MEDICATIONS

Marcy Rosendale

VASOPRESSIN

Synonyms. Antidiuretic hormone (ADH) is available as Pitressin (Monarch) and Vasopressin Injection (American Pharmaceutical Partners, American Partners).

Sources. Vasopressin is obtained from bovine (arginine vasopressin) and porcine (lysine vasopressin) posterior pituitary glands. Vasopressin is available in solution for injection. In humans, vasopressin is used in the treatment of diabetes insipidus, to stimulate peristalsis, and as adjunct treatment of acute, massive hemorrhage.[1] In veterinary medicine, vasopressin is used in the diagnosis and treatment of diabetes insipidus.

Toxicokinetics. Vasopressin is a polypeptide hormone produced by the hypothalamus. Vasopressin is destroyed in the gastrointestinal tract when given orally and is therefore given intranasally or parenterally. In dogs and cats, vasopressin has been administered via subcutaneous, intramuscular, and intravenous routes.[2] Intranasal absorption is poor in humans. Following absorption, vasopressin is distributed in extracellular fluid and is not thought to bind to plasma proteins. Small amounts of vasopressin are eliminated in the urine unchanged, with most being degraded in the liver and kidney. Subcutaneous administration of vasopressin in humans resulted in 5% of the total dose being excreted unchanged in the urine after 4 hours. Intravenous administration may result in urinary excretion of 5% to 15% of the unchanged hormone.[1] Peptidases in the liver and kidney rapidly inactivate vasopressin, resulting in a plasma half-life of 17 to 35 minutes.

Mechanism of Action. Vasopressin binds to receptors on the surface of cells in a variety of tissues throughout the body. The effects of vasopressin on many of these tissues are not completely understood. Receptors are currently categorized into V_{1a}, V_{1b}, and V_2 types. V_{1a} receptors are found in a number of different tissue types, including vascular smooth muscle. Hormone binding at these receptors is thought to mediate the pressor effects of vasopressin by causing vasoconstriction. Other tissues with V_{1a} receptors include the bladder, myometrium, gastrointestinal smooth muscle cells, adipocytes, hepatocytes, spleen, testis, CNS, and platelets. Activation of vasopressin receptors on platelets increases circulating factor VIII and von Willebrand factor. V_{1a} receptors are also found on the epithelial cells of the renal cortical collecting duct and in the vasa recta. V_{1b} receptors are found in the adenohypophysis. V_2 receptors are found on cells in the renal collecting duct and are responsible for increasing water permeability in the collecting ducts.[3]

Toxicity and Risk Factors. Any species of animal in which vasopressin is being used therapeutically or as a diagnostic tool is at risk of developing adverse effects. Accidental exposure of animals with access to medication containers is also possible. Because vasopressin is inactivated in the stomach, toxicity following ingestion is not expected. However, it is possible that some absorption may occur through mucous membranes proximal to the stomach, especially in the case of exposure to large amounts of the medication. No particular species or breed of animal is known to be at greater risk of adverse effects or toxicity following vasopressin use or overdose. In humans, pediatric and geriatric populations are thought to be more sensitive to the effects of vasopressin.

Clinical Signs. Little information regarding vasopressin overdose exists in the veterinary or human literature. Clinical signs exhibited following an overdose are expected to be exaggerations of known physiologic responses to the hormone. Hypertension may be caused by peripheral vasoconstriction. Gangrene has been seen in humans following the administration of large doses of vasopressin. Increased gastrointestinal activity and compromised coronary circulation have also been seen in humans.[3] If excessive amounts of water are ingested following ADH use, signs of cerebral edema may be seen. Dogs treated with vasopressin after being water loaded developed signs consistent with water intoxication. Signs included lethargy, vomiting, increased body weight, coma, and cerebral and pulmonary edema. Ataxia, weakness, and seizures are also possible signs of water intoxication.[4]

Clinical Pathology.   Administration of excessive doses of vasopressin may cause hyponatremia when water intake is not restricted.[5] Hyponatremia caused by inappropriate endogenous ADH secretion is associated with plasma hyposmolality with high urine osmolality. Urine sodium concentrations are expected to be high. In humans, urine sodium concentrations are generally greater than 20 mEq/L and urine osmolality may be greater than 300 mOsm/kg.[4]

Lesions.   Acute overdoses of vasopressin may cause cerebral edema and associated CNS lesions. The brain may appear enlarged and softened with flattened gyri and narrowed sulci. Ventricular cavities may be compressed and herniation of the brain may be noted.[6] Osmotic demyelination syndrome may theoretically be seen in vasopressin overdose. Osmotic demyelination syndrome is associated with brain dehydration that has been seen in dogs and humans following rapid correction of hyponatremia and hypoosmolality. Myelin loss in the thalamus was noted in dogs several days after the correction of hyponatremia.[4]

Diagnostic Testing.   Plasma arginine vasopressin levels may be measured by radioimmunoassay.[7] Vasopressin levels are not useful in making treatment decisions in cases of overdose.

Treatment.   Because of the poor oral bioavailability and short half-life, efforts to decontaminate by inducing emesis or administering activated charcoal following oral exposure to vasopressin are expected to be of little benefit. Additionally, the induction of emesis in cases involving small amounts of liquid medication may not result in the retrieval of appreciable amounts of medication in the vomitus. Spontaneous emesis may occur as a direct effect of vasopressin on the smooth muscle of the stomach. Additional emetics should not be administered if spontaneous emesis has occurred.

Initial treatment of vasopressin overdose should consist of restricting free water intake while monitoring serum sodium levels and blood pressure. Hypertonic saline is recommended in the human literature for severe, acute hyponatremia following vasopressin overdose.[5] Prophylactic use of hypertonic saline is not recommended. Use of direct-acting vasodilators such as sodium nitroprusside or hydralazine may be considered when severe hypertension is seen. With an estimated half-life of 17 to 35 minutes, a majority of clinical signs are expected to resolve within approximately 2 to 3 hours and may not require treatment other than water restriction.

Prognosis.   Experience with vasopressin overdose in domestic animals is limited. Prognosis is expected to be dependent on the severity of hyponatremia and neurologic signs.

DESMOPRESSIN ACETATE

Synonyms.   1-(3-mercaptopropionic acid)-8-D-arginine vasopressin monoacetate (salt) trihydrate, is available as DDAVP (Aventis Pharmaceuticals), Stimate, and Desmopressin Acetate Rhinal Tube (Ferring Pharmaceuticals).[8]

Sources.   Desmopressin has a variety of uses in human medicine. It is used in the treatment of central diabetes insipidus, transient trauma, or surgery-induced polyuria and polydipsia of the pituitary gland, and primary nocturnal enuresis. Desmopressin is also used in the treatment of hemophilia A and von Willebrand's disease (type 1). It is available as nasal spray, aqueous solution for injection, aqueous solution for intranasal use, and tablets.[1] No desmopressin products are labeled for veterinary use. In veterinary medicine, desmopressin is used in the diagnosis and treatment of central diabetes insipidus in the dog and cat. It is also used in the treatment of von Willebrand's disease in the dog. In addition to the aforementioned routes of administration, desmopressin nasal spray may be administered in the conjunctival sac in the dog and cat.[2]

Toxicokinetics.   Desmopressin is a synthetic polypeptide that is similar in structure to arginine vasopressin. Kinetics vary with the route of administration. The metabolism and route of elimination of desmopressin have not been determined.

Desmopressin may be administered as an intranasal spray where it is absorbed through the nasal mucosa. It is estimated that 10% to 20% of an intranasal dose is absorbed in humans. Peak plasma concentrations are seen within 40 to 45 minutes of intranasal administration in humans. Antidiuretic effects in humans may occur within 15 minutes, with peak effects in 1 to 5 hours that may persist for 5 to 21 hours. Increased levels of factor VIII and von Willebrand factor are seen within 30 minutes of administration in humans, with peak effects in about 1.5 hours. The half-life of intranasal desmopressin in humans is 3.3 to 3.5 hours.

Desmopressin tablets are poorly absorbed from the gastrointestinal tract with peak plasma levels in humans occurring in 0.9 to 1.5 hours. Antidiuretic effects are first seen at about 1 hour after ingestion and may peak at about 4 to 7 hours in humans with a half-life of 1.5 to 2.5 hours.

Peak plasma levels of factor VIII are seen in humans 1.5 to 3 hours after intravenous administration of desmopressin. The terminal half-life in humans is 75.5 minutes following intravenous administration, with a range of 0.4 to 4 hours. Intravenous administration of desmopressin causes about 10 times the antidiuretic effect of intranasal administration.[1]

Mechanism of Action.   Desmopressin is a selective V_2 receptor agonist causing increased water permeability in the collecting ducts of the kidney. Desmopressin also causes the release of von Willebrand factor and factor VIII from storage sites in the body. Desmopressin does not have the pressor effects of vasopressin at therapeutic doses.[9] Desmopressin may have V_1 pressor effects in overdose situations.[10]

Toxicity and Risk Factors.   Any species of animal in which desmopressin is being used therapeutically or as a diagnostic tool is at risk of developing adverse effects. Accidental exposure of animals with access to medication containers is also possible. Serious adverse effects may occur with therapeutic doses of desmopressin, giving the drug a relatively narrow margin of safety. Individuals with no need for an antidiuretic receiving therapeutic doses of desmopressin are at risk of water intoxication and hyponatremia. A human hemophiliac receiving an intravenous desmopressin dose of 0.5 µg/kg (a published therapeutic dose is 0.3 µg/kg) developed excessive water retention.[1] A canine therapeutic dose of desmopressin for treatment of von Willebrand's disease is 1 µg/kg administered as a subcutaneous injection.[2] Intranasal doses in humans ranging from 0.3 to 2.4 µg/kg have caused hyponatremia and seizures.

Young children may be at increased risk of developing hyponatremia and seizures. In humans, chlorpropamide, clofibrate, and indomethacin may prolong the action of desmopressin, whereas carbamazepine may prolong its action. Also in humans, lithium, epinephrine, demeclocycline, heparin, and alcohol may cause a decreased antidiuretic response to desmopressin.[11] No particular species or breed of animal is known to be at greater risk of adverse effects or toxicity following desmopressin use or overdose.

Clinical Signs. Little information regarding desmopressin overdose exists in the veterinary literature. In humans myocardial infarction secondary to arterial thromboses, seizures secondary to hyponatremia, and pulmonary edema may be seen following the therapeutic use of desmopressin. Other adverse effects reported in humans include headache, nausea, abdominal cramps, and vulval pain following parenteral use. Following intranasal use, dizziness, conjunctivitis, ocular edema, lacrimation, and rhinitis may be seen in addition to the aforementioned signs.[11] Increased blood pressure or decreased blood pressure with an increased heart rate have been seen infrequently in humans following use of desmopressin.[8] Cerebral edema secondary to overhydration and hyponatremia may cause a variety of signs, including salivation, vomiting, depression, ataxia, and seizures.[12] A dog that ingested a total desmopressin dose of 2.3 mg/kg in tablet form developed tachycardia within approximately 20 minutes of ingestion (maximum reported heart rate of 268 beats per minute), mild hyponatremia (142 mEq/L, reference range of 145 to 158), and hypertension (maximum reported blood pressure was 202/119). Recovery was noted approximately 36 hours after exposure.[10]

Clinical Pathology. Hyponatremia may be seen in humans, usually when water intake is not restricted following therapeutic desmopressin use.[11] Decreased plasma osmolality is rarely seen in humans.[8] An increased packed cell volume was seen in a dog that ingested a 2.3-mg/kg dose of desmopressin tablets.[10]

Lesions. Desmopressin toxicosis may cause cerebral edema with CNS lesions typical of swelling in the brain. The brain may appear enlarged and softened with flattened gyri and sulci. Ventricular cavities may be compressed and herniation of the brain may be noted.[6] Osmotic demyelination syndrome may theoretically be seen in

desmopressin overdose. Osmotic demyelination syndrome is associated with brain dehydration that has been seen in dogs and humans following rapid correction of hyponatremia and hypoosmolality. Myelin loss in the thalamus was noted in dogs several days after the correction of hyponatremia.[4] Juvenile lambs treated with 10 µg of desmopressin for 13 weeks resulted in increased volume of the renal medulla and decreased volume of the renal cortex. The renal pelvis was enlarged by 29% compared with control kidneys.[13]

Diagnostic Testing. Desmopressin plasma levels may be obtained by radioimmunoassay. Desmopressin levels that correspond to clinical signs of toxicosis have not been determined and therefore cannot be used to make treatment decisions.[11]

Treatment. Decontamination should be performed in most cases of desmopressin tablet overdose. Emesis may be attempted within the first 15 minutes of ingestion when there are no contraindications. Emesis is not recommended if the dog is showing clinical signs of toxicosis. Activated charcoal and a cathartic should be administered as soon as possible up to 2 hours after exposure. In cases in which large numbers of pills were ingested, gastric lavage may be considered if emesis was not performed. The induction of emesis in cases involving small amounts of liquid medication may not result in the retrieval of appreciable amounts of medication in the vomitus. Additional emetics should not be administered if spontaneous emesis has occurred.

No specific antidote for desmopressin is available. Treatment of clinical signs should consist of supportive care until those signs resolve. Initial treatment of desmopressin overdose should consist of restricting free water intake while monitoring serum sodium levels, blood pressure, and heart rate. In cases of severe hyponatremia, furosemide and oral salt supplementation have been recommended in the human literature. No guidelines were given for salt supplementation.[11] Administration of hypertonic saline as recommended for vasopressin overdose may be a safer means of correcting sodium imbalance. Care should be taken to prevent overcorrection of hyponatremia. Prophylactic use of either oral sodium or hypertonic saline is not recommended. Use of direct-acting vasodilators such as sodium nitroprusside or hydralazine may be considered if severe hypertension is seen. Vasodilators should be used with caution because of the possibility that desmopressin can also cause transient hypotension. CNS signs associated with hyponatremia and hyposmolality should be treated by providing supportive care until the underlying cause can be corrected. Adverse effects may last for approximately 24 hours.

Prognosis. Experience with desmopressin overdose in domestic animals is limited. Prognosis is expected to be dependent on the severity of clinical signs.

INSULIN

Synonyms. The availability of specific insulin preparations is subject to frequent change. A list of insulin preparations is provided in Box 24-4.

REGULAR (CHRYSTALLINE ZINC OR UNMODIFIED) INSULIN

Insulin, regular purified pork (Novo Nordisk)
Iletin II, regular purified pork (Lilly)

ISOPHANE (NEUTRAL PROTAMINE HAGEDORN OR NPH) INSULIN

Iletin II, NPH puified pork (Lilly)
Insulin, NPH purified pork (Novo Nordisk)

INSULIN ZINC (LENTE INSULIN)

Iletin II, Lente purified pork (Lilly)
Insulin, Lente purified pork (Novo Nordisk)

INSULIN HUMAN

Humulin U Ultralente (Lilly)
Humulin R (Lilly)
Novolin R (Novo Nordisk)
Humulin R U-500 (Lilly)
Novolin R PenFill (Novo Nordisk)
Novolin R Prefilled (Novo Nordisk)
Velosulin BR Human (Novo Nordisk)
Humulin L (Lilly)
Novolin L (Novo Nordisk)
Humulin N (Lilly)
Novolin N (Novo Nordisk)
Novolin N PenFill (Novo Nordisk)
Novolin N Prefilled (Novo Nordisk)
Humulin 70/30 (Lilly)
Novolin 70/30 (Novo Nordisk)
Humulin 50/50 (Lilly)
Novolin 70/30 PenFill (Novo Nordisk)
Novolin 70/30 Prefilled (Novo Nordisk)

INSULIN LISPRO

Humalog (Lilly)

Sources. Insulin is produced in the beta cells of the mammalian pancreas. Insulin is available by prescription for parenteral use in patients with diabetes mellitus and may be of synthetic, semisynthetic, or animal origin. Semisynthetic preparations are modified pork insulin. Animal preparations are currently of porcine origin. Beef insulin, alone or in combination, is no longer commercially available in the United States. Human insulin preparations are synthetic in nature and are not extracted from the human pancreas.[1] No veterinary-approved insulin preparations are currently available.[2]

Toxicokinetics. Insulin is a protein hormone composed of two chains with a molecular weight of approximately 6000. Little species variation exists in the amino acid sequence of insulin. Porcine insulin is identical to canine insulin and human insulin differs from porcine insulin by only one amino acid. Human insulin differs from bovine insulin by three amino acids.[14] Feline insulin is most similar to bovine insulin.[7]

Insulin is degraded in the gastrointestinal tract. Ingestion of a parenteral preparation is not expected to cause toxicosis. Insulin preparations may be administered by subcutaneous intramuscular or intravenous injection. When injected via subcutaneous or intramuscular injection, insulin is absorbed into the bloodstream. Insulin administered by intramuscular injection may be absorbed more rapidly than when administered by subcutaneous injection, although a variety of other factors, including the site of injection, may also affect the rate of absorption. The type of insulin, as well as the volume and concentration, affects the rate of absorption in humans. Once absorbed into the bloodstream, insulin is distributed throughout the extracellular fluids of the body.

The liver is the major site of insulin metabolism, with the kidneys and muscle tissue playing lesser roles in breaking down the hormone. The enzyme glutathione insulin transhydrogenase is responsible for the metabolism of insulin in the liver. About 60% of the insulin reabsorbed from glomerular filtrate is metabolized in cells lining the proximal convoluted tubule of the kidney. Most of the remaining insulin is returned to the bloodstream, with only about 2% being excreted in the urine.[1]

The onset of action varies depending on the type of insulin administered. Regular insulin has an immediate effect when administered intravenously. When given by either intramuscular or subcutaneous injection, the onset of action is 10 to 30 minutes. The peak effects and duration of effects vary by route of exposure, with peak effects following IV administration occurring at 0.5 to 2 hours and effects lasting between 1 and 4 hours. Peak effects following subcutaneous administration of regular insulin occur at 1 to 5 hours with a duration of 4 to 10 hours.

Protamine zinc insulin (PZI) is administered by subcutaneous injection with an onset of action at 1 to 4 hours, a maximum effect of 3 to 12 hours, and duration of 12 to 24 hours in the cat. The duration of effect may be longer in dogs. Isophane (NPH) insulin is also administered by subcutaneous injection and has an onset of action of 0.5 to 3 hours, a maximum effect of 2 to 8 hours, and a duration of action of 6 to 12 hours in cats and 18 hours in dogs. Lente insulin takes effect immediately after subcutaneous injection and has maximum effects of 2 to 6 hours and duration of action of 8 to 14 hours in the cat.[15]

Mechanism of Action. Insulin has a wide variety of anabolic effects on the body, with the regulation of glucose transport into the cell being its most clinically relevant function. Insulin facilitates the entry of glucose into the cell. After insulin binds to specific receptors on the surface of target cells, a cascade of intracellular reactions is triggered, which result in the movement of glucose transporters to the plasma membrane of the cell and entry of glucose into the cell.[9] Insulin also facilitates the intracellular movement of potassium by stimulating Na/K-ATPase. Excessive doses of insulin may cause hypoglycemia and hypokalemia secondary to the intracellular movement of glucose and potassium.[1] In some cases when large doses of insulin are given to diabetic animals, the resultant precipitous decrease in blood glucose concentration triggers a physiologic response that results in hyperglycemia. This physiologic response is thought to be due to the stimulation of glucose production by the liver and insulin antagonism at the insulin receptor. This insulin-induced hyperglycemia is called the *Somogyi phenomenon*.[7]

Toxicity and Risk Factors. Any species of domestic animal may be affected by the administration of excessive doses of insulin. Insulin is degraded in the gastrointestinal tract, making signs of toxicosis unlikely in the event that the injectable formulation is ingested. A minimum toxic insulin dose has not been determined. Clinical signs secondary to hypoglycemia may be seen at therapeutic insulin doses. An overdose of 10 times the therapeutic dose resulted in permanent neurologic damage in a cat. Therapeutic doses of insulin vary widely depending on the species being treated, insulin type, and medical condition of the individual patient. The results of one retrospective study indicate that diabetic cats may be more likely than dogs to receive insulin overdose. In the same retrospective study, obese diabetic cats were found to be at increased risk of insulin overdose compared with diabetic cats of normal weight. Advanced age and length of insulin treatment are associated with increased risk of hypoglycemia in humans.[16] Care should be taken in selecting the correctly calibrated syringe for the particular concentration of insulin being administered to avoid an insulin overdose.

Clinical Signs. Clinical signs secondary to hypoglycemia may include ataxia, weakness, personality changes, coma, and seizures. A rapid decrease in serum glucose in small animals may cause nervousness, hunger, weakness, vomiting, tremors and tachycardia. Diarrhea, pacing, and blindness were less common signs of insulin overdose in dogs, whereas vocalizing, panting, circling, and urination were additional signs seen less commonly in cats.[16]

Clinical Pathology. Hypoglycemia is the most likely clinical pathologic abnormality to be noted following large doses of insulin. Hypoglycemia as low as 10 mg/dl in diabetic cats and 24 mg/dl in diabetic dogs has been reported in a retrospective study of 28 cases of insulin overdose. Hypokalemia was seen more frequently in diabetic cats than in dogs, with the lowest recorded serum potassium level of 2.3 mEq/L seen in cats and 2.5 mEq/L in dogs.[16]

Lesions. Death secondary to acute hypoglycemia is not expected to cause cerebral lesions. Prolonged coma secondary to hypoglycemia is associated with severe neuronal degeneration.[17]

Diagnostic Testing. Insulin assays are available; however, plasma insulin levels are not useful in the treatment of insulin overdose. In humans, plasma insulin levels may be used to help diagnose insulin overdose. Plasma insulin levels do not correlate with the severity of hypoglycemia in humans.[11]

Treatment. The treatment of insulin overdose is supportive, with the prompt administration of glucose being of primary importance. Owners should be instructed to feed their diabetic pet if early signs of hypoglycemia are noticed. If

the pet cannot eat, a sugar solution may be rubbed on the gums until veterinary care can be obtained. Patients with severe neurologic signs should receive intravenous dextrose. Supportive care of seizures includes the use of diazepam or a barbiturate in addition to dextrose. Glucagon may be used when hypoglycemia does not respond to the administration of dextrose and other supportive care. Hypokalemia should be treated with oral or intravenous potassium. In a retrospective study of insulin overdoses in dogs and cats, the median hospital stay was 20 hours with a range of 30 minutes to 10 days.[16]

Prognosis. The prognosis for insulin toxicosis depends on multiple factors, including the dose administered, overall health of the patient, and length of delay in appropriate treatment.

Prevention and Control. Care should be taken in selecting the correctly calibrated syringe for the particular concentration of insulin being administered to avoid insulin overdose. Owners should be cautioned to avoid excessive exercise in the animals that may precipitate hypoglycemia. Sudden large increases in the insulin dose should be avoided.

SULFONYLUREAS

Synonyms. Several sulfonylurea agents are listed in Box 24-5.

Sources. The sulfonylureas are prescription medications. Sulfonylureas are available only in tablet form for oral administration.

Toxicokinetics. The sulfonylurea antidiabetic drugs are chemically similar to the sulfonamide antibiotics, but have no antibiotic properties. Sulfonylureas are rapidly absorbed in the gastrointestinal tract. They are highly protein-bound, metabolized primarily in the liver, and excreted in the urine.

BOX 24-5	**SULFONYLUREA AGENTS**
GENERIC NAME	**TRADE NAME (MANUFACTURER)**
Acetohexamide	Acetohexamide Tablets (Barr)
Chlorpropamide	Diabinese (Pfizer)
Glimepiride	Amaryl (Hoechst Marion Roussel)
Glipizide (glydiazinamide)	Glucotrol (Pfizer)
	Glucotrol XL (Pfizer)
Glyburide (glibenclamide, glybenclamide, glybenzcyclamide)	DiaBeta (Hoechst Marion Roussel)
	Micronase (Pharmacia & Upjohn)
	Glynase PresTab (Pharmacia & Upjohn)
Tolazamide	Tolinase (Pharmacia & Upjohn)
Tolbutamide	Orinase (Pharmacia & Upjohn)

The kinetic information in Table 24-3 is obtained from the human literature. Kinetic information regarding the sulfonylurea medications has not been established in domestic animals.

Mechanism of Action.   The sulfonylureas are thought to act by a variety of mechanisms to ultimately cause the release of endogenous insulin. Sulfonylureas may also enhance insulin receptor binding.[11] Chlorpropamide potentiates the effect of vasopressin in the renal tubules and may also stimulate vasopressin secretion.[1]

Toxicity and Risk Factors.   Toxic doses have not been established. Severe hypoglycemia has been seen at therapeutic doses. A therapeutic dose for chlorpropamide in the dog and cat of 10 to 40 mg/kg once per day has been suggested in the treatment of diabetes insipidus. Glipizide has been prescribed at a dose range of 0.25 to 0.5 mg/kg for diabetes mellitus in the cat.[2] Glyburide has been used in the diabetic cat at a dose of 0.625 mg/kg/day.[7]

Beagle dogs have survived hypoglycemia following long-term daily doses of glimepiride at 320 mg/kg/day. Dogs also survived long-term daily chlorpropamide doses of 100 mg/kg with no mention of clinical signs in this study.[8] Doses of just 0.1 mg/kg of glipizide have caused hypoglycemia in the dog.[18] Glipizide has a published LD_{50} of greater than 4 g/kg, although the species is not identified. Glipizide has been associated with mild fetotoxicity in rats at doses of 5 to 50 mg/kg. The fetotoxicity is thought to be directly related to the hypoglycemia caused by the drug.[8] This particular category of diabetic medications should be considered to have a narrow margin of safety.

Clinical Signs.   Most signs of sulfonylurea toxicosis are expected to be secondary to hypoglycemia. Hypoglycemia may be seen in both euglycemic individuals and diabetic patients. Clinical signs secondary to hypoglycemia of other causes have included ataxia, weakness, behavioral changes, and coma.[16] Four of 50 cats treated with 2.5 mg of glipizide twice daily developed jaundice, increased total bilirubin concentration, and liver enzymes within 4 weeks of starting treatment. Other adverse effects seen in this prospective study included anorexia and vomiting. Signs resolved within 5 days of discontinuing the glipizide.[19] Tolbutamide and tolazamide have positive inotropic and arrhythmogenic effects on the cardiovascular system of dogs.[20]

TABLE 24-3 Sulfonylurea Pharmacokinetics

Agent	Peak Plasma Concentration (hours)	Half-life (hours)	Duration of Signs (hours)
Acetohexamide	Within 2	5-6 (range 2-12)	12-18
Chlorpropamide	2-4	36 (range 25-60)	24-72
Glimepiride	2-3	5-9	—
Glipizide	1-3	3-4.7 (range 2-7.3)	16-24
Glyburide	2-4	—	18-24
Tolazamide	4-8	—	16-24
Tolbutamide	3-5	—	6-10

Clinical Pathology.   All sulfonylureas are capable of causing severe hypoglycemia.

Lesions.   Even though specific lesions attributable to sulfonylurea toxicosis have not been described, severe hypoglycemia leading to prolonged coma has been associated with severe neuronal degeneration.[17]

Diagnostic Testing.   Even though it is possible to determine serum levels of the sulfonylurea drugs, those levels have not correlated with the clinical response to the drug in humans.[11]

Treatment.   No specific antidote for the sulfonylurea drugs exists. Treatment of sulfonylurea toxicosis consists of supportive care and close monitoring. Decontamination may be useful in some instances. Emesis may be safely attempted within the first 30 minutes of most exposures. However, clinical signs may be seen within 30 minutes of exposure to glipizide, so emesis may not be advisable in glipizide exposures unless initiated within the first few minutes of exposure. Severe hypoglycemia may precipitate weakness or loss of consciousness, making aspiration possible during emesis with a resultant risk of aspiration. Activated charcoal may be useful if administered within the first hour of exposure and possibly up to 2 hours after exposure if a large number of pills was ingested.

Blood glucose levels should be monitored for a minimum of 24 hours in an overdose of any sulfonylurea except chlorpropamide, which can have a 72-hour duration of effect. Delayed onset of signs up to 12 hours after sulfonylurea overdose has been seen in humans.[11] Exposures at or below a therapeutic dose can sometimes be managed by providing small, frequent meals. Blood glucose levels should be checked if weakness or other CNS signs occur. If the pet cannot eat, a sugar solution may be rubbed on the gums until veterinary care can be obtained. Hypoglycemia that is unresponsive to feeding or that is accompanied by CNS signs should be treated with intravenous dextrose.

Supportive care of seizures includes the use of diazepam or a barbiturate in addition to dextrose. Glucagon may be used when hypoglycemia does not respond to the administration of dextrose and other supportive care. Hypertonic saline may be used if hyponatremia is seen.

Prognosis.   Prognosis is usually good, as long as timely supportive care is provided for hypoglycemia and severe, prolonged neurologic signs are not seen.

Prevention and Control.   Blood glucose levels should be monitored when treating diabetic animals with the sulfonylurea antidiabetic agents.

BIGUANIDES

Synonyms.   Metformin, phenformin, and buformin are biguanide antidiabetic agents. Metformin (dimethylbiguanide hydrochloride) is currently available as Glucophage tablets (Bristol-Myers Squibb). Phenformin is no longer available in the United States.[1]

Sources. The biguanide antidiabetic agents are synthetic oral prescription medications labeled for use in the treatment of non–insulin-dependent diabetes mellitus in humans.

Toxicokinetics. In humans, metformin is slowly absorbed over a period of about 6 hours from the gastrointestinal tract, with an oral bioavailability of approximately 50% to 60%. Food has been found to decrease or delay metformin absorption. Peak plasma levels are attained in 2 to 4 hours. Metformin is negligibly bound to plasma proteins and is widely distributed in the body. Metformin is distributed into the milk of lactating rats at levels comparable to those in plasma. The plasma half-life of metformin in humans ranges from 3 to 6 hours. Metformin is not metabolized in the liver, nor is it excreted in bile. It is eliminated unchanged in the urine and feces, with 20% to 33% of an oral dose excreted in the feces in 4 to 7 days. Glomerular filtration and secretion by the proximal convoluted tubule eliminates between 35% and 52% of the total metformin dose.[1] In a pharmacokinetic study of healthy cats, intravenous metformin at 25 mg/kg had a mean oral bioavailability of 48% (range 3% to 67%), and a terminal half-life of 11.5 hours with 84% being excreted unchanged in the urine.[21]

Mechanism of Action. The biguanides lower postprandial glucose levels in type 2 diabetics. Although the exact mechanism of action is uncertain, it is thought that this group of drugs improves peripheral and hepatic sensitivity to insulin. Phenformin and, to a lesser degree, metformin have been associated with excess production of lactic acid that is thought to be secondary to an increased conversion of glucose to lactose.[1] Buformin has also been associated with lactic acidosis in humans.[11]

Toxicity and Risk Factors. No toxic doses have been established for the biguanides in humans or companion animals. Lactic acidosis has been seen following therapeutic use and overdose. In humans, geriatric patients and individuals with decreased renal function, severe hepatic insufficiency, or any condition in which hypoxemia or hypoperfusion may occur are at increased risk of developing adverse effects at therapeutic doses of the biguanides. Insufficient caloric intake and strenuous exercise that is not accompanied by food intake associated with metformin use may cause adverse effects in humans. Rats and rabbits given 600 mg/kg of metformin daily in reproductive studies did not reveal signs of fetotoxicity.[1] Severe vomiting and diarrhea were seen in a cat treated with a 250-mg daily dose of metformin. Gastrointestinal signs were not seen in a cat treated with a 125-mg/day metformin dose.[22]

Clinical Signs. Biguanide use or overdose is not expected to cause hypoglycemia except in individuals with inadequate caloric intake or following excessive exercise with insufficient food intake. Gastrointestinal upset is common in humans following therapeutic biguanide use[1] and was seen in a cat treated with metformin.[22]

Lactic acidosis has been seen in humans following both therapeutic use and in overdoses of the biguanides. Lactic acidosis was seen more frequently with phenformin than with metformin use. Lactic acidosis associated with biguanide use is associated with a high mortality rate in humans (50% to 75%). Early clinical signs of lactic acidosis in humans include vomiting, diarrhea, and abdominal pain. An acute onset of changes in consciousness and hyperventilation have also been seen in humans with lactic acidosis.[11]

Clinical Pathology. A high anion-gap metabolic acidosis determined by arterial blood gases and electrolyte levels has been seen in humans with lactic acidosis. Increased lactate levels (greater than 4 mg/dl) have also been seen in humans with lactic acidosis.[1] Serum potassium levels should be monitored when bicarbonate treatment for lactic acidosis is instituted because hypokalemia may occur as a result of alkalinization.[11]

Lesions. Specific lesions attributable to biguanide toxicosis have not been described.

Diagnostic Testing. Monitoring plasma metformin levels is possible, but has little clinical value when treating toxicosis. Gas-liquid chromatography, HPLC, and mass fragmentography have been used to measure metformin levels in humans.[11]

Treatment. No known antidote is available for the biguanide diabetic medications. Treatment of toxicosis involves decontamination and supportive care for any clinical signs of toxicosis. Decontamination may help limit the total dose if instituted soon after exposure. There is some concern in the human literature that emesis may be contraindicated because of biguanide-induced gastric mucosal irritation. Gastric lavage may be a safer alternative to emesis.[11] Emesis may be warranted if instituted shortly after an overdose, especially if there is likely to be a delay of an hour or more before lavage can be performed. An emetic should not be administered if spontaneous vomiting has occurred. Activated charcoal may bind the biguanides and should be given in cases of large overdose. The extent to which biguanides bind to activated charcoal has not been determined.

Lactic acidosis should be treated with intravenous sodium bicarbonate. In humans, 1 to 2 mEq/kg of bicarbonate has been recommended with bicarbonate being repeated as needed.[11] Lactated Ringer's solution should be avoided when choosing maintenance fluid therapy. Fluid diuresis is not recommended to enhance drug elimination.

Additional supportive care should be instituted as necessary. Sucralfate may be of benefit for gastric irritation caused by biguanide toxicosis. Cimetidine should be avoided because it can reduce metformin excretion.[1]

Prognosis. Prognosis following overdose is generally good unless lactic acidosis develops.

Prevention and Control. Pet owners should be advised to report signs of acidosis or periods of prolonged anorexia in pets receiving therapeutic doses of metformin.

ALPHA-GLUCOSIDASE INHIBITORS

Synonyms.   Acarbose is the only alpha-glucosidase inhibitor currently available in the United States. It is available as Precose (Bayer).

Sources.   Acarbose is an oligosaccharide produced by the fermentation of *ctinoplanes utahensis*. It is available in tablet formation for oral use in the treatment of type 2 diabetes mellitus in humans.[8]

Toxicokinetics.   Acarbose is poorly absorbed from the gastrointestinal tract with less than 2% of the active drug being absorbed in one human study. Peak plasma levels of active drug are obtained 1 hour after exposure. Acarbose is metabolized within the gastrointestinal tract by bacteria and digestive enzymes, with about 34% of the inactive metabolites being systemically absorbed. Peak plasma concentrations of radioactivity were seen in humans between 14 and 24 hours of receiving ^{14}C-labeled acarbose, representing the absorption of inactive metabolites. Less than 2% of the total, oral active dose was recovered in the urine, with a plasma half-life of approximately 2 hours. When the drug was given intravenously, 89% of the dose was eliminated in the urine. Also in humans, 51% of a radiolabeled acarbose dose was eliminated in the feces.[8]

Mechanism of Action.   Acarbose is a competitive inhibitor of alpha-glucosidase enzymes in the brush border of the intestine. These enzymes hydrolyze ingested carbohydrates. Alpha-glucosidase enzyme inhibition delays the digestion of carbohydrates, reducing postprandial hyperglycemia.[1]

Toxicity and Risk Factors.   Individuals of any species taking acarbose therapeutically or ingesting overdoses of acarbose are at risk of developing transient gastrointestinal upset. Doses of 200 mg given twice daily to healthy dogs caused loose stools and weight loss.[23] Diabetic dogs treated with 50 or 100 mg of acarbose twice daily also developed loose stools.[24] An acarbose dose of 480 mg/kg used in a reproductive study in rats did not reveal impaired fertility or fetotoxicity. Use of acarbose is not recommended in humans with significant renal dysfunction because of increased plasma acarbose concentrations in this group of patients.[8]

Clinical Signs.   Healthy dogs were treated with twice-daily acarbose doses of 25, 50, 100, and 200 mg for 1 week. One of 5 dogs developed loose stools at the 25- and 100-mg doses. Four of 5 dogs developed loose stools at the 200-mg acarbose dose. Two dogs exhibited weight loss.[23] Diabetic dogs also exhibited loose stools and weight loss at 50- and 100-mg twice-daily doses.[24] In addition to diarrhea, acarbose has caused abdominal pain and flatulence in humans.[8]

Clinical Pathology.   Hypoglycemia was not seen in healthy dogs treated with acarbose.[23] Hypoglycemia is not expected in humans following either therapeutic doses or overdoses of acarbose. Therapeutic use of acarbose has been associated with elevated AST and ALT levels in humans that resolved with discontinuation of the drug. Individuals with elevated liver enzymes were asymptomatic and had no other signs of liver dysfunction.[8]

Lesions.   No specific lesions are associated with acarbose toxicosis.

Diagnostic Testing.   No diagnostic tests are of clinical value in the treatment of acarbose toxicosis.

Treatment.   No antidote for acarbose exists. Treatment of any signs of toxicosis is supportive. Decontamination may be warranted in cases of large overdoses and emesis may be induced if initiated within approximately 2 hours of ingestion. Activated charcoal may aid in the removal of acarbose from the gastrointestinal tract. Acarbose treatment should be discontinued in animals that develop elevated liver enzymes at therapeutic doses. Gastrointestinal irritation should be treated supportively, which may include the use of bland diet, gastrointestinal protectants, and fluid therapy if dehydration is present.

Prognosis.   Prognosis is usually good following acarbose toxicosis. Discontinuation of the drug and supportive care generally result in the complete resolution of signs.

Prevention and Control.   Liver enzymes should be monitored when pets are placed on therapeutic doses of acarbose. The drug should be withdrawn if levels exceed normal limits to prevent possible liver damage.

THIAZOLIDINEDIONES

Synonyms.   Pioglitazone hydrochloride (Actose by Takeda), rosiglitazone maleate (Avandia by SmithKline Beecham), and troglitazone (Rezulin by Parke-Davis) are thiazolidinedione antidiabetic agents. Troglitazone has been discontinued.

Sources.   The thiazolidinediones are oral antidiabetic medications used in the treatment of type 2 diabetes mellitus in humans. They are available in tablet formation only.

Toxicokinetics.   Thiazolidinediones are peroxisome proliferator-activated receptor-gamma (PPARγ) agonists. Pioglitazone has peak plasma concentrations in humans within 2 hours of administration on an empty stomach. Food delays absorption by 1 to 2 hours. Rosiglitazone absorption is not significantly affected by ingesta, with peak plasma concentrations in humans seen about 1 hour after administration. Both pioglitazone and rosiglitazone are highly protein bound and are thought to be metabolized in the liver. The drugs and their metabolites are eliminated in the urine and feces. The half-life of pioglitazone is 3 to 7 hours, with the active metabolites having a half-life of 16 to 24 hours. The half-life of radiolabeled rosiglitazone and metabolites ranged from 103 to 158 hours, with most of the metabolites being inactive.[8]

Mechanism of Action. The thiazolidinediones improve insulin sensitivity by activating PPARγ nuclear receptors, which ultimately leads to increased insulin sensitivity in the liver, muscle, and adipose tissues.[8]

Toxicity and Risk Factors. There are no known species or breed sensitivities to the thiazolidinediones. Toxicosis has occurred with therapeutic use of thiazolidinediones. Women may have a lower rosiglitazone clearance rate and greater therapeutic response to rosiglitazone. Liver disease has also been found to prolong rosiglitazone clearance rates. Therapeutic use of troglitazone has been associated with idiosyncratic hepatotoxicity, liver failure, liver transplants, and death in humans.[8] Death secondary to heart dysfunction occurred in rats treated with 160 mg/kg of pioglitazone daily for 1 year.

Clinical Signs. Little information is available regarding signs caused by acute overdoses of the thiazolidines in humans or animals. Adverse effects in humans reported during clinical trials of rosiglitazone and pioglitazine include edema, upper respiratory tract infection, sinusitis, and headache. Back pain, fatigue, and diarrhea were also reported in clinical trials of rosiglitazone.[8] Anorexia, nausea, malaise, and jaundice was reported in humans with hepatic disease caused by troglitazone.[25]

Clinical Pathology. Anemia has been seen in humans receiving both pioglitazone and rosiglitazone, with decreases in hemoglobin and hematocrit levels. ALT levels were increased greater than 3 times the upper limit of normal in 0.2% of the rosiglitazone-treated human patients and in 0.43% of the pioglitazone patients during controlled trials. Sporadic cases of transient elevations of creatine phosphokinase levels were seen during pioglitazone clinical trials. Hypoglycemia and hyperglycemia have been noted in human diabetics treated with the thiazolidines.[8] Hypoglycemia is not expected following overdoses of the thiazolidines in the normal animal.

Lesions. Ventricular hypertrophy has been noted in the mouse, rat, dog, and monkey following chronic use of large doses of pioglitazone and rosiglitazone and is thought to be caused by volume expansion.[8] Troglitazone use in human diabetics was associated with severe hepatocellular damage 3 to 7 months after treatment was initiated.[25]

Diagnostic Testing. No diagnostic tests are clinically relevant in treating thiazolidinedione toxicosis.

Treatment. No antidote is available for the thiazolidinediones. Treatment of overdose involves decontamination and supportive care for any clinical signs of toxicosis. Decontamination may be warranted in cases of large overdoses and emesis may be induced if initiated within approximately 30 minutes of ingestion of rosiglitazone and within 1 hour of pioglitazone ingestion. Activated charcoal may aid in the removal of the thiazolidinediones from the gastrointestinal tract. Therapeutic use should be discontinued in animals that develop elevated liver enzymes. Liver enzymes should be monitored in cases of large overdoses or in cases of preexisting liver disease.

Prognosis. Prognosis following thiazolidinedione overdose is generally considered to be good in the healthy patient.

Prevention and Control. When the thiazolidinediones are used therapeutically, animals should be monitored for signs of possible hepatotoxicity and heart enlargement.

HYPERTONIC PHOSPHATE ENEMA

Joseph D. Roder

Synonyms. These products are also known as Fleet enemas or dibasic sodium phosphate enemas and are available to the consumer OTC.

Mechanism of Action. Hypertonic phosphate enemas increase the osmolality of the colon. Water then enters into the colon to equilibrate the ionic load. The mechanism of toxicosis relates to the absorption of the phosphate ions in animals and humans.[1,2]

Toxicity and Risk Factors. Cats and small dogs are at greatest risk of intoxication. Cats develop signs of poisoning after administration of 60 ml of a hypertonic phosphate enema. Animals that have underlying renal or hepatic disease are predisposed to toxicosis.[1]

Clinical Signs. Cats poisoned with a hypertonic phosphate enema may present with vomiting, depression, ataxia, bloody diarrhea, or sudden death.[1,3]

Clinical Pathology. Alterations of serum electrolyte concentrations may include hypokalemia, hyperphosphatemia, and hypocalcemia.[1,3] Additionally, animals may have a profound elevation in the serum glucose concentration and commonly have a metabolic acidosis.[1]

Lesions. No lesions were noted in experimental studies of hypertonic phosphate enema intoxication of cats.

Treatment. Administration of intravenous fluids is essential in management of acute intoxication. Fluid therapy should be continued until serum concentrations of potassium, phosphate, and calcium return to normal. The acid-base status should be monitored closely.

Prognosis. Early and aggressive fluid therapy increases the chance of complete recovery.

Prevention and Control. Other types of enemas should be used in small animals. Hypertonic phosphate enemas should not be given to animals with renal disease.

HYPOTHYROID MEDICATIONS

Marcy Rosendale

Synonyms.   Thyroxine (T_4 or 3,5,3′,5′-tetraiodo-L-thyronine) and triiodothyronine (T_3 or 3,5,3′-triiodothyronine) are endocrine hormones produced by the thyroid gland. Several formulations of these hormones are used to treat hypothyroidism in the domestic animal.[1]

A natural preparation of powdered thyroid gland (desiccated thyroid, thyroid extract) is available as Armour Thyroid (Forest Pharmaceuticals, Inc.) and is approved for use in humans. Each 65-mg desiccated thyroid tablet is approximately equivalent to 100 µg or less of levothyroxine sodium, or 25 µg of liothyronine sodium.

Levothyroxine sodium (L-thyroxine sodium, thyroxine sodium, T_4, or T_4 thyroxine sodium) is the synthetic sodium salt of thyroxine. Human-approved levothyroxine sodium products are available as Levothroid (Forest), Levoxyl (Jones Pharma), Synthroid (Knoll Pharmaceutical Company), and Levothyroxine Sodium for Injection (American Pharmaceutical Partners).[2] Veterinary levothyroxine sodium products include formulations approved for dogs: Soloxine (Daniels Pharmaceuticals, Inc.), Thyro-Tabs (Vet-A-Mix), Thyroxine Tablets (Anthony), Thyro-Form (Vet-A-Mix Animal Health), and Heska Chewable Thyroid Supplement for Dogs (Heska). Thyro-L (Vet-A-Mix) is approved for horses.

Liothyronine sodium (sodium L-triiodothyonine, L-triiodothyronine, or T_3 thyronine sodium) is the synthetic sodium salt of triiodothyronine. Cytobin (Pfizer, Inc.) is a liothyronine sodium formulation approved for dogs.[3] Human approved liothyronine sodium products are available as Cytomel (Jones Pharma) and Tiostat (Jones Pharma).

Liotrix (T_3/T_4 liotrix) is a synthetic formulation containing both levothyroxine sodium and liothyronine sodium; Thyrolar (Forest). Liotrix is a human approved product.[2]

Sources.   Natural and synthetic thyroid hormone preparations are available by prescription for the treatment of hypothyroidism in humans, dogs, cats, and horses. Natural preparations of thyroid hormones contain desiccated thyroid glands obtained from slaughterhouses and are available in tablet formulation. Sodium levothyroxine (synthetic T_4) and sodium liothyronine (synthetic T_3) are available in tablet and injectable forms. A preparation containing both synthetic thyroxine and triiodothyronine is available in tablet formulation.[4]

Toxicokinetics.   Levothyroxine is absorbed from the gastrointestinal tract with most of the absorption occurring in the small intestine. Between 40% and 80% of a levothyroxine oral dose is absorbed from the human gastrointestinal tract. Intestinal absorption may be less in the dog. Therapeutic doses of levothyroxine in the adult human are approximately one tenth those of the dog, suggesting that less of the drug is absorbed into the general circulation.[1] The presence of plasma proteins, soluble dietary factors, ferrous sulfate, aluminum hydroxide, sucralfate, or bile acid se-

questrants in the gut may inhibit the absorption of levothyroxine. Absorption is increased with fasting and may be decreased in individuals with malabsorptive states. In contrast, liothyronine is approximately 95% absorbed in the human intestine. In humans, the absorption of the natural thyroid hormones contained in formulations of desiccated thyroid gland is similar to the absorption of the respective synthetic hormones.

Thyroxine is widely distributed in the body, with the highest concentrations found in the liver and kidneys. Thyroid hormones do not cross the placenta readily and minimal amounts are distributed into the milk. Both thyroxine and triiodothyronine are highly protein bound, with thyroxine being more extensively and firmly bound than triiodothyronine.[2]

Thyroxine is deiodinated in peripheral tissues, forming the more metabolically active hormone, triiodothyronine. Tissues containing the highest amounts of the deiodinases are the liver, kidneys, muscle, brain, and heart. When the triiodothyronine found in the peripheral tissues is totally deiodinated, portions of the remaining hormone are metabolized into acetic, lactic, and pyruvic acids. In humans, about 35% of the thyroxine that enters the circulation is deiodinated in the peripheral tissues.[5] In addition to deiodination, the thyroid hormones may also be conjugated to form soluble glucuronides and sulfates that are excreted into the bile or urine. Enterohepatic recirculation of conjugated hormones in the intestines is possible. In the dog, substantial amounts of the thyroid hormones are eliminated in the feces daily, with losses of more than 50% of the thyroxine and approximately 30% of the triiodothyronine.

The plasma half-life of thyroxine is estimated to be between 8 and 16 hours in the dog, 11 hours in the cat, and 7 days in the human. The half-life of triiodothyronine is thought to be 5 to 6 hours in the dog and cat.[4] Peak plasma levels of levothyroxine have been reported to occur between 4 and 12 hours after oral administration in the dog. Peak plasma levels of liothyronine in the dog occur 2 to 5 hours after oral administration.[3]

Mechanism of Action.   Thyroid hormones cause a variety of responses in the body that usually begin with the binding of the hormone to specific receptors (especially nuclear receptors), ultimately leading to protein synthesis. Thyroxine has a lower affinity for nuclear receptors than does triiodothyronine. Thyroid hormones also bind to sites on the mitochondria and can have direct effects on the plasma membrane and the cellular cytoarchitecture. Physiologic responses to the thyroid hormones include the increase in calorigenesis via the stimulation of several organs. The heart, skeletal muscles, liver, and kidneys account for most of the calorigenic effects, ultimately leading to an increase in oxygen consumption in those tissues. Increased cardiac contractility accounts for 30% to 40% of the increase in oxygen consumption attributed to the thyroid hormones.[6] Increased contractility is the result of the direct positive inotropic effects of the hormones as well as an enhanced responsiveness to endogenous catecholamines as a result of the production of increased numbers of beta-adrenergic receptors in the heart. Thyroid hormones also increase the number of beta-adrenergic receptors in skeletal muscle, adipose tissue, and lymphocytes and decrease the number of alpha-adrenergic receptors in cardiac and vascular tissues. Normal circulating levels of the thyroid hormones result in the maintenance of adequate calorigenesis, thus determining the basal or resting metabolic rate. Adequate levels of thyroid hormones are also necessary for normal growth and development, especially in the fetus and neonate.[4]

Toxicity and Risk Factors. Any species of animal that is treated with or accidentally exposed to excessive amounts of thyroid medication is potentially at risk of developing thyroid toxicosis. Dogs are especially prone to consuming large amounts of thyroid pills, frequently consuming entire bottles of thyroid hormones.[7] Alterations of endogenous thyroid hormone production have occurred in horses exposed to excessive amounts of iodine or iodide in medication or feed. Some individual horses may respond to excess iodine by decreasing the amount of thyroid hormone production. In other cases, increased thyroid hormone is produced. Increased thyroid hormone production resulting from excess iodine exposure is referred to as *Jodbasedow thyrotoxicosis.*[8]

Although toxic doses for thyroid hormones have not been established, enough material involving dogs has been published to provide guidelines for assessing exposures in that species. In one study, a group of healthy, euthyroid beagle dogs given oral levothyroxine at doses of 0.5 mg/m² twice daily for 8 weeks did not develop signs of hyperthyroidism.[9] Accidental, acute oral overdoses of less than 0.5 mg/kg of levothyroxine in dogs did not cause clinical signs when decontamination was performed. Mild signs of thyrotoxicosis were seen in a dog accidentally ingesting a single dose of 1.5 mg/kg of levothyroxine.[10] Subcutaneous injections of levothyroxine at 0.13 mg/kg/day for 1 week did not cause signs of hyperthyroidism in a group of mixed breed dogs. When doses in the same group of dogs were increased to 0.67 to 1.01 mg/kg/day over a period of 3 to 4 weeks, a hyperthyroid state was finally induced.

Signs of hyperthyroidism were not observed in a group of four mixed-breed dogs that were fed 300 to 400 mg/kg/day (approximately equivalent to 0.46 to 0.67 mg/kg/day of levothyroxine or 0.12 to 0.17 mg/kg/day of liothyronine) of desiccated thyroid powder over a period of 18 weeks. A separate group of dogs given 500 mg/kg/day (approximately equivalent to 0.8 mg/kg/day of levothyroxine or 0.2 mg/kg/day of liothyronine) for 1 week did not develop signs of hyperthyroidism, but when the dose was increased to 900 to 1000 mg/kg/day (approximately equivalent to 1.4 to 1.7 mg/kg/day of levothyroxine or 0.35 to 0.4 mg/kg/day of liothyronine), significant signs of hyperthyroidism were exhibited.[11] Even though it appears that most dogs are tolerant of acute levothyroxine doses at least 10 to 20 times that of a therapeutic dose (0.022 mg/kg/day or 0.5 mg/m² is usually recommended as a starting dose of levothyroxine for hypothyroidism in dogs[3]), some individual dogs have reportedly developed thyrotoxicosis at much lower doses.[1]

Less is known about potentially toxic doses of triiodothyronine. Estimated triiodothyronine doses from the aforementioned study using desiccated thyroid powder

demonstrated that acute triiodothyronine doses in excess of 20 times a therapeutic dose did not cause signs of thyrotoxicosis in that group of dogs.[11] Ten dogs given 1 mg/kg of subcutaneous triiodothyronine once daily for 14 days in a different study developed signs of hyperthyroidism during the course of treatment. All 10 dogs survived the 14-day treatment period.[12] Therapeutic doses of triiodothyronine for the hypothyroid dog range from 4 to 6 μg/kg per by mouth every 8 hours, with almost complete absorption of the hormone.[3]

Although many of the signs of thyrotoxicosis are similar regardless of species, the dog appears to be at lesser risk of developing cardiac hypertrophy following excessive doses of thyroid hormones than the cat, rat, and pig. Large doses (1 mg/kg/day) of subcutaneous triiodothyronine for 14 days resulted in signs of hyperthyroidism, but did not cause cardiac hypertrophy in dogs. Similar doses for only 7 days caused significant hypertrophy in the cat, rat, and pig, as well as in humans.[12] Thyroid storm is a rare condition causing multiple organ system dysfunction in humans following massive overdoses of thyroid hormones, or in cases of untreated or undertreated hyperthyroidism.[13] Thyroid storm has not been reported in the cat despite hyperthyroidism being the most commonly diagnosed endocrine disease in cats.[14] Older animals and individuals of any age with cardiac disease may be at higher risk of developing thyrotoxicosis following thyroid hormone overdose.[10]

Clinical Signs. Clinical signs of hyperthyroidism reported for the horse include muscle tremors, excitability, tachycardia, sweating, and weight loss.[8] Similar signs, except sweating, have been reported in the dog and cat. In addition, aggressive behavior, polydipsia, polyuria, polyphagia, vomiting, voluminous soft stools, weakness, poor hair coat, heat intolerance, and panting have been reported in the dog and cat. Premature cardiac contractions, heart murmurs, gallop rhythms, and cardiomyopathy (predominantly hypertrophic cardiomyopathy) have been reported in hyperthyroid cats but are not associated with hyperthyroid states in the dog. Long-term use of excessive levothyroxine doses in the dog has caused the same signs as those commonly seen in hyperthyroid states.[1] Acute oral overdoses of thyroid hormones in dogs have produced hyperactivity, tachycardia, tachypnea, dyspnea, abnormal pupillary light reflexes, vomiting, and diarrhea. Lethargy was also noted in some cases.[10] Cats, rats, and pigs given triiodothyronine doses of up to 1 mg/kg for 7 days developed significant cardiac hypertrophy.[12] Acute overdoses of thyroid medications are not expected to cause the poor hair coat or significant weight loss seen in hyperthyroid states. Even though hyperthermia is seen in human cases of thyrotoxicosis, it is not well documented in domesticated animals.

Clinical Pathology. Long-term overdoses of thyroid hormones may result in abnormalities that resemble hyperthyroid states. Clinical pathologic abnormalities seen in some hyperthyroid cats that may be attributed to excessive thyroid hormones include mild to moderate elevations in liver enzymes, mild elevations in the packed cell volume, and a stress leukogram.

Significant abnormalities in routine clinical pathology are not expected following acute overdoses of thyroid hormones. An increased red blood cell count has been seen in dogs given large doses of thyroid hormones.[1] Abnormalities in CBC and serum chemistry values were not noted in a dog exhibiting clinical signs of thyrotoxicosis along with elevated serum thyroid hormone levels following an acute overdose of levothyroxine sodium.[10]

Lesions. Specific pathologic lesions are not expected in most cases of acute thyroid hormone overdose in the dog. Ventricular hypertrophy has been seen in cats, rats, and pigs after 7 consecutive days of triiodothyronine overdoses, but not in dogs.[12] Hypertrophy of the heart as well as chronic passive congestion of the lungs and liver were seen in three dogs that died of apparent cardiac failure during an 18-week course of thyroid hormone-induced thyrotoxicosis.[11] Centri-lobular fatty infiltration and mild hepatic necrosis or degeneration have been seen in histologic samples from hyperthyroid cats.[15]

Diagnostic Testing. Acute overdoses of thyroid hormones are expected to cause elevations of serum triiodothyronine and thyroxine values. Serum triiodothyronine and thyroxine values were obtained from a dog following an acute over-dose of up to 10.12 mg/kg of levothyroxine sodium tablets. Both triiodothyronine and thyroxine levels were elevated within 3 and 9 hours after ingestion, with values slowly declining into the normal range over the course of 6 and 36 days, respectively. The initial serum thyroxine concentration in this case was 4900.9 nmol/L (normal range of 5.3 to 26.7 nmol/L).[10] Most veterinary commercial laboratories use human radioimmunoassay (RIA) kits to determine serum triiodothyronine and thyroxine levels. Both triiodothyronine and thyroxine are relatively stable and resistant to degradation. Serum or plasma (heparinized or EDTA) samples may be stored for up to 8 days at room temperature. Sending frozen serum samples on cold packs is the preferred method for thyroid hormone measurement.[1] Although elevated thyroid hormone levels may confirm an exposure, the results may not correlate to the severity of signs and should not influence the treatment protocol.

Treatment. Treatment of thyroid hormone overdoses includes prompt decontamination and supportive care until signs resolve. Oral overdoses that are equal to or greater than 10 times the therapeutic dose of either hormone warrant decontamination within approximately 1 hour of a triiodothyronine ingestion and within 2 hours of a thyroxine ingestion in healthy adult dogs and cats. Exposures that involve large numbers of pills may benefit from decontamination several hours after ingestion because of delayed breakdown and absorption of pills. Emesis that is productive and performed shortly after the exposure may be sufficient decontamination in most cases of oral overdoses. Individuals with large overdoses that approach or exceed 25 times a therapeutic dose of either hormone should also receive one dose of activated charcoal and a cathartic. In cases of delayed decontamination, activated charcoal and a cathartic without emesis are recommended, especially when clinical

signs are evident. Although enterohepatic recirculation is possible, repeat doses of activated charcoal are not usually necessary given the low morbidity and mortality following most thyroid hormone overdoses. Individuals that are geriatric or suffer from cardiac disease may warrant more aggressive decontamination at lower overdose amounts.

Individuals receiving overdoses of the thyroid hormones should be monitored for appropriate signs of thyrotoxicosis. Signs in dogs generally occur within a few hours of ingestion of either hormone. Signs in humans may be delayed for as much as several days following an overdose of thyroxine. Delayed reactions to acute overdoses of thyroid hormones are not common in the dog. Given the difference in the half-lives of the thyroid hormones in humans compared with those in dogs and cats, delayed signs are less likely in these species.

Supportive care should be provided in cases with significant clinical signs. Sedation may be necessary when agitation or hyperactivity is present. Phenobarbital has been used to sedate human pediatric patients with thyrotoxicosis.[5] Intravenous propranolol may be used to control tachycardia in cases when the heart rate exceeds 160 to 180 beats per minute but should be avoided in cases of cardiovascular compromise. Animals with preexisting health conditions showing signs of thyrotoxicosis should be closely monitored and given any necessary supportive care.

Prognosis. The prognosis in most cases of acute thyroid hormone overdose is good in healthy adult dogs and cats receiving appropriate medical treatment.

Prevention and Control. Thyroid medications should be kept away from pets. Dermal and oral exposure of horses to products containing large amounts of iodine should be limited when possible and discontinued if signs of thyrotoxicosis occur.

METHYLXANTHINES

Jay C. Albretsen

Synonyms. Theophylline, caffeine, and theobromine are three closely related alkaloids that occur naturally in many plants. They are methylated xanthine derivatives.[1,2] The solubility of these methylxanthines is low, but is enhanced by the formation of complexes. One of the most notable is the complex of theophylline and ethylenediamine to form the drug aminophylline. Other methylxanthine complex productions are oxtriphylline (a theophylline complex) and dyphylline.

Sources. Methylxanthines are naturally occurring alkaloids in several foods and beverages all over the world as well as in some veterinary and human medications. Table 24-4 lists several products and the range of methylxanthines found in those products.

Methylxanthines are found in the leaves of *Thea sinonis* (used to make tea), in the seeds of *Theobrema cacao* (used to make chocolate), the fruit of *Coffea anabrica* (used to

TABLE 24-4 **Methylxanthine Content in Various Products**

Product	Caffeine	Theobromine	Other Comments
Coffee and Tea			
Regular coffee	8-30 mg/oz		
Decaffeinated coffee	0.4-1 mg/oz		
Tea brewed	1.8-10 mg/oz		
Tea instant	2.4-6.2 mg/oz		
Candy			
Chocolate covered candy bar	2-7 mg/oz	16-58 mg/oz	
Milk chocolate	6 mg/oz	44-56 mg/oz	
Dark chocolate	5-35 mg/oz	134 mg/oz	
Semisweet chocolate	22 mg/oz	138 mg/oz	
White chocolate	0.85 mg/oz	0.25 mg/oz	
Chocolate Cakes and Cookies			
Chocolate frosted	240 mg/cake		About 12 pieces/cake
Unfrosted	120 mg/cake		About 12 pieces/cake
Oreos	2.4 mg/cookie	15 mg/cookie	
Soft Drinks			
Colas	2.5-3.8 mg/oz		
Diet colas	0.2-4.8 mg/oz		
Decaffeinated	Trace		
Other caffeinated soft drinks	3.7-6 mg/oz		
Other Drinks			
Hot chocolate	0.33-1.33 mg/oz	75 mg/6 oz	
Chocolate milk	0.25-0.875 mg/oz	40 mg/8 oz	
Chocolate syrup	5 mg/serving	69 mg/serving	1 oz (2 Tbsp)/serving
Other Products			
Cocoa	5-42 mg/oz	130-737 mg/oz	
Baking chocolate	8-118 mg/oz	393 mg/oz	
Coffee beans	1%-2%		
Cocoa Bean Hulls	0.5%-0.85%		
Guarana	3%-5%		

Data from references 2, 3, 4, 7.

make coffee), and the nuts of *Cola acuninata* (extracts in soft drinks).[1] To be more specific, theophylline is found in tea and in medications. Caffeine is present in coffee, tea, chocolate, colas, the herb guarana, and some human stimulant drugs. Theobromine is available in chocolate, cocoa beans, cocoa bean hulls, cola, and tea.[2,3]

Toxicokinetics. In general, methylxanthines are absorbed readily after oral, rectal, or parenteral administration.[1,4] The type of preparation of theophylline can affect the absorption of these medications. For example, sustained-release preparations of theophylline are usually not completely absorbed for 6 to 8 hours after ingestion. In overdoses of sustained-release theophylline, absorption can take up to 24 hours. No significant presystemic clearance (first pass effect) exists.[4]

Food generally slows the rate of theophylline absorption. Food also can affect (by either increasing or decreasing) the bioavailability of sustained-release forms of theophylline.[1]

In people, sleep or recumbency may reduce the rate of theophylline absorption.[1] Caffeine absorption is relatively unaffected by food. However, in people, peak plasma levels are not achieved for 30 to 60 minutes after ingestion.[4]

TABLE 24–5 **Methylxanthine Elimination Half-Lives in Several Species**

	Theophylline	Caffeine	Theobromine
Dogs	5.7 hr	4.5 hr	17.5 hr
Humans	7-10 hr	3-60 hr	
Human neonates	20-36 hr	1.5-6 days	
Cats	7.8 h		
Rats		1.5-2 hr	
Mice		1.5 h	
Rabbits		3.8 hr	

Data from references 1-4, 7.

Methylxanthines are distributed to all body compartments. The apparent volume of distribution of caffeine and theophylline is similar, between 0.4 and 0.6 L/kg. Theophylline is bound to plasma protein to a greater extent than caffeine. The fraction bound to proteins decreases as the concentration of methylxanthines increases. In normal healthy humans at therapeutic doses, theophylline is 60% protein bound.[1] Methylxanthines do cross the placenta and are passed into the milk.[1]

The liver is the primary site of methylxanthine metabolism. Methylxanthines and their metabolites, in general, can be eliminated in bile and urine, depending on species, age, and health of the animal.[1,3,4] Age variations play a part in theophylline excretion. Theophylline is primarily excreted in the urine of neonates.[4] Less than 15% of theophylline and 5% of caffeine are eliminated unchanged in the urine of humans.[1] Most caffeine is eliminated by bile in rabbits.[5] Enterohepatic recirculation and reabsorption from the urinary tract have been reported for methylxanthine compounds.[1,4] In rabbits, mice, hamsters, and dogs, 60% to 89% of an oral theobromine dose was eliminated in the urine.[6] Elimination half-lives are variable between species. Half-lives are prolonged in overdose situations, and they seem to be age dependent.[4,7] Table 24-5 lists half-lives of caffeine, theobromine, and theophylline in several species.

Mechanism of Action. Several mechanisms of action have been proposed for methylxanthines in the body. Currently, the mechanism with the most clinical relevance is the competitive antagonism of adenosine receptors by methylxanthines. Evidence suggests that these cellular adenosine receptors are blocked at both therapeutic and toxic doses of methylxanthines.[1,2,4] Adenosine is a bronchoconstrictor, an anticonvulsant, and a regulator of cardiac rhythm. These are considered opposite many methylxanthine effects.[2] Adenosine receptors are linked to cAMP through guanine nucleotide binding regulatory proteins (G proteins), as well as to other intracellular effector systems.

A second clinically relevant theory regarding the mechanism of action of methylxanthine is that it affects intracellular calcium levels. Methylxanthines increase the amount of calcium entering cells. They also inhibit the uptake and sequestration of calcium by the sarcoplasmic reticulum of striated muscle,[2,4] causing increased strength and contractility of skeletal muscles.[2]

Another theory is that methylxanthines inhibit cellular phosphodiesterase, causing an increase in intracellular cAMP. Many things are affected by increased cAMP, including the regulation of potassium channels.[1,4] However, at therapeutic levels, theophylline causes negligible inhibition of phosphodiesterase in humans.[4] The levels of methylxanthines capable of inhibiting phosphodiesterase in vivo are probably only achieved in overdose situations.[6]

Sympathetic nervous system stimulation is also a proposed mechanism of methylxanthine action. At therapeutic levels of theophylline, increased levels of the circulating catecholamines epinephrine and norepinephrine are found.[4] Increases in circulating catecholamines have been directly related to hypokalemia, metabolic acidosis, and cardiac disturbances in dogs poisoned with theophylline.[4] The clinical significance of this effect is unclear.

Toxicity and Risk Factors. Animal poisonings caused by methylxanthines are common, usually due to dogs ingesting chocolate; however, all animals can be affected by methylxanthines. Occasionally, inappropriate use of methylxanthine products in animals has been reported. Caffeine has been used in horses to enhance their racing abilities, but it is illegal to do so.[2] Table 24-6 lists lethal and toxic oral doses of the most common methylxanthines in humans, dogs, cats, and rats.

In people, older and younger patients are at a greater risk of developing toxicosis after chronic theophylline use, even at therapeutic doses.[4] This age difference is not present in acute overdoses and does not seem to be a factor with other methylxanthines.

Clinical Signs. The clinical signs associated most frequently with each methylxanthine are listed below. Often (as with chocolate ingestion), more than one methylxanthine has been ingested and is responsible for the signs that develop.

Caffeine. The most common signs of caffeine toxicosis in animals are vomiting, restlessness, hyperactivity, tachycardia, and tachypnea. These initial signs can lead to muscle tremors, seizures, cyanosis, and other cardiac arrhythmias.[2,7]

Theobromine. In dogs, the usual signs of theobromine poisoning are vomiting, diarrhea, polyuria, hyperactivity, cardiac arrhythmias (e.g., tachycardia or premature ventricular contractions), hyperthermia, tremors, and seizures. The signs may also include hematuria, muscle weakness, bradycardia, dehydration, coma, and death.[2,7]

Theophylline. The signs and symptoms of theophylline intoxication can be separated into four body systems. The first body system, and usually the most sensitive to theophylline, is the gastrointestinal system. Theophylline overdoses cause nausea and vomiting. Second, theophylline

TABLE 24–6 Toxic Oral Dosages of Methylxanthines in Several Species

	Theobromine	Theophylline	Caffeine
Dog	250-500 mg/kg (LD$_{50}$)	290 mg/kg (LD$_{50}$)	140-150 mg/kg (MLD)
Human	115 mg/kg (MLD) 26 mg/kg (MTD)	5 mg/kg/day (MTD)	150-200 mg/kg (MLD)
Cat	200 mg/kg (LD$_{50}$)	800 mg/kg (LD$_{50}$)	100-150 mg/kg (MLD)
Rat	1265 mg/kg (LD$_{50}$)	225 mg/kg (LD$_{50}$)	174-210 mg/kg (LD$_{50}$)

Data from references 1, 2, 4, 7, 9. *MTD*, Minimum toxic dose; *MLD*, minimum lethal dose; *LD$_{50}$*, lethal dose in 50% of tested animals.

affects the musculoskeletal system, causing tremors and weakness. The third body system affected by theophylline is the cardiovascular system. Hypotension, tachycardia, premature ventricular contractions, and other cardiac arrhythmias can occur. These signs may be life threatening to the animal if the signs are not controlled. The fourth body system is the neurologic system. Theophylline overdoses cause agitation, seizures, hyperactivity, and other behavioral abnormalities.[2,4,7]

Clinical Pathology. No specific clinical pathology abnormalities have been reported for caffeine and theobromine overdoses. In human patients, theophylline overdoses are often associated with hyperglycemia and hypokalemia.[4] In addition, metabolic acidosis, hypomagnesemia, and hypophosphatemia have been reported in human theophylline toxicoses.[4]

Lesions. No specific lesions produced by methylxanthines occur.

Diagnostic Testing. Methylxanthines and their metabolites can be measured in several different samples. Serum, plasma, various tissues, urine, and even stomach contents can be used.[2,4] However, methylxanthine screening may not be part of the normal tests run at every diagnostic laboratory. The local diagnostic laboratory should be consulted regarding this matter before samples are sent for analysis.[2,4] Methylxanthines are stable in serum or plasma for 14 days and for 4 months, respectively. They are also excreted in milk.[2]

Treatment. No antidote for methylxanthine toxicosis is available. Consequently, when treating a methylxanthine poisoning, four areas of therapy should be considered: (1) decontamination, (2) basic life support, (3) symptomatic care, and (4) hastening elimination.

Decontamination is best accomplished by emesis, gastric lavage, and administration of activated charcoal. In any case, decontamination *should not be done* if the animal is showing significant clinical signs. It is important to take care of any life-threatening signs before decontaminating the animal. Emesis is most successful when the methylxanthine ingestion was within the past 2 hours. Hydrogen peroxide (1 tsp/5 lb), syrup of ipecac (1 to 2 ml/kg in dogs, and 3.3 ml/kg in cats), apomorphine (0.03 mg/kg intravenously, 0.04 mg/kg intramuscularly [generally only used in dogs]), and xylazine (1.1 mg/kg intramuscularly or subcutaneously) are examples of emetics.[8] In the case of chocolate poisoning, the chocolate can form a ball or lump in the stomach of the animal. This lump may remain in the stomach for several hours. Consequently, emesis may be of value in dogs more than 2 hours after the chocolate was ingested; however, these lumps of chocolate may be difficult to remove.[2] Gastric lavage may be performed, but a large-bore tube should be used with copious amounts of water. To safely perform gastric lavage, the animal must be unconscious or lightly anesthetized, and an endotracheal tube should be used to protect the respiratory tract.[8]

Activated charcoal can be given to prevent absorption of the methylxanthines. The recommended dose in all animals is 1 to 4 g/kg by mouth. Activated charcoal adsorbs the methylxanthines, but if it remains in the intestinal tract for a long period of time, it could release the methylxanthines and allow them to be absorbed by the animal. To prevent this, activated charcoal is often mixed with a cathartic (such as 70% sorbitol, magnesium, or sodium sulfate at a dose of 250 mg/kg).[8] Multiple doses of activated charcoal have been recommended in dogs because of the long half-life of theobromine in dogs. Enterohepatic recirculation may occur, and it is thought that the charcoal, when given multiple times, acts as a sink to bind methylxanthine metabolites and prevent them from being accessible to the bacteria in the lower intestinal tract. These bacteria may take methylxanthine metabolites and alter them in such a way as to allow them to be reabsorbed by the animal.[2]

Basic life support is the most important care to be given in symptomatic animals. Initially, respiratory and cardiovascular health should be monitored. If necessary, artificial ventilation and fluid therapy should be given to control respiratory difficulties and shock. If the animal is seizuring, diazepam (0.5 to 2 mg/kg intravenously), phenobarbital (2 to 6 mg/kg intravenously slowly), other barbiturates, or gas anesthetics can be used to control the convulsions if necessary.[2]

Symptomatic care includes treating other clinical signs of methylxanthine overdose. Tremors can often be controlled with diazepam (0.5 to 2 mg/kg intravenously) or methocarbamol (50 to 220 mg/kg intravenously slowly, not to exceed 330 mg/kg/day). An ECG of the animal should be done if possible. Bradycardias can be treated with atropine (0.01 to 0.02 mg/kg intravenously). Tachyarrhythmias can be controlled using a beta-blocker such as propranolol or metoprolol (0.04 to 0.06 mg/kg intravenously; the rate of administration should not exceed 1 mg/2 minutes when given intravenously). Because propranolol reduces theophylline clearance in humans, metoprolol is preferred over propranolol in cases of theophylline toxicosis. Other drugs that may affect methylxanthine clearance include erythromycin, corticosteroids, and cimetidine.[1] Consequently, the use of these drugs should be avoided. Ventricular tachyarrhythmias in dogs can also be treated with lidocaine (1 to 2 mg/kg intravenously followed by a 0.1% solution administered at 30 to 50 µg/min).[2] Lidocaine should not be used in cats. Other clinical signs can be treated as they arise.

Finally, to help speed elimination, multiple doses of activated charcoal are indicated as discussed previously.[4] Activated charcoal (1 to 4 g/kg orally) can be given up to every 3 hours for as long as 72 hours.[2] A cathartic should be given daily as long as the animal does not already have diarrhea. It may also be advantageous to catheterize the bladder. Methylxanthines and their metabolites can be reabsorbed in the urinary tract from the urine.[2]

Prognosis. It is rare for deaths to occur following caffeine and theobromine overdoses because of the large quantities of these methylxanthines that animals must consume to reach a lethal dose. In animals that develop clinical signs of methylxanthine toxicosis, most recover within 24 to 48 hours if the signs are controlled. If the signs are not controlled, the prognosis is guarded to poor.

TABLE 24–7 **Summary of Mechanism and Signs of Toxicosis Related to Skeletal Muscle Relaxants**

Agent	Proposed Mechanism of Action	Signs of Toxicosis
Neuromuscular Blocking Agents		
Depolarizing		
Succinylcholine	Depolarizes motor endplate of myoneural junction by acting as acetylcholine agonist	Prolonged paralysis, apnea
Nondepolarizing		
Atracurium Cisatracurium Doxacurium Mivacurium Pancuronium Rocuronium Tubocurarine Vecuronium	Competitively block access of acetylcholine to motor endplate receptors of myoneural junction	Prolonged paralysis, apnea
Centrally Acting Skeletal Muscle Relaxants		
Baclofen	Presynaptic gamma-amino butyric acid (GABA) agonist	Depression, agitation, vocalization, ataxia, hyporeflexia, hypothermia, respiratory depression, bradycardia, hypotension, hypertension, tachycardia, coma, seizure
Carisoprodol Chlorphenesin carbamate Chlorzoxazone Metaxalone Methocarbamol	General central nervous system sedation; mechanism of muscle relaxation is unknown but is not due to direct effect on muscle	Stupor, coma, hypotension, respiratory depression
Cyclobenzaprine	Related to tricyclic antidepressants; potentiation of norepinephrine; anticholinergic effect	Similar to tricyclic antidepressants: tachycardia, hyperactivity, cardiac arrhythmias, seizures, anticholinergic effects
Orphenadrine	Antimuscarinic agent; may affect cerebral motor centers; also has antihistaminic and local anesthetic action	Anticholinergic effects: tachycardia, weakness, gastrointestinal disturbances, agitation, seizures
Agents with Direct Effect on Skeletal Muscle		
Dantrolene	Reduces release of calcium from the sarcoplasmic reticulum, decreasing muscle contraction	Paralysis, respiratory compromise, crystalluria, hepatopathy

Prevention and Control. Keep candy and other sources of methylxanthines away from animals.

MUSCLE RELAXANTS

Sharon Gwaltney-Brant

Synonyms. Skeletal muscle relaxants encompass a wide range of drugs with different mechanisms of action. Skeletal muscle relaxants may be peripherally acting or centrally acting. Peripherally acting relaxants include dantrolene, which acts directly on skeletal muscle, and the neuromuscular blockers, atracurium besylate (Tracrium), decamethonium bromide (Syncurine, C-10), gallamine (Flaxedil), metocurine (Metubine),

pancuronium bromide (Pavulon), rocuronium bromide (Zemuron), succinylcholine (Anectine, Quelicin, Sucostrin), tubocurarine chloride (Tubarine), and vecuronium bromide (Norcuron). Centrally acting skeletal muscle relaxants include baclofen (Lioresal) carisoprodol (Soma), chlorphenesin carbamate (Maolate), chlorzoxazone (Parafon Forte) , cyclobenzaprine (Flexeril), guaifenesin (Gecolate), metaxalone (Skelaxin), methocarbamol (Robaxin, Robaxin-V), and orphenadrine (Norflex). A summary of the different classes of skeletal muscle relaxants is listed in Table 24-7. Diazepam (Valium), a benzodiazepine, is also used as a skeletal muscle relaxant in some instances, but it is not included in this discussion.

Sources. Neuromuscular blocking agents are used primarily as adjuncts for surgical anesthesia of human and veterinary patients when significant muscle relaxation is desired.[1] Because consciousness and pain sensation are not affected by these agents, they are not to be used as sole anesthetic agents for surgical procedures.[2,3] Dantrolene is used in humans for the treatment of upper motor neuron disorders such as multiple sclerosis and cerebral palsy. In both human and veterinary medicine, dantrolene is used to prevent and treat malignant hyperthermia. Additional uses of dantrolene in veterinary medicine include treatment of functional urethral obstruction in dogs and cats, prevention and treatment of equine postanesthetic myositis, treatment of equine exertional rhabdomyolysis, treatment of small animal black widow spider envenomation, and treatment of porcine stress syndrome.[3] Oral skeletal muscle relaxants (e.g., baclofen, carisoprodol, methocarbamol) are used in human medicine to relieve muscle spasms and discomfort from trauma and dyskinetic disorders. Guaifenesin is used in veterinary medicine as an adjunct to anesthesia in large and small animals, and it is present in many human cold or cough medications in which it is used as an expectorant.[1,3] Methocarbamol is approved for use in veterinary medicine for reduction of muscle spasms and as a treatment for traumatic and inflammatory skeletal muscle disorders.[3]

Toxicokinetics. Neuromuscular blockers are ionized at physiologic pH and therefore are poorly absorbed from the gastrointestinal tract.[2] For this reason, neuromuscular blocking agents are only administered by intravenous or, occasionally, intramuscular injection. Following injection, neuromuscular blocking agents distribute throughout the extracellular space, concentrating at myoneural junctions.[2] Most of these agents have a short duration of action resulting from redistribution to other extracellular compartments (e.g., tubocurarine) or rapid inactivation by plasma esterases and spontaneous degradation (e.g., atracurium).[2] Some, such as pancuronium, are excreted unchanged in the urine, and renal insufficiency can prolong their duration of action.[2] Vecuronium is metabolized in the liver and excreted in the bile; hepatic insufficiency or drug overdose may result in cumulative effects with repeated doses.[2]

Succinylcholine is rapidly hydrolyzed by plasma pseudocholinesterase to succinylmonocholine, which has some activity.[2] This metabolite is further degraded into succinic acid and choline, which can be used by the body for normal cellular metabolism. Species variability in sensitivity to succinylcholine may be due to species differences in activity of pseudocholinesterases.[2]

Dantrolene is poorly (35%) absorbed from the gastrointestinal tract and reaches peak plasma levels in 4 to 6 hours after ingestion.[4] Dantrolene has a relatively wide volume of distribution and is metabolized by the liver.[5] In humans, dantrolene has a half-life of 6 to 8 hours.[4]

Guaifenesin has poor oral absorption and large oral doses must be administered for therapeutic effect.[3] For this reason, when used for its muscle relaxant effects, guaifenesin is usually administered parenterally, most often intravenously. In horses, guaifenesin induces recumbency within 2 minutes of intravenous administration and the duration of action of a single dose is 10 to 20 minutes.[3] Guaifenesin is metabolized in the liver and excreted through the urine. The half-life of guaifenesin in ponies is 60 to 85 minutes.[3]

Baclofen is well absorbed orally and reaches peak blood levels within 2 hours,[4] although at high doses, complete absorption may be prolonged over several hours.[6] Baclofen has low protein binding and a wide volume of distribution; baclofen crosses the placenta but does not cross the blood-brain barrier at therapeutic levels.[4] Up to 80% of the drug is eliminated unchanged in the urine, with less than 20% undergoing hepatic metabolism.[4] The half-life of baclofen in humans is 2.5 to 4 hours, but in overdose situations, the half-life has been reported to increase to as much as 34 hours as a result of saturation of metabolic and elimination mechanisms.[4]

Carisoprodol is well absorbed orally and reaches peak plasma levels within 2 hours.[5] Carisoprodol is rapidly distributed to the CNS. The drug is metabolized via dealkylation, hydroxylation, and conjugation in the liver.[5] The major metabolite is meprobamate, which has sedative activity; most metabolites are excreted in the urine.[5] Chlormezanone is structurally similar to carisoprodol and has similar kinetics.[4]

Chlorzoxazone is rapidly absorbed from the gastrointestinal tract and has a rapid onset of action.[4] The drug has a small volume of distribution and a short half-life (1 hour in humans). Chlorzoxazone is metabolized in the liver, and metabolites are excreted in the urine.[4]

Cyclobenzaprine has slow oral absorption, with peak levels occurring in 3 to 8 hours after ingestion. Cyclobenzaprine is highly (93%) protein bound, exhibits a first pass hepatic metabolism, and may undergo enterohepatic recirculation.[5] Cyclobenzaprine is excreted through the urine almost entirely as inactive metabolites. The half-life of cyclobenzaprine in humans is 24 to 72 hours.[5]

Metaxalone is rapidly absorbed from the gastrointestinal tract, with onset of action within 1 hour and peak plasma levels within 2 hours of ingestion.[1] It is not known whether metaxalone crosses the placenta or enters the milk.[1] Metaxalone undergoes hepatic metabolism and metabolites are excreted in the urine.[1] In humans, the duration of action at therapeutic levels is 4 to 6 hours and the half-life is 2 to 3 hours.

Methocarbamol and chlorphenesin are structurally related. Both drugs are rapidly absorbed orally, and onset of action is within 30 minutes after ingestion.[4] These drugs have wide volumes of distribution, hepatic metabolism, and urinary excretion of metabolites (guaifenesin is a minor metabolite of these drugs). Half-lives range from 1 hour for methocarbamol to 2 to 5 hours for chlorphenesin.[4]

Orphenadrine is rapidly and completely absorbed from the gastrointestinal tract, with peak levels occurring 2 to 4 hours after an oral dose. Delayed absorption may occur as a result of the anticholinergic effects of orphenadrine.[4] Orphenadrine has low protein binding and reaches high concentrations in the liver and lungs.[5] Orphenadrine is metabolized in the liver to at least eight metabolites, which are excreted in the urine or bile; orphenadrine undergoes significant enterohepatic recirculation.[4] The half-life of orphenadrine in humans is 15 hours for a single dose and may increase to 40 hours with long-term dosages.[5]

Mechanism of Action. Neuromuscular blocking agents are classified as depolarizing or nondepolarizing, depending on the mechanism by which they affect postsynaptic receptors.

Depolarizing agents such as succinylcholine and deca-methonium bind to and cause initial depolarization of the postsynaptic membrane similar to the endogenous neuro-transmitter acetylcholine.[2] Unlike acetylcholine, which is rapidly hydrolyzed to allow repolarization of the neuronal membrane, succinylcholine and similar drugs remain at the postsynaptic receptors, resulting in prolonged membrane depolarization. Inhibition of further impulse transmission causes flaccid paralysis of the muscle. The initial de-polarization from succinylcholine results in transient muscle fasciculation before paralysis; this effect may not be apparent in animals that are anesthetized before succinylcholine administration.[2] Succinylcholine increases serum potassium levels as a result of efflux of potassium from cells, and it increases intraocular, intracranial, and intragastric pressures.[7]

Nondepolarizing neuromuscular blockers include the curare family of drugs (e.g., tubocurarine, atracurium). These drugs occupy acetylcholine receptors on the nicotinic cholinergic receptors on skeletal muscle cells, thereby com-petitively inhibiting acetylcholine-mediated signal trans-mission.[2] None of the neuromuscular blocking agents cross the blood-brain barrier to enter the CNS; therefore, no central effects occur and animals treated with these agents remain conscious and able to feel pain. For this reason, the use of neuromuscular blockers as sole "anesthetic" agents for surgical procedures is considered inappropriate and inhumane.[2] Some neuromuscular blockers (e.g., succinyl-choline, atracurium) can trigger histamine release.[2]

Dantrolene exerts its effects directly on skeletal muscle by inhibiting the release of calcium by the sarcoplasmic reticulum, decreasing the force of muscle contraction.[4] This effect does not occur in cardiac or smooth muscle.

Baclofen mimics GABA within the spinal cord, blocking excitatory responses to sensory input. Once considered to be a GABA agonist,[4] baclofen is now thought to act at a unique site on the nerve terminal.[5] At therapeutic levels, baclofen has virtually no CNS effect as a result of its inability to cross the blood-brain barrier; however, in overdose situations, CNS effects are obvious.[4] When administered intrathecally, baclo-fen is also an inhibitor of substance P, a stimulatory com-pound within the brain stem, and it reduces myocardial epinephrine and norepinephrine content.[5]

Carisoprodol and chlormezanone are related to the sedative drug meprobamate. These drugs appear to depress postsynaptic spinal reflexes, but much of the skeletal muscle relaxation properties are due to their sedative effects.[4] Similarly, the mechanism of muscle relaxation from chlor-zoxazone and metaxalone is not clear, but it may be related to the CNS depressant effects of these drugs.

Cyclobenzaprine is structurally related to amitriptyline, a tricyclic antidepressant.[4] Its skeletal muscle relaxation activity is related to its anticholinergic effects, because it inhibits central and peripheral muscarinic activity.[5]

Methocarbamol, chlorphenesin, and guaifenesin act by blocking nerve impulse transmission within the brain stem, spinal cord, and subcortical levels of the brain. At least part of the skeletal muscle relaxant effects of these drugs are due

to their sedative effects.[4] Guaifenesin blocks polysynaptic reflexes more effectively than monosynaptic reflexes.[2] Gua-ifenesin has marked sedative and hypnotic effects resulting from depression of the reticular formation of the brain stem.[2]

Orphenadrine is structurally related to diphenhydramine and has prominent anticholinergic effects.[4] Orphenadrine depresses myocardial contraction and cardiac conduction, produces peripheral cholinergic blockade, has central de-pressant activity, and has some degree of histaminic and local anesthetic activity.[5]

Toxicity and Risk Factors.   There are few established toxic doses for skeletal muscle relaxants in animals. Baclofen has produced significant clinical signs in dogs at estimated doses of less than 5 mg/kg,[6] and ingestion of 150 mg in adult humans has been associated with serious intoxication.[5] Guaifenesin reportedly has a margin of safety of 3 times the therapeutic dose, resulting in a potential minimum toxic dose of approximately 132 mg/kg in dogs, 165 mg/kg in cattle and horses, 132 mg/kg in swine, and 198 mg/kg in goats.[3]

Variation exists between species in their relative sensitivity to succinylcholine, with bovines and canines being more sensitive, and equines and porcines being more resistant. These differences are likely due to species differences in activity of pseudocholinesterases. Aminoglycoside antibiotic exposure, organophosphate exposure, and prior treatment with cholinesterase inhibitors have been reported to prolong the effects of succinylcholine.[13] In addition, conditions such as chronic anemia, hepatic disease, and malnutrition may decrease plasma cholinesterase levels and result in pro-longation of muscle relaxation induced by succinylcholine.[7] Elevations in serum potassium levels from succinylcholine may result in severe hyperkalemia in animals with severe burns, trauma, or neuromuscular disease.[3,7]

Animals with preexisting cardiovascular disease may be particularly sensitive to the potential cardiovascular effects of drugs such as succinylcholine, atracurium, baclofen, and orphenadrine.[5] Hepatic or renal dysfunction may delay metabolism or excretion of many skeletal muscle relaxants.[1]

Clinical Signs.   Neuromuscular blocking agents cause flaccid paralysis, beginning with the head, neck, and tail. The paralysis is progressive and affects the limbs, laryngeal muscles, abdominal muscles, intercostals, and diaphragm, in order. Signs of paralysis resolve in a reverse sequence.[2] Rapid administration of tubocurarine may cause hypotension in dogs.[2] At therapeutic levels, these agents can cause malignant hyperthermia, rhabdomyolysis, hypersalivation, hyperkalemia, bradycardia, tachycardia, hypertension, hypo-tension, arrhythmias, and histamine release, resulting in urticaria, dermal flushing, and bronchospasm.[3]

Toxic effects of dantrolene include gastrointestinal upset, CNS depression, muscle weakness, hypotension, and chem-ical hepatopathy (most commonly associated with chronic use but sometimes seen with high single doses).[5] The hepatic effects range from reversible hepatitis to acute fulminant hepatic necrosis. Very large doses may result in crystalluria, with resulting renal injury. Humans have low mortality from dantrolene overdose.[5]

In general, toxicosis from centrally acting skeletal muscle relaxants presents as depression, hypotension, and hypothermia; in severe cases, coma and respiratory muscle depression requiring ventilatory support may result.[4] In dogs, signs of baclofen overdose include hypertension, bradycardia, tachycardia, vomiting, respiratory depression, muscular hypotonia, vocalization, miosis, seizures, and coma. Signs have been reported to persist up to several days after exposure.[6] Overdose of guaifenesin may result in paradoxical muscle rigidity, apneustic breathing, nystagmus, and hypotension.[3] In humans with carisoprodol toxicosis, tachycardia, CNS depression, agitation, myoclonus, respiratory depression, coma, and death have been reported.[5,8] Because of its structural similarity to TCAs, cyclobenzaprine might be expected to behave similarly to TCAs in an overdose situation. In humans, the most commonly reported effects of cyclobenzaprine overdose included tachycardia, hypertension, hypotension, lethargy, and signs of cholinergic blockade (agitation, confusion, and hallucination); deaths from cyclobenzaprine toxicosis are uncommon in humans.[5] Orphenadrine has marked anticholinergic effects and, in humans, orphenadrine toxicosis resembles TCA toxicosis, resulting in tachycardia, cardiac arrhythmia, hypotension, hypothermia, seizures, and coma.[5]

Clinical Pathology. Few specific clinical pathologic alterations are expected with most skeletal muscle relaxant toxicoses. Baseline liver and kidney values should be obtained to determine whether preexisting disorders exist that may interfere with drug elimination. Succinylcholine has been reported to exacerbate hyperkalemic states at therapeutic doses,[3] so electrolyte monitoring would be recommended in cases involving this drug. Orphenadrine toxicosis in humans has been associated with hypokalemia, hypoglycemia, elevations in liver enzymes, and coagulopathy.[5]

Lesions. No specific lesions are expected in animals succumbing to skeletal muscle relaxant toxicosis. In humans with orphenadrine overdose, pathologic lesions include cerebral edema, pulmonary edema with hemorrhage, hepatic necrosis, and renal congestion.[5]

Diagnostic Testing. Many skeletal muscle relaxants and their metabolites can be measured qualitatively and quantitatively in blood or urine by spectrophotometry or chromatography, but these values are of no value in managing clinical cases.[5,9]

Treatment. Treatment goals include patient stabilization, decontamination, and supportive care. In comatose animals, respiration should be monitored closely and ventilatory support should be provided. In some cases, this entails endotracheal intubation and mechanical ventilation.[5] Body temperature should be closely monitored in comatose animals to prevent hypothermia.

Diazepam is the preferred drug for most skeletal muscle relaxant-induced seizures. Because of the potential for exacerbating CNS depressants, barbiturates should be reserved only for serious seizures that are refractory to other anticonvulsants.[4] Diazepam was also successful in managing baclofen-induced agitation in dogs.[6]

Cardiac status should also be monitored and arrhythmias treated as needed. In many cases, mild arrhythmias resolve with the institution of intravenous fluid therapy. Bradycardia from cyclobenzaprine or orphenadrine should not be treated with atropine because of the risk of exacerbating anticholinergic effects. In humans, catecholamines have been used to successfully treat orphenadrine-induced bradycardia.[5]

Neostigmine, physostigmine, and edrophonium are anticholinesterase drugs that may be used to treat the effects of neuromuscular blocking agents.[7] These drugs inhibit acetylcholinesterase, allowing buildup of acetylcholine at the neuromuscular junction. As acetylcholine levels increase, the competitive antagonism of the neuromuscular blocker is overridden and neuromuscular transmission is resumed. The anticholinesterase drugs can induce bradycardia; therefore, pretreatment with glycopyrrolate or atropine is recommended.[7] Because these anticholinesterase drugs have short duration of action and their effects may wear off before the neuromuscular blocker has been eliminated, animals should be closely monitored for the return of paralysis after their use.

No specific antidotes exist for the centrally acting skeletal muscle relaxants. In humans, the use of physostigmine for toxicosis from drugs such as baclofen and orphenadrine has had mixed results. Because of the potential for serious adverse effects from physostigmine, its use in treating skeletal muscle relaxants is usually restricted to severe cases with life-threatening signs.[5] Flumazenil, a GABA antagonist, has been successfully used to manage human carisoprodol toxicosis,[10] but its efficacy in managing toxicosis from other skeletal muscle relaxants is questionable.[5]

Decontamination consists of emesis or gastric lavage followed by activated charcoal with a cathartic. Because many of these drugs have a rapid onset of signs, emesis should be performed under veterinary supervision. The risk of anesthesia furthering the CNS depression induced by muscle relaxants must be seriously considered when a gastric lavage is performed. Repeated doses of activated charcoal may be of benefit with drugs that undergo enterohepatic recirculation, such as orphenadrine or cyclobenzaprine.[4,5]

Intravenous fluid therapy is essential to maintain cardiovascular support and promote urine flow. Whereas fluid diuresis may assist in the elimination of baclofen,[5,8] many other skeletal muscle relaxants require metabolism before elimination, and diuresis does not enhance their elimination. Blood pressure monitoring should be instituted. Although baclofen-induced hypertension in a dog was successfully treated with sodium nitroprusside, in many cases specific antihypertensive therapy may not be needed.[8] Treatment should continue until all signs of toxicosis have been resolved for 24 hours. In the case of comatose animals requiring ventilatory support, assisted ventilation may be required for up to several days.[4,5] Electrolyte and blood gas status should be monitored and any abnormalities corrected as needed.

Prognosis. Animals with mild to moderate signs of skeletal muscle toxicosis have a good prognosis as long as they receive prompt veterinary attention.[8] Comatose or seizuring animals have a more guarded prognosis. Comatose animals may require several days to recover, but if provided proper respiratory, cardiovascular, and thermoregulatory support, even these animals have a chance to fully recover.

Prevention and Control. Neuromuscular blocking agents such as succinylcholine should be used with care in animals, and proper precautions should be taken to ensure that preexisting conditions that might contribute to the toxicity of these agents (e.g., exposure to organophosphate compounds) have been taken into consideration. Proper ventilatory support equipment should be available any time these products are used.

Exposure of animals to centrally acting skeletal muscle relaxants is generally related to accidental overdose. All medications should be stored in areas well away from pets. Owners should be made aware of signs of adverse reactions or overdoses in pets that are on skeletal muscle relaxants. Human and veterinary drugs should be stored separately to avoid accidental mixup of medication, and pets should be kept out of the area while a human medication is being taken to avoid ingestion of dropped pills by pets. Children should be watched closely while they take their medications to ensure that they are not "slipping" the medication to a pet. Likewise, if medication for one pet is put into food, the pet should be closely observed to be sure that another pet does not "steal" the medication.

VITAMINS

Joseph D. Roder

VITAMIN A

Sources. Vitamin A intoxication is a chronic disease that is generally due to improperly mixed feeds or incorporation of feedstuffs that contain high concentrations of vitamin A (raw liver, fish).

Mechanism of Action. Increased concentrations of vitamin A induce chondrocytes to produce more extracellular matrix proteins. The additional matrix proteins produced a framework for mineralization.[1]

Toxicity and Risk Factors. All animals are susceptible. Cattle have been poisoned following long-term consumption of 30,000 IU/kg body weight[2] and rabbits had reproductive failures following consumption of a diet containing greater than 100,000 IU/kg vitamin A.[3]

Clinical Signs. Animals may exhibit anorexia, weight loss, lameness, bone pain, and rigidity.[4] Pregnant animals that are suffering from hypervitaminosis A may have reproductive failures.

Lesions. The physeal regions of long bones may be fused at an earlier age.[5] Exostoses and fusion of the vertebrae and sternum may be observed. In rabbits, fetal resorptions, abortions, and stillbirths have been reported. The fetuses had cleft palate, hydrocephalus, and microencephaly.[3]

Diagnostic Testing. Radiographs of affected animals may show exostoses and premature closure of physeal plates.[4] Chemical analysis for vitamin A can be performed on the feed, serum, or liver.

Treatment. No specific treatment for this disease is available.

Prognosis. The bony changes are permanent and do not resolve following removal of elevated vitamin A levels in the diet.

VITAMIN D

Animals may be exposed to high concentrations of vitamin D from multivitamins, improperly mixed feeds, or from overzealous supplementation. Other sources include cholecalciferol-containing rodenticides, consumption of calcinogenic plants, or ingestion of a topical psoriasis medication for humans that contains calcipotriene, a vitamin D analogue.

The mechanism of action, clinical signs, and treatment are essentially the same regardless of the source of vitamin D. A detailed discussion of vitamin D toxicosis can be found in Chapter 26 in the section "Cholecalciferol Rodenticides."

VITAMIN K$_3$

Synonyms. Vitamin K$_3$ is also known as menadione, menadione sodium bisulfite, K Thrombin, and Vikaman.

Mechanism of Action. The mechanism of vitamin K$_3$ intoxication is not clearly delineated. Menadione has been shown to cause cytotoxicosis through the formation of reactive oxygen species and oxidative stress, which can be modulated by antioxidants.[6,7]

Toxicity and Risk Factors. Horses are reported to have been poisoned at therapeutic doses (2 to 8 mg/kg) given parenterally.[8]

Clinical Signs. The clinical signs may include colic, depression, anorexia, and dehydration. Signs indicating hemolytic anemia are also seen and include hematuria.

Clinical Pathology. Poisoned animals may have elevated serum urea nitrogen and creatinine, as well as hematuria, hyponatremia, and hyperkalemia.

Lesions. The kidneys may be enlarged and pale. Histologic evaluation of the kidney shows renal tubular nephrosis.

Treatment. No specific antidote is available. Animals must be treated symptomatically for renal disease and electrolyte imbalances.

Prognosis. The prognosis is guarded depending on the degree of renal damage.

Prevention and Control. Vitamin K_3 parenteral products should not be used in horses because of the possibility of intoxication.

REFERENCES

Analgesics

NONSTEROIDAL ANTIINFLAMMATORY AGENTS

1. Ricketts AP et al: Evaluation of selective inhibition of canine cyclooxygenase 1 and 2 by carprofen and other nonsteroidal anti-inflammatory drugs, *Am J Vet Res* 59:1441, 1998.
2. Vane JR, Botting RM: Anti-inflammatory drugs and their mechanism of action, *Inflamm Res* 47(suppl 2):S78, 1998.
3. MacPhail CM et al: Hepatocellular toxicosis associated with administration of carprofen in 21 dogs, *J Am Vet Med Assoc* 212:1895, 1998.
4. Dow SW et al: Effects of flunixin and flunixin plus prednisone on the gastrointestinal tract of dogs, *Am J Vet Res* 51(7):1131, 1990.
5. Dye TL: Naproxen toxicosis in a puppy, *Vet Hum Toxicol* 39:157, 1997.
6. Snow DH et al: Phenylbutazone toxicosis in Equidae: a biochemical and pathophysiological study, *Am J Vet Res* 42:1754, 1981.
7. MacAllister CG et al: Comparison of adverse effects of phenylbutazone, flunixin meglumine, and ketoprofen in horses, *J Am Vet Med Assoc* 202:71, 1993.
8. Reimer ME et al: The gastroduodenal effects of buffered aspirin, carprofen, and etodolac in healthy dogs, *J Vet Intern Med* 13:472, 1999.
9. Meschter CL et al: The effects of phenylbutazone on the morphology and prostaglandin concentrations of the pyloric mucosa of the equine stomach, *Vet Pathol* 27:244, 1990.
10. Ramirez S et al: Renal medullary rim sign in 2 adult quarter horses, *Can Vet J* 39:647, 1998.
11. Spyridakis LK et al: Ibuprofen toxicosis in a dog, *J Am Vet Med Assoc* 189:918, 1986.
12. Abrams KL: Hypocalcemia associated with administration of sodium bicarbonate for salicylate intoxication in a cat, *J Am Vet Med Assoc* 191:235, 1987.
13. Baggot JD: Drug therapy in the neonatal foal, *Vet Clin North Am Equine Pract* 10: 87, 1994.

ACETAMINOPHEN

14. Savides MC et al: The toxicity and biotransformation of single doses of acetaminophen in dogs and cats, *Toxicol Appl Pharmacol* 74(l):26,1984.
15. Court MH, Greenblatt DJ: Molecular basis for deficient acetaminophen glucuronidation in cats. An interspecies comparison of enzyme kinetics in liver microsomes, *Biochem Pharmacol* 53:1041, 1997.
16. Villar D et al: Ibuprofen, aspirin and acetaminophen toxicosis and treatment in dogs and cats, *Vet Hum Toxicol* 40:156, 1998.
17. Nash SL et al: The effect of acetaminophen on methemoglobin and blood glutathione parameters in the cat, *Toxicology* 31(3-4):329, 1984.
18. Savides MC et al: Effects of various antidotal treatments on acetaminophen toxicosis and biotransformation in cats, *Am J Vet Res* 46:1485, 1985.
19. Rumbeiha WK et al: Comparison of *N*-acetylcysteine and methylene blue, alone or in combination, for treatment of acetaminophen toxicosis in cats, *Am J Vet Res* 56:1529, 1995.
20. Rolband GC, Marcuard SP: Cimetidine in the treatment of acetaminophen overdose, *J Clin Gastroenterol* 13(1):79, 1991.
21. Panella C et al: Effect of ranitidine on acetaminophen-induced hepatotoxicity in dogs, *Dig Dis Sci* 35:385-391,1990.

Anticonvulsants

BARBITURATES

1. Dayrell-Hart B et al: Hepatotoxicity of phenobarbital in dogs: 18 cases (1985-1989), *J Am Vet Med Assoc* 199:1060, 1991.
2. Poffenbarger EM, Hardy RM: Hepatic cirrhosis associated with long-term primidone therapy in a dog, *J Am Vet Med Assoc* 186:978,1985.
3. Bunch SE et al: Compromised hepatic function in dogs treated with anticonvulsant drugs, *J Am Vet Med Assoc* 184:444, 1984.
4. Jacobs G et al: Neutropenia and thrombocytopenia in three dogs treated with anticonvulsants, *J Am Vet Med Assoc* 212:681, 1998.

BROMIDE

5. Gayer PT: Toxic mechanism of bromate poisoning in a dog: a case study, *Vet Hum Toxicol* 36:208, 1994.
6. Knight HD, Reina-Guerra M: Intoxication of cattle with sodium bromide-contaminated feed, *Am J Vet Res* 38:407, 1977.
7. Trepanier LA et al: Therapeutic serum drug concentrations in epileptic dogs treated with potassium bromide alone or in combination with other anticonvulsants: 122 cases (1992-1996), *J Am Vet Med Assoc* 213:1449, 1998.

Antidepressants

TRICYCLIC ANTIDEPRESSANTS

1. Pentel PR et al: In Haddad LM et al, editors: *Clinical management of poisoning and overdose,* ed 3, Philadelphia, 1998, WB Saunders.
2. Wismer TA: Antidepressant drug overdoses in dogs, *Vet Med* 95:520, 2000.
3. Plumb DC: *Veterinary drug handbook,* ed 3, Ames, Iowa, 1999, Iowa State University Press.

SEROTONERGIC DRUGS

4. Mahmood I et al: The pharmacokinetics and absolute bioavailability of selegiline in the dog, *Biopharm Drug Dispos* 15:653, 1994.
5. Gwaltney-Brant SM et al: 5-Hydroxytryptophan toxicosis in dogs: 21 cases (1989-1999), *J Am Vet Med Assoc* 216:1937, 2000.
6. Brent J: In Haddad LM et al, editors: *Clinical management of poisoning and overdose,* ed 3, Philadelphia, 1998, WB Saunders.
7. Li Kam, Wa TC et al: A comparison of the renal and neuroendocrine effects of two 5-hydroxytryptamine renal prodrugs in normal man, *Clin Sci* 85:607, 1993.
8. *American Hospital Formulary Service,* Bethesda, Md, 1999, American Society of Health System Pharmacists.
9. Sanders-Bush E, Mayer ST: In Hardman JG et al, editors: *The pharmacologic basis of therapeutics,* ed 9, New York, 1996, McGraw-Hill.
10. Mills KC: Serotonin syndrome, a clinical update, *Crit Care Clin* 13:763, 1997.
11. Landsberg G, Ruehl W: Geriatric behavioral problems, *Vet Clin North Am Small Anim Pract* 27:1537, 1997.
12. King JN et al: Pharmacokinetics of clomipramine in dogs following single-dose and repeated-dose oral administration, *Am J Vet Res* 61:80, 2000.
13. Overall KL: In Dodman NH, Shuster L, editors: *Psychopharmacology of animal behavior disorders,* Malden, Mass, 1998, Blackwell Science.
14. Tollefson GD: In Schatzberg AF, Nemeroff CB, editors: *Textbook of psychopharmacology,* Washington, DC, 1995, American Psychiatric Press.

Antihistamines

1. Babe KS, Serafin WE: In Hardman JG et al, editors: *The pharmacologic basis of therapeutics,* ed 9, New York, 1996, McGraw-Hill.
2. Adams HR: In Adams HR, editor: *Veterinary pharmacology and therapeutics,* ed 7, Ames, Iowa, 1995, Iowa State University Press.

3. Plumb DC: *Veterinary drug handbook,* ed 3, Ames, Iowa, 1999, Iowa State University Press.
4. Kirk MA: In Haddad LM et al, editors: *Clinical management of poisoning and overdose,* ed 3, Philadelphia, 1998, WB Saunders.
5. Otto CM, Greentree WF: Terfenadine toxicosis in dogs, *J Am Vet Med Assoc,* 205:1005, 1994.
6. Scott DW, Buerger RG: Nonsteroidal anti-inflammatory agents in the management of canine pruritus, *J Am Anim Hosp Assoc* 24:425, 1988.
7. Clark JO, Dorman DC: In Bonagura, editor: *Kirk's current veterinary therapy XIII,* Philadelphia, 2000, WB Saunders.
8. Campbell A: In Campbell A, Chapman M, editors: *Handbook of poisoning in dogs and cats,* Oxford, England, 2000, Blackwell Science.

Antimicrobials

SULFONAMIDES

1. Weiss DJ, Klausner JS: Drug-associated aplastic anemia in dogs: eight cases (1984-1988), *J Am Vet Med Assoc* 196(3):472, 1990.
2. Morgan RV, Bachrach A Jr: Keratoconjunctivitis sicca associated with sulfonamide therapy in dogs, *J Am Vet Med Assoc* 180(4):432, 1982.
3. Collins BK et al: Sulfonamide-associated keratoconjunctivitis sicca and corneal ulceration in a dysuric dog, *J Am Vet Med Assoc* 189(8):924, 1986.
4. Scott DW et al: Drug eruption associated with sulfonamide treatment of vertebral osteomyelitis in a dog, *J Am Vet Med Assoc* 168(12):1111, 1976.
5. Bunch SE: Hepatotoxicity associated with pharmacologic agents in dogs and cats, *Vet Clin North Am Small Anim Pract* 23(3):659, 1993.
6. Twedt DC et al: Association of hepatic necrosis with trimethoprim sulfonamide administration in 4 dogs, *J Vet Intern Med* 11(1):20, 1997.
7. Thomas HL, Livesey MA: Immune-mediated hemolytic anemia associated with trimethoprim-sulphamethoxazole administration in a horse, *Can Vet J* 39(3):171, 1998.
8. Gookin JL et al: Clinical hypothyroidism associated with trimethoprim-sulfadiazine administration in a dog, *J Am Vet Med Assoc* 214(7):1028, 1999.
9. Poirier LA et al: An FDA review of sulfamethazine toxicity, *Regul Toxicol Pharmacol* 30(3):217, 1999.

PENICILLINS

10. Robbins RL et al: Immune-mediated haemolytic disease after penicillin therapy in a horse, *Equine Vet J* 25(5):462, 1993.
11. Blue JT et al: Immune-mediated hemolytic anemia induced by penicillin in horses, *Cornell Vet* 77(3):263, 1987.
12. Rehg JE et al: Toxicity of cecal filtrates from guinea pigs with penicillin-associated colitis, *Lab Anim Sci* 30(3):524, 1980.
13. Chapman CB et al: The role of procaine in adverse reactions to procaine penicillin in horses, *Aust Vet J* 69(6):129, 1992.

TETRACYCLINES

14. Gross DR et al: Adverse cardiovascular effects of oxytetracycline preparations and vehicles in intact awake calves, *Am J Vet Res* 42(8):1371, 1981.
15. Gyrd-Hansen N et al: Cardiovascular effects of intravenous administration of tetracycline in cattle, *J Vet Pharmacol Ther* 4(1):15, 1981.
16. Amacher DE, Martin BA: Tetracycline-induced steatosis in primary canine hepatocyte cultures, *Fundam Appl Toxicol* 40(2):256, 1997.
17. Riond JL et al: Cardiovascular effects and fatalities associated with intravenous administration of doxycycline to horses and ponies, *Equine Vet J* 24(1):41, 1992.
18. Moalli MR et al: Oxytetracycline-induced nephrotoxicosis in dogs after intravenous administration for experimental bone labeling, *Lab Anim Sci* 46(5):497, 1996.
19. Lairmore MD et al: Oxytetracycline-associated nephrotoxicosis in feedlot calves, *J Am Vet Med Assoc* 185(7):793, 1984.
20. Vaala WE et al: Acute renal failure associated with administration of excessive amounts of tetracycline in a cow, *J Am Vet Med Assoc* 191(12):1601, 1987.
21. Vivrette S et al: Hemodialysis for treatment of oxytetracycline-induced acute renal failure in a neonatal foal, *J Am Vet Med Assoc* 203(1):105, 1993.

FLUOROQUINOLONES

22. Vancutsem PM et al: The fluoroquinolone antimicrobials: structure, antimicrobial activity, pharmacokinetics, clinical use in domestic animals and toxicity, *Cornell Vet* 80:173, 1990.
23. Gunther T et al: *In vitro* evidence for a Donnan distribution of Mg2+ and Ca2+ by chondroitin sulphate in cartilage, *Arch Toxicol* 71(7):471, 1997.
24. Ball P et al: Comparative tolerability of the newer fluoroquinolone antibacterials, *Drug Saf* 21(5):407, 1999.
25. Machida M et al: Toxicokinetic study of norfloxacin-induced arthropathy in juvenile animals, *Toxicol Appl Pharmacol* 105(3):403, 1990.
26. Yoshida K et al: Pharmacokinetic disposition and arthropathic potential of oral ofloxacin in dogs, *Vet Pharmacol Ther* 21(2):128, 1998.
27. Burkhardt JE et al: Ultrastructural changes in articular cartilages of immature beagle dogs dosed with difloxacin, a fluoroquinolone, *Vet Pathol* 29(3):230, 1992.
28. Burkhardt JE et al: Morphologic and biochemical changes in articular cartilages of immature beagle dogs dosed with difloxacin, *Toxicol Pathol* 20(2):246, 1992.

AMINOGLYCOSIDES

29. Uzuka Y et al: Threshold changes in auditory brainstem response (ABR) due to the administration of kanamycin in dogs, *Exp Anim* 45:325, 1996.
30. Frazier DL et al: Gentamicin pharmacokinetics and nephrotoxicity in naturally acquired and experimentally induced disease in dogs, *J Am Vet Med Assoc* 192:57, 1988.
31. Crowell WA et al: Neomycin toxicosis in calves, *Am J Vet Res* 42:29, 1981.
32. Green SL et al: Effects of hypoxia and azotaemia on the pharmacokinetics of amikacin in neonatal foals, *Equine Vet J* 24:475, 1992.
33. Garry F et al: Enzymuria as an index of renal damage in sheep with induced aminoglycoside nephrotoxicosis, *Am J Vet Res* 51:428, 1990.
34. Rivers BJ et al: Evaluation of urine gamma-glutamyl transpeptidase-o-creatinine ratio as a diagnostic tool in an experimental model of aminoglycoside-induced acute renal failure in the dog, *J Am Anim Hosp Assoc* 32(4):323, 1996.
35. Davies C et al: Effects of a prostaglandin E1 analogue, misoprostol, on renal function in dogs receiving nephrotoxic doses of gentamicin, *Am J Vet Res* 59:1048, 1998.
36. Brashier MK et al: Effect of intravenous calcium administration on gentamicin-induced nephrotoxicosis in ponies, *Am J Vet Res* 59:1055, 1998.

CHLORAMPHENICOL

37. Watson AD, Middleton DJ: Chloramphenicol toxicosis in cats, *Am J Vet Res* 39:1199, 1978.
38. Settepani JA: The hazard of using chloramphenicol in food animals, *J Am Vet Med Assoc* 184:930, 1984.

LINCOMYCIN

39. Keir AA et al: Outbreak of acute colitis on a horse farm associated with tetracycline-contaminated sweet feed, *Can Vet J* 40(10):718, 1999.
40. Rehg JE, Pakes SP: Implication of *Clostridium difficile* and *Clostridium perfringens* iota toxins in experimental lincomycin-associated colitis of rabbits, *Lab Anim Sci* 32:253, 1982.
41. Borriello SP, Carman RJ: Association of iota-like toxin and *Clostridium spiroforme* with both spontaneous and antibiotic-associated diarrhea and colitis in rabbits, *J Clin Microbiol* 17:414, 1983.
42. Raisbeck MF et al: Lincomycin-associated colitis in horses, *J Am Vet Med Assoc* 179:362, 1981.
43. Maiers JD, Mason SJ: Lincomycin-associated enterocolitis in rabbits, *J Am Vet Med Assoc* 185:670, 1984.
44. Bartlett JG et al: Antibiotic-induced lethal enterocolitis in hamsters: studies with eleven agents and evidence to support the pathogenic role of toxin-producing clostridia, *Am J Vet Res* 39(9):1525, 1978.

TILMICOSIN

45. Jordan WH et al: A review of the toxicology of the antibiotic MICOTIL 300, *Vet Hum Toxicol* 35:151, 1993.
46. Main BW et al: Cardiovascular effects of the macrolide antibiotic tilmicosin, administered alone and in combination with propranolol or dobutamine, in conscious unrestrained dogs, *J Vet Pharmacol Ther* 19(3):225, 1996.
47. McGuigan MA: Human exposures to tilmicosin (MICOTIL), *Vet Hum Toxicol* 36:306, 1994.

KETOCONAZOLE

48. Cummings AM et al: Ketoconazole impairs early pregnancy and the decidual cell response via alterations in ovarian function, *Fundam Appl Toxicol* 40(2):238, 1997.
49. Rodriguez RJ, Acosta D Jr: Comparison of ketoconazole- and fluconazole-induced hepatotoxicity in a primary culture system of rat hepatocytes, *Toxicology* 96(2):83, 1995.
50. Plumb DC: *Veterinary drug handbook,* ed 3, Ames, Iowa, 1999, Iowa State Press.
51. Medleau L, Chalmers SA: Ketoconazole for treatment of dermatophytosis in cats, *J Am Vet Med Assoc* 200:77, 1992.
52. Greene CE et al: Trichosporon infection in a cat, *J Am Vet Med Assoc* 187:946, 1985.

AMPHOTERICIN B

53. Hoitsma AJ et al: Drug-induced nephrotoxicity. Aetiology, clinical features and management, *Drug Saf* 6(2):131, 1991.
54. Rubin SI et al: Nephrotoxicity of amphotericin B in dogs: a comparison of two methods of (AmBisome) in beagle dogs, *Pharm Res* 16(11):1694, 1999.
55. Plumb DC: *Veterinary drug handbook,* ed 3, Ames, Iowa, 1999, Iowa State Press.
56. Bekersky I et al: Safety and toxicokinetics of intravenous liposomal amphotericin B administration, *Can J Vet Res* 53(1):23, 1989.

GRISEOFULVIN

57. De Carli L, Larizza L: Griseofulvin, *Mutat Res* 195:91, 1988.
58. Rottman JB et al: Bone marrow hypoplasia in a cat treated with griseofulvin, *J Am Vet Med Assoc* 198:429, 1991.
59. Levy JK: Ataxia in a kitten treated with griseofulvin, *J Am Vet Med Assoc* 198:105, 1991.
60. Kunkle GA, Meyer DJ: Toxicity of high doses of griseofulvin in cats, *J Am Vet Med Assoc* 191:322, 1987.
61. Scott FW et al: Teratogenesis in cats associated with griseofulvin therapy, *Teratology* 11:79, 1975.
62. Shelton GH et al: Severe neutropenia associated with griseofulvin therapy in cats with feline immunodeficiency virus infection, *J Vet Intern Med* 4:317, 1990.
63. Schutte JG, van den Ingh TS: Microphthalmia, brachygnathia superior, and palatocheiloschisis in a foal associated with griseofulvin administration to the mare during early pregnancy, *Vet Q* 19:58, 1997.

Antineoplastics

ANTIMETABOLITES

1. Plumb DC: *Veterinary drug handbook,* ed 3, White Bear Lake, Minn, 1999, Pharma Vet Publishing.
2. Dorman DC et al: 5-Fluorouracil toxicosis in the dog, *J Vet Intern Med* 4(5):254, 1990.
3. Okeda R et al: Subacute neurotoxicity of 5-fluorouracil and its derivative, carmofur, in cats, *Acta Pathol Jpn* 38(10):1255, 1988.

ALKYLATING AGENTS

4. Plumb DC: *Veterinary drug handbook,* ed 3, White Bear Lake, Minn, 1999, Pharma Vet Publishing.
5. Peterson JL et al: Acute sterile hemorrhagic cystitis after a single intravenous administration of cyclophosphamide in three dogs, *J Am Vet Med Assoc* 201:1572, 1992.
6. Laing EJ et al: Treatment of cyclophosphamide-induced hemorrhagic cystitis in five dogs, *J Am Vet Med Assoc* 193:233, 1988.
7. Kitchell BE, Dhaliwal RS: In Bonagura JD, editor: *Kirk's current veterinary therapy XIII,* Philadelphia, 2000, WB Saunders.

MITOTIC INHIBITORS

8. Plumb DC: *Veterinary drug handbook,* ed 3, White Bear Lake, Minn, 1999, Pharma Vet Publishing.
9. Kitchell BE, Dhaliwal RS: In Bonagura JD, editor: *Kirk's current veterinary therapy XIII,* Philadelphia, 2000, WB Saunders.
10. Todd GC et al: Animal models for the comparative assessment of neurotoxicity following repeated administration of vinca alkaloids, *Cancer Treat Rep* 63:35, 1979.
11. Zemann BI et al: A combination chemotherapy protocol (VELCAP-L) for dogs with lymphoma, *J Vet Intern Med* 12:465, 1998.
12. Hamilton TA et al: Vincristine-induced peripheral neuropathy in a dog, *J Am Vet Med Assoc* 198:635, 1991.

ANTIBIOTIC ANTINEOPLASTICS

13. Muller I et al: Anthracycline-derived chemotherapeutics in apoptosis and free radical cytotoxicity (Review), *Int J Mol Med* 1:491, 1988.
14. Plumb DC: *Veterinary drug handbook,* White Bear Lake, Minn, 1999, Pharma Vet Publishing.
15. Ogilvie GK et al: Acute and short-term toxicoses associated with the administration of doxorubicin to dogs with malignant tumors, *J Am Vet Med Assoc* 195:1584, 1989.
16. Kanter PM et al: Comparison of the cardiotoxic effects of liposomal doxorubicin (TLC D-99) versus free doxorubicin in beagle dogs, *In Vivo* 7:17, 1993.
17. Eschalier A et al: Study of histamine release induced by acute administration of antitumor agents in dogs, *Cancer Chemother Pharmacol* 21(3):246, 1988.
18. Seifert CF et al: Dexrazoxane in the prevention of doxorubicin-induced cardiotoxicity, *Ann Pharmacother* 28:1063, 1994.

CISPLATIN

19. Lacy CF et al: *Drug information handbook,* ed 7, Hudson, Ohio, 1999, Lexi-Comp.
20. Plumb DC: *Veterinary drug handbook,* ed 3, White Bear Lake, Minn, 1999, Pharma Vet Publishing.
21. Knapp DW et al: Cisplatin toxicity in cats, *J Vet Intern Med* 1:29, 1987.
22. Moore AS et al: Evaluation of butorphanol and cyproheptadine for prevention of cisplatin-induced vomiting in dogs, *J Am Vet Med Assoc* 205:441, 1994.
23. Forrester SD et al: Prevention of cisplatin-induced nephrotoxicosis in dogs, using hypertonic saline solution a: the vehicle of administration, *Am J Vet Res* 54:2175, 1993.
24. Thamm DH, Vail DM: Preclinical evaluation of a sterically stabilized liposome-encapsulated cisplatin in clinically normal cats, *Am J Vet Res* 59:286, 1998.

Antiparasiticals

PIPERAZINE DERIVATIVES

1. Lovell RA: Ivermectin and piperazine toxicoses in dogs and cats, *Vet Clin North Am Small Anim Pract* 20:453, 1990.
2. Hamilton RG et al: Dirofilaria immitis: diethylcarbamazine-induced anaphylactoid reactions in infected dogs, *Exp Parasitol* 61(3):405, 1986.

IMIDAZOTHIAZOLES

3. Hsu WH: Toxicity and drug interactions of levamisole, *J Am Vet Med Assoc* 176:1166, 1980.
4. Montgomery RD, Pidgeon GL: Levamisole toxicosis in a dog, *J Am Vet Med Assoc* 189:684, 1986.
5. Babish JG et al: Toxicity and tissue residue depletion of levamisole hydrochloride in young goats, *Am J Vet Res* 51:1126, 1990.
6. Cook WO et al: Levamisole toxicosis in swine, *Vet Hum Toxicol* 27:388, 1985.

ORGANOPHOSPHOROUS COMPOUNDS

7. Baker NF et al: Acute oral median lethal dose of haloxon and coumaphos in sheep as influenced by plasma A esterase, *Am J Vet Res* 41(11):1857, 1980.

8. Jortner BS et al: Haloxon-induced delayed neurotoxicity: effect of plasma A (aryl) esterase activity on severity of lesions in sheep, *Neurotoxicology* 4(2):241, 1983.

9. Wilson RD et al: Somatosensory-evoked response of ataxic Angora goats in suspected haloxon-delayed neurotoxicity, *Am J Vet Res* 43(12):2224, 1982.

10. Mehl A et al: The effect of trichlorfon and other organophosphates on prenatal brain development in the guinea pig, *Neurochem Res* 19(5):569, 1994.

11. Pope AM et al: Trichlorfon-induced congenital cerebellar hypoplasia in neonatal pigs, *J Am Vet Med Assoc* 189(7):781, 1986.

MACROLIDE ENDECTOCIDES

12. Yamazaki J et al: Macrolide compounds, ivermectin and milbemycin D, stimulate chloride channels sensitive to GABAergic drugs in cultured chick spinal neurons, *Comp Biochem Physiol* 93(1):97, 1989.

13. Paul AJ et al: Clinical observations in collies given ivermectin orally, *Am J Vet Res* 48(4):684, 1987.

14. Tranquilli WJ et al: Assessment of toxicosis induced by high-dose administration of milbemycin oxime in collies, *Am J Vet Res* 52(7):1170, 1991.

15. Roder JD, Stair EL: An overview of ivermectin toxicosis, *Vet Hum Toxicol* 40(6):369, 1998.

16. Beal MW et al: Respiratory failure attributable to moxidectin intoxication in a dog, *J Am Vet Med Assoc* 215(12):1813, 1999.

17. Kitagawa H et al: Clinical and laboratory changes after administration of milbemycin oxime in heartworm-free and heartworm-infected dogs, *Am J Vet Res* 54(4):520, 1993.

18. Tranquilli WJ et al: Response to physostigmine administration in collie dogs exhibiting ivermectin toxicosis, *J Vet Pharmacol Ther* 10(1):96, 1987.

DISOPHENOL

19. Penumarthy L et al: Investigations of therapeutic measures for disophenol toxicosis in dogs, *Am J Vet Res* 36:1259, 1975.

20. Martin CL: The formation of cataracts in dogs with disophenol: age susceptibility and production with chemical grade, 2,6-diiodo-4-nitrophenol, *Can Vet J* 16:228, 1975.

21. Martin CL et al: Formation of temporary cataracts in dogs given a disophenol preparation, *J Am Vet Med Assoc* 161:294, 1972.

ARSENICAL ANTIHELMINTHICS

22. Holmes RA et al: Thiacetarsemide in dogs: disposition kinetics and correlations with selected indocyanine green kinetic values, *Am J Vet Res* 47:1338, 1986.

23. Maksimowich DS et al: Effect of arsenical drugs on *in vitro* vascular responses of pulmonary artery from heartworm-infected dogs, *Am J Vet Res* 58:389, 1997.

24. Boudreaux MK, Dillon AR: Platelet function, antithrombin-III activity, and fibrinogen concentration in heartworm-infected and heartworm-negative dogs treated with thiacetarsamide, *Am J Vet Res* 52:1986, 1991.

25. Raynaud JP: Thiacetarsamide (adulticide) versus melarsomine (RM 340) developed as macrofilaricide (adulticide and larvicide) to cure canine heartworm infection in dogs, *Ann Rech Vet* 23:1, 1992.

26. Plumb DC: *Veterinary drug handbook*, ed 3, White Bear Lake, Minn, 1999, Pharma Vet Publishing.

27. Rawlings CA, McCall JW: In Bonagura JD: *Kirk's current veterinary therapy XIII*, Philadelphia, 2000, WB Saunders.

Bronchodilators

1. Boothe DM: In Adams HR, editor: *Veterinary pharmacology and therapeutics*, Ames, Iowa, 1995, Iowa State University Press.

2. Plumb DC: *Veterinary drug handbook*, ed 3, Ames, Iowa, 1999, Iowa State University Press.

3. Nelson HS: Drug therapy: (beta)-adrenergic bronchodilators, *N Engl J Med* 333:499, 1995.

4. ASPCA-National Animal Poison Control Center: Unpublished data, 1992–1999.

5. McEvoy GK: *American hospital formulary service*, Bethesda, Md, 2000, American Society of Hospital Pharmacists.

6. Petruska JM et al: Cardiovascular effects after inhalation of large doses of albuterol dry powder in rats, monkeys, and dogs: a species comparison, *Fundam Appl Toxicol* 40:52, 1997.

7. Adams HR: In Adams HR, editor: *Veterinary pharmacology and therapeutics*, Ames, Iowa, 1995, Iowa State University Press.

8. Lefkowitz RJ et al: In Hardman JG, Limbird LE, editors: *Goodman and Gilman's the pharmacological basis of therapeutics*, New York, 1996, McGraw-Hill.

9. Detweiler DK: Spontaneous and induced arterial disease in the dog: pathology and pathogenesis, *Toxicol Pathol* 17:94, 1989.

10. Padrid P: In Kirk RW: *Current veterinary therapy XII*, Philadelphia, 1995, WB Saunders.

11. Rosendale ME, Volmer PA: Albuterol inhaler toxicosis in dogs, *J Vet Emerg Crit Care* 8:255, 1998.

12. Papich MG: In Norsworthy GD, editor: *The feline patient*, Baltimore, 1998, Williams & Wilkins.

13. Du Plooy WJ et al: The dose-related hyper- and-hypokalaemic effects of salbutamol and its arrhythmogenic potential, *Br J Pharmacol* 111:73, 1994.

14. Ellenhorn MJ: *Ellenhorn's medical toxicology: diagnosis and treatment of human poisoning*, ed 2, Baltimore, 1997, Williams & Wilkins.

15. Kittleson MD, Kienle RD: *Small animal cardiovascular medicine*, St Louis, 1998, Mosby.

16. Haffner CA, Kendall MJ: Metabolic effects of beta 2-agonists, *J Clin Pharmacol Ther* 17:155, 1992.

17. Ramoska EA et al: Propranolol treatment of albuterol poisoning in two asthmatic patients, *Ann Emerg Med* 22:1474, 1993.

18. POISINDEX Editorial Staff: Albuterol (Management/treatment protocol). In Smith R et al, editors: POISINDEX System. Englewood, Colo, Micromedex (expires September 2000).

Cardiovascular Drugs

CARDIAC GLYCOSIDES

1. Erichsen DF et al: Therapeutic and toxic plasma concentrations of digoxin in the cat, *Am J Vet Res* 41(12):2049, 1980.

2. Hamlin RL: Clinical toxicology of cardiovascular drugs, *Vet Clin North Am Small Anim Pract* 20(2):469, 1990.

3. Wijnberg ID et al: Use of phenytoin to treat digitalis-induced cardiac arrhythmias in a miniature Shetland pony, *Vet Rec* 144(10):259, 1999.

CALCIUM CHANNEL BLOCKING AGENTS

4. Schoffstall JM et al: Effects of calcium channel blocker overdose-induced toxicity in the conscious dog, *Ann Emerg Med* 20(10):1104, 1991.

5. Gay R et al: Treatment of verapamil toxicity in intact dogs, *J Clin Invest* 77(6):1805, 1986.

6. Stone CK et al: Treatment of verapamil overdose with glucagon in dogs, *Ann Emerg Med* 25(3):369, 1995.

7. Kline JA et al: Insulin is a superior antidote for cardiovascular toxicity induced by verapamil in the anesthetized canine, *J Pharmacol Exp Ther* 267(2):744, 1993.

Decongestants

SYMPATHOMIMETICS

1. Means C: Ma huang: all natural but not always innocuous, *Vet Med* 94:511, 1999.

2. POISINDEX System: Toll LL, Hurlburt KM, editors: Poisindex System, Greenwood Village, Colo, Micromedex (expires December 2000).

3. Ooms TG et al: Suspected caffeine and ephedrine toxicosis resulting from ingestion of an herbal supplement containing guarana and ma huang in dogs: 47 cases (1997-1999), *J Am Vet Med Assoc* 218:225, 2001.

4. McEvoy GK et al (editors): *2000 AHFS drug information,* Bethesda, Md, 2000, Board of the American Society of Health System Pharmacists.

5. Plumb DC: *Veterinary drug handbook,* ed 3, Ames, Iowa, 1999, Iowa State University Press.

6. Lane IF: In Osborne CA, Finco DR: *Canine and feline nephrology and urology,* Philadelphia, 1995, Lea & Febiger.

7. ASPCA Animal Poison Control Center: Unpublished data, 2000.

8. Cote E: Over-the-counter human medications in small animals. Part 1. Gastrointestinal, urinary and ophthalmic drugs, *Comp Cont Ed Prac Vet* 20:603, 1998.

9. Wiley JF: In Haddad LM et al, editors: *Clinical management of poisoning and drug overdose,* ed 3, Philadelphia, 1998, WB Saunders.

Diabetes Medications

1. McEvoy GK: *American Hospital Formulary Service,* Bethesda, Md, 2000, American Society of Hospital Pharmacists.

2. Plumb DC: *Veterinary drug handbook,* ed 3, Ames, Iowa, 1999, Iowa State University Press.

3. Jackson EK: In Hardman JG, Limbird LE, editors: *Goodman and Gilman's the pharmacological basis of therapeutics,* New York, 1996, McGraw-Hill.

4. DiBartola SP: In DiBartola SP, editor: *Fluid therapy in small animal practice,* Philadelphia, 2000, WB Saunders.

5. Ober KP: In Haddad LM et al: *Clinical management of poisoning and drug overdose,* Philadelphia, 1998, WB Saunders.

6. De Girolami U et al: In Cotran RS et al: *Robbins pathologic basis of disease,* Philadelphia, 1999, WB Saunders.

7. Feldman EC, Nelson RW: *Canine and feline endocrinology and reproduction,* ed 2, Philadelphia, 1996, WB Saunders.

8. *Physician's Desk Reference,* ed 55, Montvale, NJ, 2001, Medical Economics Company.

9. Page CP et al: *Integrated pharmacology,* London, 1997, Mosby.

10. ASPCA Animal Poison Control Center: Unpublished data, 2000.

11. Ellenhorn MJ: *Ellenhorn's medical toxicology: diagnosis and treatment of human poisoning,* ed 2, Baltimore, 1997, Williams & Wilkins.

12. Duncan DC et al: In Adams HR, editor: *Veterinary pharmacology and therapeutics,* Ames, Iowa, 1995, Iowa State University Press.

13. Bizub V, Leng L: The effect of the long-term administration of vasopressin on the development of the kidneys of growing lambs, *Res Vet Sci* 62:189, 1997.

14. Hoenig M: In Adams HR, editor: *Veterinary pharmacology and therapeutics,* Ames, Iowa, 1995, Iowa State University Press.

15. Boothe DM: In Boothe DM, editor: *Small animal clinical pharmacology and therapeutics,* Philadelphia, 2001, WB Saunders.

16. Whitley NT et al: Insulin overdose in dogs and cats: 28 cases (1986-1993), *J Am Vet Med Assoc* 211:326, 1997.

17. Jubb KV, Huxtable CR: In Jubb KV et al: *Pathology of domestic animals,* San Diego, 1993, Academic Press.

18. Blayac JP et al: Kinetic aspects of the glipizide-induced hypoglycemia in the dog, *J Pharmacol* 11:463, 1980.

19. Feldman et al: Intensive 50 week evaluation of glipizide administration in 50 cats with previously untreated diabetes mellitus, *J Am Vet Med Assoc* 210:772, 1997.

20. Ballagi-Pordany G et al: Direct effect of hypoglycemic sulphonylureas on the cardiovascular system of dogs, *Diabetes Res Clin Pract* 11:47, 1991.

21. Michels GM et al: Pharmacokinetics of the antihyperglycemic agent metformin in cats, *Am J Vet Res* 60:738, 1999.

22. Greco DS: In Bonagura JD, editor: *Kirk's current veterinary therapy XIII, small animal practice,* Philadelphia, 2000, WB Saunders.

23. Robertson J et al: Effects of the alpha-glucosidase inhibitor acarbose on postprandial serum glucose and insulin concentrations in healthy dogs, *Am J Vet Res* 60:541, 1999.

24. Nelson RW et al: Effect of the α-glucosidase inhibitor acarbose on control of glycemia in dogs with naturally acquired diabetes mellitus, *J Am Vet Med Assoc* 216:1265, 2000.

25. Zimmerman HJ: *Hepatotoxicity,* ed 2, Philadelphia, 1999, Lippincott Williams & Wilkins.

Hypertonic Phosphate Enema

1. Nir-Paz R et al: Acute hyperphosphatemia caused by sodium phosphate enema in a patient with liver dysfunction and chronic renal failure, *Ren Fail* 21(5):541, 1999.

2. Atkins CE et al: Clinical, biochemical, acid-base, and electrolyte abnormalities in cats after hypertonic sodium phosphate enema administration, *Am J Vet Res* 46(4):980, 1985.

3. Jorgensen LS et al: Electrolyte abnormalities induced by hypetonic phosphate enemas in two cats, *J Am Vet Med Assoc* 187:1367, 1985.

Hypothyroid Medications

1. Feldman EC, Nelson RW: *Canine and feline endocrinology and reproduction,* ed 2, Philadelphia, 1996, WB Saunders.

2. McEvoy GK: *American Hospital Formulary Service,* Bethesda, Md, 2000, American Society of Hospital Pharmacists.

3. Plumb DC: *Veterinary drug handbook,* ed 3, Ames, Iowa, 1999, Iowa State University Press.

4. Ferguson DC: In Adams HR: *Veterinary pharmacology and therapeutics,* Ames, Iowa, 1995, Iowa State University Press.

5. Shakir KM, Ladenson PW: In Haddad LM, editor: *Clinical management of poisoning and drug overdose,* Philadelphia, 1998, WB Saunders.

6. Farwell AP, Braverman LE: In Hardman JG, Limbird LE, editors: *Goodman and Gilman's the pharmacological basis of therapeutics,* New York, 1996, McGraw-Hill.

7. ASPCA National Animal Poison Control Center: Unpublished data, 1992-1999.

8. Duckett WM: In Reed SM, Baily WM: *Equine internal medicine,* Philadelphia, 1998, WB Saunders.

9. Panciera DL et al: Administration of levothyroxine to euthyroid dogs does not affect echocardiographic and electrocardiographic measurements, *Res Vet Sci* 53:130, 1992.

10. Hansen SR et al: Acute overdose of levothyroxine in a dog, *J Am Vet Med Assoc* 200:1512, 1992.

11. Piatnek DA, Olson RE: Experimental hyperthyroidism in dogs and effect of salivariectomy, *Am J Physiol* 201:723, 1961.

12. Hoey A et al: Cardiac changes in experimental hyperthyroidism in dogs, *Aust Vet J* 68:352, 1991.

13. Ellenhorn MJ: *Ellenhorn's medical toxicology: diagnosis and treatment of human poisoning,* ed 2, Baltimore, 1997, Williams & Wilkins.

14. Foster DJ, Thoday KL: Use of propranolol and potassium iodate in the presurgical management of hyperthyroid cats, *J Small Anim Pract* 40:307, 1999.

15. Peterson ME: In Ettinger SJ, Feldman EC: *Textbook of veterinary internal medicine,* Philadelphia, 2000, WB Saunders.

Methylxanthines

1. Serafin WE: In Hardman JG, Limbird LE, editors: *Goodman and Gilman's the pharmacological basis of therapeutics,* ed 9, New York, 1995, McGraw-Hill.

2. Hooser SB et al: In Kirk RW, editor: *Current veterinary therapy IX,* Philadelphia, 1966, WB Saunders.

3. Roberts HR, Barone JJ: Biological effects of caffeine: history and use, *Food Tech,* September, 1983, 32-39.

4. Shannon MW: In Haddad LM et al, editors: *Clinical management of poisoning and drug overdose,* ed 3, Philadelphia, 1998, WB Saunders.

5. RTECS: Registry of Toxic Effects of Chemical Substances. National Institute for Occupational Safety and Health, Cincinnati, Ohio (CD-ROM Version), Micromedex, Englewood, Colo (expires December 31, 2000).

6. Rall TW: In Goodman AG et al, editors: *The pharmacological basis of therapeutics,* ed 8, New York, 1990, McGraw-Hill.

7. Booth NE: In Booth NE, McDonald LE, editors: *Veterinary pharmacology and therapeutics,* ed 6, Ames, Iowa, 1988, Iowa State University Press.

8. Dorman DC: In Bongura JD, editor: *Current veterinary therapy XII,* Philadelphia, 1995, WB Saunders.

9. Dalvi RR: Acute and chronic toxicity of caffeine: a review, *Vet Hum Toxicol* 28(2):144, 1986.

Muscle Relaxants

1. *American Hospital Formulary Service,* Bethesda, Md, 1999, American Society of Health System Pharmacists, p 1170.

2. Adams HR: In Adams HR, editor: *Veterinary pharmacology and therapeutics,* ed 7. Ames, Iowa, 1995, Iowa State University Press.

3. Plumb DC: *Veterinary drug handbook,* ed 3, Ames, Iowa, 1999, Iowa State University Press.

4. Shannon MW: In Haddad LM et al, editors: *Clinical management of poisoning and overdose,* ed 3, Philadelphia, 1998, WB Saunders.

5. Ellenhorn MJ, editor: *Ellenhorn's medical toxicology: diagnosis and treatment of human poisoning,* ed 2, Baltimore, 1997, Williams & Wilkins.

6. Hecht DV, Allenspach K: Presumptive baclofen intoxication in a dog, *J Vet Emerg Crit Care* 8:49, 1998.

7. Martinez EA: Newer neuromuscular blockers: is the practitioner ready for muscle relaxants? *Vet Clin North Am Small Anim Pract* 29:811, 1999.

8. Roth BA, Vinson DR, Kim S: Carisoprodol-induced myoclonic encephalopathy, *J Toxicol Clin Toxicol* 36:609, 1998.

9. POISINDEX Editorial Staff: Centrally-acting skeletal muscle relaxants. In Rumack BH et al, editors: *POISINDEX System,* vol 100, MICROMEDEX, Englewood, Colo (expires December 2000).

10. Roberge RJ, Lin E, Krenzelok EP: Flumazenil reversal of carisoprodol (Soma) intoxication, *J Emerg Med* 18:61, 2000.

Vitamins

VITAMIN A

1. Woodard JC et al: Pathogenesis of vitamin (A and D)-induced premature growth-plate closure in calves, *Bone* 21(2):171, 1997.

2. Woodard JC et al: Vitamin (A and D)-induced premature physeal closure (hyena disease) in calves, *J Comp Pathol* 116:353, 1997.

3. DiGiacomo RF et al: Hypervitaminosis A and reproductive disorders in rabbits, *Lab Anim Sci* 42(3):250, 1992.

4. Goldman AL: Hypervitaminosis A in a cat, *J Am Vet Med Assoc* 200:1970-1972, 1992.

5. Coates JW et al: Gastric ulceration and suspected vitamin A toxicosis in grower pigs fed fish silage, *Can Vet J* 39:167, 1998.

VITAMIN K_3

6. Morgan WA et al: The role of reactive oxygen species in Adriamycin and menadione-induced glomerular toxicity, *Toxicol Lett* 94(3 Feb):209, 1998.

7. Shertzer HG et al: Menadione-mediated membrane fluidity alterations and oxidative damage in rat hepatocytes, *Biochem Pharmacol* 43(10):2135, 1992.

8. Rebhun WC et al: Vitamin K_3-induced renal toxicosis in the horse, *Am Vet Med Assoc* 184(10):1237, 1984.

25

Plants

ALCOHOLS AND ACIDS

ASCLEPIAS

George Burrows and Ronald J. Tyrl

Sources. Two types of disease problems, cardiotoxicosis and neurotoxicosis, are produced by species of *Asclepias* (Color Plates 1 and 2). At present, only five species with whorled (verticillate) leaves have been shown to be definitely neurotoxic (Table 25-1).[1-3] In addition, *A. incarnata* L. (swamp milkweed) also appears to be somewhat neurotoxic.

Together, the six form a complex of intergrading species across the western half of North America and thus appear to be closely related. They were classified by Woodson in the subgenus *Asclepias* and series *Incarnatae* with 10 other species that lack the whorled leaf arrangement.[4] It is not known whether other species of the genus are neurotoxic as well, but all of the others that have been investigated produce cardiotoxic effects or contain potent cardiotoxins. However, many species remain to be evaluated for toxic potential. *A. subverticillata* was formerly known as *A. galioides*. The common name *Mexican milkweed* has been used for two species, which has caused confusion as to which taxon is being cited as toxic. *A. fascicularis* is found

primarily in the United States, whereas *A. mexicana* is found only in Mexico.

These taxa occur mainly in western North America: *A. fascicularis* is found in California; *A. subverticillata* grows west from the eastern slope of the Rocky Mountains; *A. pumila* occurs in sandy sites of the Great Plains, especially the southern portion; *A. incarnata* is present from the intermountain Great Basin east through much of North America; *A. verticillata* is found from the eastern portion of the Great Plains throughout the eastern U.S.; and *A. mexicana* grows in Mexico.

Toxicokinetics. The verticillate-leaved species of *Asclepias* contain little or no cardenolides and their neurotoxic effects appear to be caused by other toxins. Although they have negligible cardenolide content, they produce some minor cardiac effects.[5] Preliminary studies indicate the possibility that the toxin may be a cinnamic ester pregnane glycoside structurally similar to the cardiotoxins typical of other species of *Asclepias*.[6]

The neurotoxins appear to be rapidly absorbed from the digestive tract and are of relatively short duration of activity. Their effects are cumulative and clinical signs may appear after a single ingestion of 1% body weight of plant material. In some instances, especially with ruminants, there may be a delay of up to 12 hours between ingestion and onset of severe signs.

Toxicity and Risk Factors. Most animal species, including poultry, are susceptible to the neurotoxic effects.

Clinical Signs. Horses display signs of colic and marked uneasiness followed by incoordination, weakness, and trembling or muscle fasciculations. They may become increasingly apprehensive and try to move about or fight their weakness, with this motion leading to their falling. Body temperature may increase and there may be profuse sweating and mydriasis. The weakness and incoordination may progress to tetanic seizures with the neck bowed. The thoracic legs are flexed with paddling movements. Death is apparently due to respiratory failure associated with prolonged seizure activity. Surviving animals may be weak for several or more days.

TABLE 25-1 **Neurotoxic Species of *Asclepias***

Species Name	Common Name
A. fascicularis Decne	Narrow-leaved milkweed, Mexican milkweed
A. mexicana Cav.	Mexican whorled milkweed
A. pumila (A.Gray) Vail	Plains whorled milkweed
A. subverticillata (A.Gray) Vail	Western whorled milkweed, horsetail milkweed
A. verticillata L.	Eastern whorled milkweed, spider milkweed

In addition to exhibiting the same signs, cattle may bloat, groan, and salivate excessively between convulsive episodes. Sheep have champing of the jaws, head shaking, head pressing, and twitching of the eyelids, ears, and lips. The animal stands with a humped-up appearance and its head held elevated. When forced to move, the motion is described as an exaggerated jackrabbit-like gait with head held up.[7]

In poultry, obvious signs of intoxication occur within a few hours of ingestion. They include loss of muscular control, excitement, bizarre posturing, and periodic violent seizures with running movements.

Lesions.   Hemorrhages on the surface of the heart and other tissues may be the only gross lesions. Microscopic changes are limited to mild nonsuppurative myocardial cellular degeneration and mononuclear infiltration. Traumatic skin damage can occur secondary to violent seizures.

Treatment.   Sedatives are of value to reduce the frequency and severity of the seizures. Activated charcoal given orally may be of some value. However, it is difficult to administer oral medications in the presence of seizures or without worsening their frequency and severity.

Prognosis.   The presence of violent seizures indicates a poor prognosis. Recovery from milder signs may be followed by the presence of neurologic signs for several days.

Prevention and Control.   Prevention of animal access to plants in the pasture or in hay is the only effective means of controlling animal losses. It is particularly important to examine alfalfa hay for the presence of the distinctive flowers, pods, and whorled leaves of *Asclepias,* especially in areas where *A. fascicularis* or *A. subverticillata* may be present in hay fields.

REFERENCES

1. Marsh CD, Clawson AB: The Mexican whorled milkweed *(Asclepias mexicana)* as a poisonous plant, *USDA Bull* 969, 1921.
2. Glover GH, Newsom IE, Robbins WW: A new poisonous plant, the whorled milkweed *(Asclepias verticillata)*, *Colo Agric Exp Sta Bull* 246, 1918.
3. Marsh CD, et al: Poisonous properties of the whorled milkweeds *Asclepias pumila* and *A. verticillata* var. geyeri, USDA Bull 942, 1921.
4. Woodson RE: The North American species of *Asclepias* L, *Annals Missouri Bot Gard* 41:1, 1954.
5. Ogden L, et al: Experimental intoxication in sheep by *Asclepias,* In James LF, Keeler RF, Bailey EM Jr, Cheeke PR, Hegarty MP, editors: *Poisonous plants, proceedings of the third international symposium,* Ames, Iowa, 1992, Iowa State University Press.
6. Robinson GH, et al: Investigation of the neurotoxic compounds in *Asclepias subverticillata* (western whorled milkweed). In Garland T, Barr AC, editors: *Toxic plants and other natural toxicants,* New York, 1998, CAB International.
7. Clark JG: Whorled milkweed poisoning, *Vet Hum Toxicol* 21:431, 1979.

CICUTOXIN

Anthony P. Knight

Synonyms.   Synonyms for water hemlock include cowbane, beaver poison, musquash root, and poison parsnip.

Sources.   Water hemlocks, members of the family Apiaceae (Umbelliferae), are found throughout the world and are some of the most poisonous plants affecting humans and animals. All species of water hemlock are poisonous. Several poorly differentiated species of water hemlock occur in North America. The best known are *Cicuta douglasii*, which is found mostly in the western United States and *C. maculata,* found predominantly in the eastern United States. At least two other species are recognized in North America.[1] In Europe, water dropwort *(Oenanthe crocata)* contains a very similar potent toxin to that found in water hemlock.[2]

Water hemlock is an erect, hairless, perennial or biennial plant growing to a height of 4 to 5 feet. Stems emerge from a cluster of two to eight thick tuberous (parsnip-like) roots (Color Plate 3). At the base of the hollow stem are a series of tightly grouped partitions that may contain a pungent yellow fluid. The leaves are alternate and one to three times pinnately divided. The leaflets are 3 to 10 cm long and linear-lance, with toothed edges. The larger leaf veins terminate in the notches of the leaf margins. The flowers are white in the form of a loose, compound umbel (Color Plate 4). The flower is supported by a whorl of a few narrow bracts. The yellowish-brown seeds are oval and flattened laterally with prominent ribs.

The preferred habitat for water hemlocks includes wet meadows, riverbanks, irrigation ditches, and water edges. They often grow with their roots in water. Some species of water hemlock have adapted to altitudes as high as 8000 feet, whereas others grow at sea level.

Toxicokinetics.   All species of water hemlock should be considered highly poisonous because they contain cicutoxin $(C_{17}H_{22}O_2)$, an unsaturated long-chain alcohol that is one of the most toxic naturally occurring plant compounds.[1-5] The alcohol derivative, cicutol $(C_{17}H_{22}O)$, is relatively nontoxic.[6] Cicutoxin is present in the pungent, oily yellow fluid that exudes from the cut surface of the stem base and roots. The toxin is concentrated in the tuberous roots, but all parts of the plant, including the fluid found in the hollow stems, are toxic. The newly emerging plant in the spring is the most toxic, whereas the mature leaves in late summer seem to have minimal toxicity to cattle. The roots are highly poisonous at all times. Animals that die often have the chewed hemlock roots in the esophageal groove and anterior rumen, indicating that cicutoxin is rapidly absorbed through epithelial surfaces and kills the animal before the plant material moves far through the digestive system.

Mechanism of Action.   The site of action of cicutoxin appears to be the central nervous system, although its precise mechanism of action is unknown. Cicutoxin has similar pharmacologic properties to picrotoxin and strychnine, which act primarily by blocking the gamma aminobutyric acid (GABA) receptors, thereby affecting the major inhibitory pathways in the brain.[7,8] Seizures and generalized convulsions result. Seizures do not develop until enough of the toxin is absorbed to block sufficient GABA receptors to exceed the seizure threshold.

The severity, frequency, and duration of the seizures caused by cicutoxin have direct bearing on the degree of

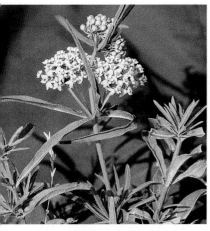

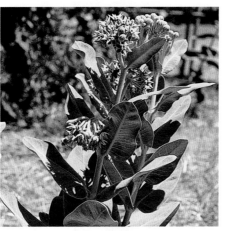

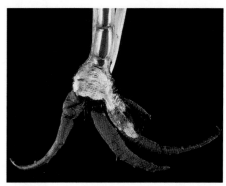

Plate 3. Sectioned stem and root crown showing partitions of the hollow stem and the tuberous roots of water hemlock *(Cicuta douglasii)*. (Photo courtesy Dr. AP Knight.)

Plate 1. A "narrow leaf" milkweed *(Asclepias* sp.). (Photo courtesy Dr. KH Plumlee.)

Plate 2. A "broad leaf" milkweed *(Asclepias* sp.). (Photo courtesy Dr. KH Plumlee.)

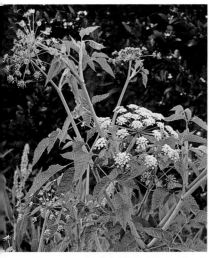

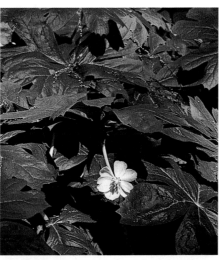

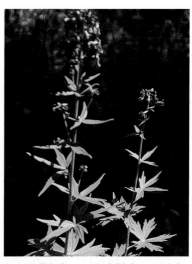

Plate 4. Water hemlock *(Cicuta maculata)*. (Photo courtesy Dr. AP Knight.)

Plate 5. Mayapple *(Podophyllum peltatum)*. (Photo courtesy Dr. WR Hare.)

Plate 6. Tall larkspur *(Delphinium* spp.*)* leaves and terminal inflorescence. (Photo courtesy Dr. AP Knight.)

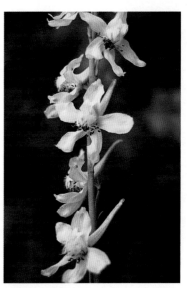

Plate 7. Low larkspur *(Delphinium nelsoni)* leaves and blue flowers. (Photo courtesy Dr. AP Knight.)

Plate 8. Larkspur flowers *(Delphinium virescens)* showing characteristic spur. (Photo courtesy Dr. AP Knight.)

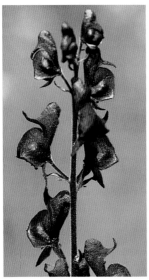

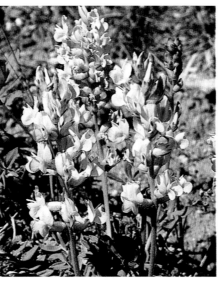

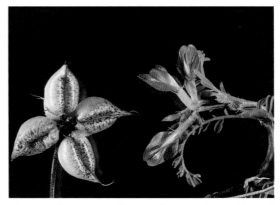

Plate 9. Monkshood flower *(Aconitum columbianum)* with characteristic "hood." (Photo courtesy Dr. AP Knight.)

Plate 10. White locoweed *(Oxytropis sericea).* (Photo courtesy Dr. AP Knight.)

Plate 11. Blue or spotted locoweed *(Astragalus lentiginosus)* showing the inflated, spotted seedpods. (Photo courtesy Dr. AP Knight.)

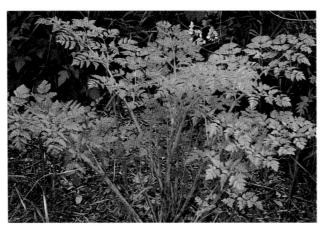

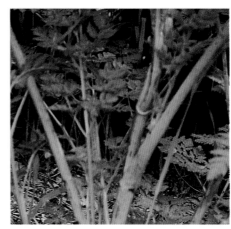

Plate 12. Poison hemlock *(Conium maculatum).* (Photo courtesy Dr. KH Plumlee.)

Plate 13. Purple splotches on stem of poison hemlock. (Photo courtesy Dr. KH Plumlee.)

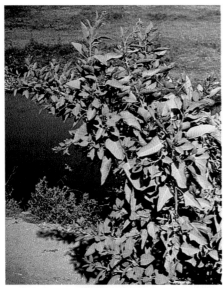

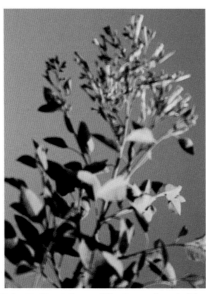

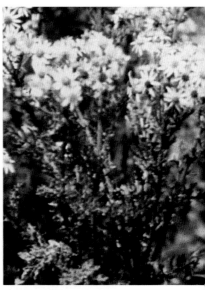

Plate 14. Tree tobacco *(Nicotiana glauca).* (Photo courtesy Dr. PC Blanchard.)

Plate 15. Tree tobacco *(Nicotiana glauca).* (Photo courtesy Dr. PC Blanchard.)

Plate 16. Tansy ragwort *(Senecio jacoba* (Photo courtesy Dr. BL Stegelmeier.)

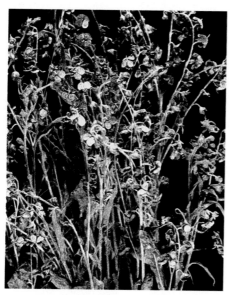

Plate 17. Houndstongue *(Cynoglossum officinale)* dry senescent plant. (Photo courtesy Dr. BL Stegelmeier.)

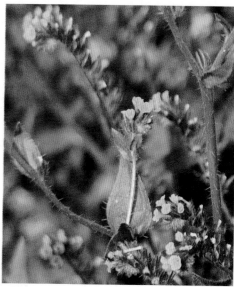

Plate 18. Fiddleneck *(Amsinckia intermedia).* (Photo courtesy Dr. KH Plumlee.)

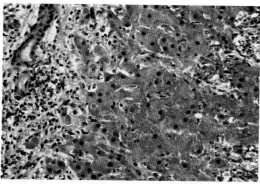

Plate 19. Photomicrograph of liver from a horse with acute pyrrolizidine alkaloid intoxication. Note the extensive necrosis and hemorrhage adjacent to biliary epithelium. (H&E stain paraffin section). (Photo courtesy Dr. BL Stegelmeier.)

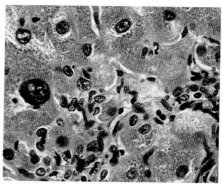

Plate 20. Photomicrograph of liver from a horse with chronic pyrrolizidine alkaloid intoxication. Note the megalocytosis with nuclear vacuolation, biliary proliferation, or oval cell proliferation (H&E stain paraffin section). (Photo courtesy Dr. BL Stegelmeier.)

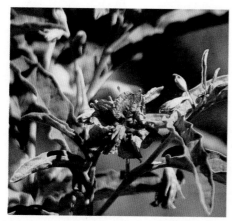

Plate 21. Nightshade *(Solanum* sp.). (Photo courtesy Dr. KH Plumlee.)

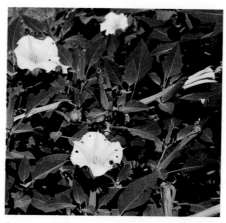

Plate 22. Jimson weed *(Datura* sp.) (Photo courtesy Dr. KH Plumlee.)

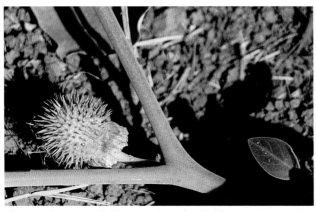

Plate 23. Jimson weed *(Datura* sp*.)* seed pod. (Photo courtesy Dr. KH Plumlee.)

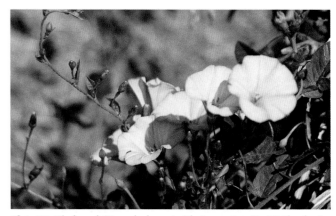

Plate 24. Bindweed *(Convolvulus* sp.). (Photo courtesy Dr. KH Plumlee.)

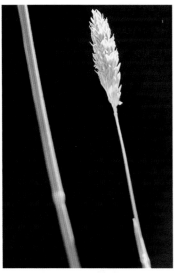

Plate 25. Canary grass *(Phalaris caroliniana).* (Photo courtesy Dr. SS Nicholson.)

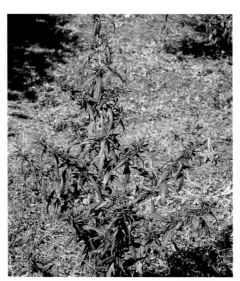

Plate 26. Cocklebur *(Xanthium* sp.). (Photo courtesy Dr. KH Plumlee.)

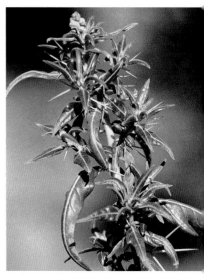

Plate 27. Cocklebur *(Xanthium* sp.). (Photo cou Dr. KH Plumlee.)

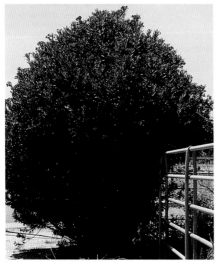

Plate 28. Oleander *(Nerium oleander).* (Photo courtesy Dr. KH Plumlee.)

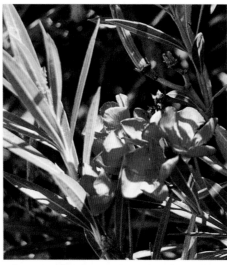

Plate 29. Oleander *(Nerium oleander).* (Photo courtesy Dr. KH Plumlee.)

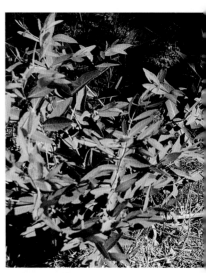

Plate 30. Dogbane *(Apocynum* sp.). (Photo cou Dr. KH Plumlee.)

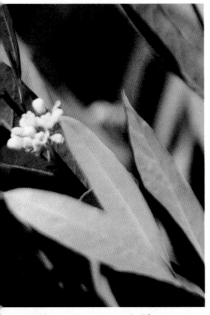

Plate 31. Dogbane *(Apocynum* sp.). (Photo courtesy KH Plumlee.)

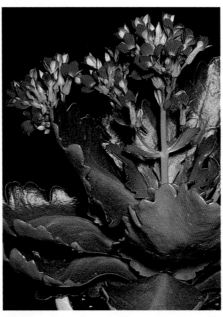

Plate 32. *Kalanchoe* sp. (Photo courtesy Dr. KH Plumlee.)

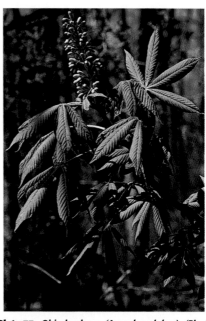

Plate 33. Ohio buckeye *(Aesculus glabra).* (Photo courtesy Dr. WR Hare.)

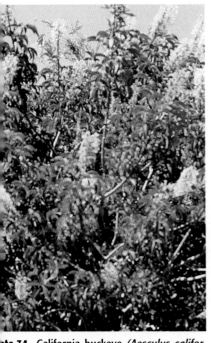

Plate 34. California buckeye *(Aesculus califorica).* (Photo courtesy Dr. KH Plumlee.)

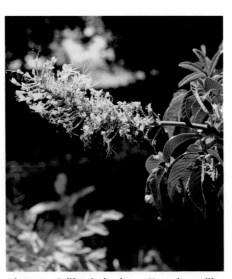

Plate 35. California buckeye *(Aesculus californica).* (Photo courtesy Dr. KH Plumlee.)

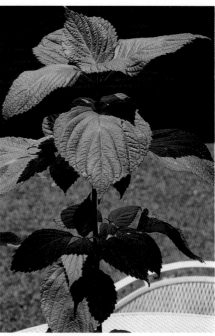

Plate 36. Perilla mint *(Perilla frutescens).* (Photo courtesy Dr. SS Nicholson.)

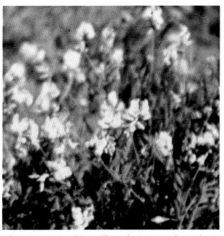

Plate 37. Columbia milkvetch *(Astragalus miser).* (Photo courtesy Dr. BL Stegelmeier.)

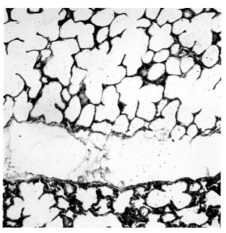

Plate 38. Photomicrograph of the lung of a cow poisoned with NPA. Note extensive interlobular and alveolar emphysema (H&E stained paraffin section). (Photo courtesy Dr. BL Stegelmeier.)

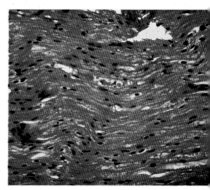

Plate 39. Photomicrograph of the lumbar spi cord of a cow poisoned with NPA. Note Wallerian axonal degeneration with diges vacuoles containing debris-laden macropha (H&E stained paraffin section). (Photo courtesy BL Stegelmeier.)

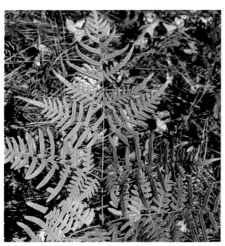

Plate 40. Bracken fern *(Pteridium aquilinum).* (Photo courtesy Dr. SS Nicholson.)

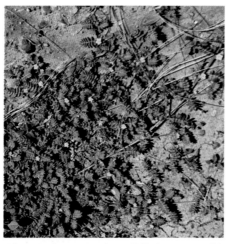

Plate 41. Puncture vine *(Tribulus terrestris).* (Photo courtesy Dr. KH Plumlee.)

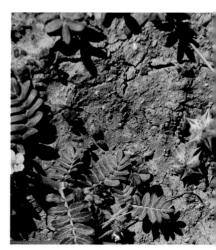

Plate 42. Puncture vine *(Tribulus terrestris).* N the detached spiny fruits in center of pho (Photo courtesy Dr. KH Plumlee.)

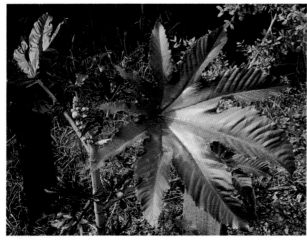

Plate 43. Castor bean *(Ricinus communis)* leaves. (Photo courtesy Dr. KH Plumlee.)

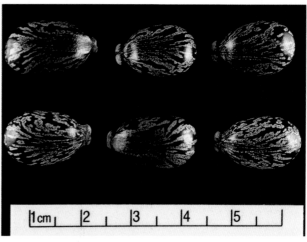

Plate 44. Castor bean *(Ricinus communis)* seeds. (Photo courtesy Dr. JC Albretsen.)

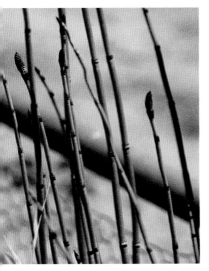

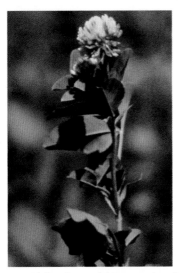

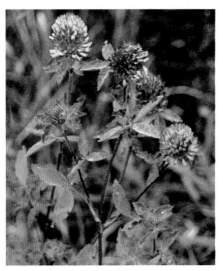

Plate 45. Horsetail (*Equisetum* sp.). (Photo courtesy KH Plumlee.)

Plate 46. Alsike clover. (Photo courtesy Dr. PA Talcott.)

Plate 47. Red clover. (Photo courtesy Dr. PA Talcott.)

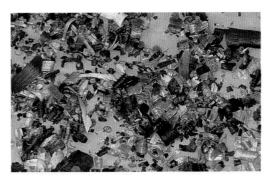

Plate 48. A variety of tree shavings used as stall bedding. The black walnut shavings are dark brown, whereas the shavings from pine and cedar are pale. (Photo courtesy Dr. KH Plumlee.)

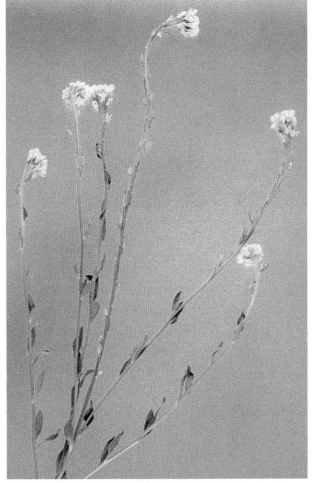

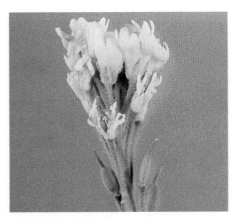

Plate 49. Hoary alyssum (*Berteroa incana*). (Photo courtesy Dr. PA Talcott.)

Plate 50. Hoary alyssum (*Berteroa incana*). (Photo courtesy Dr. PA Talcott.)

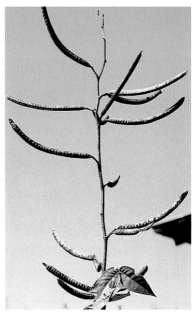

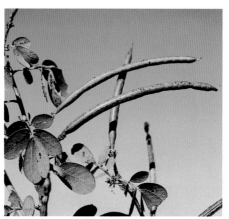

Plate 52. Sicklepod *(Senna obtusifolia).* (Photo courtesy Dr. SS Nicholson.)

Plate 51. Coffee senna *(Senna occidentalis).* (Photo courtesy Dr. SS Nicholson.)

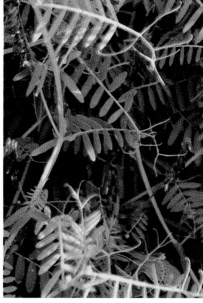

Plate 53. Vetch *(Vicia* sp.). (Photo courtesy Dr Plumlee.)

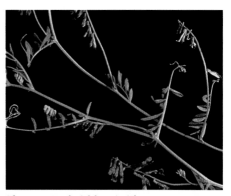

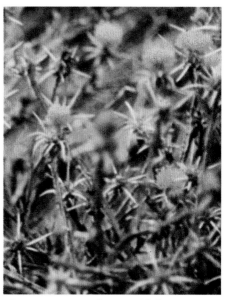

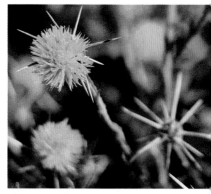

Plate 54. Vetch *(Vicia* sp.). (Photo courtesy Dr. LW Woods.)

Plate 55. Mature yellow starthistle *(Centaurea solstitialis).* (Photo courtesy Dr. PA Talcott.)

Plate 56. Yellow starthistle *(Centaurea solstiti* flowers. (Photo courtesy Dr. KH Plumlee.)

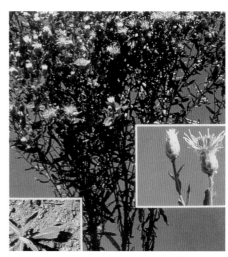

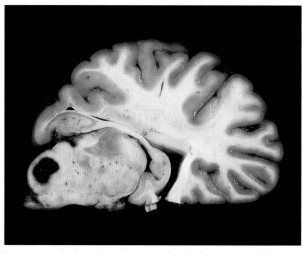

Plate 57. Russian knapweed *(Acroptilon repens).* (Photo courtesy Dr. PA Talcott.)

Plate 58. Sagittal section of equine brain depicting malacia of the globus pallidus. (Photo courtesy Dr. PA Talcott.)

myonecrosis and consequent survival of the animal.[6] Excessive motor neuron stimulation, resulting in severe seizures such as those reported in strychnine poisoning, has been shown in sheep experimentally poisoned with water hemlock.[6,8] Although the seizure activity and muscle necrosis do not appear to be caused by changes in serum potassium and calcium, cicutoxin does have strong potassium channel blocking properties in T lymphocytes.[9,10]

Toxicity and Risk Factors. Animal and human poisoning from water hemlock generally results from the consumption of the root crowns and roots. As little as 50 to 110 mg/kg body weight of the fresh water hemlock plant can induce fatal poisoning in animals.[3,10-13] The lethal dose of fresh water hemlock (*C. douglasii*) is 2 oz for adult sheep, 12 oz for adult cattle, and 8 oz for adult horses.[10] Sheep experimentally given ground hemlock tubers at 1.4 g/kg body weight developed a mild increase in salivation, nervousness, and a few muscular tremors without seizures. Sheep given 2.8 g/kg developed seizures followed by recovery. Sheep given 6.4 g/kg of tuber developed severe seizures and died within 90 minutes.[6]

Clinical Signs. Most animals die in 1 to 3 hours after consuming a lethal dose of water hemlock.[6] Signs may start within an hour of eating the plant or tuberous roots and progress rapidly to convulsive seizures and lateral recumbency. Excessive salivation, vigorous chewing movements, teeth grinding, and frequent urination and defecation can be observed in the early phase of poisoning. Depending on the quantity of toxin absorbed, animals become ataxic, uncoordinated, and develop grand mal seizures. During the violent seizures, animals have been known to chew off their tongues. Poisoned animals have dilated pupils and progress to a state of coma before dying of respiratory paralysis and asphyxia. If a sublethal dose of water hemlock has been consumed, animals often recover if not stressed.

Clinical Pathology. Clinical pathologic changes from water hemlock poisoning are variable depending on the duration and severity of the muscle convulsions induced by the cicutoxin. The serum enzymes lactic dehydrogenase, aspartate transaminase, and creatine kinase markedly increase in those animals that have frequent and prolonged seizure episodes.[6] Blood glucose may be elevated due to epinephrine release resulting from central nervous system stimulation.

Lesions. Animals that die of water hemlock poisoning have no gross pathognomonic postmortem lesions. Multifocal, diffuse myocardial degeneration is encountered in acute water hemlock poisoning.[6] In less acute poisoning, degeneration is also seen in skeletal muscles and is related to the severity of the seizures.

Diagnostic Testing. Confirming a diagnosis of water hemlock poisoning requires eliminating other causes of sudden death, identifying the plant in the animal's environment, and finding parts of the plant or roots in the esophageal groove, rumen, or stomach. Frequently, the plants are well chewed and difficult to detect; however, pieces of the root are most identifiable. Identification of characteristic plant epidermal cell structures in the gastrointestinal contents can be attempted to help confirm the diagnosis.[14] Suspect plant material recovered from the digestive track at postmortem can be analyzed using gas chromatography and matched to the known mass spectra of cicutoxin.[15] Plant samples frozen at 10° C remain stable for up to 8 months with little deterioration of cicutoxin levels.[15]

The differential diagnoses for water hemlock poisoning should include other toxic plants such as yew (*Taxus* spp.), acute nitrate and cyanide poisoning, anthrax, clostridial diseases, hypomagnesemia, and electrocution.

Treatment. It is rarely possible to treat water hemlock poisoning because of the peracute nature of the disease. No specific antidote is available for cicutoxin. However, the intravenous administration of sodium pentobarbital at the onset of seizures in sheep prevented lethal cardiac and skeletal muscle degeneration and resulted in complete recovery.[6] Laxatives may speed removal of the plant from the digestive system. Vomiting should be induced before clinical signs in dogs suspected of eating water hemlock. The use of dilute acetic acid orally in cattle has been reported to be beneficial in neutralizing the toxin. A rumenotomy to remove all plant material from the esophageal groove and rumen may be indicated if the animal is actually observed eating water hemlock.

Prognosis. Because of the potency of cicutoxin and its profound effect on the central nervous system, water hemlock poisoning has a very poor prognosis unless aggressive measures are taken early to prevent seizures and the resulting myonecrosis that causes death.

Prevention and Control. Water hemlock is one of the few plants that should be diligently removed from areas where animals have access. The plant should be dug up and burned if possible. Selectively spraying water hemlock with herbicides such as 2,4-D or glyphosate (Roundup) kills the plant; however, herbicides may make the plant more palatable before it dies. Because water hemlock grows in or adjacent to water, it is important to follow manufacturer recommendations and government ordinances regarding the use of herbicides in riparian areas.

REFERENCES

1. Mulligan GA: The genus *Cicuta* in North America, *Can J Bot* 58:1755, 1979.
2. Anet EFLG, Lythgoe B, Silk MH, Trippett S: Oenanthotoxin and cicutoxin. Isolation and structures, *J Chem Soc* 66:309, 1953.
3. Kingsbury JM: *Poisonous plants of the United States and Canada*, Englewood Cliffs, NJ, 1964, Prentice-Hall.
4. Marsh DC, Clawson AB: Cicuta, or water hemlock. *U.S. Department of Agriculture Bulletin* 69:1, 1914.
5. Payonk GS, Segelman AB: Analytical and phytochemistry of the American water hemlock, *Cicuta maculata* (Umbelliferae), *Vet Hum Toxicol* 22:367, 1980.
6. Panter KE et al: Water hemlock (*Cicuta douglasii*) toxicosis in sheep: pathologic description and prevention of lesions and death, *J Vet Diagn Invest* 8:474, 1996.

7. Haddad LM, Shannon MW, Winchester JF: *Clinical management of poisoning and drug overdose*, ed 3, Philadelphia, 1998, WB Saunders.
8. Boyd RE et al : Strychnine poisoning, *Medicine* 74:507, 1983.
9. Panter KE et al: Toxicosis in livestock from the hemlocks (*Conium* and *Cicuta* spp.), *J Anim Sci* 66:2407, 1988.
10. Strauss U et al: Cicutoxin from *Cicuta virosa*–a new and potent potassium channel blocker in T lymphocytes, *Biochem Biophysical Res Comm* 219:332, 1996.
11. James LF, Ralphs MH: Water hemlock, *Utah Science* 47:67, 1986.
12. Warwick BL, Runnels HA: Water hemlock poisoning of livestock, Ohio Agricultural Experiment Station 14:35, 1929.
13. Fleming CE, Peterson NF: The poison parsnip or water hemlock (*Cicuta occidentalis*), *Univ Nevada Agric Exp Station Bull* 100:1, 1920.
14. Potter RL, Ueckert DN: Epidermal cellular characteristics of selected livestock-poisoning plants in North America, Texas A & M University, College Station, 1997, Texas Agricultural Experiment Station.
15. Smith RA, Lewis D: Cicuta toxicosis in cattle: case history and simplified analytical method, *Vet Hum Toxicol* 29:240, 1987.

INSOLUBLE CALCIUM OXALATES

Charlotte Means

Synonyms. Some genera have numerous species; more than 200 varieties of *Philodendron* alone have been identified (Table 25-2). Because common names are shared among various genus and species, occasionally plant identification errors can occur.

TABLE 25-2 **Scientific and Common Names of Plants that Contain Insoluble Calcium Oxalates**

Genus and Species	Common Names
Aglaonema modestrum	Chinese evergreen
Alocasia antiquorum or *Colocasia*	Alocasia, elephant's ear
Anthurium spp.	Flamingo plant
Arisaema triphyllum	Jack-in-the-pulpit
Arum maculatum	Cuckoo-pint
Caladium spp.	Caladium, elephant's ear
Calla palustris	Wild calla, wild arum
Dieffenbachia spp.	Dumb cane varieties
Epipremnum (Scindapsus) spp.	Devil's ivy, pothos varieties, marble queen, variegated philodendron, taro vine
Monstera spp.	Ceriman, mother-in-law, Swiss cheese plant, hurricane plant, fruit salad plant, cutleaf philodendron, Mexican breadfruit
Philodendron spp.	Philodendron varieties
Spathiphyllum spp.	Peace lily
Symplocarpus foetidus	Skunk cabbage
Syngonium podophyllum	Nephthytis
Xanthsoma spp.	Malanga, caladium, elephant's ears
Zantedeschia aethiopica	Calla lily, arum lily

Sources. Many popular houseplants and ornamentals contain insoluble calcium oxalate crystals. Most of these plants are in the family Araceae and all the plants cause a similar clinical syndrome. Many of these plants have broad green or variegated green leaves. Most do not produce flowers or produce inconspicuous flowers. Although usually ornamentals, several species grow in wooded areas.[1,2]

Mechanism of Action. All parts of the plants are toxic, but sometimes leaves contain little or no toxin. The primary mechanism of action involves calcium oxalate crystals. The plants (primarily studied in *Dieffenbachia* spp.) contain cells known as *idioblasts*. These cells contain raphides, which are spicules of calcium oxalate crystals that are sharp and needle shaped. The crystals are packed in a gelatinous substance that contains free oxalic acid.

When the tip of the idioblast is broken during ingestion, sap from the plant or saliva from the animal enters the cell, causing the gelatinous material to swell. The swelling forces the raphides to shoot from the cell, rather like a bullet. The sharp crystals penetrate the oral mucosa, tongue, and throat, causing mechanical damage. The cells may continue to expel crystals for a significant amount of time, even after a piece of plant material is swallowed. Some species also contain proteolytic enzymes, which stimulate the release of kinins and histamines by the body. The rapid inflammatory response aggravates the mechanical damage caused by the crystals.[1,3, 4]

Clinical Signs. The onset of clinical signs is rapid and can occur immediately or up to 2 hours after ingestion. Therefore, pain and irritation can be immediate on chewing. The pain may be expressed by head shaking and intense hypersalivation. A change in vocalization can occur, usually sounding weak or hoarse. Depression and anorexia are often present. Swelling of the mucous membranes of the oral cavity, pharynx, and tongue are generally present. If significant swelling occurs, it is possible for dyspnea to develop but actual obstruction of the airway is rare.

Nausea and vomiting are common responses to the irritation of the crystals in the stomach and diarrhea may develop. Because of the immediate irritant effect, large ingestions are uncommon. In case of a massive ingestion, vomiting and diarrhea may be severe enough to cause dehydration, electrolyte imbalances, and shock. Reports of cardiac arrhythmia, mydriasis, coma, and death are in the literature. However, it is unlikely that severe clinical signs will be seen.[1,4,5]

Treatment. Treatment is primarily symptomatic and supportive. Most cases can be managed at home. The mouth should be rinsed with water. Offering a small quantity of milk, yogurt, or cottage cheese frequently provides some relief from oral pain, possibly by precipitating some of the calcium oxalate crystals. An antihistamine, such as diphenhydramine (2 to 4 mg/kg by mouth or intramuscularly every 8 hours as needed[6]) helps reduce oral swelling. A mild gastrointestinal protectant, such as kaolin/pectin (dogs and cats: 1 to 2 ml/kg four times daily; small birds: 1 drop twice daily; large birds: 1 ml up to four times daily[6]) or sucralfate (dogs weighing >20 kg: 1 g three to four times daily; dogs weighing <20 kg: 0.5 g three to four times daily; cats: 0.25 g two to three times daily[6]), can help reduce irritation in the stomach and intestines.

If dyspnea occurs, the animal should be observed at a veterinary clinic until the pharyngeal swelling resolves and the animal is breathing normally. When persistent vomiting and diarrhea occur, intravenous (IV) fluids and gastrointestinal protectants should be administered.[4]

Prognosis. Clinical signs usually persist for a few hours and should be completely resolved within 24 hours. In almost all cases, a complete recovery is expected.

Prevention and Control. Including lists of potentially toxic plants in new kitten and puppy kits, as well as plants to avoid in aviaries, can help educate pet owners to potential toxic plant hazards.

REFERENCES

1. Spoerke DG, Smolinske SC: *Toxicity of houseplants,* Boca Raton, Fla, 1990, CRC Press.
2. Frohne D, Pfander HJ: *A colour atlas of poisonous plants,* London, 1983, Wolfe Publishing.
3. Cheeke PR: *Natural toxicants in feeds, forages, and poisonous plants,* ed 2, Danville, Ill, 1998, Interstate Publishers.
4. Osweiler GD: *Toxicology,* Philadelphia, 1996, Williams & Wilkins.
5. Beasley VR, Dorman DC et al: *A systems affected approach to veterinary toxicology,* Urbana, Ill, 1999, University of Illinois.
6. Plumb DC: *Veterinary drug handbook,* ed 3, Ames, Iowa, 1999, Iowa State University Press.

ISOCUPRESSIC ACID

Patricia A. Talcott

Synonyms. The disease "pine needle abortion" has been associated with the ingestion of *Pinus ponderosa, Pinus contorta, Juniperus communis,* and *Cupressus macrocarpa* in cattle and buffalo.

Sources. *P. ponderosa* (i.e., ponderosa pine, western yellow pine, yellow pine, pondosa pine, blackjack pine, bull pine) has been classically associated with pine needle abortion in the bovine. This pine tree is prevalent throughout the western United States. It is a large deciduous tree, up to 230 feet tall, with 4- to 10-inch needles distributed mostly in threes. During early growth, the bark is dark-brown or black. As the tree ages, the bark becomes cinnamon-red, very thick, and divided into large plates that break off freely.

P. contorta (i.e., lodgepole pine, black pine, scrub pine, shore pine, coast pine, tamarack pine) is found along the western coast of the United States from Alaska to Baja, California, and east to Colorado, North and South Dakota, and Alberta and Saskatoon, Canada. These are tall, slender trees, reaching heights up to 100 feet, and have 1- to 2.5-inch needles that are typically distributed in twos. The brown-gray bark is thin and scaly, and the cones can be orange-red or yellow-brown in color. These trees are more

adapted to high mountain slopes at elevations of 6000 feet or higher.

Several varieties of *J. communis* (i.e., common juniper, mountain juniper) exist. They are small (<7 feet tall) sprawling bushes, mostly located in lowland woods to mountain valleys and open rocky alpine slopes. These bushes have scalelike to needle-like leaves arranged in twos or threes and small green or brown berries. *Cupressus macrocarpa,* the Monterey cypress, commonly found in New Zealand, is not native to the United States.

Toxicokinetics. Isocupressic acid was first hypothesized as being the abortifacient agent present in the resin of ponderosa pine needles.[1] Since then, isocupressic acid has been found in lodgepole pines, junipers, and the Monterey cypress (all trees associated with premature parturition and abortion in cows). This compound has since been shown experimentally to cause premature parturition or abortion in late term cows following both oral and intravenous administration.[2] Subsequent metabolism studies have isolated various metabolites of isocupressic acid. It is currently unknown whether any or all of these metabolites are active abortifacient agents. Since these initial studies, it has further been suggested that acetyl- and succinylisocupressic acid are the naturally present compounds found in pine needles and that they are rapidly converted to isocupressic acid following ingestion.[3]

Isocupressic acid, in vitro, is metabolized to imbricatoloic acid, to a structurally uncharacterized isomer of imbricatoloic acid, and to dihyroagathic acid.[4] In liver homogenate preparations, isocupressic acid is oxidized to agathic acid.[4] Following IV infusion, agathic acid was identified as the major metabolite; however, after oral administration, dihydroagathic acid was identified as the major metabolite.[4,5]

One group of investigators has suggested that myristate and laurate esters of 1,14-tetradecanediol and 1,12-dodecanediol may be responsible for the abortifacient activity.[6] These lipidlike compounds were first isolated from *P. ponderosa* needles and were shown to have potent vasoconstrictive activity in an in vitro placentome perfusion assay. However, to the author's knowledge, these compounds have not been shown to cause abortions in vivo.

Mechanism of Action. The exact biochemical mechanism of action of isocupressic acid is still under investigation. The current hypothesis suggests that the active metabolites cause a reduction in uterine blood flow to the fetus as a result of an increase in vascular tone.[7,8] The decrease in uterine arterial blood flow may result from activation of α_2-adrenergic receptors, which could then facilitate the extracellular uptake of calcium through the potential sensitive Ca^{++} channels, directly resulting in decreased arterial diameter and blood flow. This reduction in blood flow, with subsequent reduction in nutrients and oxygen to the fetus, would then stimulate the release of fetal cortisol, the direct stimulus for parturition in cows.

Toxicity and Risk Factors. Cows in the last 3 months of pregnancy are at greatest risk. As the stage of gestation progresses, the incidence of abortion increases. Cows appear to be most susceptible after the eighth month of gestation. Toxic properties have been found in the needles, bark, and new growth tips; however, it is the needles that present the greatest abortifacient risk. Cows have reportedly died following ingestion of pine needles from an apparent toxicosis thought to be due to toxins other than isocupressic acid. In addition, pine needles administered to steers intraruminally were shown to have a negative effect on nitrogen intake and digestibility, along with fluid rate of passage.[9]

The approximate daily toxic dose of isocupressic acid is 200 mg/kg body weight.[2] Assuming that a pregnant cow weighs 450 kg and the isocupressic content of the needles is 1% dry weight, then the cow would have to ingest approximately 9 kg of pine needles daily to receive a toxic dose. Pregnant cows (240 days of gestation) orally gavaged with daily doses of 4.5 to 5.5 kg lodgepole pine needles per kilogram body weight (isocupressic acid [ICA] level = 0.8% dry weight; daily dose of 62 to 78 mg ICA/kg body weight) aborted in 8 to 10 days, whereas cows receiving 4.5 to 5.5 kg common juniper needles per kilogram body weight (ICA level = 2% dry weight; daily dose of 190 to 245 mg ICA/kg body weight) aborted in 3 to 4 days.[10] All four listed trees or shrubs typically contain isocupressic acid at concentrations greater than 0.5% on a dry weight basis. Premature parturition and abortion can follow ingestion of either fresh or dry needles. Sudden weather changes (e.g., early spring snowstorms), starvation, and changes in feed management may predispose cows to ingest pine needles. Also, cows originating from pine-free areas seem to be more predisposed to problems than native cows. It has been suggested from field case reports that sheep, goats, and llamas may be susceptible as well. However, this has not been confirmed experimentally.

Clinical Signs. Premature parturition or abortion can occur as early as 48 hours after ingestion of sufficient amount of plant material, and can continue to occur for 2 weeks or more after the exposure is terminated. This variation is probably due to the gestational age of the cow, the amount of needles consumed, and the concentration of isocupressic acid present. Symptoms of premature udder development and milk production ("bagging-up"), vulvar swelling, and mucoid or hemorrhagic vaginal discharge can be observed. Retained fetal membranes are an extremely common sequela, potentially leading to septic metritis and death. Calves that are born prematurely may live, but are generally very small and weak and require extensive nursing care.

Clinical Pathology. No specific clinical pathologic abnormalities are present in cows with this disease. Elevated white cell counts, with left shifts, and elevated fibrinogens can be seen in cows with septic metritis.

Lesions. The pathologic changes in the tissues, both maternal and fetal, are nonspecific. Vasoconstriction of the caruncular vascular bed with necrosis and hemorrhage, along with reduced numbers of binucleate, trophoblastic giant cells in the placentomes, and increased numbers of necrotic luteal cells in the corpus luteum have been reported.[11,12]

Diagnostic Testing. No specific, readily available diagnostic tests exist that can confirm an isocupressic acid–induced parturition or abortion. The diagnosis is based on evidence of access to these plants (i.e., trees or shrubs in pasture, needles in manure) and eliminating infectious, nutritional, and management-related causes of abortion.

Treatment. Retained placentas are a difficult problem to address. Uterine infusions, prostaglandin, oxytocin, and collagenase have all been tried with limited success. The most conservative approach is to monitor the cow's temperature and treat the endometritis when it develops.

Prognosis. Premature calves may survive with intensive and appropriate supportive care, but complications in the cow (e.g., retained placenta, metritis, septicemia) may be fatal. Cows that survive may experience difficulty in conceiving, which can lead to lower calf weights at market. Otherwise, there are no residual effects on the cow's fertility, especially when there are no secondary complications.

Prevention and Control. The only successful management program that can be implemented to prevent this disease is to not allow pregnant cows access to the pine needles during the critical late stages of gestation. It is not known whether the concentrations of isocupressic acid vary significantly between individual trees or populations of trees, or whether factors such as time of year, weather conditions, soil conditions, or maturity of tree affect levels as well. Attempts to delay or prevent parturition through the use of progestins or prostaglandin inhibitors have met with limited success.[13]

REFERENCES

1. Gardner DR et al: Ponderosa pine needle-induced abortion in beef cattle: identification of isocupressic acid as the principal active compound, *J Agric Food Chem* 42:756, 1994.
2. Gardner DR et al: Isocupressic acid and related diterpene acids from *Pinus ponderosa* as abortifacient compounds in cattle, *J Nat Toxins* 6:1, 1997.
3. Gardner DR et al: Abortifacient activity in beef cattle of acetyl- and succinylisocupressic acid from ponderosa pine, *J Agric Food Chem* 44:3257, 1996.
4. Gardner DR et al: Pine needle abortion in cattle: metabolism of isocupressic acid, *J Agric Food Chem* 47:2891, 1999.
5. Lin SJ et al: In vitro biotransformations of isocupressic acid by cow rumen preparations: formation of agathic and dihydroagathic acids, *J Nat Prod* 61:51, 1998.
6. Al-Mahmoud MS et al: Isolation and characterization of vasoactive lipids from the needles of *Pinus ponderosa*, *J Agr Food Chem* 43:2154, 1995.
7. Ford SP et al: Effects of ponderosa pine needle ingestion on uterine vascular function in late-gestation beef cows, *J Anim Sci* 70:1609, 1992.
8. Christenson LK, et al: Effects of ingestion of pine needles (*Pinus ponderosa*) by late-pregnant beef cows on potential sensitive Ca^{2+} channel activity of caruncular arteries, *J Reprod Fertil* 98:301, 1994.
9. Pfister JA et al: Adverse effects of pine needles on aspects of digestive performance in cattle, *J Range Manage* 45:528, 1992.
10. Gardner DR et al: Abortifacient effects of lodgepole pine (*Pinus contorta*) and common juniper (*Juniperus communis*) on cattle, *Vet Human Toxicol* 40(5):260, 1998.
11. Stuart LD et al: Pine needle abortion in cattle: pathological observations, *Cornell Vet* 79:61, 1989.

12. Jensen R et al: Evaluation of histopathologic and physiologic changes in cows having premature births after consuming Ponderosa pine needles, *Am J Vet Res* 50:285, 1989.
13. Short RE et al: Endocrine responses in cows fed ponderosa pine needles and the effects of stress, corpus luteum regression, progestin, and ketoprofen, *J Anim Sci* 73:198, 1995.

PODOPHYLLIN

William R. Hare

Synonyms. Synonyms for *Podophyllum peltatum* include mayapple, American mandrake, Indian apple, wild lemon, duck's foot, and umbrella leaf.

Sources. The mayapple is a perennial herb with a simple stem and one or two large, 20 to 25 cm in diameter, round, dark-green, umbrella shaped leaves (Color Plate 5). Leaves are characterized by having five to nine lobes. The plant grows 15 to 45 cm in height from a fleshy horizontal root-stock or rhizome. The plant has a single leaf when flowerless and double leaves when flowering. Flowers are white and single, one per stem or plant, found between and under the leaves. The flower is approximately 5 cm in diameter, having six to nine petals with a short, 2.5 to 5 cm, nodding petiole. The plant usually flowers in May and then forms a large, 2.5 to 5 cm, ovoid, yellow, fleshy berrylike fruit, which ripens in July. The rootstock or rhizome is most toxic, but all parts of the plant should be considered potentially toxic. Only the ripened fruit is not known to be toxic.[1]

Mayapple can be found throughout the United States and southern Canada. It is especially prevalent in wet meadows, damp open wooded areas, and along roadside ditches.

Toxicokinetics. The toxic principle of mayapple is podophyllin. Its constituents include podophyllin resin, podophyllotoxin, picropodophyllin, quercetin, and pellatins. Podophyllin resin, in turn, is a mixture of 16 biologically active compounds further classified as lignins and flavonols. Podophyllin is known to have gastrointestinal, neurologic, and teratogenic effects. Mayapple extracts containing podophyllin have been used for hundreds of years as a "home remedy" for both its cathartic activity and for the topical treatment of warts. There are currently a number of studies and clinical investigations on the use of podophyllotoxin derivatives for the treatment of a variety of malignant conditions.[2,3]

Podophyllin is absorbed readily from the gastrointestinal tract and skin. However, very little is known about the distribution and metabolism of all the podophyllin constituents. Podophyllic acid is eliminated predominantly in the urine and has a 30-minute half-life, whereas podophyllotoxin is eliminated predominantly in the bile with approximately a 48-hour half-life.[4]

Mechanism of Action. The exact mechanism of action of podophyllin on the gastrointestinal tract is unknown. However, it is generally believed that the cathartic effect of podophyllin is secondary to gastrointestinal irritation. Podophyllin is neurotoxic; however, the exact mechanism of action on the nervous system is also unknown, but may be related to its toxic effects on cell respiration. Podophyllin has a direct toxic effect on mitochondria, reducing the activity of electron transport enzymes, cytochrome oxidase, and succinoxidase.

Podophyllin's teratogenic effects and anticancer activity are thought to be related to its toxic effects on cell division and nucleic acid synthesis. Podophyllum is a spindle poison and blocks mitosis in metaphase.[5] It binds to proteins, inhibits purine synthesis, and stops purine incorporation into RNA.[6]

Toxicity and Risk Factors. Cattle, sheep, horses, llamas, swine, dogs, cats, monkeys, and exotic and laboratory animals can all be expected to develop adverse clinical signs following significant exposure to podophyllin. Animals normally do not ingest mayapple, and clinical cases of poisoning are rare. However, there still is potential for poisoning, especially of livestock grazing in the early spring, when forage is scarce and mayapple is one of the first plants to appear. The risk of poisoning to companion animals is due to the overuse or accidental ingestion of "home remedy" preparations of mayapple extract. In humans, clinical exposure has shown a wide variation in toxicity with deaths reported following exposure to as little as 350 mg and survival following exposure to as much as 2.8 g.

Clinical Signs. Clinical signs usually appear within a few hours following exposure but may be delayed as long as 12 hours or more. Early clinical signs include vomiting, diarrhea, and anorexia. In addition, fever, hypersalivation, excess lacrimation, conjunctivitis, keratitis, mental confusion, ataxia, paralysis, coma, and death have been reported. Tachycardia and tachypnea are seen secondarily; oliguria progressing to anuria has also been reported. In most uncomplicated cases, adverse clinical signs usually resolve within 7 to 10 days.

Clinical Pathology. Metabolic and respiratory acidosis with accompanying changes in bicarbonate may be noticed. Renal failure and toxic hepatitis have been reported and supported by serum chemistries. In addition, changes in peripheral blood counts usually accompany bone marrow suppression.[6,7]

Lesions. Pathologic lesions include gastroenteritis and possibly bone marrow suppression.

Diagnostic Testing. No routine diagnostic tests to confirm mayapple poisoning are available. The identification of mayapple plant parts from stomach contents, following emesis or postmortem examination, can confirm exposure. Identification of plant material may be improved by a visual chromatographic chemical test.[8]

Treatment. No antidote is available and treatment is usually supportive. Decontamination efforts are important. Use of activated charcoal followed by gastrointestinal protectants are helpful. In cases of marked toxicosis, fluids should be administered and the acid-base status and serum electrolytes monitored. Adverse clinical signs usually resolve within 7 to 10 days, or sooner.

Prognosis.   The prognosis is generally good to fair, especially when exposure is limited and treatment is instituted early. When exposure is great and clinical signs are characterized by marked neurologic deficits or are accompanied by cardiovascular collapse, the prognosis is grave to guarded.

Prevention and Control.   Grazing animals should not have access to mayapple, especially if forage is scarce. Pastures with significant growth of mayapple can be improved with careful use of most broadleaf herbicides. Mayapple extracts found in alternative medicines and home remedies can be poisonous and must be used appropriately.

REFERENCES

1. Kingsbury JM: *Poisonous plants of the United States and Canada,* Englewood Cliffs, NJ, 1964, Prentice-Hall.
2. Damayanthi Y, Lown JW: Podophyllotoxins: current status and recent developments, *Curr Med Chem* 5(3):205, 1998.
3. Schacter L: Ectoposide phosphate: what, why, where, and how? *Semin Oncol* 23 (6 Suppl, 13):1, 1996.
4. Clark AN, Parsonabe MJ: A case of podophyllum poisoning with involvement of the nervous system, *Br Med J* 2:1155, 1957.
5. Leikin JB, Paloucek FP: *Poisoning & Toxicology Handbook,* ed 2, Hudson, 1996, Lexi-Comp.
6. Cassidy DE et al: Podophyllum toxicity: a report of a fatal case and review of the literature, *J Toxicol Clin Toxicol* 19(1):35, 1982.
7. Moher LM, Maurer SA: Podophyllum toxicity: case report and literature review, *J Fam Pract* 9(2):237, 1979.
8. But PP et al: Instant methods to spot-check poisonous podophyllum root in herb samples of clematis root, *Vet Hum Toxicol* 39(6):366, 1997.

QUINONES AND FURANOCOUMARINS

George Burrows and Ronald J. Tyrl

Sources.   Toxic quinones and furanocoumarins are associated with genera of the Apiaceae (carrot/celery family), the Clusiaceae (St. John's wort family), and the Polygonaceae (buckwheat family) (Table 25-3). These compounds cause photosensitization when plants are eaten in large quantities by livestock.

Genera of the Apiaceae known to cause photosensitization include *Ammi, Cymopterus, Heracleum,* and *Sphenosciadium.* All have the family's characteristic compound umbrella-shaped inflorescence with white petaled flowers and pinnately compound or pinnately dissected leaves. Two species of *Ammi* are present in North America. Both are erect, herbaceous annuals or biennials. They are of generally scattered occurrence, most common in the states along the Gulf Coast.

One species of *Cymopterus* is clearly recognized as toxic, although others of the several dozen species occurring in North America may also present a risk under appropriate circumstances. It is a short-stemmed perennial occurring on the western slope of the Rocky Mountains, mainly in juniper areas of southern Utah.

One native and two introduced species of *Heracleum* are present in North America. Of primary importance and concern is the native species is a robust, single-stemmed perennial with large leaves. It is found in wet habitats across the continent and is most abundant in the north.

A single species of *Sphenosciadium* exists as an erect perennial with compound leaves. It is found in wet sites in the mountains of Oregon and California and in scattered areas of the Great Basin.

In the Clusiasceae, only a few members of the genus *Hypericum* present a risk of photosensitization. The toxic species are herbaceous with showy flowers bearing bright yellow petals and tiny, punctate, translucent, or black glands on the leaves, sepals, and petals. Most North American species lack the pigment glands and are not toxic.

Mainly of historical concern because it is now little used as a forage for livestock, the single species of *Fagopyrum* is of toxicologic interest. It is an erect annual herb with scattered occurrence as naturalized populations across North America and an occasionally cultivated grain crop.

Toxicokinetics.   The effects of the quinones are cumulative with continued consumption of the plants. They are slowly eliminated from the body and their effects may persist because of the time needed for the skin lesions to heal.

Ingested furanocoumarins are metabolized in the rumen or the liver and are excreted in the urine and bile.[1,2] They may be present in milk and eggs, but the public health risk is low because the compounds are in low concentrations.[3] Like the quinones, their effects may persist for some time.

Mechanism of Action.   The quinones are type II (secondary) and furanocoumarins are type I (primary) photosensitizing agents.[4,5] The quinones include hypericin, contained in the minute glands of *Hypericum,* and fagopyrin, a derivative of hypericin found in the foliage and inflorescences of *Fagopyrum esculentum.* The furanocoumarins and related furanochromones are present in most plant parts of the members of the Apiaceae. The principal furanocoumarins are linear compounds such as psoralen, xanthotoxin, and bergapten.

In all of these plants, the toxins cause disease when ingested or, in the case of Apiaceae, also by topical exposure.

TABLE 25-3 Plants that Contain Quinones or Furanocoumarins

Scientific Name	Common Name
Ammi majus L.	Bishop's weed, greater ammi
A. visnaga L.	Bisnaga, bishop's weed, toothpick ammi
Cymopterus ibapensis M. E.Jones	Spring parsley
Heracleum lanatum Michx.	Cow parsnip
Sphenosciadium capitellatum A.Gray	White heads, ranger's button
Hypericum perforatum L.	St. John's wort, Klamath weed, goatweed
Fagopyrum esculentum Moench.	Buckwheat, common buckwheat

The quinones are activated by light wavelengths of 540 to 610 nm and cause formation of singlet oxygen, which reacts with nucleic acids, membrane lipids, and amino acids of the capillary endothelium.[4,6] The furanocoumarins are activated by long wavelength ultraviolet light (320 to 380 nm) and cause more extensive effects (typical of type I reactions) because of cross-linking of DNA.[4] Tissue injury also may involve lipid-membrane alterations secondary to fatty acid interactions with the activated furanocoumarins.[7]

Toxicity and Risk Factors. All animal species are at risk, but herbivores more so. In cases of sheep eating *Cymopterus ibapensis*, the greatest risk is starvation of nursing lambs. Because of the painful lesions of the mammary gland skin, the mothers may not allow the lambs to suckle.[8]

Toxin levels in *Hypericum* peak in midsummer but this is offset by decreased palatability at this time. Considerable variation in toxin concentrations exists in plants across North America.

Clinical Signs. Similar signs are produced by all of these photosensitizing taxa. They include erythema and edema of the skin in areas of minimal pigmentation or areas less protected by wool or feathers. Severe pruritus is common. Blisters may form, with subsequent exudation and sloughing of the skin of the teats, udder, and escutcheon. A striking demarcation in distribution of the lesions coincides with lighter colored areas of the skin. Photophobia with inflammation of the cornea and conjunctiva can occur. Systemic signs such as diarrhea and restlessness may accompany the skin changes.

Lesions. Skin and eye changes are the most prominent lesions. In some animals there may also be mild histopathologic changes such as renal tubular dilation with flattened epithelia and hepatic fatty change and necrosis.

Diagnostic Testing. Incrimination of a specific plant may be aided by the use of an in vitro microbiologic assay of photosensitivity potential.[9]

Treatment. If sloughing occurs, the skin lesions require topical treatment. Antibiotics for secondary bacterial infections may be necessary. Nursing offspring of affected mothers should be given supplemental feeding. Animals should be provided shelter from the sun until the lesions resolve.

Prognosis. Typically, the skin lesions resolve when the animal is prevented access to the offending plants, although healing may require several weeks or months.

REFERENCES

1. De Wolff FA, Thomas TV: Clinical pharmacokinetics of methoxsalen and other psoralens, *Clin Pharmacokinetics* 11:62, 1986.
2. Kolis SJ, Williams TH, Postma EJ et al: The metabolism of 14C-methoxsalen by the dog, *Drug Metab Disp* 7:220, 1979.
3. Pangilinan NC et al: Fate of [14C] xanthotoxin (8-methoxypsoralen) in laying hens and a lactating dairy goat, *J Chem Ecol* 18:253, 1992.
4. Dodge AD, Knox JP: Photosensitizers from plants, *Pesticide Sci* 17:579, 1986.
5. Clare NT: *Photosensitization in diseases of livestock*, Bucks, England, 1952, Commonwealth Agricultural Bureaux, Farnham Royal.
6. Sheard C, Caylor HD, Schlotthauer C: Photosensitization of animals after ingestion of buckwheat, *J Exp Med* 47:1013, 1928.
7. Specht KG, Kittler L, Midden WR: A new biological target of furacoumarins: photochemical formation of covalent adducts with unsaturated fatty acids, *Photochem Photobiol* 47:537, 1988.
8. Binns W, James LF, Brooksby N: *Cymopterus watsonii*: a photosensitizing plant for sheep, *Vet Med Small Anim Clin* 59:375, 1964.
9. Rowe LD, Norman JO: Detection of phototoxic activity in plant specimens associated with primary photosensitization in livestock using a simple microbiological test, *J Vet Diagn Invest* 1:269, 1989.

SOLUBLE OXALATES

John A. Pickrell and Fred Oehme

Sources. Beets and dock (*Rumex* sp.), halogeton, and lambs quarter (*Chenopodium* sp.) are scattered throughout the United States.[1-6] Halogeton is widely spread over arid desert in the western intermountain regions. Greasewood (*Sarcobatus* sp.) is found mostly in the alkaline flood plains of the western range, where soil is intermittently moist. It is most palatable in the spring.[2,3,5] Rhubarb (*Rheum* sp.) is a perennial garden plant with edible tart leaves.[2] *Chenopodium* and *Rumex* have oxalate crystals in their leaves and stems.[7]

Oxalate concentrations are highest in the most rapidly growing plants. Leaves contain considerably higher concentrations of oxalates than seeds or stems. At peak concentrations, oxalate in leaves is about 30%, whereas seeds have approximately one third of this concentration and stems have approximately one tenth.[4] Soursob (*Oxalis cernua*) contains sufficient soluble oxalate to intoxicate animals after a dry, hot summer.[8] Tropical grasses such as *Setaria* and *Kochia* are distributed throughout the United States and contain moderate amounts (approximately 5%) of oxalate.[9,10]

Toxicokinetics. Sodium and potassium oxalate are so rapidly absorbed from the gastrointestinal tract that acute disease may occur as early as 2 hours after ingestion.[1,2] Oxalate is readily excreted.

Mechanism of Action. Soluble oxalates complex with serum calcium to form calcium oxalate, resulting in as much as a 20% depletion of ionized calcium and a functional hypocalcemia.[1,2] Although moderate amounts of calcium oxalate are excreted, it may crystallize in the kidneys as polarizing rosettes associated with fatal renal tubular necrosis.[2,11] In vitro renal cell culture suggests that free radicals may be partly responsible for the kidney cell damage, as indicated by reversal with free radical scavengers.[12]

Toxicity and Risk Factors. One-time consumption of the plant is sufficient to cause acute toxicoses. However, oxalate toxicosis depends on the rate of consumption, the amount of other feed consumed concurrently, and the total amount of oxalate consumed.[1-6] For example, an amount of greasewood that would be lethal if ingested at one time after a short fast can be tolerated without harmful effects if ingested over the course of several hours or if ingested with other food.[6]

Clinical Signs. Clinical disease occurs more commonly in sheep than in cattle. Early clinical signs of oxalate-induced hypocalcemia may occur 2 to 6 hours after ingestion. One group of sheep showed signs 40 hours after being allowed to graze a pasture with rumex.[6] The signs included dullness, rumen atony, bloat, twitching, ataxia, teeth grinding, and tetany or seizures. Bradycardia, slobbering, weakness, and incoordination preceded an inability to rise and coma 1 to 2 hours after onset of symptoms.[1-6,13] Animals that do not die acutely may demonstrate vomiting, depression, weight loss, diarrhea, and death within 1 to several days.[1-6]

Clinical Pathology. Calcium oxalates cause hypocalcemia. Blocked renal tubules can result in hyperkalemia. Blood urea nitrogen (BUN) level increases when animals take several days to die.[2]

Lesions. Postmortem findings include excess abdominal and thoracic fluid, diffuse petechiae throughout the digestive tract and on serosal membranes surrounding the heart, and emphysema of the lungs. Sheep dying acutely have polarizing calcium oxalate crystal rosettes in the kidney tubular lumen, lumen distention, and a flattened degenerated tubular epithelium consistent with tubular nephrosis.[2] In animals that live longer, the cortex and medulla of the kidney are dark, often separated by a gray line of oxalate accumulation that has a gritty consistency when cut.[3]

Diagnostic Testing. Plant identification and the occurrence of calcium oxalate crystals in the kidneys support a diagnosis. Measurement of oxalate concentrations in forage and kidney can be performed at some laboratories.[1,2,4,9]

Treatment. Dicalcium phosphate: sodium chloride (1:3) may bind soluble oxalates in the gut. Treatment with electrolytes for hypocalcemia and with fluid therapy for renal nephrosis is frequently not successful.

Prognosis. Advanced clinical signs signal a poor prognosis.[1,2,5,6]

Prevention and Control. Control is mostly a function of range and feeding management to limit exposure to plants that contain soluble oxalates and to provide plenty of other forage. Well-fed animals can tolerate considerably greater doses of ingested oxalate than animals with restricted feed and water intake.

REFERENCES

1. Murphy M: *A field guide to common animal poisons,* Ames, Iowa, 1996, Iowa State University Press.
2. Osweiler GD: *Toxicology,* Philadelphia, 1996, Williams & Wilkins.
3. Kingsbury JM: *Poisonous plants of the United States and Canada,* Englewood Cliffs, NJ, 1964, Prentice-Hall.
4. Hulbert LC, Oehme FW: *Plants poisonous to livestock,* Manhattan, Kan, 1968, Kansas State University.
5. Blodgett D: Renal toxicants. In Howard JL, Smith RA: *Current veterinary therapy, food animal practice 4,* Philadelphia, 1999, WB Saunders.
6. Panciera RJ et al: Acute oxalate poisoning attributable to ingestion of curly dock (*Rumex crispus*) in sheep, *J Am Vet Med Assoc* 196:1981, 1981.
7. Rehkis J: The poisonous plant *Oxalis cernua, Vet Hum Toxicol* 36:23, 1994.
8. Cheeke PR: Endogenous toxins and mycotoxins in forage grasses and their effects on livestock, *J Anim Sci* 73:909, 1995.
9. Rankins DL, Smith GS: Nutritional and toxicological evaluations of kochia hay (*Kochia scoparia*) fed to lambs, *J Anim Sci* 69:2925, 1991.
10. Miller C et al: Oxalate toxicity in renal epithelial cells: characteristics of apoptosis and necrosis, *Toxicol Appl Pharmacol* 162:132, 1999.
11. Scheid C et al: Oxalate toxicity in LLC-PK1 cells: role of free radicals, *Kidney Int* 49:413, 1996.
12. Doaigey AR: Occurrence, type, and location of calcium oxalate crystals in leaves and stems of 16 species of poisonous plants, *Am J Bot* 78:1608, 1991.
13. Angus KW et al: Acute nephropathy in young lambs, *Vet Rec* 124:9, 1989.
14. Aiello S, editor: *The Merck veterinary manual (toxicology),* Whitehouse Station, NJ, Merck.

TANNIC ACID

Konnie H. Plumlee

Synonyms. The disease is known as oak poisoning or acorn poisoning. In years past, calves born with certain deformities (especially shortened diaphyses and enlarged epiphyses of the forelimbs) were known as "acorn calves" because the deformities were thought to be caused by ingestion of acorns by the dams during gestation. However, it is now believed that other factors, such as dam malnutrition, are the actual cause of "acorn calves."[1,2]

Sources. Oak trees and shrubs are found nearly worldwide, and oak poisoning has been reported in most countries. Hundreds of species of oak exist and all should be considered potentially toxic. Toxicosis occurs from ingestion of buds, twigs, leaves, and acorns. However, most incidents of toxicosis result from ingestion of immature leaves in the spring or freshly fallen acorns in the autumn.[3-5]

Mechanism of Action. Historically, oak tannins (tannic acid) were believed to be the toxic principal in oak because the highest concentrations of tannic acid are found in immature oak leaves and in freshly fallen acorns, which are the sources of most incidents of toxicosis.[6,7] However, the disease could not be reliably reproduced in cattle and rats given tannic acid, so this idea fell out of favor for many years.[7] In the 1960s, toxicosis was produced during a series of experiments in rabbits given tannic acid and its metabolites, gallic acid and pyrogallol, orally.[7,8] The findings in these rabbit studies have been overinterpreted in subsequent years by other authors and applied to other species, especially ruminants, when in fact the gross pathology lesions were not described in great detail and no histopathology was performed on the rabbit tissues.

Experimentally, commercial tannic acid was found to be mainly hepatotoxic when given parenterally to mice, rats, dogs, rabbits, guinea pigs, cattle, and goats. Liver disease occurred following oral administration of tannic acid in rats, rabbits, and dogs in some studies but not others. Oral administration of tannic acid caused periacinar coagulative and hemorrhagic necrosis of the liver in mice.[9]

Attempts to reproduce oak toxicosis in ruminants by administering commercially produced tannic acid have been unsuccessful. Tannic acid given to sheep orally resulted in methemoglobinemia, whereas tannic acid given intraperitoneally to sheep and mice resulted in liver injury.[9] However, tannic acid given to sheep via the abomasum resulted in severe abomasal damage and mild-to-severe necrosis of the liver.[10] Kidney lesions, when present, were focal and not of the magnitude or same nature as those found in cattle that die of oak poisoning.[10] In another study, cattle were given tannic acid orally and developed methemoglobinemia, but no clinical signs or clinical pathology changes similar to those found with oak poisoning.[3]

In summary, administration studies demonstrate that tannic acid is responsible for gastrointestinal lesions in both monogastrics and ruminants. Liver disease can occur in monogastrics and in ruminants when the rumen is bypassed. However, the classic signs and lesions associated with oak poisoning in cattle have not been reproduced so far with tannic acid.

Toxicity and Risk Factors. Few reports of oak toxicosis in horses are found in the literature; most cases are reported in cattle. Predisposing factors include abnormally large acorn production in some years, access to trimmed oak branches when no other forage was available, or severe weather conditions that prevented normal foraging with subsequent acorn or oak bud ingestion.[5,11-15]

Clinical Signs. In cattle, constipation and brown-colored urine are early signs. The discolored urine is transient, sometimes lasting for less than 24 hours, and so may be unnoticed.[3] Significant renal disease may be present by the time anorexia, depression, and rumen atony are observed.[3] Other signs that have been reported include roughened haircoat, hemorrhagic diarrhea, and abdominal rigidity.[3,5]

In monogastrics, the primary signs are related to gastrointestinal disturbances. Horses with mild cases of oak poisoning develop colic, reduced peristaltic sounds, depression, and constipation. Horses with more severe cases exhibit colic, rectal tenesmus, and hemorrhagic diarrhea. Hemoglobinuria, hematuria, and icterus have also been reported. Acorn husks are often observed in the feces of horses with acorn poisoning.[11-15]

Clinical Pathology. Cattle given oak developed elevated BUN and creatinine values. Protein, glucose, and blood were evident in the urine. The enzymes aspartate aminotransaminase (AST) and sorbitol dehydrogenase were transiently elevated. The complete blood count remained normal.[3] However, some of the calves from a group of 16 with varying stages of oak toxicosis also had leukocytosis, hypocalcemia, hyperphosphatemia, hyponatremia, hyperkalemia, and hypochloremia.[5]

One case report of fatal acorn poisoning in a horse listed marked dehydration, mildly elevated creatine kinase, azotemia, hypoproteinemia, and hyperglycemia about 7 hours before death. This horse also had decreased serum calcium and chloride, but elevated phosphorus. Total bilirubin and the liver enzymes were normal. The urine was concentrated, but contained protein, occult blood, and hemoglobin casts. The prothrombin time, the activated partial thromboplastin, and fibrin degradation products were increased, presumably because of disseminated intravascular coagulopathy.[11]

Lesions. In general, ruminants typically develop kidney disease and gastrointestinal lesions, whereas monogastric animals primarily develop gastrointestinal disease.

Cattle develop perirenal edema, retroperitoneal edema, ascites, and hydrothorax.[3] The kidneys appear pale and swollen with small white foci and petechial hemorrhages scattered throughout the cortices.[16] Gastrointestinal lesions can range from a mild multifocal rumenitis to severe congestion of the rumen, abomasum, small intestine, large intestine, and mesentery. Ulcerations and hemorrhage may be observed anywhere within the gastrointestinal tract, including the mouth, pharynx, and esophagus.[4,16] Desquamated necrotic tissue and mucus may also be observed within the lower gastrointestinal tract.[16]

Histopathologic lesions of the bovine kidney can include severe nephrosis, secondary nephritis, cortical interstitial edema, dilated tubules, and thickened mesangium of the glomeruli. The dilated tubules have low cuboidal, tall columnar, or nonexistent epithelium and may contain homogenous or granular, pink proteinic material.[3]

The most prominent findings in horses are hemorrhagic enteritis and severe edema of the mesentery, cecum, and large intestine.[11,13-15] Acute peritonitis, rupture of the stomach, and bowel obstruction caused by acorns have also been reported.[13] In one horse, a large amount of bright-yellow fluid was found in the pericardial sac, thorax, and abdomen, which are lesions typically found in ruminants. This horse also had mucosal edema and petechiation extending from the stomach to the rectum with coalescing ulcers in the cecum and colon. The kidneys were pale and swollen with petechiae scattered throughout the cortices. Histopathology revealed moderately severe nephrosis.[11]

Rabbits that were given oral gallic acid isolated from shin oak developed hemorrhagic gastritis and stomach ulcers with occasional subserosal hemorrhage and edema extending into the duodenum. The renal cortices were usually pale with congestion or hemorrhage under the capsule, giving the kidney a mottled appearance. Some rabbits had swollen kidneys and a few had congested kidneys. Most rabbits had pale livers with congested areas and prominent lobules. Some rabbits had fluid in the thoracic and abdominal cavities.[7]

Diagnostic Testing. Pyrogallol, a metabolite of tannic acid, can be found in serum and urine of cattle given either oak leaves or commercial tannic acid.[17] However, pyrogallol is only detectable during a transient period of time early in the course of the disease and can no longer be detected by the time that most abnormal clinical signs and clinical pathology findings occur.[3] Therefore, the usefulness of diagnostic testing is limited.

Treatment.   Treatment is limited to symptomatic and supportive care for gastrointestinal and renal disease.

Prognosis.   The prognosis for monogastrics depends on the severity of the gastrointestinal lesions. Morbidity for cattle can be high. However, many cattle that survive the acute toxicosis and continue to eat make a complete recovery.[5] In one study, steers that recovered from oak bud toxicosis had increased rate of weight gain and efficiency of feed conversion as compared to normal herdmates in a feedlot, indicating that a compensatory weight gain occurred.[18]

Prevention and Control.   Oak toxicosis often follows an episode of feed deprivation after a spring snowstorm or after acorns have fallen in the autumn. Animals forage on oak buds and acorns when adequate feed sources are not available. Therefore, the best method of prevention is to provide supplemental feed immediately after snowstorms and in the fall when grass is diminished.

Calcium hydroxide has been shown experimentally to bind to tannins. Calcium hydroxide prevented toxicosis in rabbits when given concurrently with tannic acid in a 1:6 ratio.[19] Calcium hydroxide as 9% to 15% of supplemental feed decreased the occurrence of toxicosis in calves fed oak buds and leaves.[20] Similar results were found when calcium hydroxide was supplemented to goats fed plants, besides oak, that contained tannins.[21] However, oak toxicosis is usually sporadic; therefore, calcium hydroxide supplementation as a preventive measure on a herd basis may not be economically feasible.

REFERENCES

1. Barry MR, Murphy WJB: Acorn calves in the Albury district of New South Wales, *Aust Vet J* 40:195, 1964.
2. Hart GH et al: Acorn calves: a nonhereditary congenital deformity due to maternal nutritional deficiency, *Bull 699,* California Agricultural Experiment Station, 1947.
3. Plumlee KH et al: Comparison of disease in calves dosed orally with oak or commercial tannic acid, *J Vet Diagn Invest* 10:263, 1998.
4. Kasari TR et al: Oak *(Quercus garryana)* poisoning of range cattle in southern Oregon, *Compend Contin Educ* 8:F17, 1986.
5. Spier SJ et al: Oak toxicosis in cattle in northern California: clinical and pathologic findings, *J Am Vet Med Assoc* 191:958, 1987.
6. Harper KT et al: In James LF et al: *The ecology and economic impact of poisonous plants on livestock production,* Boulder, Colo, 1988, Westview Press.
7. Pigeon RF et al: Oral toxicity and polyhydroxyphenol moiety of tannin isolated from *Quercus havardi* (shin oak), *Am J Vet Res* 23:1268, 1962.
8. Dollahite JW et al: The toxicity of gallic acid, pyrogallol, tannic acid, and *Quercus havardi* in the rabbit, *Am J Vet Res* 23:1264, 1962.
9. Zhu J et al: Tannic acid intoxication in sheep and mice, *Res Vet Sci* 53:280, 1992.
10. Zhu J, Filippich LJ: Acute intra-abomasal toxicity of tannic acid in sheep, *Vet Human Toxicol* 37:50, 1995.
11. Anderson GA et al: Fatal acorn poisoning in a horse: pathologic findings and diagnostic considerations, *J Am Vet Med Assoc* 182:1105, 1983.
12. Duncan CS: Oak leaf poisoning in two horses, *Cornell Vet* 51:159, 1961.
13. Wharmby MJ: Acorn poisoning, *Vet Rec* 99:343, 1976.
14. Broughton JE: Acorn poisoning, *Vet Rec* 99:403, 1976.
15. Daniels MG: Acorn poisoning, *Vet Rec* 99:465, 1976.
16. Neser JA, et al: Oak *(Quercus rubor)* poisoning in cattle, *J South African Vet Assoc* 53:151, 1982.
17. Tor ER et al: GC/MS determination of pyrogallol and gallic acid in biological matrices as diagnostic indicators of oak exposure, *J Agric Food Chem* 44:1275, 1996.
18. Ostrowski SR et al: Compensatory weight gain in steers recovered from oak bud toxicosis, *J Am Vet Med Assoc* 195:481, 1989.
19. Dollahite JW, Camp BJ: Calcium hydroxide: an antidote for tannic acid poisoning in rabbits, *Am J Vet Res* 23:1271, 1962.
20. Dollahite JW et al: Calcium hydroxide, a possible antidote for shin oak poisoning in cattle, *Southwest Vet* 17:115, 1963.
21. Murdiati TB et al: Prevention of hydrolysable tannin toxicity in goats fed *Clidemia hirta* by calcium hydroxide supplementation, *J Appl Toxicol* 10:325, 1990.

TREMETONE

Gavin L. Meerdink, Richard L. Fredrickson, Jr., and Gary O. Bordson

Synonyms.   At least three plants are known to contain the tremetone group of toxins. White snakeroot is the common name for *Eupatorium rugosum* (synonyms are *E. urticaefolium, Ageratina altissima* L.). Other common names include richweed, Indian sanicle, white sanicle, deerwort, boneset, poolwort, squawweed, white top, stevia, and sow thoroughwort. Rayless goldenrod or jimmyweed are common names for *Haplopappus heterophyllus* (synonyms are *Applopappus heterophyllus, Iscoma wrightii,* and *Bigelowia rusbeyi).* Burroweed, *Haplopappus tenuisectus* (synonym is *Isocoma tenuisecta),* is the third plant recognized to contain tremetone. (*H. fruticosus* and *H. hartwegii* are closely related with similar habitats and may also contain the same toxic principle.[1-4])

Sources.   White snakeroot is a perennial with an erect stem, 2 to 4 feet tall, that may be branched near the top. Leaves are opposite (with each ascending pair perpendicular to the next) and are large (3 to 6 inches in length), heart shaped, and serrated. The plant is crowned with white composite-head flowers. The roots are white, branched, and fibrous. The plant can be found in the eastern half of the United States and Canada in the shade of open, moist timber areas. Several varieties of *E. rugosum* exist. Other species, such as *E. serotinum* (late eupatorium), which grows in open sunlight, are not known to contain the toxic agent.

Rayless goldenrod is a low-growing, shrublike plant with erect stems rising from a woody crown to a height of 2 to 4 feet. Leaves are narrow and alternate with entire or slightly toothed margins. The flowers mature to a crop of seeds with numerous short, white bristles. The plant is common in the Southwest, particularly along roadsides and moist areas near rivers and irrigation canals.

Burroweed is a woody half-shrub, about 1 to 2 feet tall, with leaves that are alternate, narrow, and pinnately divided into linear lobes. The leaves are resinous and sticky. Yellow flowers are in small, dense heads. The deep tap root permits survival during critical droughts. The plant grows on southwestern plains, mesas, and hillsides from 2000 to 5500 feet in elevation. It is most abundant on depleted ranges and from a distance can be differentiated from sage by its deeper green color.[3]

Toxicokinetics. Tremetol was the name given to an impure mixture isolated from white snakeroot by Couch in 1927. Four ketones (tremetone, dehydrotremetone, dihydrotremetone, and hydroxytremetone) were later identified; the primary toxic component was called tremetone.[5] However, tremetone does not cause intoxication until microsomal activation by cytochrome P-450 occurs.[6] Tremetone is readily converted or decomposes to dehydrotremetone that is not toxic even after microsomal activation. The efficient conversion of tremetone to dehydrotremetone may explain why the activity of white snakeroot plant extracts vary.[4]

The kinetic details for these compounds are not known. Reports suggest slow excretion of the toxins. However, 22 cases of suspected poisoning in cattle and horses from 1997 through 1999 were reviewed and toxins were detected in only nine of the case submissions. The evidence from these diagnostic submissions suggests that tissue samples from animals that survive more than a few days following their last known exposure to the plants are negative for any of the four metabolites. Limited evidence from urine sample analyses suggests that these compounds disappear from urine soon after exposure ceases.[7] Although the effects of these toxins may be prolonged, there is no experimental documentation of retarded excretion.

This group of compounds is structurally similar to the insecticide rotenone. Although not proven, this relation suggests the possibility of a shared mechanism.[4]

Toxicity and Risk Factors. Poisoning from tremetone-containing plants, particularly white snakeroot, has been observed in humans, cattle, horses, sheep, goats, mules, hogs, fowl, dogs, cats, and a variety of laboratory animals. Generally, morbidity is low, which is likely a reflection of individual selective grazing.[1,2]

Data are insufficient to determine differences in species sensitivity or to predict a toxic dose. In a study on white snakeroot, clinical signs were observed after the horse ingested approximately 20 pounds of green plant tops over a period of several days.[8] An estimate from field observations suggested that ingestion of 0.5% to 1.5% body weight of plant material over 1 to 3 weeks for horses, cattle, and sheep leads to the onset of clinical signs.[1] Generally, white snakeroot poisoning in animals requires several days for the appearance of signs of toxicosis. Because of the required hepatic microsomal activation of tremetone and the degradation of the active toxin to an inactive form, the amount of plant material needed for intoxication is variable and unpredictable. Lactating animals are likely less susceptible to poisoning because of the excretion of this toxin via the milk.

A hazard of poisoning from these plants is that at least some animals evidently consume these plants without the coercion of hunger. White snakeroot stays green and succulent into the fall; toxicity does not appear to be reduced by frost. Poisoning from dried white snakeroot in hay has occurred; however, the toxin is apparently reduced after drying.[2]

The historical infamy of white snakeroot is its relation to human health via the ingestion of milk (or dairy products) from cows that have grazed on the plant. From early Colonial times in North America to the late nineteenth century, "trembles" or "milk fever" in people, especially children, and calves caused significant problems. The association of this plant's ingestion by cows resulting in toxic milk was not made, and in some instances, entire settlements were evacuated. Calves, humans, and cats have been poisoned via milk. The suckling offspring can develop clinical signs before evidence of intoxication is manifested by the lactating parent.

Clinical Signs. The onset of signs may be slow to develop and not particularly distinctive at first. The disease course depends on the quantity of plant toxin consumed over time. Because the toxin is readily excreted in milk, clinical signs may appear in a suckling offspring before they are observed in the dam. The onset appears similar in all animals and varies more with dose than species.

A reluctance to move, with slow, sluggish behavior is usually the first evidence of intoxication. Stiffness of gait and ataxia soon follow. When forced to move, the animal may stand with a wide stance to maintain balance. Horses have been observed to cross legs. Muscle tremors (particularly about the flank and hind legs) and weakness increase in severity and become more generalized. This is a prominent feature of the disease and resulted in the term *trembles*. Animals may then become recumbent, usually sternal, with the head extended. When relaxed, the trembling usually subsides, but it resumes if the animal is forced to stand. Constipation, nausea, vomiting, slobbering, loss of appetite, ventral edema, urinary incontinence, and labored or accelerated respiration may also be observed in some cases. With sufficient dose and severity, an animal remains recumbent, sometimes struggling periodically, and eventually lapses into a coma and dies. An odor of acetone may be noted on the breath.[1,2] Abortion is not a consistent feature of this disease. Some animals have aborted during the poisoning incident, while other survivors have carried their fetuses to a normal delivery.

Muscle tremors may be more pronounced in cattle, whereas horses have more sweating and cardiovascular effects. Intermittent profuse sweating, sometimes in a patchy pattern associated with the shoulders or limb muscles, is often observed. In documented cases, the pulse and respiratory rates were increased; respiration was labored and shallow. The capillary refill time was increased (>3 seconds) and eyes were dilated with sluggish pupillary light responses. The sclera and conjunctiva were icteric with vascular congestion.[9] Urine has been observed as dark red-brown in color that is probably from myoglobinuria. Cardiac arrhythmia and distention of the jugular veins provide evidence of the effects on the myocardium. Electrocardiographic studies of cases have revealed increased atrial rates, variable QRS complexes, prominent ST segment depression, and premature ventricular beats.[10]

Clinical Pathology. Clinical chemistry results reflect muscle and liver damage. Serum creatine kinase (CK) enzymes are routinely elevated from the effects on muscle. Serum alkaline phosphatase (AP), AST, and alanine aminotransferase (ALT) are elevated. Glucose is increased, especially with severe poisoning. Blood pH values are often decreased and the P_{CO_2} is usually elevated.[9]

Lesions.   Focal areas of pallor, often linear, of the myocardium and occasionally skeletal muscles may be the only obvious gross findings observed on necropsy. Myocardial hemorrhage and pericardial effusion may also be found. The lesions have been found in the left ventricular papillary muscles and interventricular septum and occasionally in the right ventricular myocardium. Pericardial fluid accumulation has also been described from some cases. Myocardial lesions are more common in horses than in cattle. Skeletal muscle pallor foci sometimes can be found in the major muscles of the shoulders and possibly the gluteal muscles. The liver, kidneys, spleen, and lungs usually are diffusely dark-red, firm, and markedly congested. Dark-colored urine (myoglobin or hemoglobin) might be found in the bladder or renal pelvis.

Histologically, the pale foci of cardiac and skeletal muscle are areas of myofiber degeneration and necrosis. Besides congestion, the kidneys may contain pigment consistent with myoglobin or hemoglobin (pigmentary nephrosis). Variable amounts of tubular epithelial degeneration and regeneration may be present depending on the severity and acuteness of the exposure. Hepatic changes include retention of bile, congestion, and diffuse hepatocellular swelling and cytoplasmic vacuolation. Centrilobular degeneration, which is described occasionally, might be a result of hypoxia. Pulmonary edema is common along with vascular congestion.[9,10]

Lesions in aborted fetuses have not been observed or described by others.

Diagnostic Testing.   Some veterinary diagnostic laboratories offer testing for this group of toxins. The toxins have been detected most often from liver and kidney. Toxins may be found in urine if the sample is collected soon (probably within a day or two) of plant ingestion. In one case, dehydrotremetone was detected in aborted equine fetal liver and kidney tissues. In the nine positive cases reviewed in diagnostic laboratory records, evidence of toxins was not detected in cardiac muscle, lung, serum, or stomach contents.[7]

Differential diagnoses include ionophores, myocardial plant toxins (e.g., oleander), vitamin E deficiency, and selenium deficiency.

Treatment.   An antidote is not known. Oral administration of activated charcoal (1 g/kg body weight) may limit absorption. Although full recovery may take a few weeks, supportive care with ample food and water to recumbent animals is often successful.

Prognosis.   Depending on the severity of the intoxication, animals can recover following a long period of decreased appetite and muscular weakness. Recumbent cattle may eventually recover if left with feed and water and quiet rest. Horses that have not exhibited severe cardiac affects (tachycardia or arrhythmia) or muscle tremors have a favorable prognosis for recovery to normal activity within a couple of weeks with quiet stall rest and supportive care. However, the likelihood of permanent cardiac damage affecting future performance is not known.

Prevention and Control.   Avoidance of exposure to these plants is the simple prevention. Herbicide control or physical removal or range management such as timed grazing may be used to avoid or limit ingestion.

REFERENCES

1. Kingsbury JM: *Poisonous plants of the United States and Canada,* Englewood Cliffs, NJ, 1964, Prentice-Hall.
2. Panter KE, James LF: Natural plant toxicants in milk: a review, *J Anim Sci* 68:892, 1990.
3. Schmutz EM et al: *Livestock-poisoning plants of Arizona,* Tuscon, Ariz, 1968, University of Arizona Press.
4. Beier RC et al: Isolation of the major component in white snakeroot that is toxic after microsomal activation: possible explanation of sporadic toxicity of white snakeroot plants and extracts, *Natural Toxins* 1:286, 1993.
5. Bonner WA, DeGraw JI Jr: Ketones from "white snakeroot" *Eupatorium urticaefolium, Tetrahedron* 18:1295, 1962.
6. Beier RC, et al: Microsomal activation of constituents of white snakeroot (*Eupatorium rugosum* Houtt), to form toxic products, *Am J Vet Res* 48(4):583, 1987.
7. Bordson GO, Meerdink GL: White snakeroot: analysis and case reports (abstract), *Proceedings of AOAC International, Midwest Section,* 2000.
8. Doyle LP, Walkey FL: *White snakeroot poisoning in livestock, SB No. 270,* Purdue University Agricultural Experiment Station, 1949.
9. Olsen CT et al: Suspected trematol poisoning in horse, *J Am Vet Med Assoc* 185(9):1001, 1984.
10. Smetzer D et al: Cardiac effects of white snakeroot, *Equine Pract* 5(2):26, 1983.

ALKALOIDS

CEVANINE ALKALOIDS

Kip E. Panter

The *Veratrum* and *Zigadenus* spp. in the family Liliaceae contain nitrogenous steroidal alkaloids termed *azasteroids.* These alkaloids can be divided into several different groups, two of which have significant veterinary importance: jervanine and cevanine. The jervanine alkaloids are found in *Veratrum* spp., which have been associated with teratogenic effects in livestock and are discussed in a separate section. The cevanine group of alkaloids, which affect the nervous system, are found in both *Veratrum* and *Zigadenus* spp.

Synonyms.   Ten species of *Zigadenus* include *Z. paniculatus* (foothill death camas), *Z. venenosus* (meadow death camas), *Z. nuttallii* (Nuttall's death camas), *Z. gramiineus* (grassy death camas), *Z. elegans* (white death camas), *Z. fremontii, Z. densus* (black snakeroot or crow poison), *Z. graberrimus, Z. glaucus* (white camas), and *Z. leimanthoides.*

Common names for *Veratrum* include false or western hellebore, white hellebore, California false hellebore, wild corn, skunk cabbage, and corn lily.

Sources.   Death camas grows in various habitats from the rocky desert foothills to the more moist meadows and grassy plains. Species of death camas grow throughout the United States and Canada but most livestock losses occur in the West. The five most common species associated with poisoning include *Z. paniculatus, Z. venenosus, Z. nuttallii, Z. gramiineus,* and *Z. elegans.*

The leaves of death camas resemble broad blades of grass and frequently grow densely in grassy areas often grazed by sheep and cattle. Furthermore, death camas appears earlier in the spring than most grasses and may be heavily grazed, often with disastrous consequences.[1]

V. californicum usually grows at elevations of 1500 to 3000 m and is found in the mountain valleys of the Pacific Coast and Northern Rocky Mountain states. *V. viride* is found at lower elevations throughout the United States. The other species grow at lower elevations. *V. album* grows in European countries and, although not widespread in the United States, it does grow in Alaska.

Mechanism of Action. The cevanine group of steroidal alkaloids includes zygadenine, veramarine, veracevine, sabine, protoverine, and germine. These neurotoxic alkaloids bind open selected voltage-sensitive Na^+ channels, which allows increased movement of Na^+, Ca^{++}, and K^+ through the membrane. The overall result is a delay of repolarization and increased repetitive activity. All excitable cells are affected, but especially the vagal afferent fibers and endings, such as epimyocardial receptors.

The primary effects are on the cardiovascular system: decreased heart rate, peripheral vasodilation, and hypotension. The amplitude and frequency of respiration increase and the heart stops in diastole.[2] It is believed the drop in blood pressure is due to reflex peripheral vasodilation and the reduced heart rate is due to a neural reflex.

Toxicity and Risk Factors. All parts of the plant are toxic, particularly the leaves and bulbs. Young plants are more toxic than mature plants. Plant feeding experiments in which various *Zigadenus* species were fed to sheep produced symptoms of poisoning at levels of 0.2% to 1% of the animal's body weight and lethal poisoning at 0.5% to 2.5%, confirming the highly toxic nature of these plants. Table 25-4 lists toxic and lethal doses of five species of death camas in sheep.

Most death losses are reported in sheep; however, horse and cattle poisonings have been recorded under range conditions. Sheep appear to be more susceptible than cattle, horses, chickens, and swine; however, this may be because sheep are more likely to graze these types of plants.

TABLE 25-4 **Toxicity of Five *Zigadenus* Species to Sheep**

Zigadenus spp.	Mean Minimum Toxic Dose (g/kg body weight)	Mean Minimum Lethal Dose (g/kg body weight)
Z. paniculatus	10.09 (3.57*)	25.2 (6.59*)
Z. venenosus	4.00	20.16
Z. nuttallii	2.02	5.04
Z. gramineus	4.00	6.04
Z. elegans	20.16	60.49

Adapted from Kingsbury JM: *Poisonous plants of the United States and Canada,* Englewood Cliffs, NJ, 1964, Prentice-Hall.
*Data from Panter KE et al: Death camas poisoning in sheep: A case report, *Vet Human Toxicol* 29:45, 1987.

Clinical Signs. Clinical signs of toxicosis appear 1 to 8 hours after ingestion with excess salivation, ataxia, muscular trembling, incoordination, increased respiration, dyspnea, cyanosis, weakness, depression, reduced body temperature, nausea, abdominal pain, vomition, collapse, coma, and death. Often animals are found dead in a sternally recumbent position with no signs of struggling. Death may occur quickly (<12 hours) or in 2 to 3 days. Clinical signs of pneumonia-like symptoms may manifest in sublethal cases and require treatment.[1,3]

Swine vomit soon after ingestion and generally do not show overt signs of toxicosis.

Lesions. Grossly, lesions include severe pulmonary congestion, hemorrhage, hydrothorax and edema, congestion of the kidneys, inflammation of the gastrointestinal tract, and areas of degeneration of skeletal muscles and myocardium. Microscopic lesions include those of pulmonary congestion and edema.[1]

Diagnostic Testing. Diagnosis of poisoning is usually associated with identification and availability of plants and history of ingestion. Confirmation may be possible from analysis of stomach contents for plant fragments or analysis for steroidal alkaloids in the blood, liver, kidney, or rumen contents.

Treatment. Initial treatment for *Zigadenus* poisoning, depending on the species of animal, may consist of gastric lavage, rumenotomy, induced emesis, or oral administration of activated charcoal and saline cathartic. Atropine can be used to reverse the hypotension and bradycardia followed by sympathomimetics or ganglionic blocking drugs to reverse the hypotension from reflex peripheral vasodilation.

No prescribed treatment is available for *Veratrum* toxicosis; however, no cases of death from natural poisoning with *Veratrum* have been reported.[4] When clinical signs occur, animals generally stop grazing because of gastrointestinal upset and muscular weakness and subsequently recover spontaneously.

Prognosis. The prognosis for mild intoxications is good if animals are left alone and stress from handling is kept to a minimum. Prognosis for recovery is poor if animals are recumbent because bloat and aspiration pneumonia occur. Animals that survive apparently recover completely.

Prevention and Control. Death camas is usually ingested in the early spring before grasses and quality forbs are available. Therefore, delaying grazing until grasses and quality forbs are available prevents most poisonings. Death camas may be controlled with herbicide treatment including 2,4-D, Dicamba, or Picloram.[5] However, because death camas is often widespread on ranges, the economics of control often precludes herbicide treatment.

REFERENCES

1 Panter KE et al: Death camas poisoning in sheep: a case report, *Vet Human Toxicol* 29:45, 1987.

2. Spoerke DG, Spoerke SW: Three cases of *Zigadenus* (death camas) poisoning, *Vet Human Toxicol* 21:346, 1979.
3. Kingsbury JM: *Poisonous plants of the United States and Canada*, Englewood Cliffs, NJ, 1964, Prentice-Hall.
4. Binns W et al: A congenital cyclopia-type malformation in lambs induced by maternal ingestion of a range plant *Veratrum californicum*, *Am J Vet Res* 24:1164, 1963.
5. Klingman DL et al: Systemic herbicides for weed control, *Bull AD-BU-2281*, University of Minnesota Extension Service, 1983.

COLCHICINE

Charlotte Means

Sources.   The autumn crocus (*Colchicum autumnale*) and the glory lily (*Gloriosa* spp.) are the two plants that contain colchicine in significant quantities. Autumn crocus is frequently grown as a house or garden plant. However, in Europe it grows in meadows, and livestock poisonings have been reported.[1] The leaves appear in the spring, die back, and then the flowers bloom. The flowers closely resemble spring-blooming crocuses. Glory lilies are generally grown in gardens in Florida and Hawaii, but can be grown in pots anywhere. Glory lilies are considered a climbing perennial.[2]

Toxicokinetics.   Colchicine is rapidly absorbed and peak effects are reached within 10 hours of ingestion. Colchicine is metabolized in the liver and is excreted into the bile, allowing enterohepatic recirculation. Most is excreted in the urine (either unchanged or as metabolites), although a small percentage is excreted in the feces.[3,4]

Mechanism of Action.   Colchicine is an antimetabolite, which inhibits spindle formation during normal cell division. Rapidly dividing cells are the most sensitive.

Toxicity and Risk Factors.   All parts of these plants are toxic, with the alkaloids being most concentrated in the corms or tubers, and the seeds. Glory lily tubers contain about 0.3% colchicine. Autumn crocus seeds contain about 0.8% colchicine and the corms contain 0.6%. Flowers may contain 0.1% colchicine. Drying a plant does not decrease the toxicity. Generally, a few seeds of an autumn crocus are considered potentially lethal and about 2 to 5 g of a glory lily tuber is potentially lethal.[3,5]

Clinical Signs.   Clinical signs involve multiple organ systems. Initial clinical signs include nausea, vomiting, diarrhea, gastrointestinal hemorrhage, hypotension, and leukocytosis. Many people report a burning sensation in the mouth, and stomatitis can develop. As signs progress, seizures, neuropathies, cardiac arrhythmias, and renal and hepatic failure develop. In animals surviving the first few days, coagulopathies and myelosuppression are possible.[3,6]

Treatment.   For a recent ingestion, emesis should be induced and multiple doses of activated charcoal given. A chemistry panel, including electrolytes, should be monitored for 3 to 4 days. A complete blood count should be done on days 7, 10, and 14 after ingestion to ensure myelosuppression does not occur.

Treatment is symptomatic and supportive. Fluid therapy is critical to maintain hydration status. Gastrointestinal protectants, such as sucralfate, may be necessary. Diazepam can be used for seizures. Cardiac function should be monitored. When leukocytosis is present, a broad-spectrum antibiotic may be necessary.[3,4,7] If myelosuppression results in anemia or leukopenia, erythropoietin (100 IU/kg subcutaneously) or filgastrim (5 μg/kg) may be administered.[8]

Goat serum colchicine-specific Fab fragments have been used successfully for human colchicine toxicoses. Fab fragments have resulted in a rapid reversal of life-threatening hemodynamic instability. This is currently considered an investigational drug and is only available in Europe.[4]

REFERENCES

1. Chareyre S et al: Acute poisoning of cows by autumnal crocus, *Vet Human Toxicol* 31:261, 1989.
2. Frohne D, Pfander HJ: *A colour atlas of poisonous plants*, London, 1983, Wolfe Publishing.
3. POISINDEX System Editorial Staff: Plants: Colchicine. In: Toll LL, Hurlbut KM, editors: *POISINDEX System*, Englewood, Colo, Micromedex (edition expires December 2000).
4. Donovan JW: In Haddad LM et al: *Clinical management of poisoning and drug overdose*, ed 3, Philadelphia, 1998, WB Saunders.
5. Spoerke DG, Smolinske SC: *Toxicity of houseplants*, Boca Raton, Fla, 1990, CRC Press.
6. Ogilvie GK: Hematopoietic growth factors: tools for a revolution in veterinary oncology and hematology, *Comp Cont Ed Pract Vet* 13:851, 1993.
7. Beasley VR, Dorman DC et al: *A systems affected approach to veterinary toxicology*, Urbana, Ill, 1999, University of Illinois.
8. Plumb DC: *Veterinary drug handbook*, ed 3, Ames, Iowa, 1999, Iowa State University Press.

DITERPENE ALKALOIDS

Anthony P. Knight

Sources.   Diterpenoid alkaloids that are toxic to animals are found principally in the plant family Ranunculaceae (buttercup family) and mostly in the genera *Delphinium* and *Aconitum*. Other genera containing diterpenoid alkaloids include *Garrya*, *Inula* (Compositae), and *Anopterus* (Grossulariaceae). The C_{19} and C_{20} norditerpenoid alkaloids with many substituted and esterified hydroxyl and methoxyl groups are the most biologically active and most toxic.[1-3]

Larkspur.   At least 80 species of larkspur (*Delphinium* spp.) grow in North America, most of which are found in the western states extending from Alaska and the Canadian Provinces south to Mexico.[3-6] Larkspur poisoning of cattle has been attributed to relatively few species of *Delphinium* that include *D. barbeyi*, *D. bicolor*, *D. geyeri*, *D. glaucescens*, *D. glaucum*, *D. nuttallianum*, *D. occidentale*, *D. tricorne*, and *D. virescens*.[3] It is probably wise to assume that all larkspurs are potentially poisonous, including those that are cultivated as ornamentals.

Larkspurs can be arbitrarily grouped for descriptive purposes into tall, low, and plains (foothills) varieties according to their growth habit. Tall larkspurs (*D. barbeyi*. and *D. occidentale*, *D. glaucescens*, *D. glaucum*) (Color Plate 6) grow in deep, moist, and highly organic soils at high altitudes, often attaining heights of 7 feet.[4,7] The plants emerge as the snows recede and, once established, form long-lived dense stands. The tall larkspurs generally grow in mountain forests, especially where snowdrifts occur perennially. Low larkspurs (D. nuttallianum, D. nelsoni, D. bicolor, and D. virescens) (Color Plate 7) grow at high as well as lower elevations in drier range land, seldom growing more than 2 to 3 feet tall. Low larkspur species emerge early in the spring and die off in early summer as the soil dries out. Plains or foothills larkspur (D. geyeri) is common in the foothills of the Rocky Mountains and short-grass prairies and is intermediate in its growth habit, attaining a height of 3 to 4 feet when in flower.

Larkspurs are erect herbs arising from a single or clustered, often woody rootstock. Most indigenous species are perennials, whereas introduced species tend to be annuals. The leaves are clustered at the base of the plant and are simple, alternate, petioled, and palmately lobed into three to five divisions. In some species, especially the plains and low species, the leaves are further deeply divided. The leaves have relatively long petioles compared to those of monkshood. The stems are hollow, unlike those of monkshood (Aconitum spp.), which are filled with pith. The showy flowers, generally blue to purple but ranging from white to occasionally red, are produced on terminal erect racemes. Flowers have five sepals and four petals, with the upper sepal and pair petals being elongated to form a characteristic spur that protrudes backward (Color Plate 8). Seedpods are erect, containing three to five cells, and split down the inside ridge to release numerous dark seeds.

Monkshood. Several common species of monkshood grow in North America. The most important are A. columbianum (western monkshood), A. uncinatum (Pennsylvania to Georgia), A. reclinatum (Eastern states and west to Ohio), and A. lutescens (Idaho to New Mexico). Monkshood is generally found growing in rich, moist soils of meadows and open woods. Western monkshood (A. columbianum) often grows in the same areas as tall larkspur (Delphinium) species found at high altitude.

Monkshood (Aconitum spp.) are perennial herbaceous plants with tall leafy stems growing to 5 feet in height. The leaves are alternate, palmately lobed, and similar to those of larkspurs and geraniums that often grow in the same habitat. Monkshood can, however, be differentiated from larkspur even if the flowers are not present because the leaves have very short petioles and because the stems of monkshood and wild geranium are not hollow like those of larkspur. The flowers are usually deep blue-purple, but occasionally white or yellow, and are produced on simple racemes or panicles. The flowers are perfect and zygomorphic, with five petal-like sepals. The upper sepal is larger and forms a characteristic helmet or hood that conceals two to five petals (Color Plate 9). Numerous stamens and two to five pistils are present in each flower. The fruit consists of three to five pods (follicles) that spread apart when mature to release the brown seeds.

Toxicokinetics

Larkspurs. These plants contain many toxic and nontoxic norditerpenoid alkaloids. Forty alkaloids have been identified in the larkspur species that are most frequently associated with cattle poisoning.[3,8,9] Individual species of larkspur may contain more than 15 separate alkaloids, with toxicity being attributed exclusively to the methylsuccidimido anthranoyllycoctine group.[10] To date the most toxic of these alkaloids isolated from tall larkspurs are 14-deactylnudicauline (DAN) and methyllycaconitine (MLA).[3,10,11] Although the former alkaloid is more toxic, greater than 15 times as much MLA is produced in the plant, making it the most important toxic component of the tall larkspurs.[12] The plains larkspur (D. geyeri) and the low larkspur (D. nuttallianum) have been shown to contain MLA as well as the highly toxic alkaloid nudicauline.[13] The diterpenoid alkaloids are rapidly absorbed from the digestive tract and are not degraded in the rumen.[10] The toxicity of the different larkspur species is most likely due to the quantity and the combined effects of the alkaloids present in the plants, the rate at which they are absorbed from the digestive tract, and the means by which they are metabolized and excreted from the animal. The metabolism and excretion of the alkaloids are poorly understood.

Monkshood. These plants contain a variety of polycyclic diterpenoid alkaloids including aconitine, mesaconitine, and hypaconitine that have similar toxicity to those found in *Delphinium* and *Garrya* species.[1]

Mechanism of Action.

The alkaloids act principally at the neuromuscular junction (postsynaptic nicotinic and cholinergic receptors), causing a curare-like blockade with resulting muscle weakness and paralysis.[14,15] The alkaloids reversibly bind to and block the action of nicotinic acetylcholine receptors at the neuromuscular junction, thus competing with acetylcholine for the receptors.[16] Acetylcholine receptors in the brain are also blocked by MLA.[17] The neuromuscular blocking effect of MLA alkaloids is similar to that of nicotine and the snake toxin bungertoxin.[18] If sufficient receptors are blocked by MLA, DAN, and other larkspur alkaloids, the muscle does not respond to the effects of acetylcholine and does not contract. Binding affinity of the larkspur alkaloids to the cholinergic receptors varies markedly with the tissue and among species.[19] Cattle cholinergic receptors are more susceptible to diterpenoid alkaloids than are those of sheep, which explains the refractoriness of sheep to larkspur poisoning.[20]

Toxicity and Risk Factors

Larkspur. Cattle are the most susceptible to larkspur poisoning, whereas sheep are refractory to the effects of the alkaloids.[5] Sheep tolerate about four to five times the amount of larkspur alkaloids that would be fatal to cattle.[4] Sheep can be used as biological controls in the management of tall larkspur because they can be used to graze the larkspur before cattle, thereby reducing the risk to cattle.[21] Horses are susceptible to larkspur poisoning but to a much lesser degree than cattle.

The alkaloid content of larkspurs varies depending on the species and stage of growth.[12,22] Individual plants and certain stands of larkspur appear to be more toxic than others. Larkspur poisoning "hot spots" are recognized by ranchers who frequently anticipate losses when cattle are herded in these areas. The alkaloid content of tall larkspurs also appears to be consistently higher in plants growing in full sun as opposed to those growing in the shade. Tall larkspur species have the highest alkaloid content in their early growth stage before starting to elongate their flower spikes.[12] Studies with *Delphinium barbeyi* have shown it to be the most toxic of the larkspurs.[4,5,23] The alkaloid content steadily declines as the plant matures, although the green seedpods contain significant quantities of the alkaloids.[12] The toxicity attributed to the tall larkspur species cannot be assumed to hold true for the low or foothills larkspur species. Unlike the tall larkspurs, the foothills larkspur (*D. geyeri*) is readily eaten by cattle in the early spring before it flowers, causing significant death loss. By the time it flowers, the foothills larkspur is not consumed in a significant quantity, pre-sumably because cattle generally have plenty of other forage available.

The concentrations of MLA and DAN alkaloids in immature tall larkspur ranges from 5 to 12 mg/g and 0.2 to 0.8 mg/g dry weight, respectively.[23] The alkaloid content of the seeds and pods is 12 mg/g . The dose of tall larkspur that will pro-duce signs of poisoning in cattle depends on the quantity of total alkaloid in the plant and the rate at which the plant is consumed. Experimentally it has been determined that the total oral toxic dose of the alkaloids MLA and DAN from tall larkspur (*D. barbeyi*) is 11.2 mg/kg body weight.[23] The lethal dose 50 (LD_{50}) for the total toxic alkaloids can be extrap-olated from this and is 25 to 40 mg/kg body weight.[23] Experimentally it has been shown that 17 g/kg body weight of the green plant of *D. barbeyi* is lethal to cattle.[12,24] As-suming a concentration of 5 mg/g dry weight of MLA and DAN in the plant, a 450-kg cow would need to rapidly eat 1.8 kg dry weight (6.5 kg wet weight) of tall larkspur to develop clinical signs.[23] The lethal dose of larkspur is more difficult to determine because it is not only dependent on the alkaloid content, but it is also related to the rate at which rumen bloat develops and the amount of stress to which the animal is subjected.

No correlation between alkaloid concentration and pala-tability of the plant was observed in cattle regardless of whether the plant was fresh or dried.[25] Sheep avoid eating the plants in the preflowering stage when the alkaloid con-tent is highest, but readily eat the flower stalks and buds as they mature. In drought years, the consumption of tall larkspur by cattle almost entirely ceases; therefore, mortality from larkspur poisoning is lowest during droughts.[23,25] Graz-ing studies have also shown that cattle self-regulate the consumption of larkspur if they consume more than 25% larkspur in their daily diet for 1 to 2 days. Following these periods of high larkspur consumption, cattle eat very little larkspur for several days, apparently enabling their system to clear the toxic alkaloids.[25-27] Death from larkspur poisoning, therefore, appears to be related to the rapid ingestion of a lethal dose of larkspur, as seems to occur in the as yet unexplained phenomenon of the gluttonous consumption of tall larkspur by cattle in a short period of time following a summer rain storm.[28]

Monkshood.   Native and cultivated monkshood species should be considered toxic to animals and humans.[1] All parts of the plant are toxic, especially the roots, seeds, and leaves. Although no extensive documentation of the toxicity of monkshood exists in humans, poisoning due to the misuse of medicinal extracts of aconitine is well recognized.[29] Horses have been reported to be fatally poisoned after eating 0.075% of their body weight in green plant.[30] In the western United States, most suspected cases of *Aconitum* poisoning in cattle are more likely to be due to tall larkspur poisoning because it grows more abundantly in the same area and is more toxic than monkshood.[30]

Clinical Signs

Larkspur.   The most frequently observed sign of larkspur poisoning is the sudden death of cattle on rangeland populated with larkspur, because cattle frequently die within 3 to 4 hours of consuming a lethal dose of larkspur. When observed in the early stages of poisoning, cattle show the effects of impaired neuromuscular function, including uneasiness, increased excitability, and muscle weakness that causes stiffness, staggering, and a basewide stance.[5,31,32] The front legs may be affected first, causing the animal to kneel before finally becoming recumbent. Muscle weakness may cause the animal to suddenly collapse, especially if it is stressed; frequent attempts to stand are uncoordinated and result in rapid exhaustion.[33] Muscle twitching, abdominal pain, regurgitation, and constipation are common clinical findings.

Bloating is common as a result of the neuromuscular blocking effect of the alkaloids on the esophagus, impairing the ability of the animal to eructate. Bloat also develops rapidly because larkspurs, being succulent and high in pro-tein, are highly fermentable by rumen microorganisms, thereby increasing the rate of gas production in the rumen. Once laterally recumbent, inhalation of regurgitated rumen contents commonly leads to fatal inhalation pneumonia. Death probably results from the combined effects of res-piratory muscle paralysis, bloat, and inhalation of regur-gitated rumen contents.

Monkshood.   Monkshood poisoning resembles that of larkspur poisoning. Symptoms begin within a few hours of cattle ingesting a toxic quantity of the plant, with death following a few hours to a few days later, depending on the dose of toxic alkaloids ingested. Affected animals initially become restless, salivate excessively, develop muscle weak-ness, have a weak, erratic heart rhythm, and have difficulty in breathing before collapsing into lateral recumbency.[30] Bloat-ing is a common problem in ruminants once they become recumbent. Cardiac conduction disturbances and arrhyth-mias are common clinical signs.

Diagnostic Testing.   No pathognomonic signs of larkspur poisoning are found on postmortem examination. The absence of diagnostic pathology and evidence of larkspur having been grazed by cattle are often the only means of arriving at a diagnosis of larkspur poisoning. Bloat and the presence of rumen contents in the bronchi are supportive of a diagnosis of larkspur poisoning.[5] Similarly, rumen contents may be examined microscopically for characteristic larkspur epidermal cell structure indicating larkspur consumption.[34] A mouse bioassay method developed for Dunce cap larkspur (*Delphinium occidentale*) relating total alkaloid to growth stage of the plant may prove useful in determining the toxicity of other larkspur species.[35] However, electrospray atmospheric pressure chemical ionization and sequential tandem mass spectrometry now enable rapid and accurate determination of different alkaloids in large numbers of plant samples.[36]

Treatment

Larkspur. Treatment myths abound in the early literature and have involved the use of a variety of compounds, including atropine, potassium permanganate, turpentine, bacon fat, chewing tobacco, whiskey, and prophylactic tail vein phlebotomy.[37,38] Most of these early remedies have little scientific basis and have not proven to be effective. The use of turpentine and bacon fat given orally may have helped reduce the severity of the bloat that develops with larkspur poisoning. Apparent claims of successes with unique remedies are most likely due to the variability in toxicity of the larkspurs under different growing conditions, time of year, and quantity of total toxic alkaloid consumed. If less than a lethal dose of larkspur is consumed, an animal will likely recover no matter what the treatment.

Because the principal effect of the toxic larkspur alkaloids is to compete for acetylcholine receptors at the neuromuscular junction, the logical approach to treatment is to increase the accumulation of acetylcholine at the neuromuscular junction by inhibiting cholinesterase. Inhibitors of cholinesterase, such as physostigmine and possibly neostigmine, are effective in reversing some of the effects of the larkspur alkaloids. Cattle given physostigmine (0.4 to 0.8 mg/kg body weight) rapidly intravenously while in sternal or lateral recumbency resulting from tall larkspur poisoning recover within a few minutes.[39] Because the effects of physostigmine are short-lived, relapse may occur, especially if the animal is stressed. Treatment should be repeated as needed over several hours until clinical signs have abated. It should be emphasized that physostigmine is not approved for use in animals and should be used only under the direction of a veterinarian in accordance with the regulations pertaining to the use of extralabel drugs.

Neostigmine (0.04 mg/kg) appears to have some effectiveness in reversing some of the effects of the larkspur alkaloids but is not as effective as physostigmine for treating larkspur poisoning. Neostigmine is, however, approved for use in cattle. Some organophosphate compounds with anticholinesterase activity may have potential for the treatment of larkspur poisoning.

Early recognition of larkspur poisoning is essential for successful treatment. Stress and excitement of the affected animal should be avoided because they will exacerbate respiratory distress and hasten death of the animal. It is therefore often better to quietly herd affected range cattle away from the area where larkspur is being grazed rather than to catch and restrain an animal to treat it. Affected animals should be kept sternal if they become recumbent, and bloat should be relieved by passing a stomach tube to remove excess rumen gas and reduce respiratory difficulty. Trocarization of the rumen to relieve the bloat may be less stressful than trying to pass a stomach tube.

Monkshood. No proven treatment for monkshood poisoning is available. Affected animals should be stressed as little as possible, and possibly have a better chance of survival if they are herded away from the source of the plants without stressful attempts at treatment. Symptomatic treatment with intravenous fluids and relief of rumen bloat may be undertaken as necessary.

Prognosis.
Cattle that are in lateral recumbency and bloated when first observed with larkspur poisoning have a poor prognosis. Stressing the animal to treat it is frequently sufficient to kill it. Animals showing early signs of muscle tremors and ataxia have a reasonably good prognosis if they can be removed from the larkspur without undue stress. Treatment with physostigmine is often not necessary if the animal can be allowed to quietly detoxify and excrete the alkaloids.

Prevention and Control.
Although larkspur poisoning can be prevented by denying cattle access to the plants, this is not feasible under most ranching conditions because it would be uneconomical to eliminate vast areas of rangeland for livestock grazing. Strategies for effectively using rangeland infested with larkspur must therefore be developed by understanding the phenology and toxicity characteristics of larkspurs. Cattle tend to eat larkspur at certain stages of its growth and eat very little of the plants at other times. Extensive observations of cattle on tall larkspur range have shown that they eat virtually no larkspur before it initiates its flower spikes.[12,26,40,41] This means that tall larkspurs are unpalatable to cattle when they are most toxic, because the highest concentrations of the toxic diterpenoid alkaloids are in the leaves and stems before flowering.[12,23] Knowing the times when tall larkspurs are most toxic and when cattle find the plants most palatable, it is possible to manage cattle so that they are kept away from the larkspur during a "toxic window" when the probability of poisoning is highest.[12] This toxic window occurs from when the tall larkspur elongates its flower stems until the seedpods are mature. After that period, the larkspur is minimally toxic and palatability is high. In essence, this means that tall larkspur range can be grazed relatively safely before the plants begin to flower, but the cattle must be removed from the larkspur during the flowering period and until the seedpods have matured. To effectively manage cattle using this toxic window, the tall larkspur must be closely observed to determine when the plants start to elongate their flower spikes. As soon as this occurs and cattle start to eat the flower shoots, they should be removed from the larkspur areas. This management strategy is only valid when there are plenty of other forages available and the cattle are not forced into a situation in which they must eat larkspur because they are without adequate food. Early season grazing and the use of the toxic window principle are only relevant to tall larkspur and should not be attempted with the foothill or low larkspurs that seem to be quite palatable in the early spring when they are highly toxic.

With the advent of accurate and rapid testing methods, it will be possible to sample larkspur and determine the alkaloid content before turning cattle onto range that has a high potential for larkspur poisoning.[36] By knowing the amount of alkaloid in the larkspur, it will be possible to determine high-risk years or growth phases of the plant and to manage the cattle accordingly.

Sheep can be used to reduce the availability of larkspur if they are allowed to graze the plants before cattle.[21,42] In the case of tall larkspur, sheep may be particularly effective in grazing the flower shoots and trampling the plants, thereby reducing the availability of the larkspur for cattle. To be effective biologic controls, large flocks of sheep need to be used and herded into those areas where the larkspur is abundant so that sufficient larkspur is eaten and trampled to reduce its consumption by cattle.

Providing adequate calcium, phosphorus, and mineralized salts for cattle has been recommended as a preventive measure for larkspur poisoning. However, mineral supplementation of cattle grazing rangeland infested with tall larkspur has been shown to have no effect in reducing the amount of larkspur consumed.[43] A balanced mineral supplement should be provided to cattle to prevent mineral deficiencies, but should not be relied on as a preventive measure for larkspur poisoning.

Larkspurs can be controlled and their populations reduced with herbicides, but it is economically prohibitive to do so on a wide scale.[43-47] Herbicide spraying of larkspur can be effective in reducing cattle losses, particularly where larkspur hot-spots are a perennial problem. The tall larkspurs can be controlled using a variety of currently available herbicides including picloram (Tordon), metsulfuron (Escort), and glyphosate (Roundup).[48,49] These herbicides are effective because they kill the root and not just the vegetative portion of the plant. The use of 2-4,D (2,4-dichlorohenoxy acetic acid) to control larkspur is not very effective because only a temporary dieoff of the vegetative parts of the plants occurs. Surfactants enhance the efficacy of herbicides because they enhance the absorption of the chemicals through the waxy surface of the leaves. The most effective time to apply herbicides is in the early vegetative or leaf stage before the flower stalks begin to form.[48] A second application of the herbicide should be applied to any plants that survive the first application. Newer application methods such as carpeted rollers also help to apply the herbicides to the tall larkspur without affecting lower growing beneficial plants and grasses and use less chemical than conventional spraying methods. It should be noted that herbicides increase the alkaloid content of larkspur and therefore the plants should not be grazed after spraying until the plants have completely died off.[48,49] Herbicidal control of tall larkspur may result in significant increases in grasses for at least 5 years after spraying.[49]

Under some ranch management systems, it is possible to train cattle not to eat larkspur, using the principle of food aversion.[50-52] Cattle do not form a natural aversion to eating larkspur, but they do form a strong aversion to eating larkspur if they are given repeated intraruminal infusions of lithium chloride.[50-53] Training cattle to avoid eating larkspur can be accomplished by harvesting and feeding fresh larkspur to cattle. As soon as an animal has started eating the larkspur, it is restrained and given lithium chloride (100 mg/kg body weight) via stomach tube. Lithium is a potent irritant and emetic that induces abdominal pain that the animal associates with the last thing it was eating,

namely larkspur. The averted cattle can then be returned to the grazing area and closely observed for a day or two to be sure all have developed an aversion to larkspur. Those that have not should be retreated intraruminally with lithium. Once cattle have developed an aversion to larkspur, they retain this aversion from year to year, as long as they are not exposed to cattle that are eating larkspur.[51,53,54] Aversed cattle relearn to eat larkspur by observing other cattle doing so, a process of social facilitation.[53] To maintain a herd with an aversion to larkspur requires constant vigilance so that any animal that starts re-eating larkspur is either immediately retreated with lithium or is removed from the herd. Induced aversion to eating larkspur has potential in some closed herd situations in which averted cattle can be closely observed and managed.[54,55]

Other possibilities for the control of larkspur include the use of insect biological controls. The larkspur myrid (*Hopplomachus affiguratus*) that devitalizes tall larkspur by sucking fluids from the plant tissues has shown potential as an insect control.[56] Plants devitalized by the myrids become stunted, fail to produce flowers and seeds, and appear to be unpalatable to cattle. In time, the larkspur stands may become sufficiently weakened to reduce their potential for poisoning cattle. The success of the myrid as an insect biological control will depend on whether or not it can sustain itself in large numbers on larkspur stands to reduce the plant population, without itself becoming victim to its own predators that will predictably increase as the myrid population increases.

REFERENCES

1. Pelletier SW, Keith LH: Diterpenoid alkaloids from *Aconitum, Delphinium,* and *Garrya* species. In Manske RHF, Holmes HL, editors: *The alkaloids* ,Vol XII, New York, 1970, Academic Press.
2. Jaycno JM: Chemistry and toxicology of the diterpenoid alkaloids. In Blum MS, editor: *Chemistry and toxicology of diverse classes of alkaloids,* Fort Collins, Colo, 1996, Alaken.
3. Olsen JD, Manners GD: Toxicology of diterpenoid alkaloids in rangeland larkspur (*Delphinium* spp.). In Cheeke PR, editor: *Toxicants of plant origin,* Vol 1, Alkaloids, Boca Raton, Fla, 1989, CRC Press.
4. Cronin EH, Nielsen DB: Tall larkspur and cattle on high mountain ranges. In Keeler RF, Van Kampen KR, James LF, editors: *Effects of poisonous plants on livestock,* New York, 1978, Academic Press.
5. Kingsbury JM: *Poisonous plants of the United States and Canada,* Englewood Cliffs, NJ, 1964, Prentice-Hall.
6. Pfister JA et al: Larkspur (*Delphinium* spp.) poisoning in livestock, *J Nat Toxins* 8:81, 1999.
7. Olsen JD: Tall larkspur poisoning in cattle and sheep, *J Am Vet Med Assoc* 173:762, 1978.
8. Olsen JD et al: Poisonous properties of larkspur (*Delphinium* spp.), *Collectanea Botanica* (Barcelona) 19:141, 1990.
9. Grina JA et al: Alkaloids from *Delphinium geyeri.* Three new C20 Ä diterpenoid alkaloids, *J Organic Chem* 51:390, 1986.
10. Manners GD et al: Toxicity and chemical phenology of norditerpenoid alkaloids in tall larkspurs, *J Agric Food Chem* 41:96 1993.
11. Manners GD et al: Structure-activity relationships of norditerpenoid alkaloids occurring in toxic larkspur (*Delphinium*) species, *J Nat Prod* 58:863, 1995.
12. Pfister JA et al: Effects of phenology, site, and rumen fill on tall larkspur consumption by cattle, *J Range Manage* 41:509, 1988.

13. Manners GD et al: The toxic evaluation of norditerpenoid alkaloids in three tall larkspur *(Delphinium)* species. In Collegiate SM, Dorling PR, editors: *Plant associated toxins: agricultural, photochemical and ecological aspects,* Wallingford, Oxford, UK, 1994, CAB International.

14. Pfister JA et al: Cattle grazing tall larkspur on Utah mountain rangeland, *J Range Manage* 41:118, 1988.

15. Nation PN et al: Clinical signs and studies of the site of action of purified larkspur alkaloid, methyllycaconitine, administered parenterally to calves, *Can Vet J* 23:264, 1982.

16. Dobelis P et al: Effects of *Delphinium* alkaloids on neuromuscular transmission, *J Pharm Exp Ther* 291:538, 1999.

17 Dobelis P et al: Antagonism of nicotinic receptors by *Delphinium* alkaloids, *Neuroscience* 631, 1993 (abstract).

18. Kukel CF, Jennings KR: Delphinium alkaloids as inhibitors of α-bungeratoxin binding to rat and insect neural membranes, *Can J Physiol Pharmacol* 72:104, 1994.

19. Ward JM et al: Methyllycaconitine: a selective probe for neuronal α-bungerotoxin binding sites, *FEBS Lett* 270:45, 1990.

20. Olsen JD, Sisson DV: Toxicity of extracts of tall larkspur *(Delphinium barbeyi)* in mice, hamsters, rats, and sheep, *Toxicology* 56:33, 1991 (letter).

21. Ralphs MH, Browns JE: Utilization of larkspur by sheep, *J Range Manage* 44:619, 1991.

22. Aiyar VN et al. The principal toxin of *Delphinium brownii* Rydb, and its mode of action, *Experientia* 35:1367, 1979.

23. Pfister JA et al: Toxic alkaloid levels in tall larkspur *(Delphinium barbeyi)* in western Colorado, *J Range Manage* 47:355, 1994.

24. Olsen JD: Larkspur toxicosis: a review of current research. In Keeler RF, Van Kampen KR, James LF, editors: *Effects of poisonous plants on livestock,* New York, 1978, Academic Press.

25. Pfister JA, Cheney CD: Operant behavioral analysis of acute tall larkspur *(Delphinium barbeyi)* intoxication in cattle, *Behavior* 4:43, 1998.

26. Pfister JA et al: Tall larkspur ingestion: can cattle regulate intake below toxic levels? *J Chem Ecol* 23:759, 1997.

27. Olsen JD, Sisson DV: Description of a scale for rating the clinical response of cattle poisoned by larkspur, *Am J Vet Res* 52:488, 1991.

28. Ralphs MH et al: Storms influence cattle to graze larkspur: an observation, *J Range Manage* 4:275, 1994.

29. Chang TKY et al: Aconitine poisoning due to Chinese herbal medicines: a review, *Vet Hum Toxicol* 36:452, 1994.

30. Kingsbury JM: *Poisonous plants of the United States and Canada,* Englewood Cliffs, NJ, 1964, Prentice-Hall.

31. Olsen JD et al: Poisonous properties of larkspur *(Delphinium* spp.), *Collectanea Botanica* (Barcelona)19:141, 1990.

32. Olsen JD: Larkspur poisoning: as we now know it and a glance at the future, *The Bovine Practitioner* 28:157, 1994.

33. Flemming CE et al: The low larkspur *(Delphinium andersonii), Bull 105,* University of Nevada Agriculture Experiment Station, 1923.

34. Potter RL, Ueckert DN: Epidermal cellular characteristics of selected livestock-poisoning plants in North America, Texas A & M University, College Station, 1997, Texas Agricultural Experiment Station.

35. Olsen JD: Rat bioassay for estimating toxicity of plant material from larkspur *(Delphinium* spp.), *Am J Vet Res* 38:277, 1977.

36. Gardner DR et al: Analysis of toxic norditerpenoid alkaloids in *Delphinium* species by electrospray, atmospheric pressure chemical ionization, and sequential tandem mass spectrometry, *J Agric Food Chem* 47:5049, 1999.

37. Chestnut VK, Wilcox EV: The stock-poisoning plants of Montana, *Bull 26 USDA,* 1901.

38. Knight AP, Pfister JA: Larkspur poisoning in livestock: myths and misconceptions, *Rangelands* 19:10, 1997.

39. Pfister JA et al: Reversal of tall larkspur *(Delphinium barbeyi)* poisoning in cattle with physostigmine, *J Vet Hum Toxicol* 36:511, 1994.

40. Pfister JA et al: Grazing risk on tall larkspur-infested rangelands, *Rangelands* 19:12, 1997.

41. Pfister JA et al: Early season grazing by cattle of tall larkspur-infested range lands, *Larkspur Symposium Proceedings.* Colorado State University Cooperative Extension, 1996.

42. Ralphs MH, Olsen JD: Prior grazing by sheep reduces waxy larkspur consumption by cattle: an observation, *J Range Manage* 45:136, 1992.

43. Pfister JA, Manners GD: Mineral salt supplementation of cattle grazing tall larkspur infested range land during drought, *J Range Manage* 44:105, 1991.

44. Nielsen DB et al: Economic considerations of poisonous plants on livestock. In James LF, Ralphs MH, Nielsen DB, editors: *The ecology and economic impact of poisonous plants on livestock production,* Boulder, Colo, 1988, Westview Press.

45. Nielsen DB, Cronin EH: Economics of tall larkspur control, *J Range Manage* 30:434, 1997.

46. Nielsen DB et al: Economic feasibility of controlling tall larkspur on rangelands, *J Range Manage* 47:369, 1994.

47. Cronin EH et al: Cattle losses, tall larkspur, and their control, *J Range Manage* 29:364, 1976.

48. Ralphs MH et al: Timing of herbicide applications for control of larkspurs *(Delphinium* spp.), *Weed Science* 40:264, 1992.

49. Ralphs MH: Long term impact of herbicides on larkspur and associated vegetation, *J Range Manage* 48:459, 1994.

50. Olsen JD, Ralphs MH: Feed aversion induced by intraruminal infusion of larkspur extract in cattle, *Am J Vet Res* 47:1829, 1986.

51. Ralphs MH, Olsen JD: Comparison of larkspur alkaloid extract and lithium chloride in maintaining cattle aversion to larkspur in the field, *J Anim Sci* 70:1116, 1992.

52. Olsen JD et al: Aversion to eating larkspur plants induced in cattle by intraruminal infusion of lithium chloride, *J Anim Sci* 65(suppl 1):218, 1987.

53. Lane MA et al: Conditioned taste aversion: potential for reducing cattle loss to larkspur, *J Range Manage* 43:127, 1990.

54. Ralphs MH, Cheney CD: Influence of cattle age, lithium chloride dose level, and food type in the retention of food aversions, *J Anim Sci* 71:373, 1993.

55. Ralphs MH: Continued food aversion: training livestock to avoid eating poisonous plants, *J Range Manage* 45:46, 1992.

56. Ralphs MH et al: Biological agents to control larkspur or reduce risk of poisoning, *Proc Larkspur Symposium,* Colorado Cooperative Extension, 1996.

INDOLIZIDINE ALKALOIDS

Anthony P. Knight

The genera of plants discussed in this section have been associated with three general syndromes of livestock poisoning caused by three different poisons. Some species may contain one or more of the toxicants and consequently may cause a combination of clinical signs in animals that have eaten them. The three toxicants are indolizidine alkaloids, nitropropanol glycosides, and selenium. The nitropropanol glycosides and selenium are discussed in separate sections.

Synonyms. The *Astragalus* and *Oxytropis* plants are commonly called locoweeds, vetches, or milkvetches. The neurologic disease is referred to as locoism, the Spanish word for *crazy.*

Sources. Indolizidine alkaloids are cyclic organic compounds containing nitrogen that are present in a variety of plants in the family Fabaceae (Leguminosae) found growing in many parts of the world. The best known plant genera containing toxic indolizidine alkaloids are *Swainsona, Astragalus, Oxytropis,* and *Castanospermum.* Some fungi, especially *Rhizoctonia leguminocola,* also produce indolizidine alkaloids with similar toxic properties to those found in plants.[1]

The most important indolizidine alkaloid with respect to its toxic effect on animals is swainsonine. It was first isolated from *Swainsona canescens* (gray swainson pea) in Australia.[2,3] The *Swainsona* species are leguminous herbs mostly confined to Australia and are closely related to plants in the genus *Astragalus* found in other parts of the world.[4] In North America, swainsonine has been found in a variety of plants of the genera *Astragalus* and *Oxytropis*[5-7] (Box 25-1). Castanospermine, present in the seeds of the Australian chestnut tree *(Castanospermum australe),* and slaframine, which is produced by the fungus *Rhizoctonia leguminicola,* are structurally and biologically similar to swainsonine.[8] *Rhizoctonia leguminicola* is also capable of synthesizing swainsonine.[1,8]

In North America, about 370 species of *Astragalus* and *Oxytropis* have been identified, a fraction of the 2000 species known to exist throughout the world.[9] Many species of *Astragalus* and *Oxytropis* in North America are not poisonous and are useful forage plants for livestock and wildlife. Some species, such as *A. cicer* and *A. tenellus,* are nontoxic and are useful forages for range animals.[10] However, the more common species that are found in vast areas of western North America, such as *A. lentiginosus, A. mollissimus,* and *O. sericea,* are poisonous and cause considerable economic losses to the livestock industry annually. In an extensive global survey of 1690 species of *Astragalus,* 221 (13%) tested positive for toxic nitropropanol glycosides, which are discussed in a separate section.[11]

Astragalus and *Oxytropis* species are indigenous wild flowers found throughout North America; they are especially well adapted to the drier areas of the West and Southwest. These members of the legume family are perennials arising from a deep taproot and with alternate and pinnately compound leaves. Some species are densely haired, giving the leaves a bluish color. *Astragalus* species are often multistemmed with a sprawling habit, whereas *Oxytropis* species have very short stems with basely grouped leaves (Color Plate 10). The pealike flowers are produced in axillary racemes and, depending on the species, vary in color from white to yellow to purple. Unlike the *Astragalus* species, the *Oxytropis* species have a pointed keel, giving rise to their common name of point vetch or point locoweed. Seedpods are pealike, although some are distinctly inflated or bladderlike (Color Plate 11). Numerous seeds are produced that remain viable in the soil for as long as 50 years.[12]

Toxicokinetics. Swainsonine, the principal toxic indolizidine alkaloid, has been detected in 16 species of *Astragalus* and *Oxytropis*[13] (see Box 25-1). The alkaloid is found in all parts of the plant with highest concentration in the leaves, flowers, and seedpods.[14] Swainsonine plays the major role in the pathogenesis of locoweed poisoning that is commonly referred to as locoism. Other alkaloids present in the plants may have an as yet unidentified role in the poisoning of animals.

Swainsonine is a relatively small and stable molecule that is readily absorbed from the digestive tract of simple stomached and ruminant animals. It is rapidly distributed throughout all tissues and crosses the placenta to affect the fetus.[15] Swainsonine is secreted through the milk, thereby adding to the amount of alkaloid a suckling animal may acquire from ingesting the plant directly.[16,17] The levels of swainsonine in milk decline rapidly and are not detectable after 24 hours following a single experimental injection of swainsonine.[8] However, cows that have grazed locoweed may have residual plant in the rumen for 2 to 3 days that could result in milk swainsonine levels persisting for several days.

Swainsonine is apparently excreted unchanged through the urine, because urine from locoweed-fed sheep is toxic to rats.[18] The half-life of swainsonine in the blood of cattle and sheep is 16 to 20 hours.[19] Clearance from the liver and kidney is about 60 hours.[20] With this longer tissue half-life, animals that are to be used for human consumption should be withheld from any source of swainsonine for at least 25 days before slaughter.[20,21]

Mechanism of Action. Swainsonine inhibits the action of two lysosomal enzymes, alpha-*D*-mannosidase and Golgi mannosidase II, which are important in the metabolism of saccharides and the formation of glycoproteins.[22,23] The inhibition of alpha-mannosidase causes cells to accumulate oligosaccharides.[19] The second enzyme, Golgi mannosidase II, when inhibited, affects the normal structure of glycoproteins because of the disruption of *N*-asparagine-linked glycoprotein synthesis.[8,23] As a result, oligosaccharide-glycosylated proteins accumulate in the cells of the brain and many other organs, interfering with normal cellular function.[24-26] In effect, swainsonine causes a generalized lysosomal storage disease similar to the genetically transmitted disease mannosidosis described in humans and cattle.[26-28] Alteration of glycoprotein metabolism has a generalized effect on a variety of hormones, cytokines, and receptors that cause hormone and endocrine dysfunction,

BOX 25-1	***ASTRAGALUS*** **AND** ***OXYTROPIS*** **SPECIES THAT CONTAIN SWAINSONINE**
Astragalus allochrous	*A. oxyphysus*
A. argillophilus	*A. playanus*
A. assymetricus	*A. praelongus*
A. bisulcatus	*A. pubentissumus*
A. didymocarpus	*A. pycnostachysus*
A. dyphysus	*A. tephrodes*
A. earlei	*A. thurberi*
A. emoryanus	*A. wootonii*
A. flavus	*Oxytropis besseyi*
A. humistratus	*O. campestris*
A. lentiginosus	*O. condensata*
A. lonchocarpus	*O. lambertii*
A. mollissimus	*O. saximontana*
A. missouriensis	*O. sericea*
A. nothoxys	

Data from references 5, 6, 46.

reproductive failure, decreased immune system function, heart failure, and impairment of nutrient absorption from the digestive system.[29]

Toxicity and Risk Factors.   Horses, cattle, sheep, goats, elk and domestic cats are naturally and experimentally susceptible to the toxic effects of swainsonine.[30-33] All animals, however, should be considered vulnerable to the toxic effects of the alkaloid.

The palatability of locoweed does not have any relationship to the quantity of swainsonine in the plant.[34] Although horses, cattle, and sheep have been reported to develop a preference for locoweeds, there is no dependence on the plants as if the animals were addicted.[34,35] Consumption of locoweed appears to be related to the availability of the plant, lack of other forages, and the fact that locoweeds are palatable and nutritious. Locoweeds have similar nutrient value as alfalfa, which may explain why animals may eat locoweed even when normal forages are present. Some animals also learn to eat locoweeds through the phenomenon of social facilitation, whereby they learn to eat the plants through observation of other animals that are eating locoweed.[36,37]

The quantity of swainsonine in locoweeds varies according to the species, stage of growth, and the growing conditions of the plants. The succulent growing plants appear to be the most palatable, although cattle relish the flowers and immature seedpods.[14] The concentration of swainsonine in locoweed (0.09% to 0.23% dry weight) varies with the stage of growth. The highest concentrations of swainsonine are found in the flowers and seeds (0.28% and 0.36%, respectively) and consequently the quantity of plant that an animal has to eat to receive a toxic dose varies.[19]

Experimentally, locoism can be produced by feeding 0.75 to 1 lb/day of dried locoweed to horses and cattle for 75 to 85 days.[33,38] Decreased weight gains, one of the first observable signs of locoweed poisoning, can be induced in sheep fed as little as 0.2 mg/kg swainsonine for 30 days.[21] Consumption of greater quantities of locoweed over shorter periods would likely decrease the time before clinical signs of locoism become evident. However, there appears to be a threshold at which an increasing dose of swainsonine does not increase the extent or severity of the toxicity.[19,21] Young animals are most severely affected by swainsonine, because maturing and rapidly growing cells are more vulnerable to the effects of the toxin, and the suckling animal is likely to get additional swainsonine from its dam's milk.

Clinical Signs.   Livestock poisoning attributable to locoweeds has been recognized since the early part of this century and continues to be the major cause of loss to the livestock industry over all other plant-induced toxicities combined.[39-43] The locoweeds and vetches have been associated with three general syndromes of livestock poisoning. The best known is that of locoism caused by the effects of the alkaloid swainsonine.[39,44] In addition, the locoweeds and vetches cause respiratory problems and peripheral nerve degeneration caused by the effects of nitropropanol glycosides.[45,46] A third syndrome is caused by chronic selenium toxicosis.[44] Some species of *Astragalus* may contain one or

more of the toxicants and consequently may cause a combination of clinical signs in animals that have eaten them.[44,46] The following discussion is limited to those clinical signs attributed to the indolizidine alkaloids.

Neurologic disease.   The clinical signs of locoweed poisoning are usually not observed until the animal has eaten the locoweed over several weeks, and even then the signs can be easily mistaken for those of other disease syndromes. Affected animals may exhibit a variety of signs, including depression, circling, incoordination, ataxia, and unpredictable behavior, especially if the animal is stressed or excited.[30-33,39,43] Some horses become totally unpredictable in their response to handling and may fall down when being haltered or ridden. Poor vision, proprioceptive deficits, and sudden changes in behavior such as rearing and falling over backward make "loco" horses dangerous and unsafe to ride. Horses appear to show the nervous signs of locoweed poisoning more commonly than do cattle or sheep. Cattle may become nervous and aggressive when handled and may refuse to enter a chute as they would normally. Sheep develop a stargazing behavior, appear blind, and lose the normal flocking instinct. Weight loss, despite ample forage and grain being available, is typical.[47] Weight loss and poor growth rates of young animals may be a result of nervous system depression, inability to eat normally, and impaired digestion and absorption. Horses in particular become more depressed over time and may appear to be asleep. Death eventually results when the animal is too weak to stand and succumbs to convulsions and coma.

Infertility and reproductive failure.   The reproductive problems and congenital defects commonly associated with locoweeds most probably result from the effects of swainsonine on the pituitary gland, ovaries, uterus, and fetus.[24,25,48] Progesterone levels decrease and prostaglandin levels increase from the effects of swainsonine on the luteal cells.[49] Swainsonine also affects the placenta by inhibiting cellular mannosidases.[25] The resulting accumulation of oligosaccharides in the cells impairs the function of the placenta, allowing swainsonine to directly affect the developing fetus. The placenta appears to be most susceptible to the effects of locoweed during the first 90 days of pregnancy, but is vulnerable at any stage.[50] Normal placentation may be affected, causing fetal resumption, abortions, infertility, hydrops allantois subcutaneous edema in the fetus, and fetal deformities.[50-56] Cows with hydrops may carry the pregnancy to term, but more frequently abort or become recumbent and unable to rise owing to the massive weight of the fluid in the uterus. Retention of fetal membranes and subsequent infertility are common sequelae to hydrops.

Lambs and calves born to locoweed-poisoned dams may be born alive but weak and often die after a few days. Others may be smaller than normal, or have deformities of the limbs or head.[50,57] The formation of congenital abnormalities such as crooked legs is probably due to fetal immobilization induced by the locoweed.[58] Pregnant mares that consume quantities of woolly loco (*A. mollissimus*) in early gestation may produce foals with crooked legs due to deformity of the bones of the fetlocks.[59]

The effects of swainsonine on male fertility can be profound and significantly affect the fertility of rams and bulls. Rams having consumed locoweed (*A. lentiginosus*) for prolonged periods have been observed to develop testicular atrophy with decreased spermatogenesis.[60] The formation of abnormal sperm with proximal droplets and decreased motility of sperm are attributable to the accumulation of oligosaccharides in the cells of the seminiferous tubules, epididymis, and vas deferens.[61] Libido and normal breeding behavior is also affected. The effects of swainsonine on the male reproductive organs are transitory and normal spermatogenisis returns after 70 days of a locoweed-free diet.[62]

Heart failure.   A correlation exists between the incidence of "high mountain disease" or congestive right-sided heart failure in cattle and the consumption of a locoweed (*O. sericea*) at high altitude.[63-66] Cytoplasmic vacuolation characteristic of swainsonine toxicosis has been observed in the lungs of cattle eating locoweed and which developed congestive right ventricular failure.[64-66] Experimentally, the fetuses of ewes fed locoweed for 2 to 3 months developed heart irregularities and right ventricular hypertrophy, suggesting there may also be a direct effect of swainsonine on the heart.[56,58] The effects of swainsonine on the myocardium and lungs in combination with the hypoxia of high altitude can result in a high incidence of congestive right-sided heart failure in cattle. Cattle also genetically predisposed to pulmonary hypertension are likely to be especially compromised if they consume locoweed growing at high altitudes.

Weight loss and poor performance.   The continuous consumption of locoweeds by calves over the course of the growing season and even when the plants are dry or dormant during the winter can result in stunted, poor-growing calves. Poor growth rates and loss of weight are probably due to the combined effects of swainsonine on the nervous system, causing suppression of appetite, difficulty in finding and prehending food, decreased growth hormone production, and decreased intestinal glycosidases, which is important in food utilization.[67] Calves with locoweed poisoning appear clinically similar to, and can be mistaken for, calves that have been affected by bovine virus diarrhea. Affected calves have significantly lower weaning weights and gain very poorly during the first 6 to 8 weeks when placed on a concentrate ration under feedlot conditions.[68] However, once the effects of swainsonine have diminished after calves have been off of all sources of locoweed for about 60 days, compensatory weight gains can be expected.

Locoweed-poisoned animals often appear to have a greater incidence of common diseases such as foot rot, pneumonia, warts, and other infections, suggesting that affected animals may have a compromised immune system. Swainsonine at low doses has been shown to increase lymphocyte function in vitro.[69,70] At sustained high doses, swainsonine depresses lymphocyte blastogenesis and lysosomal function.[71] Evidence for this is detectable in sheep that, when repeatedly fed locoweed, had lymphocytes with decreased responsiveness to mitogens.[71] Peripheral lymphocytes in the affected sheep contain cytoplasmic vacuoles characteristic of swainsonine toxicity. Calves chronically eating locoweed and which are vaccinated with modified live

virus vaccines do not develop good titers to the vaccine. Once normal lymphocytes are repopulated after the calves have been free of swainsonine for at least a month, a normal immune response to vaccination can be expected.[68]

Clinical Pathology.   Owing to the generalized effects of swainsonine on lysosomal function, affected animals may have elevated levels of the serum enzymes and altered hormone levels that can be useful in the clinicopathologic diagnosis of locoweed poisoning. Serum alpha-mannosidase levels decline significantly from the inhibition of the enzyme by swainsonine.[19] The inhibitory activity of alpha-mannosidase can be determined spectrophotometrically using commercial jackbean alpha-*D*-mannosidase and *p*-nitrophenyl mannoside as a substrate with swainsonine as the assay standard.[72] Mannosidase activity returns to normal in 6 days once the animal is prevented from eating more locoweed.[19]

The serum enzymes alkaline phosphatase, aspartate aminotransferase, and lactate dehydrogenase increase from the effects of the swainsonine on the liver and other tissues, whereas serum protein and albumin tend to be decreased.[71,73-75] Mean thyroid levels (T_4 and T_3) are usually decreased in animals eating locoweed.[19]

The presence of vacuoles in the cytoplasm of peripheral lymphocytes may be seen in locoweed poisoning.[33,71] The vacuolated lymphocytes often persist in the circulation for several weeks after an animal has ceased eating locoweed, making this a useful diagnostic finding when coupled with other findings.

Lesions.   No gross postmortem lesions are characteristic of locoweed poisoning. Emaciation, occasional stomach ulcers, thyroid hypertrophy, and pale coloration to the liver and kidneys have been reported.[24,25,75]

The detection of cytoplasmic vacuoles in the cells of the brain, liver, kidney, lymphocytes, and other tissues is characteristic of locoweed (swainsonine) poisoning. The vacuoles seen histologically are the site of the accumulated oligosaccharides that are removed during the staining process of the tissues for histopathology. In animals exhibiting neurologic signs of locoism, cytoplasmic vacuolation of neurons in the brain is characteristic. Similar vacuolation is often present in pituitary gland, thyroid, pancreas, kidneys, liver, and other exocrine glands.[24,25,33] Marked cytoplasmic vacuoles are also present in the retina and other structures of the eye.[76] Experimentally, vacuoles can be first demonstrated in the kidney tubules 4 days after initiating locoweed feeding. Vacuoles in the neurons are detectable by day 8, and placental lesions developed in 8 to 16 days after the start of feeding locoweed.[76,77]

Animals with chronic locoweed poisoning, which have not eaten locoweed for more than a month, have vacuolation restricted to hepatocytes and neurons of the brain.[33] Vacuoles may be visible in the Purkinje cells of the cerebellum for more than a year. Noticeable loss of Purkinje cells over time accounts for the residual neurologic abnormalities typical of locoweed poisoning.[37] The vacuoles present in cells that are characteristic of swainsonine toxicosis are similar to those found with other lysosomal storage diseases in animals such as alpha- and beta-*D*-mannosidosis reported in cattle and goats.[27,78,79]

Diagnostic Testing.   Locoweed poisoning may be tentatively diagnosed in animals by demonstrating the presence of swainsonine in the serum, coupled with decreased serum alpha-mannosidase activity.[73] The half-life of swainsonine in the serum is approximately 16 to 20 hours.[19] This means that an animal suspected of locoweed poisoning must have blood sampled within 2 days of eating locoweed for there to be detectable levels of swainsonine. Similarly, serum alpha-mannosidase activity can only be reliably assayed within 6 days of the last time the animal would have eaten locoweed before enzyme activity returns to normal.[19] Examining feces or rumen contents for characteristic plant epidermal cells can be useful in confirming that an animal has recently eaten locoweed.[80]

A profile of decreased alpha-mannosidase activity, increased aspartate aminotransferase, and detectable swainsonine levels in the serum of a live animal is diagnostic of locoweed poisoning. A diagnosis of locoweed poisoning is best made in a dead animal by demonstrating the presence of characteristic cytoplasmic vacuoles in the cerebellar Purkinje cells, lymphocytes, liver, thyroid gland, and various other tissues.[19,24,25,33,73] In chronic cases it is important to submit the brain for histopathologic diagnosis in that lesions persist the longest in the neurons.

Treatment.   No proven effective treatment for locoweed poisoning has been established. Fowler's solution and reserpine, once recommended for treating locoism, are unwarranted in light of current knowledge regarding the etiology of locoweed poisoning.[81] Because of the short half-life of swainsonine, recovery from the effects of the alkaloid are rapid as long as the symptoms are not of long duration and animals are removed from the locoweed before extensive cellular degeneration has occurred in the brain. Other organs tend to recover rapidly once no further locoweed consumption occurs. Animals that have aborted generally will conceive in subsequent reproductive cycles as long as they do not develop severe secondary infections of the reproductive system. Compensatory weight gains can also be anticipated in animals once they are removed from locoweed and are fed a balanced, nutritious diet. Further consumption of locoweed should be prevented immediately and in subsequent years as animals retain a preference for the plants from year to year.

Prognosis.   Complete recovery from locoweed poisoning usually occurs as long as the animals are not chronically affected. Cell populations such as lymphocytes, intestinal epithelium, and glandular tissue with rapid turnover respond quickly to the removal of swainsonine. Weight gains, reproductive performance, and antigen processing by the immune system return to normal in 1 to 2 months. However, regeneration of affected neurons in the brain and spinal cord of chronically affected animals does not occur. Horses in particular may have permanent neurologic deficits that make

them a liability to human safety.[33] The prognosis for horses should always be guarded.

Prevention and Control.   The most effective management strategy for the prevention of locoweed poisoning is to deny animals access to the plants when they are most palatable. It is therefore important to recognize the growth characteristics of locoweeds and the conditions under which livestock prefer to graze the plants. Cattle and probably other herbivores eat locoweed particularly when grazing pressure is high and other forages are unavailable.[82-84] However, livestock voluntarily eat locoweed when it is in the flower and early seedpod stages.[85] Although this corresponds to when swainsonine levels are highest in the plant, it is not the swainsonine level in the plants that makes them palatable. The early seedpod stage coincides with the highest levels of protein and carbohydrate in the plant, which may increase palatability.[86] It is therefore wise to remove livestock from the locoweed areas when the plants are in the flower and pod stage, and until other forages are available. When other forages become available in the spring and summer, cattle usually stop eating locoweed until grasses are depleted.[85] Overgrazing obviously increases the probability of locoweed being grazed. Increased rainfall can mean more growth of locoweed populations, making more plants available both in the summer and winter.[87] In mild winters when there is little snow cover, locoweed grazing continues and poisoning occurs when least expected. Although less toxic, locoweeds retain some of their toxicity even when dried.

Experimentally it has been shown that cattle naive to locoweed greatly increase their consumption of locoweed when placed with locoweed eaters.[88] This phenomenon, referred to as *social facilitation*, means that animals learn to eat certain plants by observing the eating habits of others. Social facilitation is the reason that, over a period of seasons, the percentage of cattle grazing locoweed in the herd increases exponentially. Locoweed grazing by livestock is not an addictive problem as was once thought, because consumption voluntarily stops when other, more palatable forages are available.[89] Animals do, however, develop a preference for locoweed, much as animals develop a liking for alfalfa.

By rotating livestock from locoweed to non-locoweed–infested pastures, effective use of the rangeland can be accomplished without severely poisoning the animals. Sheep and cattle should be left on the locoweed areas for less than 4 weeks at a time to avoid the development of locoweed poisoning that affects performance.[90] Studies in sheep showed that a 4-week period of locoweed feeding induces neurologic abnormalities that require 6 weeks to resolve, indicating that a 4-week rotational grazing plan may not give sufficient time for animals to fully recover from the effects of the locoweed poisoning.[90]

A variety of herbicides can be effectively used to control both *Astragalus* and *Oxytropis* species, including the chemicals clopyralid, dicamba, picloram, and triclopyr.[91] The phenoxy herbicide 2,4-D is marginally effective as long as it is applied when the plants are actively growing. In all cases, it is most important to ensure the herbicide being used is approved for use in the area and that the manufacturer's recommendations are followed. Seeds of many locoweeds can persist in the soil for at least 50 years, requiring repeated application of appropriate herbicides periodically to control locoweed reemergence.[92]

Conditioned food aversion is a method that has been used successfully to teach cattle to not eat locoweed.[93] Aversion is accomplished by associating locoweed with something distasteful that causes temporary abdominal pain or discomfort. The plants are collected and fed to cattle, which then receive a bolus of lithium chloride. This very irritating substance causes the animal to develop "colic," which it associates with eating locoweed. This aversion to eating the locoweed persists through subsequent growing seasons as long as the animals are not mingled with locoweed eaters. Through social facilitation, the cattle relearn to eat locoweed from the locoweed eaters.[94] Conditioned food aversion has potential in the management and prevention of locoweed poisoning in certain limited and well-managed herds.

Although various mineral and protein supplements have been recommended for the prevention of locoweed poisoning in livestock, it has not been proven that mineral supplementation will prevent locoweed poisoning or reduce the consumption of the plants.[95,96] However, animals that are deficient in protein and micronutrients will benefit nutritionally from such supplements.

REFERENCES

1. Broquist HP: The indolizidine alkaloids, slaframine and swainsonine: contaminants in forages, *Ann Rev Nutr* 5:391, 1985.
2. Huxtable CR, Dorling PR: Poisoning of livestock by *Swainsona* spp: current status, *Aust Vet J* 59:50, 1982.
3. Dorling PR et al: Isolation of swainsonine from *Swainsona canescens*: historical aspects. In James LF, Elbien AD, Molyneux RJ, Warren CD, editors:. *Swainsonine and related glycosidase inhibitors,* Ames, Iowa, 1989, Iowa State University Press.
4. Hartley WJ: A comparative study of darling pea (*Swainsona* spp) poisoning in Australia with locoweed (*Astragalus* and *Oxytropis* spp) poisoning in North America. In Keeler RF, Van Kampen KR, James LF, editors: *Effects of poisonous plants on livestock,* New York, 1978, Academic Press.
5. Molyneux RJ, James LF: Loco intoxication: indolizidine alkaloids in spotted locoweed (*Astragalus lentiginosus*), *Science* 216:190, 1982.
6. Molyneux RJ et al: The occurrence and detection of swainsonine in locoweeds. In James LF, Elbein LD, Molyneux RJ, Warren CD, editors: *Swainsonine and related glycosidase inhibitors,* Ames, Iowa, 1989, Iowa State University Press.
7. Smith GS et al: Swainsonine content in New Mexican locoweeds, *Proceedings Western Section, Am Soc Anim Sci* 43:405, 1992.
8. Broquist HP: Livestock toxicosis, slobbers, locoism, and indolizidine alkaloids, *Nutr Rev* 44:317, 1986.
9. Williams MC, Barneby RC: The occurrence of nitrotoxins in North American *Astragalus* (Fabaceae), *Brittonia* 29:310, 1997.
10. James LF: The effects of *Astragalus tenellus* in sheep, *J Range Manage* 24:161, 1971.
11. Williams MC: Nitro compounds in foreign species of *Astragalus, Weed Sci* 29:261, 1981.
12. Ralph MH, Cronin EH: Locoweed seed in soil: density, germination, and viability, *Weed Sci* 35:792, 1987.
13. Molyneux RJ et al: Analysis and distribution of swainsonine and related polyhydroxyindolizidine alkaloids by thin layer chromatography, *Phytochem Anal* 2:125, 1991.
14. Ralphs MH, Molyneux RJ: Livestock grazing locoweed and the influence of swainsonine on locoweed palatability and habituation. In James LF, Elbien AD, Molyneux RJ, Warren CD, editors: *Swainsonine and related glycosidase inhibitors,* Ames, Iowa, 1989, Iowa State University Press.
15. Hartley WJ, James LF: Fetal and maternal lesions in pregnant ewes ingesting locoweed (*Astragalus lentiginosus*), *Am J Vet Res* 36:825, 1975.
16 James LF, Hartley WJ: Effects of milk from animals fed locoweed on kittens, calves and lambs, *Am J Vet Res* 38:1263, 1977.
17. Molyneux RJ et al: Polyhydroxy alkaloid glycosidase inhibitors from poisonous plants of global distribution: analysis and identification. In Colegate SM, Dorling PR, editors: *Plant-associated toxins,* Wallingford, UK, 1994, CAB International.
18. James LF, Van Kampen KR: Effects of locoweed toxin on rats, *Am J Vet Res* 37:845, 1976.
19. Stegelmeier BL et al: Serum swainsonine concentration and alpha-mannosidase activity in cattle and sheep ingesting *Oxytropis sericea* and *Astragalus lentiginosus* (locoweeds), *Am J Vet Res* 56:149, 1995.
20. Stegelmeier BL et al: Tissue swainsonine clearance in sheep chronically poisoned with locoweed (*Oxytropis sericea*), *J Anim Sci* 76:1140, 1998.
21. Stegelmeier BL et al: The pathogenesis and toxicokinetics of locoweed (*Astragalus* and *Oxytropis* spp.) poisoning in livestock, *J Nat Toxins* 8:35, 1999.
22. Dorling PR et al: Inhibition of lysosomal alpha-mannosidase by swainsonine, an indolizidine alkaloid isolated from *Swainsona canescens, Biochem J* 191:649, 1980.
23. Tulsiani DR et al: The similar effects of swainsonine and locoweed on tissue glycosidases and oligosaccharides of the pig indicate that the alkaloid is the principal toxin responsible for locoism, *Arch Biochem Biophys* 232:76, 1984.
24. Van Kampen KR, James LF: Pathology of locoweed poisoning in sheep, *Pathol Vet* 6:413, 1969.
25. Van Kampen KR, James LF: Pathology of locoweed poisoning in sheep: sequential development of cytoplasmic vacuolization in tissues, *Pathol Vet* 7:503, 1970.
26. Dorling PR et al: Lysosomal storage disease in *Swainsona* spp. toxicosis: an induced manosidosis, *Neuropathol Appl Neurobiol* 4:285, 1978.
27. Jolly RD, Hartley WJ: Storage diseases of domestic animals, *Aust Vet J* 53:1, 1977.
28. Leipold HW et al et al: Mannosidosis of Angus calves, *J Am Vet Med Assoc* 175:457, 1979.
29. Stegelmeier BL et al: In Garland T, Barr AC, editors: *Toxic plants and other natural toxicants,* New York, 1998, CAB International.
30. James LF et al: Locoweed (*Astragalus lentiginosus*) poisoning in cattle and horses, *J Am Vet Med Assoc* 155:525, 1969.
31. Oehme F et al: *Astragalus mollissimus* (Locoweed) toxicosis of horses in western Kansas, *J Am Vet Med Assoc* 152:271, 1968.
32. Wolfe GJ, Lance WR: Locoweed poisoning in a northern New Mexico elk herd, *J Range Manage* 37:59, 1984.
33. James LF, Van Kampen KR: Acute and residual lesions of locoweed poisoning in cattle and horses, *J Am Vet Med Assoc* 158:614, 1971.
34. Ralphs MH et al: Feed preferences and habituation of sheep poisoned by locoweed, *J Anim Sci* 68:1354, 1990.
35. Ralphs MH et al: Grazing behavior and forage preference of sheep with chronic locoweed toxicosis suggest no addiction, *J Range Manage* 44:208, 1991.
36. Ralphs MH et al: Social facilitation influences cattle to graze locoweed, *J Range Manage* 47:123, 1994.
37. Ralphs MH, James LF: Locoweed grazing, *J Nat Toxins* 8:47, 1999.
38. Stegelmeier BL et al: The lesions of locoweed (*Astragalus mollissimus*), swainsonine, and castanospermine in rats, *Vet Pathol* 32:289, 1995.
39. Marsh CD et al: The locoweed disease, *U.S. Department of Agriculture Bull* 1054:1, 1919.
40. Mathews FP: Locoism in domestic animals, *Texas Agric Exp Station Bull* 456:5, 1932.
41. Mathews FP: The toxicity of red-stemmed peavine (*Astragalus emoryanus*) for cattle, sheep, and goats, *J Am Vet Med Assoc* 97:125, 1940.

42. Nielson DB: The economic impact of poisonous plants on the range livestock industry in the 17 western states, *J Range Manage* 31:325, 1978.

43. James LF et al: *The ecology and economic impact of poisonous plants on livestock production,* Boulder, Colo, 1988, Westview Press.

44. James LF et al: Syndromes of *Astragalus* poisoning in livestock, *J Am Vet Med Assoc* 178:146, 1981.

45. Williams CB, Barneby RC:The occurrence of nitro-toxins in North American *Astragalus* (Fabaceae), *Brittonia* 29:310, 1977.

46. Cheeke PR: *Natural toxicants in feeds, forages and poisonous plants,* Danville, Ill, 1998, Interstate Publishers.

47. Kirkpatrick JG, Burrows GE: Locoism in horses, *Vet Hum Toxicol* 32:168, 1990.

48. Panter KE et al: Locoweeds: effects on reproduction in livestock, *J Nat Toxins* 8:53, 1999.

49. Ellis LC et al: Reduced progesterone and altered cotyledonary prostaglandin levels induced by locoweed (*Astragalus lentiginosus*) in sheep, *Am J Vet Res* 46:1903, 1985.

50. Balls LD, James LF: Effect of locoweed (*Astragalus* spp) on reproductive performance of ewes, *J Am Vet Med Assoc* 162:291, 1973.

51. Hartley WJ, James LF: Fetal and maternal lesions in pregnant ewes ingesting locoweed (*Astragalus lentiginosus*), *Am J Vet Res* 36:825, 1975.

52. Hartley WJ, James LF: Microscopic lesions in fetuses of ewes ingesting locoweed (*Astragalus lentiginosus*), *Am J Vet Res* 34:209, 1973.

53. James LF et al: Sequence in the abortive and teratogenic effects of locoweed fed to sheep, *Am J Vet Res* 30:377, 1969.

54. James LF et al: Abortive and teratogenic effects of locoweed on cattle and sheep, *Am J Vet Res* 28:1379, 1967.

55. James LF: Effect of locoweed on fetal development: preliminary study in sheep, *Am J Vet Res* 33:835, 1972.

56. Panter KE et al: Ultrasonographic imaging to monitor fetal and placental developments in ewes fed locoweed (*Astragalus lentiginosus*), *Am J Vet Res* 48:686, 1987.

57. James LF: Lesions in neonatal lambs resulting from maternal ingestion of locoweed, *Cornell Vet* 61:667, 1971.

58. Bunch TD et al: Ultrasound studies of the effects of certain poisonous plants on uterine function and fetal development in livestock, *J Anim Sci* 70:1639, 1992.

59. McIlwraith CW, James LF: Limb deformities in foals associated with ingestion of locoweed by mares, *J Am Vet Med Assoc* 181:255, 1982.

60. James LF, Van Kampen K: Effects of locoweed intoxication on the genital tract of the ram, *Am J Vet Res* 32:1253, 1971.

61. James LF, Panter KE: Locoweed poisoning in livestock. In James LF, Elbien AD, Molyneux RJ, Warren GC, editors:. Swainsonine and related glycosidase inhibitors, Ames, Iowa, 1989, Iowa State University Press.

62. Panter KE, Hartley WJ. Transient testicular degeneration in rams fed locoweed (*Astragalus lentiginosus*), *Vet Hum Toxicol* 30:318, 1989.

63. James LF et al: Relationship between ingestion of locoweed *Oxytropis sericea* and congestive right-side heart failure in cattle, *Am J Vet Res* 2:254, 1983.

64. James LF et al: Locoweed (*Oxytropis sericea*) poisoning and congestive heart failure in cattle, *J Am Vet Med Assoc* 189:1549, 1986.

65. Panter KE et al: The relationship of *Oxytropis sericea* (green and dry) and *Astragalus lentiginosus* with high mountain disease, *Vet Hum Toxicol* 30:318, 1988.

66. James LF et al: Swainsonine-induced high mountain disease in calves, *Vet Hum Toxicol* 33:217, 1991.

67. Stegelmeier BL et al: Serum swainsonine concentration and alpha-mannosidase activity in cattle and sheep ingesting *Oxytropis sericea* and *Astragalus lentiginosus* (locoweeds), *Am J Vet Res* 56:149, 1995.

68. Knight AP, Greathouse G: *Locoweed in northern Colorado: its effects on beef calves. Locoweed and broom snakeweed research update,* Albuquerque, NM, 1996, New Mexico State University.

69. Das PC et al: Activation of resident tissue specific macrophages by swainsonine, *Oncology Res* 7:425, 1995.

70. Galustian C et al: Swainsonine, a glycosylation inhibitor, enhances both lymphocyte and tumor susceptibility in LAK and NK cytotoxicity, *Immunopharmacology* 27:165, 1994.

71. Sharma RP et al: Effect of repeated locoweed feeding on peripheral lymphocytic function and plasma proteins of sheep, *Am J Vet Res* 10:2090, 1984.

72. Miller PR et al: Alpha-mannosidase inhibitory activity of locoweed extracts after incubation in rumen fluid. In James LF et al, editors: *Poisonous plants: proceedings of the third international symposium,* Ames, Iowa, 1992, Iowa State University Press.

73. Stegelmeier BL et al: Serum alpha-mannosidase activity and the clinicopathologic alterations of locoweed (*Astragalus mollissimus*) intoxication in range cattle, *J Vet Diagn Invest* 6:473, 1994.

74. James LF, Binns W. Blood changes associated with locoweed poisoning, *Am J Vet Res* 28:1107, 1967.

75. James LF et al: Physiopathologic changes in locoweed poisoning of livestock, *Am J Vet Res* 31:663, 1970.

76. Van Kampen KR, James LF: Ophthalmic lesions in locoweed poisoning of cattle, sheep, and horses, *Am J Vet Res* 32:1293, 1971.

77. Van Kampen KR: Sequential development of the lesions in locoweed poisoning, *Clin Toxicol* 5:575, 1972.

78. Jones MZ et al: Caprine beta-mannosidosis: clinical and pathological features, *J Neuropathol Exp Neurol* 42:268, 1983.

79. Abbitt M et al: Beta-mannosidosis in 12 Salers calves, *J Am Vet Med Assoc* 198:109, 1991.

80. Potter RL, Ueckert DN: *Epidermal cellular characteristics of selected livestock-poisoning plants in North America,* Texas A&M University, College Station, 1997, Texas Agricultural Experiment Station.

81. Staley EE: An approach to treatment of locoism in horses, *Vet Med Small Anim Clin* 73:1205, 1978.

82. Ralphs MH: Cattle grazing white locoweed: influence of grazing pressure and palatability associated with phenological growth stage, *J Range Manage* 40:330, 1987.

83. Ralphs MH et al: Social facilitation influences cattle to graze locoweed. *J Range Manage* 47:123, 1994.

84. Ralphs MH et al: Seasonal grazing of locoweeds by cattle in northeastern New Mexico, *J Range Manage* 46:416, 1993.

85. Ralphs MH et al: Cattle grazing white locoweed: diet selection patterns of native and introduced cattle, *J Range Manage* 40:333, 1987.

86. Ralphs MH et al: Utilization of white locoweed (*Oxytropis sericea* Nutt.) by range cattle, *J Range Manage* 39:344, 1986.

87. Taylor CA, Ralphs MH: Reducing livestock losses from poisonous plants through grazing management, *J Range Manage* 45:9, 1992.

88. Ralphs MH et al: Cattle grazing white locoweed in New Mexico: influence of grazing pressure and phenological growth stage, *J Range Manage* 47:270, 1974.

89. Ralphs MH et al: Grazing behavior and forage preference of sheep with chronic locoweed toxicosis suggest no addiction, *J Range Manage* 44:208, 1991.

90. Pfister JA et al: Operant analysis of chronic locoweed intoxication in sheep, *J Anim Sci* 74:2622, 1996.

91. Ralphs MH, Cronin EH: Locoweed seed in soil: density, longevity, germination, and viability, *Weed Sci* 35:792, 1987.

92. Ralphs MH, Ueckert DN: Herbicide control of locoweeds: a review, *Weed Technol* 2:460, 1988.

93. Ralphs MH: Conditioned food aversion: training livestock to avoid eating poisonous plants, *J Range Manage* 45:46, 1992.

94. Ralphs MH et al: Creating aversions to locoweed in naïve and familiar cattle. *J Range Manage* 50:361, 1997.

95. James LF,Van Kampen KR: Effect of protein and mineral supplementation on potential locoweed (*Astragalus* spp.) poisoning in sheep, *J Am Vet Med Assoc* 164:1042, 1974.

96. Bachman SE et al: Early aspects of locoweed toxicosis and evaluation of a mineral supplement or clinoptilolite as dietary treatments, *J Anim Sci* 70:3125, 1992.

JERVANINE ALKALOIDS

Kip E. Panter

The *Veratrum* and *Zigadenus* spp. in the family Liliaceae contain nitrogenous steroidal alkaloids termed *azasteroids*. These alkaloids can be divided into several different groups, two of which have significant veterinary importance: jervanine and cevanine. The jervanine group consists of a variety of alkaloids found in *Veratrum* spp., which has been associated with teratogenic effects in livestock. The cevanine group of alkaloids, which affect the nervous system, are found in both *Veratrum* and *Zigadenus* spp. and are discussed in a separate section.

Synonyms.   Common names for *Veratrum* include false or western hellebore, white hellebore, California false hellebore, wild corn, skunk cabbage, and corn lily.

Sources.   *Veratrum californicum* usually grows at elevations of 1500 to 3000 m and is found in the mountain valleys of the Pacific coast and northern Rocky Mountain states. *V. viride* is found at lower elevations throughout the United States. The other species grow at lower elevations. *V. album* grows in European countries and, although not widespread in the United States, it does grow in Alaska where it has been suspected to cause toxicosis in Alpacas.[1]

Toxicokinetics.   Steroidal alkaloid toxins have been identified in *Veratrum* spp. and have been responsible for great losses to the livestock industry. Since the 1930s, more than 100 alkaloids have been identified; some of these are pharmacologically active, most are toxic, and some possess teratogenic activity.[2] The teratogenic jervanine alkaloids include cyclopamine, cycloposine, jervine, and veratrobasine.[3] Little information is available on the disposition of these alkaloids in mammals.

Mechanism of Action.   The mechanisms of action of *Veratrum*-induced malformations include inhibited cellular movement during differentiation. Cyclopamine interferes with intercellular signals that regulate cellular identity, patterning, and tissue interactions during embryogenesis and organogenesis. Thus, the function in a multitude of developmental processes ranging from neural tissue specification to bone morphogenesis is altered.

Toxicity and Risk Factors.   *Veratrum californicum*, *V. viride*, and *V. album* are the species most commonly encountered by grazing livestock. All parts of the plant are toxic; however, the alkaloids are found in higher concentrations in the roots and rhizomes. Roots and rhizomes are used in isolation of the toxins for experimental purposes but are seldom eaten by livestock. Highest risk for induction of birth defects in sheep is in the fall because of the association of breeding season, susceptibility of early embryos, and availability of the plants. Cattle seldom ingest these plants and natural cases of *Veratrum*-induced birth defects are rare. Toxicosis has been experimentally produced in cattle, sheep, goats, and rabbits.[4]

Clinical Signs.   *Veratrum* ingestion causes craniofacial defects that are frequently accompanied by increased incidence of shortened limbs, tracheal stenosis, and increased embryonic loss.[5] Feeding ewes *Veratrum* roots and leaves from day 12 to day 30 of gestation induces cleft palate and lip, brachygnathia, hypermobility of hocks, syndactylism, and shortened metacarpals and metatarsals.[6] Experimental feeding during gestation days 30 to 36 results in hypoplasia and shortened metacarpal and metatarsal bones. Craniofacial defects such as cyclops in sheep are associated with ingestion on day 14, limb and tracheal defects during days 28 to 33 of gestation, and increased embryonic death at days 14 to 19.[5]

Clinical Pathology.   Serum biochemistry and blood profiles have not been characterized for *Veratrum* poisoning.

Diagnostic Testing.   Diagnosis of poisoning is based on identification and availability of the plant, history of ingestion, and clinical signs.

Prevention and Control.   Prevention of birth defects can easily be accomplished by manipulating the breeding season to avoid maternal exposure to *Veratrum* during critical stages of pregnancy. Short- and long-term herbicide control of *Veratrum* has been accomplished with 2,4-D, and Picloram.[7]

REFERENCES

1. Leach JB III, Big Lake Veterinary Hospital, Alaska: Personal communication, 1995.
2. Rahman AU et al: New steroidal alkaloids from rhizomes of *Veratrum album, J Nat Prod* 55:565, 1992.
3. Keeler RF: In Nes WD et al, editors: *Isopentenoids in plants, biochemistry and function*, New York, 1984, Marcel Dekker.
4. Binns W et al: Chronologic evaluation of teratogenicity in sheep fed *Veratrum californicum, J Am Vet Med Assoc* 147:839, 1965.
5. Keeler RF, Stuart LD: The nature of congenital limb defects induced in lambs by maternal ingestion of *Veratrum californicum, Clin Toxicol* 25:273, 1987.
6. Binns W et al: Congenital deformities in lambs, calves, and goats resulting from maternal ingestion of *Veratrum californicum*: hare lip, cleft palate, ataxia and hypoplasia of metacarpal and metatarsal bones, *Clin Toxicol* 5:245, 1972.
7. Williams MC: Twenty-year control of California false-hellebore, *Weed Tech* 5:40, 1991.

LYCORINE

Charlotte Means

Synonyms.   Table 25-5 lists the most common plants.

Sources.   These plants generally are planted in the fall for spring blooms. Some are forced for indoor blooming during the winter and spring. They are generally perennials with narrow, flat leaves and lilylike flowers on leafless stalks. Amaryllis is very popular as a potted plant in December. Narcissus is one of the first flowers to bloom in spring.

TABLE 25-5 **Plants in the Amaryllidaceae Family**

Genus Name	Common Name
Narcissus spp.	Daffodil, jonquil, paper whites
Clivia spp.	Clivia lily, Kaffir (or caffir) lily
Galanthus nivalis	Snowdrop
Ismene calithina	Filmy lily, basket lily, spider lily, hymenocallis
Hippeastrum spp.	Barbadoes lily, fire lily
Amaryllis spp.	Amaryllis, naked lady, Aztec lily, belladona lily, orchid lily, jacobean lily, and other terms

Toxicity and Risk Factors. These plants contain a variety of alkaloids; at least 15 have been identified in daffodils alone. The most important alkaloid is lycorine (also known as narcissine). The bulbs contain the highest concentration of lycorine, especially in the outer epidermis.[1,2]

Most of the plants also contain galanthamine, which is a cholinesterase inhibitor. Narsiclasine has colchicine-like effects at 0.5 to 0.9 mg/kg.

Clinical Signs. Although all parts of the plant are toxic, ingesting small amounts of foliage generally only results in drooling, vomiting, and diarrhea. The plant has a definite purgative action. The animal may appear depressed and be anorectic. With larger ingestions, hypotension is not uncommon and weakness or ataxia may occur. Clinical signs generally occur within 1 hour of ingestion and most cases resolve within a few hours. It is unusual to see more than mild signs if foliage of amaryllis or Barbadoes lilies is ingested.[3]

Ingestion of bulbs or large quantities of foliage can result in muscle tremors and seizures. Ingestion of a part of a bulb may be lethal to a small dog.[1-3] Hepatic damage has been reported in animals in older references, but there are no recent reports of hepatic damage.

Treatment. For a recent exposure, emesis is induced and activated charcoal administered. If a small amount of foliage was consumed, the animal may be monitored at home. The animal should not be given food or water for 2 to 3 hours. If significant vomiting occurs, intravenous fluids should be administered to replace electrolytes and correct dehydration. Metoclopramide may be given as an antiemetic at 0.1 to 0.5 mg/kg intramuscularly. Gastrointestinal protectants such as sucralfate can be soothing to the mucosa. Seizures may be treated with diazepam, 0.5 to 1 mg/kg intravenously in increments of 5 to 10 mg to effect.[3,4]

Prevention and Control. Dogs will eat bulbs laid out in preparation for planting. Bone meal, blood meal, or other fertilizers are frequently mixed in the soil when planting. Dogs eat the soil for the bone meal and may ingest the bulb at the same time. Owners should be cautioned to plant bulbs where pets cannot dig them up.

REFERENCES

1. Spoerke DG, Smolinske SC: *Toxicity of houseplants*, Boca Raton, Fla, 1990, CRC Press.
2. POISINDEX System Editorial Staff: Plants: colchicine. In Toll LL, Hurlbut KM, editors: *POISINDEX System*, Englewood, Colo, Micromedex (edition expires December 2000).
3. Beasley VR, Dorman DC et al: *A systems affected approach to veterinary toxicology*, Urbana, Ill, 1999, University of Illinois.
4. Plumb DC: *Veterinary drug handbook*, ed 3, Ames, Iowa, 1999, Iowa State University Press.

PIPERIDINE ALKALOIDS

Kip E. Panter

Conium maculatum, Nicotiana spp., and *Lupinus* spp. contain piperidine alkaloids, which are basic compounds that are derivatives of piperidine (hexahydropyridine, $C_5H_{11}N$) and most are derived from biosynthetic pathways with lysine, acetate, or mevalonate as the precursor.[1,2]

Synonyms. Common names for *Conium maculatum* include poison-hemlock, hemlock, spotted hemlock, California or Nebraska fern, and poison fool's parsley[3] (Color Plates 12 and 13). This plant should not be confused with water hemlock (*Cicuta*). Common names for *Nicotiana* include burley tobacco (*N. tabacum*), wild tree tobacco (*N. glauca*), wild tobacco (*N. trigonophylla*), and coyote tobacco (*N. attenuata*).

Sources. Piperidine alkaloids are widely distributed in nature. Hundreds of piperidine alkaloids have been identified in plants, microorganisms, insects, and animals. For a review of the chemistry and list of numerous piperidine alkaloids, see reference 4 (Schneider, 1996). This section discusses the piperidine alkaloids causing toxicoses in livestock and limits the discussion to *Conium* (poison-hemlock), *Nicotiana* spp. (tobaccos), and a limited number of *Lupinus* spp. Pyridine alkaloids predominate in *Nicotiana* spp. and are discussed in more detail in the next section. Likewise, quinolizidine alkaloids constitute the majority of alkaloids in lupines, with piperidine alkaloids found in relatively few species. Quinolizidine alkaloids and lupines containing these alkaloids are also discussed later.

Conium maculatum. *Conium maculatum* (poison-hemlock) is native to Europe and Asia and has become naturalized in North America. Contamination of hay with vegetative parts and grains with seeds of *Conium* has resulted in large losses.[5-7]

Nicotiana spp. Although burley tobacco (*N. tabacum*) is an introduced plant, it is widely cultivated in the mideastern, central, and mid-Atlantic United States. The significance of burley tobacco in livestock poisoning comes from its association with livestock toxicoses and teratogenicity in sows and newborn pigs in Kentucky and Missouri in the late 1960s and early 1970s.[8-10] Initially, nicotine was believed to be the toxin causing the birth defects, but it was later confirmed that anabasine (α-pyrido-piperidine) was the teratogen.[11] *N. glauca* was reported to cause toxicosis in cattle and anabasine was the putative toxin.[12]

Outbreaks of malformations associated with tobacco resulted from a practice of feeding discarded burley tobacco stalks to pregnant sows.[8] Once the source was established and the practice discontinued, no further outbreaks were reported. The structural significance is that anabasine meets piperidine structural characteristics considered to be essential for induction of terata, that is, a piperidine alkaloid with a side chain of three carbons or more (in this case, a pyridine ring) attached next to the N atom. This structural importance was established by Keeler and Balls[13] and further research has supported this theory and expanded on other important structural components.[14]

Whereas nicotine is a true pyridine, anabasine may be referred to as a pyridine or a piperidine because it contains both a pyridine (C_5H_5N) and a piperidine ($C_5H_{11}N$) moiety.

Lupinus spp.   Lupines are widespread throughout the world and more than 500 species have been identified. Two hundred to 300 species are found in North America, with 150 species in the intermountain west and 95 species in California.[15-17]

Although most lupines contain quinolizidine alkaloids, a few contain piperidine alkaloids *(L. arbustus, L. argenteus)* and some contain both piperidine and quinolizidine alkaloids *(L. formosus)*. The piperidine alkaloids in *L. formosus* include ammodendrine, *N*-methyl ammodendrine, and *N*-acetyl hystrine. *Lupinus arbustus* contains ammodendrine and *N*-methyl ammodendrine.

Toxicokinetics.   Toxicity of *Conium*, like most plants, varies depending on stage of plant growth, location, and environment. Available data on toxicity of *Conium* are listed in Tables 25-6 and 25-7. Five principal alkaloids have been found in *Conium maculatum:* coniine, *N*-methyl coniine, γ-coniceine, conhydrine, and pseudoconhydrine. Although specific pharmacokinetic data are limited for most of the piperidine alkaloids in these plants, data on the absorption and elimination pattern of piperidine alkaloids from *Lupinus formosus* have been reported.[18] Similar absorption and elimination profiles probably occur for *Conium* and *Nicotiana*. Briefly, ammodendrine and *N*-methyl ammodendrine are rapidly absorbed and appear in blood within 30 minutes after oral gavage of ground plant. Maximum alkaloid levels occurred about 24 hours after administration. Plasma elimination was rapid for *N*-methyl ammodendrine and *N*-acetyl hystrine ($t_{1/2}$ <30 min) whereas ammodendrine was much slower ($t_{1/2}$ ~12 hours).[18] Similar studies should be done to characterize the blood absorption and elimination profiles for piperidine alkaloids in *Conium* and *Nicotiana*. Toxicity of individual alkaloids is related to structural characteristics and comparison of nine of these alkaloids is made in Table 25-6.

Mechanism of Action.   The predominant action of piperidine alkaloids from *Conium* is nicotinic in nature, consisting of initial transient stimulation followed by a more persistent depression of the autonomic ganglia, neuromuscular junctions, and medulla.[19,20] Pharmacologic investigations with coniine have it to be a a neuromuscular blocking agent. Peripheral actions on smooth muscle are caused by initial ganglionic stimulation and subsequent blockage in cats,

TABLE 25-6 Comparative Toxicity of Nine Toxic Alkaloids with Similar Structural Characteristics from *Lupinus*, *Conium*, and *Nicotiana*

Piperidine Alkaloid*	Plant	LD$_{50}$ (mg/kg)†	95% CI
γ-Coniceine	*C. maculatum*	2.52	2.33-2.73
Coniine	*C. maculatum*	11.41	9.55-13.64
N-methyl coniine	*C. maculatum*	20.54	19.12-22.08
Anabaseine	*N. glauca*	1.05	1.048-1.057
Anabasine	*N. glauca*	1.62	1.5-1.75
N-Methyl anabasine	*N. glauca*	12.46	10.06-15.43
N-Acetyl hystrine	*L. formosus*	29.7	27.81-31.73
Ammodendrine	*L. formosus*	134.38	128.34-140.71
N-Methyl ammodendrine	*L. formosus*	110.68	103.19-118.7

Adapted from Panter KE et al: In Garland T, Barr AC, editors: *Toxic plants and other natural toxicants*, New York, 1998, CAB International.
*Those alkaloids with a single unsaturation adjacent to the N (i.e., γ-coniceine, anabaseine, and *N*-acetyl hystrine) are most toxic.
†Using a mouse bioassay and intravenous injection of alkaloids.

mice, guinea pigs, and rats.[20] Coniine produces blockade of spinal reflexes, which has been attributed to the increased permeability of membranes to potassium ions. The pharmacologic properties of γ-coniceine and *N*-methyl coniine are similar to those of coniine except that γ-coniciene is more stimulatory to autonomic ganglia and *N*-methyl coniine has a greater blocking effect.[20] Similar structure activity relationships exist for the *N*-methyl and unsaturated derivatives of the *Lupinus* piperidine alkaloid ammodendrine and the *Nicotiana* piperidine alkaloid anabasine.[14] These piperidine alkaloids are neuromuscular blockers preventing normal fetal movement during critical stages of gestation, resulting in contractures and cleft palate.[21,22]

Toxicity and Risk Factors.   In comparing the toxicity of the three predominant alkaloids in *Conium*, γ-coniceine was found to be about seven times more toxic than coniine and about 13 times more toxic than *N*-methyl coniine.[14,19] A similar relationship occurs with three of the main active alkaloids—(anabasine, anabaseine, and *N*-methyl anabasine) from *N. glauca* and three of the main alkaloids (ammodendrine, *N*-acetyl hystrine, and *N*-methyl ammodendrine) from *Lupinus formosus* (see Table 25-7).[14]

Comparative toxicities of nine alkaloids with structural similarities from *Conium*, *Nicotiana*, and *Lupinus* are represented in Table 25-6. Toxicoses from *Conium* and *Nicotiana* in livestock are infrequent and risk is relatively low. Availability of good-quality forage generally determines the propensity of the livestock to graze these plants. Lupine, however, is frequently grazed as part of the diet and toxicosis generally only occurs when hungry animals are placed in dense lupine patches or when the quality grasses and forbs are depleted or mature. Lupine seedpods are high in protein and other nutrients and thus provide important nutrients during late season grazing.

Clinical Signs.   All animal species fed dosages of poison-hemlock high enough to induce obvious clinical signs developed muscular weakness, trembling, ataxia, slobbering, a rapid pulse, dilated pupils, frequent urination and defecation, and a characteristic musty mousy odor on the breath and in the urine (see Table 25-7). The initial stimulation is followed by an analgesic-like depression. Horses exhibit the most remarkable signs of ataxia and staggering. Pigs, goats, sheep, and cattle may experience a temporary partial loss of vision caused by the nictitating membranes of the eye covering the pupil, with pigs most severely affected. Birds (turkeys, quail, and geese) exhibit ataxia and an inability to fly.[23,24]

The greatest risk to livestock occurs in cattle because moderate lupine ingestion has been associated with large outbreaks of "crooked calf disease."[25] *Conium* and *Nicotiana* have also been shown to induce similar birth defects in livestock following experimental feeding trials. In the field, *Conium* has been implicated in crooked calf disease in cattle and *N. tabacum* in skeletal malformations and cleft palate in pigs.[8,13] The susceptible stages of gestation for maternal exposure to these plants and their alkaloids for cattle are 40 to 100 days for skeletal contractures and cleft palate or 40 to 50 days for cleft palate only; in pigs, 30 to 60 days for contractures and cleft palate and 30 to 40 days for cleft palate only; in sheep and goats, 30 to 60 days for skeletal defects and cleft palate and 35 to 41 days for cleft palate only (see Table 25-7).

Historically, poison-hemlock has been associated with human poisoning. Most recently, Frank and colleagues reported successful treatment of poison-hemlock poisoning in a 6-year-old boy and his father.[26] Whereas numerous poisonings are referenced in the literature, Daugherty reviewed one of the most famous, that being the execution of the philosopher Socrates in 399 BC using an extract (tea) of poison-hemlock.[27] Apparently, this same poison-hemlock–based tea was regularly used to execute criminals during Socrates' time.

Lesions. Few lesions are associated with poisoning of adult animals from piperidine alkaloids and are not diagnostic. Histologically, lesions are not pathognomonic. In human poisonings resulting in death, congestion of the lungs and liver was reported.[28] Histologically, rhabdomyolysis with coarse vacuolizations of myocyte, multifocal necrosis of myocytes. and macrophage infiltration were reported in three patients.[29]

These piperidine alkaloids are associated with birth defects, that is, contracture-type skeletal malformations and cleft palate. Pathologically, arthrogryposis, scoliosis, kyphosis, torticollis, and cleft palate in neonates of cattle, sheep, horses, goats, and pigs are suggestive of maternal exposure to plants containing these types of alkaloids. Whereas bone development is apparently normal, the skeletal malformations are contracture-type, associated with a lack of fetal movement in utero during critical stages of gestation.[21] Likewise, cleft palate is induced because of mechanical interference of palatal shelf closure by the tongue associated with piperidine-induced inhibition of fetal movement.[22]

Diagnostic Testing. In livestock, diagnosis is based on history of plant ingestion and clinical signs, supported by chemical analysis of blood (serum or plasma), stomach contents, liver, or kidney. Diagnosis of poisonous plant toxi-

TABLE 25-7 **Oral Toxicity of *Conium maculatum* and *Coniine***

Animal Species	Oral Dosage: Moderate to Severe Clinical Signs	Lethal Dose	Plant Type*,†	Teratogenic
Cattle	3.3-6.6 mg/kg	5 g/kg	Coniine	MCC
	0.9-1.9 g/kg		Fresh plant	MCC
Sheep	44 mg/kg	6 g/kg	Coniine	No
	5.4-5.8 g/kg		Fresh plant	MCC
Goats	3.1 g/kg	4.1 g/kg	Seed	CP, MCC
	7.8-10.8 g/kg		Fresh plant	CP, MCC
Swine	7 g/kg		Fresh plant, Illinois spring	No
	5.1 g/kg		Fresh plant, Illinois fall	CP, MCC
	0.5 g/kg		Illinois seed	CP, MCC
		11.43 g/kg	Utah spring growth	CP, MCC
	1 g/kg		Utah seed	CP, MCC
Horses	15.5 mg/kg		Coniine	
	4.6 g/kg		Fresh plant	No data

Data adapted from references 13, 23, 32-36.
*Toxicity of fresh plant varies depending on stage of plant growth, environment, locations, season of the year, soil, and moisture.
†Alkaloid content: *Fresh plant*: fall growth (Illinois): total alkaloid 0.014 % (98% γ-coniceine, 2% unidentified); spring growth (Illinois): total alkaloid 0.029% (19.8% γ-coniceine, 0% coniine, 80.2% unidentified); spring growth (Utah): total alkaloid 0.023% (98% γ-coniceine, 2% unidentified), *Seed*: Illinois: total alkaloid 0.92% (51% coniine, 49% γ-coniceine); Utah: total alkaloid 0.217% (50% γ-coniceine, 50% unidentified).
CP, Cleft palate; *MCC*, skeletal deformities.

coses from these plants generally relies on clinical history, identifying the plant availability, proof of plant ingestion, clinical signs observed, confirmatory plant fragment identification in the rumen or toxin identification in the stomach contents, blood, urine, liver, or kidney. Development of methods for detection of toxins in tissues is advancing.[30,31]

Treatment.   No specific treatment for poisoning exists. In human poisoning cases, gastric lavage, respiratory support, and symptomatic treatment with careful monitoring of vital signs resulted in full recovery.[26] In animals, potential treatment includes gastric lavage, activated charcoal, and support of respiration. However, in livestock, the added excitement and stress related to restraint and treatment may exacerbate the toxic effects and result in death. Recommendations include careful monitoring of animals and assisted respiration if necessary, while avoiding overexcitement and stress to the animal.

Prognosis.   If acute poisoning does not progress to respiratory failure and death, the prognosis for full recovery is good.

Prevention and Control.   Many of these plants can be controlled with broadleaf herbicide treatment. Good control of lupines can be accomplished with 2,4-D and glyphosate and excellent control with Dicamba and Picloram.[37,38] No specific treatments are recommended for the tobaccos, but it is presumed that broadleaf herbicides similar to those already mentioned would give good control. In most cases, grazing of these plants is avoided by livestock if good-quality forage or feed is available. However, lupine pods are high in protein and often an accepted feed for cattle and sheep, especially once grasses and other quality forbs have matured and dried. Once conditioned to eat plants such as poison-hemlock, certain livestock and wildlife species return to the same areas where poisoning occurred and seek out more plants. This behavior has been reported in pigs, elk, and wild geese.[24,32,38]

REFERENCES

1. Leete E: Biosynthesis of hemlock and related piperidine alkaloids, *Acc Chem Res* 4(3):100, 1971.
2. Leete E, Olson JO: Biosynthesis and metabolism of the hemlock alkaloids, *J Am Chem Soc* 94(15):5472, 1972.
3. Kingsbury JM: *Poisonous Plants of the United States and Canada,* Englewood Cliffs, NJ, 1964, Prentice-Hall.
4. Schneider MJ: In Pelletier SW, editor: *Alkaloids: chemical and biological perspectives,* vol 10, New York, 1996, Elsevier.
5. Anonymous: Unusual case of hemlock poisoning in swine, *The California Veterinarian* 2:26, 1951.
6. Kubik IM et al: Outbreak of hemlock poisoning in cattle, *Veterinarstvi* 30:157, 1980.
7. Galey FD et al: Toxicosis in dairy cattle exposed to poison hemlock (*Conium maculatum*) in hay: isolation of *Conium* alkaloids in plants, hay, and urine, *J Vet Diagn Invest* 4:60, 1992.
8. Crowe MW: Skeletal anomalies in pigs associated with tobacco, *Mod Vet Pract* 69:54, 1969.
9. Menges RW et al: A tobacco related epidemic of congenital limb deformities in swine, *Environ Res* 3:285, 1970.
10. Crowe MW, Swerczek TW: Congenital arthrogryposis in offspring of sows fed tobacco (*Nicotiana tabacum*), *Am J Vet Res* 35:1071, 1974.
11. Keeler RF et al: Teratogenic effects of *Nicotiana glauca* and concentration of anabasine, the suspect teratogen in plant parts, *Cornell Vet* 71:47, 1981.
12. Plumlee KH et al: *Nicotiana glauca* toxicosis of cattle, *J Vet Diagn Invest* 5:498, 1993.
13. Keeler RF, Balls LD: Teratogenic effects in cattle of *Conium maculatum* and *Conium* alkaloids and analogs, *Clin Toxicol* 12:49, 1978.
14. Panter KE et al: In Garland T, Barr AC, editors: *Toxic plants and other natural toxicants,* New York, 1998, CAB International.
15. Cronquist A et al: *Intermountain flora, vascular plants of the intermountain west, USA,* vol 3B, New York, 1989, New York Botanical Garden.
16. Wink M et al: Patterns of quinolizidine alkaloids in 56 species of the genus *Lupinus. Phytochemistry* 38:139, 1995.
17. Riggins R, Sholars R: In Hickman JC, editor: *The Jepson manual, higher plants of California,* Berkley, Calif, 1993, University of California Press.
18. Gardner DR, Panter KE: Ammodendrine and related piperidine alkaloid levels in the blood plasma of cattle, sheep and goats fed *Lupinus formosus, J Nat Toxins* 3(2):107, 1994.
19. Bowman WC, Sanghvi IS: Pharmacological actions of hemlock (*Conium maculatum*) alkaloids, *J Pharm Pharmacol* 15:1, 1963.
20. Fodor GB, Colasanti B: In Pelletier SW: *Alkaloids: chemical and biological perspectives,* vol 3, New York, 1985, John Wiley and Sons.
21. Panter KE et al: Multiple congenital contractures (MCC) and cleft palate induced in goats by ingestion of piperidine alkaloid-containing plants: reduction in fetal movement as the probable cause, *Clin Toxicol* 28:69, 1990.
22. Panter KE, Keeler RF: Induction of cleft palate in goats by *Nicotiana glauca* during a narrow gestational period and the relation to reduction in fetal movement, *J Nat Toxins* 1:25, 1992.
23. Frank AA, Reed WM: Comparative toxicity of coniine, an alkaloid of *Conium maculatum* (poison hemlock), in chickens, quails, and turkeys, *Avian Dis* 34(2):433, 1990.
24. Converse K: National Wildlife, Madison, Wis: Personal communication, 1989.
25. Panter KE et al: Observations of *Lupinus sulphureus*-induced "crooked calf disease," *J Range Manage* 50:587, 1997.
26. Frank BS et al: Ingestion of poison hemlock (*Conium maculatum*), *West J Med* 163:573, 1995.
27. Daugherty CG: The death of Socrates and the toxicology of hemlock, *J Med Biography* 3:178, 1995.
28. Drummer OH et al: Three deaths from hemlock poisoning, *Med J Aust* 162:592, 1995.
29. Rizzi D et al: Rhabdomyolysis and acute tubular necrosis in coniine (hemlock) poisoning, *Lancet* 2:1461, 1990.
30. Holstege DM et al: Rapid multiresidue screen for alkaloids in plant material and biological samples, *J Agric Food Chem* 43:691, 1995.
31. Lee ST et al: Development of enzyme-linked immunosorbent assays for toxic larkspur (*Delphinium* spp.) alkaloids, *J Agric Food Chem* 48:4520, 2000.
32. Keeler RF et al: Teratogenicity and toxicity of coniine in cows, ewes and mares, *Cornell Vet* 70:19, 1980.
33. Panter KE: *Toxicity and teratogenicity of Conium maculatum in swine and hamsters,* Doctoral thesis, University of Illinois, 1983.
34. Panter KE et al: Induction of cleft palate in newborn pigs by maternal ingestion of poison hemlock (*Conium maculatum*), *Am J Vet Res* 46:1368, 1985.
35. Panter KE et al: Congenital skeletal malformations induced by maternal ingestion of *Conium maculatum* (poison hemlock) in newborn pigs, *Am J Vet Res* 46:2064, 1985.
36. Panter KE et al: Maternal and fetal toxicity of poison-hemlock (*Conium maculatum*) in sheep, *Am J Vet Res* 49:281, 1988.
37. Klingman DL et al: Systemic herbicides for weed control, *Bull AD-BU-2281,* University of Minnesota Extension Service, 1983.

38. Ralphs MH et al: Herbicide control of poisonous plants, *Rangelands* 13:73, 1991.

39. Jessup DA et al: Toxicosis in tule elk caused by ingestion of poison hemlock, *J Am Vet Med Assoc* 189:1173, 1986.

PYRIDINE ALKALOIDS

Kip E. Panter

Synonyms. Common names for *Nicotiana* include burley tobacco *(N. tabacum)*, wild tree tobacco *(N. glauca)*, wild tobacco *(N. trigonophylla)*, and coyote tobacco *(N. attenuata)* (Color Plates 14 and 15). Common names for *Lobelia* include Indian tobacco, eye-bright, asthma-weed, bladderpod *(L. inflata)*, wild tobacco *(L. nicotianaefolia)*, cardinal flower *(L. cardinalis)*, blue cardinal flower, great blue lobelia *(L. siphilitica)*, lobelia *(L. berlandieri)*, and water lobelia *(L. dortmanna)*, among others.

Sources. Pyridine alkaloids are heterocyclic nitrogenous compounds with a basic structural core (C_5H_5N). Pyridine alkaloids are widespread in the plant kingdom and found in many plant genera, including *Nicotiana* and *Lobelia*.[1] Australia has 19 native species of *Nicotiana* and 19 species of *Lobelia*.[2] Worldwide, more than 100 species of *Nicotiana* and 200 to 300 species of *Lobelia* exist.[2,3]

The *Nicotiana* spp. responsible for poisoning in the western United States include *N. glauca* (tree tobacco), *N. trigonophylla* (wild tobacco), *N. tabacum* (cultivated tobacco, burley tobacco), and *N. attenuata* (coyote tobacco, wild tobacco). *N. glauca* grows in the southern United States, Mexico, Argentina, and Hawaii in waste places at or below 1000 meters. *N. trigonophylla* grows in arid and semiarid habitats in southern Nevada, Utah, Colorado to California, western Texas, Mexico, and Central America. *N. tabacum* is cultivated in the eastern and southeastern United States. *N. attenuata* grows in dry sandy or gravelly soils along stream beds from Wyoming to Washington State, south to California and Mexico. In South Africa and California, *N. glauca* has caused poisoning and in Australia several of the 19 native species as well as *N. tabacum* have been implicated in livestock poisoning episodes.[2,4,5]

Lobelias are widely distributed in the eastern United States and Canada with distribution of some species into the southern and midwestern states. Growth habitat is diverse but includes meadows, pastures, and cultivated fields and waste areas where adequate moisture can support growth. Some *Lobelia* species require high moisture habitats and grow in shallow water along streams, lakes, and ponds. Although *L. purpurascens* has been suspected of poisoning livestock in Australia and is reported to contain alkaloids, definitive evidence for poisoning is lacking.[2]

Mechanism of Action. Of the 20 or so alkaloids studied from tobacco, nicotine is the most prevalent and often exhibits the most potent effects on certain organ systems. Nornicotine is the second most prominent alkaloid in burley tobacco and is two to three times more toxic than nicotine in several animal species including rat and rabbit models. The main alkaloids in *Lobelia* are lobeline, lobelanidine, and the di-ketone, lobelanine. Lobeline has pharmacologic activity similar to that of nicotine but that is less intense. The other *Lobelia* alkaloids, including lobelanine, lobelanidine, and lobelidine, exert similar but weaker effects.

Both lobeline and nicotine are classified as ganglionic stimulants. Nicotine mimics acetylcholine at sympathetic and parasympathetic ganglia, at neuromuscular junctions of skeletal muscle, and at some synapses in the central nervous system (CNS).[6] Nicotine-induced initial stimulation of all autonomic ganglia is usually followed by a persistent ganglionic and neuromuscular blockade.

The pharmacologic effects of nicotine and other tobacco alkaloids are complex, unpredictable, and variable depending on the organ system affected.[6] These alkaloids induce multiple pharmacologic effects via initial stimulation of ganglionic nicotinic receptors with subsequent ganglionic blockade. Nicotinic ganglionic blockade occurs as a two-phase process.[6]

Low doses cause depolarization and stimulation of receptors similar to acetylcholine. Higher doses cause stimulation followed by blockage at autonomic ganglia and myoneural junctions of skeletal muscle. Death is a result of respiratory failure from neuromuscular blockade.

Both nicotine and lobeline increase cardiac output as well as systolic and diastolic blood pressure through positive inotropic and chronotropic effects on the myocardium. Stimulation of sympathetic ganglion and the adrenal medulla leads to a release of catecholamines affecting the cardiovascular system. In the adrenal medulla, nicotine causes an initial surge of catecholamines, but subsequently the normal release of catecholamines in response to nerve stimulation is blocked.

Effects on the CNS result in tremors and, at larger doses, convulsions. The effects of nicotine on the chemoreceptor zone and emetic center cause nausea and vomiting. Gastrointestinal effects result from parasympathetic stimulation leading to increased tone and motor activity.

Toxicity and Risk Factors. Toxicoses in livestock are rare, but have occurred from ingestion of domesticated tobaccos and wild tobaccos.[5,7] *Lobelia* species, especially *L. inflata* and *L. berlandieri*, have been implicated in livestock poisoning, but incidents are rare.[8,9] Relative risk of poisoning is low if good quality forages are available and animals are not forced to graze undesirable plants because of overgrazing, introduction of hungry animals into concentrated patches, and the like.[9,10] Poisoning caused by cultivated tobacco *(N. tabacum)* has occurred when horses were kept in tobacco barns and when livestock have accidentally entered fields of cultivated tobacco. Pregnant sows were poisoned eating tobacco stalks.[7]

Although more than 40 pyridine alkaloids have been found in tobacco as a result of the intensive chemical studies on this plant, nicotine is by far the predominant alkaloid and accounts for greater than 93% of the total alkaloid content.[11] Feeding experiments with *N. glauca* showed it to be toxic to sheep at about 1% of body weight. Pharmacologic studies performed with nornicotine, a minor *N. tabacum* alkaloid, have shown similar effects and roughly the same potency as nicotine in a number of animal systems but two to three times the toxicity in rabbits and mice.

The entire *Lobelia* plant is toxic, with roots and seeds considered most toxic. Alkaloid content varies from 0.13% to 0.63%, with highest levels reported just before and after flowering. Flower stalks are reported to contain 0.9% to 1.1% lobeline.

Clinical Signs.   The pattern of clinical signs from nicotine toxicity includes excitement, fine motor tremors, elevated respiration, ataxia, weakness, prostration, coma, paralysis, and death caused by respiratory paralysis. Cattle, horses, and sheep fed *N. trigonophylla*, *N. attenuata*, and *N. tabacum* exhibited a variety of nervous symptoms including tremors, ataxia, staggering, weakness, and prostration.[8] Onset of clinical effects is rapid (15 to 45 minutes after exposure) and progression of the syndrome occurs in minutes to a few hours depending on dosage.[7,12] Duration of signs may be 1 to 2 hours in mild cases, extending to 24 hours or more following severe intoxication.

Early signs are excitation, tachypnea, salivation, lacrimation, emesis, and diarrhea followed by muscle weakness, twitching, depression, tachycardia, shallow and slow respiration, collapse, coma, cyanosis, cardiac and respiratory arrest, and death. Rapid but weak pulse accompanies erratic heart action; abdominal pain accompanied by diarrhea and vomition are often observed, as is difficulty in breathing. Death may occur within minutes or up to several days after ingestion and seems to be caused by respiratory failure or suffocation from inhaled vomitus.[8]

Symptoms reported from field poisoning of cattle by other *Nicotiana* species in Australia include ataxia, unwillingness to move, uncoordinated gait, and arching of the back. The animals often become recumbent, first sternally, then laterally as the severity increases, and they often kick violently with all four limbs while lying on their sides.[2] Sheep exhibit similar clinical signs of toxicosis.

Clinical signs of *L. berlandieri* toxicosis in cattle include profuse salivation, dilation of pupils, and collapse. *L. berlandieri* poisoning in cattle and sheep caused sluggishness, excessive salivation, diarrhea, anorexia, ulceration around the mouth, nasal discharge, coma, widely distributed hemorrhage, and mild gastroenteritis.[8]

Lesions.   Lesions of *Nicotiana* poisoning are nonspecific. Necropsy reveals congestion and hemorrhage in the abomasum, small and large intestine, and sometimes in the gall bladder. Congestion in the kidneys and lining of the eye socket is also frequently observed.[2] Widely distributed hemorrhage with subcutaneous hemorrhage, subdural edema, and cerebral congestion was reported in cases of *L. berlandieri* poisoning in cattle.[9]

Diagnostic Testing.   Diagnosis is made based on history of exposure, signs, and relative absence of lesions. Poisoning may be confirmed by chemically identifying nicotine or other nicotine-like alkaloids in urine, blood, liver, kidney, or gastrointestinal contents.[13]

Treatment.   Administration of an emetic or enterogastric lavage may be helpful in appropriate species. Most cases involve livestock, and decontamination is limited to administration of activated charcoal to slow or prevent further absorption. Atropine may be used if parasympathetic effects are present but the dosage should be titrated to the response. Artificial respiration and fluid therapy may be administered for support until recovery is complete. However, handling and stress of treatment may exacerbate toxic effects in livestock.

Prognosis.   When sublethal doses are ingested, recovery is often complete without intervention. When larger doses are ingested, prognosis is poor.

Prevention and Control.   Prevention of poisoning is accomplished by providing adequate quality forage or feed, managing livestock to prevent high numbers in areas where poisonous plants occur, and prevention of accidental exposure. Specific control recommendations for *Nicotiana* spp. are not available but it is presumed that broadleaf herbicides would be effective. Recommended herbicides for *Lobelia* include 2,4-D and Dicamba.[14] Swine should not be fed tobacco waste or discarded stocks.

REFERENCES

1. Marion L: In Manske RHF, Holmes HL: *The alkaloids: chemistry and physiology,* New York, 1950, Academic Press.
2. Everest SL: *Poisonous plants of Australia,* Melbourne, Australia, 1981, Angus and Robertson.
3. Judd WS et al: *Plant systematics: a phylogenetic approach,* Sunderland, Mass, 1999, Sinauer Associates.
4. Kellerman TS et al: *Plant poisonings and mycotoxicoses of livestock in Southern Africa,* Cape Town, 1988, Oxford University Press.
5. Plumlee KH et al: *Nicotiana glauca* toxicosis of cattle, *J Vet Diagn Invest* 5:498, 1993.
6. Fodor GB, Colasanti B: In Pelletier SW, editor: *Alkaloids: chemical and biological perspectives,* vol. 3, New York, 1985, John Wiley and Sons.
7. Crowe MW: Skeletal anomalies in pigs associated with tobacco, *Mod Vet Pract* 69:54, 1969.
8. Kingsbury JM: *Poisonous plants of the United States and Canada,* Englewood Cliffs, N.J., 1964, Prentice-Hall.
9. Bailey EM: In Howard JL, editor: *Principle oisonous plants of the Southwestern USA.* Philadelphia, 1986, WB Saunders.
10. Dollahite JW, Allen TJ: Poisoning of cattle, sheep, and goats with *Lobelia* and *Centaurium* species, *Southwest Vet* 15:126, 1962.
11. Leete E: In Pelletier SW, editor: *Alkaloids, chemical and biological perspectives,* vol. 1, New York, 1983, Wiley-Interscience.
12. Panter KE et al: Multiple congenital contractures (MCC) and cleft palate induced in goats by ingestion of piperidine alkaloid-containing plants: reduction in fetal movement as the probable cause, *Clin Toxicol* 28:69, 1990.
13. Holstege DM et al: Rapid multiresidue screen for alkaloids in plant material and biological samples, *J Agric Food Chem* 43:691, 1995.
14. Klingman DL et al: Systemic herbicides for weed control, *Bull AD-BU-2281,* University of Minnesota Extension Service, 1983.

PYRROLIZIDINE ALKALOIDS

Bryan Stegelmeier

Synonyms.   Seneciosis, hepatic cirrhosis, and venoocclusive disease are common names for the disease caused by pyrrolizidine alkaloids (PA)s.

Sources. More than 350 PAs have been identified in more than 6000 plants in the Boraginaceae, Compositae, and Leguminosae families. About half of the identified PAs are toxic and several are carcinogenic. PA-containing plants are found throughout the world and they are the most common poisonous plants affecting livestock, wildlife, and humans. Plants that commonly cause poisonings are listed in Table 25-8.

Compositae family. Of more than 3000 *Senecio* species, more than 30 have been established as causing livestock and human poisonings. Diseases known as "stomach staggers," "walking disease," "Pictou disease," "Winton disease," "Molteno," "dunziekte," "sirasyke," and several other unnamed diseases have proven to be *Senecio* intoxication.[1,2] The following short descriptions are of the *Senecio* species that most commonly poison livestock. Many other plant species have been suspected of poisoning, but their toxicity has not been confirmed.

Senecio jacobaea, or tansy ragwort, is a common western European weed (Color Plate 16) that was inadvertently introduced into eastern Europe, South Africa, Australia, New Zealand, and North America.[3-5] As with most PA-containing plants, tansy is unpalatable and generally not eaten by livestock. Poisoning occurs when plants or seeds contaminate feeds, when grazing animals cannot easily differentiate the early rosette from grasses and clovers, or when no other forages are available. *S. jacobaea* contains six toxic alkaloids.[6-8] The chronic lethal dose in cattle is approximately 2.5 mg total PA/kg body weight for 18 days. Because the average PA concentration found in tansy ragwort is about 0.2% of the plant dry weight, a 300-kg cow would need to eat approximately 0.4 kg of dry plant or nearly 1.7 kg of fresh plant per day for several weeks to obtain a lethal dose. Such PA concentrations have been found contaminating feeds. Higher doses cause acute hepatocellular necrosis and liver failure, but these poisonings are rare because such doses are

TABLE 25-8 Compositae, Leguminosae, and Boraginaceae Plants that Have Been Associated with Pyrrolizidine Alkaloid Poisoning

Family	Animal	Family	Animal
Compositae		*S. vernalis*	Goats
		S. vulgaris	Horses, rodents
Senecio abyssinicus	Rats		
S. alpinus	Cattle	**Leguminosae**	
S. bipinnatisectus	Calves		
S. brasiliensis	Cattle	*Crotalaria anagyroides*	Cattle
S. burchelli	Cattle	*C. assamica*	Mice
S. cisplatinus	Livestock	*C. equorum*	Horses
S. desfontainei	Poultry	*C. goreensis*	Chickens
S. douglasii var. *longilobus*	Cattle, rodents	*C. incana*	Humans
S. errraticus	Cattle, horses, sheep	*C. juncea*	Cattle, horses, pigs
S. glabellus	Livestock, rats	*C. laburnoides*	Humans
S. heterotrichius	Cattle	*C. mucronata*	Sheep, cattle
S. integerrimus	Livestock	*C. nana*	Humans, rats
S. jacobaea	Livestock, rodents, poultry	*C. retusa*	Poultry, pigs
S. latifolius	Cattle	*C. sagittalis*	Horses
S. lobatus	Cattle	*C. saltiana*	Goats, mice, calves
S. lautus	Cattle	*C. spectabilis*	Livestock, rodents, poultry
S. leptolobus	Cattle	*C. verrucosa*	Humans
S. madagascariensis	Horses		
S. montevidensis	Cattle	**Boraginaceae**	
S. oxyphyllus	Cattle		
S. pampeanus	Cattle	*Amsinckia intermedia*	Livestock, rodents
S. plattensis	Horses	*Cynoglossum officinale*	Cattle, horses
S. quadridentatus	Cattle	*Echium plantagineum*	Livestock, rodents
S. raphanifolius	Yaks	*Heliotropium amplexicale*	Cattle
S. retrorsus	Wildlife	*H. dasycarpum*	Sheep
S. riddellii	Livestock	*H. europaeum*	Livestock, poultry, rodents
S. sanguisorbae	Sheep	*H. lasocarpium*	Humans
S. selloi	Cattle	*H. ovalifolium*	Sheep, goats
S. spartioides	Livestock	*H. scottae*	Mice
S. spathulatus	Cattle	*H. supinum*	Rats
S. subalpinus	Cattle	*Symphytum officinale*	Humans, rodents
S. tweediei	Cattle	*S. peregrinum*	Poultry
		Trichodesma ehrenbergii	Poultry

Data from references 1, 4, 5, 12, 13, 16, 18, 19, 20, 22, 23, 27, 28, 30, 31, 33, 34, 48, 52, 55, and 67-127.

unpalatable.[6] Several recent reviews of livestock and human poisonings have been written.[9-11]

S. riddellii, or Riddell's groundsel, is found in Nebraska, New Mexico, Texas, Colorado, and Wyoming.[12,13] *S. riddellii* differs from other *Senecio* species in that it contains a single major alkaloid, riddelliine.[12] Alkaloid concentrations in plants vary greatly, with measured concentrations ranging between 0.2% and 18.0% (dry weight).[2] *S. riddellii* is toxic to cattle at doses of 15 mg PA/kg body weight for 20 days.[12] At 18% PA of the dry matter, 33 g dry or 176 g fresh *S. riddellii* per day would be toxic for a 300-kg cow. Although riddelliine is less toxic than PAs from other *Senecio* species, the plant can contain more toxin, making the whole plant highly toxic. Recent experimental studies have also shown riddelliine to be carcinogenic to rodents.[14]

Senecio douglasii var. *longilobus* (threadleaf or woolly groundsel) is a perennial, branched, woody shrub that is often found on abused or degraded arid rangelands. Found in several southwestern states,[15] it contains four alkaloids with concentrations that vary from 0.63% to 2.02% of the plant dry weight.[16] Doses of 10 to 13 mg PA/kg body weight for 15 days are lethal for cattle.[16] At PA concentrations of 2%, doses of about 150 g dry plant or 750 g green plant per day for 15 days would poison a 300-kg cow. That is about one third the toxicity of *S. riddellii*.

Senecio vulgaris, or common groundsel, is an erect annual or biennial. It has been used for several medicinal purposes including a remedy for intestinal parasites, disordered liver function, and irregular menstruation, as a laxative, and as an ingredient of a soothing lotion.[17] Livestock poisonings have been sporadic, and feeds contaminated with *S. vulgaris* have poisoned horses.[18,19]

Leguminosae family. *Crotalaria* species, introduced as soil-enriching cover crops, are often found along fence rows and ditch banks where they may spread and contaminate fields. Most have long, kidney-shaped seeds that rattle in mature dry pods, resulting in the common name "rattle pod." Their seeds are often harvested with grains, thus contaminating feed and food. *C. sagittalis* has induced Missouri "Bottom disease," causing animals to become slow, emaciated, weak, and stuporous with hepatic degeneration. Most animals died within a few weeks.[21] Horses, which are highly susceptible, have often been poisoned in *C. sagittalis*–infested stubble fields.[20] *Crotalaria* seeds contaminating grain have poisoned both livestock and poultry.[21]

Boraginaceae family. *Cynoglossum officinale*, or hound's tongue, an annual or biennial European plant, is a noxious weed found in many Western pastures, rangelands, and fields (Color Plate 17). Generally unpalatable to livestock, cattle and horses are poisoned when they are fed contaminated feed.[22-24] Hound's tongue contains four PAs, with heliosupine being the most abundant and toxic.[25] PA concentrations are highest in immature plants and range from 0.5% to 2.2%. Approximately 10 to 15 mg PA/kg body weight for 14 days was lethal for cattle and horses. A lethal dose for a 300-kg cow would be 136 g dry plant or 680 g green plant per day for 14 days.[24,26]

Both *Echium* and *Heliotropium* species intermittently poison Australian livestock.[27,28] *E. plantagineum*, commonly called Patterson's curse or Salvation Jane, is a noxious weed that can replace nutritious forages and poison livestock. Sheep are relatively resistant, but horses and other livestock are susceptible.[29,30]

Heliotropium poisoning, especially *H. europaeum* poisoning, has also been reported in Australian pigs, cattle, and sheep.[31-33] Although *Heliotropium* spp. are found in the southern United States, poisoning is rarely reported. A Mediterranean annual that is commonly called *heliotrope*, it can invade fields and contaminate feeds and food. Transfer of PAs to honey and wildlife intoxications have renewed interest in *Echium* and *Heliotropium* toxicity.

Amsinckia intermedia, commonly called tarweed or fiddleneck, is an annual weed that grows in waste areas and fields (Color Plate 18). *Amsinckia is* not highly toxic, but it has been reported to cause "walking disease" in horses and "hard liver disease" in cattle and swine.[20,34-36]

Symphytum officinale, or comfrey, has been used as both forage and a medicinal herb. It contains several PAs, which cause disease in both experimental animals and humans.[37,38] Low doses of comfrey have been shown to produce hepatic neoplasms in rodents.[39] Several countries have restricted its sale and most herbal companies no longer market comfrey-containing products. Nonetheless, comfrey continues to be used in herbal preparations on an individual basis.

Several other plants, including members of the *Borago* and *Trichodesma* genera, also contain small amounts of PAs (see Table 25-8). Although some are used as medicinal plants and herbs, there is little information concerning the effects of low-dose PA exposure associated with these plants.

Toxicokinetics. PAs are not directly toxic, but require bioactivation to the toxic dehydropyrrolizidine alkaloids ("pyrroles") (Step 1, Fig. 25-1). This bioactivation occurs primarily in the liver by the action of several different mixed function oxidases.[1] Metabolism includes mechanisms to both activate and detoxify PAs. The nontoxic metabolites are quickly excreted and the toxic species either damage the liver or are transported to other tissues.

Mechanism of Action. With appropriate leaving groups on carbons 7 and 9, pyrroles are potent electrophiles. Some pyrroles are bifunctional electrophiles possessing carbon-centered electrophiles at the 7 and 9 positions. These can cross-link DNA, proteins, amino acids, and glutathione.[40] Cellular defense mechanisms including soluble nucleophiles, such as glutathione, may react with pyrroles, allowing rapid excretion.[41] Other pyrroles may polymerize, becoming harmlessly sequestered, or excreted (Step 6). However, many react with cellular nucleophilic compounds including proteins and nucleic acids (Step 7). Depending on the extent, as well as the importance or location of the damage, these adducts are responsible for the cytotoxic and antimitotic effects of poisoning.

Some pyrrole-tissue adducts may persist for months or years, and little is known about their ultimate fate. The progressive nature of PA-induced hepatotoxicity suggests pyrrolic adducts are recycled, reacting with new nucleophiles and inciting further cellular damage (Step 8). PAs or their pyrrole metabolites may also be hydrolyzed, producing alcoholic dehydronecines (Step 2). These may be de-

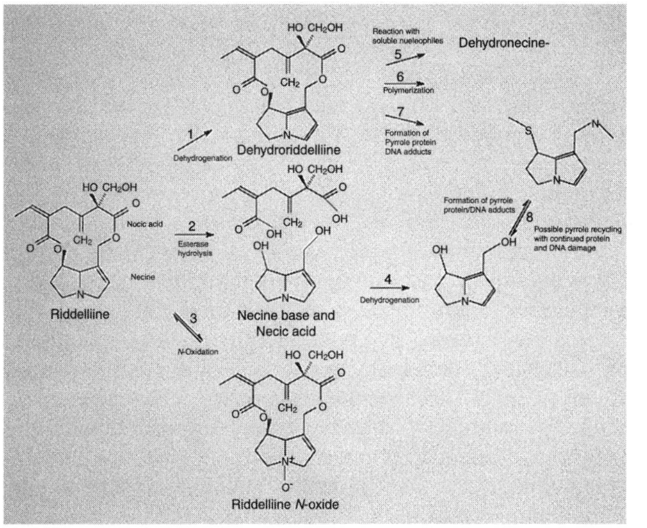

Fig. 25-1. Structure and metabolism of pyrrolizidine alkaloids (riddelliine is shown as an example). Pyrrolizidine alkaloids (PAs) are composed of a necine base that is esterified to one or several necic acids. It may be metabolized by several liver mixed function oxidases, producing both toxic and nontoxic metabolites. Dehydrogenation *(Step 1)* produces toxic dehydronecine. This may react with soluble nucleophiles, such as glutathionine, to be excreted *(Step 5)*; it may polymerize *(Step 6)*; or it may alkylate other cellular nucleophiles including proteins and nucleic acids *(Step 7)*. These dehydronecine or pyrrolic adducts may remain in tissue long after exposure and little is known of their ultimate metabolism. It is speculated that pyrroles may be recycled *(Step 8)*. Although not proven, recycled pyrroles released as proteins and nucleic acids are catabolized, and could react with other cellular nucleophiles resulting in continued cellular damage. This is supported by the progressive nature of chronic PA intoxication, in that hepatic damage continues long after PA exposure is discontinued. PAs may also be hydrolyzed *(Step 2)*, producing free necine base and necic acids. Although less toxic than many PAs, necines may also be reduced to produce dehydronecine *(Step 4)*. The third metabolic path involves oxidation of the necine nitrogen, producing the N-oxide *(Step 3)*. These are more soluble and are easily excreted. However, after excretion or in other tissues, N-oxides may be reduced and reabsorbed.

hydrogenated (Step 4), but the resulting pyrrolic metabolites are less reactive, less toxic, more water soluble, and more easily excreted than the dehydro-PAs. Pyrrolizidine alkaloids and activated pyrroles may be further oxidized to form N-oxides (Step 3). These are excreted, but may be reduced to the basic alkaloid in some tissues or in the intestinal tract to be reabsorbed and metabolized again.[1] Plant PA alkaloids are composed of both the free base and N-oxides, and both should be analyzed and included when determining plant toxicity.[1]

Toxicity and Risk Factors. Despite similar structures, acute PA toxicity is highly variable. Toxicity and the tissue damage are pyrrole specific.[42] Reactive metabolites of seneciphylline and retrorsine are primarily hepatotoxic. Less reactive PAs, such as trichodesmine and monocrotaline, form more stable pyrrole intermediates, resulting in fewer hepatic changes with extensive extrahepatic lesions.[43] Hepatotoxic

PAs, such as retrorsine, develop high liver pyrrole concentrations that peak about 2 hours after a single PA dose. Hepatic pyrrole concentrations decrease slowly over the next 24 hours, but residues can be detected days later. Nonhepatotoxic PAs such as rosmarinine have lower hepatic pyrrole production and are removed from the liver much more rapidly.[1]

Susceptibility to poisoning is influenced by species, age, sex, and temporary factors such as biochemical, physiologic, and nutritional status. Different animal species have vastly different susceptibilities to PAs. For example, the toxic doses of some plants were 20 times higher for sheep than those that killed cattle. For this reason, sheep and goats have been used to graze pastures that are dangerous to horses and cattle.[44] Horses appear to be about as sensitive to PA toxicity as cattle, but pigs are reported to be the most sensitive animal species. The reported toxicity indexes are pigs = 1; chickens = 5; cattle and horses = 14; rats = 50; mice = 150; sheep and goats = 200.[44]

Rumen transfaunation studies, in vitro rumen culture studies, and infusion studies (injecting purified PAs into portal and systemic circulation) all suggest that at least a portion of species susceptibility to PA toxicity is due to rumen metabolism.[45-47] Additional work suggests species susceptibility is more closely related to liver metabolism. Different species have different rates of both pyrrole activation and detoxification.[48,49] Varying amounts and rates of urinary excretion of N-oxide metabolites have also been detected in different species.[50] It is likely that species susceptibility is a complex interaction involving alkaloid and animal specific differences in both preabsorption and postabsorption metabolism. For example, guinea pigs are highly resistant to the toxicity of most PAs, but they are very susceptible to jacobine. Chung and Buhler[51] found that this specific toxicity is likely due to the guinea pig's ability to quickly produce jacobine pyrroles and conversely their relatively slow hydrolysis of jacobine esters and slow oxidation to form the jacobine N-oxide. The ultimate inference is that toxicity information from one species is of little use to predict toxicity in other species.

Age and gender play a large role in determining an animal's response to PAs. Young animals are generally more susceptible to poisoning than are aged adults.[52] Neonatal and nursing animals and humans have been reported to develop fatal hepatic disease while their lactating mothers were unaffected.[53-56] Gender differences are seen, in that PA toxicity in male rats is much higher than that seen in females.[57] These differences have been linked to metabolic rates.[52] It has been postulated that toxicity is linked to both the ability of the liver to synthesize pyrroles as well as the hepatocyte proliferation rates, or growth and metabolic rates.

The physiologic state of the animal also contributes to toxicity. Nutritional status is important especially relating to nutrients that rely heavily on hepatic metabolism, such as copper and molybdenum.[33,58] As a result, animals that have marginal nutrition are more likely to develop disease. For example, PA-poisoned sheep are more likely to develop copper toxicosis than normal animals.[58] As mentioned previously, pyrrolic esters may react with nucleophilic scavengers such as glutathione with consequent excretion of the glutathione adduct. Therefore, animals with increased hepatic glutathione might be expected to be more resistant to PA toxicosis.[41,59-60] Hepatic bioactivation of PAs can be promoted or inhibited by treatments that upregulate, enhance, or otherwise alter hepatic microsomal activity (e.g., phenobarbital, chloramphenicol).[59,61]

Plant and plant-animal interactions also contribute to toxicity. Palatability, which reflects the amount and rate that animals eat, varies with season, location, weather, and availability of other forages. PA concentration in plants varies with the environment, plant phenotype, and site. Usually plants are most toxic in the early bud stage when beginning to flower. Nonetheless, there are large variations in PA concentrations from year to year and from site to site.[62] This makes it difficult to predict when a particular group of plants will contain toxic PA concentrations.[1]

Clinical Signs.   Animals with acute toxicosis show signs of acute liver failure, including anorexia, depression, icterus, visceral edema, and ascites.

Animals with chronic toxicosis show clinical signs such as photosensitivity, icterus, or increased susceptibility to other hepatic diseases such as lipidosis or ketosis. Animals may show no clinical signs for several months or even years after PA ingestion. With loss of hepatic function, poisoned animals often do poorly. When such hepatic cripples are subjected to normal stresses such as pregnancy or lactation, they develop clinical liver failure.

Clinical Pathology.   Serum biochemical changes associated with acute intoxication include massive elevations in aspartate aminotransferase (AST), sorbitol dehydrogenase (SDH), alkaline phosphatase (ALP), and gamma-glutamyltransferase (GGT) activities with increased amounts of bilirubin and bile acids. However, with chronic poisoning, serum biochemistries may be normal for several months or even years after PA ingestion. Animals develop only transient elevations in serum enzymes (AST, SDH, ALK, and GGT). They may have mild elevations in serum bilirubin and bile acids.

Lesions.   Cellular indications of PA intoxication are first seen as hepatocyte swelling that is dose dependent. With continuing damage, cellular degeneration continues with ultimate loss of cellular homeostasis and necrosis or cell death. The lesions of PA toxicosis are dose dependent and have been histologically characterized as acute and chronic changes. High PA doses ingested quickly cause acute intoxication with pan-lobular hepatocellular necrosis accompanied by hemorrhage and minimal inflammation (Color Plate 19).

Chronic poisoning is caused by lower PA doses of longer duration. Hepatic biopsies often have focal hepatocyte necrosis (piecemeal necrosis), minimal peribiliary fibrosis, and mild bile duct proliferation. With time, damaged hepatocytes often develop into large megalocytes (Color Plate 20). Hepatocellular damage may continue, resulting in continued hepatocyte necrosis with subsequent inflammation, fibrosis, and ultimately cirrhosis.

Diagnostic Testing.   Because clinical signs of poisoning are often delayed, it is often difficult to document exposure to PA-containing plants. Initial kinetic studies found such

animals to have low concentrations of tissue-bound pyrroles that may not be detectable.[63] This makes diagnosis difficult.

Many diagnoses are made using histologic changes alone (hepatic necrosis, fibrosis, biliary proliferation, and megalocytosis). However, these are nonspecific changes and a definitive diagnosis is difficult. The ubiquitous nature of PA-containing plants suggests that PA intoxication is under-diagnosed.

Chemical methods using both spectrophotometry and gas chromatography/mass spectrometry have been developed to detect tissue-bound pyrroles (PA metabolites).[64,65] Although these have proven to be useful in identifying exposed animals, they lack sensitivity and they are not quantitative. Hopefully, improved sensitive diagnostics, including enzyme-linked immunosorbent assay–based immunodiagnostics, will provide better information on pyrrole kinetics, possible pyrrole recycling, or the cumulative effects of poisoning.

Treatment.   The progressive nature of chronic PA intoxication suggests that low, chronic PA exposure has cumulative effects. Little is known about what doses or durations are damaging, or the effect of subclinical intoxication on growth or productivity. Although various treatments and diet supplements have been suggested, none have proven to be effective in livestock.[66]

Prognosis.   Poisoned animals that show clinical signs rarely recover.

Prevention and Control.   Prevention is the best control measure. Because most poisonings are attributed to contamination of forages or feed, careful inspection of feed is recommended. Contaminated feeds should be discarded or fed to less susceptible species. Inspection of fields before harvest provides the best chance of detecting PA-containing plants. Although most PA-containing plants are not highly palatable, it is also recommended that plants be eliminated from pastures and ranges. Species-specific herbicide regimens have been developed for most plants and they are widely available through county weed and extension services.

REFERENCES

1. Mattocks AR: *Chemistry and toxicology of pyrrolizidine alkaloids,* Orlando, Fla, 1986, Academic Press.
2. Johnson AE et al: Senecio: a dangerous plant for man and beast, *Rangelands* 11:261, 1989.
3. Ford EJ et al: Serum changes following the feeding of ragwort *(Senecio jacobea)* to calves, *J Comp Pathol* 78:207, 1968.
4. Thorpe E, Ford EJ: Development of hepatic lesions in calves fed with ragwort *(Senecio jacobea), J Comp Pathol* 78:195-205, 1968.
5. Giles CJ: Outbreak of ragwort *(Senecio jacobaea)* poisoning in horses, *Equine Vet J* 15:248, 1983.
6. Johnson AE: Changes in calves and rats consuming milk from cows fed chronic lethal doses of *Senecio jacobaea* (tansy ragwort), *Am J Vet Res* 37:107, 1976.
7. Goeger DE et al: Effect of tansy ragwort consumption on dairy goats and goat milk transfer of pyrrolizidine alkaloids *Senecio jacobaea,* intoxication. In Cheeke PR, editor: *Symposium on pyrrolizidine (Senecio) alkaloids: toxicity, metabolism, and poisonous plant control measures,* Corvallis, Ore, 1979, Nutrition Research Institute, Oregon State University.

8. Johnson AE, Smart RA: Effects on cattle and their calves of tansy ragwort *(Senecio jacobaea)* fed in early gestation, *Am J Vet Res* 44:1215, 1983.

9. Cheeke PR, Pierson-Goeger ML: Toxicity of *Senecio jacobaea* and pyrrolizidine alkaloids in various laboratory animals and avian species, *Toxicol Lett* 18:343, 1983.

10. Cheeke PR: More threats from an old foe: tansy ragwort, *Senecio jacobaea* talks explain human hazards poisonous to humans as well as cattle and horses, pyrrolizidine alkaloids, *Oreg Agric Prog* 25:4, 1979.

11. Craig AM et al: Serum liver enzyme and histopathologic changes in calves with chronic and chronic-delayed *Senecio jacobaea* toxicosis, *Am J Vet Res* 52:1969, 1991.

12. Johnson AE et al: Toxicity of Riddell's groundsel *(Senecio riddellii)* to cattle, *Am J Vet Res* 46:577, 1985.

13. Molyneux RJ et al: Toxicity of pyrrolizidine alkaloids from Riddell groundsel *(Senecio riddellii)* to cattle, *Am J Vet Res* 52:146, 1991.

14. Chan PC et al: Toxicity and carcinogenicity of riddelline following 13 weeks of treatment to rats and mice, *Toxicon* 32:891, 1994.

15. Mathews FP: Poisoning of cattle by species of groundsel, *Bull 481:*1, Texas Agriculture Experiment Station, 1933.

16. Johnson AE, Molyneux RJ: Toxicity of threadleaf groundsel *(Senecio douglasii* var. longilobus) to cattle, *Am J Vet Res* 45:26, 1984.

17. Mitich LW: Common groundsel *(Senecio vulgaris)*, *Weed Tech* 9:209, 1995.

18. Lessard P et al: Clinicopathologic study of horses surviving pyrrolizidine alkaloid *(Senecio vulgaris)* toxicosis, *Am J Vet Res* 47:1776, 1986.

19. Mendel VE et al: Pyrrolizidine alkaloid-induced liver disease in horses: an early diagnosis, *Am J Vet Res* 49:572-578, 1988.

20. Kingsbury JM: *Poisonous plants of the United States and Canada*, Englewood Cliffs, N.J., 1964, Prentice-Hall.

21. Williams MC, Molyneux RJ: Occurrence, concentration, and toxicity of pyrrolizidine alkaloids in *Crotalaria* seeds, *Weed Sci* 35:476, 1987.

22. Knight AP et al: *Cynoglossum officinale* (hound's-tongue)—a cause of pyrrolizidine alkaloid poisoning in horses, *J Am Vet Med Assoc* 185:647, 1984.

23. Baker DC et al: Hound's-tongue *(Cynoglossum officinale)* poisoning in a calf, *J Am Vet Med Assoc* 194:929, 1989.

24. Stegelmeier BL et al: Pyrrole detection and the pathologic progression of *Cynoglossum officinale* (houndstongue) poisoning in horses, *J Vet Diagn Invest* 8:81, 1996.

25. Pfister JA et al: Pyrrolizidine alkaloid content of houndstongue *(Cynoglossum officinale* L.), *J Range Manage* 45:254, 1992.

26. Baker DC et al: *Cynoglossum officinale* toxicity in calves, *J Comp Pathol* 104:403, 1991.

27. Seaman JT, Dixon RJ: Investigations into the toxicity of *Echium plantagineum* in sheep. 2. Pen feeding experiments, *Aust Vet J* 66:286, 1989.

28. Seaman JT et al: Investigations into the toxicity of *Echium plantagineum* in sheep. 1. Field grazing experiments, *Aust Vet J* 66:279, 1989.

29. Seaman JT: Patterson's curse, *Echium plantagineum* is a curse for horses poisoning the liver, *Agric Gaz N S W* 89(5):43, 1978.

30. Giesecke PR: Serum biochemistry in horses with *Echium* poisoning, *Aust Vet J* 63:90, 1986.

31. McLennan MW et al: Heliotropium poisoning in cattle, *Aust Vet J* 48:480, 1972.

32. Jones RT et al: *Heliotropium europaeum* poisoning of pigs [letter], *Aust Vet J* 57:396, 1981.

33. Peterson JE et al: *Heliotropium europaeum* poisoning of sheep with low liver copper concentrations and the preventive efficacy of cobalt and antimethanogen, *Aust Vet J* 69:51, 1992.

34. McCulloch EC: Nutlets of *Amsinckia intermedia* toxic to swine, horses and cattle, *Madrono* 5:202, 1940.

35. McCulloch EC: The experimental production of hepatic cirrhosis by the seed of *Amsinckia intermedia, Science* 91:95, 1942.

36. Woolsey JHJ et al: Two outbreaks of hepatic cirrhosis in swine in California, with evidence incriminating the tarweed, *Amsinckia intermedia, Vet Med* 47:55 1952.

37. Brauchli J et al: Pyrrolizidine alkaloids from *Symphytum officinale* L. and their percutaneous absorption in rats, *Experientia* 38:1085, 1982.

38. Furmanowa M et al: Mutagenic effects of aqueous extracts of *Symphytum officinale* L. and of its alkaloidal fractions medicinal plants, *J Appl Toxicol* 3:127, 1982.

39. Hirono I et al: Carcinogenic activity of *Symphytum officinale, J Natl Cancer Inst* 61:865, 1978.

40. Woo J et al: DNA interstrand cross-linking reactions of pyrrole-derived bifunctional electrophiles: evidence for a common target site in DNA, *J Am Chem Soc* 115:3407, 1993.

41. Yan CC, Huxtable RJ: Relationship between glutathione concentration and metabolism of the pyrrolizidine alkaloid, monocrotaline, in the isolated, perfused liver, *Toxicol Appl Pharmacol* 130:132, 1995.

42. Huxtable RJ: Human health implications of pyrrolizidine alkaloids and herbs containing them. In Cheeke PR, editor: *Toxicants of plant origin,* Boca Raton, Fla, 1989, CRC Press.

43. Van-Zwanenberg D: A "singular calamity," *Med Hist* 17:204, 1973.

44. Hooper PT: Pyrrolizidine alkaloid poisoning: pathology with particular reference to differences in animal and plant species. In Keeler RF et al, editors: *Effects of poisonous plants on livestock,* New York, 1978, Academic Press.

45. Craig AM et al: Metabolism of toxic pyrrolizidine alkaloids from tansy ragwort *(Senecio jacobaea)* in ovine ruminal fluid under anaerobic conditions, *Appl Environ Microbiol* 58:2730, 1992.

46. Wachenheim DE et al: Characterization of rumen bacterial pyrrolizidine alkaloid biotransformation in ruminants of various species, *Vet Human Toxicol* 34:513, 1992.

47. Craig AM, Blythe LL: Review of ruminal microbes relative to detoxification of plant toxins and environmental pollutants. In Colegate SM, Dorling PR, editors: *Plant associated toxins: agricultural, phytochemical, and ecological aspects,* Wallingford, Oxford, UK, 1994, CAB International.

48. Peterson JE, Jago MV: Toxicity of *Echium plantagineum* (Patterson's curse). 2. Pyrrolizidine alkaloid poisoning in rats, *Aust J Agric Res* 35:305, 1984.

49. Winter CK et al: Species differences in the hepatic microsomal metabolism of the pyrrolizidine alkaloid senecionine, *Comp Biochem Physiol C* 90:429, 1988.

50. Chu PS, Segall HJ: Species difference in the urinary excretion of isatinecic acid from the pyrrolizidine alkaloid retrorsine, *Comp Biochem Physiol C* 100:683, 1991.

51. Chung WG, Buhler DR: Major factors for the susceptibility of guinea pig to the pyrrolizidine alkaloid jacobine, *Drug Metab Disp* 23:1263, 1995.

52. Chauvin P et al: An outbreak of *Heliotrope* food poisoning, Tadjikistan. November 1992-March 1993, *Sante* 4:263, 1994.

53. Stillman AE et al: Hepatic veno-occlusive disease due to pyrrolizidine *(Senecio)* poisoning in Arizona, *Gastroenterology* 73:349, 1977.

54. Roulet M et al: Hepatic veno-occlusive disease in newborn infant of a woman drinking herbal tea, *J Pediatr* 112:433, 1988.

55. Small AC et al: Pyrrolizidine alkaloidosis in a two month old foal, *Zentralbl Veterinarmed A* 40:213, 1993.

56. Sperl W et al: Reversible hepatic veno-occlusive disease in an infant after consumption of pyrrolizidine-containing herbal tea, *Eur J Pediatr* 154:112, 1995.

57. Williams DW et al: Bioactivation and detoxication of the pyrrolizidine alkaloid senecionine by cytochrome P-450 enzymes in rat liver, *Drug Metab Disp* 17:387, 1989.

58. Seaman JT: Hepatogenous chronic copper poisoning in sheep associated with grazing *Echium plantagineum, Aust Vet J* 62:247, 1985.

59. Petry TW, Sipes IG: Modulation of monocrotaline-induced hepatic genotoxicity in rats, *Carcinogenesis* 8:415-419, 1987.

60. Yan CC, Huxtable RJ: Effects of monocrotaline, a pyrrolizidine alkaloid, on glutathione metabolism in the rat, *Biochem Pharmacol* 51:375, 1996.

61. Chung WG et al: A cytochrome p4502b form is the major bioactivation enzyme for the pyrrolizidine alkaloid senecionine in guinea pig, *Xenobiotica* 25:929, 1995.

62. Johnson AE et al: Chemistry of toxic range plants. Variation in pyrrolizidine alkaloid content of *Senecio, Amsinckia,* and *Crotalaria* species, *J Agric Food Chem* 33:50, 1985.

63. Stegelmeier BL, USDA/ARS PPRL, Logan, Utah: Unpublished data, 2000.

64. Mattocks AR, Jukes R: Recovery of the pyrrolic nucleus of pyrrolizidine alkaloid metabolites from sulphur conjugates in tissues and body fluids, *Chem Biol Interact* 75:225, 1990.

65. Schoch TK et al: GC/MS/MS detection of pyrrolic metabolites in animals poisoned with the pyrrolizidine alkaloid riddelliine, *J Nat Toxins* 9(2):197, 2000.

66. Johnson AE: Toxicity of tansy ragwort to cattle. In Cheeke PR, editor: Symposium on pyrrolizidine (*Senecio*) alkaloids: toxicity, metabolism, and poisonous plant control measures, Corvallis, Ore, 1979, Nutrition Research Institute, Oregon State University.

67. Niggli U: Control of *Senecio alpinus* (L.) Scop. [Toxic plant for cattle, Switzerland]. Die Bekampfung von Alpenkreuzkraut (*Senecio alpinus* (L.) Scop.). Schweiz-Landwirtsch-Monatsh. Bern : Gesellschaft Schweizerischer Landwirte 60(11):448, 1982.

68. Candrian U et al: Stability of pyrrolizidine alkaloids in hay and silage, *J Agric Food Chem* 32:935, 1984.

69. Tokarnia CH, Dobereiner J: Experimental poisoning of cattle by *Senecio brasiliensis, Pesquisa Veterinaria Brasileira* 4:39, 1984.

70. Nazario W et al: Role of *Senecio brasiliensis* in toxic incidents in cattle in Sao Paulo State, *Pesquisa Agropecuaria Brasileira* 23:537, 1988.

71. Robertson W: Cirrhosis of the liver in stock in cape colony produced by two species of *Senecio* (*Senecio burchelli* and *Senecio latifolius), J Comp Pathol Therapeut* 19:97, 1906.

72. Habermehl GG et al: Livestock poisoning in South America by species of the *Senecio* plant, *Toxicon* 26:275, 1988.

73. El-Sergany MA et al: Studies on blood cytology, serum enzymes and the histopathology of the liver in chicks fed dried *Senecio desfontainei, Archiv fur Geflugelkunde* 48:77, 1984.

74. Araya O, Fuentealba IC: Chronic hepato-toxicity of *Senecio erraticus* in calves from two 50-day feeding periods in consecutive years, *Vet Hum Toxicol* 32:555, 1990.

75. Morton JF: Ornamental plants with poisonous properties, *Proc Florida State Hort Soc* 71:372, 1958.

76. Goeger DE et al: Comparison of the toxicities of *Senecio jacobaea, Senecio vulgaris,* and *Senecio glabellus* in rats, *Toxicol Lett* 15(1):19, 1983.

77. Mendez M-del-C et al: Intoxication with *Senecio* spp. (*Compositae)* in cattle in Rio Grande do Sul, *Pesquisa Veterinaria Brasileira* 7:51, 1987.

78. Hansen AA: Indiana plants injurious to livestock. In *Indiana Agriculture Experiment Station Circular,* West Lafayette, Ind, 1930, Purdue University.

79. Bredenkamp MW et al: A new pyrrolizidine alkaloid from *Senecio latifolius* DC, *Tetrahedron Lett* 26:929, 1985.

80. Bredenkamp MW: The isolation, structure and chemistry of the major pyrrolizidine alkaloids of *Senecio latifolius* DC, *Dissert Abst Int B* 48:135, 1987.

81. Kidder RW: Is bitterweed (*Senecio lobatus)* killing glades cattle, *Florida Grower* 60:14, 1952.

82. Noble JW et al: Pyrrolizidine alkaloidosis of cattle associated with *Senecio lautus, Aust Vet J* 71:196, 1994.

83. Driemeier D, Barros CSL: Experimental poisoning in cattle by *Senecio oxyphyllus* (*Compositae), Pesquisa Veterinaria Brasileira* 12:33, 1992.

84. Lilley CW: Pyrrolizidine alkaloid toxicosis *Senecio plattensis,* equine practice, *Vet Pract* 2(2):6, 1980.

85. McCain JW et al: *Indiana plants poisonous to livestock and pets,* West Lafayette, Ind, 1985, Cooperative Extension Service, Purdue University.

86. Dickson J, Hill R: Cotton fireweed (*Senecio quadridentatus)* poisoning of cattle, *Proc Aust Vet Assoc* 1:92, 1977.

87. Winter H et al: Pyrrolizidine alkaloid poisoning of yaks: diagnosis of pyrrolizidine alkaloid exposure by the demonstration of sulphur-conjugated pyrrolic metabolites of the alkaloid in circulating haemoglobin, *Aust Vet J* 70:312, 1993.

88. Basson PA: Poisoning of wildlife in southern Africa, *J South Afr Vet Assoc* 58:219, 1987.

89. Rosiles-M R, Paasch LH: Hepatic megalocytosis in sheep. Short communication [*Senecio sanguisorbae,* toxicity]. Megalocitosis hepatica en ovinos, *Vet Mex* 13:151, 1982.

90. Odriozola E et al: Pyrrolizidine alkaloidosis in Argentinian cattle caused by *Senecio selloi, Vet Human Toxicol* 36:205, 1994.

91. Davis CL: *Senecio* poisoning in livestock, *West Vet* 5:28, 1958.

92. Smith RA, Panariti E: Intoxication of Albanian cattle after ingestion *of Senecio subalpinus. Vet Hum Toxicol* 37:478, 1995.

93. Mendez MC, Riet-Correa F: Intoxication by *Senecio tweediei* in cattle in southern Brazil, *Vet Hum Toxicol* 35:55, 1993.

94. Hippchen C et al: Experimental studies with goats on the hepatotoxicity of *Senecio* alkaloids from *Senecio vernalis, Praktische Tierarzt* 67:322, 1986.

95. Tokarnia CH, Dobereiner J: Experimental poisoning of cattle with *Crotalaria anagyroides* (Papilionoideae), *Pesquisa Veterinaria Brasileira* 3:115, 1983.

96. Chan MY et al: A comparative study on the hepatic toxicity and metabolism of *Crotalaria assamica* and *Eupatorium* species, *Am J Clin Med* 17:165, 1989.

97. Theiler A: Jaagzeikte in horses (*Crotalariosis equorum), Res Rep 5-6:1-56,* South African Department of Agriculture, Veterinary Education, 1918.

98. Norton JH, O'Rourke PK: Toxicity of *Crotalaria goreensis* for chickens, *Aust Vet J* 55:173, 1979.

99. Schmeda-Hirschmann G et al: A magic use of *Crotalaria incana* pods, *J Ethnopharmacol* 21:187, 1987.

100. Zhang XL: Toxic components of the seeds of *Crotalaria juncea* and their toxicity for pigs, *Chin J Vet Sci Technol [Zhongguo Shouyi Keji]* 7:13, 1985.

101. Nobre D et al: *Crotalaria juncea* intoxication in horses, *Vet Hum Toxicol* 36:445, 1994.

102. Heath D et al: A pulmonary hypertension-producing plant from Tanzania, *Thorax* 30:399, 1975.

103. Laws L: Toxicity of *Crotalaria mucronata* to sheep, *Aust Vet J* 44:453, 1968.

104. Tokarnia CH, Dobereiner J: Experimental poisoning of cattle by *Crotalaria mucronata* (Leguminosae Papilionoideae) Brazil. [Intoxicacao experimental por *Crotalaria mucronata* (Leg. Papilionoideae) em bovinos], *Pesqui Vet Bras Braz J Vet Res* 2:77, 1982.

105. Tandon BN et al: Ultra-structure of liver in veno-occlusive disease due to *Crotalaria nan Burm, Ind J Med Res* 68:790, 1978.

106. Shrivastava AB et al: Haematological study on toxicity of *Crotalaria nana* in rats, *Ind J Anim Sci* 55:255, 1985.

107. Hooper PT, Scanlan WA: *Crotalaria retusa* poisoning of pigs and poultry, *Aust Vet J* 53:109, 1977.

108. Alfonso HA, Sanchez LM: Intoxication due to *Crotalaria retusa* and *C. spectahbilis* in chickens and geese, *Vet Hum Toxicol* 35:539, 1993.

109. Barri ME, Adam SE: The toxicity of *Crotalaria saltiana* to calves, *J Comp Pathol* 91:621, 1981.

110. Barri ME et al: Effects of *Crotalaria saltiana* on Nubian goats, *Vet Hum Toxicol* 26:476, 1984.

111. Piercy P-LaV, Rusoff L-L: Livestock poisoning by *Crotalaria spectabilis,* Baton Rouge, La, 1945, Louisiana State University and Agricultural and Mechanical College, Agricultural Experiment Station.

112. McGrath JP et al: *Crotalaria spectabilis* toxicity in swine: characterization of the renal glomerular lesion, *J Comp Pathol* 85:185, 1975.

113. Figueredo M-de-los-A et al: Pathomorphology of acute experimental poisoning with *Crotalaria spectabilis* and *C. retusa* in broilers, *Revista Cubana de Ciencias Veterinarias* 18:63, 1987.

114. Arseculeratne SN et al: Studies on medicinal plants of Sri Lanka: occurrence of pyrrolizidine alkaloids and hepatotoxic properties in some traditional medicinal herbs *Crotalaria verrucosa, Holarrhena antidysenterica, Cassia auriculata, J Ethnopharmacol* 4:159, 1981.

115. Schoental R et al: Islet cell tumore of the pancreas found in rats given pyrrolizidine alkaloids from *Amsinckia intermedia* Fisch and Mey and from *Heliotropium supinum* L, *Cancer Res* 30:2127, 1970.

116. Glover PE, Ketterer PJ: Blue heliotrope kills cattle, *Queensland Agricultural Journal* 113:109, 1987.

117. Ketterer PJ et al: Blue heliotrope *(Heliotropium amplexicaule)* poisoning in cattle, *Aust Vet J* 64:115, 1987.

118. Muratov DS: Enzyme activity in blood serum of sheep poisoned with *Heliotropium dasycarpum, Sbornik Rabot Uzbekskogo Vet Instit* 21:272, 1973.

119. Tandon HD et al: An epidemic of veno-occlusive disease of the liver in Afghanistan. Pathologic features, *Am J Gastroenterol* 70:607, 1978.

120. Culvenor CCJ et al: *Heliotropium lasiocarpum* Fisch and Mey identified as cause of veno-occlusive disease due to herbal tea, *Lancet* 1:978, 1986.

121. Abu-Damir H et al: The effects of *Heliotropium ovalifolium* on goats and sheep, *Br Vet J* 138:463, 1982.

122. Wahome WM et al: An acute toxicity study of *Heliotropium scottae* Rendle in mice, *Vet Hum Toxicol* 36:295, 1994.

123. Awang DVC et al: Echimidine content of commercial comfrey *(Symphytum* spp.–Boraginaceae), *J Herbs Spices Med Plants* 2:21, 1993.

124. Mossoba MM et al: Application of gas chromatography/matrix isolation fourier transform infrared spectroscopy to the identification of pyrrolizidine alkaloids from comfrey root *(Symphytum officinale* l), *J Aoac Int* 77:1167, 1994.

125. Lei ZY et al: Studies on toxicity of alkaloids in *Symphytum peregrinum* Leded. 3. Effects of pyrrolizidine alkaloids on chicken, *Grassland of China Zhongguo Caoyuan* 21:26, 59, 1984.

126. Shevchenko NKh et al: [*Trichodesma* poisoning in poultry], *Veterinariia* 49:99, 1973.

127. Wassel G et al: Toxic pyrrolizidine alkaloids of certain *Boraginaceous* plants, *Acta Pharmaceutica Suecica* 24:199, 1987.

QUINOLIZIDINE ALKALOIDS

Kip E. Panter

More than 150 quinolizidine alkaloids have been identified in the Leguminosae family.[1] Most of the known quinolizidine alkaloids have been found in several genera of this very large plant family, especially *Lupinus, Laburnum, Cytisus,* and *Thermopsis.* Most species of *Lupinus* contain quinolizidine alkaloids, but a few contain both or predominantly piperidine alkaloids. For example, *Lupinus formosus* contains both quinolizidine and piperidine alkaloids, whereas *L. arbustus* contains only piperidine alkaloids.

Three different clinical syndromes are attributed to quinolizidine alkaloids:

1. *Teratogenesis* has been reported in cattle that ingest the *Lupinus* species that contain anagyrine when the ingestion occurs during days 38 to 70 of gestation. The clinical signs and pathogenesis are the same as those caused by the piperidine alkaloids.
2. *Myopathy* in cattle is caused by *Thermopsis montana,* which contains quinolizidine alkaloids such as thermopsine.
3. *Acute neurologic disease,* primarily in sheep and sometimes in cattle, is caused by quinolizidine alkaloids from *Lupinus, Laburnum,* and *Cytisus* spp. The disease caused by these three genera is the same. *Lupinus* is discussed below in greatest detail, as the representative plant for this group.

Synonyms. Many of these plants have common names associated with some taxonomic feature of the plant or location: *Lupinus sulphureus,* yellow lupine; *L. leucophyllus,* velvet or woolly-leaved lupine; *Laburnum,* golden chain; and *Cytisus,* Scotch broom. *Thermopsis rhombifolia* or *T. montana* is often referred to as false lupine, yellow bean, or golden banner.

Sources. More than 500 species of annual, perennial, or soft, woody, shrublike lupines exist worldwide: 200 to 300 species in North and South America, including 150 species in the Intermountain West of the United States and 95 species in California.[2-4] *Laburnum anagyroides* is referred to as golden chain, bean tree, or laburnum, and grows in most regions of the United States and Great Britain. It is planted for its ornamental and aesthetic value. *Cytisus scoparius,* Scotch broom, grows on the East Coast and West Coast in sandy soils along roadsides and in waste places. *Thermopsis* is widespread in pastures, fields, and uncultivated areas throughout the western United States and Canada.

Lupine poisoning of livestock has been reported in Australia, South Africa, Europe, and the United States. The largest number of quinolizidine alkaloid poisoning episodes have occurred as a result of animals consuming various lupines in the western United States. Not all lupines are toxic; some species have been selected for low alkaloid content (sweet lupines), and are cultivated as nutritious feed for animals and foods for humans and are valued for their ability to fix nitrogen in the soil. These "sweet" lupines do not survive in the wild. Toxicosis (lupinosis) from sweet lupines has occurred but is not associated with alkaloids but rather peptide mycotoxins (phomopsins) produced by fungal parasites *(Diaporthe toxica;* anamorph *Phomopsis* spp.) growing on the stubble.[5]

Toxicokinetics. More than 70 quinolizidine alkaloids have been identified in range and domestic lupines.[6,7] These alkaloids contain the basic structural quinolizidine ring system $(C_9H_{18}N)$. They may be represented by the simplest alkaloids such as lupinine $(C_{10}H_{19}NO)$, which is homologous with cytisine $(C_{11}H_{14}N_{20})$, an alkaloid common in *Cytisus.* The tetracyclic quinolizidine alkaloids are represented by sparteine, lupanine, and anagyrine $(C_{15}H_{20}N_{20})$. Anagyrine is the most well known in livestock poisoning and is recognized as a teratogen causing "crooked calf disease."[8-10]

The alkaloid extract from *Thermopsis* contains predominantly *N*-methylcytisine, cytisine, 5,6-dehydrolupanine, thermopsine, and anagyrine, whereas the extracts from *Lupinus* and *Laburnum* contain predominantly anagyrine and cytisine, respectively. Therefore, anagyrine and cytisine alone cannot account for the clinical effects of *Thermopsis.* Thermopsine from *Thermopsis* is a diastereomer of anagyrine, but it causes different clinical effects and is not associated with birth defects.[11] Quinolizidine alkaloids with an α-pyridone A-ring may be responsible for the lesions and individual α-pyridones such as thermopsine may have cumulative effects.[12]

Recent research on the in vivo disposition of quinolizidine alkaloids is limited. In humans, lupanine and 13-hydroxylupanine half-life of elimination as measured in the urine after oral administration was 6.5 and 5.9 hours, respectively, and 95% to 100% of the total alkaloid administered was recovered in the urine unchanged within 72 hours of administration.[13,14]

Alkaloid absorption and serum elimination profiles for a single oral dose of *Lupinus caudatus* or *Lupinus formosus* have been reported in cattle, sheep, and goats.[15,16] The quinolizidine alkloids from *L. caudatus* were detected in plasma by 30 minutes after ingestion, peaked by 3 to 8 hours depending on the alkaloid, and, in the case of 5,6-dehydrolupanine and lupanine, remained high in the plasma for 28 hours, at which time a relatively sharp decline in the serum was reported ($t_{1/2}$ = 14 hours).[15] The piperidine alkaloids from *L. formosus* showed similar patterns of absorption and elimination as those reported for *L. caudatus*.[16] Alkaloids were detected within 30 minutes of ingestion, peaked in 8 hours, remained relatively high for up to 24 hours in all three animal species, then declined with a $t_{1/2}$ of about 12 hours.[16]

Mechanism of Action.   Little is known about individual alkaloid toxicity; however, 14 quinolizidine alkaloids isolated from *Lupinus albus, L. mutabilis,* and *Anagyris foetida* were analyzed for their affinity to muscarinic and nicotinic acetylcholine receptors.[1] Table 25-9 shows comparative binding affinities.

Lupanine, 13-hydroxylupanine, and sparteine all block ganglionic transmission, decrease cardiac contractility, and increase motility and tone of the uterine smooth muscle.[13] In another assay system, lupanine and sparteine blocked nicotinic cholinergic receptor activity, and both compounds were weak antagonists of the muscarinic cholinergic receptor.[17]

Toxicity and Risk Factors.   Seeds and seedpods contain the highest concentrations of alkaloids. Alkaloids are translocated from the vegetative parts to seeds. The toxicity of lupanine administered intraperitoneally in a mouse bioassay was less than sparteine with an LD_{50} equal to 175 mg/kg vs 36 mg/kg, respectively.[17]

The nutrient content of the seeds often overrides the toxicity, especially in late summer or early fall when grasses become less palatable. Sheep are especially likely to eat seed heads. Cases involving loss of more than 1000 head of sheep have been reported, and lupines have been responsible for the greatest losses of sheep in the states of Montana, Idaho, and Utah.[18] Today, large losses are rare because the sheep flocks and numbers have been reduced on mountain ranges and the practice of feeding lupine hay has ceased.[18]

Clinical Signs

Lupinus.   The early clinical signs of poisoning in sheep include labored breathing and depression, followed by coma and death within a day or sometimes several days later. In other cases, severe breathing difficulty occurs rapidly, but rather than exhibiting depression, the animal throws itself around violently, sometimes butting other animals or pressing against a fence or other solid object. Death occurs from respiratory paralysis after periods of trembling and apparent convulsion-like signs or following a brief comatose period. Weak pulse and slow respiration usually precede death in those cases in which symptoms are delayed.

Clinical signs of poisoning in cattle begin with excessive salivation (frothing) and grinding of the teeth, progressing to ataxia, muscular weakness, and recumbency. If the dosage is high enough, death occurs from respiratory failure.[19] Cattle are rarely acutely poisoned, but lupine-induced crooked calf disease continues to be a serious problem for cattle producers in the West.

Thermopsis.   Cattle are reluctant to move and walk with a stiff gait. Muscle tremors develop if the animals are forced to move.[11,12,20] Other signs can include depression, anorexia, and swollen eyelids. Following large ingestions, cattle become recumbent and die.

Clinical Pathology.   Calves fed *Thermopsis* alkaloid extracts had elevated serum CK and AST when compared with calves fed alkaloid extracts from *Lupinus* or *Laburnum*. Serum CK and AST were greatest on day 4 of gavaging

TABLE 25-9 **Binding Affinities of Quinolizidine Alkaloids to Nicotinic and Muscarinic Acetylcholine Receptors**

Nicotinic Receptor*		Muscarinic Receptor*	
IC_{50}	Alkaloid	IC_{50}	Alkaloid
0.05 μM	*N*-Methylcytisine	11 μM	13 α-Tigloyloxylupanine
0.14 μM	Cytisine	21 μM	Sparteine
5 μM	Lupanine	25 μM	Angustifoline
155 μM	17-Oxosparteine	33 μM	Albine
160 μM	13 α-Tigloyloxylupanine	47 μM	Multiflorine
190 μM	3 α-Hydroxylupanine	74 μM	3 α-Hydroxylupanine
193 μM	Albine	114 μM	Lupanine
310 μM	Tetrahydrorhombifoline	118 μM	17-Oxosparteine
331 μM	Sparteine	129 μM	Tetrahydrorhombifoline
490 μM	13 β-Hydroxylupanine	132 μM	Anagyrine
>500 μM	Angustifoline	140 μM	13 β-Hydroxylupanine
>500 μM	Multiflorine	190 μM	Lupinine
>500 μM	Lupinine	400 μM	Cytisine
2096 μM	Anagyrine	417 μM	*N*-Methylcytisine

Adapted from Schmeller et al: Binding of quinolizidine alkaloids to nicotinic and muscarinic acetylcholine receptors, *J Nat Prod* 57:1316, 1994.
*Binding affinities (IC_{50}) indicate the concentration of a particular quinolizidine alkaloid that displaces 50% of the specifically bound radiolabeled ligand, ^{3}H-nicotine for nicotinic receptors and ^{3}H-quinuclidinyl benzilate (QNB) for muscarinic receptors.

and increased approximately fortyfold and sixfold, respectively, compared to control calves or calves fed *Lupinus* and *Laburnum* extracts.[12]

Lesions. Apart from the teratogenesis in cattle (multiple congenital contractures and cleft palate) lesions from *Lupinus* are not diagnostic. Likewise, no diagnostic lesions are associated with toxicosis from *Cytisis* and *Laburnum*.

Thermopsis does not produce diagnostic gross lesions. However, degeneration of skeletal muscles is apparent histologically. Myocardial degeneration is not typical.[12,20]

Diagnostic Testing. Chemical analysis for alkaloids in blood, liver, kidney, or stomach contents with history of consumption may be diagnostic for animals with acute neurologic disease.

Treatment

Lupinus. No treatment exists for acute neurologic disease in sheep beyond general supportive and symptomatic care. Stress may exacerbate the clinical signs and may contribute to the cause of death. Acute toxicoses and death losses in cattle are rare, and severe clinical signs are infrequently reported in the field. More commonly, calves with skeletal contracture defects and cleft palate are observed.

Thermopsis. Treatment of animals with moderate-to-severe myopathies induced by *Thermopsis* is often futile. For valuable animals, feeding ground hay and grain while assisting animals to stand and exercise may facilitate recovery after a period of time.

Prognosis. If ingestion is not lethal from acute neurologic disease then recovery is usually complete. Treatment for severe limb contractures is futile and the prognosis for survival is poor. Calves born with mild contractures of the front legs often recover and grow normally.

Prolonged recumbency is a severe sequela of toxicosis in cattle and horses following ingestion of *Thermopsis montana.*[11,12,20] Once animals become recumbent, prognosis for recovery is poor.

Prevention and Control. Prevention of teratogenic effects involves managing grazing to avoid ingestion of lupines during susceptible stages of gestation. *Lupinus* and *Thermopsis* can be controlled using broadleaf herbicides, specifically 2,4-D, Dicamba, Picloram, Triclopyr, or combinations thereof.[21,22] This is usually based on economic benefit and the significance of the infestation.

REFERENCES

1. Schmeller T et al: Binding of quinolizidine alkaloids to nicotinic and muscarinic acetylcholine receptors, *J Nat Prod* 57:1316, 1994.
2. Wink M et al: Patterns of quinolizidine alkaloids in 56 species of the genus *Lupinus*, *Phytochemistry* 38:139, 1995.
3. Cronquist A et al: *Intermountain flora, vascular plants of the intermountain west, USA,* vol 3B, New York, 1989, The New York Botanical Garden.
4. Riggins R, Sholars R: In Hickman JC, editor: *The Jepson manual, higher plants of California,* Berkeley, Calif, 1993, University of California Press.
5. Allen JG, Cousins DV: In Garland T, Barr AC, editors: *Toxic plants and other natural toxicants,* New York, 1998, CAB International.
6. Kinghorn AD, Balendrin MF: In Pelletier SW, editor: *Alkaloids: chemical and biological perspectives,* New York, 1984, John Wiley and Sons.
7. Keeler RF: In Cheeke PR, editor: *Toxicants of plant origin, vol 1. Alkaloids,* Boca Raton, Fla, 1989, CRC Press.
8. Keeler RF: Lupine alkaloids from teratogenic and nonteratogenic lupins. II. Identification of the major alkaloids by tandem gas chromatography-mass spectrometry in plants producing crooked calf disease, *Teratology* 7:31, 1973.
9. Keeler RF: Lupin alkaloids from teratogenic and nonteratogenic lupins. III. Identification of anagyrine as the probable teratogen by feeding trials, *J Toxicol Environ Health* 1:887, 1976.
10. Davis AM, Stout DM: Anagyrine in western American lupines, *J Range Manage* 39:29, 1986.
11. Keeler RF et al: Toxicity of *Thermopsis montana, Cornell Vet* 76:1157, 1986.
12. Keeler RF, Baker DC: Myopathy in cattle induced by alkaloid extracts from *Thermopsis montana, Laburnum anagyroides* and a *Lupinus* spp, *J Comp Pathol* 103:169, 1990.
13. Mazur M et al: Pharmacologic studies of lupanine and 13-hydroxylupanine, *Acta Physiologica Polonica* 17:299, 1966.
14. Petterson DS et al: Disposition of lupanine and 13-hydroxylupanine in man, *Xenobiotica* 24:933, 1994.
15. Gardner DR, Panter KE: Comparison of blood plasma alkaloid levels in cattle, sheep and goats fed *Lupinus caudatus, J Nat Toxins* 2(1):1, 1993.
16. Gardner DR, Panter KE: Ammodendrine and related piperidine alkaloid levels in the blood plasma of cattle, sheep and goats fed *Lupinus formosus, J Nat Toxins* 3(2):107, 1994.
17. Yovo K et al: Comparative pharmacological study of sparteine and its ketonic derivative lupanine from seeds of *Lupinus albus, Planta Medica* 50:420, 1984.
18. Chestnut VK, Wilcox EV: The stock poisoning plants of Montana: a preliminary report, *Bull 26,* Washington, DC, 1901, U.S. Dept. of Agriculture.
19. Panter KE et al: Teratogenic and fetotoxic effects of two piperidine alkaloid-containing lupines *(L. formosus* and *L. arbustus)* in cows, *J Nat Toxins* 7:131, 1998.
20. Baker DC, Keeler RF: Myopathy in cattle caused by *Thermopsis montana, J Am Vet Med Assoc* 194:1269, 1989.
21. Klingman DL et al: Systemic herbicides for weed control, *Bull AD-BU-2281,* 1983, University of Minnesota Extension Service.
22. Ralphs MH et al: Herbicide control of poisonous plants, *Rangelands* 13:73, 1991.

TAXINE ALKALOIDS

Stan W. Casteel

Sources. *Taxus* spp. are evergreen trees or shrubs with thin, scaly, purple to reddish-brown bark covering the trunk and alternate branchlets.[1] Branches of some species are somewhat flattened in appearance with flattened 1- to 2-cm needle-like leaves in opposite pairs. A fleshy scarlet cup (aril) surrounds green to black seeds. Western or Pacific yew *(Taxus brevifolia)* is a medium-sized tree (5 to 10 m) with a straight or contorted trunk. Japanese yew *(T. cuspidata),* Hicks yew *(T. media), T. capitata,* and English yew *(T. baccata)* are common ornamental shrubs, and ground hemlock *(T. canadensis)* is a native eastern United States species. Florida yew *(T. floridana)* is restricted to Florida.

Mechanism of Action.   Taxine alkaloids are a complex mixture of cardiotoxins isolated from yew that can induce fatal conduction disturbances with direct action on cardiac myocyte ion channels.[2] The many compounds isolated from yew have given rise to a confusing proliferation of nomenclature.[3] Examples of isolated compounds and their derivatives include taxicatin; taxicin I and II; taxine; taxine A, B, C, I, and II; taxinine; taxinine A, B, E, H, J, K, and L; taxusin; and taxol. Many of these names do not refer to alkaloids (taxinines), and a number of them are not derivatives of the basic taxane nucleus. The contribution of individual compounds to the toxicity of this shrub has not been ascertained. An extract of alkaloids from *T. baccata* slowed atrial and ventricular rates of isolated frog heart in a dose-dependent manner.[4] At higher concentrations, the rate-depressing effect was most pronounced on the ventricle. These in vitro experimental results are consistent with cardiotoxic effects in poisoned livestock. The mechanism of these effects may result from calcium and sodium current inhibition.[5]

Taxol, an antimicrotubule cancer chemotherapeutic agent first isolated from *T. brevifolia,* has been synthesized and extracted from other *Taxus* species.[6] Side effects of the drug in humans include bradycardia, atrioventricular block, and ventricular tachycardia. Because of the limited quantities of naturally occurring taxol in yews, its contribution to animal toxicoses from plant ingestion is presumably small.

Toxicity and Risk Factors.   All parts, except the aril portion (fleshy red structure surrounding the seed), are considered toxic. Specific toxicity information is limited and is presumably affected by growing conditions and time of year. Mature leaves are reportedly most toxic in the winter.[7] Because *Taxus* is toxic, green or dry[8] clippings must be disposed of by composting or burning. Sublethal doses of toxin are secreted via the milk, thereby posing a possible human health hazard.[3] The safety of meat consumption from dead livestock has not been determined and must be considered with discretion. Animal intoxication from Pacific yew ingestion has not been reported, but a case report of a poisoned child demonstrates the toxic potential of this species.[9] Estimated fatal doses of yew leaves are variable and imprecise because of a lack of experimental data. An aqueous slurry of 160 g of ground Japanese yew was fatal to a pony within $1\frac{1}{4}$ hours of oral ingestion.[10] Other estimates indicate that ingestion of 0.2% to 0.5% of body weight[2] is fatal to cattle, and the fatal dose in horses is 0.05% of body weight.[8]

Exposure to yew foliage most often is associated with disposal of clippings in pastures adjacent to residential areas or when livestock have access to landscaped plots. Most poisonings have involved cattle[8,11-14] or horses[15]; however, sheep,[16] deer,[17] poultry,[16] game bird,[18] pet bird,[19,20] and canine[21] intoxications have been reported.

Clinical Signs.   Clinical signs in poisoned livestock primarily reflect conduction disturbances in the heart. Acute intoxication often results in sudden death within hours of ingestion of yew. Electrocardiography in intoxicated human patients reveals depressed or absent P-waves with atypical bundle branch block and increased QRS duration.[22,23]

Clinical poisoning in cattle is characterized by anxiety, bradycardia, jugular pulse, dyspnea, hypothermia, trembling, weakness, ataxia, recumbency, and sometimes diarrhea in subacute cases. Forced movement of normally appearing livestock may result in collapse to lateral recumbency followed by brief struggling, agonal respiratory efforts, and death in minutes. Cows have collapsed so suddenly and died that owners often describe them as appearing gunshot. Other animals sometimes return to standing position only to collapse and die later.

Onset of clinical signs is expectedly variable and may be delayed in ruminants when compared with monogastrics. Signs of intoxication and death of cattle began within 2 to 3 hours of initial exposure to English yew clippings.[14] Of 43 steers and heifers, 35 died within 11 hours after exposure; most died within 4 hours. Japanese yew killed 2 of 8 steers in a pasture when yard trimmings were thrown over the fence.[8] The first steer was found dead the next day and the second was trembling. Thirty-six hours later, that steer collapsed and died while being restrained for treatment. One Angus cow and two calves were found dead in a residential yard containing yew.[12] Three other cows were removed from the yard, but died during the following 3 days.

In the winter of 2001, the author became aware of a herd of 70 third trimester cows turned into a new pasture. Nine cows were dead the following morning. Three more cows collapsed and died before they could be removed from the pasture. Five more cows were dead by the end of the following day. Four cows aborted late-term dead calves within 4 days of yew ingestion. The owner had removed yew bushes from around the house 2 months earlier and deposited them in a ditch in the pasture to slow erosion. Several had taken root and were still green at the time of the poisoning.

The onset of intoxication in horses may occur within an hour of ingestion. A pony given 120 g of an aqueous slurry of Japanese yew showed signs of intoxication within 1 hour.[10] The lips and tail were atonic, and the pulse was not palpable from the external maxillary artery. The pony became progressively ataxic and paretic, trembled, developed an audible respiratory grunt, and collapsed to lateral recumbency. The course of clinical intoxication lasted less than 45 minutes. Similarly, rapid onset and short clinical courses have been corroborated from field observations. In one case, two horses were found dead in their paddock and a third collapsed and died while being led to another location.[24]

A case of suspected Japanese yew intoxication has been reported in a dog.[21] Clinical signs preceding initial presentation included 1 week's duration of intermittent vomiting, seizuring, and aggressive behavior. Signs resolved during hospitalization but resumed when the dog was returned to its home. This puppy had a history of chewing yew branches in the yard and the problems resolved after the shrubs were removed.

The toxic potential of *Taxus* has been evaluated in canaries[19] and budgerigars.[20] Two canaries given a total dose of 240 mg (12 g/kg body weight) of an aqueous slurry of ground *Taxus media* died less than 2 hours after showing signs of regurgitation, dyspnea, depression, and weakness. One of four budgies died after two doses of 250 mg of *Taxus media* given 90 minutes apart. Two hours after the initial dose, all four budgies showed signs of intoxication including repeated attempts to vomit, wide-based stance, dyspnea, and ataxia. One of the four died within 15 minutes of onset, showing signs of cyanosis of the eyelids and feet. The remaining budgies were ataxic for 2 to 4 more hours but recovered completely within 24 hours. It was concluded that budgerigars are less susceptible than canaries to yew intoxication.

Lesions. Diagnosis of yew poisoning is commonly based on a history of sudden death in livestock having had access to yard shrubs from clippings or after escape from the pasture. Necropsy lesions are not diagnostic; however, close examination of stomach or rumen contents for the flattened, evergreen needles is highly significant and often the basis for diagnosis. Gross and microscopic lesions are rarely identified, although congestion of the abomasum and moderate congestion and interlobular edema of the lungs have been reported.[14] Inflammation of the stomach and small intestines is more likely seen in monogastrics and animals surviving beyond a few hours.

Diagnostic Testing. Taxine alkaloids are difficult to isolate; however, extracts of gastrointestinal contents from poisoned animals can be compared to plant extracts. Reported methods for detection include mass spectrometry,[25] thin layer chromatography,[6] gas chromatography,[26] and liquid chromatography/mass spectrometry.[27]

Treatment. Successful treatment has not been experimentally demonstrated. Restraint necessary for treatment may precipitate cardiac arrest and therefore must be minimized. Administration of activated charcoal to bind the toxic alkaloid-like compounds from yew may require mixing with a palatable feed to allow passive ingestion by exposed livestock. Alternatively, three intoxicated goats survived after being treated by rumenotomy, disposal of contents, and replacement with mineral oil, electrolytes, activated charcoal, and alfalfa pellets.[13] Removal of the *Taxus*-containing rumen contents and instillation of activated charcoal (1 to 2 g/kg body weight) probably would have produced comparable results.

Prognosis. Simple-stomached animals are likely to die within 12 hours. Full recovery is expected in those that survive beyond this time. Ruminants, because of their anatomic differences and the associated retention of forage in the rumen, may die up to 3 days after ingestion of yew.

Prevention and Control. As with other ornamental plant poisonings, access must be denied to landscaped yards and discarded clippings. Yew clippings should be composted, burned, or sent to a landfill.

REFERENCES

1. Turner N.J., Szczawinski AF: *Common poisonous plants and mushrooms of North America*, Portland, Ore, 1991, Timber Press.
2. Wilson CR et al: Taxines: a review of the mechanism and toxicity of yew *(Taxus* spp.) alkaloids, *Toxicon* 39:175, 2001.
3. Miller RW: A brief survey of *Taxus* alkaloids and other taxane derivatives, *J Nat Prod* 43:425, 1980.
4. Tekol Y: Negative chronotropic and atrioventricular blocking effects of taxine on isolated frog heart and its acute toxicity in mice, *Plant Med* 5:357, 1985.
5. Tekol Y: Electrophysiology of the mechanisms of action of the yew toxin, taxine, on the heart, *Arzneimmittelforschung* 37:428, 1987.
6. Witherup KM et al: *Taxus* spp. needles contain amounts of taxol comparable to the bark of *Taxus brevifolia*; analysis and isolation, *J Nat Prod* 53:1249, 1990.
7. Puyt JD et al. Yew, poisonous plant no. 2, *Point Veterinaire* 13:86, 1982.
8. Alden CL et al: Japanese yew poisoning of large domestic animals in the Midwest, *J Am Vet Med Assoc* 170:314, 1977.
9. Cummins RO et al: Near-fatal yew berry intoxication treated with external cardiac pacing and digoxin-specific FAB antibody fragments, *Ann Emerg Med* 19:38, 1990.
10. Lowe JE et al: *Taxus cuspidata* (Japanese yew) poisoning in horses, *Cornell Vet* 60:36, 1970.
11. Thomson GW, Barker IK: Japanese yew *(Taxus cuspidata)* poisoning in cattle, *Can Vet J* 19:320, 1978.
12. Kerr LA, Edwards WC: Japanese yew: a toxic ornamental shrub, *Vet Med/Small Anim Clin* 76:1339, 1981.
13. Casteel SW, Cook WO: Japanese yew poisoning in ruminants, *Mod Vet Pract* 66:875, 1985.
14. Panter KE et al: English yew poisoning in 43 cattle, *J Am Vet Med Assoc* 202:1476, 1993.
15. Karns PA: Intoxication in horses due to ingestion of Japanese yew *(Taxus cuspidata). Equine Pract* 5:12, 1983.
16. Orr AB: Poisoning in domestic animals and birds, *Vet Rec* 64:339, 1952.
17. Kohler H, Grunberg W: Yew poisoning in a kangaroo, *Archiv Fur Experimentelle Veterinarmedizin* 14:1149, 1960.
18. Jordan WJ: Yew *(Taxus baccata)* poisoning in pheasants *(Phasianus colchicus), Tijdschrift voor Diergeneeskunde* 89(suppl 1):187, 1964.
19. Arai M et al: Evaluation of selected plants for their toxic effects in canaries, *J Am Vet Med Assoc* 200:1329, 1992.
20. Shropshire CM et al: Evaluation of selected plants for acute toxicosis in budgerigars, *J Am Vet Med Assoc* 200:936, 1992.
21. Evans KL, Cook JR: Japanese yew poisoning in a dog, *J Am Anim Hosp Assoc* 27:300, 1991.
22. Schulte T: Lethal intoxication with leaves of the yew tree *(Taxus baccata), Arch Toxicol* 34:153-158, 1975.
23. Van Ingen G et al: Sudden unexpected death due to *Taxus* poisoning. a report of five cases, with review of the literature, *Forensic Sci Internatl* 56:8, 1992.
24. Rook JS: Japanese yew toxicity, *Vet Med* 89:950, 1994.
25. Smith RA: Comments on diagnosis of intoxication due to *Taxus, Vet Hum Toxicol* 31:177, 1988.
26. Sinn LE, Porterfield JF: Fatal taxine poisoning from yew leaf ingestion, *J Forensic Sci* 36:599, 1991.
27. Kite GC et al: Detecting *Taxus* poisoning in horses using liquid chromatography/mass spectrometry, *Vet Human Toxicol* 42:151, 2000.

TROPANE ALKALOIDS

John A. Pickrell, Fred Oehme, and Shajan A. Mannala

Sources. *Datura* spp (Jimson weed, Angel's trumpet) occurs as a weed in gardens, crop fields, and dry lots where livestock are confined (Color Plates 22 and 23). Although it grows throughout the United States, *Datura* grows best in fertile soils often located in the eastern half of the United States. *Atropa belladonna* (belladonna) grows throughout the United States and is cultivated in gardens.[1] Convolvulus (bindweed) is fast becoming the predominant plant along the front range of the Rocky Mountains[2,3] (Color Plate 24).

Toxicokinetics.   Belladonna alkaloids include atropine, hyoscyamine, and hyoscine. *Datura* contains hyoscyamine, atropine, and scopolamine.

The toxic level is 0.15 mg/kg body weight of alkaloid. Cattle may be killed from ingestion of plants at 0.06% to 0.09% of body weight.[4] The course of disease may be as short as minutes or hours and is usually less than 1.5 days.

Mechanism of Action.   These alkaloids are anticholinergic, causing a parasympatholytic action ("red as a beet, dry as a bone, mad as a hen, and crazy as a calf on jimsonweed").[1,4-6] They are competitive antagonists of acetylcholine at muscarinic cholinergic receptors.

Toxicity and Risk Factors.   Although the toxin is present in all parts of the plant, it is most concentrated in the seeds.[1] *Datura* (Jimson weed) is unpalatable and is eaten only by hungry animals.[7]

Clinical Signs.   Pigs are most frequently affected, but all species are susceptible. Initially animals show thirst and have flushed skin. Second, they develop mydriasis and have visual disturbances resulting in insensible wandering or blindness. Restlessness and muscular twitching progress to incoordination, paralysis, and delirium (hallucinations). Respiratory paralysis may occur and results in death. At low doses, signs are parasympatholytic: dry mucous membranes, gastrointestinal atony and tympany, tachycardia, convulsions, and a reduction in urine output.[1,4-6]

Clinical Pathology.   Changes are nonspecific, reflecting the condition of the animal.

Lesions.   No significant visible lesions are noted.[1,4-6]

Diagnostic Testing.   Presence of the plant in the gastrointestinal contents or in the pasture or hay plus the relevant clinical signs are used to diagnose this intoxication.[1,4-6] Care should be taken to differentiate this condition from rabies and encephalitic disease.[4] The tropane alkaloids can be found in urine or gastrointestinal contents, but testing is not routinely available in many diagnostic laboratories.[8]

Treatment.   Treatment is limited to controlling the signs of the animal. Mania can be controlled only with tranquilizers (diazepam or phenobarbital) or anesthesia (pentobarbital). Occasionally large doses of parasympathetic drugs may be of use.[5] However, arecoline and pilocarpine are not recommended because they tend to depress breathing.[7]

Prognosis.   Death may occur within minutes to hours at high exposure levels.[4] At lower levels, prognosis is considered to be guarded.

Prevention and Control.   Remove animals from the source of the plant.[6]

REFERENCES

1. Osweiler GD: *The National Veterinary Medical Series Toxicology,* Philadelphia, 1996, Williams & Wilkins.

2. Schultheiss PC et al: Toxicity of field bindweed (*Convolvulus arvense*) to mice. *Vet Hum Toxicol* 37:452, 1995.

3. Todd FG et al: Tropane alkaloids and toxicity of *Convolvulus arvensis, Phytochemistry* 39:301, 1995.

4. Murphy M: *A field guide to common animal poisons,* Ames, Iowa, 1996, Iowa State University Press.

5. Fowler M: *Poisonous plants: a veterinary guide to toxic syndromes* (a CD-ROM), Davis, Calif, 1996, University of California.

6. Pickrell JA et al: *Poisonous plant collection* (a CD-ROM), Manhattan, Kan, 1999, Kansas State University.

7. Hulbert LC, Oehme FW: *Plants poisonous to livestock.* Manhattan, Kan, 1968, Kansas State University.

8. Ori K, Mikata H, Tsuromori T: A rapid determination method for scopolia extract in gastrointestinal drugs by capillary electrophoresis, *Yakugaku Zasshi* 119:868, 1999 (ABS, Japanese).

TRYPTAMINE ALKALOIDS

Steven S. Nicholson

Synonyms.   Canary grass poisoning, phalaris grass toxicosis, and phalaris staggers are names for the disease caused by tryptamine alkaloids.

Sources.   The toxicity of phalaris grasses is associated with the presence of tryptamine alkaloids in the plants. *Phalaris* spp. reported to have induced toxic effects in cattle and sheep include *P. angusta* in Argentina, *P. caroliniana,* and *P. minor* in the United States, as well as *P. aquatica* (formerly tuberosa), *P. arundinacea* (reed canary grass), and *P. canariensis* in several countries including Australia, New Zealand, Norway, and South Africa (Color Plate 25). Signs and lesions of chronic phalaris toxicosis were reported in feedlot lambs, some of which had no known exposure to phalaris grasses, and low levels of tryptamine alkaloids were detected in the feed.[1] *P. coerulescens* (blue canary grass), which contains alkaloids related to tryptamine alkaloids, is associated with sudden deaths of horses in Australia.[2]

Toxicokinetics.   Three alkaloids (*N,N*-dimethylated indole-alkylated amines) in *Phalaris* spp. are related to the neurotransmitter serotonin (5-hydroxy-tryptamine). These alkaloids are thought to be responsible for the neurologic signs and lesions of canary grass poisoning. Administration of tryptamine alkloids orally or parenterally to sheep has reproduced the acute toxicosis.

Horses fed reed canary grass may excrete the substituted tryptamine compound bufotenine in the urine.[3]

Mechanism of Action.   Tryptamine alkaloids appear to act directly on serotonergic receptors in specific brain and spinal cord nuclei. Effects in certain cranial nerve cell bodies may be the cause of prehensile malfunction of the lips and tongue sometimes seen in cattle.

Toxicity and Risk Factors.   Phalaris grasses are valuable cool season forages. They may be planted for pasture and seeds may be introduced in hay or as contaminants in ryegrass, wheat, or oat seed. Alkaloid content may increase during rapid growth after rainfall. Toxicosis has been reported in sheep and cattle. However, young lambs that are nursing affected ewes have not developed clinical signs. Horses grazing pastures toxic to ruminants are apparently not affected.

Clinical Signs. In sheep, a peracute toxicosis causes ventricular fibrillation, respiratory distress, and cyanosis. Sudden death may occur even before onset of neurologic signs.

Excitability, muscle tremors, uncoordinated gait, knuckling, staggering, and falling occur in the acute form of phalaris toxicosis in cattle and sheep. Head nodding and a stiff rabbit-hopping gait may be noted. Forcing the animals to move enhances the clinical signs. Handling an affected animal may induce convulsions, which include paddling and tetany. Left alone, signs diminish and the affected animal may stand up and return to the group. Recovery from acute canary grass poisoning in cattle and sheep generally occurs within a few days if the animals are slowly and quietly moved away from the source. Signs may persist in some sheep for several weeks. Relapse in sheep up to 5 months later has been reported.[4,5]

Chronic canary grass toxicosis in sheep and cattle is called *phalaris staggers*. The signs develop gradually and usually appear during the first 1 to 4 months of grazing. However, a striking feature of chronic toxicosis in some cattle and sheep is the delayed onset of signs up to 5 months after last grazing phalaris grass. Signs, which resemble those of acute poisoning, persist for weeks after removal from the forage. Chronic poisoning in cattle may begin with trembling and an un-coordinated gait, which progresses to a wasting condition caused by the inability to prehend forage or feed. Attempts to lick the muzzle or eat cause the tongue to dart out one side of the mouth. Rear limb ataxia and stiffness are reported. Morbidity rates vary from 5% to 50% in reported outbreaks and mortality is high. Recovery may occur in young cattle.

Clinical Pathology. Increased serum creatine kinase is attributed to partial recumbency. Greenish intracytoplasmic granules have been observed within macrophages of the cerebrospinal fluid (CSF) of sheep. Mildly increased protein concentration and increased small mononuclear cells in CSF have been reported.

Lesions. Lesions may be minimal or not present in early peracute or acute deaths. Macroscopic lesions include green-ish pigment in the renal cortex and in transverse sections of fixed CNS specimens. Focal, well-demarcated, bilaterally symmetrical, greenish-gray discoloration was seen in the midbrain corresponding to the pontine, lateral geniculate, or red nuclei, and within the medulla oblongata. Similar pig-mentation was found throughout the length of the spinal cord in the ventral horns.

Microscopic lesions include numerous neurons through-out the brain stem and spinal cord that contain varying amounts of greenish-brown to black intracytoplasmic (usually perinuclear) granular pigment. Electron micrograph of a neuronal perikaryon showed the granules confined within lysosomes. Degenerative lesions are in the medial longitudinal fasciculus and throughout the spinal cord within the ventral, lateral, and ventromedial areas of white matter.

In the most severely affected areas, lesions consisted of widespread individual axon sheath swelling, with axonal necrosis and loss, demyelination, macrophage infiltration within some axon sheaths, and diffuse marked gemistocytic and fibrillary astrocytosis.

Diagnosis. A history of grazing *Phalaris* spp., the presence of clinical signs of acute or chronic phalaris toxicosis, the elimination of other tremorogenic toxicoses (ryegrass stag-gers, paspalum staggers, bermuda grass tremors), and the presence of compatible histopathologic lesions confirm diag-nosis. Pitfalls in recognition of phalaris toxicosis include the possible 4- to 5-month delay of signs and relapses of acute cases, especially in sheep.

Treatment. Affected animals should be removed slowly and quietly from the source of the toxin. Handling or forced movement may induce convulsions or sudden death from cardiac or respiratory failure, especially in sheep.

Prognosis. Some sheep and cattle may recover from acute phalaris grass toxicosis within a few days of being removed from the toxic forage. Mortality may be high in chronic cases. The potential for delayed onset of signs and relapse must be considered.

Prevention and Control. *Phalaris* spp. are often grazed extensively by sheep and cattle, without harm. If clinical signs develop, the animals should be removed from the pasture. Supplemental cobalt in sheep, by drench or in heavy cobalt rumen pellets, is a preventive measure used for phalaris staggers in Australia.

REFERENCES

1. Lean IJ et al: Tryptamine alkaloid toxicosis in feedlot sheep, *J Am Vet Med Assoc* 195:768, 1989.
2. Colegate SM et al: Suspected blue canary grass *(Phalaris coerulescens)* poisoning of horses, *Aust Vet J* 77:537, 1999.
3. Hintz HF: Reed canary grass and bufotenine, *Equine Pract* 12:17, 1990.
4. Nicholson SS et al: Delayed phalaris grass toxicosis in sheep and cattle, *J Am Vet Med Assoc* 195:345, 1989.
5. East NE, Higgins RJ: Canary grass *(Phalaris* sp) toxicosis in sheep in California, *J Am Vet Med Assoc* 192:667, 1988.

GLYCOSIDES

CALCINOGENIC GLYCOSIDES

Petra A. Volmer

Synonyms. Calcinosis, enzootic calcinosis, espichamento, espichacao, and enteque seco are terms that have been used to describe the disease syndrome resulting from exposure to these plants. Naalehu disease in Hawaii and Manchester wasting disease in Jamaica are associated with similar clinical and pathologic findings as with the calcinogenic plants. The etiology for these diseases is not clear, although mineral imbalances in the soil and, in the case of Manchester wasting disease, the pasture grass *Stenotaphrum secundatum* have been implicated.[1]

Sources.   Several members of the Solanaceae family contain vitamin D–like compounds. *Solanum malacoxylon* (synonym *S. glaucophyllum*) is the calcinogenic plant responsible for the disease enteque seco in Argentina and espichamento or espichacao in Brazil. Common names for *S. malacoxylon* include American egg plant and Sendtner. *S. verbascifolium* and *S. torvum* have also demonstrated vitamin D–like activity.[2] *Nierembergia veitchii* is a Solanaceous plant that has caused enzootic calcinosis of livestock in Brazil. *Cestrum diurnum* (day-blooming jessamine, wild jasmine, day cestrum, king-of-the-day, Chinese inkberry), another member of this family, is associated with enzootic calcinosis in cattle and horses in Florida. These plants should not be confused with other members of the Solanaceae family, especially the *Solanum* species (nightshades), which cause gastrointestinal irritation and affect cholinergic nerve transmission.

Although the previously described plants are considered undesirable weeds, another calcinogenic plant has some value as a pasture crop. *Trisetum flavescens* (golden oatgrass, yellow oatgrass), a member of the Poaceae family, is responsible for enzootic calcinosis in cattle, goats, and horses in the Alpine regions of Germany and Austria. *Trisetum* is used as a forage crop in mountain pastures at altitudes of greater than 1000 meters.

Mechanism of Action.   The calcinogenic plants contain a glycoside of 1,25-dihydroxycholecalciferol (calcitriol) or a calcitriol-like compound. Calcitriol is the active form of vitamin D (cholecalciferol) and acts to increase calcium absorption from the gastrointestinal tract, increase bone resorption of calcium, and decrease renal calcium excretion. Excess calcitriol overwhelms normal calcium feedback mechanisms, resulting in hypercalcemia and hyperphosphatemia. Prolonged elevations of serum calcium and phosphorus, with calcium × phosphorus products greater than 60 mg/dl, can result in soft tissue calcification. Mineralization of vital organ systems such as cardiac, pulmonary, renal, and gastrointestinal often results in the demise of the animal by interfering with normal physiologic processes.

Toxicity and Risk Factors.   Experiments with the plants *Solanum malacoxylon, Cestrum diurnum, Trisetum flavescens,* and *Nierembergia veitchii* indicated average vitamin D contents of 82,800, 63,200, 12,000, and 16,400 IU/kg, respectively.[3] Animals grazing infested pastures with limited access to other food sources are at risk. Grazing for prolonged periods (weeks or more) may result in hypercalcemia, hyperphosphatemia, and subsequent calcification.

Clinical Signs.   Cattle, horses, sheep, goats, and pigs have been affected. The disease is progressive, and may take weeks to manifest. Early signs often go unnoticed. At later stages, animals exhibit depression, weakness, weight loss, stunted growth, infertility, anorexia, cardiac arrhythmias or tachycardia, impaired or stilted gait, walking or grazing on knees, and frequent recumbency.[4-8] Most of these signs can be attributed to hypercalcemia and subsequent soft tissue calcification. Death may result from emaciation and weakness, as well as from cardiac and pulmonary insufficiency.[9] Administration of *S. malacoxylon* to rabbits suggests that the calcinogenic principle may pass through the placenta to the fetus.[9]

Clinical Pathology.   During the time of ingestion, animals develop a hypercalcemia and hyperphosphatemia. These levels may decrease within days after removal from the offending plant material, resulting in normal calcium and phosphorus levels despite mineralization and persistent clinical signs.[4] As soft tissue calcification progresses, elevations in blood urea nitrogen (BUN) and creatinine may be noted on serum chemistry analyses. Radiology may reveal calcification of multiple organs, including the vascular walls of the limbs.[4]

Lesions.   Gritty, white-tan deposits are apparent on the surfaces or within the parenchyma of various organs such as kidney, intestines, stomach, heart, great vessels, bones, tendons, ligaments, and lungs. The extent of tissue change is related to the duration of the hypercalcemia.[10] Histopathology may reveal degranulation of thyroid C cells and accumulation of secretory granules of parathyroid chief cells early in the course of the disease. Following several weeks of exposure, hyperplasia of thyroid C cells and atrophy of the parathyroids may be noted.[11] Basophilic granular material (mineralization) may be found in the renal basement membranes, glomerular tufts, Bowman's capsule, pulmonary alveolar septa, bronchiolar epithelium, endocardium, gastric and intestinal musculature, and other tissues.

Diagnostic Testing.   Elevated levels of 1,25-dihydroxycholecalciferol may be detectable in serum of recently exposed animals.

Treatment.   Animals should be removed from the plant source and given clean feed. Any supplemental vitamin D preparations should be discontinued. Individual treatment of animals to decrease serum calcium and phosphorus, such as the use of furosemide, prednisolone, saline diuresis, and calcitonin or pamidronate, is usually not practical in herd situations. Addition of aluminum sulfate in the diet of rabbits experimentally exposed to *S. malacoxylon* prevented the absorption of phosphate and reduced the incidence of calcified lesions.[12]

Prognosis.   The prognosis is poor once extensive calcification has occurred. Soft tissue calcification may gradually resorb to a small degree, but surviving animals usually remain chronically poor-doers. In one study, sheep spontaneously poisoned by *N. veitchii* were monitored for up to 17 months following removal from an infested pasture. Spontaneous death occurred within months 13 and 17 of the study. Postmortem examination revealed gross and histopathologic lesions similar to those described for enzootic calcinosis, but there was evidence of a slight decrease in the degree of arterial calcification. There was no evidence of regression in arterial intimal proliferation, osseous and cartilaginous metaplasia of arteries and cardiac valves, or in bones or the thyroid gland. Spontaneous deaths were attributed to pulmonary edema secondary to left-sided congestive heart failure.[13] In a similar study, rabbits examined at intervals up to 26 months following the calcinogenic insult exhibited limited reversibility of calcification in lung, kidney, and aortic wall. Aortic wall and tendons had the least tendency to demineralize.[14]

Prevention and Control. Toxicoses are more likely to occur when other nutritious forage is not available. Elimination of *Solanum*, *Cestrum*, and *Nierembergia* species may require herbicidal or manual removal of the plant stands. It is recommended to cut *Trisetum flavescens* hay after blooming because calcinogenicity decreases with maturity of this plant.[4] Concentration of 1,25-dihydroxycholecalciferol in *Trisetum* also decreases during the drying process, so calcinosis can be controlled by harvesting dry hay instead of haylage.[4] Ensiling does not destroy the calcinogenic activity of *Trisetum flavescens*.[15] *Trisetum*-infested pastures can be plowed and reseeded with other forage crops.[4]

REFERENCES

1. Arnold RM, Fincham IH: Manchester wasting disease: a calcinosis caused by pasture grass *(Stenotaphrum secundatum)* in Jamaica, *Trop Anim Health Prod* 29:174, 1997.
2. Boland RL: Plants as a source of vitamin D_3 metabolites, *Nutr Rev* 44:1, 1986.
3. Mello JRB, Habermehl GG: Qualitative and quantitative studies on the effects of calcinogenic plants, *Dtsch Tierarztl Wochenschr* 105:25, 1998.
4. Braun U et al: Enzootic calcinosis in goats caused by golden oat grass *(Trisetum flavescens)*, *Vet Rec* 146:161, 2000.
5. Campero CM, Odriozola E: A case of *Solanum malacoxylon* toxicity in pigs, *Vet Hum Tox* 32:238, 1990.
6. Durand R et al: Intoxication in cattle from *Cestrum diurnum*, *Vet Hum Tox* 41:26, 1999.
7. Krook L et al: Hypercalcemia and calcinosis in Florida horses: implication of the shrub, *Cestrum diurnum*, as the causative agent, *Cornell Vet* 65:26, 1975.
8. Krook L et al: *Cestrum diurnum* poisoning in Florida cattle, *Cornell Vet* 65:557, 1975.
9. Gorniak SL et al: Evaluation in rabbits of the fetal effects of maternal ingestion of *Solanum malacoxylon*, *Vet Res Comm* 23:307, 1999.
10. Dammrich K et al: Skeletal changes in cattle poisoned with *Solanum malaxocylon*, *Zentralblatt fur Veterinarmedizin-A* 22: 313-, 1975.
11. Collins WT et al: Ultrastructural evaluation of parathyroid glands and thyroid C cells of cattle fed *Solanum malacoxylon*, *Am J Path* 87:603, 1977.
12. Wase AW: Effect of *Solanum malacoxylon* on serum calcium and phosphate in laboratory animals, *Fed Proc* 31:708, 1972.
13. De Barros SS et al: Clinical course and reversibility of enzootic calcinosis caused by *Nierembergia veitchii* in sheep, *Pesquisa Veterinaria Brasileira* 12:1, 1992.
14. Hanichen T, Hermanns W: The question of reversibility of tissue calcification in enzootic calcinosis of cattle and in experimental hypervitaminosis D, *Dtsch Tierarztl Wochenschr* 97:479, 1990.
15. Heinritzi K et al: Investigations on the calcinogenic activity of ensiled yellow oat grass *(Trisetum flavescens)*, *Zeitschrift Tierphysiologie, Tierernahrung Futtermittelkunde* 39:139, 1977.

CARBOXYATRACTYLOSIDE

John A. Pickrell, Fred W. Oehme, and Shajan A. Mannala

Sources. Carboxyatractyloside is a diterpenoid glycoside that occurs naturally in plants found in Europe, Africa, South America, and Asia. It may be present at 600 ppm in dried plants.[1] This toxin is found in *Xanthium* (cocklebur), an annual plant that grows throughout the United States (Color Plates 26 and 27). Cocklebur grows readily from a spiny 1.5-cm bur in floodplains or moist rich soils.[2,3]

Toxicokinetics. The toxin is water soluble, readily absorbed, and acts quickly. Death may occur in a few hours. Alternatively, the course of disease may be protracted for as long as 2 to 3 days.[2-4]

Mechanism of Action. Carboxyatractyloside is a glycoside that competitively inhibits the adenine nucleoside carrier in mitochondria and oxidative phosphorylation. This action blocks adenosine triphosphate (ATP) transport into mitochondria. In vitro, proximal tubular cells are unusually sensitive to atractyloside.[1,2,4]

Toxicity and Risk Factors. The toxin is present in the seeds and in the recently generated cotyledons (seed leaves) and is stable to drying. Seeds contain higher amounts of toxin than dicotyledonary seedlings. However, most animals do not eat seeds unless they are softened. Although cattle and sheep are affected, most cases occur in swine.[2-5] Cotyledonary seedlings fed at 0.75% to 3% of body weight or ground bur fed at 20% to 30% of the ration caused acute depression, convulsions, and death.[1-4,6]

Clinical Signs. Depression, abdominal pain and tenderness, anorexia, salivation, vomiting, and dyspnea can occur. Nervous signs include fasciculations, extensor rigidity, spasmodic contractions of the limbs and neck muscles, convulsions, opisthotonus, paddling, prostration, coma, and death.[2-5] Hyperexcitability, blindness, and acute death have been reported.[4,6]

Clinical Pathology. Changes indicate severe liver involvement: increased γ-glutamyltransferase (GGT), bile acids, aspartate aminotransferase (AST), or alanine aminotransaminase (ALT).[4] Marked hypoglycemia and elevated liver enzymes occur in pigs fed cocklebur seedlings, ground bur, or atractyloside.[7]

Lesions. Lesions include gastrointestinal irritation, a firm, pale liver, and hepatic centrilobular hemorrhages on the cut surface, as well as moderate to massive histologic necrosis. Acute nephritis was indicated by mild to moderate tubular degeneration. Occasionally, seedlings, seeds, or burs may be found in the gastrointestinal contents.[2,4-6]

Diagnostic Testing. Access to plants and appropriate signs or lesions are typically used to make the diagnosis. Atractyloside measurement is not routinely available in United States diagnostic laboratories.

Treatment.   Treatment is limited to supportive care.

Prognosis.   The prognosis is guarded to poor for pigs consuming toxic amounts of dicotyledonary atractyloside. Pigs that are initially unaffected may develop liver disease at a later date.[2,4,5]

Prevention and Control.   Prevention is limited to denying animals access to the plants or destroying the plants with herbicides.[2-5]

REFERENCES

1. Obatomi DK, Bach PH: Biochemistry and toxicology of the diterpenoid glycoside atractyloside, *Food Chem Toxicol* 36:335, 1998.
2. Osweiler GD: *The National Veterinary Medical Series Toxicology,* Philadelphia, 1996, Williams and Wilkins.
3. del Carmen Mendez M: Intoxication by *Xanthium cavanillesii* in cattle and sheep in southern Brazil, *Vet Hum Toxicol* 40:144, 1998.
4. Murphy M: *A field guide to common animal poisons,* Ames, Iowa, 1996, Iowa State University Press.
5. Hulbert LC, Oehme FW: *Plants poisonous to livestock,* Manhattan, Kan, 1968, Kansas State University,.
6. Witte ST et al: Cocklebur toxicosis in cattle associated with the consumption of mature *Xanthium strumarium, J Vet Diagn Invest* 2:263, 1990.
7. Stuart BP, Cole RJ, Gosser HS: Cocklebur (*Xanthium strumarium,* L. var. strumarium) intoxication in swine: review and redefinition of the toxic principle, *Vet Pathol* 18:368, 1981.

CARDIAC GLYCOSIDES

Francis D. Galey

Sources.   Oleander *(Nerium oleander)* is an ornamental evergreen shrub with leathery, dark-green leaves (Color Plates 28 and 29). A native of the Mediterranean region, the bush is a member of the Apocyanacea family. That family also includes laurel *(N. indicum),* yellow oleander *(Thevetia peruviana),* and dogbane *(Apocynum* spp.) (Color Plates 30 and 31). Other plants that contain cardiac glycosides include foxglove *(Digitalis* spp.), lily-of-the-valley *(Convallaria majalis),* some species of milkweed *(Asclepias* spp.), and *Kalanchoe* spp. (Color Plate 32).

Oleander is cultivated widely in the southern United States, including most of California, as well as in many other parts of the world.[1-3] Rose laurel is found in Hawaii,[3] and yellow oleander is found in Australia and Florida.[4,5] Dogbane is a common weed that is indigenous to the United States.[5]

All parts of oleander are toxic, and ingestion of clippings from the plant is a common cause of poisoning in animals.[6] Because this plant is most commonly involved in poisonings, it is discussed in most detail.

N. oleander is an evergreen bush that can grow 20 feet tall.[1,3,7] Oleander bark is smooth and remains green until it is several years old. The leathery, simple, oblong-lanceolate, pointed leaves are long and narrow (10 to 30 cm × 3 cm). They are dark gray-green and are arranged in whorls of three or may rarely be opposite. The leaves have a prominent midrib with parallel veins that extend to the periphery from the midrib. Distinctive stomata exist on the leaves that can

be used for identification.[7,8] The flowers are borne in terminal clusters of dark-red, pink, or white blossoms in the spring and early summer. Yellow oleander has a yellow flower and a milky sap. The fruit of oleander is a long, narrow pod with many hairy seeds.

Dried and fresh leaves of oleander are considered to be highly toxic to animals because of glycosidal toxins that cause sudden death with gastroenteritis and heart failure. A major cause of oleander poisoning in livestock is hedge trimmings tossed into dry lots or hidden in hay. Otherwise, the plant is bitter to farm animals and frequently avoided. Animals have reportedly been poisoned following ingestion of water into which plant material has been placed.[9] Companion animals such as dogs are also reportedly susceptible to oleander poisoning from ingestion of plant, leaves, or water in which oleander has soaked.

Toxicokinetics.   The toxicity of oleander results from several cardiac glycosides, the most prominent of which is oleandrin (the aglycone is oleandrigenin) and neriine.[1] Little is known about the kinetics of oleander in animals. Experimentally, oleander is rapidly absorbed. Massive doses of the leaves may kill an animal within 1 hour. More commonly, however, the toxic signs may appear 8 to 24 hours after exposure.[10] Evidence of oleandrin was observed in the milk of a dairy cow that died of oleander toxicosis.[10] However, testing of milk from herd mates and the bulk tank revealed no oleander toxin at 5 days after the last possible time of exposure in that case.

Mechanism of Action.   Cardiac glycosides cause poisoning by inhibiting Na^+/K^+ ATPase, which is essential for cardiac function. This effect is similar to that of digitalis glycosides.[1,11] Intravenous injection of oleandrin in dogs and cats led to direct autonomic effects, including vagal stimulation in the first 24 hours and beta-sympathetic stimulation after 24 hours.[11] The beta-sympathetic effect was unmasked by administration of atropine to block vagal effects. Animals ingesting oleander plant material also suffered from central (bleating and convulsing) and peripheral nervous system effects (tremors).[1] Livestock exposed to oleander may have diarrhea and can have large amounts of fluid in the bowel.[6]

Inhibition of sodium-potassium ATPase can lead to accumulation of potassium outside the cell and sodium within. The accumulation of potassium can lead to a cascade of calcium release, positive inotropy, and high-grade heart block caused by interference with vagal tone.[11,12] Animals with digitalis-type toxicosis have electrocardiographic abnormalities of slowed AV conduction, followed by dropped beats, and ST segment changes with progressive escape beats and ventricular arrhythmias.[10,12] If vagal effects are ablated, direct effects of oleander toxins on the sympathetic system may become apparent, leading directly to the tachyarrhythmias.[11] This direct effect on the sympathetic nervous system was demonstrated using blockade by propranolol after pretreatment of experimental dogs with atropine to ablate the vagal effects.[11]

Oleandrin given via IV injection resulted in increased aortic systolic, aortic mean, and left ventricular pressures while reducing overall cardiac output within 15 minutes of injection in dogs.[13]

Toxicity and Risk Factors. Oleander is an extremely toxic plant. As little as 0.005% of an animal's body weight in dry oleander leaves may be lethal (10 to 20 leaves for an adult horse or cow).[3] More recently, studies have determined median toxic doses of ground oleander leaves in horses and crossbred beef heifers.[10] The median toxic dose of oleander in the horse was estimated to be 26 mg/kg of plant per body weight (approximately seven average-sized leaves). The median toxic dose of oleander was estimated to be 45 mg/kg of plant per body weight for cattle, a level equivalent to approximately 12 average-sized leaves. One heifer that was given 1 g of plant/kg of body weight died within 45 minutes after ingestion without any evidence of lesions.

Oleander is toxic when dry. Most poisonings occur in animals that are exposed to clippings or to fallen and dried leaves. Thus, a significant risk factor for livestock can be the misguided feeding or mishandling of clippings from a trimmed or cut hedge of oleander. Other sources of oleander have included a variety of accidental inclusions in forages such as beet and other vegetable greens, as well as in hay.

Clinical Signs. Animals exposed to oleander are often found dead. If found alive, they present with rapidly developing, nonspecific signs that may resemble colic.[1,6] Clinical signs, if observed, develop 2 to 8 hours after exposure and may include abdominal pain, weakness, rumen atony, vomiting in some species, and excessive salivation.[1,3,8] Initially, bradycardia may be present for up to 24 hours, followed by a weak, irregular, fast pulse with tachycardia and ventricular arrhythmia.[1,3,8,10,11] Gallop rhythms have been reported in cattle with oleander toxicosis.[8] Affected animals may also develop lethargy, uneasiness, mydriasis, tremors, and increased urination, cyanosis, followed by excitement, intermittent convulsions, depression, dyspnea, and coma before death.[1,3] Abortion has been reported in monkeys.[14] Cardiac arrhythmias lead to death within 2 to 48 hours after the onset of signs.

The horses experimentally given 20 mg/kg of plant per body weight (total dose of approximately 6 medium-sized leaves) developed either no or mild signs.[10] However, horses given twice that amount of oleander in that experiment developed clinical signs of toxicosis within 8 hours after dosing. Initial signs included lethargy and mild colic. Diarrhea and weakness followed. By 24 hours after administration, horses developed a wide variety of cardiac arrhythmias including various AV conduction blocks and ventricular arrhythmias. Measurement of cardiac physiology parameters revealed no primary abnormalities until arrhythmias led to a decrease in function.

Two heifers given 25 mg/kg of ground oleander plant per body weight and 1 of 4 cattle given 50 mg/kg of plant per body weight were unaffected.[10] Three of 4 heifers given 50 mg/kg of plant per body weight and all animals given 100 mg/kg of body weight of oleander developed clinical poisoning. Affected cattle became weak and ataxic by 12 hours after administration. By 24 hours after administration of the higher levels, diarrhea, weakness, and lethargy were present. Most animals had audible dropped heartbeats, pulse deficits, and tachycardia by 24 hours after administration. In one heifer, one beat was skipped every third heartbeat at 12 hours after administration with 50 mg/kg of plant per body weight. All of the animals that developed signs were dead by 48 hours after administration. An animal exposed to a massive dose died within minutes without evidence of signs or lesions.

Clinical Pathology. Clinical chemistry changes in animals with oleander poisoning largely are those associated with colic. Hyperkalemia (up to twice normal in monkeys) occurring late in the toxic syndrome is most likely associated with damage to cardiac myocytes.[14] Alterations in electrolytes and cardiac physiology were not found to be significant in horses until cardiac arrhythmias led to a decrease in cardiac function.[10]

Lesions. Postmortem lesions reported for animals with oleander toxicosis vary from fluid in the bowels and cardiac congestion with myocardial necrosis to no lesions at all in cases of sudden death after a massive dose.* Lesions in horses include mild pulmonary edema, large amounts of fluid in the pericardium and body cavities, and histologic evidence of multifocal myocardial degeneration and necrosis.[6,10] Other changes in the heart can include mural thrombi and hemorrhage under the epicardial surface of many sections.[10] Affected cattle have variably large volumes of fluid in the bowels and varying degrees of thrombosis and hemorrhage in the heart.[10] Histologically, heart tissue has evidence of multifocal myocardial inflammation, degeneration, and necrosis. Mild renal tubular lesions have also been reported. Organ weights for the pancreas were decreased and for the adrenal glands were increased in monkeys given high levels of oleander.[14]

Diagnostic Testing. Diagnosis in some lethal cases may be facilitated by finding leaves in the environment, feed, or ingesta. However, leaves may be macerated beyond identification or passed into the posterior gastrointestinal tract. Leaf identification can be facilitated by identification of characteristic venation pattern and stomata in leaves.[6-8]

Historically, oleander glycosides have been tested using various immunoassay methods originally developed for monitoring digoxin-based medications based on the possibility of cross reaction between the different types of cardiac glycosides.[4,15,16] More recently, assays have been developed to identify oleandrin in ingesta and body fluids.[6,10] The new methods involve the use of two-dimensional thin layer chromatography (TLC) and high-performance liquid chromatography (HPLC). This two-dimensional TLC method has proved to be very useful for detection of oleandrin in gastrointestinal contents at a 0.02 ppm limit of detection.[6] The limit of detection for oleandrin using HPLC was 0.05 ppm. Replicate fortifications of stomach contents (n = 6) revealed a mean recovery of 85%.[17] More recently, high performance liquid chromatography with mass spectrometric detection has been employed to confirm oleander poisoning.[18]

---

*References 1, 3, 6, 8, 10, 14.

The TLC method was not found to be of sufficient sensitivity to consistently identify oleandrin in urine, although it was found on a few occasions. One Holstein dairy cow was found to have detectable (by TLC) oleandrin in milk after exposure to oleander leaves from a hay source.[10] Repeat testing of milk from previously affected survivors and the bulk tank at 5 days after exposure revealed no oleandrin. Oleandrin is not always expected in the upper gastrointestinal tract, but is usually present in the cecal or fecal material. Testing of feces has enabled diagnosis in horses on an antemortem basis.

Treatment. Exposed animals should be removed from the source. Very early after exposure, the gut should be evacuated using emesis (if appropriate). Otherwise, adsorption of the toxin using cholestyramine resins or activated charcoal has been suggested.[12] Repeated use of adsorbents may hasten toxin elimination by blocking enterohepatic recirculation of cardiac glycosides.[12] The use of potassium in fluids should be used only if hyperkalemia is demonstrated to be absent.[12] Calcium-containing solutions and quinidine should be avoided.

Atropine may be useful in treating bradyarrhythmias that may be observed in the first 24 hours after exposure.[11,12,19] Extreme care should be exercised when using atropine in the horse because fatal gut stasis may result. If its use is necessary, atropine can be slowly dripped intravenously to the horse, stopping immediately when desired effect (e.g., normalized heart rate) appears or if the gut begins to slow. Propranolol has been used experimentally to treat tachyarrhythmias because sympathetic nervous system effects predominate after 24 hours.[11,19] Lidocaine and phenytoin also may be useful to treat the tachyarrhythmias.[11,12,19] Additionally, the administration of anticardiac glycoside Fab antibodies has been suggested and used therapeutically for digitalis toxicosis[20] and in one case of oleander poisoning in a human.[16] The use of flunixin was useful in treating horses that had colic and diarrhea due to oleander poisoning in my experience.

Prognosis. Animals poisoned with oleander are often found dead. Despite early treatment, animals with oleander poisoning frequently die within hours to 2 days. In animals that survive sufficiently long to receive treatment, signs may persist for 24 hours or longer after the plant material is evacuated from the gut.[21] The possibility of permanent cardiac damage must be considered.

REFERENCES

1. Everist SL: *Poisonous plants of Australia*, ed 2, London, 1981, Angus and Robertson.
2. Kellerman TS et al: *Plant poisonings and mycotoxicoses of livestock in South Africa*, Cape Town, South Africa, 1988, Oxford University Press.
3. Kingsbury JM: *Poisonous plants of the United States and Canada*, Englewood Cliffs, NJ, 1964, Prentice-Hall.
4. Ansford A, Morris H: Oleander poisoning, *Toxicon* 3(suppl):15, 1983.
5. Knight AP: Oleander poisoning, *Compend Cont Ed Pract Vet* 10:262, 1988.
6. Galey FD et al: Diagnosis of oleander poisoning in livestock, *J Vet Diagn Invest* 8:358, 1996.
7. Frohne D, Pfander JH: *A colour atlas of poisonous plants* (Bisset NG, English translation), London, 1984, Wolfe Publishing.
8. Mahin L et al: A case report of *Nerium oleander* poisoning in cattle, *Vet Hum Toxicol*, 26:303, 1984.
9. Vahrmeijer J: *Poisonous plants of Southern Africa that cause livestock losses*, Cape Town, South Africa, 1981, Tafelberg Publishers.
10. Galey FD et al: In Garland T, Barr AC, editors: *Toxic plants and other natural toxicants*, New York, 1998, CAB International.
11. Szabuniewicz JD et al: Treatment of experimentally induced oleander poisoning, *Arch International Pharm* 189:12, 1971.
12. Adams HR: In Booth NH, McDonald LE, editors: *Veterinary pharmacology and Therapeutics*, ed 6, Ames, Iowa, 1988, Iowa State University Press.
13. Deavers SI et al: Effects of oleandrin on cardiovascular hemodynamics in the dog, *Am J Vet Res* 40:1421, 1979.
14. Schwartz WL et al: Toxicity of *Nerium oleander* in the monkey (*Cebus apella*), *Vet Pathol* 11:259, 1974.
15. Osterloh J et al: Oleander interference in the digoxin radioimmunoassay in a fatal ingestion, *J Am Med Assoc* 247:1596, 1982.
16. Shumaik GM et al: Oleander poisoning: treatment with digoxin-specific Fab antibody fragments, *Ann Emerg Med* 17:732, 1988.
17. Tor E et al: Determination of oleander glycosides in biological matrices by high performance liquid chromatography, *J Agric Food Chem* 44:2716, 1996.
18. Tracqui A et al: Confirmation of oleander poisoning by HPLC/MS, *Int J Legal Med* 111:32, 1998.
19. Szabuniewicz JD et al: Experimental oleander poisoning and treatment, *Southwest Vet* 25:105, 1972.
20. Haber E: Antibodies and digitalis: the modern revolution in the use of an ancient drug, *J Am College Cardiol* 5:111A, 1985.
21. Fowler ME: *Plant poisoning in small companion animals*, St Louis, 1980, Ralston Purina Company.

COUMARIN GLYCOSIDES

Anthony P. Knight

Synonyms. Synonyms for dicoumarol are dicoumarin, dicumarol, or dicumarin.

Sources. Many hundreds of coumarin glycosides are found in a wide variety of plant species of the genera Apiaceae, Fabaceae, Rutaceae, Compositae, and several smaller genera. One of these glycosides, the lactone of coumarinic acid (*o*-hydroxycinnamic acid) produces the pleasant, sweet, vanilla-like smell of a newly mown hay meadow. It is the high coumarin content in sweet vernal grass that produces its desirable smell. Well-known plants that contain significant amounts of coumarin include sweet clovers (*Melilotus* spp.), daphne (*Daphne* spp.), holygrass (*Heirochloe odorata*), and sweet vernal grass (*Anthoxanthum odoratum*).[1,2] Ferns (Polypodiaceae) and some pines (Pinaceae) also contain coumarins.[3] Coumarin glycosides present in the Mediterranean plant *Ferula communis* have also been associated with poisoning in sheep.[4]

The sweet clovers are the most important coumarin-containing plants associated with poisoning in animals. Yellow sweet clover was introduced to North America as a forage crop because of its drought-resistant properties, tolerance of saline-soils, and comparable nutritive value to that of alfalfa. It has subsequently become widely established as a common weed in many states throughout North America. Seven species of sweet clover are present in North America with about 20 species worldwide. The primary species that have become naturalized in North America include *Melilotus officinalis* (yellow sweet clover), *M. alba* (white sweet clover), and *M. indica* (sour clover, Indian melilot). White sweet clover is a larger, coarser plant with thicker stems, making it less desirable than the yellow species for hay making purposes.

Toxicokinetics. Although a useful forage for livestock, it was noted in 1924 that when cattle were fed moldy sweet clover hay or silage, they developed a fatal hemorrhagic syndrome known as sweet clover poisoning.[5] It was later established that certain soil fungi growing in the stems of sweet clover convert coumarin to dicoumarol, the active toxin responsible for sweet clover poisoning.[6] The most common fungi capable of converting coumarin glycosides to dicoumarol include *Aspergillus fumigatus*, *A. niger*, and members of the genera *Arthrobacter*, *Penicillium*, *Humicolor*, *Fusarium*, and *Mucor*.[7] Improperly cured hay with high moisture content promotes the growth of these soil fungi, particularly in the stems of the plants. The hay may therefore have no outward appearance of being moldy. At other times when moisture content is high the hay may be black and have a musty odor.[8] However, not all moldy sweet clover hay necessarily contains toxic levels of dicoumarol.

Dicoumarol (3,3″-methylen-bis-4-hydroxycoumarin), the primary toxin, is produced by fungi in the stems of the plants through a complex process whereby *o*-coumaric and melilotic acid glucosides are converted to beta-hydroxy-melilotic acid, then to 4-hydroxycoumarin, and finally to toxic dicoumarol.[3,6] The liver is the primary site of dicoumarol metabolism where it is oxidized in the liver mitochondria.[9,10] Salicylates, barbiturates, and diphenylhydantoin decrease the action of dicoumarol by displacing it from plasma proteins and inducing dicoumarol-metabolizing systems in the liver.[6,10] Coumarin compounds are primarily excreted through the kidneys.

Mechanism of Action. Coumarin itself is minimally toxic to animals, and only after prolonged feeding of the compound to dogs and laboratory animals has it been shown to cause liver damage.[9] Baboons fed large amounts of coumarin (67.5 mg/kg/day) for 2 years did not develop liver damage. Hepatotoxicity caused by coumarin has not been observed in other animals.

Dicoumarol, however, is readily absorbed from the digestive tract and interferes with vitamin K function by competitively inhibiting the epoxide reductase enzyme essential for regenerating the active form of vitamin K.[11] Common anticoagulant rodenticides also inhibit the same enzyme.[12] Vitamin K functions as a cofactor in the modification of specific glutamyl residues in the vitamin K–dependent plasma proteins to γ-carboxyglutamyl residues essential for the interaction of clotting factors with phospholipid surfaces.[13] In the absence of adequate vitamin K, there is marked reduction in the activation of prothrombin, and vitamin K–dependent factors VII, IX, and X are consumed, which results in a hemorrhagic diathesis.[3,6] Already formed clotting factors in the bloodstream are not affected, and it may take several days for these to be depleted. Therefore a delay of 2 to 14 days often occurs between the feeding of dicoumarol-

containing hay and the appearance of the hemorrhagic syndrome typical of sweet clover poisoning.

Toxicity and Risk Factors. Cattle are most frequently affected by eating moldy sweet clover hay containing high levels of dicoumarol, although horses and other livestock can be similarly affected.[14-16] Sheep are reported to be less susceptible to dicoumarol than are cattle.[17] Most poisoning from sweet clover occurs during the winter when animals are fed moldy sweet clover hay or silage. The highest levels of dicoumarol (165 ppm) occur in hay with the highest protein content.[18] Coumarin levels of 20 to 30 ppm cause severe coagulation defects.[19] Prolonged consumption of moldy sweet clover hay containing 10 ppm of dicoumarol leads to partial depletion of clotting factors and a hemorrhagic syndrome.[17] Animals usually have to consume the toxic hay for 4 to 5 weeks to sufficiently deplete their coagulation factors before the hemorrhagic syndrome can occur. Dicoumarol may remain toxic in hay for several years, whereas properly prepared sweet clover silage tends to have much lower levels of dicoumarol.[18]

Clinical Signs. Often the first indication of sweet clover poisoning in cattle is prolonged hemorrhaging from surgical sites following castration and dehorning. Death is a common outcome as a result of severe blood loss. Large subcutaneous hematomas, especially over bony protuberances following relatively mild trauma are common. Hematomas may develop in the mesentery, causing severe colic.[2] The amount of resulting blood loss into these subcutaneous or abdominal hematomas can be fatal. Some animals may present with swollen joints and a progressive stiffness leading to recumbency and death.[20] Hemorrhaging from the vagina, epistaxis, and the presence of blood in the feces may also be evident. Other cattle may be found dead as a result of hemorrhaging subcutaneously or into body cavities, pericardial sac, and the cranium. Animals with severe anemia may exhibit abnormal neurologic behavior resulting from the effects of hypoxia. "Downer" cattle have been reported as a result of hemorrhaging into the spinal cord following the larval migration of *Hypoderma bovis*.[21]

Cows may abort as a result of intrauterine hemorrhaging, fetal hypoxia, and may produce stillborn calves.[18] Prolonged hemorrhaging from the umbilicus of newborn calves may result in neonatal death.[2,16] Newborn calves may be severely affected while their dams may have only minimal depletion of their clotting factors.[22] Depending on the severity of the anemia, general weakness, pale mucous membranes, tachycardia, and tachypnea are evident on physical examination.[1,8,22]

Clinical Pathology. The prothrombin time (PT) and the activated partial thromboplastin time (aPTT) are characteristically prolonged in dicoumarol poisoning.[23] Platelet numbers are not affected. Coagulation factors IX and X activity are reduced from normal ranges of 50% to 150% and 80% to 175%, respectively.[24] Depending on the duration and severity of the depletion of the vitamin K–dependent factors, affected animals often have a marked reduction in the packed cell volume and total protein caused by hemorrhaging. Large hematomas and hemothorax may cause mild icterus. Other diseases that can result in prolonged PT and aPTT include anticoagulant rodenticide poisoning and hepatic failure.[25]

Lesions.   Animals that die of sweet clover poisoning typically show evidence of extensive hemorrhaging and anemia. Subcutaneous hemorrhages and hematomas over bony protuberances are common. Hemorrhaging into body cavities, muscle masses, joints, the intestinal lumen, and organ surfaces are generally evident. Other than general pallor to the organs and tissues, there are usually no other distinctive gross lesions visible.[1,22] Histologic examination of tissues generally shows evidence of recent hemorrhaging and mild degenerative changes in hepatocytes, possibly as a result of hypoxia.[20]

In the differential diagnosis of cattle exhibiting signs of abnormal blood clotting and resulting hemorrhaging, poisoning from anticoagulant rodenticides should be considered.[26] Bracken fern *(Pteridium aquilinum)* poisoning in cattle induces thrombocytopenia and a syndrome of petechiation and hematuria that may resemble dicoumarol poisoning. Dicoumarol poisoning does not affect thrombocyte numbers, thus helping to differentiate it from bracken fern poisoning and disseminated intravascular coagulopathy (DIC). Clostridial infections caused by *Clostridium hemolyticum* (bacillary hemoglobinuria) and *Cl. novyii* (Black's disease) may also resemble dicoumarol poisoning and may be differentiated by culturing of the bacteria from the affected tissues. A hemorrhagic syndrome attributable to type II bovine virus diarrhea can mimic the clinical signs of dicoumarol toxicity.[27]

Diagnostic Testing.   Samples of suspect hay or silage, particularly containing the stems of the plants, should be submitted for the detection of dicoumarol by TLC or HPLC.[20,28] Several hay samples should be submitted from different hay bales because levels of dicoumarol can vary markedly between bales.[18] In large, round bales, samples should be collected from the center as well as the outer layers of the bale. Moldy sweet clover hay containing less than 20 µg/g (ppm) is not likely to cause poisoning in cattle.[18,19] However, sweet clover hay containing 20 to 30 µg/g (ppm) of dicoumarol causes poisoning if fed for 130 days. Dicoumarol levels exceeding 50 µg/g (ppm) are likely to cause severe poisoning.[19] Levels of dicoumarol as high as 165 µg/g (ppm) have been reported in sweet clover hay that was high in protein.[18] When hay or silage containing high levels of dicoumarol is fed to cattle, the clotting factors may be depleted and signs of hemorrhaging may occur in less than 15 days. Dicoumarol levels may remain high in hay for several years.

Dicoumarol may also be detected and quantified in liver samples using TLC and mass spectrometry/mass spectrometry.[28] Dicoumarol levels in the livers of calves with sweet clover poisoning have ranged from 1 to 5 ppm.[16,20,29] Dicoumarol can be detected in the serum of cattle using HPLC as long as 13 days after the animals have stopped being fed sweet clover silage.[8]

Treatment.   Once a diagnosis of dicoumarol poisoning is confirmed, all feeding of the suspect hay or silage should be stopped, and the animals provided good quality grass or alfalfa hay. Affected animals should not be stressed or traumatized to avoid the risk of inducing hemorrhaging. The most effective treatment in severe cases is whole blood transfusions to immediately replace the depleted blood coagulation factors and red blood cells. Several liters of whole blood (5 L for an adult cow with a packed cell volume less than 20) or 10 ml/kg of plasma should be administered, and repeated as necessary. Vitamin K_1 should be administered at a dose of 1 to 5 mg/kg body weight either subcutaneously or intramuscularly, depending on the severity of poisoning and whether the animal has been transfused.[29] Vitamin K_1 therapy may be needed for 1 to 2 weeks.

Vitamin K_3 is not effective in the treatment of dicoumarol poisoning in cattle.[29] Horses with dicoumarol poisoning should not be treated with vitamin K_3 because they may develop acute tubular nephrosis.[30]

Prevention and Control.   Grossly moldy hay or silage should not be fed to livestock. Hay containing yellow sweet clover and sweet vernal grass should be tested for dicoumarol levels if there is a question as to how well the hay or silage was prepared relative to the moisture content. Fungal growth in hay and silage can be prevented by adding 2 ppm of propionic acid during the curing process.[31] Similarly, ammoniation with anhydrous ammonia inhibits fungal growth in sweet clover hay, thereby decreasing dicoumarol concentrations in the hay.[32] Cultivars of yellow sweet clover with low and high levels of coumarin have been identified, with as much as a twentyfold difference in dicoumarol levels existing between them.[31] The yield of hay per acre is, however, less for the low coumarin varieties.

Whenever elective surgical procedures are contemplated for cattle that have been fed sweet clover hay or silage in the previous month, the procedures (dehorning, castration, branding) should be delayed until the PT can be evaluated. Prolonged PT may take several weeks to return to normal after further consumption of dicoumarol has ceased. Pregnant cows should not be fed sweet clover hay within 1 month of calving to avoid hemorrhaging problems at calving.[23]

Prevention of sweet clover poisoning by feeding vitamin K_3 to cattle is not effective.[28,33,34]

REFERENCES

1. Pritchard DG et al: Haemorrhagic syndrome of cattle associated with the feeding of sweet vernal *(Anthoxanthum odoratum)* hay containing dicoumarol, *Vet Rec* 113:78, 1983.
2. Bartol JM et al: Hemorrhagic diathesis, mesenteric hematoma and colic associated with ingestion of sweet vernal grass in a cow, *J Am Vet Med Assoc* 216:1605, 2000.
3. Murray RDH, Mendez J, Brown SA, editors: *The natural coumarins,* New York, 1982, John Wiley and Sons.
4. Tligui N, Ruth GR: *Ferula communis* variety *brevifolia* intoxication in sheep, *Am J Vet Res* 55:1558, 1994.
5. Schofield FW: Damaged sweet clover: the cause of a new disease in cattle simulating hemorrhagic septicemia and blackleg, *J Am Vet Med Assoc* 64:553, 1924.

6. Kosuge T, Gilchrist D: Chemistry of coumarin and related compounds. In Wyllie TD, Morehouse LG, editors: *Mycotoxic fungi, mycotoxins, mycotoxicoses* New York, 1977, Marcel Dekker.

7. Bellis DM, Spring MS, Stoker JR: The biosynthesis of dicoumarol, *Biochem J* 103:202, 1967.

8. Puschner B et al: Sweet clover poisoning in dairy cattle in California, *J Am Vet Med Assoc* 212:857, 1998.

9. Cohen AJ: Critical review of the toxicology of coumarin with special reference to interspecies differences in metabolism and hepatotoxic response and their significance to man, *Food Cosmet Toxicol* 17:277, 1979.

10. Christensen F: Metabolism of dicoumarol by liver microsomes from untreated and phenobarbital treated rats, *Biochem Pharmacol* 21:2303, 1972.

11. Ren P et al: Mechanism of action of anticoagulants: correlation between the inhibition of prothrombin synthesis and the regeneration of vitamin K_1 from vitamin K_1 epoxide, *J Pharm Exp Ther* 201:541, 1977.

12. Bell RG: Metabolism of vitamin K and prothrombin synthesis: anticoagulants and the vitamin K-epoxide cycle, *Proc Soc Exp Biol Med* 37:2599, 1978.

13. Nelsestuen GL, Zytkovitz TH, Howard JB: The mode of action of vitamin K. Identification of γ-carboxyglutamic acid as a component of vitamin K, *J Biol Chem* 249:6374, 1974.

14. DeHoogh W: Dicoumarol toxicity in a herd of Ayrshire cattle fed moldy sweet clover, *Bovine Pract* 24:173, 1989.

15. McDonald GK: Moldy sweet clover poisoning in a horse, *Can Vet J* 21:250, 1980.

16. Blakely BR: Moldy sweet clover (dicoumarol) poisoning in Saskatchewan cattle, *Can Vet J* 26:357, 1985.

17. Linton JH et al: Dicoumarol studies: oral administration of synthetic dicoumarol to various classes of sheep and cattle, *Can J Anim Sci* 43:344,1963.

18. Benson ME, Casper HH, Johnson LJ: Occurrence and range of dicoumarol concentrations in sweet clover, *Am J Vet Res* 42:2014, 1981.

19. Casper HH, Alstad AD, Monson SB: Dicoumarol levels in sweet clover toxic to cattle, *Proc Ann Meet Assoc Vet Lab Diagn* 25:41, 1982.

20. Yamini B et al: Dicoumarol (moldy sweet clover) toxicosis in a group of Holstein calves, *J Vet Diagn Invest* 7:420, 1995.

21. Meads EG, Taylor PA, Pallister WA: An unusual outbreak of sweet clover poisoning in cattle, *Can Vet J* 5:65,1964.

22. Fraser CM, Nelson J: Sweet clover poisoning in newborn calves, *J Am Vet Med Assoc* 135:283, 1959.

23. Radostits OM, Searcy GP, Mitchall KG: Moldy sweet clover poisoning in cattle, *Can Vet J* 21:155, 1980.

24. Morris DD: Alterations in the clotting profile. In Smith BP, editor: *Large animal internal medicine*, ed 2, St Louis, 1996, Mosby.

25. Morris DD: Diseases of the hematopoietic and hemolymphatic systems. In Smith BP, editor: *Large animal internal medicine*, ed 3, St Louis, 2002, Mosby.

26. Petterino C, Paolo B: Toxicology of various anticoagulant rodenticides in animals, *Vet Human Toxicol* 43:353, 2001.

27 Walz PH et al: Effect of experimentally induced type II bovine viral diarrhea virus on platelet function in calves, *Am J Vet Res* 60:1396, 1999.

28. Braselton WE, Neiger RD, Poppenga RH: Confirmation of indandione rodenticide toxicosis by mass spectrometry/mass spectrometry, *J Vet Diagn Invest* 4:441, 1992.

29. Alstad AD, Casper HH, Johnson LJ: Vitamin K treatment of sweet clover poisoning in calves, *J Am Vet Med Assoc* 187:729, 1985.

30. Rebhun WC et al: Vitamin K_3-induced renal toxicosis in the horse, *J Am Vet Med Assoc* 184:1237, 1984.

31. Sanderson MA, Meyer DW, Casper HH: Dicoumarol concentrations in sweet clover hay treated with preservatives and in spoiled hay of high and low coumarin cultivars of sweet clover, *Anim Feed Sci Tech* 14:221, 1986.

32. Sanderson MA, Meyer DW, Casper HH: Dicoumarol concentrations and quality of sweet clover forage treated with propionic acid or anhydrous ammonia, *J Anim Sci* 61:1243, 1985.

33. Goplen BP, Bell JM: Dicumarol studies IV: antidotal and antagonistic properties of vitamin K_1 and vitamin K_3 in cattle, *Can J Anim Sci* 41:91, 1967.

34. Casper HH et al: Evaluation of vitamin K_3 feed additive for the prevention of sweet clover disease, *J Vet Diagn Invest* 1:116, 1989.

CYANOGENIC GLYCOSIDES

John A. Pickrell and Fred Oehme

Sources. Cyanogenic glycosides are found in pitted fruits in the *Prunus* genus (cherries, peaches, almonds, and apricots), in unpitted fruits (elderberry), grasses (Johnson grass, sorghum, sudan), and corn. Depending on growth conditions, cyanogenic glycoside sources may be further amplified and the toxins can also be found in vetch (*Vicia sativa*), white clover (*Trifolium repens*), birdsfoot trefoil (*Lotus*), and arrowgrass (*Triglochin*).[1-6]

Toxicokinetics. Once cyanogenic glycosides, such as amygdalin and prunasin, are converted to cyanide, they are rapidly absorbed from the gastrointestinal or respiratory tracts.[1-4,7,8]

Mechanism of Action. Cyanide combines with iron in cellular cytochrome oxidase to prevent terminal electron transfer and blocks cellular respiration so that oxyhemoglobin cannot release oxygen for electron transport in the cytochrome system.[1,2,4,7,9] Cyanide severely depresses most hemodynamic and metabolic functions, leading to buildups of organic acid.[1,4,10] Thus, erythrocytes can accumulate oxygen as oxyhemoglobin and even become supersaturated so that the blood is a bright cherry red, but cannot deliver the oxygen to the tissues. The hemoglobin in this situation is more than 99% saturated with oxygen, but no oxygen is passed to the cells.[1,2]

Toxicity and Risk Factors. A high nitrogen to phosphorus ratio in soil favors increased cyanogenic glycoside formation. The most rapidly growing plants have the greatest concentrations of cyanide. Cyanogenic glycosides are stored in different plant compartments from their metabolizing enzymes. The glycosides can be converted to cyanide when the plant or seed integrity is compromised by chewing, by mechanical grinding, or by being ground in the crop of a bird.[1,4] Environmental stresses such as drought, frost, or wilting can cause the formation of additional cyanogenic glycosides and can interrupt the integrity of seeds, leaves, bark, stems, or fruits of plants.[1-4]

Although forage cyanide concentrations of 50 ppm are suspicious, those that exceed 200 ppm are considered to be high enough to deliver a dose of 2 mg hydrogen cyanide/kg body weight and to produce clinical signs.[1,4] Wilted forage or forage with high free cyanide content is more toxic than forage with intact seeds and leaves.

A hard freeze can make wilted cherry tree leaves available to insects. Insects such as tent caterpillars can nearly strip cherry tree leaves and rapidly excrete much of the cyanogenic glycosides into the surrounding forage. This leads to focused toxicity from cyanogenic glycosides.[5] Although tent caterpillars do reduce the cyanide content during digestion of the leaves, the effect of excreting cyanide rapidly or of large numbers of caterpillars remains to be determined.[6]

Clinical Signs.   Signs develop quickly, often within 10 to 60 minutes. Principal signs from acute cyanide intoxication include hyperventilation, decreased blood pressure, hypoxemia-induced convulsions, coma, shock, respiratory failure, and death. The progression after the onset of convulsions is rapid. Even though the patient is still alive, tissues and mucous membranes are a characteristic bright cherry red.

Clinical Pathology.   No specific clinical pathologic changes occur.[1-4]

Lesions.   No lesions are specific for cyanide intoxication because of the rapidity of death. The blood is bright cherry-red immediately after death. As postmortem time increases, this color darkens over the next 2 to 6 hours, depending on environmental temperature. Stress-induced petechial hemorrhages may occur in the abomasum, subendocardium, and subepicardium. Although the odor of "bitter almonds" has been reported, the ability to detect this odor is genetic and the odor disappears with time.[1,2,4]

Diagnostic Testing.   Most diagnoses are made based on clinical signs and evidence of consumption of appropriate plants. The suspect plants can be analyzed for cyanide content.[1-4,10] Those with more than 200 ppm cyanide have sufficiently high concentrations to acutely produce clinical signs.[1,2,4]

Treatment.   Optimum treatment is rapid administration of either sodium nitrite (20% solution, 10 to 20 mg/kg) or methylene blue (1% to 4% solution, 2 to 3 g/500 lb body weight). Both should not be administered. The purpose of either nitrite or methylene blue is to create methemoglobin, which removes cyanide from the cytochrome oxidase to form cyanmethemoglobin.[1-4,8,9]

Administering 20% thiosulfate solution (<600 mg/kg) intravenously provides sulfur donors.[12] When thiosulfate is given, rhodanese helps exchange cyanide with thiosulfate to form thiocyanate, which is water soluble and rapidly excreted in the urine.[1-4,8,9] Experimental sulfur donors (diethyl tetrasulfide, diallyl tetrasulfide, and diisopropyl tetrasulfide) have been shown to protect mice against exposure to twice the lethal dose 50 (LD_{50}) concentration of cyanide.[12]

Cobalt salts have been recommended as therapy because they penetrate into cells and complex cyanide to form the nontoxic cyanide cobalt.[13] Cobalt salts have not been approved for use in animals in the United States.

Prognosis.   Prognosis is fair with optimum treatment that is received before severe respiratory distress. Because of the sudden onset of signs, most animals have a poor-to-grave prognosis.[1-4]

Prevention and Control.   Animals should not be allowed to access plants and fruit pits that may contain the toxic glycosides.[1-6] During hazardous growth conditions, suspect forage should be assayed before allowing herbivores to graze.

REFERENCES

1. Osweiler GD: *Toxicology,* Philadelphia, 1996, Williams & Wilkins.
2. Murphy M: *A field guide to common animal poisons,* Ames, Iowa, 1996. Iowa State University Press.
3. Hulbert LC, Oehme FW: *Plants poisonous to livestock,* Manhattan, Kan, 1968, Kansas State University.
4. Fitzgerald KT: Cyanide. In Peterson ME, Talcott PA, editors: *Small animal toxicology,* Philadelphia, 2001, WB Saunders.
5. Anonymous: Caterpillars, cherry trees may take blame for foal deaths in Kentucky, *J Am Vet Med Assoc* 219:13, 2001.
6. Fitzgerald TD, Jeffers PM, Mantella D: Depletion of host-derived cyanide in the gut of the eastern tent caterpillar, *J Chem Ecol* 28:257, 2002.
7. Kingsbury JM: *Poisonous plants of the United States and Canada,* Englewood Cliffs, NJ, 1964, Prentice-Hall.
8. Aiello S, editor: *The Merck veterinary manual (Toxicology),* Whitehouse Station, NJ, Merck.
9. Nicholson SS: Cyanogenic plants. In Howard JL, editor: *Current veterinary therapy: food animal practice 3,* Philadelphia, 1993, WB Saunders.
10. Casteel SW: Principal toxic plants of the midwestern and eastern United States. In Howard JL, Smith RA, editors: *Current veterinary therapy: food animal practice 4,* Philadelphia, 1999, WB Saunders.
11. Breen PH et al: Combined carbon monoxide and cyanide poisoning: a place for treatment, *Anesth Analg* 80:671, 1995.
12. Baskin SI et al: In vitro and in vivo comparison of sulfur donors as antidotes to acute cyanide intoxication, *J Appl Toxicol* 19:173, 1999.
13. Astier A, Baud FJ: Complexation of intracellular cyanide by hydroxocobalamin using a human cellular model, *Hum Exp Toxicol* 15:19, 1996.

CYCASIN

Jay C. Albretsen

Synonyms.   Cycad palms are known as sago palms *(Cycas cirinalis),* Japanese cycad *(Cycas revoluta),* cardboard palms *(Zamia furfuracea),* coontie plants *(Zamia pumila),* or simply by their genus *Cycads, Zamias,* or *Macrozamia.*[1-4]

Sources.   The members of the Cycadales order include three families: Cycadaceae (with one genus, *Cycas*), Stangeriaceae (with a single species, *Stangeria eriapus),* and Zamiaceae (with eight genera, of which *Zamia* species are encountered most frequently in the United States).[3-6] These plants are palmlike in appearance and are native to tropical and subtropical climates around the world. They have been used for many years as a food source and for medicinal purposes.[7] Lately, their increased use as ornamental houseplants has made them available all over the world.[6,8] The Cycadales order includes both male and female plants in each species, and only the female plant produces the nuts (seeds).[1,2,4]

Toxicokinetics.   Cycad palms have three types of toxins.[1,2,4,8]

1. Cycasin is the major glycoside present in Cycads. Cycasin is converted to its aglycone methylazoxymethanol (MAM) by β-glucosidases. These β-glucosidases can be found in the skin of newborn animals or in the gastrointestinal tract of most other animals.

2. β-methylamino-*L*-alanine   (BMAA) is a neurotoxic amino acid.

3. An unidentified toxin with a high molecular weight.

No specific information is known about the kinetics of the cycad toxins in humans or animals. However, signs of toxicosis in dogs usually occur within 12 to 24 hours of ingestion.[3,8,9] In cattle, the hindlimb paralysis may take several days to appear. These neurologic signs also require long-term ingestion of the cycad plants.[1,8] In sheep fed *Macrozamia redlei* nuts, chronic liver disease developed over a period of 3 to 11 months.[1]

Mechanism of Action. Cycasin irritates the gastrointestinal tract and causes hepatic necrosis.[1,8] This glycoside is also carcinogenic, mutagenic, and teratogenic.[1,2,4,8] The toxic amino acid BMAA causes ataxia in rats, but is not the cause of hindlimb ataxia in cattle.[4] Rats given high doses of BMAA developed necrosis of the neurons in the cerebellum, causing the rats to become ataxic.[1,10] Although the mechanism is not known, BMAA has also been implicated as the cause of Guam disease in humans. The third major toxin in cycad palms is unknown at this time. This toxin is suspected of causing axonal degeneration in the central nervous system (CNS).[2,4,8]

Toxicity and Risk Factors. Because of the multiple toxins inherent in cycads and the varying habits of each animal species, different syndromes are caused by cycad ingestion. Cattle prefer to eat leaves, but sheep and dogs are known to consume leaves and seeds.[7-9] In fact, dogs have consumed all parts of the cycad plant, including the roots.[9] Sheep frequently ingest seeds and leaves and often ingest large amounts at a time.

Cycasin is thought to be responsible for the hepatic and gastrointestinal signs seen in sheep and dogs after the plants are eaten.[1,4] Nuts (seeds) contain a higher amount of the glycosides (cycasin) than do other parts of the plant. Dogs that develop signs most often ingest seeds or have been chewing on the plants and roots.[9] As few as two seeds ingested by dogs can cause signs.[11]

BMAA has caused ataxia in rats but is unlikely to be involved in the cause of zamia staggers in cattle.[10] The doses of BMAA used in rats to cause ataxia were a very large amount compared to what an animal might be exposed to when eating the whole cycad plant. Its effect in causing disease in most animals is unknown.[1,10]

The unidentified toxin in cycads is thought to be the cause of hindlimb paralysis in cattle resulting from axonal degeneration in the central nervous system.[1,4] Cattle usually must consume the plants for extended periods of time before any signs appear.[7-9]

Clinical Signs. Most animals are affected by either the gastrointestinal and hepatic disease syndrome or the ataxia and central nervous disease syndrome. These differences in disease are probably a result of the different doses consumed by the animals, their duration of exposure, and the parts of the cycad plant ingested.[1,7,9]

In dogs, the most commonly reported clinical sign following cycad ingestion is vomiting (with or without blood).[9] Depression, diarrhea, and anorexia have also been reported frequently. Seizures did occur in some cases, but the seizures were usually thought to be secondary to hepatic damage. Even though deaths have been reported, most dogs survived with appropriate supportive care.[9]

The customary signs reported after sheep have ingested cycads are lethargy, anorexia, weight loss, and gastroenteritis (which may or may not be hemorrhagic).[1,7] Both dogs and sheep consume more of the cycad glycosides.[7-9] Massive outbreaks of disease in sheep have been reported and death occurs frequently.[1]

In cattle, frequently reported signs include weight loss, weakness, ataxia, and paresis (a syndrome called *zamia staggers*). However, the cattle have often been exposed for several days, which made determining the etiology of the disease difficult.[1,7] Although cattle are more frequently affected by CNS disease, it is still possible to see hepatic damage in cattle after cycad ingestion.[1,7]

Clinical Pathology. Elevated serum ALT, AST, and alkaline phosphatase are commonly reported in dogs ingesting cycads. Hyperbilirubinemia and electrolyte abnormalities are also often noted. Increased BUN and leukocytosis have occasionally been reported in dogs.[9]

Clinically affected ruminants may develop leukocytosis, hypoalbuminemia, and elevations of AST, alkaline phosphatase, and GGT. Hypocholesterolemia and decreased triglyceride levels were also noted in several heifers after the consumption of cycad plants for an undetermined amount of time.[7]

Lesions. Gastrointestinal lesions in dogs with cycad poisoning include hemorrhage and necrosis of gastrointestinal mucosa.[8] Focal necrosis and ulceration of the abomasum have been reported in sheep.[1] Dairy heifers exposed to cycad plants did not develop any gastrointestinal lesions.[7]

Histologic lesions in the liver of dogs ingesting cycad plants include cirrhosis, marked focal centrolobular, and midzonal coagulation necrosis.[8] The principal hepatic lesions in ruminants ingesting cycad plants are megalocytosis, periacinar necrosis, and fibrosis.[1]

Some animals with hepatic disease caused by cycad ingestion may develop hepatic encephalopathy. Characteristic nervous signs and spongy degeneration of the central nervous system may be present.[1] Other brain and spinal cord lesions include demyelination and axonal degeneration in brain, spinal cord, and dorsal root ganglia.[7]

Diagnostic Testing. Often identifiable fragments of the cycad plant or seeds are found in the stomach or intestinal contents of poisoned animals. Although cycasin and BMAA can be found in the liver of animals that ingest cycad palms, no diagnostic laboratories routinely test for these compounds.

Treatment. Emesis and activated charcoal help prevent signs in animals that have recently ingested cycads. However, if it has been longer than 2 to 4 hours since the plant material was ingested, emesis is not likely to have any benefit because the stomach is probably empty by then.[9] In addition, inducing emesis in a symptomatic animal is often contraindicated. If the ingestion occurred less than 12 hours earlier, activated charcoal prevents further absorption of the cycad toxins.[9,11] In some cases, multiple doses of activated charcoal may be beneficial.

No antidote for any of the cycad toxins is available. Consequently, treatment of poisoned animals focuses on supportive and symptomatic care. Companion animals can be given gastrointestinal protectants such as sucralfate (1 g in large dogs, 0.5 g in small dogs orally every 8 hours), H_2 blockers such as cimetidine (5 to 10 mg/kg intravenously or by mouth every 8 hours), or misoprostol (1 to 3 µg/kg).[12] Fluid and electrolyte support is beneficial and should be used as needed. The fluid of choice for animals with hepatic damage is 5% dextrose.[13] Blood transfusions may be necessary if gastrointestinal tract hemorrhage is severe.[9,13,14]

Prognosis.   The prognosis is good if the animal is decontaminated before the onset of clinical signs. Prognosis is guarded when animals are showing signs. Surviving cattle with neurologic signs have remained ataxic and have had secondary atrophy of hindlimb musculature for the remainder of their lives.[7] The disease could lead to lifelong hepatic support in animals with hepatic damage.[7,8,9]

Prevention and Control.   The young leaves of cycad plants are considered to be very palatable. Cattle and sheep preferentially seek out the cycad palms.[3,7,8,11] All animals should be denied access to areas that contain cycad palms, or the palms should be destroyed.

REFERENCES

1. Hooper PT: In Keeler RF, VanKampen KR, James LF, editors: *Effects of poisonous plants on livestock,* New York, 1978, Academic Press.
2. Kinghorn D: In Keeler RF, Tu AT, editors: *Handbook of natural toxins: plant and fungal toxins,* vol 1, New York, 1983, Marcel Dekker.
3. Botha CJ et al: Suspected cycad *(Cyas revoluta)* intoxication in dogs, *J S Afr Vet Assoc* 62:189, 1991.
4. Cheeke PR: *Natural toxicants in feeds, forages, and poisonous plants,* Danville, Ill, 1998, Interstate Publishers.
5. Hall WT: Cycad (zamia) poisoning in Australia, *Aust Vet J* 64:149, 1987.
6. Tustin RC: Notes on the toxicity and carcinogenicity of some South African cycad species with special reference to that of *Encephalartos lanatus, J S Afr Vet Assoc* 54:33, 1983.
7. Reams RY et al: Cycad *(Zamia puertoriquentis)* toxicosis in a group of dairy heifers in Puerto Rico, *J Vet Diagn Invest* 5:488, 1993.
8. Senior DF et al: Cycad intoxication in the dog, *J Am Anim Hosp Assoc* 21:103, 1985.
9. Albretsen J et al: Cycad palm toxicosis in dogs: 60 cases (1987-1997), *J Am Vet Med Assoc* 213:99, 1998.
10. Seawright AA et al: In Watters D, Lavin M, Maguire D et al: *Toxins and targets: effects of natural and synthetic poisons on living cells and fragile ecosystems,* Lausanne, Switzerland, 1992, Hardwood Academic Publishers.
11. Knight MW, Dorman DC: Selected poisonous plant concerns in small animals, *Vet Med* 92:260, 1997.
12. Plumb D: *Veterinary drug handbook,* Ames, Iowa, 1995, Iowa State University Press.
13. Leveille-Webste CR: In Morgan RV, editor: *Handbook of small animal practice,* ed 3, Philadelphia, 1997, WB Saunders.
14. Center SA: In Ettinger SJ: *Textbook of veterinary internal medicine,* ed 3, Philadelphia, 1989, WB Saunders.

ESCIN SAPONINS

William R. Hare

Synonyms.   More than 25 different species of *Aesculus* grow worldwide,[1] and all species should be regarded as being potentially poisonous if ingested. The most common synonyms are buckeye and horse chestnut. Other names include bongay, conquerors, conquor, fish poison, and blackeyes. Names for specific species include *A. glabra,* Ohio buckeye; *A. pavia,* red buckeye; *A. octandra,* marsh or yellow buckeye; *A. flava,* sweet or yellow buckeye; *A. californica,* California buckeye; and *A. hippocastanum,* common horse chestnut.

The common horse chestnut, *A. hippocastanum,* is not related to the edible American chestnut, *Castanea* spp.

Sources.   *Aesculus* spp. are represented as deciduous trees or shrubs. The genus is easily recognized by the characteristic opposite, palmately compound, 20 to 40 cm long, oblong, serrate, dark-green, usually stalkless, leaflets. The blossom clusters are located at the ends of branches and bloom in April and May. The fruit consists of a seedpod capsule that covers smooth, glossy, bright-brown seeds (one to three), which have a distinctive white or tan scar (hence the name buckeye). The seedpods vary in size and shape depending on the species of *Aesculus,* but are approximately 2 to 4 cm in diameter, appear in July and August, and drop to the ground in September and October.

A. glabra, Ohio buckeye, is a medium-sized tree, growing 25 to 30 meters in height with foliage composed of five to seven palmate leaflets approximately 20 to 25 cm long (Color Plate 33). It has a spiny seedpod capsule and yellowish flowers with noticeable gland dots. The Ohio buckeye is native to North America and ranges from western Pennsylvania through southern Michigan to Nebraska and southward to Texas. It grows well on fertile soil, within wood lots, along riverbanks, and is a common inhabitant of fence-rows.

A. hippocastanum, common horse chestnut, is a moderately large tree, growing 30 to 35 m in height with foliage composed of five to seven palmate leaflets approximately 30 cm long. It has a spiny seedpod capsule and whitish flowers with characteristic red and yellow gland dots. It is a European native that has become well established and naturalized in North America. It grows within a large geographic area and can be found from Maine to California and southern Canada to Florida. Hybrid forms are available commercially and it has become a popular ornamental shade tree throughout the United States.

A. pavia, red buckeye, is a moderately large shrub growing 3.5 to 4.5 m in height with foliage composed of five to seven palmate leaflets, a smooth seedpod capsule, and red flowers. It is native to North America and ranges from the southeastern states and westward to eastern Texas. It grows well on fertile soil and can be found growing within woodlots, along side streams, or within fence-rows.

A. octandra and *A. flava,* marsh buckeye, and sweet buckeye, are medium-sized trees, growing 25 to 28 meters in height with foliage composed of five to seven palmate leaflets approximately 20 to 24 cm in length. It has a smooth seedpod capsule and usually yellow flowers (sometimes purplish) with noticeable gland dots. Both of these species are also referred to as yellow buckeyes. They are native to North America and range from southern Pennsylvania to Georgia and westward as far as eastern Texas. It grows abundantly in the southeastern states and can be found alongside mountain streams and marshes.

A. californica, California buckeye, is a moderately sized tree growing 3 to 12 m in height, with relatively broad branches (Color Plates 34 and 35). The foliage is composed of five stalked, palmate leaflets approximately 18 cm long. The seedpod is small, pear shaped, and has a smooth capsule. The flowers are usually a whitish pale-pink color. It is native to California and can be found in greatest abundance on the dry hillsides and canyons of the Pacific Coast range and the Sierra Nevada foothills. It does not grow at high elevations, but prefers the hillsides to the valley floor.

Toxicokinetics. *Aesculus* spp. have many toxic principles, some of which are esculin (a coumarin glycoside), escin (a mixture of saponins identified as Ia, Ib, IIa, IIb, IIIa, IIIb, IV, V, VI[2,3]), and frangula (an anthroquinone). In animals that use intestinal microbes for digestion, esculin may be hydrolyzed to the aglycone form, thereby becoming a systemic toxin. All of these compounds cause gastrointestinal effects and the aglycone of esculin causes neurologic effects.

Although specific toxicokinetic studies in animals have not been carried out for *Aesculus* spp. or their extracts, there are sufficient clinical and experimental reports to draw some conclusions on absorption and elimination. Saponins in general are poorly absorbed from the gastrointestinal tract and not absorbed topically. Because they are irritating to the gastrointestinal mucosa, they produce inflammation and improve their absorption. Adverse clinical signs usually appear within 1 to 3 hours after ingestion of seeds, foliage, or extract preparations.[4] Absorption kinetics may vary somewhat by animal species, because gastrointestinal microbes can carry out conversion of poorly absorbable saponins to more readily absorbable aglycones,[5] and because of simple anatomic differences. In ruminants, absorption may be delayed 6 to 12 hours, with most animals exhibiting adverse clinical signs 12 to 18 hours after exposure.[6] Adverse effects appear to peak at 24 to 28 hours after exposure. No information is available on the distribution or metabolism of the toxic principles, but clinical and experimental reports suggest that they are primarily eliminated in the urine and milk, with approximately a 24-hour half-life.

Mechanism of Action. The exact mechanism of the toxic principles is unknown. However, saponins in general are gastrointestinal irritants and can produce marked inflammation and severe gastroenteritis. Escin is a mixture of triterpenoid saponins. On hydrolysis they can yield sterol-like compounds that are biologically active and 1,2,7-trimethyl naphthalene. Naphthalenes are cytotoxic compounds and responsible for enterotoxic, neurotoxic, and hematotoxic abnormalities. Esculin is known to be cytotoxic and may produce neurotoxic effects through this action. Frangula is an anthraquinone, which acts to stimulate the colon by increasing fluid secretion into the small and large intestine and directly increasing intestinal motility by activation of the myenteric plexus.

Toxicity and Risk Factors. Cattle, sheep, horses, mules, pigs, llamas, dogs, cats, monkeys, fish, birds, bees, exotic, and laboratory animals could all be expected to develop signs associated with poisoning following exposure. Animals usually do not forage on buckeyes or horse chestnuts unless nutritionally deprived. Therefore, clinical cases of poisoning are rare. However, grazing animals could be particularly at risk in the early spring and late fall, when sufficient forage may be lacking. Alternative medicine preparations of *Aesculus* spp. no longer appear to be popular and are not as much of a risk to companion animals as the ingestion of seeds or the chewing of bark.

The new young leaves, the terminal shoots at the end of branches, the flowers, and the bark are most toxic. The seeds can also be very toxic and are most commonly associated with poisoning. Seed toxicity appears to peak in July and August when they are just beginning to form within the seedpods and then gradually decreases. The flowers of *A. hippocastanum* have been reported to be toxic to bees; the honey made from their nectar is also toxic.[1]

Toxicity varies with each species of *Aesculus.* The horse chestnut is the most toxic to the greatest number of animal species, but all species of *Aesculus* should be regarded as potentially toxic. One or two buckeyes or horse chestnut seeds may be sufficient to produce toxicosis in small animals; however, most large animals require a greater exposure. Adult horses may require the ingestion of more than 20 horse chestnut seeds or the chewing and ingestion of a significant amount of the tree's bark to produce a significant toxicosis. Cattle ingesting *Aesculus octandra*'s seeds, bark, or new terminal shoots in amounts greater than 0.5% of body weight produce a severe toxicosis, and ingestion of greater than 1% body weight produces death.[6]

Clinical Signs. Gastrointestinal signs vary and may not be present in some clinical cases. Vomiting and diarrhea may appear 1 to 3 hours after ingestion. Noticeable irritation to the buccal cavity may be present. Colic is the main problem associated with ingestion of *Aesculus* by horses. Pulse and respiration are dependent on the animal's level of activity and excitement. The body temperature is normal.

If the exposure is great or repeated over a period of time, CNS signs can occur: depression, mental confusion with periods of excitement, ataxia, walking in a stiff-legged manner, muscle twitching, loss of balance, spontaneous tonic-clonic spasms, seizures, bilateral-medial-dorsal strabismus, first sternal then lateral recumbency, opisthotonos, head flopping, and death.[4,6-8]

Clinical Pathology. Most of the clinical pathology alterations are related to stress. However, hyperglycemia or hypoglycemia, glycosuria, ketonuria, proteinuria, and increased serum urea nitrogen levels may accompany decreased hepatic function and glomerular leakage due to toxic insult.[6] The urine is often described as appearing red as a result of the presence of the toxin in alkaline urine.

Lesions. Gross pathology lesions tend to be unremarkable. However, histopathology of the liver usually indicates a mild degenerative process characterized by centrilobular vacuolization with swelling of individual hepatocytes, as well as the finding of occasional hepatocytes at various stages of cellular necrosis.[6] Sometimes, a widely disseminated focal hepatic necrosis is reported. Histopathologic lesions of the kidney are usually absent.

Diagnostic Testing. Some of the toxins may be detected in the urine or serum using HPLC[9] or TLC[10] methods. However, routine testing is not available to confirm buckeye or horse chestnut poisoning. The identification of *Aesculus* plant parts from stomach contents, following emesis or found at postmortem, can help confirm exposure.

Treatment. No antidote exists; therefore, treatment is usually supportive and directed at preventing absorption. Decontamination efforts are important, but use of cathartics is often not necessary. Treatment with activated charcoal, with or without a laxative, followed by gastrointestinal protectants can be helpful. In cases of marked toxicosis, treatment with diazepam should help control seizure activity and muscle spasms. Intravenous fluids containing appropriate electrolytes should be administered. Renal function, the acid-base status, and electrolytes should be monitored. Use of parenteral vitamin complexes and antioxidant preparations may help protect the liver.

Prognosis. The prognosis for cases exhibiting severe neurologic signs accompanied by seizures and renal failure is poor to guarded. However, cases exhibiting predominantly a gastrointestinal syndrome with mild signs of neurologic deficits have a good prognosis. Most cases of poisoning resolve within 72 to 96 hours, if not sooner. But it is not uncommon for neurologic deficits to take from 2 to 3 weeks to 12 to 18 months to resolve.

Prevention and Control. Grazing animals should not be allowed access to *Aesculus* trees and shrubs. These plants are most toxic in the spring, but most poisonings occur from ingesting fallen seeds in September and October. Ingestion of leaves and seeds following a summer thunderstorm is also a common means of poisoning for large and small animals. Home remedy preparations containing *Aesculus* extract should be used with extreme caution to prevent accidental ingestion by companion animals.

REFERENCES

1. Kingsbury JM: *Poisonous plants of the United States and Canada,* Englewood Cliffs, NJ, 1964, Prentice-Hall.
2. Yoshikawa M et al: Bioactive saponins and glycosides. III. Horse chestnut, *Chem Pharm Bull* 44(8):1454, 1996.
3. Matsuda H et al: Effects of eschins Ia, Ib, IIa, and IIb from horse chestnut, the seeds of *Aesculus hippocastanum* L., on acute inflammation in animals, *Biol Pharm Bull* 20(10):1092, 1997.
4. Williams MC, Olsen JD: Toxicity of seeds of three *Aesculus* spp. to chicks and hamsters, *Am J Vet Res* 45(3):539, 1984.
5. Allison MJ: The role of ruminant microbes in the metabolism of toxic constituents from plants. In Keller RJ, VanKampen KR, James LF, editors: *Effects of poisonous plants on livestock,* 1978, Academic Press.
6. Magnusson RA et al: Yellow buckeye *(Aesculus octandra* Marsh) toxicity in calves, *Bovine Pract* 18:195, 1983.
7. Casteel SW, Wagstaff DJ: *Aesculus glabra* intoxication in cattle, *Vet Hum Toxicol* 34(1):55, 1992.
8. Kornheiser KM: Buckeye poisoning in cattle, *Vet Med Small Anim Clin* 78:769, 1983.
9. Yoshikawa M et al: Bioactive saponins and glycosides. XIII. Horse chestnut. Quantitative analysis of escins Ia, Ib, IIa, and IIb by means of high performance liquid chromatography (HPLC), *J Pharm Soc Japan* 119(1):81, 1999.
10. Gocan S, Cimpan G, Muresan L: Automated multiple development thin layer chromatography of some plant extracts, *J Pharm Biomed Anal* 14:1221, 1996.

FURANS

Steven S. Nicholson

Synonyms. Perilla mint is also called beefsteak plant and mint weed (Color Plate 36).

Sources. Perilla ketone from the mint plant *Perilla frutescens* and 4-ipomeanol from moldy sweet potatoes *(Ipomoea batatas)* cause atypical interstitial pneumonia, primarily in cattle. This disease has also been associated with *F. oxysporum* and *F. semitectum* in peanut-vine hay and green beans.[1]

Perilla mint is widespread in the southern United States where it is a major toxic plant. It has a distinct odor. Perilla may be found around corrals and hog pens, but more often in shaded areas in light woods along creeks and rivers. It is an erect, branching, herbaceous annual that grows 1 to 5 feet tall, has square and sometimes dark-red–brown stems, and has oval, serrated leaves that are 2 to 4 inches wide. Small white flowers are produced on spikes. The underside of the leaves may have a purple tint. Ornamental varieties are purple. In late summer, large numbers of round seeds about 1 mm in diameter are produced.

A stress metabolite (4-hydroxymyoporone) is produced in sweet potatoes infected with the molds *Fusarium solani and F. oxysporum.* A potent pulmonary toxin, 4-ipomeanol, is not produced by the sweet potato but by fungal metabolism of the stress metabolite.

Mechanism of Action. Perilla ketone and 4-ipomeanol damage endothelial cells and type I pneumocytes, resulting in subsequent formation and proliferation of type II pneumocytes.

Toxicity and Risk Factors. Perilla mint is most toxic during the flower and seed stages in late summer when availability of good-quality forage may be limited. Cattle may coexist with perilla for years without grazing it. Cattle held overnight in corrals or small pastures where the weed is plentiful are apt to eat the plant. Several pounds of the green plant may be lethal to a cow within 1 to 2 days. Perilla baled in hay retains some toxicity.

Access to mold-damaged sweet potatoes has occurred when cattle were fed culls from a cannery, when fed potatoes spoiled in storage, and when grazing plowed fields.

Clinical Signs. Atypical interstitial pneumonia is characterized by acute onset of dyspnea, extension of the head and neck, and an expiratory grunt. Froth from pulmonary edema may be present around the mouth and nose. Coughing is minimal. Subcutaneous emphysema under the skin of the neck and back may be present.

Lesions. The lungs are distended and rib imprints are visible on the surface. All lobes of the lung may have severe interstitial and alveolar emphysema; bullae are common. Slight to marked edema of the lungs may be present. Emphysema may extend into the mediastinal space and subcutaneously over the cervical, thoracic, and lumbar areas. Portions of perilla stems and leaves, with their characteristic odor, may be recognizable in rumen contents. Perilla seeds, minus the black seed coat, are white, 1 mm in diameter, and may be found in the contents of the rumen, omasum, abomasum, and feces.

Histopathologic lesions are those of acute interstitial pneumonia and include dilated and ruptured alveoli. Flat squamous epithelial cells (type I pneumocytes) lining the alveoli are replaced by cuboidal cells (type II pneumocytes). Many alveoli are edematous and interlobular septa contain air and fluid.

Treatment. Antibiotics, antihistamines, flunixin meglumine, corticosteroids, and diuretics may not significantly alter the outcome of atypical interstitial pneumonia cases. Severely dyspneic animals may collapse and die during handling and restraint.

Prognosis. Cattle with mild to moderate perilla mint toxicosis generally recover within 7 to 10 days. The prognosis is good if they do not die within 2 to 3 days. Mortality rate is high when sweet potatoes are the source of the toxin.

Prevention and Control. Temporary elimination of perilla mint by mowing or herbicide application before the seed stage is effective in some situations.

REFERENCES

1. Roberson JR et al: Acute respiratory distress syndrome in adult beef cattle fed peanut hay, *Vet Med* 92:644, 1997.

GLUCOSINOLATE

John A. Pickrell and Fred Oehme

Sources. Annual plants of the mustard family, including rape and kale, flower early in the spring and may be the first available green plants.[1] Plant oximes are converted into glucosinolates, which animals metabolize into thiocyanates and isothiocyanates that are toxic to livestock.[1-4]

Toxicokinetics. Clearance of alpha-isothiocyanate is rapid, with 5% or less of the isothiocyanate remaining in the tissues after 24 hours. Clearance for mice is 70% to 80% in urine, 13% to 15% in exhaled air, and 3% to 5% in feces.[5]

Mechanism of Action. Plants metabolize oximes to glucosinolates, which are concentrated in leaf protoplasts, to reduce consumption by herbivores.[2,3,6] Glucosinolates are hydrolyzed to aglycones, including thiocyanates and isothiocyanates. Isothiocyanate concentrates in the liver, kidneys, and blood.[4]

The cytochrome P-450–dependent S-oxidative pathway is probably related to isothiocyanate toxicity as indicated by inhibition of hepatotoxicity by SKF-525A, a metabolic inhibitor, and hepatotoxicity stimulation by phenobarbital, a P-450 enhancer.[7]

Toxicity and Risk Factors. Toxins are present in all plant parts, but are most concentrated in the seeds.[1]

Clinical Signs. Isothiocyanate is toxic to the gastrointestinal tract as indicated by the clinical signs of fluid to hemorrhagic diarrhea that can be severe.[1] Within 3 to 4 hours, domestic and wild herbivores that received moderate to high doses of glucosinolate developed anorexia and colic. Over the next 4 to 5 days, they developed fluid to hemorrhagic diarrhea of varying severity. Some animals weakened and died. Abortions were possibly related to clinical condition or effects.[1,8] Cattle receiving one fourth of this glucosinolate exposure (16 mg/kg/day) had blood at the end of urination, mild colic, and palpably normal kidneys, uteri, and urinary bladders. Within 24 hours after removing the offending plant from the ration, urine was clear of blood and cattle were clinically normal.[8]

Clinical Pathology. Liver enzymes may be elevated.[9,10] A high glucosinolate meal in chicks produced a mild serum AST increase that paralleled a mild liver lesion.[11]

Lesions. Domestic and wild herbivores receiving sufficiently high doses of glucosinolate to produce fatalities from 1 day's exposure had massive submucosal edema of the forestomachs, especially the rumen.[8] Liver lesions in domestic and wild herbivores were sufficient to produce pathology. Experimentally, chicks receiving a high glucosinolate meal had mild liver lesions and increased serum AST.[11]

Diagnostic Testing. The presence of mustards and gastrointestinal clinical signs, especially hemorrhage, supports this diagnosis. Measurements of glucosinolate in ruminal and duodenal digesta, urine, and milk are possible, but are not available routinely in veterinary diagnostic laboratories.[8,10]

Treatment. After low to moderate exposures, removal of glucosinolate-containing feed and forage or a change to low glucosinolate levels in feed may be sufficient to alleviate clinical signs.[8] If treatment is required, supportive therapy for diarrhea with fluids and electrolytes may be helpful.[1] Rarely, in cases of major blood loss, transfusion may be required.

Prognosis. The prognosis is guarded to fair, depending on how much glucosinolate was consumed and over what time period. In a situation in which 100% of the hay was *Thlapsi*, half of the beef cows had signs in a few hours and 4% died by 4 to 5 days, despite removal of the *Thlapsi* hay and symptomatic treatment. When 25% of the hay was *Thlapsi* (16.25 mg/kg isothiocyanate/day), dairy heifers had less severe signs, which disappeared 1 day after removing the *Thlapsi* hay.[8]

Prevention and Control. Animals should be removed from pastures or hay containing glucosinolate and provided high-quality diets.[1,8] Extraction procedures and biotechnological approaches are being developed to reduce glucosinolate in meals.[12,13] In addition, the ensiling process reduces forage glucosinolate to the point where it can substitute for grass silage in lambs.[9]

REFERENCES

1. Osweiler GD: *Toxicology,* Philadelphia, 1996, Williams and Wilkins.
2. Hansen CH et al: CYP83B1 is the oxime-metabolizing enzyme in the glucosinolate pathway in *Arabidopsis, J Biol Chem* 276:24790, 2001.
3. Yui YH, Smith RA, Spoerke DG: *Foodborne disease handbook: plant toxicants,* vol 3, ed 2, New York, 2001, Marcel Dekker.
4. Breschi MC et al: Distribution and fate of alpha-napthl-isothiocyanate (ANIT) in the organs and body fluids of the rat, *Arzneimittelforschung* 27:122, 1977.
5. Ioannou YM, Burka LT, Matthews HB: Allyl isothiocyanate: comparative disposition in rats and mice, *Toxicol Appl Pharmacol* 75:173, 1984.
6. Chen S, Halkier BA: Characterization of glucosinolate uptake by leaf protoplasts of *Brassica napus, J Biol Chem* 275:22955, 2000.
7. Traiger GJ, Vyas KP, Hanzlik RP: Effect of inhibitors of alpha-naphthyl-isothiocyanate-induced hepatotoxicity on the in vitro metabolism of alpha-naphthylisothiocyanate, *Chem Biol Interact* 52:335, 1985.
8. Smith RA, Crowe SP: Fanweed toxicosis in cattle: case history, analytical method, suggested treatment, and fanweed detoxification, *Vet Hum Toxicol* 29:155, 1987.
9. Vipond JE et al: Effects of feeding ensiled kale (*Brassica oleracea*) on the performance of finishing lambs, *Grass Forage Sci* 53:346, 1998.
10. Subuh AMH, Rowan TG, Lawrence TLJ: Toxic moieties in ruminal and duodenal digesta in milk and hepatic integrity in cattle given diets based on rapeseed meals of different glucosinolate contents either untreated or treated with heat or formaldehyde, *Anim Feed Sci Tech* 52:51, 1995.
11. Kloss P et al: Studies on the toxic effects of crambe meal and two of its constituents, 1-cyano-2- hydroxy-3- butene (CHB) and epiprogoitrin in broiler chick diets, *Br Poul Sci* 37:971, 1996.
12. Bell JM: Nutrients and toxicants in rapeseed meal: a review, *J Anim Sci* 58:996, 1984.
13. Vageeshbabu HS, Chopra VL: Genetic and biotechnological approaches for reducing glucosinolates from rapeseed-mustard meal, *J Plant Biochem Biotechnol* 6:53, 1997.

NITROPROPANOL GLYCOSIDES

Bryan Stegelmeier

Synonyms. Nitropropanol glycoside, 3-nitropropanol, miserotoxin, 3-nitropropionic acid, and aliphatic nitrocompounds are names used to describe the toxins. Common names for *Astragalus* spp. are milkvetch and timber milkvetch. The disease caused by these toxins is sometimes referred to as cracker heels or roaring disease.

Sources. The toxic nitro compounds include 3-nitropropanol, 3-nitropropionic acid, and their glycoside derivatives (miserotoxin is the β-D-glucoside of 3-nitropropanol). These aliphatic nitrocompounds have been identified in more than 600 species of plants. Nearly 450 of these are in the Fabaceae family and contain either 3-nitropropionic acid (NPA) or 3-nitropropanol (NPOH). This has been used as a phenotype to determine *Astragalus* taxonomy. Toxic *Astragalus* species (Color Plate 37) that poison livestock are common in North and South America, with fewer reported from Europe (Table 25-10).[1,2] Other plants, including many violets (*Viola* spp.), lotus (*Lotus* spp.), indigo (*Indigofera* spp.), as well as many species of *Hippocrespo, Coronilla, Hiptage, Heteropterus, Janusia,* and *Corynocarpus,* contain toxic nitrocompounds.[3-8] NPA and NPOH can also be produced by *Aspergillus oryzae* and *A. soyae,* common fungi of fermented products.[9,10] Although not associated with NPA-containing plants of North America, NPA has contaminated feed or food, including sugar cane, and has been shown to be a potent neurotoxin.[11,12]

Toxicokinetics. Conjugates and esters of NPA and NPOH, such as miserotoxin, are rapidly hydrolyzed by rumen microbial enzymes. Monogastric animals are less susceptible to toxicosis. Monogastric animals may avoid toxic NPOH and NPA by absorbing intact glycosides that are easily excreted. The major site of NPA and NPOH absorption is from the reticulorumen in sheep and cattle.[13]

NPOH is absorbed more rapidly than NPA; however, NPA is the toxic species. Alcohol dehydrogenase quickly converts NPOH to NPA in the liver. Microbial metabolism of nitrocompounds has been studied, and microbial promotants have been used to alter microbial metabolism and subsequent NPA toxicity.[14,15] Specific rumen bacteria use NPA, NPOH, or miserotoxin as electron acceptors producing 3-aminopropanol and β-alanine.[16,17] Other minor metabolic pathways include hydrolysis forming inorganic nitrite and 3 carbon hydrocarbon. The toxic nitrite may be absorbed and oxidize hemoglobin, causing methemoglobinemia.

Mechanism of Action. NPA is a potent inhibitor of succinate dehydrogenase, fumerase, and aspartase, which are enzymes of the Krebs or tricarboxylic acid cycle.[18,19,20] Lesions appear to be due to inhibited cellular oxidative phosphorylation, decreased energy production, and loss of cellular homeostasis. Serum methemoglobin concentrations are moderately elevated in poisoned animals. Hemoglobin oxidation is probably not the cause of death in that oxidation can be inhibited with methylene blue. In treated cattle, methemoglobin does not develop, but animals continue to develop neurologic disease and die.[20]

Toxicity and Risk Factors. In cattle, acute poisoning occurred at doses of more than 27 g/kg of NPOH per body weight or 7 g of NPOH per animal (15 g miserotoxin per animal, generally about 1.5 kg fresh plant).[21] Sheep appear to tolerate much higher doses. Chronically poisoned animals exposed to lower doses over several weeks develop similar progressive disease. In both cases, when animals develop severe clinical signs, they rarely recover.

Clinical Signs. The clinical signs of poisoning are related to the dose and they vary greatly in different animal species. Poisoned cattle and sheep develop respiratory and neurologic disease; horses and rodents commonly develop neurologic disease.

TABLE 25-10 *Astragalus* Species that Commonly Poison Livestock in North America

Astragalus spp. that Contain Nitrotoxin	Location	Habitat
Astragalus atropubescens (Kelsey milkvetch)	Northwest (Idaho, Montana, Wyoming)	Annual on sandy or gravel hillsides
A. Canadensis (Canada milkvetch)	North America (indigenous)	Perennial widespread in Northwest with large population and poisonings
A. emoryanus (red stem peavine)	Southwest (Texas, New Mexico, Nevada, Arizona)	Annual with extensive population cycles that cause poisoning
A. falcatus (milkvetch)	North America (introduced)	Annual widespread in Northwest with large population and poisonings
A. miser var hylophyllus (Yellowstone milkvetch)	Wyoming, Utah, Montana	Annual found in pine forests and sagebrush
A. miser var oblongifolius (Wasatch milkvetch)	Utah, Colorado	Annual found in mountain sagebrush communities
A. miser var serotinus (Columbia milkvetch)	British Columbia	Perennial in fescue grasslands and Douglas fir zones
A. pterocarpus (winged milkvetch)	Nevada and southeastern California	Desert annual that can be locally abundant
A. tetrapterus (4-winged milkvetch)	Utah	Annual found in desert sandy soils, locally abundant
A. whitnii	California (Sierra Nevada Mountains)	Annual on stony or sandy slopes and ridges above trees
Astragalus praelongus, toanus, convallarius, and *campestris*		

Data from references 2, 27-30.

Poisoned animals develop dyspnea, rales, stridor, and muscular weakness. These animals have severe emphysema and generally die within a couple of hours. Some animals also develop pronounced neuromuscular abnormalities including abnormal gait, rear limb proprioceptive defects, and goose-stepping. The gait abnormalities can cause feet lesions that are referred to as "cracker heels." Poisoned horses may be reluctant to back up. Poisoned animals become weak and emaciated and a few develop temporary blindness. As the disease progresses, animals lose condition, develop a rough, dull haircoat, and may develop rear limb paresis or paralysis. These animals generally die within several weeks. When stressed or forced to move, affected cattle may collapse and die. Lactating cattle and sheep are more commonly affected than nonlactating animals.[22]

Lesions. The distribution and extent of NPA-induced lesions are also species specific. Rats given NPA developed degeneration and malacia in the globus pallidus, entopeduncular nucleus, and substantia negra,[23] which are similar to lesions seen in horses poisoned with knapweed. Most livestock develop both respiratory and neurologic lesions.

Cattle given *A. miser* var. *hylophylus* or *A. emoryanus* develop severe emphysema with bronchiolar constriction and interlobular edema (Color Plate 38). Numerous focal hemorrhages are found throughout the CNS with focal malacia in thalamic nuclei. Axonal degeneration and spheroids with wallerian degeneration are found throughout the spinal cord (Color Plate 39). Other findings include muscle atrophy and overall wasting.[24] Sheep develop similar neurologic degeneration; however, the lung change has been characterized as that of pulmonary edema. Horses have also been poisoned, but the clinical signs and lesions have not been well described.[23]

Clinical Pathology. Poisoned animals have variable changes in hematology and serum biochemistries. Transient increases in AST, creatinine kinase, and sorbitol dehydrogenase activities have been reported, as have moderate increases in methemoglobin and mild decreases in hemoglobin. These changes are probably due to NPA-induced recumbency and nitrite hemoglobin oxidation.[25] Currently, there are no NPA-specific changes that could be used to indicate poisoning.

Diagnostic Testing. Identification of poisoned animals has been primarily associated with clinical signs, evidence of plant consumption, and finding the characteristic gross and histologic lesions. Both NPA and NPOH can be identified in the serum or plasma of poisoned animals by HPLC.[26]

Treatment and Prognosis.   Various in vitro treatments and transfaunations to enhance ruminal bacterial detoxification of NPOH have been studied; however, such techniques have yet to be adapted and proven effective in range conditions.[15] Treatments including methylene blue and thiamine have been used unsuccessfully to treat NPA poisoning.[22,27] Because animals that develop clinical disease rarely recover, current management techniques have been to avoid exposures that allow animals to become poisoned.

Prevention and Control.   Current recommendations are that cattle can safely use grasslands containing milkvetch, if adequate forage is available. Studies on Columbia milkvetch (*A. miser* var *serotinus*) showed that milkvetch consumption correlates with both abundance and palatability of other forages. Cattle avoided milkvetch and ate more palatable forages in grassland sites. This continued until the desirable species were depleted. In forested areas with similar Columbia milkvetch densities, cattle preferred milkvetch to the less palatable pine grasses. There was no evidence of addiction to Columbia milkvetch.[28]

Nitro toxin concentrations are highest in plants that are in the bud and flower. Toxin concentrations decrease rapidly as the plant matures and begins to senesce.[28] Grazing later, after the plants begin to senesce, has been recommended. Rotational grazing or flash grazing techniques have been suggested, but have not been definitively proven effective.

Rumen microbes become adapted to metabolizing nitrocompounds, allowing animals to become more tolerant to poisoning. It has been suggested that adaptation may be enhanced by certain high-protein diets and supplements.

Most of these toxic vetches are easily controlled with herbicides.[29,30] Care should be taken when using herbicides because some treated plants can become more palatable or more toxic.

REFERENCES

1. Stermitz RF, Yost GS: Analysis and characterization of nitro compounds from *Astragalus* species. In Keeler RF et al, editors: *Effects of poisonous plants on livestock*, New York, 1978, Academic Press.
2. Williams MC: 3-Nitropropionic acid and 3-nitro-1-propanol in species of *Astragalus, Can J Bot* 60:1956, 1981.
3. Williams MC: Toxic nitro compounds in Lotus, *Agron J* 75:520, 1983.
4. Williams MC: Nitro compounds in *Indigofera* species, *Agron J* 73:434, 1981.
5. Gnanasunderam C, Sutherland ORW: Hiptagin and other aliphatic nitro esters in Lotus pedunculatus, *Phytochem* 25:405, 1986.
6. Majak W, Bose RJ: Nitropropanoylglucopyranoses in *Coronilla varia, Phytochem* 16:415, 1976.
7. Moyer BG et al: 3-nitropropanoyl-*D*-flucopyranoses of *Corynocarpus laevigatus, Phytochem* 18:111, 1979.
8. Salem MA, Williams JM, Wainwright SJ, Hipkin CR: Nitroaliphatic compounds in hippocrepis comosa and other legumes in the European flora, *Phytochem* 40:89, 1995.
9. Iwasaki T, Kosikowski FV: Production of beta-nitropropionic acid in foods, *J Food Sci* 38:1162, 1973.
10. Kinosita R et al: Mycotoxins in fermented food, *Cancer Res* 28:2296, 1968.
11. Ming L: Moldy sugarcane poisoning: a case report with a brief review, *Clin Toxicol* 33:363, 1995.
12. 3-Nitropropionic acid's lethal triplet: cooperative pathways of neuro-degeneration, *Neuroreport* 9:R57, 1998.
13. Muir AD, Majak W, Pass MA, Yost GS: Conversion of 3-nitropropanol (miserotoxin aglycone) to 3-nitropropionic acid in cattle and sheep, *Toxicol Lett* 20:137, 1984.
14. Majak W: Metabolism and absorption of toxic glycosides by ruminants, *J Range Manage* 45:67, 1992.
15. Anderson RC et al: Enrichment and isolation of a nitropropanol metabolizing bacterium from the rumen, *Appl Environ Microbiol* 62:3885, 1996.
16. Anderson RA, Rasmussen MA, DiSpirito AA, Allison MJ: Characteristics of a nitropropanol-metabolizing bacterium isolated from the rumen, *Can J Microbiol* 43:617, 1997.
17. Anderson RC et al: Denitrobacterium detoxificans gen. nov. sp. nov., a ruminal bacterium that respires on nitrocompounds, *Int J Sys Evol Microbiol* 50:633, 2000.
18. Coles CJ et al: Inactivation of succinate dehydrogenase by 3-nitro-propionate, *J Biol Chem* 254:5161, 1979.
19. Alston TA et al: 3-Nitropropionate, the toxic substance of *Indigofera*, is a suicide inactivator of succinate dehydrogenase, *Proc Natl Acad Sci USA* 74:3767, 1977.
20. Williams MV, Van Kampen KR, Norris RA: Timber milkvetch poisoning in chickens, rabbits and cattle, *Am J Vet Res* 30:2185, 1969.
21. Majak W et al: Toxicity and metabolic effects of intravenously administered 3-nitropropanol in cattle, *Can J Anim Sci* 61:633, 1981.
22. James LF et al: Field and experimental studies in cattle and sheep poisoned by nitro-bearing *Astragalus* or their toxins, *Am J Vet Res* 41:377, 1980.
23. Gould DH, Gustine DL: Basal ganglia degeneration, myelin alterations, and enzyme inhibition induced in mice by the plant toxin, 3-nitropropanoic acid, *Neuropathol Appl Neurobiol* 8:377, 1982.
24. Dawson R et al: Excitotoxins, aging and environmental neurotoxins: implications for understanding human neurodegenerative diseases, *Toxicol Appl Pharmacol* 134:1, 1995.
25. Maricle B et al: Evaluation of clinicopathological parameters in cattle grazing timber milkvetch, *Can Vet J Revue Vet Canadienne* 37:153, 1996.
26. Muir AD, Majak W: Quantitative determination of 3-nitropropionic acid and 3-nitropropanol in plasma by HPLC [High-pressure liquid chromatography, *Astragalus miser*, timber milkvetch], *Toxicol Lett* 20:133, 1984.
27. Pass MA et al: Lack of a protective effect of thiamine on the toxicity of 3-nitropropanol and 3-nitropropionic acid in rats, *Can J Anim Sci* 68:315, 1988.
28. Majak W et al: Seasonal grazing of Columbia milkvetch by cattle on rangelands in British Columbia, *J Range Manage* 49:223, 1996.
29. Williams MC, Ralphs MH: Effect of herbicides on miserotoxin concentration in wasatch milkweed (*Astragalus miser* var. oblongifolius), *Weed Sci* 35:746, 1987.
30. Williams MC, James LF: Effects of herbicides on the concentration of poisonous compounds in plants: a review, *Am J Vet Res* 44:2420, 1983.

PHYTOESTROGENS

John A. Pickrell and Fred Oehme

Sources.   *Trifolium repens* (white clover) is grown in Europe and New Zealand, and *Trifolium subterraneum* (subterranean clover) is grown mostly in Australia.[1,2] Higher trifolium seed yields result in a better seeding, 3.15-fold as much subterranean clover, but decreased concentrations of the phytoestrogens: formononetin, genistein, and biochanin A.[3] *Medicago sativa* (alfalfa, Lucerne) grown in the United States produces coumesterol, which is moderately estrogenic and may cause infertility.[1] Alfalfa irrigated with human sewage increases phytoestrogen content (mostly coumesterol) from 1.5- to 15-fold, most likely depending on estrogen equivalents in the sewage.[4] *Vicia sativa* (common vetch) has a low concentration of formononetin, which raises circulating estrogen and may contribute to infertility.[5,6]

Mechanism of Action. Phytoestrogens are rapidly absorbed, bind with estrogen receptors, and lead to infertility by interfering with transport and fertility of ova, causing cystic hyperplasia of the cervix, inducing loss of libido in males, and feminizing males. All herbivores are affected, but primarily cattle and sheep.[1,6,7] Phytoestrogens can cause organizational effects in the reproductive tract during organogenesis.[8] Phytoestrogens increase weights of oviducts and testes and combs of either sex in white leghorn chickens.[9]

Toxicity and Risk Factors. Clinical effects and documented infertility as a result of estrogen-containing plants appear uncommonly proven, although often suspected.

Clinical Signs. Infertility may be the only clinical sign in females. Loss of libido and feminization may occur in males.[1,2]

Lesions. Cystic hyperplasia and increased folding of the cervix in female herbivores have been noted, especially in cattle and sheep.[1,2,6-8]

Diagnostic Testing. Infertility and reproductive abnormalities are related to elevated levels of circulating estrogen that can be measured in endocrinology laboratories.[1,6]

Treatment. Withdrawal from phytoestrogen sources often at least partially ameliorates herbivore infertility. Any additional treatment is symptomatic.[1,6]

Prognosis. Animals rarely die, although they may have permanent loss of productivity.[1,2,6-8]

Prevention and Control. Animals should be denied access to suspect plants, and irrigation with human sewage should be avoided.[4]

REFERENCES

1. Osweiler GD: *Toxicology*, Philadelphia, 1996, Williams & Wilkins.
2. Kingsbury JM: *Poisonous plants of the United States and Canada*, Englewood Cliffs, NJ, 1964, Prentice-Hall.
3. Craig AD: Pasture production of two cultivars of *Trifolium subterraneum* at Kybybolite, South Australia, *Aust J Exp Agric* 32:611, 1992.
4. Shore LS et al: Induction of phytoestrogen in *Medicago sativa* leaves by irrigation with sewage water, *Environ Exp Botany* 35:363, 1995.
5. Anonymous: Register of Australian herbage plant cultivars, *J Aust Inst Agric Sci* 38:142, 1972.
6. Shore LS et al: Relationship between peripheral estrogen concentrations at insemination and subsequent fetal loss in cattle, *Theriogenology* 50:101, 1998.
7 Adams NR: Organizational and activational effects of phytoestrogens on the reproductive tract of the ewe, *Proc Soc Exp Biol Med* 208:87, 1995.
8. Cantero A et al: Histopathological changes in the reproductive organs of manchego ewes grazing on Lucerne, *J Vet Med Series A* 43:325, 1996.
9. Mohsin M, Pal AK: Phyto-estrogen in relation to physiology of birds: effect on the development of reproductive and endocrine organs of chicken, *Ind Vet J* 54:25, 1977.

PROTOANEMONIN

George Burrows and Ronald J. Tyrl

Sources. The presence of protoanemonin as a toxicant is associated primarily with members of the Ranunculaceae or crowfoot family. The main concern is species of *Ranunculus*, but the species of several other genera either contain protoanemonin or cause problems suggestive of its presence (Table 25-11). They include *Actaea, Anemone, Caltha, Clematis, Helleborus,* and *Hydrastis.*

Plants of *Ranunculus* are herbaceous annuals or perennials, most often with glossy yellow petals. They are found across the continent in a variety of habitats ranging from relatively dry to wet soils; a few may occur in shallow water.

Mechanism of Action. Intoxications caused by *Ranunculus* are due mainly to the irritant effects of protoanemonin. Formed from glycosides such as ranunculin when plant tissues are macerated, protoanemonin is a potent vesicant that primarily irritates the mucous membranes of the digestive system.[1] Effects on the urinary system, mammary glands, and brain associated with ingestion of especially large amounts of plant material also have been reported.[2,3] Protoanemonin is subsequently polymerized to the inactive anemonin, the form found in dried plants. The irritant effects occur relatively soon after ingestion of fresh plants, although there is considerable variation in the severity of disease.[3,4] In some cases such as those involving *Ranunculus testicularis,* severe disease and numerous deaths in sheep have been reported.[5]

Toxicity and Risk Factors. For the most part, taxa of the Ranunculaceae that contain protoanemonin are early-season plants. The levels of protoanemonin and the irritant effects of plant ingestion are greatest during flowering.[1,6] Protoanemonin concentrations may be in excess of 2% dry weight in some species of the genus.[3] Most animal species are susceptible to the irritant effects.

Clinical Signs. Typical signs associated with consumption of the crowfoots are related to the blistering of the skin,

TABLE 25-11 Representative Species of *Ranunculus* Present in North America

Species Name	Common Name
R. abortivus L.	Smallflower or little leaf buttercup
R. acris L.	Tall buttercup, tall crowfoot
R. arvensis L.	Corn or field buttercup
R. flammula L.	Spearwort, creeping buttercup
R. sceleratus L.	Blister buttercup, cursed crowfoot

mouth, and irritation of the lower digestive tract. They include erythema and swelling of the muzzle and lips, weakness, vomiting, diarrhea, and colic. Hematuria, tremors, seizures, and paralysis as well as reddish, bitter milk also have been reported.[2,3,7,8]

Lesions. Most commonly, edema and reddening of the abomasum and small intestines are present with a few splotchy hemorrhages on the serosa of the intestines and moderate excess fluid in the abdomen.

Treatment. In most situations, treatment is not necessary. In severe cases, symptomatic relief of the irritant effects may be needed.

Prognosis. Except for the rare, severe case, the outcome of the disease is favorable, with recovery in a few days.

REFERENCES

1. Hill R, Van Heyningen R: Ranunculin: the precursor of the vesicant substance in buttercup. *Biochem J* 49:332, 1951.
2. Gunning OV: Suspected buttercup poisoning in a Jersey cow, *Br Vet J* 105:393, 1949.
3. Shearer GD: Some observations on the poisonous properties of buttercups, *Vet J* 94:22, 1938.
4. Griess D, Rech J: Diagnosis of acute poisoning by rannunculi *(Ranunculus acris I* and *Ficaria ranunculoides)* in horses, *Rev de Med Vet* 148:55, 1997.
5. Olsen JD et al: Bur buttercup poisoning of sheep, *J Am Med Assoc* 183:538, 1983.
6. Nachman RJ, Olsen JD: Ranunculin: a toxic constituent of the poisonous range plant bur buttercup *(Ceratocephalus testiculatus), J Agric Food Chem* 31:1358, 1983.
7. Fuller TC, McClintock E: *Poisonous plants of California,* Berkeley, Calif, 1986, University of California Press.
8. Kingsbury JM: *Poisonous plants of the United States and Canada,* Englewood Cliffs, NJ, 1964, Prentice-Hall.

PTAQUILOSIDE

Konnie H. Plumlee and Steven S. Nicholson

Synonyms. *Pteridium aquilinum* is commonly called bracken fern or brake fern (Color Plate 40). *Cheilanthes sieberi* is commonly called rock fern.

Sources. Bracken fern occurs worldwide and several varieties are recognized. In Australia and New Zealand, both rock fern and bracken fern cause similar toxicoses. Bracken is a branching fern 1 to 5 feet tall that is found in well-drained soil. Rhizomes are more toxic than fronds and stems. Bracken remains toxic in hay.

Mechanism of Action. Ptaquiloside is the compound in bracken fern long-believed to cause death of precursor cells in the bone marrow and neoplasia formation in the urinary tract. Ptaquiloside has been found in the milk of cows ingesting bracken fern, and the milk caused tumors in mice.[1]

However, one study found that some compounds found in bracken fern (including ptaquiloside, quercetin, and shikimate) have a low order of cytotoxicity and questioned their role in aplastic anemia of cattle.[2]

Toxicity and Risk Factors. Bracken fern can cause several different diseases, depending on factors such as the age of the animal, geographic location, the duration and rate of consumption, and the toxin content in the plant.[1] The disease syndromes include aplastic anemia in cattle and sheep, enzootic bovine hematuria caused by urinary tract neoplasms, tumors of the upper digestive tract, and a progressive retinal degeneration called bright blindness in sheep.[1] Bovine papillomavirus type 2 has been associated with bladder tumors induced by bracken fern, and bovine papillomavirus type 4 has been associated with squamous cell carcinoma of the upper digestive tract.[1,3]

When cattle ingest young fronds or rhizomes in recently plowed ground over 3 to 4 weeks or longer, the cumulative effect is suppression of bone marrow activity. The result is a severe pancytopenia, especially a thrombocytopenia and a leukopenia, which results in terminal anemia.[3] The risk that cattle will eat large amounts of bracken fern is increased when the animals are hungry and the plant is readily available. Drought and overstocking heavily infested pastures increase the risk. Conversely, ingestion of small amounts of bracken over several years leads to neoplasia of the urinary tract or digestive tract.

In North America, the most common syndrome is aplastic anemia in cattle, which is associated with acute toxicity.[3] One case of urinary neoplasia consistent with bracken fern toxicosis was identified in a llama in California that had long-term exposure to the plant.[3] In England and Wales, sheep develop a progressive retinal atrophy called bright blindness. Bracken fern causes fibrosarcoma of the mandible in sheep and tumors of the upper alimentary tract in cattle in England.

A retrospective pathology study revealed that bracken fern toxicosis is common in southern Brazil, with 50% of the cases being aplastic anemia, 42% being tumors of the upper digestive tract, and 8% being chronic hematuria. However, the authors noted that the incidence of chronic hematuria is probably underreported because farmers tend to cull these animals rather than have them diagnosed.[1] This same study found that, of the cows with aplastic anemia, 63% were 1 to 3 years old and 29% were older than 3 years. Of the cows with tumors of the digestive tract, 22% were 4 to 5 years old, 38% were 5 to 7 years old, and 33% were older than 7 years.[1]

Clinical Signs. An acute onset of fever, lethargy, loss of appetite, and hemorrhage occurs in cattle with the aplastic anemia syndrome. The stool contains fresh and digested blood. Hemorrhages may be visible in the vulva, mouth, conjunctiva, and anterior chamber of the eye. The urine may contain blood.

Enzootic hematuria presents as intermittent blood loss from hemorrhages and tumors of the urinary bladder, anemia, elevated heart rate, weakness, and death.

Clinical Pathology. Aplastic anemia results in bone marrow suppression. Thrombocyte and granulocyte production are affected first. Thrombocytopenia may be marked in asymptomatic herd mates that have not yet become noticeably ill.

Blood-loss anemia and blood in the urine are expected with chronic enzootic hematuria.

Lesions. Cattle that die of aplastic anemia have numerous small and large hemorrhages present on the thoracic pleura, the epicardium, the mucosa of the larynx, the serosa of viscera, and on the lining of the gall bladder and urinary bladder. In the intestines, areas of necrosis and hemorrhage 20 to 40 mm in diameter are visible.

One retrospective Brazilian study of 89 cases of tumors in the upper digestive tract over a 4-year period revealed that all were squamous cell carcinomas. Thirty-four animals had tumors at the base of the tongue or pharynx, 27 animals had tumors in the rumen, 20 had tumors in the esophagus, and eight had tumors in multiple areas. Another Brazilian study revealed 40 tumors with 21 of the tongue and pharynx, 25 in the esophagus, and 11 in the rumen. However, in the United Kingdom, tumors of the rumen and esophagus are more common.[1]

Tumors that cause enzootic hematuria may be benign or malignant and include transitional cell carcinoma, squamous cell carcinoma, papilloma, hemangioma, hemangiosarcoma, leiomyosarcoma, fibroma, and fibrosarcoma with a metastatic rate of about 10%.[3] Bladder tumors are most common in cattle, but tumors have been reported in the ureters and renal pelves.[3]

Diagnosis. A history of exposure to bracken fern over several weeks or months and appropriate clinical signs support a diagnosis of bracken fern poisoning.

Treatment. Blood or platelet transfusion might be useful in cattle with aplastic anemia. Antibiotics may prevent secondary infections.

Prognosis. The mortality rate in cattle with bone marrow failure is nearly 100%. A rising thrombocyte count suggests that recovery might occur. Otherwise, the bracken fern–related conditions are essentially not treatable.

Prevention and Control. It is risky to confine cattle and sheep to pastures where bracken fern is present in quantities sufficient to provide a significant portion of the diet for several weeks or longer. The risk is greatest in the spring when young, tender fronds are emerging and where desirable forage is limited. A repeated rotational grazing system so that cattle are exposed to bracken for 3 weeks then moved to a bracken-free pasture for 3 weeks may prevent aplastic anemia. Vaccination against bovine papillomavirus may decrease the incidence of bracken fern–induced tumors.[1]

REFERENCES

1. Gava A et al: Bracken fern *(Pteridium aquilinum)* poisoning in cattle in southern Brazil, *Vet Human Toxicol* 44:362, 2002.
2. Ngomuo AJ, Jones RS: Cytotoxicity studies of quercetin, shikimate, cyclohexanecarboxylate and ptaquiloside, *Vet Human Toxicol* 38:14, 1996.
3. Peauroi JR et al: Anemia, hematuria, and multicentric urinary neoplasia in a llama *(Lama glama)* exposed to bracken fern, *J Zoo Wildlife Med* 26:315, 1995.

STEROIDAL SAPONINS

George Burrows and Ronald J. Tyrl

Sources. Toxic steroidal saponins are present in genera of several plant families that are not closely related: *Agave* and *Nolina* in the Agavaceae, or agave, family; *Panicum* in the Poaceae, or grass, family; and *Tribulus* in the Zygophyllaceae, or creosote bush, family (Table 25-12). In addition, species of *Brachiaria* in the Poaceae and *Narthecium* in the Liliaceae or lily family cause similar problems.

Species of *Agave* are succulent, perennial, yucca-like herbs with spine-tipped leaves and flowers borne on elongate stalks. Of the numerous species of *Agave,* only one is of toxicologic significance. It is found in rocky desert sites of the Southwest, often locally abundant.

Species of *Nolina* are somewhat yucca-like but have a more tussock appearance. The leaves are long and arching, toothed in some species, and lack the thick succulent appearance of those of *Agave.* They are native to the deserts of the southwestern United States.

Panicum is the largest genus of the Poaceae. Comprising both cool- and warm-season grasses, there are more than 100 native and introduced species present in North America. Of the six species of greatest toxicologic interest, *P. virgatum* and *P. dichotomiflorum* are native to the temperate regions of North America; the others of concern are introduced from Africa or India. *P. coloratum* has been planted extensively as a livestock forage in southern Texas.

TABLE 25-12 Plants that Contain Steroidal Saponins

Scientific Name	Common Name
A. lecheguilla Torr.	Lechuguilla
N. bigelovii (Torr.) S.Watson	Sacahuista
N. microcarpa S.Watson	Smallseed nolina, sacahuista
N. texana S.Watson	Bunchgrass, sacahuista
P. antidotale Retz.	Blue panicum
P. coloratum L.	Kleingrass
P. dichotomiflorum Michx	Smooth witchgrass, fall panic grass
P. maximum Jacq.	Guinea grass
P. miliaceum L.	Common millet, broom millet, hog millet, Russian millet
P. virgatum	Switchgrass
T. cistoides L.	Burr nut
T. terrestris L.	Puncture vine, caltrop, goathead

Species of *Tribulus* are prostrate, spreading annual or perennial herbs bearing noxious fruits with stout spines, having the appearance of horns (Color Plates 41 and 42). The two species present in North America are distributed across the southern half of the continent.

Mechanism of Action. Intoxication from this group of plants is due to the inability of the liver to clear the blood of phylloerythrin, and the problem is generally known as hepatogenous photosensitization.[1] A breakdown product of chlorophyll in the digestive tract, phylloerythrin is normally absorbed and excreted by the liver.[2,3] Certain types of liver damage predispose an accumulation of phylloerythrin. When phylloerythrin is not cleared from the blood, it accumulates in sufficient quantities to function as a photodynamic agent. Singlet oxygen formed in the presence of 320 to 400 nm wavelength light reacts at the site of its formation—in the capillaries of the skin—to cause the cellular destruction typical of photosensitization.[4]

Plants containing toxic amounts of these steroidal saponins cause a unique type of liver lesion known as crystalloid or crystal-associated cholangiohepatopathy because of the presence of crystalloid structures in the bile ducts and other sites. The crystalloid material has been determined to be insoluble calcium salts of sapogenic glucuronides in *Panicum* and *Tribulus* as well as *A. lechuguilla*.[5-7] The sapogenins have not been identified in *Nolina*, but the lesions produced by the genus are consistent with those of the other genera. It is not clear whether the steroidal saponins alone are responsible for the disease.

Toxicity and Risk Factors. The range of species affected by these plants is not known, but sheep and goats are most commonly affected. Horses are occasionally affected by *Panicum*, and cattle rarely by the other genera. The susceptibility to intoxication is due in some measure to greater predisposition of sheep and goats to consume the plants or their more toxic parts. This is especially true for *Nolina*, because the buds and flowers, which are most toxic, are seldom eaten by cattle, in contrast to their ready consumption by sheep and goats. *Nolina* is a risk only in those years when large numbers of flowers are produced. *Tribulus* is also readily eaten by sheep.

In most instances, disease follows ingestion of the plants for several weeks or more. *Panicum* is mainly a risk when mature and in flower or seed, *Tribulus* anytime in the growing season, *Agave* in the winter when it is most likely to be eaten, and *Nolina* in late winter and early spring when it is in flower.

Clinical Signs. The signs produced by these compounds are similar to other causes of photosensitization with additional systemic effects related to the involvement of the liver. Depression, pruritus, reduced appetite, loss of body weight, and sometimes icterus are present. The urine may be dark, yellowish brown. The less pigmented areas of skin are reddened and swollen, and the affected areas eventually are covered with exudate and become cracked and necrotic. The sclera and cornea may be icteric or reddened and there may be some degree of photophobia. In sheep, the ears, lips, eyelids, and face around the nose are most affected and animals that recover may lose ears or rarely an eye. Swelling of affected areas occurs. When the head is involved, the disease is sometimes referred to as *bighead*.

Clinical Pathology. During the course of the disease, serum calcium may be elevated; potassium and phosphorus may be decreased. Marked elevation of bilirubin and serum hepatic enzymes, especially GGT, is present. Sulfobromophthalien clearance may be slowed but not always markedly.

Lesions. The most obvious changes are in the skin. A marked thickening with a gelatinous appearance extending into the deeper corium is obvious. Crusty and ulcerative or proliferative areas may be present. The tissues may be icteric and the liver swollen and yellowish brown.

Fatty change, zonal necrosis, and bile pigment in macrophages may be apparent microscopically in the liver. The most distinctive lesions are the polarizing crystals or needle-shaped clefts in and around bile ducts, surrounded by brownish amorphous material filling the ducts. Crystals also may be observed in other areas of the liver, in the bile, and in the renal tubules where they are accompanied by tubular necrosis.

Treatment. Affected animals should be promptly removed from the offending forage and, if possible, provided shade. Good nursing care is appropriate for the liver disease and decreased appetite.

Prognosis. If the animals are promptly removed from the offending forage, many animals may recover. However, if the liver lesions are extensive, deaths may be expected.

Prevention and Control. Zinc supplementation, such as used for facial eczyma, has been suggested as a possible preventive measure, and zinc oxide given intraruminally seemed to provide some benefit against *Nolina* intoxication.[8] This preventive approach has not been thoroughly evaluated.

REFERENCES

1. Clare NT: Photosensitization in animals, *Adv Vet Sci* 2:182, 1955.
2. Blum HF: *Photodynamic action and disease caused by light, American Chemical Society Monograph Series No 85,* New York, 1941, Reinhold.
3. Rimmington C, Quin JI: Studies on the photosensitization of animals in South Africa. VII. The nature of the photosensitizing agent in geeldikkop, *Onderstepoort J Vet Sci Anim Ind* 3:137, 1934.
4. Dodge AD, Knox JP: Photosensitizers from plants, *Pesticide Sci* 17:579, 1986.
5. Miles CO et al: Identification of the calcium salt of epismilagenin beta-D-glucuronide in the bile crystals of sheep affected by *Panicum dichotomiflorum* and *Panicum schinzii* toxicosis, *J Agric Food Chem* 40:1606, 1992.
6. Miles CO et al: Photosensitivity in South Africa. VII. Chemical composition of biliary crystals from a sheep with experimentally induced geeldikkop, *Onderstepoort J Vet Res* 61:215, 1994.
7. Camp BJ et al: Isolation of a steroidal sapogenin from the bile of a sheep fed *Agave lecheguilla*, *Vet Hum Toxicol* 30:533, 1988.
8. Rankins DL et al: Characterization of toxicosis in sheep dosed with blossoms of sacahuista (*Nolina microcarpa*), *J Anim Sci* 71:2489, 1993.

PROTEINS AND AMINO ACIDS

β-AMINO PROPRIONITRILE

John A. Pickrell and Fred Oehme

Sources. *Lathyrus* spp. (vetchling, wild pea, singletary pea) have a variety of toxic species that are grown as cover crops and forage in ranges throughout the Great Plains or grow wild in the southeastern United States.[1,2] Chick pea *(Cicer arietinum)* contains lathyrogens and can also be toxic[3]. Vetchling and chick pea are close relatives to poison vetch *(Astragalus).* Therefore, *Astragalus lentigenosus* has been wrongly assumed to produce lathyrogens.[4]

The toxic principle, β-amino proprionitrile (BAPN), occurs in various concentrations among *Lathyrus* species and is concentrated in the seeds, but is present in the green parts of the plant as well.[1]

Toxicokinetics. Although BAPN is absorbed rapidly, toxicosis is likely only if significant quantities are consumed over long periods of time.[1]

Mechanism of Action. BAPN interferes with lysyl oxidase, the enzyme responsible for cross-linking collagen, resulting in impairment of connective tissue stability and causing osteolathyrism and angiolathyrism.[3,5-8] Whereas BAPN has pronounced osteolathyritic and angiolathyritic activities, it also is neurodegenerative in vitro.[5-8] However, current attention is focused on its glutamate analog, beta-(N)-oxalyl-amino-L-alanine (3-N-oxalyl-L-2,3-diamonopropanoic acid), which when present in sufficient quantities mimics glutamate toxicity.

Neurolathyrism, osteolathyrism, and angiolathyrism are human diseases caused by overconsumption of the excitatory amino acids contained in *Lathyrus* spp.[5] Of 500 human cases of neurolathyrism in Bangladesh, 60 complained of bone pain and showed skeletal deformities suggestive of osteolathyrism.[8] Failure of fusion was found in 30- to 37-year-old humans, presenting clear evidence of osteolathyrism.[8]

Toxicity and Risk Factors. Toxicoses are only likely if large quantities are consumed over long periods of time.[1] Diets of less than 25% flour from *Lathyrus* seeds were not found to be toxic.[2] Diets of 25%, 50%, and 80% flour from seeds resulted in reduced growth, lameness, hernias, and skeletal deformities in rats (osteolathyrism).[2] BAPN (100 to 600 ppm) also produced dissecting aneurysms (angiolathyrism) in rapidly growing 1- to 10-week-old broilers and turkeys, as well as laryngeal hemiplegia in horses.[3,9-11] Broilers or turkeys growing less rapidly were less susceptible.[3,9-11]

Clinical Signs. Neurolathyrism is an acute syndrome in livestock. Cattle and sheep have a stilted gait, are weak, and shift weight from one limb to another. Horses may be more severely affected than cattle and occasionally develop laryngeal hemiplegia.[1,3]

Chronic osteolathyrism occurs less frequently and presents as lameness, but most likely has both neurologic and connective tissue deficits.[1,3,5,7-8] In growing turkeys, acute death has been reported.[3] Eggs produced by layers are usually larger and irregularly shaped. Egg production decreases significantly.[10,11]

Clinical Pathology. Nonspecific clinical pathologic changes are noted for osteolathyrism or neurolathyrism. Death is acute with angiolathyrism, with no specific changes noted.[1]

Lesions. Few gross lesions occur with neurolathyrism or osteolathyrism. Massive hemorrhage occurs when angiolathyrism results in a dissecting aneurysm of the posterior aorta. However, dissections of smaller vessels are more difficult to detect. Almost always, significant intimal thickening or a large fibrous plaque is present at the site of rupture.[3]

Diagnostic Testing. Plant identification of *Lathyrus* is the most common means of diagnosis. Measurement of BAPN in the seed or feed is usually not available with routine diagnostic laboratory analyses.[1]

Treatment. Treatment is typically limited to supportive measures.[1,3] Laryngeal hemiplegia (roaring) in horses may be corrected surgically to stabilize the affected side of the larynx to prevent dynamic collapse during exercise.[3]

Prognosis. Clinical signs are not reversible.

REFERENCES

1. Osweiler GD: *Toxicology,* Philadelphia, 1996, Williams & Wilkins.
2. Kingsbury JM: *Poisonous plants of the United States and Canada,* Englewood Cliffs, NJ, 1964, Prentice-Hall.
3. Aiello S, editor: *The Merck veterinary manual* (toxicology), Whitehouse Station, NJ, 1998, Merck.
4. Hulbert LC, Oehme FW: *Plants poisonous to livestock,* Manhattan, Kan, 1968, Kansas State University.
5. Spencer PS, Schaumberg HH: Lathyrism: a neurotoxic disease, *Neurobehav Toxicol Teratol* 5:625, 1983.
6. Capo MA et al: In vitro neuronal changes induced by beta-aminoproprionitrile, *J Environ Pathol Toxicol Oncol* 13:259, 1994.
7. Grela ER et al: [Lathyrism in people and animals.], *Med Wetery* 56:568, 2000 Polish.
8. Haque A et al: Evidence of osteolathyrism among patients suffering from neurolathyrism in Bangladesh, *Nat Toxins* 5:43, 1997.
9. Mahendar M et al: Pathology of vascular lesions induced by beta amino proprionitrile (BAPN) in chicken, *Cheiron* 3:112, 1987.
10. Chowdhury CD: Effect of feeding a lathyrus toxin on egg weight, egg production and egg malformity in laying chicken, *Asian Australasian J Anim Sci* 4:275, 1991.
11. Chowdhury CD: Effects of low and high dietary levels of beta-aminoproprionitrile (BAPN) on the performance of laying chickens, *J Sci Food Agric* 52:315, 1990.

DIMETHYL DISULFIDE

John A. Pickrell and Fred Oehme

Sources. Mustards *(Brassica* spp.) are annual plants and forage crops grown throughout the United States. They flower early in the spring and may well be the first green plants available. Mustards usually have small yellow or white four-petaled flowers, simple leaves, and dark brown seeds.[1-4]

Toxicokinetics.   These plants contain *S*-methyl cysteine sulfoxide, which is reduced by microbial fermentation to the toxic dimethyl disulfide in the intestinal tract of monogastric animals or the rumen and then absorbed into the blood. Metabolism and absorption take less than 1 day.[1,5,6]

Mechanism of Action.   Dimethyl disulfide is an oxidant, and glutathione reduces its oxidative potential to erythrocytes. However, when the quantity of dimethyl disulfide exceeds the body's glutathione reserves, erythrocytes are oxidized to form Heinz bodies, resulting in hemolysis and Heinz-body anemia.[1,5-9] Dimethyl disulfide delivered over longer time periods allows induction of more glutathione for the hepatic degradation of dimethyl disulfide.[8]

Clinical Signs. Animals may be depressed, constipated, and hemoglobinemic. Dark-brown to reddish urine (hemoglobinuria) and pale to icteric mucous membranes may be present. If anemia is severe, affected animals have tachycardia, polypnea, and possibly cyanosis.[1,2,4-7]

Clinical Pathology. The hemoglobin, number of red blood cells, and packed cell volume are significantly decreased.[1,2,4-7] Heinz bodies are present in red blood cells.

Lesions. No specific gross lesions are found. Tissues are pale, except for the kidneys, which may be dark.[1,3,4]

Diagnostic Testing. The diagnosis is typically made indirectly by the presence of *Brassica*, evidence of consumption, and appropriate clinical signs. Dimethyl disulfide is not routinely analyzed at veterinary diagnostic laboratories.[1,2]

Treatment. Treatment is mostly supportive. A transfusion may be life saving in advanced cases. Diuresis with fluids may reduce the occurrence of hemoglobin nephrosis.[1,2,4]

Prognosis. The prognosis depends on the degree of anemia. The presence of hemoglobin nephrosis reduces the chance of recovery.[1,2,4]

REFERENCES

1. Murphy M: *A field guide to common animal poisons,* Ames, Iowa, 1996, Iowa State University Press.
2. Osweiler GD: *Toxicology,* Philadelphia, 1996, Williams & Wilkins.
3. Aiello S, editor: *The Merck veterinary manual (toxicology),* Whitehouse Station, NJ, Merck.
4. Hulbert LC, Oehme FW: *Plants poisonous to livestock,* Manhattan, Kan, 1968, Kansas State University.
5. Maxwell MH: Production of Heinz body anemia in domestic fowl after ingestion of dimethyl disulfide: a hematological and ultrastructural study, *Res Vet Sci* 30:233, 1981.
6. Duncan AJ, Milne JA: Effects of oral administration of brassica secondary metabolites, allyl cyanide, allyl isothiocyanate and dimethyl disulphide on the voluntary food intake and metabolism of sheep, *Br J Nutr* 70:631, 1993.
7. Duncan AJ, Roncin B, Elston DA: The effect of blood glutathione status and breed on the susceptibility of adult female sheep to the haemolytic anaemia induced by the brassica antimetabolite, dimethyl disulphide, *Anim Sci* 60:93, 1995.
8. Siess MH et al: Modification of hepatic drug-metabolizing enzymes in rats treated with alkyl sulfides, *Cancer Lett* 120:195, 1997.
9. Mussinan CJ, Keelan ME, editors: Sulfur compounds in foods. ACS Symposium Series no 564, 1994.

LECTINS

Jay C. Albretsen

Synonyms. Lectins are proteins with affinity for sugar molecules. They are phytotoxins and are also referred to as hemagglutinins and toxalbumins. Ricin and abrin are the names of the most toxic lectins, found in *Ricinus communis* (Color Plates 43 and 44) and *Abrus precatorius,* respectively.[1-3]

Sources. Lectins are found in most beans, including soybeans, kidney, pinto, and navy beans. Other plants suspected of containing these glycoproteins are *Jatropha curcas* (coral plants, physic nuts, barbados nuts), *Robina pseudoacacia* (black locust), *Momordica charantia* (bitter gourd, bitter cucumber, African cucumber), *Hura crepitans* (monkey's dinner bell, monkey's pistol, possum wood, sandbox tree), and some species of *Sophora.* The plants considered to produce the most toxic lectins are *R. communis* (castor bean, castor oil plant, mole bean plant, palma christi, African wonder tree, coffee tree) and *A. precatorius* (jequirty, rosary pea, prayer bean, crab's eye, precatory bean, Indian bead, Seminole bead, weather plant, mieniemienie).[1-4] The toxic component in the castor bean plant is the water-soluble, heat-labile toxalbumin ricin. Castor bean oil, if properly extracted, does not contain ricin.[1,2,5]

Toxicokinetics. All lectins are poorly absorbed from the digestive tract. The actual release of the lectin may require chewing or piercing of the seed coat.[1-3] Lectins are water soluble and are destroyed by moist heat.[1] Ricin and abrin consist of two polypeptide chains cross-linked by two disulfide bonds. Other lectins have two polypeptide chains, but are not cross-linked with disulfide bonds.[1,3,6,7]

No other information on metabolism, distribution, and elimination is available for lectins. However, signs most often develop within 6 hours of castor bean ingestion in dogs.[8] Clinical signs associated with castor bean toxicosis in animals often occur several hours after ingestion of the beans.[2,5] All dogs show signs within 42 hours. The duration of signs is between 1.5 and 5.5 days in dogs.[8]

Mechanism of Action. Ricin and abrin are cellular toxins and the mechanism of toxicity in mammalian cells has been extensively studied.[3,5-7,9-12] Ricin and abrin are composed of two glycoprotein chains. The B chain facilitates endocytosis of the toxins, and then the A chain inhibits protein synthesis and causes cell death[5-7,9]

The B chain of the ricin and abrin molecules binds to galactoside-containing proteins on the cell surface, allowing internalization of the toxin. Mammalian cells possess a large number of glycoproteins and glycolipids with galactose residues that are available for the B chain of ricin to attach.[7] This ensures that most, if not all, ricin and abrin molecules present at the cell surface will enter the cells by endocytosis.

Once in the cell, some of the lectins are transported to lysosomes or back to the cell surface. In a lysosome or outside the cell, they can produce no cellular damage.[7] However, some are moved from the endosomes to the trans-Golgi network, resulting in retrograde transport of the ricin and abrin through the Golgi stack. Ultimately, the A chain is translocated into the cytosol and works its way back to the endoplasmic reticulum. Once in the endoplasmic reticulum, the A chain depurinates 28S ribosomal ribonucleic acid (rRNA) by the removal of a specific adenine residue.[5-7,12] Protein synthesis cannot occur and the cell dies.[1,2,5] Ricin also disturbs calcium homeostasis in the cardiovascular system by decreasing calcium uptake by the sarcoplasmic reticulum and increasing sodium-calcium exchange.[10,12-14]

Lectins in beans bind to cells on the intestinal wall and cause nonspecific interference of nutrient absorption. Evidence exists that lectins impair the immune system.[1] Rat IgE, but not IgG, increases after ricin administration. The cause of this effect is not known.[15]

Toxicity and Risk Factors. Poisoning has occurred in many animals, including dogs, poultry, wild fowl, pigs, horses, sheep, and goats.[1,2] Even though all parts of the ricin and abrin plants contain lectins, clinical toxicosis is most often associated with ingestion of the seeds, which are extremely toxic because they contain more lectins.[2] Most livestock poisonings are a result of seed contamination of feed grains.[1] Swine are also fed cull beans in some areas. The lectins ingested in these cases would likely be destroyed if the feed is heat-treated first.[1] In companion animals, the beans must be crushed or broken in order for the toxalbumin to be released.[5]

Ricin and abrin are some of the most deadly substances known. Ricin and abrin are much more toxic parenterally than orally and ricin has been used as a homicidal poison.[3,6] Lethal doses of ricin range from 0.025 μg given intraperitoneally in mice to 1 mg/kg orally in humans.[5,6] Less than one precatory bean, if it has been crushed, is sufficient to kill a human.[1]

Recent cases of castor bean exposure suggest that ingestion infrequently results in death despite ricin being one of the most potent toxins known.[16,17] A possible explanation for this inconsistency may be that sometimes castor beans are swallowed whole. The toxalbumins in castor beans are not likely to be released unless the seed coat is damaged or compromised.[1,2,8]

Clinical Signs. The major effects are on the intestinal mucosa. Reduced growth rate, diarrhea, decreased nutrient absorption, and increased incidence of bacterial infections are common with all ingested lectins. The more toxic lectins, such as abrin and ricin, result in more severe signs. Initially, gastrointestinal irritation results in vomiting, diarrhea, and abdominal pain. These signs often progress to hemorrhagic gastroenteritis.[1,3]

Clinical Pathology. In cases of castor bean ingestion in dogs, the most common abnormal laboratory tests are leukocytosis, increased alanine aminotransferase (ALT), and increased aspartate aminotransferase (AST) levels.[8]

Lesions. The main lesions associated with lectin ingestion are gastroenteritis. Histologically, disruption of normal microvilli in the jejunum has been reported.[1] After absorption, ricin is preferentially distributed to the liver, spleen, and muscle.[5,6,9] In these organs, ricin causes reversible liver damage, vascular endothelial injury, edema, and myalgias.[9] The deregulation of intracellular calcium homeostasis causes myocardial necrosis and cardiac hemorrhage.[10,12-14]

Treatment. No specific antidote exists for lectin toxicosis. Supportive and symptomatic care in all species is important.[5] Emesis can be beneficial in animals that can vomit if instituted early after ingestion. Activated charcoal (1 to 4 g/kg body weight orally) and a cathartic (magnesium sulfate at 250 mg/kg body weight orally or 70% sorbitol at 3 ml/kg body weight orally) can be beneficial even if given several hours after the ingestion.[18,19]

Gastrointestinal protectants such as kaolin-pectin or sucralfate (0.25 to 2 g three times a day by mouth) should be used as needed.[20] Appropriate fluid and electrolyte therapy should be considered very important because hypotension can often be controlled with balanced electrolyte solutions. Fluid administration should account for both daily requirements and ongoing fluid losses.[18] Because of the adverse effect that lectins have on the gastrointestinal tract, small amounts of a bland diet should be given frequently for several days once the vomiting is controlled. Seizures have been reported after some ricin ingestions and may be controlled with diazepam (0.5 to 1 mg/kg body weight intravenously) in companion animals.[19]

Complete blood count and serum biochemistry values are helpful. Specific elevations of liver or kidney biochemical values may not occur for 12 to 24 hours following lectin ingestion. Antibiotics, lactulose (0.1 to 0.5 mg/kg body weight three times per day orally), or dietary management along with appropriate fluid therapy can be used to correct the clinical signs associated with hepatic failure.[20] Similarly, signs of renal failure should be treated with appropriate fluid therapy and supportive care. Repeated clinical biochemistry evaluations are indicated until enzyme levels return to normal and clinical signs resolve.

The effectiveness of glucocorticoid administration in animals following lectin ingestion is not known. Dexamethasone given 3 days before ricin administration delayed death in mice challenged with lethal doses of ricin. It is postulated that dexamethasone inhibits lipid peroxidation. Because lethal ricin doses result in increased lipid peroxidation, dexamethasone could be the reason for the delayed time of death in the challenged mice.[6]

Prognosis. Because lectins are poorly absorbed and the seeds must be chewed for signs to develop, the mortality rate is low in all animals. However, because of the serious potential of ricin and abrin, all exposures could potentially be lethal. Therefore, if an animal is showing signs of lectin poisoning, the prognosis should be guarded.

Prevention and Control. Lectins are destroyed by heat. Therefore, all animal foods that contain lectins should be heat-treated before they are fed. Castor beans and rosary peas should be kept out of reach of all pets. If the plants are grown for ornamental purposes, the seeds that are produced in the fall need to be removed. Even though all parts of the plant contain lectins, castor bean poisoning in dogs is most often from the seeds.[8]

REFERENCES

1. Cheeke PR, Shull LR: *Natural toxicants in feeds and poisonous plants,* Westport, Conn, 1985, AVI Publishing.
2. Knight MW, Dorman DC: Selected poisonous plant concerns in small animals, *Vet Med* 92:260, 1997.
3. Furbee B, Wermuth M: Life threatening plant poisoning, *Med Tox* 13:849, 1997.
4. Muenscher WC: P*oisonous plants of the United States,* New York, 1975, Macmillan Publishing.
5. Ellenhorn MJ et al: *Medical toxicology: diagnosis and treatment of human poisoning,* ed 2, Baltimore, 1997, Williams & Wilkins.
6. Muldoon DF, Stohs SJ: Modulation of ricin toxicity in mice by biologically active substances, *J Appl Toxicol* 14:81, 1994.
7. Lord JM, Roberts LM: The intracellular transport of ricin: why mammalian cells are killed and how ricinus cells survive, *Plant Phys Biochem* 34:253, 1996.
8. Albretsen JC et al: Evaluation of castor bean toxicosis in dogs: 98 cases, *J Am Anim Hosp Assoc* 36:229, 2000.
9. Fu T et al: Ricin toxin contains three lectin sites which contribute to its in vivo toxicity, *Int J Immunopharmacol* 18:685, 1996.
10. Ma L et al: Ricin disturbs calcium homeostasis in the rabbit heart, *J Biochem Toxicol* 10:323, 1995.
11. Palatnick W, Tenenbein M: Hepatotoxicity due to castor bean ingestion, *Clin Toxicol* 35:528, 1997.
12. Zhang L et al: Effects of ricin administration to rabbits on the ability of their coronary arteries to contract and relax in vitro, *Toxicol Appl Pharmacol* 129:16, 1994.
13. Ma L et al: Ricin depresses cardiac function in the rabbit heart, *Toxicol Appl Pharmacol* 138:72, 1996.
14. Christiansen VJ et al: The cardiovascular effects of ricin in rabbits, *Pharmacol Toxicol* 74:148, 1994.
15. Thorpe SC et al: The effect of the castor bean toxin, ricin, on rat IgE and IgG responses, *Immunology* 68:307, 1989.
16. Challoner KR, McCarron MM: Castor bean intoxication, *Ann Emerg Med* 19:1177, 1995.
17. Alpin PJ, Eliseo T: Ingestion of castor oil plant seeds, *Med J Aust* 168:423, 1997.
18. Dorman DC: In Bonagura JD, editor: *Current veterinary therapy XII,* Philadelphia, 1995, WB Saunders.
19. Leveille-Webste CR: In Morgan RV, editor: *Handbook of small animal practice,* ed 3, Philadelphia, 1997, WB Saunders.
20. Plumb DC: *Veterinary drug handbook,* ed 3, Ames, Iowa, 1999, Iowa State University Press.

PROPYL DISULFIDE

Patricia A. Talcott

Synonyms. The plants that contain these toxins include onion, garlic, leek, shallot, and chive.

Sources. All *Allium* species belong to the Amaryllidaceae family. More than 400 species of these plants exist, all having a potent odor, and most of them perennial, rhizomatous, or bulbous herbs. Onion species can either be native or grown for food, whereas others are grown as ornamentals for flower and rock gardens. Poisonings in animals have been reported as being a result of ingestion of raw, dry, or cooked onions. Reports have implicated fresh raw onions, cull onions, onion souffle,[1] minced dehydrated onions,[2,3] cooked onions,[4] baby food containing onion powder,[5] wild onions,[6] and garlic[7] as sources of poisoning for domestic animals.

Toxicokinetics. The toxic principles are thought to be a group of structurally similar *n*-propyl disulfides and thiosulfinate compounds.[8] The hemolytic effect of sodium *n*-propylthiosulphate has been extensively studied.[9]

Mechanism of Action. The recycling of disulfides leads to the formation of oxygen free radicals, which can directly damage erythrocyte membranes and lead to an intravascular hemolysis. Free radicals can also denature hemoglobin, which precipitates out within the erythrocytes and binds to the interior of the red blood cell to form Heinz bodies. These damaged cells are ultimately removed from circulation by the reticuloendothelial system or undergo hemolysis leading to anemia.[10] The disulfides also can be reduced by glutathione and glutathione peroxidase to thiols. Oxyhemoglobin then mediates the oxidation of thiols to free radicals. During this process, methemoglobin can also be produced.[10]

Toxicity and Risk Factors. Reported toxic doses of onion plants to animals depends on the onion source (e.g., species of onion, cooked versus dried, time of year, and growing conditions) and species of animal involved. The interval between time of ingestion and onset of clinical signs is dose dependent and varies depending on whether the exposure occurred once or was continuous. Heinz body hemolytic anemia associated with ingestion of onions has been reported in several species, including dogs, cats, cattle, sheep, goats, and horses. Cats, dogs, and cattle appear to be most susceptible to the onion's toxic effects, whereas sheep and goats appear to be most resistant. This difference in susceptibility between species may be due to differences in hemoglobin structure, as well as differences in metabolism and detoxification within the gastrointestinal tract and internal tissue organs.

Experimentally induced anemia has been observed in dogs fed raw onions at dosages between 11 and 15 g/kg body weight per day.[11] The maximum clinical pathologic effect was observed 7 to 12 days after the initial exposure. The onset of clinical signs was more gradual in the dogs receiving the lower dose, whereas the dogs receiving the higher dose showed signs of hemolytic changes within 2 to 3 days. An acute hemolytic anemia was observed in a dog (body weight not reported, but possibly 40 to 50 pounds) that ingested 3 to 4 ounces of dehydrated onions (approximately 21 to 28 ounces of raw onions).[2] Dogs fed 5.5 g/kg body weight of minced dehydrated onions exhibited severe hematologic changes within 24 hours of exposure, which continued for several days thereafter.[3] Twelve to 24 hours after ingestion of 200 g of boiled onions, dogs exhibited decreases in hemoglobin concentrations while methemoglobin levels and Heinz bodies both increased.[12] Kingsbury cites the toxic dose of raw onions in dogs as being equal to or greater than 0.5% of the animal's body weight.[13] Dogs receiving 1.25 ml/kg body weight of garlic extract (5 g whole garlic per kilogram) developed decreases in erythrocyte and hemoglobin levels and increases in Heinz bodies and eccentrocytes several days after ingestion.[7] Hemolysis was not observed in any dog at any time during that study. Oral administration of 500 μmol/kg body weight of sodium n-propylthiosulphate has been associated with a Heinz body hemolytic anemia in dogs.[9] In dogs, reduction of erythrocyte glutathione concentrations enhances the oxidative damage caused by the toxins.

A study in 1998 confirmed that cats ingesting baby food containing as little as 0.3% onion powder exhibited increases in Heinz body formation.[5] Within 10 hours of being fed 28 g of raw onion per kilogram body weight daily for 3 days, cats displayed an increase in Heinz body formation and decreases in packed cell volume and red blood cell counts.[14]

An adult quarter horse receiving daily doses of between 1 and 4 pounds of wild onion tops exhibited significant clinical pathologic abnormalities, including a decrease in packed cell volume and an increase in Heinz body formation.[15]

Nonlactating dairy cows developed signs of toxicosis 24 hours after being fed approximately 0.04 kg/kg body weight of onions.[16] Signs of toxicosis were observed in calves and yearlings that ate approximately 8 to 15 kg of onions per head over a period of 5 days.[17] In 1999, Rae[10] reported a case in which five cows died and two aborted after consuming 20 kg of onions per cow per day for 6 weeks.

Even though sheep are relatively resistant to the toxic effects of onions, dosages of 50 g/kg body weight per day of onion for 15 days caused a severe Heinz body hemolytic anemia.[18] Two groups of sheep fed either 150 or 300 g of dried wild onion exhibited a Heinz body hemolytic anemia.[6]

Clinical Signs.   Onion poisoning can be caused by both acute and chronic exposures, depending on species of animal affected and dose over time. Clinical signs can appear abruptly within 24 hours of ingestion, or take several days or weeks to become apparent. The most commonly reported clinical signs include inappetence, ataxia, lethargy or recumbency, tachycardia, tachypnea or dyspnea, and pale or jaundiced mucous membranes. Vomiting and diarrhea can occur, but it is generally not persistent. A distinctive onion odor to the breath is often detected. Abortions can occur up to several days following the onset of signs. Death to the fetus is most likely due to hypoxia. Decreased rumen motility has been reported in cattle. Once the onions are removed from the diet, signs of poisoning can persist for several days.

Clinical Pathology.   The severity of changes are species, dose, and time dependent. Changes include Heinz bodies, Howell-Jolly bodies, evidence of regeneration (basophilic stippling, polychromasia), hemoglobinemia, hemoglobinuria, anemia, hyperbilirubinemia, and elevated lactate dehydrogenase activity. Heinz bodies can be observed in cases of exposure without any evidence of hemolysis, particularly in

cats. The degree of damage to the hemoglobin molecule and the erythrocyte membrane is proportional to the exposure dose. Methemoglobin levels may also be significantly increased above normal. Changes compatible with recumbency (i.e., elevated creatine kinase), renal damage (i.e., azotemia), and hepatic damage (i.e., elevated alkaline phosphatase) may be observed as well. Eccentrocytosis has also been reported.

Lesions.   The carcass may have an onion odor during necropsy. However, this odor does dissipate over time. Gross lesions include pale or jaundiced mucous membranes, dark brown-red urine, pale liver, and congested, dark red-brown spleen and kidneys. Hemoglobin casts, nephrotubular necrosis, and hepatic necrosis (periacinar, centrilobular, or midzonal) are commonly observed histologic changes. Hemosiderosis may also be observed in the renal proximal tubules, liver, and spleen.

Diagnostic Testing.   No diagnostic tests are available for the toxins associated with onion poisoning. The disease is often recognized from the history or examination of pasture and property.

Treatment.   The treatment aims are to maintain adequate cardiovascular support through intravenous fluid therapy or blood transfusions.

Prognosis.   The prognosis is highly dependent on the severity of the anemia and the species of animal affected. Abortion caused by hypoxia may occur in any pregnant animal that is experiencing significant anemia.

Prevention and Control.   Prevention in all animals can be achieved by limiting access to any potential sources of *Allium* spp. Because of the difficulties in some areas in disposing of cull onions, they have been used effectively in sheep and cattle diets. Onions are often more than 85% moisture and have similar nutritional value as barley on a dry-matter basis. From studies performed in cattle, it appears that cattle perform well on diets containing up to 25% (dry matter) onions (46% as is), which are best fed by chopping or crushing the onions into the total mixed ration.[19] Onion poisoning in cattle is most commonly seen when cattle are allowed unlimited access to onions over a period of several days or more.

REFERENCES

1. Spice RN: Hemolytic anemia associate with ingestion of onions in a dog, *Can Vet J* 17(7):181, 1976.
2. Farkas MC, Farkas JN: Hemolytic anemia due to ingestion of onions in a dog, *J Am Anim Hosp Assoc* 10:65, 1974.
3. Harvey JW, Rackear D: Experimental onion-induced hemolytic anemia in dogs, *Vet Pathol* 22:387, 1985.
4. Lees GE et al: Idiopathic Heinz body hemolytic anemia in three dogs, *J Am Anim Hosp Assoc* 15:143, 1979.
5. Robertson JE et al: Heinz body formation in cats fed baby food containing onion powder, *J Am Vet Med Assoc* 212(8):1260, 1998.
6. Van Kampen KR et al: Hemolytic anemia in sheep fed wild onion (*Allium validum*), *J Am Vet Med Assoc* 156(3):328, 1970.

7. Lee KW et al: Hematologic changes associated with the appearance of eccentrocytes after intragastric administration of garlic extract to dogs, *Am J Vet Res* 61(11):1446, 2000.

8. Block E et al: *Allium* chemistry: HPLC analysis of thiosulfinates from onion, garlic, wild garlic (Ramsoms), leek, scallion, shallot, elephant (great-headed) garlic, chive, and Chinese chive. Uniquely high allyl to methyl ratios in some garlic samples, *J Agric Food Chem* 40:2418, 1992.

9. Yamato O et al: Induction of onion-induced haemolytic anaemia in dogs with sodium n-propylthiosulphate, *Vet Rec* 142(9):216, 1998.

10. Rae HA: Onion toxicosis in a herd of beef cows, *Can Vet J* 40:44, 1999.

11. Sebrell WH: An anemia of dogs produced by feeding onions, *US Pub Health Rep* 45:1175, 1930.

12. Yamoto O, Maede Y: Susceptibility to onion-induced hemolysis in dogs with hereditary high erythrocyte reduced glutathione and potassium concentrations, *Am J Vet Res* 53(1):134, 1992.

13. Kingsbury JM: *Poisonous plants of the United States and Canada*, ed 1, Englewood Cliffs, NJ, 1964, Prentice-Hall.

14. Kobayashi K: Onion poisoning in a cat, *Fel Pract* 11:22-27, 1981.

15. Pierce KR et al: Acute hemolytic anemia caused by wild onion poisoning in horses, *J Am Vet Med Assoc* 160(3):323, 1972.

16. Van Der Kolk JH: Onion poisoning in a herd of dairy cattle, *Vet Rec* 147:517, 2000.

17. Verhoeff J et al: Onion poisoning of young cattle, *Vet Rec* 117:497, 1985.

18. Selim HM: Rumen bacteria are involved in the onset of onion-induced hemolytic anemia in sheep, *J Vet Med Sci* 61(4):369, 1999.

19. Lincoln SD: Hematologic effects and feeding performance in cattle fed cull domestic onions (*Allium cepa*), *J Am Vet Med Assoc* 200(8):1090, 1992.

THIAMINASE

John A. Pickrell and Fred Oehme

Sources.   *Pteridium aquilinum* (bracken fern) is widespread and grows in semishaded areas with moderate moisture and well-drained soil[1-4] (Color Plate 40). It grows in dense patches and spreads by underground rhizomes.

Equisetum spp. (horsetail) are found in wet areas, usually near running or standing water[1,4] (Color Plate 45). They spread by rhizomatous growth and can form dense populations.

Mechanism of Action.   Both plants contain thiaminase, which decreases dietary thiamine before it can be absorbed and participate in intermediary metabolism. Thiamine pyrophosphate is an obligate cofactor in several reactions in carbohydrate metabolism. Cellular stores of adenosine triphosphate (ATP) decline and pyruvate increases as thiamine concentrations decrease in peripheral blood.[1]

Toxicity and Risk Factors.   If horses are maintained on a diet nutritionally marginal in B vitamins, then hay with more than 20% bracken produces signs within a month.[1,3] If bracken fern is included in the diet of rats, the rats continue to gain weight for about 10 days, develop signs, and die by 30 days after first ingestion. It is nearly impossible to detect a thiamine deficiency in cattle.[3]

Equisetum spp. are not palatable and so intoxication from fresh plants is unlikely except perhaps in winter when no other green forage is available. Most poisonings occur in horses that ingest contaminated hay. Nervous signs can develop by 40 days after ingestion.[1-5]

Clinical Signs.   Horses develop anorexia, appear unthrifty, lose weight, and become emaciated. They gradually become uncoordinated, have a wide stance, develop posterior paralysis, and may be unsuccessful in their attempts to rise. Muscle fasciculations may occur if the animals are exercised. Some cases progress to terminal opisthotonus, convulsions, and death.[1-4]

Clinical Pathology.   Thiamine deficiency does not result in specific changes.

Lesions.   No specific gross lesions are found at necropsy.

Diagnostic Testing.   Response to treatment with thiamine and evidence of plant consumption supports the diagnosis. Measurement of thiamine concentrations in blood is not routinely available.[1]

Treatment.   Specific treatment is 100 to 200 mg thiamine twice on the first day and then daily for 7 to 14 days.[1-4]

Prognosis.   Early cases respond well to treatment and the prognosis is good. If the animal has advanced signs, the prognosis for recovery is poor.[2-4]

REFERENCES

1. Murphy M: *A field guide to common animal poisons*, Ames, Iowa, 1996, Iowa State University Press.

2. Osweiler GD: *Toxicology*, Philadelphia, 1996, Williams & Wilkins.

3. Kingsbury JM: *Poisonous plants of the United States and Canada*, Englewood Cliffs, NJ, 1964, Prentice-Hall.

4. Hulbert LC, Oehme FW: *Plants poisonous to livestock*, Manhattan, Kan, 1968, Kansas State University.

5. Fabre B, Geay B, Beaufils P: Thiaminase activity in *Equisetum arvense* and its extracts, *Plantes Medicinales et Phytotherapie* 26,190, 1993.

TRYPTOPHAN

John A. Pickrell and Fred Oehme

Synonyms.   The disease has been termed "fog fever" because of its association with fog and the lush green forage that results from the atmospheric moisture.[1-4] More recent names for the disease include acute bovine pulmonary edema and emphysema (ABPE) and acute respiratory distress syndrome (ARDS).

Sources.   This disease is a result of moving hungry adult cattle from dry pastures to lush forage of many grasses, alfalfa, rape, kale, turnip tops, or a host of other plants. The genus of plant is not as important as the fact that it is lush and provides the opportunity for greater exposure to L-tryptophan.

Mechanism of Action.   L-Tryptophan from plants is converted to 3-methylindole (3-MI) in the rumen, absorbed into the blood, and concentrated in the lung.[4] Most tryptophan from the rumen is absorbed in the duodenum.[5] The cytochrome P-450 system (mixed function oxidases, or MFO) primarily in the lung Clara cells and macrophages and, to a lesser degree, the type II pneumocytes, converts 3-methylindole to a reactive component, which is pneumotoxic.[3,4] The toxins destroy the Clara cells and type I pneumocytes. To restore the alveolar epithelium, type II pneumocytes quickly proliferate, but have decreased ability to synthesize and secrete surface-active phospholipids that are capable of lowering the surface tension. Without functional surfactant, the animal develops emphysema.

Toxicity and Risk Factors. Signs begin within 12 hours after consuming lush green forage.[4] Most cases occur between July and December, and arise within 2 weeks of a pasture change. Morbidity varies from 1% to 100%. Mortality may be as high as 50% to 90%, but averages approximately 30% in the first 2 to 3 days.[1-4]

Clinical Signs. Coughing is not a dominant feature. Affected animals have severe dyspnea, rapid breathing, and are reluctant to move.[3,4] To facilitate breathing, they stand with their feet wide apart, head and neck extended and lowered, and their nostrils flared.[4] Less severely affected animals are depressed, have an expiratory grunt, wheeze, and have froth flowing out their nostrils.[2-4] Mild cases can go unnoticed unless exercised. Consolidated lung sounds can be detected in the caudal dorsal region as crackles. Rumen atony often accompanies these signs. As animals progress to advanced stages, they become sternally recumbent and die during the second to third day if undisturbed. If affected animals are stressed or exercised, they can die a few hours after the onset of dyspnea.[1-4]

Clinical Pathology. No specific clinical laboratory findings relate to ARDS.[1-4]

Lesions. Macroscopically, cranial lung lobes are deep-purple, heavy, do not collapse normally, and glisten when cut.[3] Pulmonary edema is apparent, especially ventrally, with gelatinous yellow fluid oozing from the cut surfaces. Emphysematous gas bullae occur throughout the lung. In animals less severely affected, lungs are pinkish-tan, rubbery, and firm.[2-4]

Histologically, alveolar ducts are lined with hyaline membranes, edema, scattered eosinophils, neutrophils, and alveolar macrophages. Large mononuclear cells and a mixture of macrophages and epithelial cells are found in alveolar lumens.[3,4]

Diagnostic Testing. Diagnosis is typically based on history, clinical signs, and lesions.[1,2] Determination of tryptophan in pastures or animal plasma[6,7] is not routinely available in veterinary diagnostic laboratories.

Treatment. Treatment with nonsteroidal antiinflammatory agents, diuretics, bronchodilators, and antihistamines has limited success.

Prognosis. Mildly affected animals may recover most respiratory function.[2-4] Moderately affected animals that survive often become unthrifty without regaining full pul-

monary function. The prognosis for severely affected animals is poor.

Prevention and Control. Sudden introduction of lush pasture into cattle diets can be avoided by cutting the forage for hay first or by limiting the grazing time on the new pasture. Partial protection can be provided by adding an ionophore, such as monensin or lasalocid, to the diet beginning 1 week before the pasture change and continuing for 10 days after the pasture change.[1-4,8,9]

REFERENCES

1. Murphy M: *A Field guide to common animal poisons,* Ames, Iowa, 1996, Iowa State University Press.
2. Aiello S, editor: *The Merck veterinary manual (toxicology),* Whitehouse Station, NJ, Merck.
3. Breeze R, Carlson JR: Acute bovine pulmonary edema and emphysema. In Howard JL, editor: *Current veterinary therapy: food animal practice 3,* Philadelphia, 1989, WB Saunders.
4. Kerr LE, Linnabary RD: A review of interstitial pneumonia in cattle, *Vet Hum Toxicol* 31:247, 1989.
5. Hammond AC et al: Site of 3-methylindole and indole absorption in steers after ruminal administration of L-tryptophan, *Am J Vet Res* 45:171, 1984.
6. Selman IE et al: Experimental production of fog fever by change to pasture free from *Dictocaulus vivparus* infection, *Vet Rec* 14:278, 1977.
7. Mackenzie A, Heaney RK, Fenwick GR: Determination of indole and 3-methylindole in plasma and rumen fluid from cattle with fog fever or after L-tryptophan administration, *Res Vet Sci* 23:47, 1977.
8. Hammond AC, Carlson JR, Breeze RG: Prevention of tryptophan-induced acute bovine pulmonary edema and emphysema (fog fever), *Vet Rec* 107:322,1980.
9. Hammond AC, Carlson JR, Breeze RG: Monensin and the prevention of tryptophan-induced acute bovine pulmonary edema and emphysema, *Science* 201:153, 1978.

TERPENES

DITERPENE ESTERS

John A. Pickrell and Fred Oehme

Sources. More than 2 dozen *Euphorbia* spp. (toxic spurges) occur as indoor ornamental plants, garden plants, or weeds. They are worldwide and range widely over the United States in disturbed areas such as cultivated areas, roadsides, and overgrazed pastures.[1-3] They are more common throughout the Great Prairie.[3] Flowering spurges may be cultivated as ornamental plants.[2,4]

Mechanism of Action. *Euphorbia* spp. contain blistering compounds that directly irritate the skin, mucous membranes, and gastrointestinal tract on contact.[1] The toxic compounds are diterpenoid euphorbol esters that activate protein kinase C, which causes cytoskeletal damage and enzyme dysfunction.[1]

Toxicity and Risk Factors. The sap is toxic in both fresh and dried plants.[1] Honey made from *Euphorbia* flowers may be toxic to nonherbivores.[2] Ingestion of *Euphorbia* species by livestock at 1% or more of animal body weight may cause clinical signs.[1]

Most *Euphorbia* spp. are relatively mild in their toxic actions. Poinsettia (*Euphorbia pulcherrima*), despite anecdotal reports about its lethality, is less toxic than many *Euphorbia* spp. and rarely causes problems beyond mild gastrointestinal signs.[5-7] On the other hand, *Euphorbia esula* (leafy spurge) is a highly invasive pasture weed that can cause clinical signs in cattle; sheep and goats seem unaffected by the plant.

Clinical Signs. Exposures in small animals are usually minimal, so clinical signs frequently are limited to mild gastrointestinal signs: salivation, vomiting, and diarrhea.

In livestock, horses are most severely affected, but cattle and sheep are also affected.[3] Signs begin within minutes of contact. Irritation and blistering of mouth and skin as well as the mucosa are expected. Blistering can lead to salivation, irritation of the upper gastrointestinal tract, and diarrhea with or without blood. Collapse and death are not uncommon if the dose is sufficiently high.[1-3,8,9]

Clinical Pathology. No specific clinical laboratory findings are related to euphorbia.[1-3]

Lesions. Lesions are not specific and are limited to blistering of the mouth, skin, and upper gastrointestinal tract.[1-3]

Diagnostic Testing. Evidence of ingestion and appropriate clinical signs are the best diagnostic aids in live animals. Phorbols, daphanes, or ingenols are not routinely measured in veterinary diagnostic laboratories.[10]

Treatment. In small animals, ingested toxins are diluted with water or milk.[2] Mineral oil can be used in large animals. Topical exposures should be washed with alcohol. Local inflammation and necrosis can be treated with analgesics and topical ointments.[1-3]

Prognosis. Most exposures in small animals are mild and self-limiting. If large animals are displaying severe clinical signs, the prognosis is poor.

REFERENCES

1. Osweiler GD: *Toxicology*, Philadelphia, 1996, Williams & Wilkins.
2. Murphy M: *A field guide to common animal poisons*, Ames, Iowa, 1996. Iowa State University Press.
3. Hulbert LC, Oehme FW: *Plants poisonous to livestock*, Manhattan, Kan, 1968, Kansas State University.
4. Kingsbury JM: *Poisonous plants of the United States and Canada*, Englewood Cliffs, NJ, 1964, Prentice-Hall.
5. Aiello S, editor: *The Merck veterinary manual (Toxicology)*, Whitehouse Station, NJ, 1998, Merck.
6. Krenzelock EP, Jacobsen TD, Aronis JM: Plant exposures: a state profile of the most common species, *Vet Hum Toxicol* 38:289, 1996.
7. Krenzelock EP, Jacobsen TD: Plant exposures: a national profile of the most common plant genera, *Vet Hum Toxicol* 39:248, 1997.
8. Howard JL, editor: *Current veterinary therapy: food animal practice 3*, Philadelphia, 1993, WB Saunders.
9. Howard JL, Smith RA, editors: *Current veterinary therapy: food animal practice 4*, Philadelphia, 1999, WB Saunders.
10. Dimitrijevic SM et al: Analysis and purification of phorbol esters using normal phase HPLC and photodiode-array detection, *J Pharm Biomed Anal* 15:393, 1996.

GRAYANOTOXINS

Birgit Puschner

Synonyms. Andromedotoxin, acetylandromedol, rhodotoxin, asebotoxin, and polyhydroxylated diterpenes are names for the poison. Mad honey poisoning, toxic honey poisoning, azalea toxicosis, and rhododendron toxicosis are names for the disease.

Sources. Grayanotoxins are found in several members of the Ericaceae (Heath) family. The Ericaceae family contains about 1350 species that are widely distributed in all continents.[1] In the United States, members of the Ericaceae family grow naturally in acidic, moist soils and are often found along the coastal regions as well as at higher elevations in the mountain areas. Many plants of this family are grown as evergreen or deciduous garden ornamentals. The following genera typify the most common members of the Heath family and their common names: *Rhododendron* species (rhododendron, azalea, rosebay), *Kalmia* species (mountain laurel, sheep laurel, lambkill, sheepkill, dwarf laurel, calico bush), *Pieris* species (Japanese pieris, mountain pieris), *Leucothoe* species (dog hobble, dog laurel, fetter bush, black laurel), and *Lyonia* species (fetter bush, maleberry, staggerbush). Table 25-13 describes the geographic location and plant characteristics of genera found in the United States. Grayanotoxins are found in nectar, flowers, stems, and especially the leaves. Clinical signs of toxicosis may occur from ingestion of plant parts, consumption of contaminated honey, or from sucking nectar from flowers. The Heath family varies widely regarding the concentration of grayanotoxins as to whether certain members produce grayanotoxins and at what concentration. Additionally, frequent hybridization of rhododendrons has created new plants with an unknown and unpredictable concentration of grayanotoxins. Thus, analysis for grayanotoxins in plant material is often the only reliable method to determine the potential risk of certain plant species.

Toxicokinetics. Kinetics of grayanotoxins are unstudied. It is believed, however, that grayanotoxins are rapidly absorbed from the gastrointestinal tract because of a rapid onset of clinical signs after exposure. Duration of clinical signs is usually about 1 to 2 days, indicating that grayanotoxins undergo rapid metabolism and excretion.[2]

Mechanism of Action. Grayanotoxins are diterpenes with a unique tetracyclic skeleton called andromedane (Fig. 25-2). Grayanotoxins exert their effect by binding to sodium channels in excitable cell membranes of nerve, heart, and skeletal muscle. Voltage-dependent sodium channels serve as a target for many neurotoxins and are integral plasma mem-

TABLE 25-13 **Genera, Common Names, Geographic Location, and Plant Characteristics of Members of the Ericaceae Family in the United States**

Genus	Geographic Location	Plant Description
Rhododendron spp. (rhododendron, azalea, rosebay)	Pacific Northwest, California, Virginia, Georgia; cultivated widely in temperate areas of the United States	Deciduous or evergreen; alternate, elliptic leaves; flowers in terminal clusters of various colors
Kalmia spp. (Mountain laurel, sheep laurel, lambkill, sheepkill)	Pacific Northwest, California, eastern United States	Evergreen; leathery, alternate leaves; flowers in terminal umbels of various colors
Pieris spp. (Japanese pieris, mountain pieris)	Pacific Northwest, British Columbia, Virginia, Georgia, New York	Evergreen; leathery, alternate, finely toothed leaves, flowers white, small, terminal on stem
Leucothoe spp. (dog hobble, dog laurel, fetter bush, black laurel)	Southeastern United States, California	Deciduous or evergreen; alternate, glossy, serrated leaves; flowers white, small, in terminal hanging clusters
Lyonia spp. (maleberry, fetter bush, staggerbush)	Southern United States, Atlantic coastal region	Deciduous or evergreen; alternate, elliptic serrated leaves; flowers white or pink, small

brane proteins that are responsible for the generation and propagation of action potentials. Grayanotoxins increase the membrane permeability of sodium ions in excitable membranes, thus maintaining excitable cells in a state of depolarization.[3] Accumulation of intracellular sodium results in an exchange with extracellular calcium[4] and plays an important role in the control of transmitter release.[5]

Overall, the membrane effects caused by grayanotoxins account for the observed responses of skeletal and myocardial muscle, nerves, and central nervous system.

Toxicity and Risk Factors. Grayanotoxin poisoning has been reported in humans and a variety of animal species, including goats, sheep, cattle, llamas, cats, dogs, donkeys, and kangaroos. Experimentally, the effects of grayanotoxins have been studied in rats, mice, rabbits, chickens, frogs, and squid. Toxicosis is most commonly reported in goats.[6] Most animals avoid the plants of the Heath family unless other forage is lacking. Toxicosis usually occurs when animals are offered plant trimmings or stray into wooded areas during adverse weather conditions and little else is available to eat. The importance of grayanotoxins as a cause of poisoning may increase because the plants are becoming more and more popular and have spread into some marginal areas.

Numerous grayanotoxins have been found. Grayanotoxins I, III, and IV are the most toxic, with the intraperitoneal lethal dose 50 (IP LD_{50}) in mice ranging from 0.87 to 1.3 mg/kg.[7] Structure-activity relationships on certain ericaceous toxins have been carried out revealing that the toxins have characteristic activities. However, concentrations of different grayanotoxins in ericaceous plants commonly encountered in the United States have not yet been determined completely. Grayanotoxin I appears to be the most common of all grayanotoxins. The exact risk of ericaceous plants and honey derived from these plants may vary considerably among plant species.

In cattle and sheep, ingestion of grayanotoxin-containing plants in the amount of 0.2[8]% to 0.6% of the animal's body weight is considered toxic.[8] Fresh foliage in the amount of approximately 0.1% of a goat's body weight can be toxic.[9] The minimum dose resulting in clinical signs in dogs is 7 mg/kg body weight of grayanotoxin I.[10] Human reports

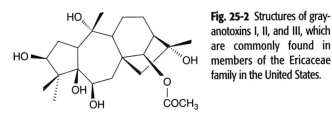

Fig. 25-2 Structures of grayanotoxins I, II, and III, which are commonly found in members of the Ericaceae family in the United States.

Grayanotoxin I

Grayanotoxin II

Grayanotoxin III

associate the development of illness after ingestion of as little as 10 g of contaminated honey.[11]

Clinical Signs.   Clinical signs of poisoning usually occur within 6 hours of exposure. Animals initially develop depression, severe salivation, abdominal pain, and vomiting or regurgitation. Diarrhea rarely occurs. The animals may then become laterally recumbent, developing seizures, tachycardia, tachypnea, and pyrexia with body temperatures of up to 106° F.[12] In severe poisonings, opisthotonus, ataxia, and convulsions can occur. Poisoning is usually not fatal, and affected animals generally recover over a period of several days. Death is most often associated with secondary aspiration pneumonia and uncontrolled convulsions. In one case, fetal mummification in a goat occurred after ingestion of *Pieris japonica* during gestation.

In humans, clinical signs of toxicosis include salivation, emesis, perioral numbness, severe hypotension, sinus bradycardia, muscular weakness, convulsions, coma, and ventricular tachycardia.[13] "Mad honey" disease has been known since 401 BC when Greek soldiers developed mass poisoning after the ingestion of contaminated honey near Trabzon, Turkey.[14]

Clinical Pathology.   Grayanotoxin exposure only leads to mild changes in clinical pathology parameters. Acidosis may develop as a result of seizures. Severe fluid loss from prolonged vomiting may lead to dehydration and electrolyte imbalances. Additionally, elevation of aspartate aminotransferase (AST) and alanine aminotransminase (ALT) has been reported in animals.[2]

Lesions.   Postmortem lesions are generally nonspecific.[6] Mild hemorrhagic enteritis, renal tubular damage, and aspiration pneumonia may be present.[2] Regurgitated material may be found in the mouth and pharynx. Sometimes, pieces of leaves of ericaceous plants are found in the gastrointestinal tract.

Diagnostic Testing.   Chromatographic methods have been developed to determine the presence of grayanotoxins in serum, urine, gastrointestinal contents, plant material, and honey. A two-dimensional thin-layer chromatography (TLC) method for qualitative analysis of grayanotoxins and other cardiotoxins is available for plant material and gastrointestinal contents.[15] If grayanotoxin poisoning is suspected, at least 10 g of gastrointestinal contents should be collected, kept frozen in a plastic container, and submitted to a diagnostic laboratory for analysis. The TLC method is rapid, providing results within 4 hours.

If gastrointestinal contents are unavailable, serum and urine can be analyzed for the presence of grayanotoxins.[16] A liquid chromatography/mass spectrometry method allows the detection at the nanogram per gram level of grayanotoxins I, II, and III in serum or urine. Grayanotoxins can be detected in urine of exposed animals up to 3 to 5 days after exposure. Serum samples should be collected in a red-top tube, separated from the clot, and kept frozen. Urine samples should be collected in a plastic vial and stored frozen until submitted for analysis.

Finding grayanotoxins in any of the submitted specimens is consistent with exposure to ericaceous plants from the environment. A diagnosis is established if clinical signs are also appropriate for grayanotoxin poisoning.

Treatment.   No specific antidote is available for grayanotoxin poisoning. If ingestion of grayanotoxin-containing plants has occurred within 3 to 4 hours, emetics should be given to animals of appropriate species if not contraindicated. Administration of activated charcoal and saline or sorbitol cathartics is recommended in animals that are alert and show no clinical signs of vomiting, regurgitation, or seizures.[6] Rumenotomy may be considered in individual animals if ingestion is known and clinical signs have not yet developed. A stomach tube may be passed if bloat occurs. Supportive therapy should include administration of intravenous fluids (sodium bicarbonate, 5% dextrose) to combat hypotension, dehydration, and metabolic acidosis.[13] Antibiotics are indicated in animals with aspiration pneumonia. Atropine should be considered in cases of severe bradycardia. Additionally, antiarrhythmics may be warranted in severely poisoned animals that do not respond to decontamination procedures and fluid therapy alone.

Prognosis.   Deaths have been reported, but the prognosis is good with supportive treatment and management of cardiac arrhythmias unless aspiration pneumonia or convulsions occur. Early gastrointestinal decontamination with activated charcoal enhances the likelihood of a fast recovery. In most cases, clinical signs of grayanotoxin toxicosis subside within 3 to 5 days after exposure.

Prevention and Control.   Prevention is primarily based on education of veterinarians and animal owners regarding the toxicity of the plants. Members of the Ericaceae family are poisonous at any time, but are usually not consumed if other feed is available. The best prevention is to keep animals away from the plants and to ensure that other feed is available. Pet owners should keep their animals away from ornamental plantings.

REFERENCES

1. Everist SL: *Poisonous plants of Australia*, ed 2, Australia, 1981, Angus and Robertson.
2. Hikino H et al: Subchronic toxicity of ericaceous toxins and *Rhododendron* leaves, *Chem Pharm Bull* 27:874, 1979.
3. Narahasi T, Seyama I: Mechanism of nerve membrane depolarization caused by grayanotoxin I, *J Physiol* 242:471, 1974.
4. Glitsch HG et al: The effect of the internal sodium concentration on calcium fluxes in isolated guinea pig auricles, *J Physiol* 209:25, 1970.
5. Zushi S et al: Effect of grayanotoxin on the frog neuromuscular junction, *J Pharm Exp Ther* 226:269, 1983.
6. Plumlee KH et al: Japanese pieris toxicosis of goats, *J Vet Diagn Invest* 4:363, 1992.
7. Hikino H et al: Structure-activity relationship of ericaceous toxins on acute toxicity in mice, *Tox Appl Pharm* 35:303, 1976.
8. Kingsbury JM: *Poisonous plants of the United States and Canada*, Englewood Cliffs, NJ, 1964, Prentice-Hall.
9. Smith MC: Japanese pieris poisoning in the goat, *J Am Vet Med Assoc* 173:78, 1978.

10. Moran NC et al: The pharmacological actions of andromedotoxin, an active principle from *Rhododendron maximum*, *J Pharm Exp Ther* 110:415, 1954.

11. Krochmal C: Poison honeys, *Am Bee J* 134:549-550, 1994.

12. Casteel SW, Wagstaff JD: *Rhododendron macrophyllum* poisoning in a group of goats and sheep, *Vet Hum Toxicol* 31:176, 1989.

13. Lampe KF: Rhododendrons, mountain laurel, and mad honey, *JAMA* 259:2009, 1988.

14. Ungan A: Şimali Anadolu'nun zehirli balı (Toxic honey of Northern Anatolia), *Tữrk Hijyen ve Tecrữbi Biyoloji Dergisi* 2:161, 1941.

15. Holstege DM et al: Multiresidue screen for cardiotoxins by two-dimensional thin layer chromatography, *J Agric Food Chem* 48:60, 2000.

16. Puschner B et al: Azalea (*Rhododendron* spp.) toxicosis in group of Nubian goats, *Proceedings of the 42nd Annual Meeting of the American Association of Veterinary Laboratory Diagnosticians*, San Diego, 1999.

MELIATOXINS

William R. Hare

Synonyms.   The most common name for *Melia azedarach* is chinaberry. Other names include Texas umbrella, white cedar, pride of India, Indian lilac, China tree, Chinese umbrella, chinatree, hoop-tree, bead-tree, cape lilac, cape syringa, and umbrella tree. However, it should not be confused with two other species of plants also known as umbrella tree, the *Schefflera* spp. and the *Musanga* spp.

Sources.   The chinaberry is a deciduous tree belonging to the Mahogany family.[1] It usually grows to a height of 6 to 12 m, but some rainforest varieties grow as high as 30 to 45 m. It is a thick and heavily branched tree with a thin, finely furrowed, grayish-brownish bark. The leaves are dark green and composed of large (2.5 to 7 cm long and 1 to 4 cm wide), serrated, lanceolate-shaped leaflets that are arranged in an alternate, bipinnate compound fashion. The small, delicate, fragrant flowers are approximately 2.5 cm across and composed of five to six petals, three to five sepals, and purplish stamen tubes. Flowers are arranged in large axillary panicles and have a rich lilaclike fragrance. The fruit consists of a small, round-to-ovoid seedpod or drupe that is approximately 1.5 cm in diameter, initially green and smooth but turning a pale yellow. There is a prolific production of these drupes with particular abundance in wet years. The fruit characteristically ripens and drops to the ground in great numbers over a short period of time.

The chinaberry is native to Persia, India, and China but has become well established worldwide and naturalized to the temperate regions of North America and coastal areas such as Hawaii and Bermuda. It is frequently planted as an ornamental shade tree and is used in contemporary landscape designs, but can also be found in thickets, open fields, and areas having recently disturbed soils.

Toxicokinetics.   The chinaberry's leaves, bark, flowers, and fruit are all potentially poisonous; however, the fruit is most toxic. The principal toxins responsible for animal poisonings are a group of tetranortriterpenes of the cytotoxic limonoid class, known as meliatoxins A1, A2, B1, and B2.[2,3] These meliatoxins are concentrated in the fruit and act as entero-

toxins and neurotoxins. However, other potentially toxic limonoids have been isolated and identified from the fruit and seeds.[4] In addition to limonoids, other potentially toxic constituents include azadarin (an alkaloid), azaridine (a resin found in the fruit), parisine (a resin found in the leaves), margosinine (a resin found in the bark), meliotannic acid, and benzoic acid.

No specific controlled toxicokinetic studies have been done in animals for chinaberry poisoning. However, information from clinical and experimental reports suggests that absorption of the toxic principles is rapid following the ingestion of fruit. Adverse clinical signs begin to appear usually within 1 to 2 hours after ingestion. Signs are progressive in nature with increasing severity. Most animals die within 48 hours following the onset of adverse clinical signs. Elimination is thought to be predominantly renal, and toxins can be found in the animal's milk.

Mechanisms of Action.   The exact mechanism involved in the action of the toxic principles is unknown. They are both enterotoxic and neurotoxic and are suspected to be responsible for pathophysiologic changes to the central nervous system, causing terminal respiratory arrest. The effects on the central nervous system are not unlike those produced by nicotine or anabasine alkaloids, with initial stimulation of sympathetic and parasympathetic ganglia followed by persistent depolarization and complete ganglionic blockade. The gastroenteritis is suspected to be predominantly the result of local irritation and inflammation, but central effects have not been ruled out.

Toxicity and Risk Factors.   Chinaberry poisoning has been reported in horses, cattle, sheep, goats, pigs, dogs, rabbits, rats, guinea pigs, and poultry.[1,5,6] Some animals such as goats, horses, donkeys, ducks, and other birds appear to be more resistant to poisoning because toxicosis was more difficult to produce even experimentally. Geographic location and climatic conditions may also affect the plant's expression or assimilation of toxic principles. Poisoning is rare, in that animals usually do not forage on fallen fruit because of its bitter taste.[7]

Feeding experiments on rabbits, pigs, and sheep have established a toxic dose for ingestion of fruit to be 5 g/kg body weight. At that level, adverse signs were noticeable at 1 to 2 hours and death at 2 to 3 days. However, larger doses produced death within 2 hours. Others have reported that ingestion of fruit equal to 0.06% to 0.07% of body weight (0.6 to 0.7 g/kg) is sufficient to produce a toxicosis. Small dogs have died following the ingestion of 5 to 6 drupe, yet goats have remained free of adverse clinical signs after ingesting more than 200 drupe.

Clinical Signs.   Adverse clinical signs usually present within 1 to 2 hours after ingestion and are characterized by vomiting or diarrhea with or without blood, colic, straining to defecate, and anorexia. Animals may show some hypersalivation. The gastrointestinal signs are soon followed by progressive nervous system abnormalities characterized by ataxia, excitement, seizures, depression, paresis, coma, and death. Death is thought to result from respiratory arrest.

Other adverse signs that have been reported include hyperthermia, hypothermia, tachycardia, bradycardia, tachypnea, apnea, dyspnea, pulmonary edema, hemorrhage, oliguria, stranguria, muscle rigidity, opisthotonus, mydriasis, miosis, and acute death.[5,6,8]

Clinical Pathology. Clinical pathology alterations have been reported, but are not consistent. The majority of abnormal values may be related to the animal's response to stress and the release of endogenous steroids. Serum chemistry abnormalities associated with hepatic insult and renal failure may be found in poisoned animals, especially when signs are of longer duration. Renal and hepatic function should be monitored during therapy, as should acid-base and electrolyte values.

Lesions. Gross pathology lesions are not pathognomonic and are usually unremarkable. However, degenerative changes of the kidney and liver characterized by congestion and hemorrhage have been reported. Nonspecific microscopic lesions of the kidney and liver characterized by fatty degeneration and occasional cellular necrosis have been noted. Usually, the longer the duration before death, the more pronounced the lesions. In natural and experimental poisoning of pigs, the most characteristic microscopic finding is a mild, diffuse cellular necrosis of the interglandular lamina propria throughout the gastrointestinal tract.[3] Other lesions that have been reported include proteinaceous casts in the renal tubules as well as moderate, diffuse, lymphoid necrosis of the mesenteric lymph nodes, spleen, and intestinal lymphoid nodules.[3] In rats, necrosis and fragmentation of skeletal muscle have been reported.[9]

Diagnostic Testing. No specific diagnostic tests are available to confirm chinaberry poisoning. The identification of ingested fruit from stomach contents can confirm exposure. Diagnosis is usually made based on a history of exposure and the characteristic clinical syndrome.

Treatment. No antidote exists. Animals suspected of ingesting chinaberry fruit should be aggressively decontaminated before signs of clinical poisoning become apparent.[6,8] If emesis is delayed and adverse clinical signs become apparent, a gastric lavage or enterogastric lavage should be administered and followed by placement of an activated charcoal slurry. The use of antiemetics, activated charcoal, and gastrointestinal protectants may be beneficial if signs of vomiting and diarrhea are already present. Rumenotomy may be indicated in ruminant species.

Use of diazepam may help to control excitement and seizures. General anesthetics may be used if deemed necessary. Intravenous corticosteroids and antibiotics are indicated, but use of aminoglycoside antibiotics is contraindicated. Fluids and appropriate electrolytes should be administered; plasma administration may also be beneficial in treatment of circulatory failure. Yohimbine, norepinephrine, or dopamine therapy may be indicated in cases of complete autonomic failure and circulatory collapse. However, none of these compounds are antidotes and all must be used with a great deal of discretion because they can potentiate seizure activity.

Prognosis. The prognosis is usually grave to poor after clinical signs progress to the nervous system. The prognosis is good if decontamination efforts are successful before the development of clinical signs.

Prevention and Control. To prevent the potential for poisoning, animal access to *Melia azedarach* or its fruit should be restricted.

REFERENCES

1. Kingsbury JM: *Poisonous plants of the United States and Canada,* Englewood Cliffs, NJ, 1964, Prentice-Hall.
2. Oelrichs PB et al: Toxic tetranortriterpenes of the fruit of *Melia azedarach, Phytochem* 22(2):531, 1983.
3. Oelrichs PB, Hill MW, Vallely PJ: The chemistry and pathology of meliatoxins A and B constituents from the fruit of *Melia azedarach* L. var *australasica.* In Seawright AA et al, editors: *Plant toxicology.* Queensland, 1985, Yeerongpilly.
4. Srivastava SD: Limonoids from the seeds of *Melia azedarach, J Nat Prod* 49(1):56, 1986.
5. Hothi DS et al: A note on the comparative toxicity of *Melia azedarach* (DHREK) berries to piglets, buffalo-calves and fowls, *J Res* 13(2):232, 1976.
6. Hare WR et al: Chinaberry poisoning in two dogs, *J Am Vet Med Assoc* 210(11):1638, 1997.
7. Vahrmeijer J: *Poisonous plants of Southern Africa that cause stock losses,* Cape Town, South Africa, 1981, Tafelberg Publishers.
8. Hare WR: Chinaberry (*Melia azedarach*) poisoning in animals. In Garland T, Barr AC, editors: *Toxic plants and other natural toxicants,* Wallingford, Oxon, UK, 1998, CAB International.
9. Bahri S, Sani Y, Hooper PT: Myodegeneration in rats fed *Melia azedarach, Aust Vet J* 69(2):33, 1992.

SESQUITERPENE LACTONES

George Burrows and Ronald J. Tyrl

Synonyms. The disease was originally called "spewing disease" because of the regurgitation or vomiting sometimes seen with subacute to chronic forms.[1]

Sources. Sesquiterpene lactones are toxins found mainly in the numerous species of *Helenium* and *Hymenoxys* in the Asteraceae or sunflower family (Table 25-14). Their heads contain yellow ray florets and disk florets of various colors.

Species of *Helenium* are widely distributed across North America. *Helenium amarum* and *H. flexuosum* are found in the eastern half, *H. autumnale* across much of the West and the East, *H. microcephalum* in the Southwest, and *H. hoopesii* at higher elevations in the western mountains. *Helenium flexuosum* and *H. hoopesii* were formerly known as *H. nudiflorum* and *Dugaldia hoopesii,* respectively.

Species of *Hymenoxys* also are taxa of the West. *H. odorata* grow in the plains and rangelands of the Southwest, and *H. odorata* and *H. richardsonii* are present in mountain areas at higher elevations.

TABLE 25-14 Species of Plants that Contain Sesquiterpene Lactones and Commonly Pose Toxicologic Risks

Scientific Name	Common Name
Helenium	
H. amarum (Raf.) H.Rock	Bitter sneezeweed, Spanish daisy
H. autumnale L.	Common sneezeweed, sneezewort, autumn sneezeweed, staggerwort, staggerweed, yellow star, ox-eye
H. flexuosum Raf.	Purplehead sneezeweed, southern sneezeweed
H. hoopesii (A.Gray)	Orange sneezeweed
H. microcephalum DC.	Smallhead sneezeweed
Hymenoxys	
H. lemmonii (Greene) Cockerell	Lemmon's hymenoxys
H. odorata DC.	Bitterweed, bitter rubberweed
H. richarsonii (Hook.) Cockerell	Colorado rubberweed, pigue

Mechanism of Action. The toxins are pseudoguaianolide type sesquiterpene lactones known as *trans*-fused helenanolides and seco-helenanolides. Helenalin is found in many species of *Helenium,* and hymenoxon is well represented in *Hymenoxys.* Other genera that contain these types of toxins include *Baileya, Psilostrophe,* and *Sartwellia.* Concentrations of the helenolides are typically in the range of 0.5% to 3% dry weight of plant, highest in the flowers.

These lactones contain highly reactive exocyclic α-methylene-γ-lactone or cyclopentanone groups that are capable of alkylating sulfhydryl groups.[2] This alkylation causes a variety of actions, but the main effect is inactivation of essential metabolic enzymes.[3,4] Also affected are oxidative phosphorylation and cyclic adenosine monophosphate.[5,6] Hymenoxon, present mainly in *Hymenoxys,* is also mutagenic.[7]

Toxicity and Risk Factors. Probably all animal species are at risk, but these plants are quite bitter tasting and typically are not eaten except under dire circumstances. Sheep are most likely to eat the plants and are at greatest risk. Toxicity is highest with mature plants and probably bitterness as well. *Helenium amarum,* which contains the very bitter lactone tenulin, is well known as a cause of milk taint.

The lethal dose for *H. microcephalum,* the most toxic species of *Helenium,* is about 0.25% of body weight of green plant material, whereas the dose of *H. hoopesii* and *H. amarum* causing illness is 1.5% of body weight daily for several days.[8,9] The acute lethal dose for species of *Hymenoxys* is about 1% to 1.5% of body weight of green plant.[10] The toxins have a cumulative effect and typically produce disease after ingestion of the plants for days or weeks.

Clinical Signs. Several forms of disease exist, depending on the plant species and quantity eaten.

In the least common acute disease form following ingestion of plants for a few days, there is depression, decreased appetite, ruminal atony, and bloat. The animal stands groaning and with its back arched. Wheezing, coughing, repeated swallowing, possibly greenish saliva, fine tremors, and terminal convulsions may occur. Death can occur in a few hours or days. Some hemorrhage from the nose may be noted in terminal animals.

In the more common subacute form following ingestion for a few weeks, similar but milder signs are seen with regurgitation and vomiting of greenish material and death after a few days or up to 2 weeks later.

The chronic form caused by ingestion of plant for weeks or months results in very poor body condition with loss of weight and dehydration.

Clinical Pathology. Hypoglycemia, metabolic acidosis, and elevation of blood lactic and pyruvic acids may be noteworthy with the acute form. Hemoconcentration, an increase in blood urea nitrogen and creatinine, and a clotting defect associated with an increase in prothrombin and partial thromboplastin times may occur. These changes are not prominent in the less acute disease forms.

Lesions. Few, if any, distinctive lesions are found. Edema and congestion of the mucosa of the stomach and small intestine perhaps with some blood or gaseous distention may be found. Congestion, edema, some hemorrhage in the lungs, a few hemorrhages on the surfaces of the heart, and excess pericardial fluid have also been reported.

Treatment. Treatment is generally limited to removal of animals from the toxic plants and to supportive nursing care. Dietary supplements are of little value once signs are apparent.

Prognosis. With onset of distinct signs of intoxication, the likelihood of recovery is poor and requires careful nursing and feeding for a prolonged time.

Prevention and Control. Because the plants are unpalatable, their consumption and development of the disease can be prevented by providing good feed. Animals seldom eat toxic amounts of these species if they are well fed. Animals at risk can be provided with a high-protein diet (soybean meal), possibly supplemented with methionine or sodium sulfate, or given antioxidants such as ethoxyquin with methionine added. These approaches, however, have produced questionable results and must be used before onset of disease signs.[11,12]

REFERENCES

1. Marsh CD et al: Western sneezeweed *(Helenium hoopesii)* as a poisonous plant, *USDA Bull* 947, 1921.
2. Hall IH et al: Antitumor agents. 21. A proposed mechanism for inhibition of cancer growth by tenulin and helenalin and related cyclopentanones, *J Med Chem* 20:333, 1977.

3. Gaspar AR et al: The effect of sesquiterpene lactones from *Geigeria* on glycolytic enzymes, *Biochem Pharmacol* 35:493, 1986.

4. Page JD et al: Inhibition of inosine monophosphate dehydrogenase by sesquiterpene lactones, *Biochim Biophys Acta* 926:186, 1987.

5. Elissalde MH, Ivie GW: Inhibition of macrophage adenylate cyclase by the α-methylene-γ-lactone moiety of sesquiterpene lactones from forage plants, *Am J Vet Res* 48:148, 1987.

6. Narasimhan TR et al: Effects of sesquiterpene lactones on mitochondrial oxidative phosphorylation, *Gen Pharmacol* 20:681, 1989.

7. MacGregor JT: Mutagenic activity of hymenovin, a sesquiterpene lactone from western bitterweed, *Food Cosmet Toxicol* 15:225, 1977.

8. Dollahite JW et al: Toxicity of *Helenium microcephalum* (smallhead sneezeweed), *J Am Vet Med Assoc* 145:694, 1964.

9. Dollahite JW et al: Toxicity of *Helenium amarum* (bitter sneezeweed) to sheep, *Southwestern Vet* 26:135, 1973.

10. Rowe LD et al: *Hymenoxys odorata* (bitterweed) poisoning in sheep, *Southwestern Vet* 26:287, 1973.

11. Calhoun MC et al: Experimental prevention of bitterweed *(Hymenoxys odorata)* poisoning in sheep, *Am J Vet Res* 50:1642, 1989.

12. Post LO, Bailey EM: The effect of dietary supplements on chronic bitterweed *(Hymenoxys odorata)* poisoning in sheep, *Vet Hum Toxicol* 34:209, 1992.

TETRADYMOL

George Burrows and Ronald J. Tyrl

Sources.   Species of *Tetradymia*, a member of the Asteraceae, or sunflower, family, are commonly known as horsebrushes because of the appearance of their heads, which bear four disk florets and no ray florets. They are common, often conspicuous plants of the intermountain region from British Columbia to Baja, California (Table 25-15).

Possibly interacting with *Tetradymia* in the induction of toxicoses are species of *Artemisia*, the sagebrushes (see Table 25-15). Also members of the Asteraceae, they are strongly aromatic herbs or shrubs, and in this discussion are only of concern when their distribution ranges overlap those of the species of *Tetradymia* in western North America.

TABLE 25-15 **Species of Plants that Are of Toxicologic Interest**

Scientific Name	Common Name
Tetradymia	
T. canescens DC.	Spineless horsebrush, common horsebrush, little gray horsebrush
T. glabrata Torr. and A. Gray	Lizard shade, littleleaf horsebrush, spring rabbitbrush, coaloil brush, rat brush, dog brush, skink brush
Artemisia	
A. filifolia Torr.	Sand sage, sand sagebrush
A. ludoviciana Nutt.	White or prairie sage
A. spinescens D.C.Eaton	Bud, button or spring sage
A. tridentata Nutt.	Sagebrush, big sagebrush

Mechanism of Action.   The toxins in *Tetradymia* are probably furanoeremphilane derivatives such as tetradymol. The toxicity of these types of compounds is enhanced by induction of hepatic biotransformation processes.[1] Thus under conditions in which hepatic biotransformation activity is increased, *Tetradymia* presents a much increased risk. This seems to be the role of *Artemisia* in occurrence of the disease. Ingestion of *Artemisia* concurrent with or immediately preceding that of *Tetradymia* may predispose injury to the liver by *Tetradymia* by increasing hepatic mixed-function oxidase activity.[2] Secondary to the liver injury, there is presumably a decrease in the ability to clear phylloerythrin, a degradation product of chlorophyll, allowing it to build up in blood. Phylloerythrin acts as a photodynamic agent causing damage in the areas of microcirculation most likely to be exposed to ultraviolet light. As with other causes of photosensitization in sheep, swelling of the head may occur, producing the disease known as "bighead." Because the liver lesions are sometimes severe, animals may die without developing the skin lesions.[3]

Toxicity and Risk Factors.   Sheep are the main animals affected because they are most likely to eat the plants. All stages of plant growth are toxic but it is the new growth early in spring when other forage is lacking that is typically eaten.[4,5] Those species, such as *T. canescens,* which begin growth later in the spring or early summer, pose less of a risk.

Clinical Signs.   Following consumption of the plants, an abrupt onset of decreased appetite, depression, tremors, incoordination, and dyspnea occurs. In a few animals, head pressing and icterus may also be present. Eventually, swelling, erythema, and peeling or sloughing of the nose and lips and the skin around the ears and eyes may occur. The severity of effects may range from minor peeling and sloughing of the skin, to loss of ears or eyes, or death in 1 to 2 days.

Clinical Pathology.   Serum hepatic enzymes are markedly elevated, perhaps as much as 10 to 20 times the normal values, and sulfobromophthalein clearance time also is much increased.

Lesions.   Grossly, the liver is tan and friable. The gallbladder is distended with bile. Microscopically, an extensive centrilobular hepatic necrosis is evident.

Treatment.   Affected animals should be promptly removed from the offending forage and, if possible, provided shade. Good nursing care with good water and feed are appropriate for the liver disease and decreased appetite.

Prognosis.   It is likely that some animals will die within a few days after plant ingestion. Those that survive require several weeks for recovery from the more obvious signs of the liver damage. Overall, with good feed and care, most animals eventually recover from the liver disease and skin lesions.

Prevention and Control. Because ingestion of the plants is most likely when new foliage is developing, control is based on providing sufficient feed during this time so that the noxious plants are not eaten.

REFERENCES

1. Johnson AE: Experimental photosensitization and toxicity in sheep produced by *Tetradymia glabrata, Can J Comp Med* 38:406, 1974.
2. Eissa FZ et al: Effects of feeding *Artemisia filifolia* and *Helenium flexuosum* on rabbit cytochrome P450 isozymes, *Vet Hum Toxicol* 38:19, 1996.
3. Jennings PW et al: Toxic constituents and hepatotoxicity of the plant *Tetradymia glabrata* (Asteraceae). In Keeler RF, Van Kampen KR, James LF, editors: *Effects of poisonous plants on livestock,* New York, 1978, Academic Press.
4. Johnson AE: Predisposing influence of range plants on *Tetradymia*-related photosensitization in sheep: work of Drs. A. B. Clawson and W. T. Huffman, *Am J Vet Res* 35:1583, 1974.
5. Clawson AB, Huffman WT: Further notes on the study of bighead, *National Wool Grower* 26;18, 1936.

TRITERPENOID SAPONINS

George Burrows and Ronald J. Tyrl

Sources. The triterpenoid saponins are quite common in plants and in some instances are the apparent cause of disease problems in animals. Taxa from several families including the Aquifoliaceae, or holly, family, the Araliaceae, or ginseng, family, the Caryophyllaceae, or pink, family, and the Phytolaccaceae, or pokeweed, family are recognized as toxic because they contain these types of toxicants. In addition, the saponins of *Medicago* (alfalfa) have been of some historical interest because of their minor role in the development of bloat in ruminants.

Species of *Ilex* in the Aquifoliaceae family are highly prized ornamental shrubs or trees, present as natives in eastern North America and cultivated as ornamentals across the continent. Most species are toxic to some degree, and representatives include *I. aquifolium* L. (English or Christmas holly), *I. opaca* Aiton (American or white holly), *I. verticillata* (L.) A.Gray (winterberry), and *I. vomitoria* Aiton (yaupon, cassena).

Although various species of *Hedera* may contain triterpenoids and represent a toxicologic risk, *H. helix* L. (English ivy, common ivy) has been the subject of most reports of adverse effects. All are climbing, woody vines cultivated extensively throughout North America to cover ground and walls.

Four genera of the Caryophyllaceae are noteworthy as causes of intoxication because they contain triterpenoid saponins: *Agrostemma, Drymaria, Saponaria,* and *Vaccaria.* In addition, other taxa such as the prized ornamentals, *Dianthus* (pink), and *Gypsophila* (baby's breath), also contain similar steroidal saponins, but have not been reported to be toxic.

A. githago L. (corn cockle, corn campion) is the only species of *Agrostemma.* It is an erect annual herb widely distributed in fields and waste areas across North America, especially the northern half.

Species of *Drymaria* are annual or perennial, often prostrate, herbs of dry stream beds of the desert Southwest. *D. arenarioides* is restricted to the Chihuahuan and Sonoran deserts of Mexico. The two species of toxicologic concern are *D. arenarioides* Humb. & Bonpl. ex Schult. (alfombrillo, drymary) and *D. pachyphylla* Wooton & Standl. (thickleaf drymary, inkweed).

S. officinalis L. (bouncing bet, soapwort) is one of three introduced species of *Saponaria* of toxicologic significance. It is an erect herb, with large, showy, white-to-pink petals. It is widely distributed in grain fields and waste areas across North America, especially in the northwestern United States and the Canadian prairie provinces.

V. hispanica (Mill.) Rauschert (cow cockle, dairy-pink) is the single species of *Vaccaria* present in North America and was formerly called *Saponaria vaccaria.* It is a sparsely branched, erect, annual common in grain fields and waste areas throughout much of North America.

P. americana L. (poke, pokeweed, pokeberry, inkberry) is the only species of *Phytolacca* of toxicologic concern in North America. It is a fleshy, perennial herb from stout roots with purplish-black berries borne in arching racemes. Native to the eastern half of North America with scattered populations further west, it is common on disturbed sites as small, localized populations.

Mechanism of Action. Pentacyclic oleanane terpenoids, often referred to as saponins, are the cause of the disease common to all of these taxa.[1,2] The risk is mainly in the fruits of *Ilex* and *Hedera;* the seeds of *Agrostemma, Saponaria,* and *Vaccaria;* the seeds, flowers, and foliage of *Drymaria;* and the leaves, roots, and berries of *Phytolacca.* Large amounts of these terpenoids cause direct irritation of the digestive tract. In most instances, the disease is of only mild-to-moderate severity and occurs several or more hours after ingestion. However, with *Drymaria,* the disease may be severe because it grows in areas often with little alternative forage. Under adverse environmental conditions, animals may be forced to eat appreciable amounts.[3]

Toxicity and Risk Factors. All animal species are at risk, including poultry.[4] In the case of seeds contaminating feed, ground feed products are more toxic because of the decreased ability of animals to select against the seeds, and because of greater likelihood of contact of the toxins with the digestive tract surfaces. Young animals are at increased risk.

Whereas most of these plants are seldom eaten because of their irritant effects, the young stems and leaves of *Phytolacca* are prized by some individuals as a potherb and sought in the spring. When improperly prepared, it is eaten sometimes with dire consequences.[5,6]

Clinical Signs. In most cases, the disease is only of mild-to-moderate severity, with transient diarrhea and perhaps vomiting. In more severe cases, signs include decreased appetite, increased salivation, bloat, colic, and hypothermia. With *Drymaria,* and rarely with the other taxa, signs of systemic involvement such as depression, labored respiration, prostration, and terminal seizures may be present.

Lesions.   In most instances, gross lesions are limited to reddening of the mucosa of the stomach and small intestines. When poultry ingest the toxic seeds and die, they exhibit severe reddening of the mouth, tongue, and pharynx with fluid accumulation around the heart. With *Drymaria*, small hemorrhages may be present on the surfaces of many organs and free blood may be present in the intestines.

Microscopically, noteworthy changes are also most apparent with *Drymaria*, with necrosis of the intestinal mucosa and renal tubular epithelium, and around the central veins of the liver.

Treatment.   The main consideration is maintenance of hydration using fluid and electrolytes. Control of the vomiting and diarrhea may be attempted, but is typically not needed. Activated charcoal given orally may be a useful adjunct to treatment.

Prognosis.   In most cases, the disease is limited to a few hours' duration and recovery is complete within 24 hours. With *Drymaria*, deaths may be anticipated because animals eating plants of this genus are often in poor condition and are not responsive to treatment, even if it is available.[7]

Prevention and Control.   Well-fed animals usually are not at serious risk of intoxication.

REFERENCES

1. Connolly JD, Hill RA: *Dictionary of terpenoids: di- and higher terpenoids,* vol 2, London, 1991, Chapman & Hall.
2. Hostettmann K, Marston A: *Saponins,* Cambridge, UK, 1995, Cambridge University Press.
3. Dollahite JW: Toxicity of *Drymaria arenarioides* for cattle, sheep and goats, *J Am Vet Med Assoc* 135:125, 1959.
4. Bierer BW, Rhodes WH: Poultry ration contaminants, *J Am Vet Med Assoc* 137:352, 1960.
5. Callahan R et al: Plant poisoning: New Jersey, *Morbidity Mortality Weekly Report* 30;65, 1981.
6. O'leary SB: Poisoning in man from eating poisonous plants, *Arch Environ Health* 9:216, 1964.
7. Mathews FP: The toxicity of *Drymaria pachyphylla* for cattle, sheep and goats, *J Am Vet Med Assoc* 83:255, 1933.

UNCLASSIFIED TOXINS

ALSIKE CLOVER AND RED CLOVER

Patricia A. Talcott

Synonyms.   "Big liver disease," "dew poisoning," and "trifoliosis" are names given for the disease syndrome produced by these plants.

Sources.   Both alsike clover and red clover are members of the Leguminosae family, subfamily Faboideae. They are hardy and palatable plants. They thrive in cool climates and are tolerant of wet, acidic, alkaline, saline, clay, and peaty soils.

Because of these positive characteristics, these two species of plants have been used in pasture mixes throughout the United States and Canada. Depending on the specific cultivar of the plant, soil, and weather conditions, the plants can act as either short-lived perennials or can live for many years. Both types of clover can be grown alone or in combination with other grasses such as orchardgrass, timothy, and fescue, or small grains.

Alsike clover has stems that can be either erect or hanging down, often growing up to 36 inches tall (Color Plate 46). The leaves are palmately trifoliate in appearance. The leaflets are oval, 1 inch long, and finely serrated along the edges. The flowers are pink to white in globose heads up to 1 inch in diameter and located on short peduncles.

Red clover has erect stems that can grow up to 36 inches tall as well (Color Plate 47). The leaves are palmately trifoliate in appearance. The leaflets are oval to obovate, 1 to $2\frac{1}{2}$ inches long, hairy, and commonly have an inverted V-shaped "water mark" on their upper surface. The stipules are large and broad at the base. The flowers are rose-purple or dark purple-red, located in dense globose heads approximately 1 inch long.

Toxicokinetics.   The toxic principle in these two plants responsible for the hepatotoxicity and secondary photosensitivity is unknown. It is not currently known whether a secondary metabolite present in the plant or a mycotoxin is the ultimate culprit, or whether the entire plant or only specific components of the plant are responsible for the disease. *Cymodothea trifolii,* a fungus that is responsible for the disease "black blotch" or "sooty blotch" in clover and alfalfa, has been linked to the development of disease in horses.[1] Other evidence from Canada suggests that an endophytic bacterium of the genus *Capnocytophaga* may play a role in the expression of the disease.

Mechanism of Action.   The biochemical mechanism of action is still unknown. The toxin causes a direct hepatotoxic insult, often resulting in skin lesions as a result of a secondary photosensitization.

Toxicity and Risk Factors.   Based on clinical case reports, the horse appears to be the only species of animal susceptible to poisoning. There appears to be no sex, age, or breed predilection. It is most commonly diagnosed in individuals with nonpigmented areas of skin, primarily because secondary photosensitization is often the first recognized symptom of illness. The incidence of disease varies tremendously from year to year, suggesting that certain environmental conditions play a major factor in the production of the toxin. Most cases in the Pacific Northwest occur between April and November, with the incidence being highest in those years with an unusually long, wet spring. However, cases of poisoning can occur year round, because toxicoses have been associated with both pasture grazing and ingestion of baled hay. Because both the toxin and the mechanism of action are unknown, it is difficult to predict how much plant material is required to be ingested in order to receive a toxic dose, or over how long a period of time.

However, as little as 20% alsike clover in the diet has been associated with hepatotoxicosis. In my experience, hepatotoxicity associated with red clover ingestion has been seen in cases when the clover has constituted greater than 50% of the total diet.

Clinical Signs. Depending on the percentage of plant material in the total diet, symptoms of the disease can occur as early as 2 to 4 weeks after initial exposure. Sometimes, months can elapse after initial exposure before symptoms begin to occur. Sunburned lesions of the nonpigmented areas of the skin, along with mucous membranes and cornea, are commonly the first symptoms to occur in affected horses. These lesions are not observed in darkly pigmented horses, and hepatic failure may appear to occur abruptly in these animals. The sunburned lesions are typically characterized by varying degrees of erythema, edema, ulceration, necrosis, and sloughing. These changes are a result of a hepatogenous or secondary photosensitization caused by the buildup of the photoreactive pigment phylloerythrin in the skin. These lesions are nonlethal and do not usually respond to traditional topical treatments until the animal is removed from sunlight and the exposure to the clover ceases.

The disease often progresses to an acute onset of neurologic signs (i.e., hepatic encephalopathy), often characterized by depression, aimless wandering, head pressing, ataxia, loss of appetite, yawning, and grinding of the teeth.[2-5] Muscle tremors, mild colic, blindness, and inability to prehend or swallow have also been reported. This can rapidly progress to recumbency, violent episodes of excitation, coma, and death. A less commonly recognized form of this disease has been termed the chronic or cachectic form, characterized by progressive loss of appetite and weight loss, loss of condition, weakness, and poor hair coat.

Clinical Pathology. The most significant clinical pathologic abnormalities observed in affected horses include increases in γ-glutamyl transferase (GGT) and alkaline phosphatase (ALP). In examining the medical records of 16 horses diagnosed with alsike clover poisoning from Idaho and Washington, all had elevations in GGT concentrations ranging from 55 to 622 IU/L (mean 191 IU/L; normal range 11 to 44 IU/L). Fifteen of the 16 patients had elevated ALP activity, ranging from 184 to 1320 IU/L (mean 436 IU/L; normal range 97 to 196 IU/L). Eleven of the 16 had elevated aspartate transaminase activity (AST), ranging from 231 to 1454 IU/L (mean 764 IU/L; normal range 184 to 375 IU/L). Less commonly seen were elevations in serum alanine aminotransferase (ALT) and sorbitol dehydrogenase (SDH). Serum bile acids, ammonia concentrations, and total bilirubin (results in 8 of 11 horses tested were elevated, ranging from 1.1 to 13.8 mg/dl with a mean of 6.5; normal range 0.6 to 2.1 mg/dl) may be elevated as well, although icterus is not a consistent feature observed in clinically affected horses. Hemograms are typically normal, and urinalyses are normal except for possible bilirubinuria.

Lesions. Grossly, the liver can be normal, enlarged, or shrunken in size. Pathologic lesions present in the liver, from either a biopsy specimen or a necropsy specimen, can be variable in severity. Typical features include bile duct proliferation and perilobular, centrilobular, or periportal fibrosis. The fibrous connective tissue typically spares the sinusoids, but gradually constricts the surrounding functional parenchymal tissue. Mild to moderate inflammation and necrosis may be observed, but hepatic lipidosis and megalocytosis are rare.

Diagnostic Testing. No specific, readily available diagnostic tests can confirm an alsike clover or red clover poisoning. The diagnosis is made by confirming the presence of compatible clinical signs, clinical pathologic abnormalities, and histologic liver lesions, combined with confirmation of dietary exposure to these plants. Identification of the intact plants in a pasture can be done by veterinary toxicologists, botanists, and agricultural extension specialists, along with others with specific training in this area. Identification of these plants in hay or silage material is more of a challenge.

Treatment. No specific treatment exists for alsike or red clover hepatotoxicosis. Other horses on the premises should be thoroughly examined, particularly assessing hepatic integrity and function. Skin lesions resulting from the secondary photosensitization can be successfully managed through basic wound therapy: cleansing, debridement, hydrotherapy, bandaging. Horses should be kept out of direct sunlight until the lesions resolve and the liver enzyme activity is back to normal.

Treatment options for the severely affected horses are limited and should be aimed at supporting liver function. These can include IV fluids, B vitamins, low-protein, high-carbohydrate diet, branched-chained amino acids, and other basic supportive care.

Prognosis. The prognosis for patients exhibiting only photosensitization lesions is excellent, as long as appropriate medical management is instituted and exposure to the plants is stopped. Patients exhibiting hepatic encephalopathy have a poor prognosis.

Prevention and Control. The only successful management program that can be implemented to eliminate this disease is to not allow horses access to either red clover or alsike clover in the diet. It is hard to accurately estimate safe levels of this forage in the diet because of the lack of knowledge concerning the toxic principle and toxic exposure dose.

REFERENCES

1. Ames T et al: Secondary photosensitization in horses eating *Cymodothea trifolii* infested clover, *Am Assoc Vet Lab Diag* 37:45, 1994.
2. Talcott PA: Alsike clover (*Trifolium hybridum*) and red clover (*Trifolium pratense*) poisonings in horses, Proceedings of the 18th Annual Meeting of the ACVIM, Seattle, 2000.
3. Colon JL et al: Hepatic dysfunction and photodermatitis secondary to alsike clover poisoning, *Cont Ed Pract Vet Comp* 18(9):1022, 1996.
4. Nation PN: Hepatic disease in Alberta horses: a retrospective study of "alsike clover poisoning," *Can Vet J* 32:602, 1991.
5. Nation PN: Alsike clover poisoning: a review, *Can Vet J* 30:410, 1989.

ANNUAL RYEGRASS

Jeremy Allen

Synonyms.   Annual ryegrass toxicity (ARGT), corynetoxin poisoning, corynetoxicosis, and tunicaminyluracyl (TMU) poisoning are names for the disease. Similar diseases are flood plain staggers (blown grass *[Agrostis avenacea]*, parasitized by the nematode *Anguina* sp., carrying the bacterium *Rathayibacter toxicus,* which produces corynetoxins) and Stewarts range syndrome (annual beard grass *[Polypogon monspeliensis]*, the nematode *Anguina* sp., the bacteria *R toxicus,* and the corynetoxins)[1]. These two diseases only occur in Australia, have a similar pathogenesis to ARGT, and are not discussed further here. Finally, a similar disease involving the association of a nematode and a grass *(Festuca rubra commutata* Gaud., *Festuca nigrescens* Lam., Chewings fescue) occurred in Oregon until about 1960, but it has not been seen since.[2]

Sources.   ARGT is an acute and often fatal neurologic disease caused by consumption of annual ryegrass (*Lolium rigidum*) seed heads infected with the bacterium *Rathayibacter toxicus* (formerly *Clavibacter toxicus* and *Corynebacterium rathayi*[3,4]). This bacterium is normally soil borne, but gains access to the plant in winter by adhering to the surface of the parasitic nematode *Anguina funesta*. It colonizes the nematode galls and the inflorescence, and produces bacterial galls.[3] *R. toxicus* produces corynetoxins, apparently only when infected by a bacteriophage,[5] during the very short period from the end of flowering, through seed set, to maturity of the seeds.[6] The bacterial galls remain toxic throughout the following summer and autumn, and, if kept dry and protected from the weather, can remain toxic for years. Animals develop ARGT when grazing toxic ryegrass, either in pastures or crop stubbles, or when provided with feed (grain, hay, crop fines) that is contaminated with toxic ryegrass.

ARGT occurs every year in the agricultural areas of western and southern Australia, and has been reported in South Africa.[1] A disease considered clinically similar to ARGT occurred in cattle grazing annual ryegrass and fescue in the Central Valley of California in 1996 and 1997.[7]

Toxicokinetics.   The corynetoxins are glycolipids that belong to a subclass of nucleoside antibiotics, collectively referred to as TMU antibiotics. TMU-based compounds are toxic to all mammalian species and occur in nature as complexes of closely related compounds. The composition of each complex is characteristic of the microorganism that produces it, and there are currently five known naturally occurring complexes. Apart from the corynetoxins produced by *R. toxicus*, there are tunicamycin, streptovirudin, and antibiotic MM19290 produced by different *Streptomyces* spp., and an unnamed complex produced by an unidentified bacterium in water-damaged wheat.[8,9]

Only 5% of ingested toxin is actually absorbed. Once in the blood, the toxin is rapidly partitioned from the plasma into red blood cells, and then out of the blood completely, presumably into the tissues. The corynetoxins are lipophilic, are retained in the tissues (at least in the short term), are biologically active within tissues for up to several months, and are cumulative toxins.[10]

Mechanism of Action.   The fundamental lesion in the brain appears to be microvascular damage with increased permeability, leading to capillary obstruction and local ischemia. The latter causes hypoxic neuronal damage and focal parenchymal necrosis. The corynetoxins are also true or intrinsic hepatotoxins.[11]

The corynetoxins specifically inhibit the enzyme uridine diphospho-*N*-acetylglucosamine:dolichol-phosphate *N*-acetylglucosamine-1-phosphate (GlcNAc-1-P) transferase, which catalyzes the initial step in oligosaccharide assembly on dolichol phosphate, a lipid carrier involved in *N*-glycosylation of protein. This results in reduced *N*-glycosylation of a wide range of glycoproteins including enzymes, hormones, structural components of the cell membrane and extracellular matrices, and membrane receptors. The pathologic alterations in the body are probably due to the depletion of essential *N*-glycosylated glycoproteins.[10,12]

Toxicity and Risk Factors.   Corynetoxins, extracts of toxic seed heads and toxic ryegrass, have proven to be lethal to all animal species exposed naturally or tested, including sheep, cattle, horses, donkeys, pigs, guinea pigs, rats, mice, and chickens.[13]

Much information on the toxicity of the corynetoxins is derived from studies with tunicamycin, which has a similar mechanism of action as the corynetoxins, produces similar clinical disease in sheep and rats, and has similar toxicity.[14-17] The minimum oral lethal dose for tunicamycin in sheep, cattle, and pigs is approximately 1 mg/kg.[18] The oral lethal dose of corynetoxins in sheep, when administered via a slurry of toxic seed heads, is 3.2 to 5.6 mg/kg.[17] The approximate lethal dose for tunicamycin or corynetoxins given by subcutaneous injection to sheep is 20 to 40 µg/kg.[17,19] Reported lethal doses by parenteral administration for nursling rats, adult male rats, and adult female rats are 110 to 160, 350, and 450 µg/kg, respectively.[15,20] The corynetoxins are cumulative toxins. The total lethal dose is the same whether given as a single dose or as repeated smaller doses up to 2 months apart.[17]

In the Southern hemisphere, most cases of ARGT in grazing livestock occur between mid-October and mid-December (late spring to early summer), after the seed heads have developed maximum toxicity and while the pastures are undergoing senescence. Reasons for the reduced prevalence of the disease after this period are not known. It may be due to livestock changing their selection of diet after the pastures have senesced or due to some loss of the bacterial galls onto the ground where they are less available for consumption. Cases of ARGT that occur later in summer and in autumn are usually associated with the introduction of livestock onto crop stubble that contains toxic ryegrass or the feeding of contaminated hay or grain.

Clinical Signs.   Clinical signs appear abruptly, usually following some external stimulation. They include tremors, ataxia, adoption of a wide-based stance, stumbling and falling over, nystagmus, convulsions while in lateral (in cattle it may occasionally be sternal) recumbency, and death. Animals may appear to recover between episodes of ataxia and convulsions. Sheep often exhibit a high-stepping gait with their forelimbs, while the head is held high. When forced to run, some sheep have a stiff-legged or "rocking horse" gait. Some cattle appear disorientated and wander aimlessly between episodes of convulsions. Signs may appear as soon as 4 days after introduction to toxic pasture or feed (shorter periods have been recorded, but the pasture the livestock were previously on may also have been toxic). Animals may continue to exhibit neurologic signs for up to 10 days after removal from toxic feed. Ewes may abort.[2,13,21]

Clinical Pathology. The activities of plasma enzymes of hepatic origin, plasma concentrations of bile acids and total bilirubin, and plasma clotting times may be increased.[17,22]

Lesions. The liver may be enlarged, and pale tan to yellowish in color. Mild jaundice may be evident. Edema and congestion of the lungs may be present, as well as hemorrhages in a range of tissues. Rats may develop gangrene of the tail and hindlimb.[13]

The most consistent microscopic finding in the brain of affected livestock is the accumulation of perivascular, eosinophilic material, particularly in the subarachnoid space of the cerebellum between adjacent folia. Purkinje cell necrosis, swelling of astrocyte processes, occasional microthrombi within capillaries, and focal degenerative changes in the neuropil are less frequently seen. In sheep that have convulsed, focal vacuolation may be found in the thalamic radiation. In the liver, there may be diffuse vacuolation and fatty infiltration of hepatocytes, necrosis of individual hepatocytes, and biliary hyperplasia.[11,13]

It is the experience of diagnostic pathologists that the macroscopic and microscopic pathology of ARGT is neither consistent nor necessarily specific. Several animals may need to be examined to see the range of changes reported for this disease. Diagnosis is based on clinical signs, history of exposure to toxic ryegrass, pathology, and supportive evidence from other laboratory tests.

Diagnostic Testing. Collection of a liver biopsy and assay for liver microsomal GlcNAC-P-1 transferase provides a very specific diagnosis of TMU poisoning. This transferase is profoundly inhibited in ARGT.[23] Fresh liver, frozen quickly, from an animal that has just died or has been euthanized, is suitable for this purpose. An enzyme-linked immunosorbent assay (ELISA) test is available that can specifically detect and quantify the presence of *R. toxicus* in feed, rumen contents, and feces.[24] Feed can also be physically examined for the presence of ryegrass seeds and bacterial galls identified in the seeds using a light box.[13] An ELISA for corynetoxins in feed has been developed.[25]

Treatment. No satisfactory treatment for ARGT is available. Animals should be removed from the source of toxic feed as slowly and quietly as possible, and provided good-quality feed and water in a shady location where they are unlikely to

be disturbed. If possible, affected animals should be separated from unaffected animals.

The intraperitoneal administration of a cyclodextrin-magnesium gluconate-magnesium sulfate formulation initially appeared to be a suitable treatment,[26] but follow-up studies have not repeated the favorable results seen earlier.

Prognosis. It is difficult to identify which affected animals will live and which will die. Most animals that die do so within 24 hours of first showing clinical signs. Animals that convulse more frequently and more violently are less likely to survive.

Prevention and Control. The main methods of prevention are to reduce ryegrass by controlling it in cropping years and to attempt to stop development, before flowering commences, of ryegrass in pasture. Both can be achieved by the strategic use of herbicides or other management strategies. With the emergence of herbicide resistance in ryegrass populations, use of other management strategies will become increasingly important. These include heavy stocking during winter and spring, cutting pasture for silage or hay at the booting stage, and collecting and burning crop residues. When pasture is cut, it should be heavily grazed to stop the regrowth of ryegrass that will become toxic. During the high-risk period, livestock on ryegrass pasture should be inspected daily and removed from the pasture immediately when clinical signs are seen.

A cultivar of *L. rigidum* that is resistant to *A. funesta* has been bred and released.[3] When sown according to recommendations, it substantially, if not completely, reduces the risk of ARGT. Unfortunately, it is not suitable for much of the lower rainfall areas where ARGT occurs. An earlier flowering variety has been developed and results have been very promising. In the first study conducted in Western Australia, the bacterial gall count was reduced from 10,361 galls/kg to 4 galls/kg after planting this new ryegrass.

Spores of the fungus *Dilophospora alopecuri* in the soil adhere to *A. funesta* and are carried onto the ryegrass plant where they germinate, and the fungus colonizes the inflorescence. In doing this, the fungus substantially reduces the number of nematode and bacterial galls that are produced in the seed head, thus greatly reducing the risk of ARGT.[3] *D. alopecuri* is being distributed throughout regions of western Australia where ARGT is a problem.

An effective experimental vaccine against ARGT has been developed.[19] Cobalt supplementation to livestock may increase the amount of corynetoxins that needs to be consumed before toxicity occurs.[22]

REFERENCES

1. Bryden WL et al: In Colegate SM, Dorling PR, editors: *Plant-associated toxins: agricultural, phytochemical and ecological aspects,* Oxon, UK, 1994, CAB International.
2. Cheeke PR: *Natural toxicants in feeds, forages, and poisonous plants,* ed 2, Danville, Ill, 1998, Interstate Publishers.
3. Riley IT: In Colegate SM, Dorling PR, editors: *Plant-associated toxins: agricultural, phytochemical and ecological aspects,* Oxon, 1994, CAB International.

4. Sasaki J et al: Taxonomic significance of 2,3-diaminobutyric acid isomers in the cell wall peptidoglycan of actinomycetes and reclassification of *Clavibacter toxicus* as *Rathayibacter toxicus* comb. nov, *Int J Systematic Bacteriol* 48:403, 1998.

5. Ophel KM et al: Association of bacteriophage particles with toxin production by *Clavibacter toxicus*, the causal agent of annual ryegrass toxicity, *Phytopathology* 83:676, 1993.

6. Stynes BA, Bird AF: Development of annual ryegrass toxicity, *Aust J Agric Res* 34:653, 1983.

7 Galey FD, University of Wyoming: Personal communication, 1998.

8. Cockrum PA et al: In James LF et al: *Poisonous plants, proceedings of the Third International Symposium,* Ames, Iowa, 1992, Iowa State University Press.

9. Edgar JA et al: In Colegate SM, Dorling PR: *Plant-associated toxins: agricultural, phytochemical and ecological aspects,* Oxon, 1994, CAB International.

10. Stuart SJ et al: In Colegate SM, Dorling PR, editors: *Plant-associated toxins: agricultural, phytochemical and ecological aspects,* Oxon, 1994, CAB International.

11. Finnie JW: In Colegate SM, Dorling PR, editors: *Plant-associated toxins: agricultural, phytochemical and ecological aspects,* Oxon, UK, 1994, CAB International.

12. Jago MV: In Seawright et al: *Plant toxicology, proceedings of the Australia-USA Poisonous Plants Symposium,* Melbourne, 1985, Dominion Press-Hedges and Bell.

13. Purcell DA: In Seawright AA et al, editors: *Plant toxicology, proceedings of the Australia-USA Poisonous Plants Symposium.* Melbourne, 1985, Dominion Press-Hedges and Bell.

14. Jago MV et al: Inhibition of glycosylation by corynetoxin, the causative agent of annual ryegrass toxicity: a comparison with tunicamycin, *Chemico-biological interactions* 45:223, 1983.

15. Vogel P et al: Corynetoxins, the causal agents of annual ryegrass toxicity shown to be closely related to the antibiotic tunicamycin, *Toxicon Suppl* 3:477, 1983.

16. Finnie JW, Jago MV: Experimental production of annual ryegrass toxicity with tunicamycin, *Aust Vet J* 62:248, 1985.

17. Jago MV, Culvenor CCJ: Tunicamycin and corynetoxin poisoning in sheep, *Aust Vet J* 64:232, 1987.

18. Bourke CA, Carrigan MJ: Experimental tunicamycin toxicity in cattle, sheep and pigs, *Aust Vet J* 70:188, 1993.

19. Than KA et al: In Garland T, Barr AC, editors: *Toxic plants and other natural toxins,* Oxon, 1998, CAB International.

20. Peterson JE et al: Permanent testicular damage induced in rats by a single dose of tunicamycin, *Reprod Toxicol* 10:61, 1996.

21. Bourke CA: In Colegate SM, Dorling PR, editors: *Plant-associated toxins: agricultural, phytochemical and ecological aspects,* Oxon, 1994, CAB International.

22. Davies SC et al: Increased tolerance to annual ryegrass toxicity in sheep given a supplement of cobalt, *Aust Vet J* 72:221, 1995.

23. Stewart PL et al: Reduction and recovery of *N*-acetylglucosamine-1-phosphate transferase activity in the liver of sheep and rats after a single dose of tunicamycin, *Aust Vet J* 76:287, 1998.

24. Gregory A et al: Agriculture Western Australia: Unpublished data, 1999.

25. Than KA et al: In Garland T, Barr AC: *Toxic plants and other natural toxins,* Oxon, 1998, CAB International.

26. Stewart PL et al: In Garland T, Barr AC, editors: *Toxic plants and other natural toxins,* Oxon, 1998, CAB International.

AVOCADO

John A. Pickrell, Fred Oehme, and Shajan A. Mannala

Sources. Avocado, *Persea americana,* is a tree or shrub with long branches arising from terminal buds. It is widely cultivated for its fruits. The Mexican, Guatemalan, and West Indian avocado are the most common varieties or races. The fruit has a glossy, dark-green exterior over a lime green to yellow flesh. It has a smooth, ovoid, solitary seed.[1-4]

Toxicokinetics. Recent research suggests that the active principle is persin, which has been isolated from avocado leaves. Persin has been identified as (Z,Z)-1-(acetoxy)-2-hydroxy-12,15-heneicosadien-4-one. Enantio-selective synthesis of persin revealed that only the R isomer is active.[5]

Toxicokinetics are currently undefined. Clinical signs are highly variable, ranging from acute deaths in rabbits, caged birds, and goats to mastitis and agalactia in cattle, rabbits, and goats. Because rabbits and goats are part of both clinical courses, it is likely that the two syndromes involve different doses.[1-3,5]

Mechanism of Action. The mechanism of action remains to be resolved.

Toxicity and Risk Factors. All above-ground parts of *Persea americana,* especially the leaves, are toxic to cattle, horses, goats, rabbits, canaries, ostriches, and fish. Doses of 60 to 100 mg/kg cause mastitis and agalactia. At doses of persin greater than 100 mg/kg, necrosis of the myocardial fibers may occur and hydrothorax may be present.[5]

Clinical Signs. Severely affected animals present with cardiopulmonary signs, whereas less severely affected lactating animals have noninfectious mastitis and agalactia.[1-3]

Lactating mares, cattle, rabbits, and goats present with noninfectious mastitis and agalactia. The mastitis can be controlled in 1 week with treatment, but the milk production remains reduced.

Rabbits, caged birds, and goats can develop cardiac arrhythmia, submandibular edema, and acute death. Intoxicated caged birds have developed respiratory distress.[1-3] Horses that eat the fruit develop colic, diarrhea, and edema of the ventral abdomen, head, and neck. The edema is painful and can cause respiratory dyspnea. Heart sounds may be muffled following development of hydrothorax.[2]

Clinical Pathology. Elevation of creatine phosphokinase (CPK) and ALT reflect cardiac muscle damage.[2]

Lesions. Rabbits, caged birds, and goats have pulmonary congestion. Caged birds have generalized congestion, subcutaneous edema, and hydropericardium. Goats experimentally poisoned with avocado leaves died within 48 hours of ingestion with degeneration and coagulative necrosis of the myocardium. The noninfectious mastitis in mares and goats is due to necrosis of the glandular epithelium of the mammary gland.[1-4,6]

Diagnostic Testing. A history of exposure to avocado with appropriate clinical signs, or finding leaves in the gastrointestinal contents is supportive evidence.[1,3,4]

Treatment. Treatment is primarily symptomatic and supportive.[1]

Prognosis. The prognosis is guarded for animals that develop cardiac and pulmonary disease.[1,3,4] Recovery is expected in animals that develop mastitis; however, the milk production rarely returns to normal.

Prevention and Control. Animals should not be allowed access to avocado.[1]

REFERENCES

1. Aiello E, Mays A, editors: *Toxicology, plants poisonous to animals: the Merck veterinary manual,* ed 8, Philadelphia, 1998, National Publishing (Merial Limited).
2. Knight AP: In Lewis LD, editor: *Equine clinical nutrition: feeding and care,* Media, Penn, 1995, Williams & Wilkins.
3. Kingsbury JM: *Poisonous plants of the United States and Canada,* Englewood Cliffs, NJ, 1964, Prentice-Hall.
4. Everist SL: *Poisonous plants of Australia,* London, 1974, Angus and Robertson Publishers.
5. Oelrichs PB et al: Isolation and identification of a compound from avocado (*Persea americana*) leaves which causes necrosis of the acinar epithelium of the lactating mammary gland and the myocardium, *Nat Toxins* 3:344, 1995.
6. Burger WP et al: Cardiomyopathy in ostriches (*Struthion camelus*) due to avocado (*Persea americana* var. guatemalensis) intoxication, *J S Afr Vet Assoc* 65:113-118, 1994.

BLACK WALNUT

Francis D. Galey

Sources. The primary clinical concern for black walnut is the ability of fresh shavings made from heartwood to cause laminitis in equines.[1,2] The syndrome is a result of the laminae of the feet becoming necrotic.[3] Black walnut–induced laminitis in horses most commonly results from exposure to shavings made from the heartwood of the tree, usually in bedding (Color Plate 48). Anecdotal reports exist of horses being poisoned from ingestion of twigs from black walnut branches.

Black walnut (*Juglans nigra*) is a hardwood tree that is native to the eastern and central United States. Wood and hulls from the tree are potentially toxic to several species of animals and other plants. Black walnut trees may grow to 100 feet in height and have alternate, deciduous, pinnately compound leaves. The bark is furrowed and dark brown to black in color. Twigs have chambered and buff-colored pith. The heartwood is a dark, purple-brown color. The wood breaks sharply when bent (breakage characteristic of most hardwoods). The seeds are encased in woody, black shells (nuts) which are enclosed by a green semifleshy fruit.[4]

Toxicokinetics. The toxin that causes laminitis has not been identified. Horses exposed to black walnut often develop clinical signs within 4 to 12 hours.

Mechanism of Action. The toxin of black walnut that causes laminitis is unknown. Juglone, a naphthoquinone, causes toxicosis in fish and laboratory animals. Juglone was demonstrated to cause blockage of oxidative phosphory-lation in corn and fish cell mitochondria.[5,6] Results from the same studies suggest that juglone does not uncouple the oxidative phosphorylation. Based on the development of liver necrosis and pulmonary edema in dogs administered juglone via IV injection, other workers suggested that juglone may be "toxic to the cell membrane."[7]

Juglone caused dilation of vessels of the ear and heart in rabbits.[8] Dogs developed no abnormalities in electrocardiograms, heart rates, or blood pressures until near the time of death at 2 to 3 hours after being given juglone at 10 mg/kg body weight IV.[7] The outstanding postmortem lesion produced in those dogs was severe pulmonary interstitial and alveolar edema with focal pulmonary atelectasis. Focal areas of portal necrosis were present in liver tissues from the dogs.[7]

Ponies given juglone via IV injection failed to develop signs following the initial administration. After subsequent administration of 250 mg and 109 mg of juglone via IV, two ponies rapidly (within 1 hour) developed severe pulmonary edema.[9] One pony (109-mg dose) was treated successfully using dexamethasone and tripelennamine. Thus, the episodes of pulmonary edema were likely to have been anaphylactic responses. The authors speculated that the juglone was acting as a hapten based on its molecular size and weight.[9]

The mechanism of action of black walnut–induced laminitis is unknown, in part because the causative toxins have not been identified. However, crude aqueous extracts made from black walnut heartwood reversibly enhanced the ability of epinephrine to cause increased contraction of isolated equine digital arteries and veins.[10] This suggests a possible role of vasospasm in the effects of black walnut in the horse.

Horses given a crude aqueous extract of black walnut heartwood via nasogastric tube developed transient leukopenia (primarily a neutropenia) and hyperthermia at 4 to 8 hours after administration.[11] This was followed by development of pounding digital pulse, dependent edema in the forelimbs, and mild lethargy by 12 hours after administration. The development of laminitis coincided with a decrease in blood perfusion to the capillaries of the laminae relative to the rest of the forefeet when measured using gamma scintigraphy.[12] This finding suggested that black walnut–induced laminitis is likely to have an ischemic component, similar to laminitis resulting from other causes such as endotoxemia.[13] Eighty-four hours after administration of the extract of black walnut, the relative distribution of perfusion to the equine dorsal lamina was higher than the control ratio, suggesting that the ischemic region may have undergone reperfusion.[11]

Toxicity and Risk Factors. Walnut hulls are known to be toxic to fungi, bacteria, plants, fish, and mammals.[14] The most well-characterized allelopathic and toxic compound in black walnut, as mentioned earlier, is juglone (5 hydroxy 1,4 naphthoquinone).[7,8,14-16] Approximately 150 ppm of juglone is present in black walnut leaves.[17] Pure juglone is most likely not, however, the laminitis-causing toxin of black walnut.[18] Studies in which pure juglone was repeatedly administered to horses via various routes produced pulmonary edema in ponies (IV administration) but not laminitis.[9] Additionally, the heartwood from the tree, which is most likely to cause laminitis, is devoid of juglone.[18]

The 96-hour median lethal concentration (LC_{50}) for juglone in fish ranged from 27 ppb in water for northern pike (*Esox lucius*) to 88 ppb for carp (*Cyprinus carpio*).[19] Toxicity was unaffected by temperature, but making the water more alkaline (from pH of 7.4 to 9) reduced the potency of juglone by 33%. Dogs given juglone at 3 mg/kg of body weight IV developed no signs or lesions.[7] However, when the same investigators gave dogs juglone at 10 mg/kg of body weight, lethal poisoning consistently developed.

Based on cases attended by this author, as little as 5% to 20% of fresh black walnut in shavings used as bedding is capable of causing laminitis. Most horses are apparently exposed to the shavings via ingestion. Attempts to reproduce the disease with fresh shavings packed around the horse's foot were unsuccessful.[1]

Clinical Signs. Black walnut–associated laminitis occurs frequently in the form of outbreaks, unlike laminitis resulting from other causes that affect a few animals at most.[1] Incidence rates of acute laminitis have ranged in various reports from less than 30% of exposed horses to 100% of exposed horses.[1] Signs reported in addition to laminitis include increased body temperatures, increased heart and respiratory rates, edema of the lower limbs, palpable increases in coronary band and hoof temperatures, and pounding digital pulses. The severity of signs varies. Ponies and some younger horses, such as foals and yearlings, appeared to be somewhat resistant, although there were exceptions; and those younger animals that were affected recovered more quickly than adults.[1] Conversely, a few of the older horses developed rotated third phalanx (severe laminitis) and had to be euthanized.[1]

Clinical Pathology. A transient neutropenia developed in horses given an aqueous extract of black walnut at approximately 4 hours before the onset of the initial stages of laminitis.[11] An increase in plasma cortisol levels, which was sustained beyond that which may be expected for a normal diurnal rhythm, also developed in severely affected horses at about 4 to 8 hours after dosing with black walnut extract.

Lesions. No remarkable gross lesions were found on postmortem examination of horses with black walnut toxicosis induced by administration of an aqueous extract of black walnut heartwood.[11] Histologically, the dorsal laminae from those horses with laminitis at 12 hours after administration contained vacuolated epithelial cells near the tips of primary laminae. Severe laminitis in horses at 84 hours after administration was characterized by necrosis of dermal tips of dorsal primary epidermal laminae.[11] A proliferative epithelial response in those laminae was distinguished by numerous mitotic figures and clumping of epithelial cells. These findings were also consistent with the idea that black walnut–induced laminitis is, at least in part, an ischemic disease of the laminae.

Diagnostic Testing. An increased incidence of laminitis, especially in the form of an epizootic, along with evidence of

exposure of the affected animals to black walnut shavings, is suggestive of black walnut toxicosis. Black walnut heartwood can be tentatively identified using a dissecting microscope based on its purple-black color, grainy texture with crystals in grooves, and breakage pattern that is consistent with a hardwood. Absolute identification should be left to a specialist in wood science.

Treatment. Horses exposed to black walnut shavings should be removed from the suspected bedding immediately. If exposure seems to be substantial and animals can be treated before the onset of clinical signs, administration of activated charcoal via nasogastric tube may be beneficial.

Unless severe, laminitis in horses caused by black walnut toxicosis is readily reversed using traditional therapy such as phenylbutazone administered via IV injection combined with good nursing care.[1] Experimentally, changes in the distribution of perfusion caused by black walnut were at least transiently reversed using the alpha$_1$ adrenoceptor antagonist, prazocin hydrochloride.[12] Thus, further study of this agent in the treatment of horses with laminitis may be warranted.

Prognosis. Most horses with black walnut toxicosis recover completely following timely and appropriate therapy for the laminitis and removal from the suspected shavings. Severely affected horses, especially if treatment with phenylbutazone is delayed, may develop severe sequelae of laminitis caused by sinking or rotation of the third phalanx. The prognosis is grave for such animals.

Prevention and Control. Prevention of black walnut poisoning centers on avoidance of exposure. Shavings should be scrutinized for the presence of black walnut before use. Although not proven as a cause of laminitis, fallen branches from black walnut trees should be removed from the paddock. It has been suggested that drying or time decreases the toxicity of black walnut shavings because shavings which at one time caused laminitis failed to cause laminitis when reused.[1] This author, however, recommends against any use of shavings with black walnut as a bedding for Equidae.

REFERENCES

1. True RG et al: Black walnut shavings as a cause of acute laminitis, *Proc Ann Mtg AAEP*, 24:511, 1978.
2. Peterson DE: Equine laminitis associated with black walnut toxicity, *Minnesota Vet* 24:38, 1984.
3. Ganjam VK, Garner HE: Summary, proceedings of First Equine Endotoxemia/Laminitis Symposium. *Am Assoc Equine Pract Newsletter* 2:156, 1982.
4. Brockman CF: In Zimm HS, editor: *Trees of North America*, Racine, Wis, 1979, Golden Press, Western Publishing.
5. Koeppe DE: Some reactions of isolated corn mitochondria influenced by juglone, *Physiologia Plantarum* 27:89, 1972.
6. Ohta A et al: Isolation of naphthazarin from walnut "onigurumi" and its inhibitory action on oxidative phosphorylation in mitochondria, *Toxicon* 11:235, 1973.
7. Boelkins JN et al: Effects of intravenous juglone in the dog, *Toxicon* 6:99, 1968.
8. Auyong TK et al: Pharmacological aspects of juglone, *Toxicon* 1:235, 1963.

9. True RG, Lowe JE: Induced juglone toxicosis in ponies and horses, *Am J Vet Res* 41:944, 1980.

10. Galey FD et al: Effect of an aqueous extract of black walnut *(Juglans nigra)* on isolated equine digital vessels, *Am J Vet Res* 51:83, 1990.

11. Galey FD et al: Black walnut *(Juglans nigra)* toxicosis: a model for equine laminitis, *J Comp Pathol* 104:313, 1991.

12. Galey FD et al: Gamma scintigraphic analysis of the distribution of perfusion of blood in the equine foot during black walnut *(Juglans nigra)*-induced toxicosis, *Am J Vet Res* 51:688-, 1990.

13. HoodDM et al: Equine laminitis I: Radioisotopic analysis of the hemodynamics of the foot during the acute disease, *J Equine Med Surg* 2:439, 1978.

14. Gries GA: Juglone: the active agent in walnut toxicity, *Northern Nut Growers Assoc Report* 32:52, 1943.

15. Massey AB: Antagonism of the walnuts *(Juglans nigra* L. and *J. cinera* L.) in certain plant associations, *Phytopathol* 15:773-, 1925.

16. Westfall BA et al: Depressant agents from walnut hulls, *Science* 134:1617, 1961.

17. Coder KD: Seasonal changes of juglone potential in leaves of black walnut *(Juglans nigra* L.), *J chemical Ecol* 9:1203, 1983.

18. MinnickPD et al: The induction of equine laminitis with an aqueous extract of black walnut *(Juglans nigra)*, *Vet Hum Toxicol* 29:230, 1987.

19. Marking LL: Juglone (5-hydroxy-1,4-naphthoquinone) as a fish toxicant, *Transcripts Am Fish Soc* 99:510, 1970.

FORAGE-INDUCED PHOTOSENSITIZATION

Stan W. Casteel

Sources.   Forages such as alfalfa or red clover are sporadically associated with secondary photosensitization outbreaks

TABLE 25-16 **Forage and Plants Associated with Photosensitization of Uncertain Pathogenesis**

Plant	Class of Photosensitization
Avena sativa (oats)	Uncertain
Brassica napus/Triticale (rape,wheat/rye hybrid pasture)	Hepatogenous
Medicago sativa (moldy alfalfa hay)	Hepatogenous
Sorghum spp. (sudan grass)	Unknown
Trifolium hybridum (alsike clover)	Unknown
Trifolium pratense (red clover)	Hepatogenous
Triticum aestivum (wheat)	Unknown
Triticum aestivum (moldy wheat straw)	Hepatogenou
Setaria sp./Dactylis glomerata (foxtail/orchardgrass hay)	Hepatogenous

Data from references 3, 5, 7, 11-18.

in cattle, particularly when grown during unusual environmental conditions such as a period of excessive rainfall.[1-3] Forages that have been associated with photosensitization are listed in Table 25-16.

Mechanism of Action.   Cutaneous photosensitization is the manifestation of hyperreactivity of the skin to sunlight. Photosensitization is either a symptom of liver disease (secondary photosensitization) or a primary condition caused by ingestion of a unique photosensitizing compound (primary photosensitization). The photosensitizing agent is usually of plant origin, but may also be in certain drugs or industrial chemicals. In ruminants, clinical photosensitization is usually secondary to diffuse liver disease and may be more appropriately labeled a forage-induced liver disease. Phylloerythrin, derived from chlorophyll, is the photoreactive compound in plants responsible for secondary photosensitization.

At the molecular level, photosensitization is a reaction in which a photoreactive molecule is activated by the absorption of an appropriate wavelength or narrow band of light. The activated molecule then initiates a detrimental cascade of events that often results in cell death. Specific biochemical and functional effects of photosensitization reactions include formation of photoadducts with DNA and proteins, peroxidation of lipids, photooxidation of membrane proteins, inhibition of transport of essential metabolites, and leakage of lysosomal enzymes.[4] The photoreactive molecule, also called a photosensitizer, functions as an energy transducer, facilitating the change of light energy into molecular electronic energy in the form of excited chemical species. The photosensitizer may or may not be consumed in the reaction, but it consistently lowers the light energy required to produce skin lesions.

Toxicity and Risk Factors.   Photosensitization of uncertain pathogenesis is frequently reported in livestock, especially cattle.[3,5-10] This classification is reserved for cases with minimal understanding of etiology. Cases usually originate from field observations of clinical photosensitivity in livestock. The transient nature, sporadic occurrence, and difficulty in reproducing these conditions preclude timely investigative procedures necessary to clarify complete understanding. Etiologic agents are rarely demonstrated, and vague associations between suspect forage and clinical photosensitization are the norm. Even when photosensitization is reproduced with incriminated forage in feeding trials, the specific photosensitizer is not identified.

In many cases, a mycotoxin-related etiology is implied. However, samples of suspect forage screened for known mycotoxins are consistently negative. Growth and harvesting of normally acceptable forage during times of excessive rainfall presumably support the growth of a toxigenic fungus or else are conducive to the elaboration of hepatotoxic mycotoxins by normal fungal flora. Another plausible explanation is that viable forage mounts a phytoalexic response to fungal infection, with the phytoalexin being hepatotoxic for cattle.

Clinical Signs.   Clinical photosensitization resembles severe sunburn of the areas of the skin that have little or no hair (nose, udder) and of areas that have light-colored skin and, therefore white hair. The tongue, especially the tip and the underside, can be affected. The progressive clinical manifestation of photosensitization consists of lacrimation, photophobia, erythema, pruritus, cutaneous edema, fissuring of the epithelium, necrosis, and sloughing of nonpigmented exposed skin. Corneal edema also is evident in some cases.

This forage-induced condition in cattle is best characterized as a cholestatic liver disease. Clinical signs consistent with liver damage such as icterus commonly are seen with secondary photosensitization in ruminants. When bilirubin levels elevate rapidly, severe depression and anorexia are also characteristic.

Clinical Pathology.   Serum liver enzymes such as AST and serum alkaline phosphatase tend to increase primarily in the acute stage of liver injury and may not be grossly elevated at the time of clinical photosensitization. Gamma-glutamyl-transferase is an exception, having a more sustained elevation when bile duct or canalicular epithelium is damaged. In cattle, a substantial increase in these liver enzymes occurs within days of consumption. Hundred-fold increases in GGT activity sustained for several days to a few weeks are not uncommon. Clinical recognition of severe hepatobiliary disease is usually concurrent with a substantial increase in conjugated bilirubin.

Lesions.   Intrahepatic cholestasis and skin lesions characterize forage-associated liver disease. In cattle, lesions vary from mild-to-severe periportal fibrosis with mild-to-moderate bile duct hyperplasia. Mild histopathologic change has little correlation with the striking serum elevation of GGT activity that normally suggests severe damage to the biliary system.[3]

Diagnostic Testing.   Diagnosis of photosensitization is based on typical clinical signs and lesions restricted to lightly pigmented areas with sparse hair covering. Pasture type, recent weather conditions, and conditions surrounding forage harvesting should be noted. Unusually wet weather resulting in delayed harvesting of over-mature alfalfa or red clover is often associated with epizootics.

Treatment.   Supportive and symptomatic care are the only options. Secondary skin infections may be prevented with antibiotics. Animals should be provided ample shade or should be sheltered during the day.

Prognosis.   Cattle with photosensitization secondary to liver disease have a guarded chance for recovery. Cattle exposed to hepatotoxic alfalfa or red clover hay often develop a chronic progressive liver disease that is fatal.

REFERENCES

1. Casteel SW et al: Forage-associated mycotoxicosis, *Proc XVII World Buiatrics Congress,* St Paul, Minn, 1992, .
2. Casteel SW et al: Hepatotoxicosis in cattle induced by consumption of moldy forage, *Proc 6th International Congress EAVPT,* Edinburgh, 1994.
3. Casteel SW et al: Liver disease in cattle induced by consumption of moldy hay, *Vet Human Toxicol* 37:248, 1995.
4. Spikes JD: Photosensitization. In Smith KC, editor: *The science of photobiology,* ed 2, New York, 1988, Plenum.
5. Bagley CV et al: Photosensitization associated with exposure of cattle to moldy straw, *J Am Vet Med Assoc* 183:802, 1983.
6. Berry JM, Merriam JG: Phototoxic dermatitis in a horse, *Vet Med Small Anim Clin* 65:251, 1970.
7. Putnam MR et al: Hepatic enzyme changes in bovine hepatogenous photosensitivity caused by water-damaged alfalfa hay, *J Am Vet Med Assoc* 189:77, 1986.
8. Martin T, Morgan S: What caused the photosensitivity in these dairy heifers? *Vet Med* 82:848, 1987.
9. McKenzie RA et al: Smartweeds (*Polygonum* spp) and photosensitization of cattle, *Aust Vet J* 65:128, 1988.
10. Pfister JA et al: Photosensitization of cattle in Montana: is *Descurainia pinnata* the culprit? *Vet Hum Toxicol* 31:225, 1989.
11. Sippel WL, Burnside JE: Oat dermatitis, *Georgia Vet* 6:3, 1954.
12. Wikse SE et al: Hepatogenous photosensitization in beef cows grazing a combination rape/triticale pasture, *Proc 9th Annual Western Conferenc for Food Animal Disease Research,* Moscow, Idaho, 1988.
13. Scruggs DW, Glue GK: Toxic hepatopathy and photosensitization in cattle fed moldy alfalfa hay, *J Am Vet Med Assoc* 204:264, 1994.
14. Howarth JA: Sudan grass as a photosensitizing agent causing dermatitis in sheep, *North Am Vet* 12:29, 1931.
15. Cheeke PR, Shull LR: Glycosides. In *Natural toxicants in feeds and poisonous plants,* Westport, Conn, 1985, AVI Publishing.
16. Burnside JE: Photosensitization in cattle, a case report, *Georgia Vet* 5:10, 1953.
17. Schmidt H: Swell-head in sheep and goats, *Ann Report Texas Agric Exp Sta* 44:11, 1931.
18. Witte ST, Curry SL: Hepatogenous photosensitization in cattle fed a grass hay, *J Vet Diagn Invest* 5:133, 1993.

GUTIERREZIA

George Burrows and Ronald J. Tyrl

Sources.   A large genus with numerous annual and perennial species generally known as the broomweeds, *Gutierrezia* is a member of the Asteraceae, or sunflower, family. Some taxa of the genus have been placed in the genera *Xanthocephalum* and *Amphiachyris*. Only two perennial species are of toxicologic interest. *G. microcephala* occurs in the Southwest, whereas *G. sarothrae* is found throughout western North America (Table 25-17).

Toxicokinetics.   The perennial species of *Gutierrezia* have long been considered the cause of an acute systemic disease and decreased weight gain in cows and ewes as well as a

TABLE 25-17 *Gutierrezia* **Species that Are Toxic**

Species Name	Common Name
G. microcephala (DC.) A.Gray	Threadleaf snakeweed, small-headed matchweed, small-headed matchbrush, sticky snakeweed
G. sarothrae (Pursh) Britton and Rusby	Snakeweed, broom snakeweed, matchweed, matchbrush, turpentine weed, coyaye, perennial broomweed, slinkweed

cause of abortion and birth of premature calves and lambs.[1-3] When consumed over 3 to 5 days, 3% to 10% body weight of green plant material was lethal to cows and ewes, whereas the risk was lower for goats. Given to pregnant cows for several weeks, 0.5 kg/day resulted in abortions or the birth of small, weak calves. These toxins were at one time thought to be saponins, but more recent evidence indicates the probability of diterpenes similar to those of *Pinus* as the likely cause.[4]

Toxicity and Risk Factors. Cattle, sheep, and, to a lesser extent, goats are the species at risk, although other herbivores eating large quantities of the plants may also be susceptible. Losses occur mainly in areas with sandy soils and heavy infestations of the plants.

Clinical Signs. The nasal pad becomes crusted with a nasal discharge. The appetite decreases, and the animal becomes weak and listless. Icterus may also be present. Digestive disturbance appears as either diarrhea or constipation with foul-smelling mucoid feces. A stringy mucoid secretion from the vulva is typical, along with mammary development and swelling of the vulva. Within a short time, pregnancy terminates with abortion, stillbirth, or birth of small, weak neonates and retention of placental membranes. In some animals, the signs may not be prominent.

Clinical Pathology. Serum cholesterol and iron are decreased; creatinine, direct bilirubin, and indirect bilirubin are increased. Serum hepatic enzymes are mildly increased.

Lesions. Gross lesions include icterus, pale, swollen kidneys, mottled yellowish liver, and possibly reddened mucosa of the stomach and small intestine.

Microscopically, the renal tubular epithelium is mildly to moderately flattened and the tubules dilated. Hepatic necrosis is also present.

Treatment. No specific treatment is required. Good nursing care with a high level of nutrition is important.

Prognosis. Small, weak neonates have poor survival prospects. Adults, if fed well after signs develop, may recover fully.

Prevention and Control. Supplemental feeding to reduce ingestion of *Gutierrezia* is the key to preventing development of disease while allowing some use of pasture rangeland.[5] Safflower oil has provided beneficial effects in laboratory animals.[6]

REFERENCES

1. Dollahite JW, Anthony WV: Experimental production of abortion, premature calves and retained placentas by feeding a species of perennial broomweed, *Texas Agr Exp Sta Prog Report* 1884:3, 1956.
2. Dollahite JW, Anthony WV: Poisoning of cattle with *Gutierrezia microcephala,* a perennial broomweed, *J Am Vet Med Assoc* 130:525, 1957.
3. Mathews FP: The toxicity of broomweed (*Gutierrezia microcephala*) for sheep, cattle and goats, *J Am Vet Med Assoc* 88:54, 1936.
4. Roitman JN, James LF, Panter KE: Constituents of broom snakeweed (*Gutierrezia sarothrae),* an abortifacient rangeland plant. In Colegate SM,

Dorling PR, editors: *Plant-associated toxins, agricultural, phytochemical and ecological aspects,* Wallingford, UK, 1994, CAB International.
5. Staley EC et al: Decreased reproductive effects from snakeweed (*Gutierrezia microcephala*) in Sprague-Dawley rats with increased dietary snakeweed consumption, *Vet Hum Toxicol* 38:259, 1996.
6. Smith GS et al: Safflower seed oil improved embryo-fetal tolerance of toxins in snakeweed foliage ingested by rats, *J Anim Sci* 71:445, 1993 (abstract).

HOARY ALYSSUM

Patricia A. Talcott

Sources. Hoary alyssum, *Berteroa incana,* is a member of the mustard family (Brassicaceae). It can grow as an annual, biennial, or short-lived perennial, reproducing by seeds. The name "hoary" is derived from the rough, star-shaped hairs present on the stems, leaves, and seedpods. The stems are gray-green, erect, 1 to 3 feet tall, and branch near the top of the plant (Color Plate 49). The leaves are alternate, oval to oblong, narrow, gray-green, $\frac{1}{2}$ to 3 inches long, with smooth edges. The plant has numerous white flowers, 3 to 5 mm long, with four deeply divided petals located on long terminal racemes (Color Plate 50). The seedpods are hairy, oblong, 5 to 8 mm long and 3 to 4 mm wide, and somewhat flattened with a short beak on the end. There are three to six seeds per locule, brown, round, and narrowly winged. This can be a fairly aggressive plant, found in meadows, pastures, along roadsides and railroad tracks, and in disturbed lands and waste areas. This plant can be found throughout the northern United States.

Mechanism of Action. The toxin responsible for this disease is unknown.

Toxicity and Risk Factors. The exact toxic dose is unknown and often difficult to determine from field cases because of the nonuniform distribution of the plant throughout the pasture or hay bales. Anywhere from less than 10% to greater than 90% of the plant in hay bales has been associated with illness.[2]

Horses appear to be the primary species affected. Despite concern that cattle or other livestock may be sensitive as well, no case reports of these species being affected have been documented. No age, sex, or breed predilection has been noted. Case reports of illness have been associated with grazing the plant in pasture settings, as well as ingesting contaminated hay. The palatability of the plant is unknown. However, in three different free-choice grazing trials, grazing lambs consistently rejected hoary alyssum.[1]

Clinical Signs. Clinical signs are commonly observed within 12 to 36 hours of ingesting sufficient quantities of the plant. Early signs of illness include some or all of the following: lethargy, fever, distal edema of any or all limbs, and laminitis. Abdominal pain and short-term diarrhea are less commonly reported. Early parturition was reported in a group of pregnant mares following exposure to hoary alyssum–containing hay, and scrotal and testicular edema was reported in an exposed stallion.[3] Acute and severe gastrointestinal distress (moderate to profuse bloody diarrhea, abdominal pain), intravascular hemolysis, and late-term abortion were associated with hoary alyssum exposure in a herd of 29 broodmares.[4]

In some horses exposed to high concentrations in the diet (30% to 70%), deaths have been documented following signs associated with worsening of the aforementioned symptoms, shock, dehydration, acute renal failure, severe laminitis with distal phalangeal rotation, and possible endotoxemia or disseminated intravascular coagulation.

Clinical Pathology.   Complete blood counts, serum chemistry profiles, and urinalyses are commonly normal in mildly to moderately affected horses. Severely affected horses have displayed the following abnormalities: anemia, neutropenia or neutrophilia with a left shift, hematuria, methemoglobinemia, and elevated creatinine, blood urea nitrogen, phosphorus, total bilirubin, ALP alkaline phosphatase, AST, creatine kinase (CK), and SDH.[2,4,5]

Lesions.   Necropsy findings in severely affected horses have included marked perirenal hemorrhage, hemoperitoneum, hemothorax, serosal petechiae, and ecchymoses.[2] Congestion and edema of multiple organs, portal hepatitis, hemosiderin-filled splenic and hepatic macrophages, along with renal tubular casts, have been reported.[2] Limb edema is commonly observed, as is rotation of the distal phalanx of one or more limbs.

Diagnostic Testing.   Because the toxic principle is unknown, confirmation of poisoning relies heavily on eliminating other etiologic agents along with the temporal association and confirmation of ingestion of the plant. This is sometimes difficult to do because of the nonuniform distribution of this plant in the diet. In evaluating pastures following documented cases of poisonings, investigators have found that the plant can be found diffusely throughout the field at low concentrations, or can inhabit a few isolated acres at heavy concentrations.

Treatment.   Part of the initial treatment plan is to recognize and remove the offending plant from the diet. The remainder of the treatment regimen includes symptomatic and supportive care. Some treatment options used in reported clinical cases include oral activated charcoal or mineral oil, IV DMSO and lactated Ringer's solution, intramuscular flunixin meglumine, antibiotics (sodium ampicillin, ceftiofur sodium), phenylbutazone, sucralfate, and cool water hydrotherapy or icing of the limbs.

Prognosis.   Clinical signs of illness typically subside within 2 to 4 days after removal of contaminated feed and empirical treatment. More severely affected animals may require longer treatment regimens, depending on the severity of the signs and secondary complications.

Prevention and Control.   Accurate identification of the plant and recognition of this problem in horses by owners are essential for the prevention of this disease.

REFERENCES

1. Becker RL et al: Hoary alyssum: toxicity to horses, forage quality, and control, *Bulletin AG-FS-5567-A, Minnesota Extension Service,* 1991.
2. Geor RJ et al: Toxicosis in horses after ingestion of hoary alyssum, *J Am Vet Med Assoc* 201(1):63, 1992.
3. Ellison SP: Possible toxicity cause by hoary alyssum (*Berteroa incana*), *Vet Med* 87(5):472, 1992.
4. Hovda LR, Rose M: Hoary alyssum (*Berteroa incana*) toxicity in a herd of broodmare horses, *Vet Hum Toxicol* 35(1):39, 1993.
5. Kanara EW, Murphy MJ: Ingestion of hoary alyssum as a cause of laminitis in horses, *Proc 13th ACVIM Forum,* Lake Buena Vista, Fla, 1995.

HOPS

William R. Hare

Synonyms.   *Humulus lupulus* is known as common hops, but other names include lupulin, European hops, simple hops, and beer hops. Some specific names for other species of hops include *H. americanus* and *H. neomexicanus,* American or wild hops; and *H. japonicus,* Japanese hops.[1,2]

Sources.   Hops are climbing, perennial, herbaceous type plants with generally rough stems, usually having twin vines, and growing from 3 to 10 meters in length.[3] The leaves are usually opposite, palmately lobed (three to four compound leaflets), veined, and serrated. They are darker green dorsally and lighter and grayish ventrally. The plant flowers in July and August with petalless clusters arranged as axillary panicles having five sepals and stamens arranged as conelike spikes. The small, green, conelike fruit, or achenes, containing one seed each are approximately 2 to 3 cm long and appear from August through October.

H. lupulus is native to North America, Europe, and Asia and grows throughout the temperate areas of the world. *H. lupulus, H. americanus,* and *H. neomexicanus* can be found growing throughout the United States. *H. lupulus* is grown commercially on the Pacific coast, but also can be found growing wild on fertile soils, in pastures, woodlands, fencerows, among thickets, and along open marshy areas.

Toxicokinetics.   The exact toxic principle responsible for poisoning has not been identified.[4] However, hops do contain a number of constituents that are potentially toxic. They include essential oils, phenolic compounds, resins, and various biologically active nitrogenous compounds. The three primary essential oils found in hops are humulene (α-caryophyllene), myrcene (β-caryophyllene), and farnesene. These oils are particularly unstable and may be oxidized to humulene epoxide, humulenol, humulol, and humuladienone. Their sulfur-containing components include various thiols, sulfides, thioesters, thiophenes, and episulfides. At least 20 different phenolic acid compounds have been identified in hops, including coumaric acid, gallic acid, and caffeic acid.

No specific controlled toxicokinetic studies have been performed in animals for hops or hops extract. Adverse clinical signs are usually exhibited within 3 to 6 hours after ingestion. Therefore, absorption of the toxic principles is rapid. Clinical signs tend to resolve within 24 to 48 hours in survivors. Clinical reports suggest a urinary route of elimination.

Mechanism of Action. The exact mechanism of action remains unknown. However, the clinical signs suggest a mechanism that inhibits electron transfer, such as uncouplers of oxidative phosphorylation, or agents that cause critical alteration of mitochondrial activity.

Toxicity and Risk Factors. Animals do not normally ingest hops plants, and clinical cases of poisoning are rare. However, dogs are attracted to hops used in the home-brewing of beer. Therefore, dogs are at most risk, especially dogs of the greyhound breed or mixed breed dogs with some greyhound ancestry.

Clinical Signs. Adverse clinical signs are characterized by severe hyperthermia.[4] The signs in dogs mimic malignant hyperthermia and may be due to initiation of a malignant hyperthermia-like syndrome. The animal's body temperature quickly reaches 41° to 43° C. Animals appear anxious, restless, pant continuously, pace, have a tense abdomen, and have bright-red mucous membranes. They usually are vocal, with intense and continuous whimpering. The heart rate and respiratory rate progressively increase. Seizures and apnea may develop. Most dogs die within 3 hours after the development of clinical signs. They usually have dark-brown colored urine.

Clinical Pathology. CK activity is markedly elevated. Hematology values and blood gas concentrations remain unremarkable. Urine is a dark-brown color in most instances of poisoning.

Lesions. Gross pathology is unremarkable with no specific lesions noticed on necropsy. Rigor mortis occurs quickly and is often evident within 10 to 15 minutes.

Diagnostic Testing. No test is available to confirm hops poisoning. The identification of plant parts in stomach contents can confirm exposure.

Treatment. No antidote exists; treatment is supportive and symptomatic. Aggressive decontamination efforts should be carried out before the onset of clinical signs. If emesis is delayed, gastric lavage or enterogastric lavage should be performed. Activated charcoal and a cathartic should be given. IV fluids should be administered to increase urine output and to help prevent myoglobin- or hemoglobin-induced renal failure. Acid-base balance and electrolyte levels should be monitored. Ice packs and cold water baths may be used to help lower body temperature. Steroids and an antibiotic may be helpful. Diazepam or general anesthetics can be used to control the excitement or seizures that accompany poisoning. IV use of dantrolene may be helpful in treating this malignant hyperthermia-like syndrome.

Prognosis. The prognosis is poor to guarded. Most animals die 3 to 12 hours after the development of clinical signs. Animals that survive usually recover within 48 to 72 hours.

Prevention and Control. Animals should not be allowed access to hops plants, commercially available plugs, or discarded hops from home-brewing beer.

REFERENCES

1. Stevens R: The chemistry of hop constituents, *Chem Rev* 67:19, 1967.
2. Westbrooks RG, Preacher JW: *Poisonous plants of Eastern North America,* Columbia, SC, 1986, University of South Carolina Press.
3. Burgess AH: *Hops-botany, cultivation, and utilization,* London, 1964, Leonard Hill.
4. Duncan KL, Hare WR, Buck WB: Malignant hyperthermia-like reaction secondary to ingestion of hops in five dogs, *J Am Vet Med Assoc* 210(1):51, 1997.

HYPOCHAERIS

George Burrows and Ronald J. Tyrl

Sources. Species of *Hypochaeris,* members of the Asteraceae, or sunflower, family, have heads somewhat similar in appearance to those of *Taraxacum,* the common dandelion. *H. radicata* L. (spotted cat's-ear, hairy cat's-ear, rough cat's-ear, flatweed, gosmore) is the only species of toxicologic interest. A native of Eurasia, *H. radicata* is an invader of disturbed sites and fields of the Pacific states mainly west of the Sierra Nevada and Cascade Mountains. It is widely scattered in eastern North America.

Mechanism of Action. This disease of equids is referred to as Australian stringhalt, which is a reversible, outbreak-type of stringhalt with selective degeneration of peripheral nerves.[1] The toxin is unknown, and it is questionable whether *H. radicata* is truly a cause of the disease, although the clinical signs it produces are similar to those of the diseases caused by *Lathyrus* and *Pisum.*[2] Reported from the Pacific Coast states of the United States as well as Australia, the disease develops over a period of 2 to 3 weeks, primarily in the late summer and early fall.[3,4] The distal portions of large myelinated nerves are mainly affected, starting with the pelvic limbs.[5] Eventually, the left recurrent laryngeal nerve is most severely affected. The signs are related to aberrations in the reflex arc from muscle spindles.[6]

Clinical Signs. An abrupt onset occurs of sudden involuntary flexion and delayed extension of the hocks, which is especially noticeable when backing or turning. When severe, the legs strike against the abdomen during flexion. Stumbling with the thoracic limbs results in toe scuffing. Animals may recover spontaneously in a few weeks or not for years.

Lesions. No gross lesions are seen. Microscopically, wallerian degeneration of peripheral nerves such as the sciatic, peroneal, and recurrent laryngeal occurs with subsequent atrophy of fibers of the digital extensors and lateral deep flexors.[7]

Treatment. Although specific reversal of the lesions is not possible, an oral paste of phenytoin (15 mg/kg body weight) daily for 2 weeks or baclofen may provide some benefit.[2,8] Tenotomy of the lateral digital extensor also has been used to provide some benefit.

Prognosis.   The prognosis is guarded; however, the possibility of spontaneous reversal of the disease process exists.

REFERENCES

1. Pemberton DH, Caple IW: Australian stringhalt in horses, *Vet Annual* 20:167, 1980.
2. Mayhew IG: Neurologic patients, IV. I Stringhalt, lathyrism, and shivering, In *Large animal neurology*, Philadelphia, 1989, Lea & Febiger.
3. Galey FD et al: Outbreaks of stringhalt in northern California, *Vet Hum Toxicol* 33:176-177, 1991 (letter).
4. Gay CC et al: *Hypochoeris*-associated stringhalt in North America, *Equine Vet J* 25:456, 1993.
5. Cahill JI et al: Stringhalt in horses: a distal axonopathy, *Neuropathol Appl Neurobiol* 12:459, 1986.
6. Cahill JI, Goulden BE: Stringhalt: current thoughts on aetiology and pathogenesis, *Equine Vet J* 24:161, 1992.
7. Slocombe RF et al: Pathological aspects of Australian stringhalt, *Equine Vet J* 24:174, 1992.
8. Huntington PJ et al: Use of phenytoin to treat horses with Australian stringhalt, *Aust Vet J* 68:221, 1991.

KARWINSKIA

George Burrows and Ronald J. Tyrl

Sources.   A member of the Rhamnaceae, or buckthorn, family, *Karwinskia* is represented in the United States by a single species, *K. humboldtiana* (buckthorn, coyotillo, tanglefoot, tullidora). It is a shrub or small tree, the fruits of which are drupes with two or three stones, each containing a seed. Occurring in arroyos and rocky hillsides, *K. humboldtiana* is found in southwestern Texas and south into Mexico as well as in Baja, California, and adjacent Sonora.

Toxicokinetics.   Consumption of *K. humboldtiana* causes a progressive polyneuropathy with ascending systemic paralysis several days or weeks later.[1] The seeds are the most toxic, but all plant parts pose a risk to animals and humans.[2,3] A single ingestion of seeds or daily ingestion of leaves may result in expression of the disease.

The cause of disease is a series of complex anthracenes referred to as T-496, T-514, T-516, and T-544.[4] Generally called tullidinol, T-544 is a mixture of four isomers.[5] Concentrations of these anthracenes are highest in the seeds. Toxins clear rapidly, but there is probably some residual neuronal binding and damage.

Mechanism of Action.   These toxins interfere with neuronal synthesis and axonal transport of proteins in the long axons, especially of the large motor nerves.[6] Degeneration of the axon begins distally at the myoneural junction and extends retrograde to the proximal portion, resulting in axoplasmal disruption, wallerian degeneration, and myelin degeneration.[7-9] Some axonal regeneration and remyelination may also occur. The liver and lung may be affected, especially with a large dose of the toxins.

Toxicity and Risk Factors.   All animal species are at risk, including cats, rats, chickens, monkeys, cattle, sheep, and goats.[2,3] The fruits with seeds represent the highest risk, but all plant parts are toxic if eaten for a sufficient time.

Clinical Signs.   A rapid onset of hypersensitivity to touch and sounds, tremors, and increased alertness occurs. This leads to a stumbling gait, dragging of the limbs, and finally to loss of motor control, spasmodic limb movements, and flaccid paralysis. Death is due to respiratory arrest. Sensory and autonomic functions are not affected; therefore, eating, drinking, urination, and defecation remain essentially normal.

Lesions.   Gross lesions are not present. Microscopically, the main changes are wallerian degeneration, demyelination, and swelling and degeneration of Schwann cells of the peripheral nerves, especially large motor axons. The Purkinje cells and spinal cord axons may be swollen.

Treatment.   The main emphasis of treatment is to nurse the animal through the paralysis period. Some regeneration may occur, and the animal may recover at least partial function. Daily thiamine HCL may be of some benefit.[10]

Prognosis.   The prognosis is not good, but nerve regeneration and compensation for the loss of function may allow at least partial recovery.

REFERENCES

1. Bermudez MV et al: Experimental intoxication with fruit and purified toxins of buckthorn (*Karwinskia humboldtiana*), *Toxicon* 24:11, 1986.
2. Joiner GN et al: A spontaneous neuropathy of free-ranging Japanese macaques, *Lab Anim Sci* 25:232, 1975.
3. Marsh CD et al: Coyotillo (*Karwinskia humboldtiana*) as a poisonous plant, *USDA Tech Bull* 29:26, 1928.
4. Dreyer DL et al: Toxins causing noninflammatory paralytic neuronopathy. Isolation and structure elucidation, *J Am Chem Soc* 97:4985, 1975.
5. Kim HL, Stipanovic RD: Isolation of karwinol A from coyotillo (*Karwinskia humboldtiana*) fruits. In Garland T, Barr AC, editors: *Toxic plants and other natural toxicants*, New York, 1998, CAB International.
6. Munoz-Martinez EJ et al: Depression of fast axonal transport produced by tullidora, *J Neurobiol* 15:375, 1984.
7. Charlton KM et al: A neuropathy in goats caused by experimental coyotillo (*Karwinskia humboldtiana*) poisoning. II. Lesions in the peripheral nervous system, *Pathol Vet* 7:385, 1970.
8. Charlton KM et al: A neuropathy in goats caused by experimental coyotillo (*Karwinskia humboldtiana*) poisoning. V. Lesions in the central nervous system, *Pathol Vet* 7:435, 1970.
9. Heath JW et al: Buckthorn neuropathy in vitro: evidence for a primary neuronal effect, *J Neuropath Exp Neurol* 41:204, 1982.
10. Weller RO et al: Buckthorn (*Karwinskia humboldtiana*) toxins. In Spencer PS, Schaumburg HH, editors: *Experimental and clinical neurotoxicology*, Baltimore, 1980, Williams & Wilkins.

LIGUSTRUM

George Burrows and Ronald J. Tyrl

Sources.   A genus of shrubs and small trees, *Ligustrum* is a member of the Oleaceae, or olive, family (Table 25-18).

TABLE 25-18 *Ligustrum* Species of Toxicologic Interest

Species Name	Common Name
L. japonicum Thunb.	Japanese privet, wax-leaf privet
L. lucidum Aiton.f.	Glossy privet, tree privet, large-leaf privet
L. ovalifolium Hassk.	California privet
L. sinense Lour.	Chinese privet
L. vulgare L.	Privet, common privet, privet hedge

These species are widely cultivated in North America, often as hedging or screening plants. These ornamentals occasionally escape cultivation and become naturalized in open woodlands, especially in the eastern states. They may also persist at abandoned farm homesites.

Toxicity and Risk Factors. Few reports of intoxications caused by *Ligustrum* and no experimental data to substantiate the risk are in the literature. The toxins have not been identified but pentacyclic terpenoid glycosides such as ligustrins are present, which could at least account for the digestive problems.[1]

Probably all animal species are susceptible, and all plant parts represent some risk, which in most instances is low. Differences in toxicity may exist between the parts of the plant, such as the leaves and berries. New plant growth in the spring may pose a greater risk.

Clinical Signs. The signs cited vary among reports; however, they indicate the potential for digestive disturbance, cardiac effects, and possible neurologic involvement.[2,3]

Generally some degree of digestive disturbance is seen, ranging from cessation of rumination to severe diarrhea. In some cases, diarrhea is a prominent sign, whereas in others there are few distinctive signs but animals nevertheless die.[4,5] Other signs noted include colic, vomiting, ataxia, greenish nasal discharge, and recumbency bordering on paralysis. In at least one instance, the signs were suggestive of a grass tetany–like disease. The effects of extracts of leaves and cases involving berries in humans suggest the possibility of cardiotoxins capable of causing cardiopulmonary arrest.[2,3]

Lesions. Few lesions have been reported other than reddening of the mucosa of the stomach and small intestine in some, but not all, cases.

Treatment. The principal feature of treatment is maintenance of hydration using fluids and electrolytes. Administration of oral activated charcoal may provide some benefit.

Prognosis. Because in most instances the disease was well advanced when treatment was attempted and the animal response was poor, it is difficult to evaluate the prognosis. However, in most instances, prognosis must be considered poor.

REFERENCES

1. Connolly JD, Hill RA: *Dictionary of terpenoids, di- and higher terpenoids,* vol 2, London, 1991, Chapman & Hall.
2. Damirov IA: Chemical and pharmacological study of leaves of the Japanese privet grown in Apsheron, *Sbornik Trudov Azerbaidzhan Med Inst* 8:342, 1960 (Chem Abstracts 56;9376b, 1962).
3. Kozlov VA, Gylyava TN: Poisoning by the fruit of privet hedge, *Sudebno-Meditsinskaia Ekspertiza* 26:56, 1983.
4. Cooper MR, Johnson AW: *Poisonous plants and their effects on animals and man,* London, 1984, Her Majesty's Stationery Office.
5. Kerr LA, Kelch WJ: Fatal privet (*Ligustrum amurease*) toxicosis in Tennessee cows, *Vet Human Toxicol* 41:391, 1999.

LILY

Jeffrey O. Hall

Synonyms. Easter lily (*L. longiflorum*), tiger lily (*L. tigrinum*), Japanese show lily (*L. hybridum*), rubrum lily (*L. rubrum*), numerous *Lilium* hybrids, and day lilies (*Hemerocallis* sp.) have been associated with poisonings. The resultant syndrome from each of these plants has been termed lily poisoning or lily-induced nephrotoxicosis.

Sources. Since the first reported cases of Easter lily toxicosis,[1] it has been found that cats are uniquely sensitive to the nephrotoxic syndrome caused by ingestion of species from both the *Lilium* and *Hemerocallis* genera of plants.[2-6] Because only limited data are available, ingestion of any *Lilium* sp. or *Hemerocallis* sp. plants should be considered potentially lethal to cats.

Species from both the *Lilium* and *Hemerocallis* genera are commonly used ornamental plants. These plants are brought into homes as both potted plants and in numerous types of flower arrangements. This allows housecats easy access for plant ingestion. The plants also are used in flower beds and gardens, which allows access for outdoor cats, but toxicosis from outdoor plant exposure has not been documented.

Toxicokinetics. Because the toxins of these lily species has not been identified, true toxicokinetic data are not available. However, the fairly rapid onset of clinical signs indicates a rapid absorption rate for the toxins. Metabolism, being unknown, may play a role in the species specificity of the toxic syndrome, but tissue effects may be the cause of this difference. As far as elimination, one could surmise that the elimination is via the kidneys and is relatively quick. This could be predicted because 24 hours of fluid diuresis can prevent the lethal effects of the plants. But identification of the toxic agents is required before true kinetic parameters can be measured.

Mechanism of Action. The primary mechanism of action of these lily species is one of nephrotoxicity. Renal tubular epithelial cells are damaged, resulting in sloughing of the tubular cells. This renal insult is severe, with most cases culminating in anuric renal failure.

The mechanism of renal tubular damage is not known. However, the nephrotoxic syndrome requires two components. The first component is a polyuric renal failure that begins at 12 to 24 hours after the plant material is ingested. This results in the second component, which is a severe dehydration. The dehydration is required for development of anuric renal failure, which is associated with the lethality of these plants. Thus, prevention of the dehydration is a critical component in the management of these cases.

Toxicity and Risk Factors.

Leaves and flowers from plants of the *Lilium* and *Hemerocallis* genera are highly toxic to cats. Deaths have been reported from ingestion of as little as two leaves. Thus, the causative agent in the plant material is either at a high concentration or highly toxic. Furthermore, because the toxic principle has not been identified, it cannot be determined whether the toxin varies with maturity of the plant or varies between individual plants.

The lily-induced nephrotoxic syndrome only has been observed in cats, with no age or breed predilection identified. In rats, rabbits, and dogs that ingested plant material from the lilies, the nephrotoxic syndrome did not occur even with very large ingestions.

Interestingly, in all cases followed up by this author, all cats have been exclusively indoor cats. Thus, exposure to outdoor plants in these genera, theoretically, would be of lower risk for poisoning. This may be due to outdoor cats selectively chewing on other available green plants instead of these toxic plants. Or, if outdoor cats are poisoned by these

genera of plants, they may not be found or had necropsies performed to provide suggestive evidence of poisoning.

Clinical Signs.

Clinical signs of lily toxicosis predominantly reflect gastrointestinal and renal effects that follow a fairly consistent time course (Table 25-19); the only syndrome observed in species other than cats was a mild, short-term gastrointestinal upset in dogs.[1-4] In cats, the initial syndrome consists of vomiting, salivation, depression, and anorexia. The anorexia is characterized as a complete refusal of food and water. The depression and anorexia are continuous for the duration of the clinical syndrome. In contrast, the initial vomiting and salivation generally subside in 4 to 6 hours. This leads owners and veterinarians to believe that a cat is recovering from a mild gastrointestinal upset and can result in the delay of appropriate treatment.

In most cases, the clinical syndrome progresses into the more life-threatening phase of the syndrome, an anuric renal failure. Preceding the anuria, cats develop a polyuric renal failure that causes severe dehydration. This polyuria has been observed by 12 hours after ingestion. The resultant dehydration is a required component of the syndrome for a cat to progress into anuric renal failure. Cats with anuric renal failure have a recurrence of vomiting, become weak then recumbent, and in most cases die by 3 to 7 days after ingestion. Death is a result of the renal failure.

Clinical Pathology.

Although not greatly different from other causes of acute renal failure, clinical pathologic changes may assist in the diagnosis of lily poisoning, but the timing of sample collection plays a role in the identification of abnormalities (see Table 25-19). Many cats have a stress leukogram as the only CBC finding. Greater changes are observed with the serum biochemistries, with moderate to severe increases in blood urea nitrogen (BUN), creatinine, phosphorus, and potassium. In the final portion of the syndrome, AST, ALT, and ALP can be increased.

The most important finding that can serve to indicate a lily poisoning is a disproportionate increase in creatinine as compared to BUN. Numerous cases have been investigated in which the creatinine was 15 to 20 mg/dl or more at the time the anuria was identified, with BUN being only 75 to 200 mg/dl. Other cases have had serum creatinine values of greater than 30 mg/dl. This disproportionate increase in creatinine has been used as a marker for questioning owners about lily exposure and has aided in diagnosing the cause of renal failures by verifying plant ingestion.

Urinalysis can provide evidence of renal damage even before serum chemistry changes have occurred. Glucosuria and proteinuria are common findings in isosthenuric urine. Urine sediment generally contains numerous tubular epithelial casts. Early in the syndrome, these casts maintain enough cellular detail that the nuclei of the cells are visible. As the casts begin to degenerate, they become granular casts. It is important to note that crystalluria does not occur with this type of poisoning.

Lesions.

Gross pathology is limited to systemic congestion and renal lesions. Mild to severe pulmonary and hepatic con-

TABLE 25-19 **Onset and Duration of Common Clinical Signs and Clinical Pathologic Changes that Occur with Lily Poisoning in Cats**

Clinical Sign/Parameter	Onset	Duration from Onset
Vomiting	0-3 hr	4-6 hr
Salivation	0-3 hr	4-6 hr
Anorexia	0-3 hr	Throughout syndrome
Depression	0-3 hr	Throughout syndrome
Proteinuria	12-24 hr	Until anuria develops
Urinary casts	12-24 hr	Until anuria develops
Glucosuria	12-24 hr	Until anuria develops
Isosthenuria	12-24 hr	Until anuria develops
Polyuria	12-30 hr	12-24 hr
Dehydration	18-30 hr	Until corrected
Serum chemistry changes	>24 hr	Until corrected
Vomiting reoccurs	30-72 hr	Through remainder of syndrome
Anuria	24-48 hr	Through remainder of syndrome
Weakness	36-72 hr	Through remainder of syndrome
Recumbency	48-72 hr	Through remainder of syndrome
Death	3-7 days	

gestion commonly are identified. Swollen kidneys with abundant perirenal edema are found in almost all cases. In addition, the stomach and small intestinal tract are generally empty.

Pulmonary, hepatic, and renal lesions are identified with histopathologic evaluation. Vascular congestion is common. Mild hepatocellular swelling adjacent to central veins is occasionally observed.

Moderate to severe, diffuse acute renal tubular necrosis is the most prominent lesion. These lesions are often limited to the proximal tubular segments in the milder cases, but can occur distal into the collecting ducts in the more severely affected cases. Granular and hyaline casts are commonly observed in the collecting ducts. In all cases, the basement membrane is found to be intact and mitotic figures are often present. This finding indicates that tubular damage may be reparable if the animal can be kept alive and maintained long enough.

Diagnostic Testing. The toxic principles of these plants have not been identified, making analytical diagnosis impossible. Verification that one of the toxic lilies has been ingested, along with compatible clinical signs and clinical pathologic changes, is the only means of diagnosis. When postmortem lesions suggest lily poisoning, verification of plant exposure or consumption and appropriate clinical signs are required to arrive at a tentative diagnosis of lily poisoning.

Treatment. Early intervention with gastrointestinal decontamination and fluid therapy is necessary for a favorable prognosis. Commonly, cats will have vomited before clinical presentation, but further gastrointestinal decontamination should be performed to minimize further systemic exposure to the plant toxins. Induction of vomiting to remove plant material from the stomach is indicated in cats that have not vomited on their own. Activated charcoal with a cathartic should be given to assist in the gastrointestinal decontamination. For cats with protracted vomiting, it may be necessary to administer an antiemetic to prevent vomition and aspiration of the activated charcoal.

The most critical treatment is the initiation of fluid therapy before the development of anuria. Because dehydration is a critical component in the development of the anuric renal failure, initiation of fluid therapy is essential in preventing lethal effects. Fluid diuresis with normal saline at 2 to 3 times maintenance that was initiated before 24 hours after ingestion (or before development of anuria) has prevented development of the anuric renal failure in all cases for which the author is aware. This rate of fluid administration should be maintained for 24 hours.

After the development of anuric renal failure, peritoneal dialysis or hemodialysis are the only possible means of treatment. The use of drugs that are commonly employed to initiate or promote urine production, such as dopamine, furosemide, hypertonic dextrose, thiazides, and mannitol, have been unsuccessful in lily-poisoned cats. The author is aware of two cats in which peritoneal dialysis for 10 to 14 days resulted in the return of renal function. Appropriate protocols and dialysate solutions must be used, because inappropriate dialysis can be as lethal as the plant poisoning itself.

Prognosis. Cats that have ingested one of the toxic lilies and received no treatment warrant a grave prognosis. Cats treated with the protocol outlined herein before the onset of anuric renal failure have a good prognosis. Cats that have progressed into the anuric phase of the syndrome warrant a poor prognosis unless dialysis is initiated. Even with the initiation of peritoneal dialysis or hemodialysis, only a fair prognosis could be justified.

Prevention and Control. The best preventive measure for this type of poisoning is total avoidance of exposure. Because these genera of plants come in various shapes, sizes, and colors, owners should inquire specifically about *Lilium* and *Hemerocallis* genera when purchasing floral decorations to which cats may be exposed.

REFERENCES

1. Hall JO: Are Easter lilies toxic to cats? *NAPINet Rep* 3(2):1, 1990.
2. National Animal Poison Control Center (NAPCC) Computerized Case Database: University of Illinois College of Veterinary Medicine, 1987 to 1992.
3. Gathers TM: Acute renal failure in a cat. Was it tiger lily? *NAPINet Rep* 3(2):2, 1991.
4. Hall JO: Nephrotoxicity of Easter lily *(Lilium longiflorum)* when ingested by the cat, Proceedings of the Annual Meeting of the American College of Vet Internal Med, May 28-31, 1992, San Diego, Calif (abstract).
5. Mullaney TP et al: Easter lily associated nephrotoxicity in cats, North Central Conference of Veterinary Laboratory Diagnosticians, July 1993, Madison, Wis (abstract).
6. Carson TL et al: Acute nephrotoxicosis in cats following ingestion of lily *(Lilium* sp.), *Proc Annu Meet Am Assoc Vet Lab Diagn* 37:43, 1991 (abstract).

MACADAMIA NUTS

Konnie H. Plumlee

Sources. *Macadamia integrifolia* and *Macadamia tetraphylla* trees produce these nuts, which were introduced into Hawaii in the late 1800s.[1] However, toxicosis can occur anywhere that the nuts are imported.

Mechanism of Action. The toxin and mechanism of action are unknown.

Toxicity and Risk Factors. Dogs have been experimentally poisoned with 20 g of nuts per kilogram body weight.[1] The actual toxic dose has not been determined; however, clinical signs have been reported in dogs that ate an estimated 2.4 g of nuts per kilogram body weight.[1] The disease has occurred in many different dog breeds, ranging in size from Chihuahuas to Labrador retrievers.[1] Toxicosis has not been reported in other species of animals.

Clinical Signs. The onset of clinical signs is less than 12 hours, and the duration of clinical signs is typically less than 24 hours, with all dogs appearing to recover completely by 48 hours.[1] Weakness, especially of the hindlimbs, is the most common sign. Other signs that are frequently observed include depression, vomiting, ataxia, and tremors (especially of the hindlimbs). Hyperthermia, abdominal pain, lameness, pallor, recumbency, and stiffness have been reported occasionally. Sequelae and deaths have not been reported.[1]

Clinical Pathology. Serum triglycerides increase mildly, peak at 3 to 8 hours after ingestion, and return to normal by 8 to 12 hours after ingestion. Serum lipase peaks at 24 hours, but returns to normal by 48 hours after ingestion. Cholesterol and serum amylase are not affected. Elevations in alkaline phosphatase and white blood cells have been reported.[1] However, at this time, none of these changes can be directly attributed to the mechanism of the disease.

Lesions. Deaths have not been reported in clinical cases, and necropsies have not been performed following experimentally induced toxicosis. Therefore, lesions have not been described.

Treatment. Only supportive care is required until clinical signs resolve. Dogs should be kept in an enclosed environment until they are able to walk normally, so that they do not fall or injure themselves.

Prognosis. The prognosis is excellent. Dogs usually recover completely within 48 hours.

REFERENCES

1. Hansen SR et al: Weakness, tremors, and depression associated with macadamia nuts in dogs, *Vet Human Toxicol* 42:18, 2000.

MISTLETOE

George Burrows and Ronald J. Tyrl

Sources. A member of the Viscaceae, or Christmas-mistletoe, family, *Phoradendron* is a genus of evergreen, semiparasitic, woody epiphytes (Table 25-20). Capable of photosynthesis, members of the genus occur on a variety of tree hosts that provide water and inorganic nutrients via haustoria, which penetrate the host tree's vascular system.

Examples of tree species serving as hosts include junipers for *P. juniperum;* leguminous shrubs of the Sonoran deserts for *P. californicum;* deciduous trees such as oaks, willows, and poplars for *P. tomentosum;* and a variety of trees of the eastern deciduous forests for *P. leucarpum.* The last species

TABLE 25-20 *Phoradendron* **Species of Toxicologic Interest**

Species Name	Common Name
P. californicum Nutt.	Acacia or desert mistletoe
P. juniperum A.Gray	Juniper or cedar mistletoe
P. leucarpum (Raf.) Reveal & M.C.Johnst.	Eastern or Christmas mistletoe
P. tomentosum (DC.) Engelm. ex A.Gray	American or hairy mistletoe
P. villosum (Nutt.) Nutt.	Oak mistletoe

is the commonly encountered mistletoe of the eastern half of North America and includes *P. flavescens* and *P. serotinum,* taxa formerly recognized as distinct species.

Toxicity and Risk Factors. The potential for species of *Phoradendron* to cause toxic effects is still uncertain. Although these taxa have had a reputation for oxytocic activity, digestive problems, and causing collapse, there are few actual reports of toxicity.[1] Attempts to experimentally reproduce intoxications have been negative.[2] In a few instances, ingestions of leaves or berries by humans have resulted in digestive disturbance, hypotension, drowsiness, and collapse, but most exposures have not produced untoward signs.[3,4] This may be due in part to variations in mistletoe toxicity when growing on different host plants.[5]

Several potential toxicants are present in *Phoradendron,* including glycoprotein lectins that have low potency for inhibition of protein synthesis; small basic proteins called phoratoxins that decrease the rate and force of cardiac contraction and cause hypotension; and phenethylamino compounds that have possible hypertensive activity.[6-9] Despite the presence of these toxic components, the risk of intoxications from eating leaves or berries is low. If adverse effects occur, they most likely will be in the digestive tract. Animal species truly at risk are not known.

Clinical Signs. Vomiting and diarrhea are the most likely signs to be encountered, although very rarely hypotension and weakness may be present.

Treatment. A conservative approach to ingestion and possible intoxication would include oral activated charcoal as well as fluids and electrolytes. If weakness is prominent, sympathomimetics for control of hypotension may be indicated.

Prognosis. Most ingestions do not result in adverse effects.

REFERENCES

1. Crawford AC: The pressor action of an American mistletoe, *J Am Med Assoc* 57:865, 1911.
2. Cary CA et al: Poisonous plants of Alabama, *Alabama Polytechnic Institute Extension Service Circular* 71:10, 1924.
3. Krenzelok EP et al: American mistletoe exposures, *Am J Emerg Med* 15:516, 1997.
4. Moore HW: Mistletoe poisoning, *J South Carolina Med Assoc* 59:269, 1963.
5. Chesnut VK: Plants used by the Indians of Mendicino County, California. *USDA, Div Botany, Contributions U.S. National Herbarium* 7:295, 1902.
6. Endo Y et al: The mechanism of action of the cytotoxic lectin from *Phoradendron californicum,* the RNA *N*-glycosidase activity of the protein, *FEBS Lett* 248:115, 1989.
7. Graziano MN et al: Isolation of tyramine from five species of Loranthaceae, *Lloydia* 30:242, 1967.
8. Hanzlik PJ, French WO: The pharmacology of *Phoradendron flavescens* (American mistletoe), *J Pharmacol Exp Ther* 23:269, 1924.
9. Rosell S, Samuelsson G: Effect of mistletoe viscotoxin and phoratoxin on blood circulation, *Toxicon* 4:107, 1966.

PIGWEED

Steven S. Nicholson

Synonyms. Redroot pigweed, pigweed, and careless weed are common names for some *Amaranthus* spp.

Sources. *Amaranthus retroflexus* is an annual, herbaceous weed. It grows 2 to 3 feet tall and the lower stems are red or red-streaked with the color continuing down the taproot. It is widely distributed in cultivated soils, gardens, cattle lots, and waste areas.

Toxicity and Risk Factors. *Amaranthus* spp. are potential nitrate accumulators and may contain some soluble oxalates. Ruminants are at risk of nitrate poisoning if large amounts of immature pigweed stems high in nitrates are consumed.

Redroot pigweed also contains an unknown toxicant that causes renal tubular nephrosis. Toxic nephropathy, without oxalate crystals, has been reported in cattle, pigs, sheep, goats, and, rarely, in horses.[1] The plants are often browsed lightly without harm, and poisoning is rare. The risk of toxic tubular nephrosis seems to be associated with ingestion of large amounts of the green plant by animals that are not accustomed to eating it. This happens after introducing a herd or group of animals to a pasture or field where the plant is abundant, but desirable forage is not. Swine have been poisoned when fed redroot pigweed and by grazing it.

Clinical Signs. In a typical incident, cattle or swine become recumbent within 5 to 10 days after ingesting large amounts of pigweed. Depression, weakness, trembling, and incoordination may be noted initially. Signs may suggest hypocalcemia in cows, and some animals respond briefly to IV calcium. Two 300-kg steer calves had fluid-distended abdomens and extensive ventral subcutaneous edema suggesting urolithiasis.[2] Duration of illness among affected cattle ranged from 1 to 14 days in one report.[2] New cases may continue to develop for 5 to 10 days after removal from the source.

Clinical Pathology. Hypocalcemia and hyperphosphatemia with elevated CK, urea nitrogen, and creatinine are reported.

Lesions. Ascites and perirenal edema are common lesions in cattle and pigs at necropsy. The kidneys may be swollen and pale. Microscopic lesions are those of toxic nephrosis and include widespread necrosis of proximal and distal tubules in cattle and pigs. Coagulative necrosis of the proximal and distal straight tubules is also reported in cattle.[2] Oxalate crystals are seldom seen.

Diagnosis. Characteristic gross and microscopic lesions support the diagnosis. Extensively grazed stands of pigweed should be recognizable in the fields, lots, or pastures where the animals were confined in the previous 2 to 3 weeks. Strands of white fibrous plant material from mature pigweed stalks may be found in rumen contents.

Treatment. Toxic nephrosis in cattle and pigs has already occurred by the time clinical signs become apparent. Treatment with IV calcium and magnesium solutions may correct the serum electrolyte values, but cattle may remain in sternal recumbency or respond briefly.[3]

Prognosis. Prognosis is poor in most cases.

Prevention and Control. Preventing exposure and possible ingestion of large amounts of the plant, especially by cattle or pigs unaccustomed to eating it, is recommended. Control of pigweed in pastures and holding pens with herbicides may be practical. However, certain hormone-type herbicides (such as 2,4-D) may make pigweed more attractive to cattle.

REFERENCES

1. Torres MB et al: Redroot pigweed *(Amaranthus retroflexus)* poisoning of cattle in southern Brazil, *Vet Human Toxicol* 39:94, 1997.
2. Casteel SW et al: *Amaranthus retroflexus* (redroot pigweed) poisoning in cattle, *J Am Vet Med Assoc* 204:1068, 1994.
3. Kerr LA, Kelch WJ: Pigweed *(Amaranthus retroflexus)* toxicosis in cattle, *Vet Human Toxicol* 40:216, 1998.

RED MAPLE

Valentina Merola and Petra A. Volmer

Sources. *Acer rubrum*, commonly called red, Carolina, or swamp maple, is a member of the Aceraceae family. Red maples are found throughout the eastern United States from Canada to Florida, and as far west as Texas.[1] The trees are frequently planted as ornamentals because of their vibrant fall foliage. Red maples are becoming more common as land use and forest management has changed. Maples are thriving in the altered environments and crowding out rival species.

Mechanism of Action. Consumption of dried red maple leaves in horses causes hemolytic anemia with methemoglobinemia and Heinz body formation.[2] Although the toxic principle is unknown, based on the clinical signs it is probably an oxidant. Oxidizing agents cause formation of hydrogen peroxide in red blood cells, leading to damage when cellular peroxide detoxification methods are overwhelmed. Oxidizing agents, and likewise the toxin in red maple, cause both intravascular and extravascular hemolysis. Intravascular hemolysis occurs when the membrane permeability of the red blood cell is altered, the osmotic gradient changes, and the cell lyses. Extravascular hemolysis takes place when oxidized hemoglobin precipitates inside the cell resulting in Heinz body formation. Heinz bodies attach to and damage the membrane, causing the abnormal cell to be destroyed by the spleen.[3] Both processes result in severe, progressive anemia in the patient. Hemoglobin from the ruptured cells accumulates intravascularly and is filtered in the kidneys. Hemoglobin can precipitate in the tubules and lead to renal failure.

Toxicity and Risk Factors. Red maple toxicosis occurs in horses and other equids after the ingestion of wilted or dried leaves, and the disease is commonly manifested in late summer and fall. Exposure often occurs when a storm blows a branch of red maple into an animal enclosure.

Horses, ponies, and Grevy's zebras[4] are the only known animals to be susceptible to red maple. Equids are at risk because their diet and grazing habits bring them into contact with the tree, and because they have a decreased capacity for methemoglobin reduction.[5] It is important to avoid inadvertently including red maple leaves when producing hay for horses. As little as 1.5 g/kg of dried red maple leaves has been shown to cause fatal illness in a pony.[2]

Clinical Signs. Rarely, peracute death from severe methemoglobinemia and tissue anoxia can be the only sign.[2] It is more common for the nonspecific signs such as depression and anorexia to appear on the first day of illness. Other signs that may develop in the next 1 to 2 days as the disease progresses include icterus, hemoglobinuria, and brown discoloration of mucous membranes and blood.[3] The resulting lack of oxygen can cause tachypnea, dyspnea, tachycardia, cyanosis, and death. Pregnant mares may abort before showing any signs.[6]

Clinical Pathology. Anemia is the principal finding when hematology is performed. Heinz bodies, spherocytosis, and anisocytosis may also be seen on microscopic examination of the blood. The presence of eccentrocytes has also been reported.[7] The leukogram is often normal; however, an inflammatory or a stress leukogram may be present. Urine is usually discolored red or brown, and analysis may show a large number of red blood cells and possibly the presence of protein. The chemistry panel often shows changes resulting from dehydration and renal damage such as an increase in total protein and albumin as well as BUN and creatinine. Hyperbilirubinemia secondary to the hemolysis is almost always present unless it is extremely early in the disease course. Liver enzymes such as AST and CPK may be elevated. A clotting panel is usually normal.[3,5,8]

Lesions. On gross examination, splenomegaly, renal edema, and icterus are often found. Petechiae and ecchymoses may be present on serosal organ surfaces, and some cases also have lung congestion. Microscopic findings in the kidney include diffuse tubular nephrosis and hemoglobin casts. The spleen usually has foci of erythyrophagocytosis and hemosiderin accumulation.[3,9,10]

Diagnostic Testing. No specific tests are available to diagnose red maple toxicosis so it is important to rule out other causes of hemolytic anemia. Immune-mediated disease, as well as infectious agents such as equine infectious anemia, piroplasmosis, or ehrlichiosis must be considered. Other toxic agents should also be investigated, primarily any possibility of exposure to *Allium* spp. (onion, garlic, or chives), nitrates or nitrites, naphthalenes, or *Brassica* spp. (cabbages, turnips, kale, or broccoli). Diagnosis is usually based on clinical signs and a history of exposure to red maple leaves without exposure to other oxidizing agents.

Treatment. Treatment, as for many toxins, is symptomatic and supportive. Activated charcoal may be of use if given soon after ingestion. The packed cell volume and renal function must be monitored. IV fluids are extremely important to prevent dehydration and support renal function. Blood transfusion may be necessary, and oxygen by nasal insufflation should also be considered.[8]

Nonsteroidal antiinflammatory drugs could also be considered for alleviating discomfort; however, these agents can compromise renal function. A better choice for pain relief is pentazocine (0.6mg/kg IV) and butorphanol (0.05 mg/kg IV).[8] Corticosteroids could be of use to decrease phagocytosis of red blood cells, although laminitis could result.[5]

Ascorbic acid has been used successfully in two horses to reduce methemoglobin to hemoglobin. Ascorbic acid is given at 30 to 50 mg/kg twice daily in the IV fluids; however, it does take two doses to reach adequate plasma levels.[5] Methylene blue should be used with extreme caution, if at all, in these patients; it can increase the formation of Heinz bodies and further exacerbate the problem.[8]

A new treatment to consider is Oxyglobin (purified bovine hemoglobin). Recently a miniature horse and a pony were successfully treated in separate incidents of red maple toxicosis at Tufts University with Oxyglobin and blood transfusions. Oxyglobin is an oxygen-carrying fluid that could support the animal until recovery is made, or it could be used during transit until a blood transfusion can be provided.[11]

Prognosis. Even with aggressive treatment, the prognosis for these patients is guarded.

Prevention and Control. Red maples should not be planted around any type of equine housing or pastures. Red maples must not be incorporated into bales of hay meant for equine consumption. If storms occur, pastures should be examined for debris from maple trees, which should be removed immediately.

REFERENCES

1. Burrows GE, Tyrl RJ: Toxic plants of North America, Ames, Iowa, 2001, Iowa State University Press.
2. Divers TJ et al: Hemolytic anemia in horses after the ingestion of red maple leaves, *J Am Vet Med Assoc* 180:300, 1982.
3. George LW et al: Heinz body anemia and methemoglobinemia in ponies given red maple leaves, *Vet Pathol* 19:521, 1982.
4. Weber M, Miller RE: Presumptive red maple (*Acer rubrum*) toxicosis in Grevy's zebra (*Equus grevyi*), *J Zoo Wildlife Med* 28:105, 1997.
5. McConnico RS, Brownie CF: The use of ascorbic acid in the treatment of 2 cases of red maple (*Acer rubrum*) poisoned horses, *Cornell Vet* 82:293, 1992.
6. Stair EL et al: Suspected red maple (*Acer rubrum*) toxicosis with abortion in two Percheron mares, *Vet Hum Toxicol* 35:229, 1993.
7. Reagan WJ et al: Eccentrocytosis in equine red maple leaf toxicosis, *Vet Clin Pathol* 23(4):123, 1994.
8. Semrad SD: Acute hemolytic anemia from ingestion of red maple leaves, *Compend Contin Educ* 15:261, 1993.
9. Plumlee KH: Red maple toxicity in a horse, *Vet Hum Toxicol* 33:66-67, 1991.
10. Long PH, Payne JW: Red maple-associated pulmonary thrombosis in a horse, *J Am Vet Med Assoc* 184:977, 1984.
11. Paradis MR: Tufts University: Personal communication, 2001.

SENNA

Steven S. Nicholson

Synonyms. This genus of plants was formerly called *Cassia* spp.[1] The more toxic species are *Senna occidentalis* (coffee senna), *S. obtusifolia* (sicklepod), *S. roemeriana* (twin-leaf senna), and *S. lindheimeriana.*

Sources. *Senna occidentalis* and *S. obtusifolia* are found throughout the southern and eastern parts of the United States (Color Plates 51 and 52). Sicklepod is less toxic than coffee senna but is more widespread. These weeds are found in crop fields, corrals, cattle holding pens, and pastures. Coffee senna is often found in sandy soils. *S. lindheimeriana* and *S. roemeriana* are located in Texas and New Mexico.

Mechanism of Action. The myotoxic principle remains to be identified.[2] Skeletal myopathy from coffee senna has been reported in cattle, horses, and chickens.[2] Cardiomyopathy has been reported in cattle, chickens, goats, horses, and rabbits.[2] Pigs develop myopathy of diaphragm muscles.[1]

Toxicity and Risk Factors. Naturally occurring *Senna* spp. toxicosis is primarily a problem in cattle. Sicklepod is less toxic than coffee senna, may be minimally toxic when dry, and the seeds have little toxicity. Corn silage containing more than an estimated 10% to 15% contamination with sicklepod has produced myopathy in dairy cattle.

All parts of coffee senna, especially the seeds, are toxic. Seed contamination of harvested grains is the most common route of toxicosis.[2] The consumption of seeds at 1% of body weight kills cows when consumed daily for 2 to 5 consecutive days.[2] Experimental administration of dried seeds to calves proved fatal at a total dose of 0.5% body weight, whether as a single daily dose or divided into smaller, multiple doses. Coffee senna appears to be more attractive to cattle after a killing frost. Cattle are sometimes attracted to the plant after it is damaged by clipping or trampling. The plants are toxic whether green, dried, or ensiled in corn silage.

Clinical Signs. Diarrhea usually occurs and then subsides before the onset of muscular weakness.[2] Constipation has also been reported.[2] The most prominent sign of senna myopathy is decreased muscle tone, weakness, and a slow gait that progresses to sternal recumbency within a few days.[3] Animals remain bright-eyed and alert and continue to eat and drink. The body temperature remains normal.[3] Myoglobinuria causes the urine to be coffee colored and is observed in many affected cattle. Increased respiration, hyperpnea, and increased heart rate precede death, which occurs one to several days later.

Clinical Pathology. Serum CK and aspartate aminotransferase (AST) are markedly elevated when the animal becomes recumbent. CK and AST levels decline to moderately elevated levels within 3 or 4 days.

Lesions. Pale musculature may be readily evident, especially in muscles of the hip, thigh, and shoulder regions. The lesions are similar to those of white muscle disease. Numerous pale foci 1 to 2 mm in diameter are regularly spaced along individual muscle fibers. Close observation of affected muscles containing large numbers of these fibers reveals a pale, stippled, or transversely striated appearance. Adjacent muscles may appear to be normal. Pale streaks may occur in cardiac muscle of some animals, especially the left ventricle. Subepicardial hemorrhages may be present. Lungs may be diffusely dark red and congested. Up to 500 ml of yellow, serous fluid may be in the pleural cavity. The abomasum may have a reddened mucosa. Coffee-colored urine may be seen, but the kidneys are not stained dark. Lesions may be less obvious at necropsy of an animal that was down for several days or weeks before death.

Microscopic lesions include sarcoplasmic degeneration and rupture of myofibrils of skeletal muscle. Swelling of mitochondria and disorganization and fragmentation of cristae occur in striated muscle of cattle. Less severe and less extensive lesions are found in cardiac muscle. Electron microscopy has revealed mitochondrial damage in cardiac muscle.

Treatment. Prolonged supportive care in the form of shade, water, and feed may allow an occasional animal to survive. Original studies and field experience indicate that vitamin E–selenium injection is not beneficial and seems to shorten survival time.[2]

Prognosis. The prognosis is poor in cattle that become recumbent. Additional cases may continue to appear for 4 or 5 days after removal from the source of plants.

Prevention and Control. Elimination of *Senna* spp. from hayfields, grazing areas, and holding pens is strongly recommended. Cows and calves may eat shredded leaves and seedpods of coffee senna if it is mowed while cattle are present.

REFERENCES

1. Flory W et al: The toxicologic investigation of a feed grain contaminated with seeds of the plant species *Cassia, J Vet Diagn Invest* 4:65, 1992.
2. Barth AT et al: Coffee senna *(Senna occidentalis)* poisoning in cattle in Brazil, *Vet Human Toxicol* 36:541, 1994.
3. Faz EM et al: Cassia occidentalis toxicosis in heifers, *Vet Human Toxicol* 40:307, 1998.

STIPA

George Burrows and Ronald J. Tyrl

Sources. A genus of cool season grasses, *Stipa* is represented in North America by several dozen species. Species primarily found in western North America that can sometimes dominate the range include *S. eminens* Cav. (southwestern needlegrass), *S. lobata* Swallen (littleawn needlegrass), and *S. viridula* Trin. (green needlegrass). Some species are valuable forage grasses when young. However, as the common name needlegrass implies, the sharp bases of the mature florets or awns can cause mechanical injury around the mouth of grazing livestock.

S. robusta (sleepy grass) and *S. viridula* are known to have a narcotic effect on livestock. This narcotic effect has been associated mainly with horses grazing *S. robusta* in the Sacramento and Sierra Blanca Mountains of New Mexico and *S. viridula* in the mountains of northern Mexico.[1]

Mechanism of Action. These grasses have a narcotic effect on livestock and cause animals to be docile for up to several days. The effect is to render otherwise intractable animals temporarily docile. The cause of the neurologic effects appears to be toxins produced by *Neotyphodium chisosum* (formerly known as *Acremonium chisosum*), an endophytic fungus of the family Clavicepitaceae.[2] These toxins are ergot alkaloids, especially the sedative lysergic and isolysergic acids.[3]

Toxicity and Risk Factors. Horses are mainly at risk because of the relatively low dosage required and the prolonged duration of effect; however, cattle and, to a lesser extent, sheep are also at risk. A dosage of 1% body weight in horses and cattle and 4% body weight in sheep results in a narcosis for several days in horses and of 1 day in cattle and sheep.[4] Because of the limited range of distribution of these grasses, the disease is not a significant problem.

Clinical Signs. Several hours after ingestion, animals appear to slow in their movements and to drag their feet when walking. Horses become difficult to arouse and stand with their heads held low. When forced to move, they may stagger and sweat excessively. These signs may last several days. The signs are similar but of shorter duration in cattle and those in sheep are milder.

Treatment. This is a self-limiting disease; the clinical signs subside without treatment.

Prevention and Control. The disease may be prevented by feeding small amounts of the forage before animals are allowed to graze areas with substantial amounts of *Stipa*. These grasses are of low palatability and are typically eaten only by animals that have not previously been exposed to them.

REFERENCES

1. Marsh CD, Clawson AB: Sleepy grass *(Stipa vaseyi)* as a stock-poisoning plant, *USDA Tech Bull* 114:19, 1929.
2. White JF, Halisky PM: Association of systemic fungal endophytes with stock-poisoning grasses. In James LF, Keeler RF, Bailey EM Jr, Cheeke PR, Hegarty MP, editors: *Poisonous plants, proceedings of the Third International Symposium,* Ames, Iowa, 1992, Iowa State University Press.
3. Petroski RJ et al: Alkaloids of *Stipa robusta* (sleepygrass) infected with an *Acremonium* endophyte, *Na Toxins* 1:84, 1992.
4. Smalley HE, Crookshank HR: Toxicity studies on sleepy grass, *Stipa robusta* (Vasey) Scribn, *Southwestern Vet* 29:35, 1976.

TABLE 25-21 ***Vicia* Species that Have Been Associated with Intoxication Problems**

Species Name	Common Name
V. angustifolia L.	Narrow-leaved vetch
V. faba L.	Broad bean, fava bean
V. sativa L.	Common or spring vetch
V. villosa Roth	Hairy vetch

VETCH

George Burrows and Ronald J. Tyrl

Sources. *Vicia* is a large genus of the subfamily Papilionoideae of the Fabaceae, or pea, family (Table 25-21). Of considerable economic value, species of the genus are cultivated for a variety of purposes. Except for *V. faba,* which is occasionally grown in vegetable gardens, they are widely cultivated alone or with small grains such as rye or wheat. Characterized by their viny growth and 1-pinnately compound leaves, which terminate in tendrils, species of *Vicia* are similar in appearance to members of *Lathyrus* or the pea genus (Color Plates 53 and 54).

Mechanism of Action. The most important of the diseases caused by vetch is granulomatous dermatopathy accompanied by visceral granulomatous lesions, which is associated with ingestion of the foliage of *Vicia villosa* and possibly other species.[1,2] The specific cause of the dermatitis and visceral granulomatous disease is unknown, but type IV hypersensitivity has been suggested.[2]

Growth depression in poultry and neurologic disease in cattle and other animals are related to ingestion of the seeds of various species of *Vicia.*[1,3] The toxins causing the growth depression are apparently heat labile. The cause of the neurologic effects is not known, but toxins such as β-cyanoalanine and small amounts of cyanogenic glycosides are present.[4,5] The neurologic effects in cattle produce rabies-like signs.[1]

Toxicity and Risk Factors. Of sporadic occurrence, mainly in cattle with black skin such as Angus or Holstein, the granulomatous dermatopathy follows consumption of large amounts of vigorously growing plants for 3 to 4 weeks. It has also been reported in horses on *Vicia villosa* pasture, but the numbers of animals affected have not been large enough to determine the role of color.[6,7] Morbidity is usually low, approximately 10%, but rarely may be as high as 50%. Case fatality rates are 50% or more.

Clinical Signs. Several weeks after grazing vetch, a rapidly progressive dermatitis becomes apparent with papular swellings, plaques, thickening, exudation, crusting, and pruritus of the skin. The lesions, which are independent of skin pigmentation, begin on the neck, tailhead, escutcheon, and udder and then progress to other areas. Systemic effects such as weight loss, anorexia, and fever may also be noted. Animals may appear to recover, with an increase in appetite after a week or so, but then may relapse and die in a few days.

Lesions. Grossly, in addition to the obvious skin lesions, a yellowish-gray infiltrate may be noted in the dermis, adrenals, myocardium, renal cortex, and possibly other organs such as liver. Microscopically, the infiltrate consists of macrophages, lymphocytes, plasma cells, eosinophils, and multinucleated giant cells.

Treatment. No specific treatment is successful.

Prognosis. The prognosis for affected animals is unfavorable because the case fatality rate is typically high. However, unaffected herdmates removed from the pasture are not likely to develop signs.

Prevention and Control. It is not currently possible to predict the likelihood of disease occurring. Pastures containing *V. villosa* may be grazed for many years without evidence of the disease. Care should be taken, however, if cattle breeds are changed in favor of those with black skin.

REFERENCES

1. Panciera RJ: Hairy vetch *(Vicia villosa* Roth) poisoning in cattle. In Keeler RF, Van Kampen KR, James LF, editors: *Effects of poisonous plants on livestock,* New York, 1978, Academic Press.
2. Panciera RJ et al: Hairy vetch *(Vicia villosa* Roth) poisoning in cattle: update and experimental induction of disease, *J Vet Diagn Invest* 4:318, 1992.
3. Harper JA, Ascott GH: Toxicity of common and hairy vetch seed for poults and chicks, *Poultry Sci* 41:1968, 1962.
4. Ressler C: Isolation and identification from common vetch of the neurotoxin beta-cyano-*L*-alanine, a possible factor in neurolathyrism, *J Biological Chem* 237:733, 1962.
5. Ruby ES et al: Prussic acid poisoning in common vetch *(Vicia sativa)* seed, *Proc Arkansas Acad Sci* 7:18, 1955.
6. Anderson CA, Divers TJ: Systemic granulomatous inflammation in a horse grazing hairy vetch, *J Am Vet Med Assoc* 183:569, 1993.
7. Woods LW et al: Systemic granulomatous disease in a horse grazing pasture containing vetch *(Vicia* sp.), *J Vet Diagn Invest* 4:356, 1992.

YELLOW STARTHISTLE AND RUSSIAN KNAPWEED

Patricia A. Talcott

Synonyms. The disease in horses (presumably mules and donkeys as well) has been termed equine nigropallidal encephalomalacia (ENE), or chewing disease.

Sources. Yellow starthistle (other less frequently used common names include St. Barnaby's thistle, Golden thistle, cotton-tip thistle) was accidentally introduced into the United States from the Mediterranean area of Europe in the late 1870s. Because the plant has no natural enemies and because of its nature as an aggressive competitor, the weed has taken over thousands of acres throughout California, Idaho, Oregon, Colorado, and Washington. Yellow starthistle is an annual that reproduces entirely by seed production, but occasionally acts as a biennial. The seedling plant appears in early spring, with deeply indented leaf margins and pointed tips resembling dandelion leaves. The adult plant is 2 to 4 feet tall, has rigid branching, and stems covered by fine cottony hairs (Color Plate 55). The basal leaves are deeply lobed, whereas the upper leaves are narrow, linear, sharply pointed, and intact. The flowers are bright yellow, located at the ends of the branches, with bracts armed with rigid $1/4$- to 1-inch-long thorns (Color Plate 56). This plant produces a large number of seeds (>150,000), and a small percentage may remain dormant in the environment for many years. The first case of yellow starthistle–induced nigropallidal encephalomalacia reported in the literature was in northern California in 1954.[1]

Russian knapweed was also introduced into the United States from the Mediterranean area in the 1890s, likely a contaminant of alfalfa seed. It is a deep-rooted perennial that has become well established in many areas in the western United States. Young growing plants have finely toothed leaves that are covered with fine, soft hair. The adult plant is erect, 1 to 3 feet tall (Color Plate 57). The lower leaves are deeply lobed, 2 to 4 inches long, and the upper leaves are smaller, narrow, and entire. The ray flowers are pink to lavender, and the involucral bracts are egg-shaped with papery margins.

Mechanism of Action. The toxin or toxins responsible for ENE have not been *definitively* identified. Various researchers have suggested that sesquiterpene lactones,[2,3] aspartic acid and glutamic acid,[4] and DDMP (2,3-dihydro-3,5-dihydroxy-6-methy-4[H]-pyran-4-one)[5] may be responsible for causing the clinical disease. Experimental work with DDMP using equine brain homogenates suggests that the putative toxin exerts its toxic effect through interaction with the dopamine transporter, ultimately leading to selective death of dopaminergic neurons, particularly in the substantia nigra and globus pallidus.[5]

Toxicity and Risk Factors. Experimental studies with the immature plants have reproduced the disease in horses. Although not documented in the literature, it is reasonable to assume that donkeys and mules are susceptible to developing this disease as well. Numerous unsuccessful attempts have been made to reproduce this disease in other species. No sex or breed predilection is apparent based on clinical case reports. Young animals, as well as miniature ponies, appear to be at greater risk of developing the disease. Indiscriminate foraging habits, smaller body mass, and addiction to the plant material are factors that may be responsible for this phenomenon.

Large dietary intakes for long periods of time (weeks to months) are required to produce the disease. Oral daily intakes of between 1.8 and 2.6 kg of plant material (either yellow starthistle or Russian knapweed) per 100 kg body weight leads to the production of clinical disease in horses in less than 81 days (average 3 to 11 weeks).[1,6,7] The amount of weed eaten as percent of body weight was calculated as being between 59% to 200%. The disease has been reproduced experimentally in horses by feeding freshly cut, immature plants (stems, leaves, flowers), as well as by feeding air-dried and sun-cured hay.[7]

Clinical Signs. The disease is characterized clinically by signs produced secondary to damage to specific portions of the brain; that is, affected animals lack the specific ability to move food and water to the back of the oropharynx. Despite the exposure period being long in duration, the onset of clinical signs is abrupt. Owners often report that a horse, which was apparently normal to them the previous day, *"cannot eat or drink."* Affected horses are typically dehydrated, underweight, and depressed by the time they are seen by a veterinarian. This depression is often characterized by somnolent immobility. Infrequently, these periods of drowsiness are interrupted by brief periods of agitation, confusion, and excitability.

Affected horses spend a great deal of time with their heads hanging down, often with the tip of the nose just off the ground. Because of this, pitting edema of the head region is common. Affected horses have difficulty prehending food, but once in the mouth, the horse shows rhythmic chewing and tongue movements and dysphagia, with food continually dribbling from the commissures. Frequent yawning is sometimes reported, along with hypertonic, rhythmic movements of the lips, curling of the upper lip down and over the upper incisors. The mouth is often open, the tongue partially protruding and spasmodically flicking back and forth between the teeth, although no true flaccid paralysis is observed. Bruxism is sometimes reported. Most horses can swallow normally, but can drink only by submerging their heads deeply into water buckets or troughs and then tipping their heads back. Ulceration of the tongue, lips, and gingiva has also been reported. Ataxia and muscle tremors are sometimes observed. Secondary complications are few; aspiration pneumonia has been reported.

Clinical Pathology. The only consistent clinical pathologic findings are those of dehydration (e.g., elevated packed cell volume, BUN, and total protein). Leukocytosis, neutrophilia, lymphopenia, and hyperfibrinogenemia are sometimes reported.

Lesions. Gross and histologic necropsy findings include varying degrees of emaciation, along with bilateral (rarely unilateral) symmetrical, nonprogressive foci of malacia of the substantia nigra or globus pallidus (Color Plate 58). These foci are distinct, sharply demarcated, and occur as cavities filled with a yellow gelatinous material and surrounded by thick bands of large foamy gitter cells. When the disease has been reproduced experimentally with Russian knapweed, additional lesions of necrosis in the nuclei of the inferior colliculi, mesencephalic nucleus of the trigeminal nerve, and the dentate nucleus have been observed.[6]

Diagnostic Testing. Magnetic resonance imaging has been used to confirm this disease antemortem, particularly in miniature ponies, foals, and yearlings. The lesions observed are compatible with what is seen on necropsy and typically include focal, hyperintense areas in the substantia nigra or globus pallidus.

Treatment. No treatment strategies have been successful to date. The lesions appear to be irreversible. Horses can be maintained by IV fluid therapy and gastric tube enteral feeding, but the long-term prognosis is grave.

Prognosis. Once symptoms occur, the disease is fatal, and horses die of starvation if they are not humanely euthanized. In the rare case when the disease is caught early and the signs and lesions are unilateral, the horse may be able to maintain adequate food and water intake to prevent starvation and dehydration, but the signs and lesions never completely disappear.

Prevention and Control. The only true preventive measure is to prevent animal access to these two plants. Several biological control agents, natural enemies of yellow starthistle, have been introduced into the environment to curb the plant's spread. These include the weevils *Larinus curtus, Eustenopus villosus,* and *Bangasternus orientalis,* and the flies *Urophora sirunaseva, Chaetorellia australis,* and *Chaetorellia succinea.*[8] These weevils and flies are seed head feeders, all attacking yellow starthistle at different bud stages. The larvae are laid and develop in the seed heads of the growing plant. There they feast on the developing seeds. The adult weevils also feed on the plant itself. These efforts have been largely unsuccessful in controlling the spread of this weed in many areas.

One biologic control agent, a nematode *Subanguina picridis,* has been used sporadically to control the spread of Russian knapweed with limited success.[8]

REFERENCES

1. Cordy DR: Nigropallidal encephalomalacia (chewing disease) in horses on rations high in yellow star thistle, *J Neuropathol Exp Neurol* 13:330, 1954.
2. Riopelle RJ et al: In James LF et al, editors: *Poisonous plants, proceedings of the Third International Symposium,* Ames, Iowa, 1992, Iowa State University Press.
3. Cheng CHK et al: Toxic effects of solstitialin A 13-acetate and cynaropicrin from *Centaurea solstitialis* L. (Asteraceae) in cell culture of foetal rat brain, *Neuropharmacology* 32(3):271, 1992.
4. Roy DN et al: Isolation and identification of two potent neurotoxins, aspartic acid and glutamic acid, from yellow star thistle *(Centaurea solstitialis), Nat Toxins* 3(3):174, 1995.
5. Sanders SG, Harding JW: Isolation and identification of a potential neurotoxin responsible for equine nigropallidal encephalomalacia, *Proc 18th Ann Vet Med Forum, ACVIM Abstracts,* Seattle, 2000.
6. Young S et al: Nigropallidal encephalomalacia in horses fed Russian knapweed *(Centaurea repens* L.), *Am J Vet Res* 31(8):1393, 1970.
7. Young S et al: Nigropallidal encephalomalacia in horses caused by ingestion of weeds of the genus *Centaurea, J Am Vet Med Assoc* 157(11):1602, 1970.
8. Coombs EM et al: In William RD et al, editors: *Pacific Northwest 2000 weed control handbook,* Corvallis, Ore, 2000, Oregon State University.

26

Rodenticides and Avicides

3-CHLORO-*p*-TOLUIDINE HYDROCHLORIDE

Mary Michael Schell

Synonyms. 3-CPT, Starlicide, DRC-1339, and 3-chloro-4-methylaniline (3-CMA) are alternative names.

Sources. 3-CPT is an avicide, classed as a Restricted Use Pesticide by U.S. Environmental Protection Agency (EPA) guidelines, and licensed for use only by certified applicators or those under their supervision.[1] Starlicide is available as a 0.1% ready-to-use product and as a 98% powder to be applied to various baits.

Toxicokinetics. This toxicant appears to be metabolized differently in birds and mammals.

Mechanism of Action. The mechanism of action has not been determined.

Toxicity and Risk Factors. A wide range in sensitivity to the compound exists, even among birds. Starlings, redwinged blackbirds, and crows are the most sensitive, with lethal dose 50 (LD_{50}) ranging from 1.8 to 3.8 mg/kg.

Clinical Signs. In birds, clinical signs may include decreased activity and possible increased respiratory rate with mild dyspnea. Death, which occurs 1 to 3 days after ingestion, is due to renal failure and is not preceded by tremors or seizure activity.[2]

In mammals, 3-CPT has been shown to cause methemoglobinemia, central nervous system (CNS) depression, flaccid paralysis, hypothermia, and death.[2-5] In rats, mice, and cats, methemoglobinemia is an early sign, peaking within the first hour. Mild respiratory depression, hypothermia, generalized muscle flaccidity, and respiratory arrest follow.[4]

Clinical Pathology. Findings in mammals may include methemoglobinemia, hyperkalemia, and hemoconcentration.[3] Hematuria has been reported both in laboratory animals and in humans.[3] In birds, a rapid increase in blood uric acid levels occurs.[5]

Lesions. In birds, congested or hemorrhagic kidneys are frequently seen. Generalized congestion of liver and brain has also been reported. Renal tubular degeneration has been seen in some birds.[2] Histopathology may show generalized venous congestion.

Diagnostic Testing. Kidneys of both birds and mammals may contain 3-CPT.

Treatment. No specific therapy exists. Supportive care includes providing warmth and intravenous (IV) fluids. Treating the methemoglobinemia is not indicated.

Prognosis. Prognosis is related more to the dose ingested than to any treatment given. Maintaining body temperature decreases the mortality. Once hypothermia has developed, warming to raise body temperature does not decrease the death rate at a given dose.[3]

Prevention and Control. Access by nontarget birds to bait should not be allowed. Equipment used for other feed blending should not be contaminated.

4-AMINOPYRIDINE

Mary Michael Schell

Synonyms. Alternative names include 4-AP, amino-4-pyridine, Avitrol, and Avitroland.

Sources. One of the most commonly used avicides is 4-aminopyridine, which is designated as a Restricted Use Pesticide by the EPA. It is licensed for use only by certified applicators or those under their supervision. 4-AP is usually formulated in a corn or grain bait at 0.5% to 3% active ingredient, but is also available as a powder concentrate.[1,2] When the treated grain or pelleted product is mixed per label into a larger quantity of similar materials, only a small percentage of birds that consume bait ingest the treated portion. Affected birds emit a distress cry and may perform aerial distress displays.[3] Birds consuming a lethal dose progress through seizure activity to coma and to death within about 12 to 15 minutes.[4]

Toxicokinetics.   4-AP is rapidly absorbed via the gastrointestinal tract, with signs of intoxication frequently developing within 10 to 15 minutes of ingestion.[5] It can also be absorbed across the skin and via the respiratory tract. 4-AP is rapidly metabolized by the liver, and metabolites are excreted in the urine. Because of this rapid metabolism, minimal risk exists of relay toxicosis through consumption of poisoned animals. 4-AP–poisoned blackbirds were fed to canines, rats, magpies, and three species of hawks daily and no signs were noted in the test groups over 20 days.[1,6]

Mechanism of Action.   4-AP blocks the potassium ion channel and increases release of acetylcholine at the synapse. Because of the effect of enhanced nerve transmission, signs of toxicosis resemble those of cholinesterase inhibitors or of strychnine intoxication.

Toxicity and Risk Factors.   4-AP is highly toxic to both mammals and birds. Baited blackbirds experience significant mortality with an ingestion of about 0.66 mg of 4-AP.[6] Published acute oral LD_{50} values range from 3.7 mg/kg body weight in dogs up to about 20 mg/kg in rats and mice.[7] Death has been reported in two horses that ingested about 3 mg/kg.[1] Because 4-AP is water soluble, cattle have been poisoned via contamination of their drinking water.[8]

Clinical Signs.   Salivation, hyperexcitability, tremors, incoordination, tonic-clonic seizures, and cardiac arrhythmias are reported clinical signs. Horses may experience profuse sweating, fright, convulsions, and severe fluttering of the third eyelid.[9] Both cattle and horses may walk backward.[8,9] At doses near or greater than the oral LD_{50}, initial signs often begin within 15 minutes, with death occurring within 4 hours.[2] Death is due to cardiac or respiratory arrest.[1,5]

Clinical Pathology.   Metabolic acidosis and elevated liver enzymes have developed in humans.[10] Survivors may have elevated liver enzymes for 1 to 2 weeks.

Lesions.   No specific lesions are associated with 4-AP intoxication.

Diagnostic Testing.   4-AP can be detected in suspect bait, stomach contents, liver, kidney, and urine.[9,11]

Treatment.   Treatment is directed at minimizing absorption of the agent and control of any signs. Gastric lavage followed by activated charcoal should be considered. Diazepam or barbiturates may control the seizures. Pancuronium bromide antagonizes the effect of 4-AP and may be used if respiratory support is available. Xylazine has been recommended to control the excitement and tremors in horses, but case reports do not confirm its usefulness.[1,9] Propanolol or other beta-blocking agents control life-threatening tachyarrhythmias. Intubation may help protect the respiratory tract.[1,10]

Prognosis.   Affected animals that live longer than 4 hours after the onset of signs are likely to survive with supportive care.[1,8,10]

Prevention and Control.   Poisonings generally follow accidental access to quantities of baited corn or other grains, or ingestion of contaminated water.[1,8,9] Proper handling of the pesticidal product and awareness of risk to all species, not just target species, decreases unintended poisonings.

ANTICOAGULANT RODENTICIDES

Charlotte Means

Synonyms.   Anticoagulant rodenticides are the most common type of rodenticide. Warfarin and indanedione are first-generation anticoagulant rodenticides. Warfarin is found in the following products: End-o-Rat, Final Rat and Mouse Bait, Maki Meal Bait, Ra-Mo-Cide Kills Rats and Mice, Rat Kakes, and many other brands.

Indanedione rodenticides include pindone, chlorophacinone, and difethialone. Chlorophacinone is found in products such as Black Leaf Gophercide, AC Formula 90 Rodenticide, J T Eaton Answer for Mice, Rodent Doom, and Rozol Rat and Mouse Killer. Diphacinone is formulated in products such as Assasin, Contrax-D, Ditrac, and Eagles 7 Final Bite. J T Eaton's AC Formula 50, Contrax P Formula, and Speedy Rat Killer are some of the products that contain pindone. D-Cease Mouse and Rat Bait and Generations baits contain difethialone.

Second-generation rodenticides have the same basic coumarin or indanedione nucleus but have been selected for enhanced toxicity. Two of the most common are bromadialone and brodifacoum. Bromadialone is found in products such as AC Formula 70 Rodenticide, Black Leaf Blitz One Feeding, Bootleg Rat and Mouse Bait, Contrac All Weather Blox, Eagle Rat Free, Just One Bite, Hawk Bait Chunx, Maki Mini Blocks, and Rat Eraser Rat and Mouse Bait. Brodifacoum is the most commonly used active ingredient. Brodifacoum is found in products such as Combat Mouse Killer Bait, D-Con Ready Mixed Bait Bits, D-Con Mouse Prufe II, De-Mize Kills Mice and Rats, Final Blox, Jaguar Rodenticide, and Talon G.

Warfarin products generally contain 0.025% concentration of active ingredient. The usual concentration found in difethialone products is 0.0025%, and other second-generation anticoagulants generally contain 0.005% concentration of active ingredients.

All brands are not listed, and many companies make products with different active ingredients. Veterinarians should request that animal owners bring in the packaging to verify the active ingredient and to verify that the product actually is an anticoagulant rodenticide.

Sources.   Anticoagulants are designed to kill rats, mice, gophers, and other rodents. These rodenticides are easily purchased at feed stores, grocery stores, home and garden stores, and discount stores. Professional pest control companies also place rodenticides in clients' homes.

Rodenticides are formulated as place packs (pellets), wax blocks, and tracking powders. People may also mix baits with foods such as tuna or peanut butter, hoping to attract rodents, but frequently luring pets instead. A cat's grooming behavior may increase the risk of ingestion of tracking powders.

Medications such as warfarin and bishydroxycoumarin cause the same clinical syndrome as anticoagulant rodenticides. Some plants (including herbal preparations) can cause bleeding in a similar manner as anticoagulant rodenticides. These plants include *Aesculus, Melilotus, Anthoxanthum, Gallium, Dipteryx, Trillium,* and moldy *Lespedeza.*[1]

Toxicokinetics. Anticoagulant rodenticides are well absorbed orally, and peak plasma levels usually are obtained within 12 hours of ingestion. Anticoagulant rodenticides are highly bound to plasma proteins. Warfarin is generally about 90% to 95% protein bound. Anticoagulants are metabolized in the liver and excreted in the urine. Brodifacoum concentrates in the liver and may undergo some enterohepatic recirculation. It is theorized that second generation anticoagulants bind more strongly to the liver than warfarin and thus produce more persistent effects.

The half-life ($T_{1/2}$) varies greatly among substances and species. The plasma $T_{1/2}$ of warfarin in dogs is listed as 14.5 hours. The $T_{1/2}$ of diphacinone in humans is 15 to 20 days. The $T_{1/2}$ of brodifacoum in dogs is listed as 120 days and as 6 ± 4 days. The $T_{1/2}$ of brodifacoum in horses is listed as 1.22 ± 0.22 days.

On average, duration of action lasts 14 days in warfarin toxicosis, 21 days in bromadialone toxicosis, and 30 days in brodifacoum and other second-generation anticoagulant toxicosis, although some animals have required treatment for 6 weeks or more.[2-5]

Mechanism of Action. Anticoagulants block vitamin K–dependent clotting factor synthesis by inhibiting the K 1-2-3-epoxide reductase enzyme. This halts the recycling of vitamin K. Affected clotting factors include II, VII, IX, and X. This includes the extrinsic, intrinsic, and common pathways of the coagulation system. Clinical signs generally do not appear for 3 to 7 days after ingestion of the rodenticide because the coagulation system maintains its integrity until the clotting factors already present degrade naturally.[6,7]

Toxicity and Risk Factors. The susceptibility to anticoagulant rodenticides varies widely. In general, ruminants are less susceptible than monogastrics. However, all animals are at risk. Relay toxicosis is rare unless rodents compose a significant portion of the diet; therefore, relay toxicosis is most likely to occur in barn cats or birds of prey.

Many factors contribute to susceptibility. Very young or elderly animals may have increased risk of toxicity. Underlying diseases, such as hypothyroidism, can enhance or prolong toxicity by changing metabolism. Other factors contributing to toxicity include a high-fat diet, which interferes with protein binding; prolonged oral antibiotic therapy, which reduces the synthesis of vitamin K_1 by intestinal bacteria; and preexisting hepatic disease.

Because anticoagulants can cross the placenta, teratogenicity may occur. Hemorrhage may occur in the fetus even when the dam is asymptomatic. It is possible that anticoagulants could be passed through milk.

The therapeutic dose of warfarin, used to treat thromboembolism, is 0.1 mg/kg once daily in dogs and 0.06 to 0.1 mg/kg once daily in cats. Horses receive warfarin at doses of 30 to 75 mg/450 kg when anticoagulant therapy is indicated.[5,6,8]

Clinical Signs. Initial clinical signs are vague and nonspecific. The owner might notice an unusual color such as blue-green or green in the feces because most rodenticides contain a nondigestible dye.

Coagulopathies develop as vitamin K–dependent clotting factors deplete. An animal usually is lethargic and exhibits exercise intolerance. Anorexia may be present and the animal becomes weaker. The most common presentation is acute dyspnea, which occurs with bleeding into the chest cavity. Lameness occurs if the animal bleeds into a joint cavity. Bruising (both ecchymoses and petechiae) can occur, and frank hemorrhage may be observed from the nares or rectum, although these are not common presentations. If bleeding occurs in the spinal cord or brain, neurologic signs may be present, frequently mimicking intervertebral disc disease. These signs include ataxia and proprioceptive deficits. Sudden death with no earlier reported clinical signs is not uncommon. Abortions occur with placental bleeding.

Differential diagnoses include disseminated intravascular coagulation, hemophilia, coagulopathies resulting from liver disease, and vitamin K–responsive coagulopathy in swine.[5,6,9]

Clinical Pathology. Both the prothrombin time (PT) and the activated partial thromboplastin time (aPTT) become increased. However, PT typically changes before the aPTT because factor VII has a shorter $T_{1/2}$ than the other factors. By the time activated clotting times (ACTs) are elevated, hemorrhaging has occurred. Platelet numbers, thrombin clotting times (TCT,) and fibrin-fibrinogen degradation prod-ucts (FDP) are normal until bleeding begins and these products are consumed.

PIVKA (protein induced in vitamin K antagonism) is a sensitive test whose results are elevated in rodenticide poisonings as well as other vitamin K–responsive coagulopathies.[6,7]

Lesions. No specific lesions are expected. Body cavities or the gastrointestinal tract may be filled with blood.

Diagnostic Testing. Postmortem analysis can be performed on liver. Samples should be shipped chilled or frozen.[5,6] Most veterinary diagnostic laboratories are able to test for anticoagulants.

Treatment. Because of discrepancies in reported toxicity studies with second-generation anticoagulant rodenticides, 0.02 mg/kg should be assumed as a dose to begin decontamination and treatment. A trigger dose for treating warfarin ingestions is 0.2 mg/kg.

If an animal has been recently exposed, decontamination is indicated. Vomiting may be induced if ingestion occurred within the last 4 hours. Activated charcoal is indicated in significant ingestions. Because of the delayed onset of clinical signs, a known recent ingestion is not an emergency. An owner can induce emesis at home, and wait until regular office hours to bring the pet to a veterinary clinic. An exception to this rule is ingestion by pocket pets (hamsters, rats, mice, gerbils, and guinea pigs) and other exotic animals. These species cannot vomit and activated charcoal must be administered. Hamsters should be sedated and their cheek pouches flushed.

PT or PIVKA can be monitored at baseline, 48, and 72 hours. If these tests are normal, decontamination was successful or the animal did not ingest a toxic dose. Because the PT elevates *before* the animal becomes clinically ill, this is a useful test to determine whether vitamin K_1 therapy is indicated. PT and PIVKA testing must be performed before vitamin K treatment; otherwise a false-negative result is likely.

In an asymptomatic animal, if the PT is elevated or if a potentially toxic dose of anticoagulant was ingested but timely decontamination did not occur, vitamin K_1 therapy should be initiated. Vitamin K is given orally at 1.5 to 2.5 mg/kg twice daily. Small dogs, cats, and exotic animals should be started at the higher end of the range. Large-breed dogs may be started at the low end of the range. Pocket pets can be given injectable vitamin K orally or a pharmacist may compound it. Vitamin K should be given with a small amount of food to aid absorption. Vitamin K injections are not indicated because they have the potential to cause anaphylactic reactions.

Warfarin exposures should be treated for 14 days, bromadialone for 21 days, and other second-generation anticoagulant exposures for 30 days. In all cases, a PT should be checked 48 hours after the last dose of vitamin K has been given. Emphasize the importance of following medication instructions. Clinical signs may develop within 48 hours if vitamin K_1 therapy is stopped too soon.[6,9]

Large animals, such as cattle and horses, may also be treated with vitamin K. However, when this is cost prohibitive, the animal should be stalled or confined and provided with high-quality alfalfa hay. Ruminants may be treated with vitamin K_1 at 1 to 2 mg/kg subcutaneously. Vitamin K_3 therapy is less effective in anticoagulant poisoning in ruminants. Horses are given 0.5 to 2.5 mg/kg intramuscularly. Horses may develop renal failure if vitamin K_3 therapy is used.[10]

When a symptomatic animal is presented, the animal should be stabilized if shocky or dyspneic. If significant hemorrhage has occurred, whole blood, plasma, or a synthetic blood product such as Oxyglobin should be administered. If significant bleeding in the chest occurs, a chest tube may be indicated. Serial coagulation profiles and complete blood counts should be obtained. The animal should be placed on cage rest and the caloric intake maintained. Body temperature should be monitored. Once hemorrhage has occurred, it is not unusual to require high doses of vitamin K_1. Treatment is started at 5 mg/kg and increased as needed based on PT.

Once an animal is stabilized, the owner should be advised of the need for the animal to rest. Exercise may precipitate a bleeding crisis. An owner should be instructed to monitor the pet closely and immediately return for reevaluation if clinical signs appear.

Prognosis. Prognosis is generally good with early treatment. An asymptomatic animal that is properly decontaminated or placed on vitamin K therapy generally does not develop any clinical signs. If an animal is in a hemorrhagic crisis, prompt and aggressive treatment (transfusions, maintenance of cardiac and respiratory function, control of hemorrhage) can result in a successful outcome.

Prevention and Control. Owners should be advised to keep baits in areas where animals do not frequent. Pocket pets and other exotic animals allowed to roam free in the house can get behind refrigerators and other appliances. Owners need to remember that these baits are attractive to pets. When an animal is presented for treatment, the owner should be reminded to remove all bait to prevent reingestion of the rodenticide.

BROMETHALIN

David Dorman

Synonyms. The chemical name of bromethalin is N-methyl-2,4-dinitro-N-[2,4,6-tribromophenyl]-6-[trifluoromethyl] benzeneamine. This rodenticide has been marketed under a variety of trade names including Vengeance, Assault, and Trounce, among others.

Sources. Bromethalin has been used in rodenticides since the mid-1980s.[1] Bromethalin is generally sold as tan or green grain-based pellets (active ingredient: 0.01% bromethalin) packaged in 16- to 42.5-g paper "place pack" envelopes.

Toxicokinetics. Bromethalin is rapidly absorbed from the gastrointestinal tract.[1] Peak bromethalin plasma concentrations occur within several hours after ingestion. Bromethalin is metabolized by hepatic mixed function oxygenases to the more toxic N-demethylated metabolite known as desmethylbromethalin. Species with low hepatic N-demethylase activity (e.g., guinea pigs) are more resistant to bromethalin toxicosis. Bromethalin and its primary metabolite are widely distributed within the body with detectable chemical residues found in the kidney, liver, brain, and fat.[2] Bromethalin is highly lipophilic, with the fat and brain achieving the highest tissue concentrations. Bromethalin is slowly excreted, and the plasma half-life of this chemical is approximately 5 to 6 days.[1] Biliary elimination is the primary mechanism of bromethalin excretion.

Mechanism of Action. Bromethalin and its primary N-demethylated metabolite (desmethylbromethalin) effectively uncouple oxidative phosphorylation, resulting in diminished ion channel pump activity.[1] Bromethalin also induces lipid peroxidation in the brain of rats.[3] Cerebral edema and elevated cerebrospinal fluid pressure develop in lethally poisoned animals.[1,4]

Toxicity and Risk Factors. Reported oral LD$_{50}$s for bromethalin include 13 mg/kg in rabbits and greater than 500 mg/kg in guinea pigs.[1] Oral LD$_{50}$s for bromethalin are 0.54 mg/kg in cats and 3.65 mg/kg in dogs.[4,5] Minimum lethal doses for the dog and cat are 2.5 and 0.45 mg/kg bromethalin, respectively.[4,5] It is possible that individual cats and dogs may develop severe clinical signs following exposures to even smaller doses, especially if ingested long term. Secondary poisoning of nontarget animals has not been demonstrated experimentally; however, relay toxicosis may occur in the cat.

Clinical Signs. The time to onset of clinical signs and the disease syndrome induced by bromethalin are dose-dependent.[4-6] Animals that ingest bromethalin at or above the LD$_{50}$ generally develop clinical signs within 4 to 18 hours. High-dose bromethalin exposure is characterized by severe muscle tremors, hyperthermia, extreme hyperexcitability, hyperesthesia, and focal motor or generalized seizures, which appear to be precipitated by light or noise. More commonly, dogs and cats are exposed to lower doses of bromethalin (i.e., <LD$_{50}$). In this case, clinical signs develop more slowly, with animals developing signs within 2 to 7 days of ingestion. Hindlimb ataxia and paresis develop initially, with hindlimb paralysis developing several days thereafter. This paralytic syndrome is associated with decreased to absent conscious proprioception, loss of deep pain response, patellar hyperreflexia, and upper motor neuron bladder paralysis. Animals also present with mild-to-severe CNS depression that likewise often progresses to semicoma or coma. Focal motor or generalized seizures may occur in the latter stages of this syndrome. Additional signs may include anisocoria, decerebrate body posture, and fine muscle tremors. Some animals also develop marked abdominal distention and vomiting.

Although not specific for bromethalin toxicosis, electroencephalographic abnormalities commonly occur in bromethalin-poisoned animals and may include spike and spike-and-wave activity (indicative of an irritative or seizure focus), marked voltage depression (indicative of cerebral hypoxia), and abnormal high-voltage, slow-wave activities associated with cerebral edema formation.[7,8]

Clinical Pathology. Some lethally poisoned dogs have mild hyperglycemia.[4] Alterations in routine serum electrolytes and chemistries were not observed experimentally in bromethalin-poisoned cats.[5] Bromethalin toxicosis is associated with the development of mildly to moderately increased cerebrospinal fluid pressure.[4] Examination of cerebrospinal fluid from bromethalin-poisoned dogs generally revealed normal cytology, protein concentration, specific gravity, and cell count.[4]

Lesions. Lesions are generally confined to the CNS. Gross evidence of cerebral edema may or may not be evident. Spongy degeneration of most CNS white matter tracts occurs in lethally poisoned animals.[2,9] The myelin lesion, which has been characterized ultrastructurally as intramyelinic edema, is generally not associated with an inflammatory response or neuronal cell death, and may be reversible. Other toxic causes of CNS white matter spongy degeneration include trialkyl tins, hexachlorophene, and isoniazid.

Diagnostic Testing. The diagnosis of bromethalin poisoning is typically established when an exposure history to a potentially toxic dose of bromethalin exists and appropriate clinical signs develop. Postmortem diagnoses are based on the presence of diffuse white matter vacuolization in the CNS and analytical confirmation of bromethalin residues in fat, brain, and other tissues.[2] Chemical confirmation of bromethalin residues is not widely available and false-negative results may occur, especially when tissues are collected several days after bromethalin ingestion.

Treatment. Unless otherwise contraindicated, detoxification procedures (e.g., emetics) should be used for recent (<2 hours) exposures to a potentially toxic dose of bromethalin. This should be immediately followed by the administration of activated charcoal (1 to 2 g/kg by mouth) and a saline cathartic (sodium sulfate, 250 mg/kg in five to ten times as much water, by mouth). Magnesium sulfate as a cathartic is generally not recommended in order to avoid possible magnesium-induced CNS depression in animals with compromised renal function. Experimental studies have shown that repeated administration of activated charcoal is more effective than is a single dose.[10] Smaller subsequent doses of activated charcoal (0.5 to 1 g/kg) and a saline cathartic (sodium sulfate, 125 mg/kg, by mouth) should be given every 4 to 8 hours for at least 2 to 3 days to all animals that may have consumed a potentially toxic dose.

Treatment of the symptomatic bromethalin-poisoned animal is challenging. Mannitol (250 mg/kg every 6 hours IV) and dexamethasone (2 mg/kg every 6 hours IV) may be given to dogs and cats for the control of cerebral edema. These therapies, however, have been generally ineffective in preventing the toxic syndrome or reversing the syndrome once it has developed.[5,10] Contraindications for the use of mannitol include renal disease, pulmonary edema, dehydration, and intracranial hemorrhage. Animals receiving mannitol therapy may become dehydrated during treatment. Administration of oral fluids can help minimize the risk of animals developing rebound cerebral and pulmonary edema and a worsening of clinical signs secondary to rehydration.

Other symptomatic therapies may also be required. Bromethalin-induced seizures are generally managed with diazepam (1 to 2 mg/kg IV as needed) or phenobarbital (5 to 15 mg/kg IV as needed). Many animals recovering from bromethalin toxicosis exhibit prolonged anorexia and may require supplemental feeding to maintain caloric intake. Recumbent animals should be placed in padded cages to prevent decubital ulcers.

Prognosis. Some animals may fully recover from bromethalin toxicosis. Animals that display mild clinical signs (e.g., ataxia, depression) appear to recover within 1 to 2 weeks of ingestion. Animals with more severe clinical signs, including coma or paralysis, generally have a poor prognosis for recovery.

Prevention and Control. As with other rodenticides, the most effective means of prevention of bromethalin toxicosis is restricting access of pets and other nontarget species to the bait.

CHOLECALCIFEROL

Carla K. Morrow and Petra A. Volmer

Synonyms. Cholecalciferol is the chemical name of vitamin D_3. Fig. 26-1 shows the structures of cholecalciferol and its two major metabolites, 25-hydroxycholecalciferol (calcifediol) and 1,25-dihydroxycholecalciferol (calcitriol). One international unit (IU) of vitamin D_3 is equivalent to 0.025 μg of cholecalciferol.[1] Vitamin D_3 is acquired for nutritive purposes through normal dietary intake or dermal exposure to ultraviolet light. Daily nutritional requirements of vitamin D_3 (which can also be met by vitamin D_2, ergocalciferol, for most species) are summarized in Box 26-1.

Sources. Cholecalciferol is found commercially in vitamin supplements and rodenticides. Dietary supplements with cholecalciferol (or ergocalciferol) are used as general multivitamins and with calcium supplements for osteoporosis prevention and treatment. Rodenticides are labeled for the elimination of mice, rats, ground squirrels, and pocket gophers. Table 26-1 lists some of the common trade names of cholecalciferol-containing products.

Toxicokinetics. Cholecalciferol is rapidly absorbed (hours) following oral exposure. Clinical signs and changes in clinical pathology may appear in 12 to 36 hours.[2]

Cholecalciferol and its metabolites are fat soluble and are therefore stored in adipose tissue. When circulating in plasma, they are tightly bound to vitamin D–binding protein,

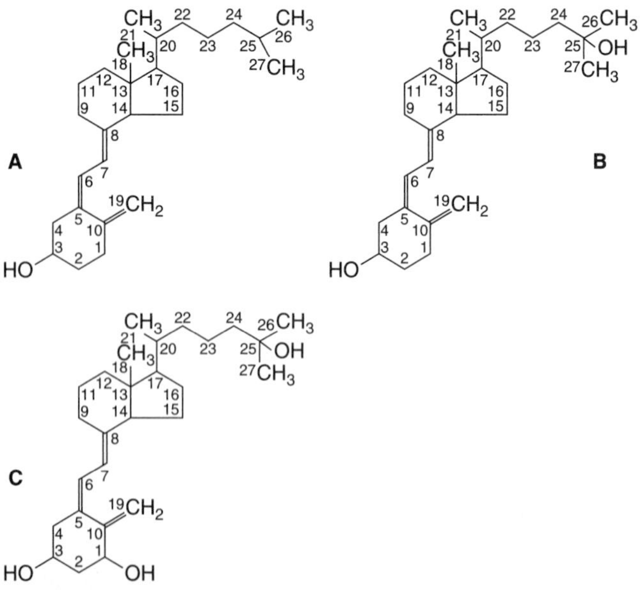

Fig. 26-1 Structure of cholecalciferol (vitamin D_3) and metabolites. **A,** Cholecalciferol. **B,** 25-Hydroxycholecalciferol (calcifediol). **C,** 1,25-Dihydroxycholecalciferol (calcitriol).

BOX 26-1	DIETARY VITAMIN D REQUIREMENTS OF ANIMALS

SPECIES	DAILY DIETARY VITAMIN D REQUIREMENT (AS D_3 OR D_2, UNLESS SPECIFIED) (DRY MATTER BASIS)
Mouse	150 IU D/kg feed
Dog	500 IU D/kg feed
Cat, guinea pig, rat	1000 IU D/kg feed
New World primates (D_3-cholecalciferol)	2000 IU D_3/kg feed
Old World primates (D_3 or D_2)	2000 IU D/kg feed
Hamster	2500 IU D/kg feed
Rabbit	3000 IU D/kg feed

Data from references 1, 20.

TABLE 26-1 Products Containing Vitamin D

Product Name	Concentration	Formulations
Quintox	0.075% Cholecalciferol	Pellets, seed mixtures, place packs
Rampage	0.075% Cholecalciferol	Pellets
Viactiv	100 IU vitamin D_2; 500 mg Ca; 40 μg vitamin K (per chew)	Milk chocolate, caramel, orange cream, mochaccino flavored chews
Multivitamins	Most products contain 400 IU of D_2 or D_3 (per tablet)	Tablets

an α_2-globulin.[3] The primary circulating metabolite is 25-hydroxycholecalciferol (calcifediol).[3] Enterohepatic recirculation of cholecalciferol and its metabolites occurs.[4]

With normal dietary intake, cholecalciferol is converted in the liver to 25-hydroxycholecalciferol (calcifediol), as seen in Fig. 26-2. There is limited negative feedback of calcifediol upon the activity of hepatic 25-hydroxylase, and its activity is not influenced by calcium and phosphorus.[3] Calcifediol becomes metabolically activated in the kidneys by renal 1-α-hydroxylase to 1,25-dihydroxycholecalciferol (calcitriol). The rate of activation by renal 1-α-hydroxylase is dependent upon plasma levels of parathyroid hormone (PTH), calcium, phosphorus, and calcitriol.[3]

With excessive or massive cholecalciferol intake, excess calcifediol is produced in the liver. Calcitriol is initially produced in the kidneys, but once a certain plasma level of calcitriol is reached, it exerts a negative feedback effect on renal 1-α-hydroxylase, and no more calcitriol is produced.[3] However, because of the limited negative feedback on hepatic 25-hydroxylase, calcifediol levels continue to increase. They become high enough to exert metabolic effects.[3]

Metabolic inactivation of calcitriol is thought to occur by an additional hydroxylation to 1,24,25-trihydroxycholecalciferol. This metabolite is further processed to the bio-

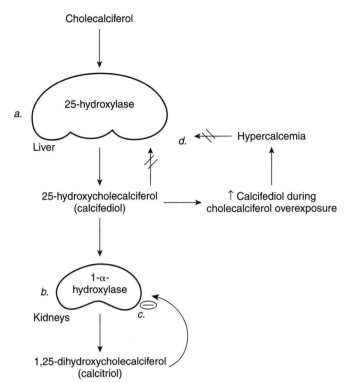

Cholecalciferol

a. 25-hydroxylase

Liver

d. ← Hypercalcemia

25-hydroxycholecalciferol
(calcifediol)

↑ Calcifediol during
cholecalciferol overexposure

b. 1-α-hydroxylase

Kidneys

c.

1,25-dihydroxycholecalciferol
(calcitriol)

Fig. 26-2 Vitamin D activation and feedback mechanisms. *a,* The first step in activating cholecalciferol is 25-hydroxylation to calcifediol. This occurs in the liver. This happens with both normal dietary ingestion and overexposures. *b,* The second step is 1-hydroxylation to calcitriol. This occurs in the kidneys. *c,* In cases of cholecalciferol overexposure, calcitriol increases to a certain level and exerts negative feedback upon renal 1-α-hydroxylase. Renal 1-α-hydroxylase activity is suppressed, and no new calcitriol is formed. *d,* Hepatic 25-hydroxylase receives minimal to no negative feedback from calcifediol, calcitriol, or calcium. In cases of cholecalciferol overexposure, calcifediol continues to be produced. Calcifediol levels become high enough to exert metabolic effects (hypercalcemia).

logically inactive calitroic acid.[3] In conditions that inhibit renal 1-α-hydroxylase (high calcitriol, high calcium, high phosphorous, low PTH), calcifediol is instead metabolized to 24,25-dihydroxycholecalciferol. This is thought to be an elimination step for calcifediol.[3] Both 1,24,25-trihydroxycholecalciferol and 24,25-dihydroxycholecalciferol have much less biologic activity than calcitriol.[3] It is unknown whether they have biologic functions other than elimination of vitamin D₃.[4]

Because of their high lipid solubility, cholecalciferol and its metabolites are eliminated slowly from the body. Cholecalciferol has a plasma $T_{1/2}$ of 19 to 25 hours and a terminal $T_{1/2}$ of weeks to months.[4] Calcifediol (25-hydroxycholecalciferol) has an experimental elimination half-life of 19 days.[4] In a clinical case of cholecalciferol toxicosis, the plasma half-life of calcifediol was 10.67 days.[5] Calcitriol (1,25-dihydroxycholecalciferol) has a plasma half-life of 3 to 5 days.[4] Elimination is primarily (96%) through the bile and feces.[3]

Mechanism of Action. The metabolic activity of vitamin D₃ and its metabolites is variable. Calcitriol is the most metabolically active form. Calcitriol binds to the vitamin D receptors (VDR) 500 times greater than calcifediol and 1000 times greater than cholecalciferol.[3]

Vitamin D₃ metabolites increase plasma calcium and phosphorus through several mechanisms. They increase the amount of intestinal calcium-binding protein (calbindin). The amount of calcium absorbed is directly related to the amount of calbindin in the enterocytes.[6] Thus, more calcium is absorbed from the intestines when calbindin is increased. Cholecalciferol metabolites also stimulate calcium and phosphorus transfer from bone to plasma.[3] Cholecalciferol metabolites, aided by PTH, cause increased renal calcium reabsorption.[3] However, during cholecalciferol toxicosis, the renal contribution to hypercalcemia is expected to be minimal compared to increased intestinal absorption and skeletal reabsorption. PTH decreases during cholecalciferol toxicosis. Without PTH, cholecalciferol metabolites have minimal renal calcium reabsorption effects.[3]

Early clinical effects (first 48 hours) are due to the direct effect of increased plasma calcium on cells. Some of these effects include altered cell membrane permeability, altered calcium pump activity, decreased cellular energy production, and cellular necrosis.[3] Specific organ effects include acute renal tubular necrosis, gastrointestinal stasis, increased gastric acid secretion, decreased skeletal muscle responsiveness, and decreased neural tissue responsiveness.[3]

With an unregulated increase in plasma calcium and phosphorus, the Ca × P product can increase to more than 70. At greater than 70, soft tissue mineralization is likely to occur. Mineralization in the kidneys, gastrointestinal tract, cardiac muscle, skeletal muscle, blood vessels, and ligaments causes structural damage that decreases the functional capacity of these tissues and organs. This loss of function contributes to continuing and end-stage clinical signs, and to long-term signs in animals that survive.[3]

Toxicity and Risk Factors. Companion animals are most at risk from exposure to cholecalciferol-containing rodenticides. Clinical signs can be seen at 0.5 mg/kg of cholecalciferol.[2] This corresponds to 6 g (79 pellets; about ½ tablespoon) of a typical (0.075%) cholecalciferol rat bait for a 20-pound dog.[7] The doses between which clinical signs and lethality occur have been reported and are narrow (less than an order of magnitude).[8] Any dose that can cause clinical signs in an individual animal should be considered serious and dangerous.

The amount of cholecalciferol (or ergocalciferol) in most vitamin supplements is not considered to be a risk for companion animals, even in cases of massive ingestion. Even though the pet may develop a self-limiting gastroenteritis, those signs can be attributed to nonspecific gastrointestinal irritation.

Relay toxicosis with cholecalciferol baits has not been reported.

Clinical Signs. In companion animals, signs of acute toxicosis develop within 12 to 36 hours after ingestion.[2] They include vomiting and diarrhea (sometimes bloody), anorexia, depression, and possibly polyuria and polydipsia.[5,9] With high doses, fulminant acute renal failure occurs by 24 to 48 hours. Complications include death from acute renal failure in severely affected animals. Animals that survive may have potential loss of renal function, loss of musculoskeletal function, and develop cardiac anomalies.[3] Signs and treatment may last for weeks as a result of the lipid storage and slow elimination of the cholecalciferol metabolites.

Clinical Pathology. In acute toxicosis, there is a rapid (12 to 72 hours after ingestion) and moderate increase in plasma phosphorus (up to 10 to 11 mg/dl), with a more severe increase in plasma calcium (up to 20 mg/dl).[5,9,10] The increase in plasma calcium often lags a few hours behind the increase in plasma phosphorus. The Ca × P product may easily exceed 130; soft tissue mineralization occurs when the Ca × P product exceeds 60. Secondary increases in blood urea nitrogen (BUN) and creatinine may also occur in this time frame. Urine specific gravity becomes isosthenuric.

Lesions. Gross lesions include diffuse soft tissue mineralization, especially of the kidneys, gastrointestinal tract, cardiac and skeletal muscles, and tendons and ligaments. Lesions secondary to azotemia may be present, including oral and gastric ulceration. Gastrointestinal hemorrhage can also be seen.[8,10]

Renal microscopic lesions include mineral crystal deposits in the cortical tubule basement membranes and Bowman capsules. Proteinaceous casts may be present.[10] Gastrointestinal lesions can include mucosal necrosis, sloughing, and hemorrhage, often next to bands of mucosal mineralization.[8,10] Cardiac lesions include necrotic, disrupted, and mineralized myocytes.[8,10] Other lesions include widespread mineralization of the tunica media of blood vessels, mineralization of skeletal muscle cells, and mineralization of bronchiolar submucosa.[8,10]

Diagnostic Testing. In companion animals, diagnostic testing needs to rule out other causes of hypercalcemia, including hypercalcemia of malignancy, chronic renal failure, primary hyperparathyroidism, feline idiopathic hypercalcemia, and ingestion of prescription skin products containing the vitamin D analogues calcipotriene or tacalcitol.

Hypercalcemia of malignancy is often due to lymphoid tumors or anal sac carcinomas, which may secrete a parathyroid hormone–related polypeptide (PTHrP).[3] PTHrP acts similarly to PTH but is not controlled by any feedback mechanisms. These tumors are often found during physical examination or with radiographic and ultrasound imaging.

In addition to elevations in BUN and creatinine, evidence for chronic renal failure may be elicited from the history (chronicity and progressiveness of polyuria or polydipsia, vomiting) and by imaging small, misshapen kidneys with radiographs and ultrasound.

Primary hyperparathyroidism has a much more chronic and progressive onset than cholecalciferol toxicosis.[11] Feline idiopathic hypercalcemia patients may have a history of being fed a urinary acidifying diet, have a normal serum phosphorus, and do not exhibit polyuria or polydipsia.[12]

Patients ingesting prescription skin products containing calcipotriene or tacalcitol present with similar clinical signs and serum chemistry abnormalities as cholecalciferol patients.[13,14] Treatment is also similar. However, definitive

TABLE 26-2 **Expected Results of PTH/PTHrP/25-Hydroxycholecalciferol Assay for Various Causes of Hypercalcemia**

Disease	PTH	PTHrP	25-Hydroxy-cholecalciferol
Cholecalciferol toxicosis	Decreased	Absent	Increased
Hypercalcemia of malignancy	Decreased	Present	Normal
Chronic renal failure	Increased	Absent	Unknown (normal)
Primary hyperparathyroidism	Increased	Absent	Unknown (normal)
Feline idiopathic hypercalcemia	Normal	Absent	Normal

Data from references 12, 15.
PTH, Parathyroid hormone; *PTHrP,* parathyroid hormone–related polypeptide.

diagnosis through chemical identification of the product is difficult (see later discussion).

Soft tissue mineralization in cholecalciferol-intoxicated patients may be detected on radiographs and ultrasound.

A PTH/PTHrP/25-hydroxycholecalciferol assay may be useful in differentiating among these causes of hypercalcemia.[15] Table 26-2 summarizes expected results. The PTH/PTHrP/25-hydroxycholecalciferol assay should detect overexposure to cholecalciferol products, in that 25-hydroxycholecalciferol (calcifediol) is elevated during cholecalciferol toxicosis. However, easy and routine assays for calcipotriene, tacalcitol, and 1,25-dihydroxycholecalciferol (calcitriol) are lacking. It is difficult to chemically confirm exposure to the synthetic analogues and calcitriol.

Postmortem samples include a full descriptive gross necropsy with full histopathology samples. If the animal was severely mineralized, determination of the underlying cause may be difficult. Elevations in 25-hydroxycholecalciferol may be detected postmortem in bile, kidney, and urine.[16]

Postmortem analysis of renal calcium to phosphorus ratio may aid in the differentiation between cases of cholecalciferol and ethylene glycol toxicosis.[16] Both of these toxins can result in renal failure with calcium precipitation in the kidneys. Patients with ethylene glycol toxicosis have a higher renal Ca-to-P ratio as a result of higher amounts of renal calcium deposition as calcium oxalate crystals.

Diagnostic laboratories should be contacted to confirm test availability. If the tests are unavailable through a clinician's usual diagnostic laboratory, then antemortem serum analysis for PTH/25-hydroxycholecalciferol, antemortem plasma for PTHrP, and postmortem bile, kidney, and urine analysis 25-hydroxycholecalciferol can be performed at Michigan State University. Send chilled samples to Animal Health Diagnostic Laboratory, Endocrine Diagnostic Section, 619 West Fee Hall B, Michigan State University, Lansing, Michigan, 48824-1315; telephone: 517-353-0621; *www.ahdl.msu.edu.*

Treatment. When exposure is recent, the animal is asymptomatic, and there are no underlying contraindications to emesis (underlying cardiac or seizure disorders; the patient is a lagomorph or rodent), standard emetic protocols can be used. All asymptomatic exposures should be given activated charcoal at 1 to 2 g/kg mixed with 50 to 200 ml water or 240 ml commercial slurry per 25- to 50-pound animal. A cathartic should be given concurrently with the activated charcoal. Many commercial slurries contain sorbitol as a cathartic, or $1/4$ teaspoon Epsom salts (magnesium sulfate) per 10 pounds of body weight can be added if the slurry does not contain a cathartic. In cases of large or massive ingestion, repeat doses of activated charcoal at one half the initial dose and without a cathartic may be given at 6- to 8-hour intervals for 48 hours. Repeat doses of activated charcoal are helpful to lessen the amount of enterohepatic recirculation of cholecalciferol and metabolites.

Baseline and daily monitoring of serum calcium, phosphorus, BUN, and creatinine are done for 96 hours (4 days). If these values stay normal and the patient remains asymptomatic, no further monitoring or treatment is necessary.[13]

In animals that develop signs or increases in serum calcium, initial treatment consists of diuresis with intravenous 0.9% saline at two to three times maintenance rates. Saline contains no calcium, and sodium ions reduce tubular calcium reabsorption, leading to increased calcium excretion.[3]

Once the animal is rehydrated, furosemide is initially given as a 5 mg/kg IV bolus and then as a 5 mg/kg/hr constant rate infusion IV[3]; oral doses of 2 to 4 mg/kg every 8 hours can also be given.[17] Furosemide causes decreased sodium and chloride reabsorption across the loop of Henle, resulting in a diminished positive potential across the tubule. This diminished potential increases renal calcium excretion.[3] Hydration status should be carefully monitored, and the amount of furosemide may need to be reduced.[3] Thiazide diuretics should not be used.[3]

Oral prednisone at 1 to 2.2 mg/kg every 12 hr is also helpful. Prednisone decreases serum calcium by decreasing bone resorption, decreasing intestinal calcium absorption, and increasing renal calcium excretion.[3]

Other supportive care measures include phosphate binders (aluminum hydroxide: Amphogel: 30 to 90 mg/kg/day divided doses, with meals) and a low-calcium, low-phosphorus diet to decrease dietary mineral absorption while the patient is being treated and monitored (generally 4 weeks).[3] Antiemetics are used as needed. Sunlight should be avoided.

Use of activated charcoal in symptomatic patients needs to be cautiously and carefully considered. The risk of aspiration in a vomiting animal may be greater than the benefit of enhanced cholecalciferol elimination.

Intravenous saline solution should be continued until serum calcium levels are normal.[13] Furosemide and prednisone can be continued for 1 to 2 weeks after cessation of IV saline and then gradually decreased.[3] Calcium levels should be monitored daily for 96 hours (4 days) after fluid cessation, then twice weekly for 2 weeks, then weekly for 2 weeks to evaluate for relapse.[3]

Severely affected animals, animals whose calcium levels do not respond to initial therapy, or who relapse after fluid discontinuation may need treatment with a bisphosphonate. The bisphosphonate pamidronate (Aredia) has been used successfully in dogs for cholecalciferol toxicosis. Pamidronate is given at 1.3 to 2 mg/kg diluted into saline and given over 2 hours IV.[18] The animal should be maintained on therapeutic IV saline until the calcium levels are normalized. Once serum calcium levels return to normal, calcium levels should

be monitored daily for 96 hours. Up to one retreatment 5 to 7 days later may be necessary.

Bisphosphonates lower plasma calcium by inhibiting bone reabsorption of calcium through blocking dissolution of hydroxyapatite and inhibiting osteoclastic bone resorption.[18] Even though bisphosphonates are expensive drugs, they may save the client money in the long run. They lower plasma calcium rapidly, within 24 to 48 hours. This allows the patient to be treated on an outpatient basis as compared to being hospitalized on IV saline for 2 to 4 weeks.

If a bisphosphonate is not available, salmon calcitonin may be used to lower serum calcium. It is given 4 to 6 IU/kg subcutaneously every 8 hours.[3] Salmon calcitonin lowers plasma calcium by inhibiting osteoclastic activity. The disadvantages of salmon calcitonin over bisphophonates are that it must be frequently administered and that patients may become refractory to it.[18]

Use of bisphosphonates and salmon calcitonin together in the same patient, either simultaneously or sequentially, is controversial. Experimental animals that received both did worse than animals receiving one or the other.[19] However, short-term use of salmon calcitonin while using a bisphosphonate is the preferred treatment of emergency hypercalcemia of malignancy in humans.[3]

Prognosis. The prognosis is good in animals that are decontaminated promptly or have serum calcium levels lowered before soft tissue mineralization takes place. The prognosis is more variable if soft tissue mineralization has occurred. Soft tissue mineralization is minimally reversible. It can lead to structural damage and decreased function of the kidneys and cardiovascular, gastrointestinal, and musculoskeletal systems. The amount of function loss, and thus the prognosis, is dependent upon the length and severity of the elevated Ca × P product. Soft tissue mineralization can occur when the Ca × P product exceeds 60 mg/dl.

Prevention and Control. Control of cholecalciferol toxicosis is dependent on controlling access to the rodent baits. Homeowners and farmstead owners should place baits where nontarget species cannot access them. If place-packs are used, they should be placed where rodents cannot drag them within reach of a pet. Homeowners and farmstead owners should also be aware of how much bait was set out and monitor its disappearance. Renters and condominium owners should request that building maintenance inform tenants when, where, and what kind of baits (and other pest control measures) are used.

SODIUM FLUOROACETATE

Kathleen Henry Parton

Synonyms. Alternative terms include compound 1080, sodium monofluoroacetate, SMFA, and fluoroacetate.

Sources. Fluoroacetate occurs naturally in a variety of plants known to poison livestock in Africa *(Dichapetalum* *cymosum* and *D. toxicarum)*, Australia *(Acacia georginae, Gastrolobium* spp and *Oxylobium* spp), and South America *(Palicourea marcgravii)*.

In the United States, fluoroacetate has been used as a rodenticide and a predacide since the 1940s. The EPA canceled all registered uses for predator control in 1972 and for rodenticides by 1990. The EPA strictly limits the use of fluoroacetate to livestock protection collars (LPCs) in those states that have registration and EPA-approved certification and training programs (Montana, New Mexico, South Dakota, Texas, and Wyoming). Livestock protection collars registered for use with sheep and goats contain 30 ml with 1% active ingredient (300 mg of fluoroacetate).[1]

The chemotherapeutic anticancer agent 5-fluorouracil and some inhaled fluorinated ethanes are metabolized to fluoroacetate.[2,3] The side effects of 5-fluorouracil and fluorinated ethanes in animals resemble 1080 toxicosis.

Toxicokinetics. Compound 1080 is readily absorbed from the gastrointestinal and respiratory tracts, abraded skin, and mucous membranes, but only slowly through intact skin. It is not known to accumulate in any one tissue. Fluoroacetate, which is considered to be nontoxic, is metabolized to monofluoroacetic acid by hydrolysis and reacts with coenzyme A to form fluoroacetyl CoA. This product combines with oxaloacetate in the Krebs cycle and is converted to fluorocitrate, a toxic metabolite. Several species, such as the Western Australian opossum, are known to be capable of rapid defluorination of fluoroacetate, which reduces the conversion of fluoroacetate to fluorocitrate. In these species, rapid defluorination and some unknown mechanism appear to afford a high degree of tolerance to fluoroacetate toxicity.[4] Fluoroacetate and fluoride ions are eliminated in the urine of rodents.[3] In sublethally poisoned animals, the elimination of fluoroacetate is usually complete within a few days.

Fluoroacetate $(CH_2FCOONa)$ is a water-soluble salt similar in appearance to flour, powdered sugar, and baking powder (Fig. 26-3). Hygroscopic when exposed to air, 1080 is insoluble in organic solvents such as kerosene, alcohol, acetone, or animal and vegetable fats and oils. The chemical structure of 1080 is essentially that of sodium acetate, with a hydrogen atom replaced by an atom of fluorine. Fluoroacetamide or 1081 (CH_2FCONH_2) is similar to fluoroacetate but less toxic and not registered for use in the United States.

Mechanism of Action. The classic theory for 1080 poisoning is the so-called "lethal synthesis" effect on the Krebs or tricarboxylic acid (TCA) cycle (Fig. 26-4). Fluoroacetate combines with acetyl CoA to form fluoroacetyl CoA, which then combines with oxaloacetate to produce fluorocitrate. Fluorocitrate inhibits aconitase and the oxidation of citric acid, resulting in the blockage of the TCA cycle, energy depletion, citrate and lactate accumulation, and a decrease in blood pH. The inhibition of aconitase interferes with

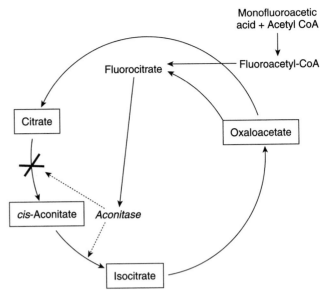

Fig. 26-4 The classic theory that fluoroacetate inhibits aconitase in the Krebs or tricarboxylic acid cycle.

cellular respiration and the metabolism of carbohydrates, fats, and proteins. Recent work suggests that fluorocitrate is converted to form 4-hydroxy-*trans*-aconitate, which binds tightly to aconitase, thereby inactivating it.[5] Citrate accumulates and binds with serum calcium. In addition, citrate accumulation leads to acidosis.

Toxicity and Risk Factors. Animals have different susceptibilities to 1080 poisoning (Table 26-3). In general, herbivores have cardiotoxic effects, carnivores have CNS effects, and omnivores have both cardiac and CNS toxicity.

TABLE 26-3 Fluoroacetate (1080) Toxicity for Various Species

Species	Oral Lethal Dose (mg/kg)	LD$_{50}$ (mg/kg)
Calves		0.22
Cat	0.3-0.5	0.20 (IV)
Cattle	0.15-0.62	0.39
Dog	0.06-0.2	0.05-1
Duck	0.91	
Fowl	10-30	4.24
Goats	0.3-0.7	
Honey bee	Highly toxic	
Horse	0.5-2.75	0.35-0.55
Human	2-5	0.7-2.1
Magpie	1.78-2.3	
Mice		8
Possum	0.3	
Pigs	0.3	0.4-1
Rabbit	0.8	
Rats		2-3
Sheep	0.25-0.5	0.25-0.5
Trout	>500	

From Bruere AN et al: Fluoroacetate, *Vet Clin Toxicol* 127:96, 1990.
IV, Intravenous.

Fig. 26-3 The structure of fluoroacetate.

$$F-\overset{\overset{\displaystyle H}{|}}{\underset{\underset{\displaystyle H}{|}}{C}}-\overset{\overset{\displaystyle }{}}{\underset{\underset{\displaystyle O}{\|}}{C}}-O-Na$$

The reason for variation in species toxicity is not known, but is apparently not due to differences in the size of the animal, the type of digestive tract, or the basal metabolic rate. Toxicity varies from an LD_{50} of 0.5 mg/kg in the dog to more than 500 mg/kg in the South African clawed toad *(Xenopis leavis)*.

Primates and birds are the most resistant species, whereas rodents and carnivores are the most susceptible. In general, the cold-blooded vertebrates are much less susceptible to 1080 than the warm-blooded vertebrates.

Sheep and goats that puncture their livestock protection collars on vegetation or by other means are unlikely to be poisoned by dermal contact. However, oral ingestion of contents of the collar could be lethal. Because tissue residues are minimal, the ingestion of muscle from a poisoned carcass is unlikely to cause toxicity. Chronic poisoning resulting from long-term ingestion of contaminated meat is rare, because 1080 does not accumulate within the body. Secondary poisoning of scavengers may occur from the ingestion of dead or dying animals, but the risk is considered low.

Compound 1080 does not yield toxic fumes, thus it is relatively safe to handle as long as the user is well trained and exercises care.

Clinical Signs. Clinical signs may appear from 30 minutes to as long as 2 hours after ingestion, depending on the dose. The variable latent period is a result of the delay in conversion of fluoroacetate to fluorocitrate and its accumulation to toxic levels. Carnivores display central nervous excitation and gastrointestinal hyperactivity. Neurologic signs in dogs include anxiety, frenzied behavior, such as running and howling, and hyperesthesia. Carnivores usually vomit, salivate, urinate, and defecate after ingesting 1080. A hypermotile gastrointestinal tract with tenesmus also occurs. Hyperthermia has been reported in dogs.

Convulsions begin after a brief period of hyperexcitability. Tonic and clonic convulsions may occur between periods of frenzied and normal behavior. Dogs in the agitated state are not responsive to external stimuli. The anoxia that occurs during convulsions leads to respiratory failure. The animal becomes weaker as the cellular energy supplies decrease. Eventually the animal becomes comatose, and death occurs from 2 to 12 hours after the appearance of clinical signs.

Cats, sheep, and pigs tend to show a combination of cardiac and central nervous responses. In addition, the pig demonstrates persistent intermittent vomiting. The poisoned cat may become depressed or excited, vocalize, and be hyperesthetic to light and touch. Hypothermia (37° C), cardiac arrhythmia, and episodes of bradycardia between convulsions have also been reported in the cat. Sheep administered an oral dose of 1 mg/kg of fluoroacetate had decreased ruminal movements, restlessness, frequent urination, muscular tremors, polypnea, and tachycardia.

Herbivores and monkeys manifest predominantly cardiac signs. Cattle may die of heart failure following ingestion of fluoroacetate. Cattle ingesting lethal quantities of fluoroacetate stagger, tremble, sweat, and show signs of gastrointestinal irritation. Horses may also show a degree of hyperesthesia to external stimuli. There are marked cardiac arrhythmias combined with ventricular alteration, myocardial depression, and terminal ventricular fibrillation. Stress or exercise often precipitates the fatal onset. Nonviolent terminal convulsions may be seen secondary to cerebral anoxia.

Animals exposed to sublethal doses show severe depression, anorexia, listlessness, teeth grinding, and weakness. Reports of dogs and cats recovering after treatment from 1080 poisoning suggest there are no lasting effects; however, livestock surviving poisoning may be unthrifty. Animals that die of 1080 intoxication develop a rapid onset of rigor mortis, with the limbs fixed in extensor rigidity.

Clinical Pathology. Clinical pathology changes include hyperglycemia, increased serum citrate, hypocalcemia (ionized), and acidosis. The increase in serum glucose may be twofold or greater. In dogs and many other species, citrate levels are elevated in serum and heart muscle and are associated with the onset of clinical signs; however, high levels are not conclusive of 1080 ingestion in that citrate is a normal occurring substance in cells. Hypocalcemia (total and ionized) is reported in association with 1080 toxicity. In cats, ionized calcium is decreased rather than total serum calcium. In the dog, only total calcium was measured and hypocalcemia was dependent on the dose of fluoroacetate and the severity of clinical signs. Electrocardiograms of cats poisoned with 1080 show a prolongation of the QT interval corresponding to a decline in ionized calcium levels. In sheep, electrocardiographic changes include arrhythmia, decreased T wave amplitude, prolonged PR intervals, and ventricular fibrillation; however, these findings are highly variable.

Lesions. Postmortem findings in animals exposed to 1080 are nonspecific. Rigor mortis is rapid in onset. If death results from sudden ventricular fibrillation there may be no lesions at all, but death occurring secondarily to hypoxia may result in general cyanosis, congestion of visceral organs, agonal petechial hemorrhages on the myocardium, and pulmonary congestion. Other findings may include an empty stomach, enteritis, and a flaccid, pale heart in diastole. Sheep and cattle show mild-to-severe lesions of the myocardium, including endocardial and epicardial petechiae, depending on dose and time of death.

Histopathologic changes of the brain may include edema and lymphocytic infiltration of perivascular tissue. The lesions are more common in the endocardium and range from inconspicuous to Zenker's necrosis and necrosis of myocardial fibers. In animals that survive for more than 12 hours, a mild inflammatory response may occur.

Diagnostic Testing. A diagnosis of 1080 poisoning is based on clinical signs, access to the poison, and the analysis of the compound in bait or vomitus. Residues of 1080 are most likely to be found in vomitus or stomach contents, a minimum of 50 g of vomitus being required for analysis. Animals that ingest a minimum lethal dose of 1080 are unlikely to have detectable levels in body tissues. In experimentally poisoned animals, tissue fluoroacetate levels were considerably less than 100 ppb.

Veterinarians should contact their local diagnostic laboratories to determine the best facility in their region for fluoroacetate analysis.

Treatment. There is no known antidote for 1080 poisoning. Because of the rapid onset of clinical signs (2 to 3 hours), it is difficult to treat animals successfully after ingestion of 1080. Recent success in Australia suggests that administering sodium bicarbonate to dogs increases the chances of survival.[7] The recommended treatment procedure is to lightly anesthetize the animal with pentobarbital sodium, insert an IV catheter, and connect the animal to a saline (0.9% NaCl) drip. Sodium bicarbonate (8.4% weight per volume) is infused through the giving port at the dose rate of 300 mg/kg over a period of 15 to 30 minutes. Alternatively, half the calculated dose is given as a bolus and the remainder infused slowly. An 8.4% sodium bicarbonate solution contains approximately 1 mEq/ml each of sodium and bicarbonate. Administration of sodium bicarbonate may worsen hypocalcemia and induce hypokalemia. Ionized calcium and potassium levels must be monitored and supplemented as necessary. Decontamination with activated charcoal is also recommended. The activated charcoal should be given via a stomach tube with the animal intubated to prevent aspiration pneumonia. Anesthesia and fluids should be maintained until the animal recovers without convulsing, usually within 24 hours if removal of fluoroacetate from the gastrointestinal tract is thorough.

Successful treatment with acetamide has been reported in New Zealand.[8] Even though administration of acetamide may be effective in the treatment of 1080 poisoning, early treatment and decontamination are important. The dose for acetamide reported for humans requires making a 10% solution of acetamide in 5% dextrose. The acetamide solution is administered at a dose of 7 to 10 ml/kg over a 30-minute period, then at 5 ml/kg every 4 hours for 24 to 48 hours. Alternatively, with the aid of a microwave oven, 15 g of acetamide granules are dissolved in 1 L of a 5% glucose solution and then administered at a rate of 10 ml/kg over 15 minutes and then reduced to 8 ml/kg/hour until the liter is finished. A second liter is made and administered at 5 ml/kg/hour. Additional acetamide is administered as needed.[8] The heart rate may greatly increase with this treatment regimen.

Glycerol monoacetate (monacetin), which was used in the treatment of fluoroacetate poisoning in humans and animals, is no longer available from chemical suppliers.

Prognosis. In general, the prognosis is poor depending on the species, the amount of 1080 ingested, and the severity of clinical signs at presentation. However, the practitioner should keep in mind that small animals with clinical signs may respond to rapid treatment.

STRYCHNINE

Patricia A. Talcott

Synonyms. Strychnine is also called gopher bait.

Sources. The strychnine alkaloid is isolated from the seeds of *Strychnos nux vomica* and *ignatii.*

Strychnine-containing baits are commonly used by homeowners, farm workers, certified applicators, and animal damage control personnel in many parts of the United States to control populations of ground squirrels, meadow and deer mice, prairie dogs, rats, porcupines, chipmunks, rabbits, and pigeons. Many baits are composed of red or green colored grain (e.g., oat, milo, corn, wheat) mixed with 0.5% to 1% strychnine sulfate. Some restricted use formulations contain much higher concentrations of the alkaloid. Some states allow over-the-counter sales of strychnine-containing products. All applications are marketed for below-ground use.

Toxicokinetics. Strychnine is rapidly absorbed from the gastrointestinal tract. Strychnine is not highly protein bound, and it is readily metabolized by hepatic enzymes.[1] Approximately 1% to 20% of an original exposure dose is excreted unchanged into the urine.[2,3] Strychnine has a wide tissue distribution and therefore only small amounts (<4 ppm) are ever detected in blood at any given time.

Mechanism of Action. Strychnine acts by blocking both the inhibitory actions of glycine on the anterior horn of the cells of the spinal cord and that of the endogenous transmitter released from the Renshaw cells.[4,5] This inhibition ultimately leads to excessive neuronal activity, producing highly exaggerated reflex arcs. Mild to severe muscle spasms result, and there is generally extreme hyperextension of the limbs and body caused by domination of the more powerful extensor muscle groups. Full tetanic convulsions will follow.

Toxicity and Risk Factors. Strychnine sulfate is a white powder and moderately soluble in water. Strychnine bait is poorly soluble in water and strongly absorbs to soil particles. Environmental persistence is not long, and more than 90% disappears from soil within 40 days. Breakdown in soil is

BOX 26-2	REPORTED ORAL LETHAL DOSE VALUES OF STRYCHNINE
SPECIES	**ORAL LD$_{50}$ OR LETHAL DOSE (mg/kg body weight)**
Dog	0.5-1.2
Cat	2
Pigs	0.5-1
Humans	30-60
Cow	0.5
Horse	0.5
Pig	0.5-1
Mule deer	17-24
Rainbow trout	2.3
Golden eagle	5-10
Sage grouse	42.5
Pheasant	8.5-24.7
Rats	2.2-14

highly dependent on the presence and growth of particular microbial or fungal soil organisms.

Strychnine is highly toxic to most animals (Box 26-2). Dogs are most frequently poisoned. Other species, such as cats, horses, cattle, and goats, are rarely exposed except under malicious circumstances. Depending on the size of the animal and concentration of strychnine present in the bait, ingestion of only a few tablespoons may be sufficient to cause death. Accidental and malicious poisoning of dogs, cats, and other companion animals with strychnine is not uncommon in many parts of the United States. Secondary poisoning resulting from ingestion of strychnine-poisoned rodents can occur, but this is infrequently encountered.

Clinical Signs. Clinical signs are similar in most species affected and generally develop within 10 to 120 minutes of ingestion. The severity of the symptoms is highly dependent on the exposure dose. Symptoms in animals exposed to low levels of strychnine may be delayed and mild (e.g., slight ataxia and muscle stiffness), whereas high-dose exposures result in rapid onset of severe muscle spasms or convulsions.

Initial symptoms commonly observed in strychnine-poisoned animals include a brief (less than 15 minutes) prodromal phase of nervousness, apprehension, anxiety, increased respiratory rate, and excessive salivation. Ataxia, muscle spasms, and stiffness gradually develop, generally beginning with the face, neck, and limb muscles. This can rapidly develop into generalized convulsions that are tonic extensor in nature (opisthotonus). The neck is usually arched back and the jaw clamped shut. These episodes may last several minutes and can be intermittent or continuous. Respiration is impaired during these episodes because of contraction of the diaphragm and thoracic and abdominal muscles. Many strychnine-poisoned patients exhibit an increased severity and frequency of these episodes following sensory stimulation (e.g., loud noise, bright light, touch). This feature, however, is not specific to strychnine, and has been observed in other types of poisonings (e.g., metaldehyde, penitrem A, roquefortine).

Typically in the early phases, the animal is conscious and aware of its surroundings. Vomiting is not commonly reported. Death is a result of medullary paralysis, most likely caused by hypoxia from impaired respiration, and can occur as quickly as 10 minutes after ingestion, or as late as 24 to 48 hours (dependent on degree of medical intervention) after ingestion. Hyperthermia caused by tremors and seizures is generally observed. Stiff, extended limbs are commonly seen terminally.

Clinical Pathology. No specific blood and serum chemistry abnormalities occur following strychnine ingestion. Poisoned animals may display changes compatible with mild dehydration (hemoconcentration) and a mild metabolic acidosis.

Lesions. No specific gross and histologic lesions are seen in strychnine-poisoned animals. Necrosis of the cerebral cortex and brain stem has been reported in strychnine-poisoned humans.[6] The exact cause of this is unclear, but it has been hypothesized that the lesions may be due to poor cerebral perfusion or cortical seizure activity.

Diagnostic Testing. The presence of strychnine in a variety of tissues can be confirmed by several analytical methods (e.g., thin layer chromatography, high-performance liquid chromatography, gas chromatography-mass spectrometry). Because strychnine-poisoned patients often do not vomit, stomach contents is the *best* tissue to select for presence of the alkaloid. Strychnine can also be found in serum, plasma, and urine, but the concentrations are much lower compared with gastrointestinal contents. Finding green or red dyed seed material in the vomitus, lavage washings, or stomach contents should encourage quantitative analysis. Liver or bile and kidney can also be used to confirm the presence of strychnine in postmortem collected tissues, but results are not as reliable because of extremely low tissue concentrations.

Treatment. Treatment options are initially directed at reducing gastrointestinal absorption, followed by appropriate symptomatic and supportive care to reverse the hyperthermia, hypoxia, and acidosis, minimize muscle spasms and convulsive activity, and maintain adequate renal output. Emetics can be used in the asymptomatic patient to evacuate the stomach. Care should be taken with the use of emetics; this type of sensory stimulation may initiate violent muscle or convulsive activity. Apomorphine (dog, cat: 0.04 mg/kg IV, 0.25 mg/kg conjunctivally) or 3% hydrogen peroxide, by mouth (1 ml/lb, up to 50 ml in the dog or 10 ml in the cat; can be repeated) can be used to induce vomiting. A more conservative approach in small animals is to perform a gastric lavage once the patient has been adequately sedated and intubated. Administration of activated charcoal with sorbitol should follow either procedure (delay a minimum of 45 minutes if emesis was induced). Strychnine is effectively bound to activated charcoal and should be considered a mainstay in the treatment of any poisoned patient.

Typically, the more urgent objectives that clinicians face in the treatment of strychnine-poisoned patients are to control the convulsions and support respiration. Barbiturates raise the threshold of spinal reflexes in animals, and because of this, pentobarbital is successfully used clinically to control strychnine-induced convulsions. Pentobarbital, 5 to 15 mg/kg IV to effect, should be administered slowly. Diazepam (dog: 0.5 to 5 mg/kg; cat: 0.5 to 1 mg/kg IV to effect), with its muscle relaxant, anxiolytic, and anticonvulsant properties, is also effective in strychnine-poisoned animals. Methocarbamol can also be used in dogs and cats at a dose of 44 to 220 mg/kg IV, not to exceed 330 mg/kg/day.[7] Methocarbamol causes skeletal muscle relaxation as well as having a secondary sedative effect. Inhalation gas anesthesia can be used initially to control seizure activity. A benefit to this choice is that a readily available, controlled source of oxygen can be provided. The chosen sedative or anesthetic depends on the severity of signs, the species of animal affected, initial response to treatment, and desired length of sedation.

Respiratory activity should be monitored frequently (rate, depth, rhythm) and respiratory assistance (e.g., mechanical ventilation) should be readily available when severe respiratory depression occurs. Intravenous fluid administration (i.e., lactated Ringer's, 0.9 % saline, saline with dextrose) can be used to correct hypovolemia, provide continuous maintenance needs, and aid in correcting any hyperthermia and acidosis. Bicarbonate can be used to correct the acidosis, but this is generally not necessary. All forms of sensory stimulation should be minimized, so patients should be kept in dark, quiet areas.

Prognosis. Most poisoned pets are continuously treated in the hospital for 24 to 72 hours. Aggressive decontamination procedures, along with 24-hour intensive care monitoring, significantly reduce the length of hospital stay and hasten recovery. Because of the rapid onset of strychnine, most patients are presented to veterinary facilities late in the progression of the disease and many die before appropriate treatment can be initiated. Prognosis for livestock and horses is poor as a result of the difficulty in effectively treating these patients in the field.

Prevention and Control. The majority of accidental strychnine poisonings are preventable if the bait is used according to label instruction. In the author's experience, free-roaming dogs are the population at greatest risk of succumbing to strychnine poisoning. Malicious poisonings also occur.

ZINC PHOSPHIDE

Jay C. Albretsen

Synonyms. Brand names include Sweeney's Poison Peanuts, ACME Gopher Killer Pellets, Bartlett Mouse Bait, Dexol Gopher Killing Pellets, Eraze Rodent Pellets, Mole Guard, ZP Tracking Powder, and many others.

Sources. Historically, zinc phosphide was a rodenticide used by certified pest control operators and has been used since the 1930s. Newer formulations, and especially those found in over-the-counter preparations, contain between 2% and 5% zinc phosphide mixed with other ingredients such as wheat, rolled oats, sugar, bread, or bran mash.[1,2] Zinc phosphide became more popular during and after World War II when red squill became difficult to obtain. As a rodenticide, zinc phosphide became popular because the rodents often died out in the open. Apparently, this is a psychologically rewarding effect to the users of the product.

Phosphine gas is widely used as a fumigant in grain storage bins and in freight ships that transport grain. It kills both insects and rodents. Phosphine gas is also used as a doping agent in silicon crystals, which are then incorporated into semiconductors.[2]

Toxicokinetics. Zinc phosphide is a crystalline, dark-gray powder. It is stable for long periods when kept dry, but degrades rapidly in damp or acidic conditions.[1,2] Its toxic activity is considered to persist for 2 weeks under average conditions.[1] Zinc phosphide rapidly forms phosphine gas when in acidic conditions. This conversion does not require any enzymes to proceed. However, phosphine gas is formed more slowly when in contact with just water.[3]

Phosphine gas is heavier than air. It has a distinct odor that has been described as similar to rotten fish or acetylene. However, odor cannot be relied on as a warning sign, because poisoning can occur at levels less than 2 ppm. The concentration at which humans can begin to detect phosphine gas is 2 ppm. Therefore, when a person can begin to detect phosphine gas, he or she is already being exposed to toxic amounts.[2,3] Zinc phosphide is usually ingested, and phosphine gas is most often inhaled.

Commercially available zinc phosphide–containing products seem to contain two fractions. The first causes a release of phosphine gas, probably related to gastric acidity. The other fraction is more slowly acted on and appears to break down later in the gastrointestinal tract.[1]

Mechanism of Action. The toxicity of zinc phosphide is fully accounted for by the phosphine gas produced after the zinc phosphide is hydrolyzed in the stomach. The exact mechanism is not clear, but phosphine has been shown to block cytochrome oxidase. Thus, oxidative phosphorylation is inhibited, blocking energy-producing processes in the mitochondria and resulting in cell death.[1,2] Phosphine also increases reactive oxygen species, resulting in peroxidation and other cellular oxidative damage.[4]

Toxicity and Risk Factors. Toxic and lethal doses of zinc phosphide vary not only between species but also depending on the acidity of the stomach or digestive tract. For example, dogs given 300 mg/kg of zinc phosphide orally can survive if they have empty stomachs. However, between 20 and 40 mg/kg is usually considered to be a lethal dose for most animals.[1,2] Box 26-3 lists specific lethal doses in several species.

Zinc phosphide has a strong tendency to induce vomiting in animals that can vomit. In addition, some zinc phosphide rodenticides also contain other emetics to help induce vomiting in animals that can vomit. Thus, the ingestion of even lethal doses of zinc phosphide does not cause consistent signs in animals. Nontarget species frequently vomit

BOX 26-3	**LETHAL DOSES OF ZINC PHOSPHIDE IN SEVERAL SPECIES**
SPECIES	**LETHAL DOSE**
Man	40 mg/kg LD_{LO}
Dog	40 mg/kg LD_{LO}
Cat	40 mg/kg LD_{LO}
Rabbit	40 mg/kg LD_{LO}
Mouse	40 mg/kg LD_{50}
Rat	12 mg/kg LD_{50}
Ruminants	60 mg/kg LD_{50}
Wild birds	23.7 mg/kg LD_{50}
Duck	37.5 mg/kg LD_{50}

From RTECS: Registry of Toxic Effects of Chemical Substances. National Institute for Occupational Safety and Health, Cincinnati, Ohio (CD-ROM Version), *Micromedex*, Englewood, Colo, (expires December 31, 2000). *LD_{LO},* Lowest reported lethal dose; *LD_{50},* lethal dose in 50% of tested animals.

the zinc phosphide recently ingested. This protective action prevents the conversion of zinc phosphide to phosphine gas. Consequently, no phosphine gas is absorbed or inhaled, and no clinical signs develop.[1,2]

Zinc phosphide can be a risk to carnivores that consume poisoned animals. In fact, relay toxicosis has been reported in dogs that ate recently poisoned rodents.[5] In cases of relay toxicosis, the zinc phosphide was believed to still be in the gastrointestinal tract of the rodents. However, carrion scavengers are unlikely to be affected by zinc phosphide–poisoned animals because zinc phosphide degrades rapidly, and very little accumulates in muscle tissues.[2,5,6]

Veterinarians and animal caretakers are also at risk when treating or handling poisoned animals. When zinc phosphide is converted to phosphine gas, the smell of phosphine gas can sometimes be evident, especially after decontaminating the animal or when the animal is necropsied. By the time humans smell phosphine gas, they are already exposed to a concentration of at least 1 to 2 ppm. The threshold limit value for phosphine gas in humans is 0.3 ppm and quickly reaches toxic doses if exposed to those levels for long. A rat inhalation LD_{50} for phosphine gas is 11 ppm over a 4-hour period of time.[3] Thus, it is important to have adequate ventilation in areas where zinc phosphide–poisoned animals are treated.

Clinical Signs. The onset of zinc phosphide poisoning is rapid. Signs can occur within 15 minutes to 4 hours after ingestion. The onset of signs is also related to when the animal last ate. Ingesting zinc phosphide on an empty stomach can delay the onset of signs. In fact, the onset of signs is reported to sometimes be delayed for as long as 12 to 18 hours. When large doses are ingested, death can occur within 3 to 5 hours after the onset of signs. It is rare for animals ingesting lethal doses to survive longer than 48 hours.[1,2]

Although there are no specific signs to characterize zinc phosphide toxicosis, it often resembles strychnine poisoning in dogs. Early signs include anorexia and depression. Next the animal develops rapid, deep, and often wheezy respirations. Vomiting is common and can contain blood.[1,2] In horses, colic and abdominal pain are common. Ruminal tympany and bloat occur in ruminants. These signs are followed by ataxia, weakness, recumbency, hypoxia, and struggling. In some cases, convulsions and hyperesthesia are seen.[1-3,6] In humans, hypotension, shock, and myocardial injury resulting in arrhythmias are seen after zinc phosphide exposures. In fact, the majority of deaths in humans are probably due to myocardial damage.[3]

Clinical Pathology. No specific clinical pathology findings occur in animals.[1]

Lesions. Zinc phosphide causes no specific lesions in animals. Organs with the greatest oxygen requirements are especially sensitive to damage from zinc phosphide toxicosis. These organs include the brain, kidneys, liver, and heart. Consequently, animals poisoned with zinc phosphide may show liver and kidney congestion. Yellow mottling is also seen in the liver of poisoned animals. In addition, it is

common to see gastritis and enteritis. Gastritis occurs most consistently in poisoned pigs. Pulmonary congestion and interlobular edema also occur.[1,2]

Histologic lesions include congestion of the liver and kidneys. Renal tubular degeneration and necrosis can be evident. Cloudy swelling and fatty degeneration are also seen in the liver.[1,2] Mononuclear infiltration and fragmentation of myocardial fibers along with inflammation of the mitral and aortic valves were reported in a 2-year-old girl poisoned with phosphine gas.[2,3]

Diagnostic Testing. Chemical detection of zinc phosphide in the stomach contents or vomitus is possible. It is also possible that zinc phosphide may be detected in the liver or kidneys.[1] However, because zinc phosphide is quickly hydrolyzed to phosphine gas, which dissipates rapidly, samples should be packed in air-tight containers and frozen to prevent phosphine loss. If possible, it is best to send the entire animal unopened to the diagnostic laboratory as quickly as possible. Even with these measures, the detection of zinc phosphide can be difficult.[1,2,6]

Treatment. Time is critical after zinc phosphide is ingested, because early decontamination can improve the prognosis.[2,3] Decontamination of animals ingesting zinc phosphide includes emesis, gastric lavage, and the use of products to increase gastric pH. Emesis in appropriate species is preferably accomplished with a centrally acting emetic (such as apomorphine or xylazine) rather than with a product such as hydrogen peroxide that must be given orally. It is also appropriate to consider using an oral aluminum or magnesium hydroxide antacid initially to slow the hydrolysis of zinc phosphide to phosphine gas. In animals that cannot vomit, activated charcoal can be beneficial, especially when mixed with an antacid (e.g., aluminum or magnesium hydroxide). A cathartic such as sorbitol or magnesium sulfate should also be added to the activated charcoal. Gastric lavage with a 5% sodium bicarbonate mixture is also recommended to help slow the hydrolysis of zinc phosphide to phosphine gas.[1-3] Zinc phosphide should be cleared from the entire gastrointestinal tract. This can be accomplished either by doing an enterogastric lavage (a "through and through") or by following gastric lavage with activated charcoal.[1]

No specific antidote for zinc phosphide or phosphine gas is available. Therapy should be directed toward correcting acidosis, solving respiratory difficulties, treating shock, and supporting animals with liver damage.[1-3] Acidosis can be corrected using calcium gluconate or sodium lactate intravenously. Respiratory problems can be helped by the administration of oxygen. Shock symptoms are often alleviated by using corticosteroids. Sodium thiosulfate (10% solution), lipotrophic agents, dextrose, B vitamins, and low-protein diets have been used to treat liver failure.[1-3] Other symptomatic and supportive care is indicated. Seizures can be controlled with diazepam, pentobarbital, methocarbamol, or gas anesethetics.[7]

Prognosis. Animals that have developed clinical signs of zinc phosphide toxicosis should be considered to have a guarded-to-poor prognosis, depending on the severity of their signs. If the animal is asymptomatic and the ingestion has been recent (within the last 1 to 2 hours), decontamination improves the prognosis.[4]

Prevention and Control.   Zinc phosphide is a commonly encountered rodenticide in over-the-counter products. It is important to read and follow all label directions. In addition, it is a good idea to keep rodenticides away from animal feeding areas and separate from animal feeds. Livestock readily consume these products because they are often pelleted or added to grains.

REFERENCES

3-Chloro-P-Toluidine Hydrochloride

1. Environmental Protection Agency: Reregistration Eligibility Decision (RED): Starlicide (3-chloro-*p*-toluidine). Includes RED Facts: *Starlicide (3-chloro-p-toluidine) fact sheet*, Government Reports Announcements & Index, Issue 12, Washington, DC, 1996.
2. Peoples SA, Westberg GL: The selective nephrotoxicity of 3-chloro-*p*-toluidine (CPT) and 2-chloro-4-acetotoluidine (CAT) is due to a difference in the metabolic handling of both compounds by the two species, *Fed Proc Fed Am Soc Exp Biol* 34(3):227, 1975.
3. Gosselin RE et al: 3-Chloro-4-methylaninline. In *Clinical toxicology of commercial products*, ed 5, Baltimore, 1981, Williams and Wilkins.
4. Borison HL et al: 3-Chloro-*p*-toluidine: effects of lethal doses in rats and cats, *Toxicol Appl Pharmacol* 31:403, 1975.
5. Hazardous Substances Data Bank (HSDB), National Library of Medicine, Bethesda, Md, (CD-ROM), Englewood, Colo, *Micromedex* (edition expires 4/30/2000).

4-Aminopyridine

1. Beasley VA: Avitrol. In *A symptomatic approach to clinical toxicology*, Urbana, Ill, 1999, University of Illinois.
2. Extension Toxicology Network (Extoxnet), 4-Aminopyridine, 1996.
3. Timm RM, editor: *Prevention and control of wildlife damage*, Lincoln, Neb, 1984, Nebraska Cooperative Extension Service, University of Nebraska.
4. Rowsell HC, Ritcey J, Cox F: *Assessment of humaneness of vertebrate pesticides*, Proceedings of 1979 CALAS Convention, University of Guelph, Ontario, June 25-28, 1979.
5. Hazardous Substances Data Bank (HSDB), National Library of Medicine, Bethesda, Md, (CD-ROM) *Micromedex*, Englewood, Colo (edition expires 4/30/2000).
6. Schafer EW, Brunton RD, Lockyer NF: Secondary hazards to animals feeding on red-winged blackbirds killed with 4-aminopyridine baits, *J Wildlife Manage* 38:424, 1974.
7. Registry of Toxic Effects of Chemical Substances (RTECS), National Institute for Occupational Safety and Health, Cincinnati, Ohio (CD-ROM), *Micromedex*, Englewood, Colo (edition expires 4/30/2000).
8. Nicholson SS: Suspected 4-aminopyridine toxicosis in cattle, *J Am Vet Med Assoc* 178:1277, 1981.
9. Ray AC et al: Clinical signs and chemical confirmation of 4-aminopyridine poisoning in horses, *Am J Vet Res* 39:329, 1978.
10. Spyker DA et al: Poisoning with 4-aminopyridine: report of three cases, *Clin Toxicol* 16:487, 1981.
11. Casteel SW, Thomas BR: A high-performance liquid chromatography method for determination of 4-aminopyridine in tissues and urine, *J Vet Diagn Invest* 2:132, 1990.

Anticoagulant Rodenticides

1. Brinker R. *Herb contraindications and drug interactions,* ed 2, Sandy, Ore, 1998, Eclectic Medical Publications.
2. Woody BJ et al: Coagulopathic effects and therapy of brodifacoum toxicosis in dogs, *J Vet Intern Med* 6:23, 1992.
3. Sheator SE, Couto CG: Anticoagulant rodenticide toxicity in 21 dogs, *J Am Anim Hosp Assoc* 35:38, 1999.
4. Boemans HJ et al. Clinical signs, laboratory changes, and toxicokinetics of brodifacoum in the horse, *Can J Vet Res* 55:21, 1991.
5. POISINDEX System: Editorial Staff: Anticoagulants: long acting. In Toll LL, Hurlbut KM, editors: POISINDEX System, Englewood, Colo, *Micromedex* (edition expires December 2000).
6. Beasley VR et al: Anticoagulant rodenticides. In *A systems affected approach to veterinary toxicology,* Urbana, Ill, 1997, University of Illinois.
7. Duncan JR et al: *Veterinary laboratory medicine,* ed 3, Ames, Iowa, 1994, Iowa State University Press.
8. Plumb DC: *Veterinary drug handbook,* ed 3, Ames, Iowa, 1999, Iowa State University Press.
9. Dorman DC: Anticoagulant, cholecalciferol, and bromethalin-based rodenticides, *Vet Clin North Am Small Anim Pract* 20:339, 1990.
10. Murphy ML: Rodenticides. In Howard JL, editor: *Current veterinary therapy 3. Food animal practice,* Philadelphia, 1993, WB Saunders.

Bromethalin

1. VanLier RBL, Cherry LD: The toxicity and mechanism of action of bromethalin: a new single-feeding rodenticide, *Fundam Appl Toxicol* 11:664, 1988.
2. Dorman DC et al: Diagnosis of bromethalin poisoning in the dog, *J Vet Diag Invest* 2:123, 1990.
3. Dorman DC et al: Effects of an extract of *Gingko biloba* on bromethalin-induced cerebral peroxidation and edema, *Am J Vet Res* 53:138, 1992.
4. Dorman DC et al: Bromethalin toxicosis in the dog, I. Clinical effects, *J Am Assoc Anim Hosp* 26:589, 1990.
5. Dorman DC et al: Bromethalin neurotoxicosis in the cat, *Prog Vet Neurol* 1:189, 1990.
6. Martin T, Johnson B: A suspected case of bromethalin toxicity in a domestic cat, *Vet Hum Toxicol* 3: 239, 1989.
7. Dorman DC et al: Quantitative and qualitative electroencephalographic changes in normal and bromethalin-dosed cats, *Prog Vet Neurol* 1:451, 1990.
8. Dorman DC et al: Electroencephalographic changes associated with bromethalin toxicosis in the dog, *Vet Hum Toxicol* 33:9, 1991.
9. Dorman DC et al: Neuropathologic findings of bromethalin toxicosis in cats, *Vet Pathol* 29:139, 1992.
10. Dorman DC et al: Bromethalin toxicosis in the dog, II. Treatment of the toxic syndrome, *J Am Assoc Anim Hosp* 26:595, 1990.

Cholecalciferol

1. Puls R: *Vitamin levels in animal health: diagnostic data and bibliographies,* Clearbrook, British Columbia,, 1994, Sherpa International.
2. Dorman DC: Anticoagulant, cholecalciferol, and bromethalin-based rodenticides, *Vet Clin North Am Small Anim Pract* 20:339, 1990.
3. Rosol T et al: In DiBartola S: *Fluid therapy in small animal practice,* ed 2, Philadelphia, 2000, WB Saunders.
4. Marcus R: In Hardman J, Limbird L, editors: *Goodman and Gilman's the pharmacological basis of therapeutics,* ed 9, New York, 1996, McGraw-Hill.
5. Dougherty SA et al: Salmon calcitonin as adjunct treatment for vitamin D toxicosis in a dog, *J Am Vet Med Assoc* 196:1269, 1990.
6. Kutchai H: In Berne R et al, editors: *Physiology,* ed 4, St Louis, 1998, Mosby.
7. Metts BC et al: In Haddad LM et al: *Clinical management of poisoning and drug overdose,* ed 3, Philadelphia, 1998, WB Saunders.
8. Talcott PA et al: Accidental ingestion of a cholecalciferol-containing rodent bait in a dog, *Vet Hum Toxicol* 33:252, 1991.
9. Fooshee SK, Forrester SD: Hypercalcemia secondary to cholecalciferol rodenticide toxicosis in two dogs, *J Am Vet Med Assoc* 196:1265, 1990.
10. Gunther R et al: Toxicity of a vitamin D3 rodenticide to dogs, *J Am Vet Med Assoc* 193:211, 1988.

11. Nelson R: In Nelson R, Couto C, editors: *Small animal internal medicine,* ed 2, St Louis, 1998, Mosby.

12. Midkiff AM et al: Idiopathic hypercalcemia in cats, *J Vet Intern Med* 14:619, 2000.

13. Volmer P: Oral toxicity of skin and eye products, American College of Veterinary Internal Medicine: 18th Annual Meeting, Chicago, 2000.

14. Hilbe M et al: Metastatic calcification in a dog attributable to ingestion of a tacalcitol ointment, *Vet Pathol* 37:490, 2000.

15. Kruger J et al: Hypercalcemia and renal failure: etiology, pathophysiology, diagnosis, and treatment, *Vet Clin North Am Small Anim Pract* 26:1417, 1996.

16. Rumbeiha W et al: The postmortem diagnosis of cholecalciferol toxicosis: a novel approach and differentiation from ethylene glycol toxicosis, *J Vet Diagn Invest* 12:426, 2000.

17. Plumb DC: *Veterinary drug handbook,* ed 3, White Bear Lake, Minn, 2000, Pharma Vet Publishing.

18. Rumbeiha W et al: Use of pamidronate disodium to reduce cholecalciferol-induced toxicosis in dogs, *Am J Vet Res* 61:9, 2000.

19. Rumbeiha W et al: The use of pamidronate disodium for treatment of vitamin D3 toxicosis in dogs, American Association of Veterinary Laboratory Diagnosticians: 40th Annual Meeting, Louisville, Ky, 1997.

20. National Research Council (NRC): *Vitamin tolerance of animals,* Washington, DC, 1987, National Academy Press.

Sodium Fluoroacetate

1. Anonymous: Reregistration Eligibility Decision (RED) Sodium Fluoroacetate. *Prevention, pesticides and toxic substances,* United States Environmental Protection Agency, 1995, Washington, DC 738-5-95-025.

2. Arellano M et al: The anti-cancer drug 5-fluorouracil is metabolized by the isolated perfused rat liver and in rats into highly toxic fluoroacetate, *Br J Cancer* 77:79, 1998.

3. Keller DA et al: Fluoroacetate-mediated toxicity of fluorinated ethanes, *Fundam Appl Toxicol* 30:213, 1996.

4. Mead RJ et al: Metabolism and defluorination of fluoroacetate in the brush-tailed possum *(Trichosurus vulpecula), Aust J Biol Sci* 32:15, 1979.

5. Lauble H et al: The reaction of fluorocitrate with aconitase and the crystal structure of the enzyme-inhibitor complex, *Proc Natl Acad Sci USA* 93:13699, 1996.

6. Bruere AN et al: Fluoroacetate, *Vet Clin Toxicol* 127:96, 1990.

7. Churchill R: 1080 Sodium fluoroacetate toxicity in dogs #3796, *Control & Therapy Series,* Postgraduate Committee in Veterinary Science of the University of Sydney 188:846, 1996.

8. McLaren J: Treatment of 1080 poisoning in dogs, *Vetscript* XII:3, 1999.

Strychnine

1. Adamson RH, Fouts JR: Enzymatic metabolism of strychnine, *J Pharmacol Exp Ther* 127:87, 1959.

2. Weiss S, Hatcher RA: Studies on strychnine, *J Pharmacol Exp Ther* 14:419, 1922.

3. Sgaragli GP, Mannaioni PF: Pharmacokinetic observations on a case of massive strychnine poisoning, *Clin Toxicol* 6:533, 1973.

4. Curtis DR et al: The specificity of strychnine as a glycine antagonist in the mammalian spinal cord, *Exp Brain Res* 12:547, 1971.

5. Curtis DR et al: A pharmacological study of the depression of spinal neurons by glycine and related amino acids, *Exp Brain Res* 6:1, 1968.

6. Heiser JM et al: Massive strychnine intoxication: serial blood levels in a fatal case, *Clin Toxicol* 30(2):269, 1992.

7. Plumb DC: *Veterinary drug handbook,* ed 3, White Bear Lake, Minn, 1999, Pharma Vet Publishing.

Zinc Phosphide

1. Osweiler GD et al: *Clinical and diagnostic veterinary toxicology,* ed 3, Dubuque, Iowa, 1985, Kendal Hunt.

2. Casteel SW, Bailey EM: A review of zinc phosphide poisoning, *Vet Hum Toxicol* 28:151, 1986.

3. Shannon MW: In Haddad LM et al: *Clinical management of poisoning and drug overdose,* ed 3, Philadelphia, 1998, WB Saunders.

4. Hsu CH et al: Phosphine-induced oxidative stress in Hepa 1c1c7 cells, *Toxicol Sci* 46:204, 1998.

5. EXTOXNET, Extension Toxicology Network, University of California, Cornell University, Michigan State University, and Oregon State University. Available at *http://ace.orst.edu/info/extoxnet/ghindex.html.*

6. Fessesswork GG et al: Laboratory diagnosis of zinc phosphide poisoning, *Vet Hum Toxicol* 36:517, 1994.

7. Plumb DC: *Veterinary drug handbook,* ed 3, Ames, Iowa, 1999, Iowa State University Press.

8. RTECS: Registry of Toxic Effects of Chemical Substances: National Institute for Occupational Safety and Health, Cincinnati, Ohio (CD-ROM), Englewood, Colo, *Micromedex* (expires December 31, 2000).

Index

A

Abamectin intoxication, 303-304

Abrin intoxication, 406-408

Absorption, 8-9, 10

Acarbose intoxication, 317-318

Acepromazine
    for ammoniated feed syndrome, 118
    for fescue toxicosis, 248
    for sympathomimetic intoxication, 310

Acer rubrum intoxication, 59t, 437-438

Acetamide, for sodium fluoroacetate intoxication, 454

Acetaminophen intoxication, 17t, 20, 59t, 62t, 284

Acetic acid, for ammonia toxicosis, 132

Acetohexamide intoxication, 315-316

Acetylandromedol intoxication, 412-414

N-Acetylcysteine, for acetaminophen intoxication, 17t, 20, 284

Acid intoxication, 55t, 139-140

Acidification, urinary, 15t, 20

Acidosis
    in biguanide intoxication, 317
    in iron intoxication, 203
    in tricyclic antidepressant intoxication, 288

Acorn poisoning, 346-348

Activated charcoal, 15-16, 15t, 20
    for acetaminophen intoxication, 284
    for albuterol intoxication, 307
    for amitraz intoxication, 178
    for analgesic intoxication, 283
    for anticholinesterase insecticide intoxication, 180
    for antihistamine intoxication, 293
    for barbiturate intoxication, 285
    for boric acid ingestion, 144
    for bromethalin intoxication, 447
    for ethylene glycol poisoning, 153
    for fertilizer ingestion, 155
    for fipronil intoxication, 184
    for metaldehyde intoxication, 183
    for methylxanthine intoxication, 325
    for organochlorine insecticide intoxication, 187
    for serotonergic drug intoxication, 290
    for strychnine intoxication, 455
    for thyroid hormone intoxication, 322
    for tricyclic antidepressant intoxication, 288
    for zinc phosphide intoxication, 457
    multiple dose, 16

Active transport, 10

Adenocarcinoma, hepatic, 67

Adenoma, hepatic, 67

Adenosine receptors, in methylxanthine intoxication, 324

Adsorbents, 15-16, 15t

Adverse event reporting, 41-44, 42b
    EPA adverse effects information reporting for, 42-43
    for pesticides, 42-43
    UPS Veterinary Practitioners' Reporting Program for, 43
    USDA Animal Immunobiologic Vigilance Program for, 43

Aesculus spp. intoxication, 394-396

Aflatoxicosis, 62t, 231-235
    clinical signs of, 233t, 234, 234t
    diagnosis of, 234-235
    in cattle, 232-233, 233t
    in swine, 233, 234t
    in trout, 234
    LD$_{50}$ in, 232, 233b
    mechanism of action of, 232
    nutritional factors in, 232-233
    pathology of, 234, 234b
    prevention of, 235
    sources of, 231
    toxicokinetics of, 231-232
    treatment of, 235

Agave spp. intoxication, 403-404

Agkistrodon intoxication, 106-111

Airways. *See also* Respiratory system.
    toxic response of, 82-83, 82f

Albuterol intoxication, 305-307

Alcohol, nervous system effects of, 72t

Aldrin intoxication, 186-188

Alfalfa, blister beetle problems in, 103

Alfalfa intoxication, 401

Algae, blue-green, 90t, 100-101

Alkali disease, 216, 216f

Alkali intoxication, 55t, 139-140

Alkalinization, urinary, 15t, 20

Alkaloid intoxication, 350-383
    cevanine, 89t, 350-351, 351t
    diterpene, 73t, 89t, 352-356
        clinical signs of, 354
        diagnosis of, 354-355
        mechanism of action of, 353
        prevention of, 355-356
        risk factors for, 353-354
        sources of, 352-353
        toxicokinetics of, 353
        treatment of, 355
    indolizidine, 73t, 357-362
        cardiac manifestations of, 360
        clinical signs of, 359-360
        diagnosis of, 361
        growth-related manifestations of, 360
        mechanism of action of, 358-359
        neurologic manifestations of, 359
        pathology of, 360-361
        prevention of, 361-362

Page numbers followed by f refer to figures; those followed by t refer to tables; and those followed by b refer to boxes.